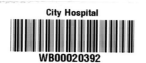

THERAPEUTIC EXERCISE

Moving Toward Function
Third Edition

Lori Thein Brody, PT, PhD, SCS, ATC
Senior Clinical Specialist, Sports and Spine Physical Therapy
UW Health
Research Park Clinic
Madison, Wisconsin
Graduate Program Director
Orthopaedic and Sports Science
Rocky Mountain University of Health Professions
Provo, Utah

Carrie M. Hall, PT, MHS
Physical Therapist
President, Movement Systems Physical Therapy
Clinical Faculty
University of Washington
Seattle, Washington

with contributors

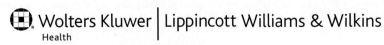

Wolters Kluwer | Lippincott Williams & Wilkins
Health

Philadelphia • Baltimore • New York • London
Buenos Aires • Hong Kong • Sydney • Tokyo

Acquisitions Editor: Emily Lupash
Product Manager: John Larkin
Marketing Manager: Allison Powell
Creative Director: Doug Smock
Compositor: SPi Technologies

Third Edition

351 West Camden Street   Two Commerce Square
Baltimore, MD 21201   2001 Market Street
                          Philadelphia, PA 19103

Printed in The People's Republic of China

Library of Congress Cataloging-in-Publication Data

Brody, Lori Thein.
    Therapeutic exercise : moving toward function / Lori Thein Brody, Carrie M. Hall.—3rd ed.
        p. ; cm.
    Hall's name appears first on the earlier edition.
    Includes bibliographical references and index.
    Summary: "Therapeutic Exercise: Moving Toward Function, Third Edition provides a conceptual framework for learning how to make clinical decisions regarding the prescription of therapeutic exercise—from deciding which exercise(s) to teach, to how to teach them, to the dosage required for the best possible outcome. Throughout this text, readers will learn how to treat, with the use of therapeutic exercise and related interventions, the impairments that correlate to functional limitations and the disability and to work toward the most optimal function possible"—Provided by publisher.
    ISBN 978-0-7817-9957-7 (hardback : alk. paper)
    1. Exercise therapy. I. Hall, Carrie M. II. Title.
    [DNLM: 1. Exercise Therapy—methods. WB 541 B8655t 2011]

    RM725.H33 2011
    615.8'2—dc22

                                                                2010023764

To purchase additional copies of this book, call our customer service department at **(800) 638-3030** or fax orders to **(301) 223-2320**. International customers should call **(301) 223-2300**.

Visit Lippincott Williams & Wilkins on the Internet: **http://www.lww.com**. Lippincott Williams & Wilkins customer service representatives are available from 8:30 am to 6:00 pm, EST.

9 8 7 6 5 4

CCS0215

To my own Fab Four:
Nathan, Louisa, Benjamin and Ethan;
And to Marc, who reminds us to have fun.
—Lori Thein Brody

I would like to dedicate this book to
my husband Glenn, whose patience, wisdom, and
support allow me to tackle such monumental projects amidst our already busy lives;
my three daughters, Caroline, Gabrielle, and Jillian,
who encourage me daily to be my best; my patients, who continously teach me about
the complexity of the movement system;
and my mother Carol,
who lived her life with courage and resolve and continues to serve as my daily inspiration.
—Carrie M. Hall

Contributors

Kimberly D. Bennett, PT, PhD
Division of Physical Therapy
Department of Rehabilitation Medicine
University of Washington School of Medicine
Consultant Olympic Physical Therapy,
Mercer Island, Washington

Dorothy J. Berg, MPT
Staff Physical Therapist
Virginia Mason Medical Center
Seattle, Washington

Janet R. Bezner, PT, PhD
Deputy Executive Director
American Physical Therapy Association
Alexandria, Virginia

Judy Dewane, PT, DSc, NCS
Assistant Professor (CHS)
Physical Therapy Program
Department of Orthopedics and Rehabilitation
    Medicine
Madison, Wisconsin

Lisa M. Dussault, OTR
Occupational Therapist, Advanced Clinician
UW Health Department of Orthopedics and
    Rehabilitation
Temporomandibular Disorders Clinic
University of Wisconsin Hospital and Clinics
Madison, Wisconsin

Rafael Escamilla, PhD, PT, CSCS, FACSM
Director of Research
Andrews-Paulos Reasearch and Education
Gulf Breeze, Florida
Professor
California State University, Sacramento
Department of Physical Therapy
Sacramento, California
Colin R. Grove, PT, MS, NCS
Department of Orthopaedics and
    Rehabilitation
Neuro Outpatient Rehabilitation
UW Health Rehabilitation Clinic
Middleton, Wisconsin

Darlene Hertling, PT, Retired
Lecturer, Division of Physical Therapy
Department of Rehabilitation Medicine
University of Washington School of Medicine
Seattle, Washington

**Carol N. Kennedy, BScPT, MCISc Manipulative
Therapy (cand), FCAMPT**
Physical Therapist
Partner, Treloar Physiotherapy Clinic
Vancouver, British Columbia

Rob Landel, PT, DPT, OCS, CSCS
Associate Professor of Clinical Physical Therapy
Director, Clinical Residency Program
Director, Orthopedic Physical Therapy
Residency Program
Department of Biokinesiology and Physical Therapy
University of Southern California
Los Angeles, California

Susan Lynn Lefever PT, MA, ATC, CPed
Physical Therapist
President, San Juan Physical Therapy, Inc
Friday Harbor, Washington

Jill McVey, DPT, ATC
Physical Therapist
Movement Systems Physical Therapy, PS
Seattle, Washington

David Musnick, MD
Peak Integrative Medical Clinic
Bellvue, Washington
Author of "Conditioning for Outdoor Fitness"

Elizabeth R. Shelly, PT, DPT, BCIA-PMDB
Physical Therapist
Specialist in Women's Health
Rock Valley Physical Therapy
Moline, Illinois

Andrew Starsky, PT, PhD
Department of Physical Therapy
Marquette University
Milwaukee, WI

M. J. Strauhal, PT
Physical Therapist
Clinical Specialist in OB-GYN and Women's Health
Providence St. Vincent Medical Center Rehabilitation Services
Portland, Oregon

Kyle Yamashiro, PT, CSCS
Owner, RESULTS Physical Therapy and Training Center
Owner, Murieta Physical Therapy
Medical Adjunct Faculty, Sacramento State University
    Department of Athletics
Oakland A's Rehabilitation Consultant

Reviewers

The publisher and authors gratefully acknowledge the many professionals who shared their expertise and assisted in developing this textbook, appropriately targeting our marketing efforts, creating useful ancillary products, and setting the stage for subsequent editions. These individuals include:

Cara Adams, PT, MS
Associate Professor
Department of Rehabilitation Sciences
Division of Physical Therapy
The University of Alabama at Birmingham
School of Health Related Sciences
Birmingham, Alabama

Patricia M. Adams, MPT
Assistant Professor of Clinical Physical Therapy
Master of Physical Therapy Program
UMDMJ
Stratford, New Jersey

Stephania Bell, PT, OCS, CSCS
Injury Analyst/Senior Writer, ESPN,
Bristol, Connecticut

Karen Blaschke OTR/L, CHT
Advance Clinical Hand and Upper Extremity Clinic
University of Wisconsin Hospital and Clinics
Madison, Wisconsin

Cynthia M. Chiarello, PT, PhD
Assistant Professor of Clinical Physical Therapy
Columbia University—Doctoral Programs in Physical Therapy
New York, New York

Lisa M. Dussault, OTR
Occupational Therapist
TMD Clinic
University of Wisconsin Hospitals and Clinics
Madison, Wisconsin

Joan E. Edelstein, PT, MA, FISPO
Director of Programming in Physical Therapy
Associate Professor of Clinical Physical Therapy
Columbia University
College of Physicians and Surgeons
New York, New York

Susan E. George, PT, MS
Associate Professor
Department of Physical Therapy
Southwest Texas State University
San Marcos, Texas

Terry Hoobler, PT, MAE
University of Alabama at Birmingham
Birmingham, Alabama

Aimee Klein, PT, MS, OCS
Clinical Assistant Professor in Physical Therapy
MGH Institute of Health Professions

Senior Rehabilitation Services
Beth Israel Deaconess Medical Center
Boston, Massachusetts

Laura Knapp, PT, MS, OCS
Clinical Assistant Professor
Division of Physical Therapy
University of Utah
Salt Lake City, Utah

Robin L. Marcus, PT, MS, OCS
Clinical Assistant Professor
Division of Physical Therapy
College of Health
University of Utah
Salt Lake City, Utah

David J. Pezzullo, PT, MS, SCS, ATC
Clinical Assistant Professor
Department of Physical Therapy
University of Pittsburgh
Pittsburgh, Pennsylvania

Paul Rockar, PT, MS, OCS
Vice President, Human Resources
CORE Network, LLC
McKeesport, Pennsylvania

Richard Ruoti, PT, PhD, CSCS
Certified WATSU Practitioner
Cofounder of Aquatic Physical Therapy section of APTA
Doylestown, Pennsylvania

Leslie Russek, PT, PhD, OCS
Associate Professor
Physical Therapy Department
Clarkson University
Potsdam, New York

Amy Schramm, PT
Senior Physical Therapist
JFK Medical Center
Edison, New Jersey

Mary Sesto, PT, PhD
Physical Therapist
Department of Occupational Medicine
University of Wisconsin
Assistant Researcher
Department of Industrial Engineering
University of Wisconsin
Madison, Wisconsin

Jamie Smith, MSPT, ATC, CSCS
Director of Physical Therapy/Instructor
Orthopedic Center for Sports Medicine and Reconstructive Surgery
Louisiana State University
Kenner, Louisiana

Gary Sutton, PT, MS, SCS, OCS, ATC, CSCS
Adjunct Clinical Assistant Professor
Department of Physical Therapy
Virginia Commonwealth University
Richmond, Virginia

C. Buz Swanik, PhD, ATC
Temple University
Philadelphia, Pennsylvania

Linda J. Tsoumas, PT, MS
Chairperson and Associate Professor of Physical Therapy
Department of Physical Therapy
Springfield College
Springfield, Massachusetts

Cynthia Watson, PT, MS, OCS
Instructor, Department of Physical Therapy
University of Texas
Southwestern Medical Center
Dallas, Texas

Nancy J. Whitby, OTR, CHT
Lead Therapist
Hospital and Clinics
University of Wisconsin
Madison, Wisconsin

Preface to the First Edition

Choosing the title of this book was not easy, but once it was decided, the choice seemed obvious. *Therapeutic Exercise: Moving Toward Function* is the title that encapsulates the premise of this book. The emergence of managed care in the United States has altered the delivery of health care. Although value has always been important, its role in today's health care management is even more critical. Value can be defined as patient satisfaction (i.e., functionally meaningful patient outcomes), divided by the financial and social costs of providing care (Kasman GS, Cram JR, Wolk SL. Clinical Applications in Surface Electromyography. Rockville: Aspen, 1998). Physical therapists are challenged daily to provide value to their patients in delivering care to improve function and quality of life. Among the many interventions available to the physical therapist, therapeutic exercise is the cornerstone in providing patients with the means to improve their functional capabilities and, ultimately, their quality of life. Although other interventions can improve these elements, it is the assumption of this book that only through careful therapeutic exercise prescription can an individual make the permanent changes necessary to maintain, optimize, or prevent future loss of function. It is the premise of this book to use therapeutic exercise for patients with musculoskeletal dysfunction for the sole purpose of achieving functionally meaningful patient outcomes.

It was our decision to write this book as a textbook and not a manual of activities and techniques. The latter deals with providing activities and techniques without the theoretic framework to make decisions about what would or could be the best possible course of treatment and the possible alternatives. *Therapeutic Exercise: Moving Toward Function* attempts to provide a conceptual framework for learning how to make clinical decisions regarding the prescription of therapeutic exercise—from deciding which exercise(s) to teach to how to teach them to the dosage required for the best possible outcome. The common thread throughout the text is to treat, with the use of therapeutic exercise and related interventions, the impairments that correlate to functional limitations and disability and to work toward the most optimal function possible.

Because this book was written primarily as a textbook, decisions were made to provide the reader and instructor with a variety of educational features:

- Extensively illustrated. Therapeutic exercise is a visual intervention. This book uses photographs and line drawings to illustrate examples of therapeutic exercises.
- Selected Interventions. Featured at the end of pertinent chapters, these are activities or techniques written for the student and are included to provide examples of application of the therapeutic exercise intervention model presented in Chapter 2. Faculty can use the Selected Interventions as models for the student to develop exercise prescriptions.

- Self-Management boxes. These are activities or techniques written for the patient. These are included as examples to show the student how to write an exercise for a patient so that all the important features of an exercise prescription are clearly understood.
- Patient-Related Instruction boxes. These are similar to Self-Management boxes. The primary difference is that these are not exercises, but rather educational features to assist in the carryover of exercise into functional activities.
- Key Points. This feature summarizes key concepts the author wants to convey in the chapter. A thorough understanding of the Key Points should be realized following the reading of each chapter.
- Critical Thinking Questions. These were provided to stimulate the reader's thinking after studying the chapter. Case Studies are used to create hypothetical situations to which concepts can be applied.
- Lab Activities. These provide examples of applied use of the concepts to practice teaching and execution of selected activities and techniques.
- Case Studies. The final unit of the book provides the reader with a description of 11 cases. These cases are used in Critical Thinking Questions and Lab Activities to provide the student with real-life situations in which to apply concepts learned in the relevant chapter.

The book is organized into seven units. The purpose of each unit is as follows:

- Unit 1 provides the foundations of therapeutic exercise, beginning with a presentation of the disablement model to provide conceptual clarity for the remainder of the book, and ending with concepts of patient management. In the second chapter, a proposed therapeutic exercise intervention model is presented. This model attempts to separate the clinical reasoning process into the individual, but cumulative steps to take in order to prescribe an effective therapeutic exercise. Chapter 3 describes two crucial elements of patient management: motor learning and self-management.
- Unit 2 provides the reader with a functional approach to therapeutic exercise for physiologic impairments. Although we attempted to include a somewhat extensive review of the scientific literature on muscle performance, balance, endurance, mobility, posture, movement, and pain, our purpose was not to publish a review of the material. Instead, we have selected pertinent literature to illustrate the concepts needed for a basic knowledge of physiologic impairments as it relates to therapeutic exercise prescription.
- Unit 3 presents special physiologic considerations to heed when prescribing therapeutic exercise. They include soft tissue injury, postoperative issues, arthritis, fibromyalgia syndrome and chronic fatigue, and obstetrics. Although

this list is not comprehensive, we chose these special considerations because of the frequency with which the clinician encounters them.

- Unit 4 provides the reader with selected methods of intervention. Although there are numerous schools of thought regarding the prescription of exercise, we chose these methods to provide the reader with examples of a variety of contrasting methods—each has its own merits. The authors have attempted to illustrate how each method can be incorporated into a cohesive program of therapeutic exercise prescription.

- Units 5 and 6 provide the reader with a regional approach to therapeutic exercise prescription. Each chapter is organized into a brief review of anatomy and kinesiology, examination and evaluation guidelines, therapeutic exercise for common physiologic impairments affecting the region, and therapeutic exercise for common medical diagnoses affecting the region. The anatomy, kinesiology, and examination and evaluation sections set the foundation for prescription of therapeutic exercise for physiologic impairments. Therapeutic exercise for physiologic impairments provides the reader with examples of exercises to improve physiologic capability and ultimately function. Therapeutic exercise for common medical diagnoses provides the reader with examples of comprehensive interventions, including therapeutic exercise for common medical conditions affecting the region.

- Unit 7 consists of 11 Case Studies, which are used in Critical Thinking Questions and Lab Activities at the end of selected chapters. Faculty can use these Case Studies for a variety of learning experiences.

- Appendices 1 and 2 give the student a quick reference for red flags of serious pathology or visceral referred symptoms and clinical actions to take in the event of serious signs and symptoms in the exercising patient.

We worked diligently to provide a comprehensive textbook designed to prepare the foundation of knowledge and skills necessary to prescribe therapeutic exercise. We urge our readers to write to us to tell us how well we accomplished our goal. We hope that subsequent editions can address your comments as well as the ever-changing needs of those involved in therapeutic exercise prescription.

Carrie M. Hall, PT, MHS
Lori Thein Brody, PT, MS, SCS, ATC

Preface to the Third Edition

Therapeutic exercise is the number one intervention provided by physical therapists. While clinicians have a variety of interventions available to them, therapeutic exercise is a key component of nearly every treatment plan. Therapeutic exercise is effectively applied across the continuum of care and throughout the lifespan. In the past, therapeutic exercise utilization by physical therapists and physical therapist assistants has focused on the rehabilitation end of the continuum. That is, the focus has been the remediation of impairments and activity limitations, and the restoration of function. While this service has been the cornerstone of physical therapist practice since the inception of the profession, *all* people can benefit from therapeutic exercise, not just those on the negative side of the continuum. The third edition of *Therapeutic Exercise: Moving Toward Function* is specifically designed to apply and appropriately dose therapeutic exercise in a variety of populations.

Health promotion and wellness have taken on an increasingly important role in our society today. Inactivity and unhealthy lifestyles have led to increases in conditions such as obesity, diabetes, heart disease, and chronic pain. According to the Centers of Disease Control, an estimated 68 million Americans age 18 and older are projected to have a diagnosis of arthritis by the year 2030. Additionally, an estimated 1 in 250 children will have been diagnosed with some form of arthritis. In 2005, an estimated 5 million Americans were diagnosed with fibromyalgia. Our role in improving the lives of patients and the vitality of our communities lies in our ability to provide leadership and expertise in the provision of and education about therapeutic exercise. Individuals living with arthritis, diabetes, heart disease, obesity, and a multitude of other health conditions can benefit from a therapeutic exercise program. Progressive increase in impairments and decline in functional abilities is not inevitable for those living with disease. The appropriate application of therapeutic exercise can significantly increase engagement in community and improve the quality of life in those living with chronic conditions. Physical therapists are ideally suited to design these therapeutic exercise programs. The Doctor of Physical Therapy graduate will be armed with the most current evidence to appropriately dose therapeutic exercise for individuals across the health continuum.

In its newly revised International Classification of Functioning, Disability and Health (ICF), the World Health Organization (WHO) emphasizes that its classification scheme is not only about people with disabilities, but is about *all people*. The WHO believes that the health and health-related status associated with *all* health conditions can be described by the ICF. This includes the continuum of people with no known disease, to those with disease-related impairments, activity limitations and participation restrictions. It includes a lifespan contiuum from pre-natal care to the very old. We embrace this vision of world, community, and individual health, advocating for physical therapists and physical therapy assistants as the providers of choice in the domain of therapeutic exercise.

Effective design and implementation of therapeutic exercise programs requires skills unique to physical therapists. Simply choosing the correct exercise is only one step of the design process. Dosing therapeutic exercise, especially in the presence of pathology, injury or disease, is challenging. Providers must make numerous clinical decisions such as mode, frequency, intensity, duration, muscle contraction type, range of motion, speed, posture, and sequence, just to name a few. Exercises must be continually modified and advanced to close the gap between the individual's current performance and their desired performance (goals) or their capacity. The third edition of *Therapeutic Exercise: Moving Toward Function* emphasizes the unique challenges and skills necessary to effectively implement therapeutic exercise programs in a variety of populations and settings. Our goal is to close the gap between an understanding of exercise fundamentals and the design and implementation of effective therapeutic exercise programs across the health continuum.

CHANGES AND ADDITIONS IN THE THIRD EDITION

The changes and additions to the third edition reflect the commitment we have to providing students and clinicians with the evidence and tools necessary to provide effective therapeutic exercise programs. The first and second editions of *Therapeutic Exercise: Moving Toward Function* utilized the Nagi disablement model as the basis for therapeutic exercise prescription. This edition utilizes the WHO International Classification of Functioning, Disability and Health (ICF) model as the starting point for discussing therapeutic exercise applications. The ICF language differs from the Nagi model in its inclusivity and focus on the continuum of health, from impairment to wellness. The reader will notice a shift in terminology and philosophy.

Many chapters included extensive information on anatomy, biomechanics, and other basic sciences. We believe that review of this material brings prior knowledge to the surface to be utilized and applied in the various chapters. However, given the limited number of pages available, we felt it more useful to move this information to the website where students can review this material as needed. This allowed more book pages to be devoted to the application of therapeutic exercise.

The chapter on fibromyalgia and chronic fatigue syndrome has been included in Chapter 10: Pain. We felt that the material in this chapter was closely tied with the content in the Pain chapter, and was more appropriately placed there. Several chapters such as Chapter 8: Balance Impairment, and Chapter 15: Proprioceptive Neuromuscular Facilitation were significantly revised with new material. All chapters were updated with new material and references. In response to feedback regarding mechanisms to help students understand exercise progression, Chapter 5: Impaired Muscle Performance was revised with more information on initial exercise dosing as well as a model of exercise progression. Many of the regional chapters include protocols for initiating and advancing therapeutic exercise programs following different injuries or surgical procedures.

We have solicited input from the users of *Therapeutic Exercise: Moving Toward Function*, and have made changes that we believe will meet their expressed needs. We believe that the application of therapeutic exercise prescription requires three dimensional consideration of a substantial number of variables, falling within the domain and expertise of medical professionals. We hope that the ideas, concepts and examples provided in this third edition will provide students with the tools they need for effective therapeutic exercise initiation and progression.

PEDAGOGICAL FEATURES

We have added several new features to deepen the learning experience. Each chapter contains "Building Blocks" and/or case study applications. These features pose scenarios or questions that engage the reader with the material, asking for application of ideas or principles after their introduction.

Rather than waiting until the end of the chapter to apply the material, the student is asked to integrate and apply the information throughout the chapter. This provides some relief from continuous reading, and asks the reader to stop and consider how the material might be applied.

New website materials also increase the depth of student learning. Applications for faculty and students include videos, powerpoint slides, sample test questions, and workbook materials. These ancillary materials are all designed to help students apply the theroretical material that forms the basis for therapeutic exercise prescription. Answers to the Building Blocks will bring the student to the website where they can find additional resources to help deepen their learning. Video clips will demonstrate exercise techniques to help visual learners understand key exercise prescription issues. Workbook materials will provide students with additional opportunities to apply therapeutic exercise, from program initiation through progressions in a variety of case-based examples. Faculty support includes powerpoint slides for each chapter, sample test questions and additional worksheets to enhance student learning. We hope that the addition of these features increases the depth and breadth of student learning in therapeutic exercise prescription.

Lori Thein Brody, PT, PhD, SCS, ATC
Carrie M. Hall, PT, MHS

Acknowledgments

In addition to all those individuals who helped create the first two editions, we wish to thank many people for their contributions to this revision. This book was made possible through the individual and collective contribution of many individuals.

We are privileged to have had so many knowledgeable and dedicated chapter contributors. We are indebted to their contribution to the original work and revisions to create an outstanding third edition. We are also acutely aware that the third edition could not have been done without input from the reviewers. We are appreciative of the insights they offered to finalize the content and design of the text. A special thanks is extended to Stephania Bell who provided additional expertise and guidance in the formation of the concepts and structure of the third edition. A book of this magnitude with its large numbers of figures, legends, displays, tables, special feature boxes, and references cannot be produced without the cohesive efforts of the talented editorial and production teams. For this we thank the editorial and production staff and art department at Lippincott, Williams & Wilkins. We would like to extend a special thanks to product manager, John Larkin, who, among many other vital functions, played the critical behind the scenes role of keeping us organized and on schedule in a professional, kind, and respectful manner.

We would like to extend our gratitude to our colleagues at the UW Health Research Park Clinic, Movement Systems Physical Therapy, P.S. in Seattle, WA, and Dave Nissenbaum, PT, ATC and the Sport and Spine Clinic for the use of their facilities. We are also grateful for the time and energy provided by the models, photographer and videographers for the revised photography and videography in this text and ancillaries.

Over the course of a person's career, many individuals assist in the development of a person's theories, knowledge, and expertise. In the years between editions, we have continued to learn from the patients, students, and teachers who perpetually challenge our thoughts and decisions, and shape our skills.

Last, but most certainly not least, we would like to especially thank our family, friends, and colleagues who offered their emotional support and generosity of time to allow us to complete this project.

Lori Thein Brody
Carrie M. Hall

Each co-author would like to extend her personal acknowledgments:

Over the course of my career, I have had the good fortune to work with some of the most highly respected individuals in physical therapy. I was most fortunate to have worked with these individuals in the formative years of my career. Now, 27 years later, I am even more acutely aware of the gratitude I feel for their mentorship role in my life. I would particularly like to thank Shirley Sahrmann, PhD, PT, FAPTA, for her incredibly insightful theories and devotion to teaching me throughout my career. Her philosophy toward exercise prescription is woven into my written word throughout this book. She is a tremendous role model in the field of physical therapy and I am immensely indebted to her for her role in making my career what it is today.

Finally, the writing of a textbook takes tremendous time and energy away from work, friends, and family. Words cannot express my appreciation for my colleagues at work and close friends whose support has been truly remarkable. I especially thank my amazing husband for his support and partnership in managing a busy household and 3 children's active schedules in order to allow me to meet the demands of a career including business owner, clinician, teacher, and book author.

Carrie M. Hall, PT, MHS

My life has been blessed with exceptional colleagues who have believed in and advocated for me as my career has wound its way through physical education, athletic training, physical therapy, preventive medicine, and adult education. My deepest gratitude goes to Peg Houglam, PT, ATC; Bill Flentje, PT, ATC; Susan Harris, PT, PhD, FAPTA; and Joseph PH Black, MDiv, PhD. These individuals provided examples of exceptional leadership and set the standard for professionalism and integrity. I am deeply grateful to them for their past and continued guidance. I also must acknowledge my sister, Jill Thein-Nissenbaum, PT, DSc,, ATC, who is always willing to provide an ear, a hand, or sage advice. I am truly blessed by her presence in my life..

I am also deeply grateful to the doctoral students at Rocky Mountain University of Health Professions. They are a remarkable group of bright, inquisitive current and future leaders who do justice to our profession. I am grateful for the opportunity to learn from each of them.

Most importantly, since the second edition I have had two more children and finally finished that last college degree. I could not have done this edition without the countless hours my husband, Marc spent telling stories, driving kids, making dinners, and taking walks. His enthusiasm for alternative ideas and fresh perspectives pushes me in new directions. I am eternally grateful.

Lori Thein Brody

Brief Contents

Contents

CHAPTER 6

Impaired Aerobic Capacity/Endurance   101
JANET R. BEZNER

CHAPTER 7

Impaired Range of Motion and Joint Mobility   124
LORI THEIN BRODY

CHAPTER 8

Impaired Balance   167
COLIN GROVE, JUDITH DEWANE AND LORI THEIN BRODY

■ UNIT 5

Functional Approach to Therapeutic Exercise of the Lower Extremities   373

CHAPTER 17

The Lumbopelvic Region   373
CARRIE M. HALL

CHAPTER 18

The Pelvic Floor   418
ELIZABETH SHELLY

CHAPTER 19

The Hip   453
CARRIE M. HALL

Foundation of Therapeutic Exercise

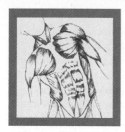

chapter 1

Introduction to Therapeutic Exercise and the Model of Functioning and Ability

LORI THEIN BRODY, CARRIE M. HALL

Among the many interventions available to physical therapists, therapeutic exercise has been shown to be fundamental to improving function and decreasing disability.[1-7] It is the premise of this text that, through carefully prescribed therapeutic exercise intervention, an individual can make significant changes in functional performance and disability, and that physical therapists have the unique educational training to be the preferred clinician for prescribing therapeutic exercise.

DEFINITION OF PHYSICAL THERAPY

The Federation of State Boards of Physical Therapy[8] defines physical therapy practice as (with updated language provided by the authors)

1. Examining, evaluating, and testing individuals with mechanical, physiological and developmental impairments, activity limitations and participation restrictions or other health and movement-related conditions in order to determine a diagnosis, prognosis, and plan of treatment and intervention, and to assess the ongoing effects of intervention.
2. Alleviating impairments, activity limitations, and participation restrictions by designing, implementing and modifying treatment interventions that may include, but are not limited to therapeutic exercise, functional training in self-care and in home community or work integration or reintegration, manual therapy including soft tissue and joint mobilization/manipulation, therapeutic massage, prescription, application, and, as appropriate, fabrication of assistive, adaptive, orthotic, prosthetic, protective and supportive devices and equipment, airway clearance techniques, integumentary protection and repair techniques, debridement and wound care, physical agents or modalities, mechanical and electrotherapeutic modalities, and patient-related instruction.
3. Reducing the risk of injury, impairment, activity limitation, and participation restriction including the promotion and maintenance of fitness, health, and wellness in populations of all ages.
4. Engaging in administration, consultation, education, and research.

It is evident from this definition that physical therapists examine, evaluate, diagnose, and intervene at the level of impairment, activity limitation, and participation restriction. The most critical message promoted by this definition is that physical therapists are primarily concerned with using knowledge and clinical skills to prevent, reduce, or eliminate impairments, activity limitations, and participation restrictions and to enable individuals seeking their services to achieve the most optimal quality of life possible.

In the past, the focus on measuring and altering impairments superseded the goals of improving function and disability. This text focuses on altering those impairments related to improving function and abilities through the use of therapeutic exercise. Instead of considering "which exercise can be prescribed to improve impairment," the physical therapist should consider "what impairments are related to reduced function and disability for *this patient* and which exercises can *improve functional performance* by addressing the appropriate impairments." Moreover, it is the physical therapist's charge to include therapeutic exercise that directly addresses the patient's function or activity limitations. Therapeutic exercises described throughout this book can remediate both impairments and activity limitations. For example, an exercise requiring the patient to move from sit to stand is an activity designed to improve a patient's transfer skills.

To understand the relationships among health conditions, impairment, activity limitation, and participation restriction, and to avoid confusion caused by misunderstood terminology, a detailed description of the classification of the components of health is necessary and is provided later in this chapter. The model is an updated version of the International Classification of Impairments, Disabilities, and Handicaps (ICIDH) first published by the World Health Organization (WHO) in 1980. The history of the original ICIDH model and the Nagi disablement model will provide the background necessary for understanding the current classification. The reader is encouraged to use this model to think about how disability relates to decisions regarding therapeutic exercise intervention.

THERAPEUTIC EXERCISE INTERVENTION

Therapeutic exercise is a health service intervention provided by physical therapists to patients and clients as part of physical therapist practice. **Patients** are persons with diagnosed impairments or activity limitations. **Clients** are persons who are not necessarily diagnosed with impairments or activity limitations but who are seeking physical therapist services for prevention or promotion of health, wellness, and fitness. Interventions for clients of physical therapists can include education regarding body mechanics provided to a group of persons involved in strenuous occupational activity, early education, and exercise prescription geared toward prevention for persons diagnosed with a musculoskeletal disease such as rheumatoid arthritis or exercise recommended for a group of high-level athletes to prevent injury or enhance performance.

Therapeutic exercise is considered a core element in most physical therapist plans of care. It is the systematic performance or execution of planned physical movements, postures, or activities intended to enable the patient/client to (1) remediate or prevent impairments, (2) enhance function, (3) reduce risk, (4) optimize overall health, and (5) enhance fitness and well-being.[9]

Therapeutic exercise may include aerobic and endurance conditioning and reconditioning; balance, coordination, and agility training; body mechanics and posture awareness training; muscle lengthening; range of motion techniques; gait and locomotion training; movement pattern training; or strength, power, and endurance training.

Although therapeutic exercise can benefit numerous systems of the body, this text focuses primarily on treatment of the musculoskeletal system. Concepts of therapeutic exercise intervention specifically for the cardiovascular/pulmonary, neurologic, and integumentary systems are not covered in this text, except as they relate to impairments of the musculoskeletal system.

Decisions regarding therapeutic exercise intervention should be based on individual goals that provide patients or clients with the ability to achieve optimal functioning in home, work (job/school/play), and community/leisure activities. To implement goal-oriented treatment, the physical therapist must

- Provide comprehensive and personalized patient management
- Rely on clinical decision-making skills
- Implement a variety of therapeutic interventions that are complementary (e.g., heat application before joint mobilization and passive stretch, followed by active exercise to use new mobility in a functional manner)
- Promote patient independence whenever possible through the use of home treatment (e.g., home spine traction, home heat or cold therapy), self-management exercise programs (e.g., in the home, fitness club, community-sponsored group classes, school-sponsored or community-sponsored athletics), and patient-related instruction.

Care must be taken to provide intervention sufficient to meet functional goals, avoid providing extraneous interventions, promote patient independence, and promote health care cost containment. In some cases, patient independence is not possible, but therapeutic exercise intervention is necessary to improve or maintain health status or prevent complications.

In these situations, training and educating family, friends, significant others, or caregivers to deliver appropriate therapeutic exercise intervention in the home can greatly reduce health care costs by limiting in-house physical therapist intervention.

THE LANGUAGE OF HEALTH: ABILITIES AND DISABILITIES

The purpose of defining a model of functioning and disability in a text on therapeutic exercise is to provide the reader with an understanding of the complex relationships of health conditions (i.e., pathology, disease, genetic anomalies), impairments, activity limitations, and participation restrictions, and to provide the conceptual basis for organizing elements of patient/client management that are provided by physical therapists. This text will use a biopsychosocial model that provides both the theoretical framework for understanding physical therapist practice and the classification scheme by which physical therapists make diagnoses.

Historically many paradigms of functioning and disability have been put forth. In traditional "medical models," disability is viewed as an individual problem caused by disease, genetics or injury, and is treated by individualized medical care. In this model, little regard is given to societal aspects of disability beyond public policy directed at health care guidelines. It is a patient-centered perspective with the individual as the focus of intervention. This contrasts "social models" which view disability as a socially created problem. Disability is created primarily by the social environment and is not an attribute of the individual. Therefore intervention and policy are not directed at individual medical care, but rather toward society at large to make environmental modifications necessary so that persons with disabilities can fully participate in all aspects of social life. A "biopsychosocial" model utilized by the WHO embraces both of these perspectives, addressing factors at the individual and social level.[10]

Evolution of the Biopsychosocial Model of Functioning and Disability

The most frequently presented models of functioning and disability have been the WHO's ICIDH[11] and a model developed by sociologist Saad Nagi[12] in the 1960s (Fig. 1-1). The original ICIDH model has been replaced with the International Classification of Functioning, Disability, and Health, known as the ICF.

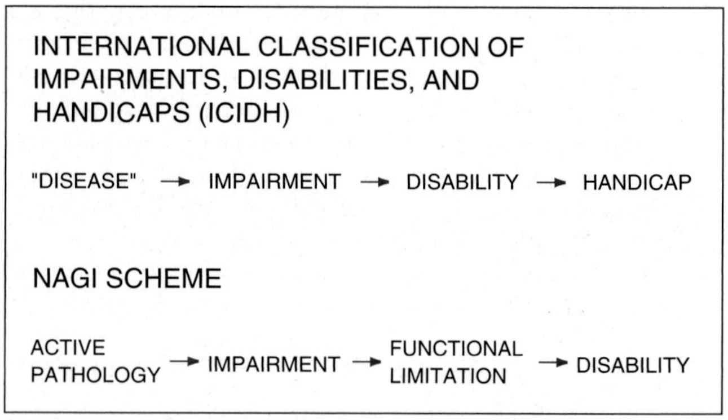

FIGURE 1-1. Two conceptual models for the disablement process.

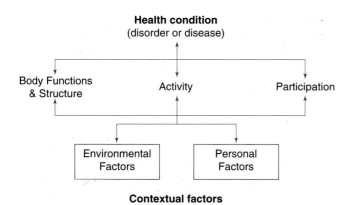

FIGURE 1-2. The WHO model of function and disability.

A review of Figures 1-1 and 1-2 demonstrates the significant differences between the original ICIDH and Nagi models and the current ICF model. In Nagi's disablement model, the central theme is the description of a process from disease or active pathology toward functional limitations and the factors limiting a person's ability to interact as a normally functioning person in society. The focus is primarily on *disability* which is reflected in the term "disablement model" used by Nagi in describing the model. However, the new ICF model focuses on both the positive and negative aspects of health, viewing health as a continuum. Rather than including only people with "disability," the ICF includes *all* people in its model. The ICF is a model of *functioning* and *disability*. Functioning is an umbrella term for body structures and function, and activities and participation (Part 1 of the ICF). It represents the positive aspects of the interaction between the individual with a health condition and that person's environmental and personal factors (Part 2 of the ICF, "Contextual Factors"). Disability is a parallel umbrella term describing the negative aspects of this same interaction. It is described by terms such as impairment, activity limitation, and participation restriction.

Nagi's model formed the basis for many of the documents produced by professional medical associations such as the American Physical Therapy Association. Many existing documents still use this language while professional associations make the transition to the ICF language. Therefore a brief discussion of the Nagi model relative to ICF language provides the reader with an understanding of the language still used in many documents and clinics, and provides a historical perspective for understanding the ICF.

Active Pathology/Health Condition

For Nagi, active pathology involves the interruption of normal cellular processes and the efforts of the affected systems to regain homeostasis. Active pathology can result from infection, trauma, metabolic imbalance, degenerative disease process, or another cause.[13] Examples of active pathology are the altered cellular processes found in osteoarthritis, cardiomyopathy, or ankylosing spondylitis. The ICF uses the term *health condition* as an umbrella term for disease, disorder, injury or trauma, as well as states such as pregnancy, ageing, congenital anomalies, or genetic predispositions.

Impairment

Impairment refers to a loss or abnormality at the tissue, organ, or body system level. The effects of disease or pathology are found in impairments of the body systems in which the pathologic state is manifest. The clinical example of a person diagnosed with rheumatoid arthritis may help to clarify the difference between pathology or health condition and impairments. Rheumatoid arthritis represents the pathology or disease diagnosis. The primary physiologic impairments associated with rheumatoid arthritis are found chiefly in the alteration of normal structure and function of bones, joints, and soft tissues of the musculoskeletal system. The impairments resulting from this disease process relevant to the musculoskeletal system may include impaired range of motion, joint mobility and integrity, or muscle performance. Body function impairments of the neuromuscular system (e.g., poor balance) or cardiovascular/pulmonary system (e.g., decreased endurance) can also be detected, usually as sequelae of the musculoskeletal system impairments.

Functional Limitation/Activity Limitation

The next level in Nagi's disablement model is functional limitation. For Nagi, this term represents a limitation in performance at the level of the whole organism or person. It appears he is referring to *components* of more complex tasks of basic activities of daily living (BADL; e.g., personal hygiene, feeding, dressing) and instrumental activities of daily living (IADL; e.g., preparing meals, housework, grocery shopping). Examples of functional limitations for Nagi might include gait abnormalities, reduced tolerance to sitting or standing, difficulty climbing the stairs, or inability to reach overhead. The ICF uses the term *activity limitation* defined as difficulties an individual may have in executing activities. These limitations range from mild to severe and are measured against a population standard.

Disability/Participation Restriction

Disability is the final element in Nagi's model. Nagi describes disability as any restriction or inability to perform socially defined roles and tasks expected of an individual within a sociocultural and physical environment. Activities and social roles associated with the term disability include[14]

- BADLs and IADLs
- Social roles, including those associated with an occupation or the ability to perform duties as a parent or student
- Social activities, including attending church and other group activities, and socializing with friends and relatives
- Leisure activities, including sports and physical recreation, reading, and travel

The ICF uses the term *participation restriction* defined as problems an individual may experience in involvement in life situations. Deficits are determined by measuring against societal standards. In the ICF, the term "disability" is reserved as an umbrella term for impairments, activity limitations, and participation restrictions.

Participation restrictions are reserved for social rather than individual functioning and people with similar activity limitations may have very different participation restrictions. For example, two persons diagnosed with the same disease with similar levels of impairment and activity limitation may have two different levels of participation restriction. One person may remain very active in all aspects of life (i.e., personal care and social roles), have support from family members in the home, and seek adaptive methods of continuing with his or her occupational tasks, whereas the other individual may choose to limit social contact, depend on others for personal care and household responsibilities, and have a job where it is not possible to use adaptive methods to participate in work tasks. Contextual factors play an important role in these differences.

The distinction between activity limitation and participation restriction is the difference between attributes and relational concepts. Attributes are phenomena that pertain to characteristics or properties of the individual. An activity limitation is primarily a reflection of the characteristics of the individual person. An activity limitation is measured at the level of the individual and compared against a population standard. Participation restriction, however, has a relational characteristic in that it describes the individual's limitation in relation to society and the environment. As the previous example demonstrated, persons with similar attribution profiles (e.g., disease, impairments, activity limitations) can present with different participation profiles. Factors such as age, general health status, personal goals, motivation, social support, and physical environment influence the level of disability the person experiences. A study of 100 patients rated at high risk for low back pain due to structural and psychosocial variables were prospectively followed for 4 to 6 years to determine the impact of these variables on disability. Psychosocial variables strongly predicted future disability whereas the structural variables had no association with future disability and medical care.[15]

INTERNATIONAL CLASSIFICATION OF FUNCTIONING, DISABILITY, AND HEALTH CLASSIFICATION

The ICF classification addresses many of the criticisms leveled at the original ICIDH and Nagi models.[10-12] Foremost among those criticisms was the focus on the disability or negative aspects of health and function. The ICF model emphasizes its ability to apply to all people, not just people with disabilities. ICF describes health and health-related states of all people, and everyone can be classified within the ICF system. Previous models were also criticized for lack of discrimination between limitations in performing societal roles and the *cause* of these limitations. In understanding the complex relationship between the individual with a health condition and that individual's response to that condition, it is important to identify the underlying cause of participation restrictions. The ICF addresses this in Part 2, "Contextual Factors." Contextual factors include environmental and personal factors.

Additionally, the language of the ICF reflects a significant change from the ICIDH. A shift has occurred, recognizing the stigmatizing and potentially negative aspects of the terms "handicap" and "disability." Therefore the WHO has decided to completely drop the term "handicap" and remove the term "disability" from a component, but retain it as the overall, umbrella term[10]. Moreover, the WHO emphasizes that the ICF is not a classification of *people* but a classification of "people's health characteristics within the context of their individual life situations and environmental impacts. It is the interaction of the health characteristics and the contextual factors that produces disability"[10].

Like the International Classification of Diseases, Tenth Revision (ICD-10)[11], the ICF uses an alphanumeric system to classify and categorize the levels of functioning and disability.[10] This enhances the system's usefulness for worldwide research and provides a common language. The letters b, s, d, and e are used to denote Body Functions, Body Structures, Activities and Participation, and Environmental Factors, *respectively*. The letters are followed by a chapter number (e.g., Chapter 7 for Body structures related to movement) followed by three or more numbers with specific descriptors and scales. Due to the complexity of the system, the details of the grading scales will not be covered in this text. For further information on this system, the reader is referred to *www.who.org*. An example of the two-level classification for *Body Structures and Body Functions* can be found in Tables 1-1 and 1-2.

The ICF classification has two major *parts*, Part 1, termed "Functioning and Disability" and Part 2, called "Contextual Factors." *Functioning* is an umbrella term indicating the positive aspects of health, used to include all body functions, activities, and participation. *Disability* is an umbrella term for the negative aspects of health, described as impairments, activity limitations, and participation restrictions. The parts are further divided into *components* with or without further division into *constructs* (see Table 1-3). A list of definitions for the essential terms can be found in Table 1-4.

TABLE 1-1   Two-Level Classification of Body Functions Related to the Motor System

NEUROMUSCULOSKELETAL AND MOVEMENT-RELATED FUNCTIONS

Functions of the joints and bones (b710–b729)
- b710 Mobility of joint functions
- b715 Stability of joint functions
- b720 Mobility of bone functions
- b729 Functions of the joints and bones, other specified and unspecified

Muscle functions
- b730 Muscle power functions
- b735 Muscle tone functions
- b740 Muscle endurance functions
- b749 Muscle functions, other specified and unspecified

Movement functions
- b750 Motor reflex functions
- b755 Involuntary movement reaction functions
- b760 Control of voluntary movement functions
- b765 Involuntary movement functions
- b770 Gait functions
- b780 Sensations related to muscles and movement functions
- b789 Movement functions, other specified and unspecified
- b798 Neuromusculoskeletal and movement-related functions, other specified
- b799 Neuromusculoskeletal and movement-related functions, unspecified

From International Classification of Functioning, Disability and Health. Geneva, Switzerland: World Health Organization, 2001.

TABLE 1-2 Two-Level Classification of Body Structures Related to the Motor System

STRUCTURES RELATED TO MOVEMENT

- s710 Structure of head and neck region
- s720 Structure of shoulder region
- s730 Structure of upper extremity
- s740 Structure of pelvic region
- s750 Structure of lower extremity
- s760 Structure of trunk
- s770 Additional musculoskeletal structures related to movement
- s798 Structures related to movement, other specified
- s799 Structures related to movement, unspecified

From International Classification of Functioning, Disability and Health. Geneva, Switzerland: World Health Organization, 2001.

Part 1: Functioning and Disability

Part 1 of the ICF deals with the majority of issues that physical therapists typically encounter in practice. The first component of this part includes the body's functions and its structures. The second component addresses activities and participation. Both the body structure and body function components have a positive and a negative aspect. This is one way in which both the "ability" and "disability" aspects of the functioning continuum are incorporated into the ICF.

Component A: Body Functions and Structures

Body functions are the physiological functions of body systems while *body structures* are the anatomical parts of the body such as organs and limbs. The body structures and the body functions components are designed to be used in parallel. For example, the body function component includes categories such as "mobility of joint functions" and the related body structures might be "joints of the shoulder region." The ICF would describe a healthy system (positive aspect) as having functional and structural integrity. The negative aspects of body functions and structures are termed impairments. *Impairments* are problems in body function or structures such as an anomaly, defect, loss, or other abnormality. They are deviations from generally accepted population standards. As with the Nagi model, impairments are not the same as pathology, but may be expressions of the pathology. However, not all impairments result from pathology. For example, congenital anatomic deformities or losses, immobilization, and faulty movement patterns can result in impairments of body structures and functions, but are not the result of pathology.

Impairments can be considered to be primary or secondary. Primary impairments result from pathology, disease or genetics. Secondary impairments arise from other impairments. For example, impairment of the muscles in the lower half of the body (e.g., paraparesis) may result in impairments of the protective functions of the skin (e.g., decubitus ulcers). Likewise, impairment of the control of voluntary movement functions (e.g., from stroke or neurological disease) may result in impairments of heart functions due to a lack of exercise, or impaired heart functions can lead to impaired respiratory functions. Secondary impairments can also lead to an additional or secondary health condition.

Impairments can be temporary or permanent, intermittent or continuous. For example, impaired joint mobility following a total knee replacement is a temporary condition, amenable to rehabilitative intervention. A joint that has been fused will have a permanent joint function impairment. Impaired joint stability such as occasional episodes of giving way following an anterior cruciate ligament tear is an intermittent impairment and may be activity related. An example of a continuous body function impairment is a shoulder that remains subluxed following a stroke. Impairments can also be described as progressing, regressing, or static.

TABLE 1-3 Overview of the ICF

COMPONENTS	PART 1: FUNCTIONING AND DISABILITY		PART 2: CONTEXTUAL FACTORS	
	BODY FUNCTIONS AND STRUCTURES	ACTIVITIES AND PARTICIPATION	ENVIRONMENTAL FACTORS	PERSONAL FACTORS
Domains	Body functions Body structures	Life areas (tasks, actions)	External influences on functioning and disability	Internal influences on functioning and disability
Constructs	Change in body functions (physiological) Change in body structures (anatomical)	Capacity: Executing tasks in a standard environment Performance: Executing tasks in the current environment	Facilitating or hindering impact of the physical, social, and attitudinal world	Impact of attributes of the person
Positive aspect	**Functioning**		Facilitators	Not applicable
	Functional and structural integrity	Activities Participation		
Negative aspect	**Disability**		Barriers hindrances	Not applicable
	Impairment	Activity limitation Participation restriction		

From International Classification of Functioning, Disability and Health. Geneva, Switzerland: World Health Organization, 2001; Table 1, p. 11.

TABLE 1-4 Relevant Definitions from the ICF

TERM	DEFINITION
Body functions	Physiological functions of body systems, including psychological functions. The standard is the statistical norm for humans.
Body structures	The structural or anatomical parts of the body such as organs, limbs, and their components classified accordingly by systems. The standard is the statistical norm for humans.
Impairment	The loss or abnormality in body structure or physiological function. Abnormality refers to a significant variation from established statistical norms.
Activity	The execution of a task or action by an individual. It is the individual perspective of functioning
Activity limitations	Difficulties an individual may have in executing activities. The limitations may range from slight to severe in terms of quality or quantity.
Participation	A person's involvement in a life situation. It is the societal perspective of functioning.
Participation restriction	Problems an individual may experience in the involvement in life situations. Participation restrictions are determined by comparing an individual's participation against what is expected of an individual without a disability in that culture or society.
Environmental factors	These make up the physical, social, and attitudinal environment in which people conduct their lives
Health condition	An umbrella term for disease (acute or chronic), disorder, injury, or trauma. It may also include other situations such as pregnancy, ageing, stress, congenital anomaly, or genetic predisposition.
Well-being	A general term encompassing the total universe of human life domains including physical, mental, and social aspects that make up a "good life." Health domains are a subset of the total universe of human life.

Component B: Activities and Participation

The second major component of the ICF Functioning and Disability portion is activities and participation. *Activity* is the execution of a task or action by an individual while *participation* is involvement in a life situation. The positive aspect of activities and participation is *functioning* implying the ability to perform individual activities and to participate in socially appropriate situations. The negative aspects are *activity limitations* and *participation restrictions*. These terms parallel the Nagi terms of *functional limitation* and *disability, respectively*.

Activity limitations are difficulties an individual may have in performing activities. These difficulties may be slight or severe. These limitations represent challenges on an individual level. Challenges at the societal level are called participation restriction and represent difficulties an individual has in a life situation. The degree of disability is determined by comparing against societal norms.

The Activities and Participation component has nine domains which encompass all life areas (Table 1-5). These domains can be used to represent abilities in activities, participation, or both. Each domain has a number associated with it, and within each domain there are several subclassifications. For example, domain 4, Mobility, has four categories with four to six more specific descriptors. An example of one category can be found in Table 1-6.

Both activities and participation have two qualifiers which represent important aspects of assessing abilities. The qualifiers are *performance* and *capacity*. Performance describes what a person actually does in his or her current environment. The performance qualifier includes all aspects of the person's situation, including psychosocial and environmental factors. Performance describes what the individual is able to do within the context (environmental and personal) of their world.

In contrast to performance, capacity is a standardized measure of an individual's ability to execute a task or action. Capacity measures attempt to capture the highest possible level of functioning that a person could attain at a given point in time. To do this, the environment and assessment procedures must be standardized. The disparity between performance and capacity provides insight into the environment's contribution to activity limitations and participation restrictions. This information can prove useful in determining how the environment can be modified to improve performance.

Part 2: Contextual Factors

Contextual factors encompass the background of the individual's personal life and environment. The two components are *environmental factors* and *personal factors*. Environmental factors reflect the external influences on functioning and disability while personal factors reflect the internal influences. These factors can have a tremendous impact on a person's health and health status. Environmental factors are those features that comprise the physical, social, and attitudinal

TABLE 1-5 Activities and Participation Domains and Qualifiers

DOMAINS		QUALIFIERS	
		PERFORMANCE	CAPACITY
d1	Learning and applying knowledge		
d2	General tasks and demands		
d3	Communication		
d4	Mobility		
d5	Self-care		
d6	Domestic life		
d7	Interpersonal interactions and relationships		
d8	Major life areas		
d9	Community, social, and civic life		

TABLE 1-6 **An Example of a Category Within the Mobility Domain of the Activities and Participation Component of the ICF**

WALKING AND MOVING (d450–d469)

- d450 Walking
- d455 Moving around
- d460 Moving around in different locations
- d465 Moving around using equipment
- d469 Walking and moving, other specified and unspecified

TABLE 1-7 **Domains of Environmental Factors Impacting Functioning and Disability**

ENVIRONMENTAL FACTORS

Chapter 1	Products and technology
Chapter 2	Natural environment and human-made changes to environment
Chapter 3	Support and relationships
Chapter 4	Attitudes
Chapter 5	Services, systems, and policies

environment in which people live and function. These factors can range from the close and personal such as the physical neighborhood in which the person lives to broader societal attitudes toward people with differing abilities. Attitudes of coworkers can impact a person's function in a work environment, and the physical structure of the neighborhood may preclude someone from walking around the block for exercise. Environmental factors can be positive, helping to improve a person's activity levels and participation, or they can be negative, producing barriers to participation. There are five categories of environmental factors (see Table 1-7).

Environmental factors are considered at two major levels, the *individual* and *societal*. The individual perspective is comprised of environmental settings such as home, school, or the workplace. The physical layout of the home, school, workplace, or environs or people encountered can support or hinder participation. The societal perspective includes both formal and informal social structures, community services, community and work organizations, government agencies, communication and transportation services, informal social networks as well as laws, regulations, and policies, both formal and informal.

The relationship among health conditions, body structures and functions, and activities and participation is a complex one,

particularly in light of environmental factors. Some work or other social structures may be positive, thereby improving a person's functioning, while others may be negative, creating barriers.

Personal factors, the second component of contextual factors, are the elements on an individual's background that are not part of the health condition or health states. Examples of these elements include gender, race, age, other health conditions, fitness, lifestyle, personal habits, coping styles, social background, education, profession, individual psychological assets, and life experiences. Like environmental factors, personal factors can have a positive or negative influence. These factors can help the person to be resilient or they can create barriers to function.

APPLICATION OF THE MODEL TO PHYSICAL THERAPIST PRACTICE

The model put forward by the ICF provides a common language and classification for describing function across a continuum of abilities. An application of this model to physical therapist practice can be found in Figure 1-3. The physical therapist practice application will be further expanded into the

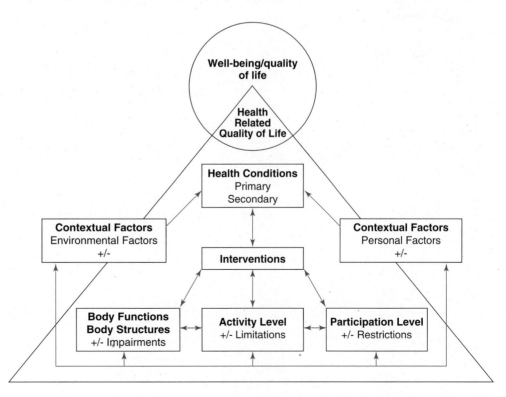

FIGURE 1-3. Modified physical therapy model of function and disability.

patient management model in Chapter 2. Physical therapists intervene at the level of impairment, activity limitation, and participation restriction. The concept of function, disability, and health refers to the "various impact(s) of chronic and acute conditions on the functioning of specific body systems, on basic human performance, and on people's functioning in necessary, usual, expected, and personally desired roles in society."[11,12] A practitioner's understanding of the factors that influence functioning and disability is fundamental to achieving the goal of restoring or improving function and reducing disability in the individual seeking services from a physical therapist. Additionally, the timing of intervention may impact psychosocial aspects of the patient's function. A study of patients with low back pain found that those patients randomized to an assess/advise/treat group demonstrated greater improvements in disability, mood, general health, and quality of life than patients in the assess/advise/wait group.[16] The authors felt that the timing of the intervention impacted the development of psychosocial features.

Therapeutic exercise intervention must not focus solely on disease, or impairments; it should additionally consider the functional loss and disability of the patient seeking physical therapist services. See Display 1-1. Although a specific therapeutic exercise intervention may be selected to remediate or prevent impairment, it must be selected in view of improving a functional outcome and the person's role in a specific sociocultural context and physical environment. Display 1-1 describes a patient with adhesive capsulitis of the shoulder. Physical examination shows impairments of body functions including mobility of the glenohumeral joint (b7100), associated shoulder girdle joints and articulations (b7101), and the scapula (b7200). The patient also lacks power of the muscles of the shoulder girdle (b7301) and has pain (b28014). A number of activities may be impacted depending upon the severity of the problem, limb dominance, and the patient's work and lifestyle. Display 1-1 lists a number of commonly limited activities, but many more possibilities exist. In this example, physical therapist interventions should be directed not only at the body function impairments (i.e., loss of mobility, loss of muscle power) but at the decreases in function such as the ability to use both arms to care for one's hair, or the ability to lift and carry loads. If full use of both upper extremities is required for

---

◆ DISPLAY 1-1

Example of ICF and ICD-10 with Coding and Descriptors of Components Relative to Patient Care

International Statistical Classification of Diseases and Related Health Problems

Primary ICD-10	m75.0	Adhesive capsulitis of the shoulder
Secondary ICD-10	m75.1	Rotator cuff syndrome
	m75.5	Bursitis of the shoulder

International Classification of Functioning, Disability, and Health

Primary ICF Codes

Body functions	b7100	Mobility of a single joint
	b7101	Mobility of several joints
	b7200	Mobility of scapula
	b7301	Power of muscles of one limb
	b29014	Pain in upper limb
Body structure	s7201	Joints of the shoulder region
	s7203	Ligaments and fasciae of the shoulder region
Activities and participation	d4300	Lifting
	d4301	Carrying in the hands
	d4302	Carrying in the arms
	d4303	Carrying on shoulders, hip, and back
	d4305	Putting down objects
	d4452	Reaching

Secondary ICF Codes

Body functions	b7401	Endurance of muscle groups
	b7800	Sensation of muscle stiffness
	b7809	Sensations related to muscles and movement functions, unspecified
	b2804	Radiating pain in a segment or region
Body structure	s7202	Muscles of the shoulder region
	s7200	Bones of the shoulder region
	s7209	Structure of shoulder region, unspecified
Activities and participation	d4201	Transferring onself while lying
	d4450	Pulling
	d4451	Pushing
	d4454	Throwing
	d4455	Catching
	d4451	Climbing
	d4550	Crawling
	d4554	Swimming
	d5100	Washing body parts
	d5202	Caring for hair
	d5400	Putting on clothes

the patient's occupation, then significant participation restrictions can result, especially if environmental factors (i.e., e330 People in positions of authority; e430 Individual attitudes of people in positions of authority; e5902 Labor and employment policies) have a negative impact. The therapist must acknowledge these factors and dialogue with the patient about the prognosis in all levels of function.

Another example is a patient with low back pain. Examination reveals that this patient has impairments associated with excessive mobility of the lumbar spine in the direction of flexion and low back pain after prolonged flexion postures and movement patterns associated with repetitive flexion. A passive or active stretch technique may be chosen to apply to the hamstrings.

Stretching the hamstrings is an intervention at the impairment level, improving the mobility of the associated joints. Improving the length of the hamstrings can increase hip range of motion and consequently improve mobility to bend forward at the hips before stressing the low back in a flexion movement pattern. Choosing to treat this impairment directly influences function by improving the mobility of a forward bend movement (i.e., a functional movement pattern) and reducing pain during an activity of daily living (e.g., bending forward to wash one's face, make the bed, set the table, reach into the refrigerator). Although weak abdominal muscles constitute a common impairment of patients with low back pain, treating weak abdominal muscles with a partial curl-up exercise, for example, may not be appropriate for that patient. The flexion force on the low back may exacerbate symptoms, and the partial curl-up may not relate to a meaningful functional movement pattern for the patient. Understanding the relationships among impairments and function for each patient enables the therapist to make sound decisions about therapeutic exercise intervention.

Health Conditions

Health conditions (disease, disorder, or condition) refers to an ongoing pathologic/pathophysiologic state that is (a) characterized by a particular cluster of signs and symptoms and (b) recognized by the patient or the practitioner as "abnormal." Health conditions are primarily identified at the cellular, tissue, and organ levels and are often the physician's medical diagnosis. It is, however, within the scope of physical therapist practice to diagnose such conditions at the tissue level using clinical tests and measures such as those outlined by Cyriax (e.g., supraspinatus tendonitis).[17] Furthermore, the complexity of the interrelationships among the components of the model of functioning and disability is indicative of the knowledge of pathology and pathophysiology necessary to perform optimal patient management. For example, in the case of a patient referred to a physical therapist with shoulder pain, the physical therapist performs an examination/evaluation to diagnose the condition. It is imperative for the physical therapist to be knowledgeable in the numerous possible causes of the patient's pain. The physical therapist's knowledge that different clusters of signs and symptoms are consistent with pathology at the tissue (e.g., tendonitis), organ (e.g., myocardial infarction), or cellular (e.g., lung cancer) level is critical for the diagnosis and management of the patient's condition. If the clinical findings on examination suggest a pathologic or pathophysiologic condition

that is not within the scope of physical therapist practice (e.g., myocardial infarction, lung cancer) that has not been addressed by the appropriate practitioner, an immediate referral is necessary (see Appendix 1). In many instances, the health condition cannot be diagnosed and the physical therapist must rely on clusters of impairments to formulate a diagnosis and intervention. A pathology-based diagnosis does not, by itself, delineate the impairments, activity limitations, or participation restrictions that will guide the physical therapist intervention (see Chapter 2). Therefore, the therapist must acknowledge the complex multidirectional and cyclical nature of the biopsychosocial model and the fact that intervention can be introduced at any component of the model, but that the more data collected regarding individual components, the more accurate the patient management will be.

Additionally, *secondary conditions* may develop as a result of a primary health condition. A secondary condition may be a type of health condition, impairment, activity limitation, or participation restriction. By definition, secondary conditions occur in the presence of a primary condition. Commonly encountered secondary conditions include pressure sores, contractures, urinary tract infection, cardiovascular deconditioning, and depression. Each of these secondary conditions can lead to additional activity limitations and participation restriction.

Impairments

Impairments are defined as losses or abnormalities of physiologic, psychologic, or anatomic structure or function. Active pathology results in impairment, but not all impairments originate from pathology (e.g., congenital anatomic deformity or loss, immobilization, faulty movement patterns). In accordance with the ICF, structural and functional impairments are differentiated throughout this text.

Physiologic Impairment

Physiologic impairment, or impairment of a body physiologic function, can be defined as an alteration in any physiologic function such as aerobic capacity, muscle performance (strength, power, endurance), joint mobility (i.e., hypomobility/hypermobility), balance, posture, or motor function (Fig. 1-4). It is an impairment of body function. Physiologic impairments also include impairment of mental function. Physical therapist practice interventions can most significantly modify physiologic impairments. Unit 2 of this text provides a more thorough discussion of each of these physiologic impairments and examples of therapeutic exercise interventions to remediate or prevent these impairments.

Structural Impairment

Structural impairment is an abnormality or loss of structure, such as hip anteversion, structural subtalar varus, structural genu varum, or congenital or traumatic loss of a limb. It is an impairment of body structure. Modifications to structural impairments can be made to improve function despite these existing impairments. The physical therapist should be aware of the presence of structural impairments to be able to provide an appropriate prognosis and determine the best plan of care. Therapeutic exercise intervention in the presence of structural impairments will be discussed in selected chapters in Units 5 and 6.

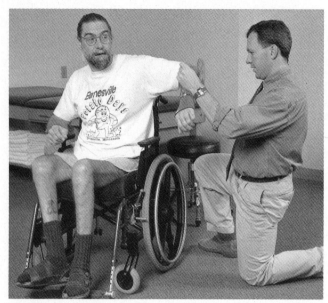

FIGURE 1-4. The patient exhibits a loss of medial rotation at the glenohumeral joint, a physiologic impairment in range of motion and joint mobility.

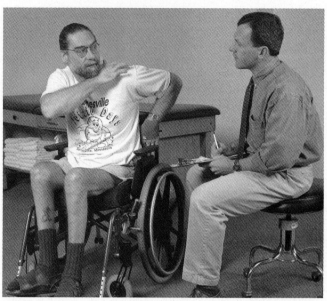

FIGURE 1-5. The activity limitation related to impaired range of motion and joint mobility is the patient's inability to transfer due to his inability to obtain appropriate shoulder range of motion to accomplish this task.

Activity Limitations, Participation Restrictions, and Quality of Life

Activity limitations and participation restrictions are limitations in individual functioning and/or functioning in society. The presence of an impairment does not necessarily mean a loss of function. For example, someone with a congenitally missing fifth finger may live a fully functioning life. In contrast, a person with a fifth metacarpal fracture in the dominant hand may be fully disabled in a job requiring hand power and dexterity. The therapist must look beyond impairments to the activity limitations to design a rehabilitation and therapeutic exercise program to address these limitations. Examples of functional activities include basic mobility (moving around, changing positions, etc.) carrying and moving objects, walking and moving and self-care (i.e., BADL, IADL) (See Figure 1-5). Examples of important categories of function from the ICF can be found in Table 1-8. Physical therapists have a strong command of therapeutic exercise to improve skills such as walking on different surfaces, moving around within the home, pushing with the lower extremities, throwing and reaching, and transfers. Exercise should focus on remediating impairments linked to activity limitations and to improving functional skills like transferring from supine to sit. Additionally, consideration must be given to the contextual factors that may impact activities and participation.

The ultimate goal for people in any health state is to maximize one's health-related quality of life (HRQL). The ICF defines well-being as an umbrella term encompassing the total universe of human life. HRQL is a subset of well-being related to health domains. It contains three major components[18,19]:

- *Physical function component,* which includes BADLs and IADLs
- *Psychologic component,* which includes the "various cognitive, perceptual, and personality traits of a person" and
- *Social components,* which involves the interaction of the person "within a larger social context or structure."

Assessments of quality of life attempt to capture how limitations in function affect physical, psychologic, and social roles as well as perceptions of health status.[20-22] A person may argue that issues related to quality of life are not distinct from disability, but quality of life is considered broader than disability, encompassing more than well being related to health such

---

TABLE 1-8 Expansion of the Categories Within the "Walking and Moving" category of the Mobility Domain

d450 Walking
- d4500 Walking short distances
- d4501 Walking long distances
- d4502 Walking on different surfaces
- d4503 Walking around obstacles
- d4508 Walking, other specified
- d4509 Walking, unspecified

d455 Moving around
- d4450 Crawling
- d4551 Climbing
- d4552 Running
- d4553 Jumping
- d4554 Swimming
- d4558 Moving around, other specified
- d4559 Moving around, other unspecified

d460 Moving around in different locations
- d4600 Moving around within the home
- d4601 Moving around within buildings other than home
- d4602 Moving around outside the home and other buildings
- d4608 Moving around in different locations, other specified
- d4609 Moving around in different locations, unspecified

d465 Moving around using equipment
d469 Walking and moving, other specified and unspecified

as education and employment. Other contextual variables contribute to an individual's sense of well being and overall quality of life. Such factors include economic status, individual expectations and achievements, personal satisfaction with choices in life, and sense of personal safety. The model (see Fig. 1-3) displays HRQL as a small part of the quality of life or well-being, and general quality of life overlaps with components of the ICF.

Contextual Factors and Interventions

The main pathway from disease to disability, including quality of life, can be modified by a host of factors such as age, gender, education, income, comorbidities, health habits, motivation, social support, and physical environment. Proper medical care and timely rehabilitation also can eliminate or reduce the impact of each component's affects on one another. Conversely, improper medical care or rehabilitation along with other aforementioned factors can magnify the impact of an impairment or limitation. Education, age, gender, disease severity, duration of illness and treatment, and comorbidity modify the functional level in persons diagnosed with rheumatoid arthritis,[22–24] and anxiety, depression, and coping style have been related to activity limitations in individuals with hip or knee osteoarthritis.[25]

Contextual factors can become risk factors if they impede progress toward full functioning in society. There are several types of risk factors:

- Demographic, social, lifestyle, behavioral, psychologic, and environmental factors
- Comorbidities (e.g., coexisting conditions)
- Physiologic impairments (e.g., short hamstrings, weak abdominal muscles, lengthened lower trapezius)
- Structural impairments (e.g., congenital scoliosis, shallow glenoid fossa, hip anteversion)
- Functional performance factors (e.g., less than optimal work station ergonomics resulting in poor posture at the work station, faulty gait kinetics or kinematics, inappropriate lifting mechanics)

The physical therapist must be aware of these factors for each individual, because they can greatly alter the individual's response to the health condition. With respect to therapeutic exercise intervention, many of these factors can directly influence the choice of activities or techniques, dosage, and expected functional outcome. An example is the scenario of two individuals involved in a motor vehicle accident and diagnosed with an acceleration injury to the cervical spine with resultant sprain or strain to the cervical soft tissues. One individual is a sedentary, 54-year-old male smoker with diabetes who has a significant forward head and thoracic kyphosis and must return to a data entry job (which he dislikes) at a poorly designed workstation. The other individual is an active and otherwise healthy, 32-year-old man who enjoys his job as a salesman and is engaged in activities such as sitting, standing, and walking throughout the day. The function and disability profiles of these two individuals are quite different, and the prognoses, therapeutic exercise interventions, and functional outcomes differ accordingly.

In addition to the risk factors present before disability, interventions (see Fig. 1-3) can alter the individual's functional level. Interventions may include extra-individual factors

(i.e., outside of the individual) such as medications, surgery, rehabilitation, supportive equipment, and environmental modifications or intra-individual factors (i.e., self-induced) such as changes in health habits, coping mechanisms, and activity modifications. The expected outcome is that interventions modify the functioning and disability profile in a positive manner. However, interventions occasionally serve as exacerbators. Exacerbators may occur in the following ways:

- Interventions may go awry.
- Persons may develop negative behaviors or attitudes.
- Society may place environmental or attitudinal barriers in the path of the individual.

Prevention and the Promotion of Health, Wellness, and Fitness

Physical therapists may prevent impairment, activity limitation, and participation restriction as well as improving the HRQL by identifying risk factors during the diagnostic process. Risk factors are typically part of the ICF profile (i.e., other health conditions, impairments, or contextual factors) that place the individual at an increased risk of disability. Identifying these factors allows the therapist to implement a prevention program. Three major types of prevention include[9]

- *Primary prevention*, which is the prevention of disease in a susceptible or potentially susceptible population through specific measures such as general health promotion efforts,
- *Secondary prevention*, which includes efforts to decrease duration of illness, severity of disease, and sequelae through early diagnosis and prompt intervention, and
- *Tertiary prevention*, which includes efforts to decrease the degree of disability and promote rehabilitation and restoration of function inpatients with chronic and irreversible diseases.

Therapeutic exercise as an intervention intends to promote primary, secondary, and tertiary prevention as well as health, wellness, and fitness. Prevention, health, wellness, and fitness must be considered critical foundational concepts of therapeutic exercise intervention (see Chapter 4).

SUMMARY

The model of **function and abilities** (see Fig. 1-3) exhibits the complexity of the relationships among health conditions, impairments, activity limitations, participation restriction, contextual factors, interventions, quality of life, and prevention, wellness, and fitness. A practitioner's understanding of this model is critical to developing a therapeutic exercise program that is effective, efficient, and meaningful for the individual seeking physical therapist services. The amount of data that can be collected during an initial examination or evaluation of an individual can be immense and often overwhelming. This model allows the physical therapist to organize data pertaining to the patient's impairments, activity limitations, and participation restrictions. It also allows the physical therapist to categorize pertinent aspects of the patient's history, the effect of prior treatment, and the presence of contextual factors. Most important, the clinical presentation can be classified in a way that identifies the impairments impeding the performance of certain functional tasks and activities, thereby focusing the treatment on only those impairments directly related to activity limitation and participation restriction. It also enables the practitioner to clarify contextual factors and interventions that may serve as impediments to improved functional performance, reduced disability, and improved quality of life, thereby serving the role of prevention, and promoting health, wellness, and fitness. With this analysis, the practitioner can develop goals that are relevant to the individual's daily life and promote health, wellness, and fitness at any level of ability.

KEY POINTS

- Physical therapists examine patients with impairments, activity limitations, and participation restrictions or other health-related conditions to determine a diagnosis, prognosis, and intervention.
- Physical therapists are involved in alleviating and preventing impairments, activity limitations, and participation restrictions by designing, implementing, and modifying therapeutic interventions.
- Therapeutic exercise intervention engages the individual to become an active participant in the treatment plan.
- Therapeutic exercise should be a core intervention in most physical therapist treatment plans.
- As the health care industry continues to change, the practitioner must recognize that the third-party reimburser for medical care is seeking health care services that are efficient and cost-effective. Prudent use of therapeutic exercise can reduce health care costs by promoting patient independence and self-responsibility.
- A thorough understanding of the process of functioning and disability can assist the practitioner in developing an effective, efficient, and cost-contained therapeutic exercise intervention, meaningful to the person seeking physical therapist services.

CRITICAL THINKING QUESTIONS

Develop a case defining each feature of the physical therapist model of functioning and disability. Given a patient with low back pain, provide a probable history of the condition. Include a brief description of each of the following features:
- Contextual factors
- Health condition
- Impairments (structural, physiologic)
- Activity limitations
- Performance restriction
- Secondary conditions

- Previous interventions (intraindividual, extraindividual, and exacerbators)

How would these elements change if the patient was a different age, had a different lifestyle, or a different occupation?

REFERENCES

1. Sayers SP, Bean J, Cuoco A, et al. Changes in function and disability after resistance training: does velocity matter?: a pilot study. Am J Phys Med Rehabil 2003;82:605–613.
2. Morey MC, Shu CW. Improved fitness narrows the symptom-reporting gap between older men and women. J Womens Health 2003;12:381–390.
3. Topp R, Mikesky A, Wigglesworth J, et al. The effect of a 12-week dynamic resistance strength training program on gait velocity and balance of older adults. Gerontologist 1993;33:501–506.
4. Rejeski WJ, Ettinger WH Jr, Martin K, et al. Treating disability in knee osteoarthritis with exercise therapy: a central role for self-efficacy and pain. Arthritis Care Res 1998;11:94–101.
5. Teixeira-Salmela LF, Olney SJ, Nadeau S, et al. Muscle strengthening and physical conditioning to reduce impairment and disability in chronic stroke survivors. Arch Phys Med 1999;80:121–128.
6. Weiss A, Suzuki T, Bean J. High intensity strength training improves strength and functional performance after stroke. Arch Phys Med Rehabil 1999;79:369–376.
7. Hiroyuki S, Uchiyama Y, Kakurai S. Specific effects of balance and gait exercises on physical function among the frail elderly. Clin Rehabil 2003;17:472–479.
8. The Model Practice Act for Physical Therapy: A Tool for Public Protection and Legislative Change. 2006: Federation of State Boards of Physical Therapy. Alexandria, VA.
9. American Physical Therapy Association. A guide to physical therapist practice, I: a description of patient management. Phys Ther 1995;75:709–764.
10. International Classification of Functioning, Disability and Health. Geneva, Switzerland: World Health Organization, 2001.
11. International Classification of Impairments, Disabilities, and Handicaps. Geneva, Switzerland: World Health Organization, 1980.
12. Nagi SZ. Disability and Rehabilitation. Columbus, OH: Ohio State University Press, 1969.
13. Verbrugge L, Jette A. The disablement process. Soc Sci Med 1994;38:1–14.
14. Pope A, Tarlov A, eds. Disability in America: Toward a National Agenda for Prevention. Washington, DC: National Academy Press, 1991.
15. Carragee EJ, Alamin TF, Miller JL, et al. Discographic, MRI and psychosocial determinants of low back pain disability and remission: a prospective study in subjects with benign persistent back pain. Spine J 2005;5(1):24–35.
16. Wand, BM, Bird C, McAuley JH, et al. Early intervention for the management of acute low back pain: a single randomized controlled trial of biopsychosocial education, manual therapy and exercise. Spine 2004;29(2):2350–2356.
17. Cyriax J. Textbook of Orthopedic Medicine. Diagnosis of Soft Tissue Lesions. 8th Ed. London, England: Bailliere Tindall, 1982.
18. Jette AM. Using health-related quality of life measures in physical therapy outcomes research. Phys Ther 1993;73:528–537.
19. Jette AM. Physical disablement concepts for physical therapy research and practice. Phys Ther 1994;74:380–386.
20. DeHaan R, Aaronson N, Limburt M, et al. Measuring quality of life in stroke. Stroke 1993;24:320–327.
21. Hollbrook M, Skillbeck CE. An activities index for use with stroke patients. Age Ageing 1983;12:166–170.
22. Mitchell DM, Spitz PW, Young DY, et al. Survival, prognosis and cause of death in rheumatoid arthritis. Arthritis Rheum 1986;29:706–714.
23. Sherrer YS, Bloch DA, Mitchell, et al. Disability in rheumatoid arthritis: comparison of prognostic factors across three populations. J Rheumatol 1987;14:705–709.
24. Mitchell JM, Burkhouser RV, Pincus T. The importance of age, education, and comorbidity in the substantial earnings and losses of individuals with symmetric polyarthritis. Arthritis Rheum 1988; 31:348–357.
25. Summers MN, Haley WE, Reville JD, et al. Radiographic assessment and psychologic variables as predictors of pain and functional impairment in osteoarthritis of the knee or hip. Arthritis Rheum 1988;31:204–207.

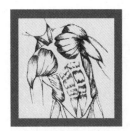

chapter 2

Patient Management

CARRIE M. HALL

INTRODUCTION

An understanding of the ICF system presented in Chapter 1 enables the clinician to provide optimal patient management by understanding the relationships between functioning and disability and environmental and personal factors. Knowledge of the ICF system enables the clinician to

- Develop comprehensive yet efficient examinations and evaluations of impairments and activity limitations relating to the patient's unique participation limitations and environmental and personal factors.
- Reach an accurate diagnosis based on logical classification of pathology, impairments, and disabilities.
- Develop a prognosis based on the evaluation and the patient's unique profile.
- Create and implement effective and efficient interventions.
- Reach a desirable functional outcome for the patient as quickly as possible.

Each patient presents with unique anatomic, physiologic, kinesiologic, psychologic, and environmental characteristics. Consideration of all these variables is necessary to develop an effective plan of care, but it can be overwhelming even for the experienced clinician. This chapter presents two additional models to assist in organizing the data and making the clinical decisions that are necessary to develop an effective and efficient therapeutic exercise intervention: the patient management model proposed by the American Physical Therapy Association[1] and a therapeutic exercise intervention model.

PATIENT MANAGEMENT MODEL

The physical therapist's approach to patient management is described as the patient management model in Figure 2-1. The physical therapist integrates these five elements of care in a manner designed to maximize the patient's outcome, which may be conceptualized as patient related (e.g., satisfaction with care) or associated with service delivery (e.g., efficacy and efficiency). The current model of patient management intends to involve the patient in decision making, which should in turn result in higher satisfaction with care. In addition, in a responsibility-focused health care system, the clinicians are called to identify and justify the hypotheses that underlie interventions, which should in turn result in improved efficiency of care and provide payers with better justification for intervention.

Examination

Examination is required before the initial intervention and is performed for all patients/clients. Examination is defined as the process of obtaining a history, performing a relevant systems review, and selecting and administering specific tests and measures to obtain data.[1] The history is expected to provide the physical therapist with pertinent information about the patient (Display 2-1).

These data can be obtained from the patient, family, significant others, caregivers, and other interested persons through interview or self-report forms, by consulting with other members of the health care team and by reviewing the medical record. Display 2-1 summarizes the data generated from the history.

The systems review is a screening process that provides information about the bodily systems involved in the patient's current disability profile. Data generated from the systems review may affect tests performed during subsequent examinations and choices regarding interventions. The systems review also assists the physical therapist in identifying possible problems that require consultation with or referral to another provider. Several major systems should be screened for involvement: cardiovascular/

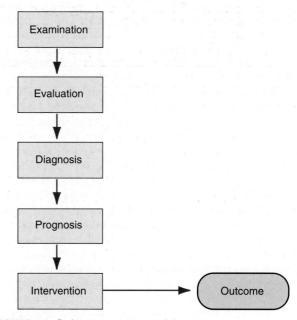

FIGURE 2-1. Patient management model.

DISPLAY 2-1
Data Generated From Client History

General Demographics
- Age
- Sex
- Race
- Primary language

Social History
- Cultural beliefs and behaviors
- Family and caregiver resources
- Social interactions, social activities, and support systems

Occupation
- Current or prior work (e.g., job, school, and play) or community activities

Growth and Development
- Hand and foot dominance
- Developmental history

Living Environment
- Living environment and community characteristics
- Projected discharge destination(s)

History of Present Condition
- Concerns that led the individual to seek the services of a physical therapist
- Concerns or needs of the individual requiring the services of a physical therapist
- Onset and pattern of symptoms
- Mechanism(s) of injury or disease, including date of onset and course of events
- Patient's, family's, or caregiver's perceptions of the patient's emotional response to the present clinical situation
- Current therapeutic interventions

- Patient's, family's, or caregiver's expectations and goals for the therapeutic intervention

Functional Status and Level of Activity
- Prior functional status, and self-care and home management (i.e., activities of daily living and instrumental activities of daily living)
- Behavioral health risks
- Sleep patterns and positions

Medications
- Medications for present condition
- Medications for other conditions

Other Tests and Measures
- Review of available records
- Laboratory and diagnostic tests

History of Present Condition
- Prior therapeutic interventions
- Prior medications

Medical or Surgical History
- Endocrine/metabolic
- Gastrointestinal
- Genitourinary
- Pregnancy, delivery, and postpartum
- Prior hospitalizations, surgeries, and preexisting medical and other health-related conditions

Family History
- Familial health risks

Social Habits (past and present)
- Level of physical fitness (self-care, home management, community, and work [e.g., job, school, and play] and leisure activities)

American Physical Therapy Association. Guide to physical therapist practice. 2nd Ed. American Physical Therapy Association. Phys Ther 2001;81:9–746.

pulmonary, integumentary, musculoskeletal, and neuromuscular. In addition, communication ability, affect, cognition, language, and learning style of the patient should be assessed. Display 2-2 summarizes the data generated from a systems review.

Depending on the data gathered from the history and systems review, the therapist may use one or more examinations in whole or in part. The examination may be as brief or lengthy as necessary to generate a diagnosis. For example, after taking the history and concluding a systems review, the physical therapist may determine that further examination is not appropriate and that the patient should be referred to another health care practitioner. Conversely, the physical therapist may determine that a detailed examination of several bodily systems is required to develop a thorough diagnosis. The specific tests and measures included in each examination generate data about the patient's impairments and activity limitations. Implementation of the examination is based on a prioritized order of tests and measures that depend on medical safety, patient comfort, and medical treatment priorities; the patient's physiologic, emotional, functional, social, and vocational needs; and financial resources. The

DISPLAY 2-2
Systems Review Data[1]

The systems review includes the following:
- Cardiopulmonary: assessment of heart rate, respiratory rate, blood pressure, and edema
- Musculoskeletal: gross symmetry, gross ROM, gross strength, height, weight
- Neuromuscular: gross coordinated movement (e.g., balance, locomotion, transfers, transitions)
- Integumentary: skin integrity, skin color, presence of scar formation
- Communication ability, affect, cognition, language, and learning style: includes the assessment of the ability to make needs known, consciousness, orientation (person, place, and time), expected emotional/behavioral responses, and learning preferences (e.g., learning barriers, educational needs)

most relevant examinations to this text that are performed by a physical therapist are listed in Table 2-1.[1]

Other information may be required to complete the examination process such as clinical findings of other health

| TABLE 2-1 | **Physical Therapy Examinations** |

- Aerobic capacity/endurance
- Anthropometric characteristics
- Assistive and adaptive devices
- Circulation (arterial, venous, lymphatic)
- Cranial and peripheral nerve integrity
- Environmental, home, and work (job/school/play) barriers
- Ergonomics and body mechanics
- Gait, locomotion, and balance
- Integumentary integrity
- Joint integrity and mobility
- Motor function (motor control and motor learning)
- Muscle performance (strength, power, endurance)
- Orthotic, protective, and supportive devices
- Pain
- Posture
- ROM (including muscle length)
- Reflex integrity
- Sensory integrity
- Ventilation and respiration/gas exchange
- Work (job/school, play), community, and leisure integration or reintegration

care professionals, results of diagnostic imaging, clinical laboratory, and electrophysiologic studies or information from the patient's place of work regarding ergonomic, posture, and movement requirements.

The examination is an ongoing process throughout the patient's treatment to determine the patient's response to intervention. Based on reexamination findings (e.g., new clinical symptoms or failure to respond in the expected manner to the intervention), the intervention may be terminated or modified. Exercise modification is discussed later in this chapter.

Evaluation

Evaluation is the dynamic process in which the physical therapist makes judgments based on data gathered during the examination. To make appropriate clinical decisions regarding the evaluation, the physical therapist must

- Determine the priority of problems to be assessed based on the medical history (and any other pertinent data collected through medical records or interactions with other health care providers) and systems review.
- Implement the examination.
- Interpret the data.

Interpretation of the examination findings is one of the most critical stages in clinical decision making. In interpreting the data to understand the sources or causes of the patient's impairments in body functions or structure, limitations in activities, restriction in participation, and environmental barriers, all aspects of the examination must be considered and analyzed to determine the following:

- Progression and stage of the signs and symptoms
- Stability of the condition
- Presence of preexisting conditions (i.e., comorbidities)
- Relationships among involved systems and sites

To remain consistent with the language of the ICF and to link the physical therapy patient management model with

the ICF model (see Fig. 1-2), the following sections provide the reader with examples of examinations and evaluations for each element of the ICF model.

Health Condition (Disorder/Disease/Injury Trauma)

Laboratory tests, imaging studies, and neurologic examinations are used to assess the presence and extent of the pathologic process at the organ, tissue, or cellular level. Because some biochemical and physiologic abnormalities may be beyond the scope of medical testing, detection often relies on the examination/evaluation of impairments. One of the frustrations for physical therapists is that often, underlying pathology associated with the impairments in body function or structure cannot be identified. Imaging, neurologic, or laboratory study results commonly are negative despite the presence of clinical signs and symptoms. However, the lack of an identifiable pathology should not lead the physical therapist to believe that an organic reason for the individual's impairments in body function or structure, activity limitations or participation restrictions is not present. Even with a diagnosis of pathology, the physical therapist should concentrate on examination and evaluation of impairments in structure and body functions, activity and participation levels, and environmental accessibility, because the pathoanatomic diagnosis cannot, in and of itself, guide the physical therapist's intervention.

Impairments in Body Function and Structure

Medical procedures to evaluate impairments in body function and structure include clinical examinations, laboratory tests, neurologic tests, imaging procedures, and the patient's medical history and symptom reports. Physical therapy procedures to examine and evaluate impairments should be based on bodily systems most treated by physical therapists including the musculoskeletal, neuromuscular, cardiovascular, pulmonary, and integumentary systems (Fig. 2-2A). Many bodily systems are not within the scope of thorough and definitive examination by a physical therapist (e.g., metabolic, renal, and circulatory). However, if pertinent to the physical therapy intervention, this information should be gathered from the patient, other medical and health care professionals, or medical records. Specific tests (e.g., pulse and blood pressure) indicating system impairments that are within the scope of therapists should be performed (Fig. 2-2B).

Examinations may reveal a list of impairments that may or may not be amenable to physical therapy treatment. It is tempting to evaluate and treat lists of impairments, but this type of practice may not be the most effective or efficient use of health care dollars. It is therefore prudent to make simultaneous decisions about whether testing or measuring any one impairment is pertinent to determining the cause(s) of the activity limitation and participation restriction. To facilitate this decision-making process, ask the following questions:

- Is the impairment related directly to a limitation in activity level or restriction in participation? For example, reduced glenohumeral range of motion (ROM) (i.e., impairment) can be directly related to an inability

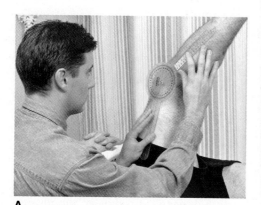

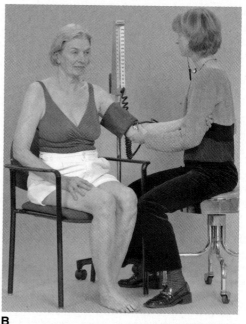

A   B

FIGURE 2-2. (A) Measurement of ROM and muscle length impairment. The patient shows signs of limited hamstring extensibility. (B) Measurement of aerobic capacity impairment. The clinician takes the patient's blood pressure.

to reach upward (i.e., limitation in activity) and perhaps paint the ceiling and therefore be unable to work as a house painter (i.e., participation restriction).

- Is the impairment a secondary condition of the primary pathology or impairment? For example, a patient has complaints of shoulder pain and loss of mobility (i.e., impairments) resulting in reduced function of the upper extremity for activities of daily living (ADL) (i.e., activity limitation) and subsequently restriction in sports or recreational activities (i.e., participation restriction). However, the source of the shoulder pain is cervical disk disease (i.e., primary pathology). Loss of mobility of the shoulder is a secondary impairment, and reduced use of the upper extremity during ADLs and sports are a secondary limitations/restrictions, both of which developed because of pain in the shoulder originating from the primary condition of cervical degenerative disk disease.
- Can the impairment be related to future limitations in activity or participation restrictions? Studies have shown that a relationship can exist between current impairment findings and future activity limitations.[2,3] For example, loss of shoulder ROM in the absence of ADL limitation may lead to limitation in the future from exaggeration of the impairment or the existing impairment leading to other impairments.
- Is the impairment unrelated to the activity limitation, participation restriction, or environmental barrier and therefore should not be assessed or treated? For example, a patient complains of shoulder pain and reduced use of the shoulder girdle during ADLs. Hypomobility of the shoulder girdle may be an obvious impairment, but it may not be related to the activity limitation. The patient's pain may occur in the midrange and be a result of impaired scapulohumeral rhythm, not hypomobility.

In summary, not all impairments result in activity limitation and participation restriction, and not all activity limitations result in participation restrictions. For the clinician to provide effective care that will ultimately affect function and reduce the potential for disability, therapeutic interventions should, in theory, target only those impairments that are related to the activity limitations. Indeed, it has been suggested that through the examination process, the clinician determines the interactions between impairments, activity limitations, participation restrictions, and environmental barriers for a patient with a given diagnosis and that this information then guides treatment.[4] Examples of cervical spine impairments include reduced range of cervical spine motion and decreased segmental joint mobility, whereas an activity limitation might be inability to rotate the head and neck sufficiently to be able to see behind. A participation restriction results when this occurs while driving an automobile in reverse. If an individual is then unable to work because his or her occupation requires automobile use that person has environmental barriers.

Activity Limitation and Participation Restriction

Rarely does the patient seen in the physical therapy department, clinic, or office describe specific complaints of weakness, loss of muscle length, or loss of joint mobility (i.e., impairments). For example, the patient is probably more concerned about his or her ability to climb a flight of stairs (i.e., activity) or get up the flight of stairs to enter his or her office (i.e., participation) than the adequate knee ROM and quadriceps force or torque production needed to climb the stairs (i.e., impairments). Furthermore, improved knee ROM and quadriceps torque production may not result in the ability to climb a flight of stairs. The inability to climb stairs may be related to other impairments, such as weak gluteal musculature, lack of ankle mobility, or psychologic impairments (e.g., fear, confidence).

One question must be addressed in daily practice and in physical therapy research, "Which and to what degree are impairments in body function and structure linked to activity limitations and participation restriction?" Many studies are attempting to establish the relationships among pathology, impairments, activity limitations, and participation restriction because this question is clinically important to physical therapists. For example, the information gained from a descriptive study of individuals with arthritis indicates correlations among pathology (i.e., arthritis), impairments (i.e., knee ROM, pain and joint stiffness, and reduced muscle performance), and activity limitations (i.e., performing ADLs including getting down to and up from the floor and ascending/descending stairs).[5] This study indicates that quadriceps muscle performance, joint pain during the activity, perceptions of functional ability, and body weight combined can predict between 39% and 56% of the variance in time to perform four functional tasks in adults with osteoarthritis of the knee. These findings appear to indicate that interventions that improve quadriceps muscle performance, reduce joint pain and body weight, and facilitate perceptions of functional ability may have a positive impact on the ability to get down to and up from the floor and ascend/descend stairs in adults with osteoarthritis of the knee.

In the ICF manual, the WHO has acknowledged that "it is difficult to distinguish between 'Activities' and 'Participation'."[6] Nevertheless, differentiation among ICF concepts and the ability to measure each clearly and distinctly is essential if the ICF is to achieve acceptance by individuals, organizations, and associations as an international classification of human functioning and disability. A crucial area of research is to improve the ICF's ability to differentiate clearly among concepts and categories within the framework and to develop sound assessment instruments that can be used to measure the various domains and qualifiers outlined in the ICF framework. Physical therapy researchers can provide important leadership in this area of research in the years ahead that, in turn, can improve our ability to provide the highest quality clinical care to our patients.

Generally, activity domain items encompass relatively simple tasks or activities (e.g., transfer from sit to stand) that an individual encounters on a frequent or daily basis. Measurement scales used for the activity domain items focus more on the ability (or perceived ability) or capacity of a person to perform each specific task or action rather than whether the individual is limited in performing them in the context of their normal daily life.

In contrast, the participation domain has been defined as the limitation the person encounters in the performance of more complex life roles. The roles contained within the participation domain refer to much more complex life activities. Participation restriction, as defined in the ICF model introduced in Chapter 1 (see Fig. 1-2), entails the social context of functional loss. Social function encompasses three domains: social interaction, social activity, and social role.[7] Each of these domains requires a certain degree of physical ability. For example, activity limitation in going up and down stairs may limit

1. A person's social interaction because of the inability to go outside the home to visit friends.
2. A person's social activity because of the inability to go to church with stairs to the front door.
3. A person's social role because of the inability to go to work and perform tasks that require going up and down stairs.

This content distinction between activity limitation and participation restriction is very consistent with the differentiation made between the functional limitations and disability domains outlined within the Nagi[8] disablement framework.

Measurement of disability requires tests that consider the complexity of variables that affect the person's ability to interact in society. With standardized tests, no single assessment instrument can measure the full range of potential impairments, activity limitations, or participation restrictions. Adequate evaluation usually must rely on a battery of appropriate instruments. It is beyond the scope of this text to discuss the various standardized tests, but a literature search on the specific population you are testing can offer explicit tests and measures for your desired purpose.[9-20]

Tests and measures of function and disability have various formats:

- The standard and most economic procedure for measuring disability is self-reports or proxy reports,[21,22] which include simple ordinal or interval scoring of the degree of difficulty in performing roles within the person's milieu.[19,23-31]
- Observation of performance of functional tasks, rating the level of difficulty (e.g., fully able, partially able, and unable), such as measuring distances, weight lifted, number of repetitions, or quality of motion based on kinesiologic standards.[23]
- Clinical tests of physical mobility (e.g., 6-minute walk test, Berg balance scale, timed up and go test, gait speeds, and timed movement battery).[32-34]
- Equipment-based evaluation of performance (e.g., use of a hand dynamometer to examine grip strength, computer-assisted assessment of balance, use of specialized grids to measure performance of closed chain activities).[24-26,35,36]

Results of a disability measure often reveal aspects of the disability that are beyond physical impairments and activity limitations. In some cases, aspects of an individual's disability are beyond the knowledge, expertise, or experience of the PT, in which case the patient should be referred to the appropriate health care professional. A simultaneous decision must be made as to whether further physical therapy intervention is appropriate or if physical therapy should be deferred until other aspects of disability are adequately dealt with. For example, a patient with low back pain may have a high level of anxiety or depression associated with the loss of function and the disability. Physical therapy may not be effective until the patient is treated for the anxiety or depression, or physical therapy concurrent with counseling may be determined to be most effective.

The time it takes to complete and interpret the self-report forms has been described as a methodologic and practical barrier to using self-reports. However, self-reports assist in determining whether activity limitations and disability exist beyond the scope of physical therapy practice and result in a referral to health care providers educated to evaluate and treat components outside the physical therapist's domain. This information may save the financial resources and time spent attempting to treat physical impairments or activity limitations that cannot be resolved without more comprehensive intervention involving other health care practitioners, family members, or significant others. The time and cost savings to the patient and the health care system justify the time spent completing and interpreting the form. It is beyond the scope of this text to discuss all of the standardized tests of disability. The Medical Outcomes Study 36-Item Short-Form Health Survey (SF-36)[37] is a multidimensional generic measure designed to assess both physical and mental health statuses. The SF-36 is a good choice for a baseline and can be complemented by a more patient population–specific disability questionnaire such as those provided in the associated reference list.[20,21,27,35,38,39]

Diagnosis

Diagnosis is the next element in the patient management model. Diagnosis is the process and end result of information obtained in the examination and evaluation. The diagnostic process includes analyzing the information obtained in the examination and evaluation and organizing it into clusters, syndromes, or categories (see Display 2-3 for definition of terms) to help determine the most appropriate intervention strategy for each patient. The diagnostic process includes the following components[1]:

- Obtaining a relevant history (i.e., examination)
- Performing a systems review (i.e., examination)
- Selecting and administering specific tests and measures (i.e., examination)
- Interpreting all data (i.e., evaluation)
- Organizing all data into a cluster, syndrome, or category (i.e., diagnosis)

The end result of the diagnostic process is establishing a diagnosis. To reach an appropriate diagnosis, additional information may need to be obtained from other health care professionals. In the event that the diagnostic process does not yield an identifiable cluster, syndrome, or category, intervention may be guided by the reduction of impairments and restoring activity and participation levels. Caution should be taken in randomly treating impairments not associated with functional outcome. The purpose of a diagnosis made by a physical therapist is not to identify all of the patient's impairments, but to focus on which impairments are related to the patient's activity and participation and therefore should be addressed by the physical therapist. To ensure optimal patient care, the physical therapist may need to share the diagnosis determined from the physical therapy examination and evaluation process with other professionals on the health care team. If the diagnostic process reveals that the condition is outside of the therapist's knowledge, experience, or expertise, the patient should be referred to the appropriate practitioner.

Diagnosis in the physical therapy patient management model is synonymous with the term clinical classification and is not to be confused with the term medical diagnosis.[40] Medical diagnosis is the identification of a patient's pathology or disease by its signs, symptoms, and data collected from tests ordered by the physician. Diagnosis established by a physical therapist is related to the primary dysfunction toward which the physical therapist directs treatment.[40-42] The ability to diagnose clusters, syndromes, or categories can foster the development of efficient treatment interventions and facilitate reliable outcomes research to present to the public, medical community, and third-party payers. For example, a common medical diagnosis of patients referred to outpatient physical therapy practices is low back pain, which is nothing more than a location of pain. If an outcomes study was performed that included all patients with the diagnosis of low back pain in a given practice, the results would not shed light on the best approach for treating low back pain because of the diverse causes, stages and severity of the condition, and comorbidities involved. Subclassification of patients based on diagnostic classification paradigms is necessary to provide more efficient patient management strategies and more meaningful outcome data.

Technologic advances (e.g., diagnostic imaging) for identifying pathology have not necessarily decreased the period in which symptoms resolve nor do they always guide physical therapy treatment. Medical diagnosis (e.g., herniated nucleus pulposus, spondylolisthesis) may not be helpful in directing successful rehabilitation of patients with low back pain.[43] The medical diagnosis, in most cases, does not provide the physical therapist with enough information to proceed with intervention. The physical therapist's diagnosis is reached only after performing a thorough examination and evaluation combined, if necessary, with the results of tests and measures ordered and performed by professionals from other disciplines and with the medical diagnosis.

Physical therapy is in the early stages of developing diagnostic classifications. After classifications are developed, much work regarding validity, reliability, and sensitivity of diagnostic classifications needs to be done.

The issue of diagnosis in physical therapy is complex and controversial. Our lack of progress toward achieving diagnostic classification schemes has been termed a diagnostic dilemma by Coffin-Zadai.[44] She describes the major components of the diagnostic dilemma as (a) the competition among new ideas, (b) the complexity of the diagnostic process and language used to describe the outcome, (c) the profession's lack of consensus regarding the diagnostic classification construct to be embraced, and (d) the rapid evolution and impact of new knowledge. The interaction of these four components results in "diagnostic disablement."[44]

The first step toward agreement regarding diagnostic classifications is to standardize the language that physical therapists use to diagnose conditions within their scope of practice. Leaders in the field of physical therapy are working toward this common language. The goal is to be able to one day correlate effective and efficient treatment with the clinical diagnosis made by physical therapists to establish more efficient and cost-effective outcomes.[40-51] Only then can

---

DISPLAY 2-3
Definitions of Terms

Cluster: A set of observations or data that frequently occur as a group for a single patient.

Syndrome: An aggregate of signs and symptoms that characterize a given disease or condition.

Diagnosis: A label encompassing a cluster of signs and symptoms commonly associated with a disorder, syndrome, or category of impairment, activity limitation, or disability.

Adapted from American Physical Therapy Association. A guide to physical therapist practice, I: a description of patient management. Phys Ther 1995;75:749–756.

physical therapists promote the efficacy of the profession in today's responsibility-focused health care environment.

Prognosis and Plan of Care

After a diagnosis has been established, the physical therapist determines the prognosis and develops the plan of care. Prognosis is the process of determining the level of optimal improvement that may be obtained from intervention, and the amount of time required to reach that level.[1] For example, an expected short-term outcome for an otherwise healthy 65-year-old person after a hip fracture treated with open reduction and internal fixation may be the ability to walk 300 ft with partial weight bearing, using a walker, in 3 days; an expected long-term outcome may be the ability to walk independently without a gait deviation in 12 to 16 weeks.

The plan of care consists of statements that specify the interventions to be used and the proposed duration and frequency of the interventions that are required to reach the anticipated goals and expected outcomes.[1] The plan of care is the culmination of the examination, diagnostic, and prognostic processes.

The prognosis and plan of care should be based on the following factors:

- The patient's health status, risk factors, and response to previous interventions
- The patient's safety, needs, and goals
- The natural history and the expected clinical course of the pathology, impairment, or diagnosis
- The results of the examination, evaluation, and diagnostic processes

To ensure the prognosis and plan of care are based on the patient's safety, needs, and goals, the physical therapist should confer with the patient and establish patient goals.[52] During this discussion, the patient must be informed of the diagnosis or prioritized impairment list if a diagnosis cannot be developed. The patient should also be provided with an explanation of the relationship between the diagnosis or impairments and the activity limitations and disability. This information can assist the patient in developing realistic goals and understanding the purpose of the selected interventions. Agreement between the patient and therapist on the long-term and short-term goals is imperative for successful treatment outcomes. When the physical therapist determines that physical therapy intervention is unlikely to be beneficial, the reasons should be discussed with the patient and other individuals concerned and documented in the medical record.

To ensure the prognosis and plan of care are based on the natural history and the expected clinical courses of the pathology, disease, or disorder the physical therapist must rely on textbooks, lectures from instructors, literature reviews, research articles, evidence-based clinical practice guidelines, and clinical experience.[53] Straus succinctly outlined the steps necessary to practice evidence-based patient management in her 1998 article[53]:

- Convert the need for information into clinically relevant, answerable questions
- Find, in the most efficient way, the best evidence with which to answer these questions (whether this evidence comes from clinical examination, published research, medical tests, or other sources)

- Critically appraise the evidence for its validity (closeness to the truth) and usefulness (clinical applicability)
- Integrate the appraisal with clinical expertise and apply the results to clinical practice
- Evaluate your performance.

Following these steps can assist the clinician in developing a sound prognosis and plan of care based on finding the best evidence available in a practical time frame.

Intervention

Intervention is defined as the purposeful and skilled interaction of the physical therapist with the patient using various methods and techniques to produce changes in the patient's condition consistent with the evaluation, diagnosis, and prognosis.[1] Ongoing decisions regarding intervention are contingent on the timely monitoring of the patient's response and the progress made toward achieving outcomes. The three major types of intervention are listed in Display 2-4. This text focuses on one aspect of direct intervention (i.e., therapeutic exercise) and patient-related instruction as it relates to therapeutic exercise.

The key to a successful intervention and patient outcome is to do the right things well.[54] To determine the right things, the physical therapist must have a thorough understanding of the patient's function/disability profile and sound clinical decision-making skills.

Clinical Decision Making for Intervention

The physical therapist is educated and trained to effectively and efficiently treat impairments in body function or structure related to activity limitations and to arrive at desirable functional outcomes for the patient. In designing the plan of care, the physical therapist analyzes and integrates the clinical implications of the severity, complexity, and acuity of pathology, disease, or disorder; the extent of the impairment of body function and structure; the types of activities and participations and the environment to which the person wishes to return. Recall that the ultimate functional goal of physical therapy is the achievement of optimal movement and functioning in the activities and participations that are unique to the individual. Physical therapists generally develop treatment interventions with the intention of restoring function and reducing disability. However, strictly impairment-based interventions often do not achieve functional goals because the focus may not be on the right impairment.

DISPLAY 2-4
Types of Physical Therapy Interventions

- Direct intervention (e.g., therapeutic exercise, manual therapy techniques, debridement, wound care)
- Patient-related instruction (e.g., education provided to the patient and other caregivers involved regarding the patient's condition, treatment plan, information and training in maintenance, and prevention activities)
- Coordination, communication, and documentation (e.g., patient care conferences, record reviews, discharge planning)

Treating the "Right" Impairments

An important clinical decision in the patient management process is to determine the impairment that most closely relates to an activity limitation or participation restriction. Physical therapists are often tempted to include impairments that are not relevant because they assume that the reduction of any or all impairments leads directly to improvement in function.[55] In reality, the treatment of impairments can only lead to improvement in function if the impairments contribute to a limitation in activity.

There is one instance, however, in which physical therapists must treat impairments that do not contribute to an identified ability limitation or participation restriction. In this instance, an impairment may not correlate with an activity limitation and participation restriction, but if left untreated, it may lead to future activity limitations. In this instance, the physical therapist may treat the impairment as a preventive measure. For example, a patient has been prescribed a prone hip extension exercise to improve gluteal strength for treatment of hip pain. However, while the patient is extending the hip, his or her lumbar spine is moving into excessive extension. If the faulty movement pattern is left untreated, low back pain may develop. Exercises need to be prescribed to improve the stability of the low back to prevent the possibility of future episodes of low back pain.

If an impairment seems to be linked to a activity limitation or participation restriction, the therapist must question whether the impairment is amenable to physical therapy intervention. To help determine the answer, the physical therapist should ask several questions:

- Will the patient benefit from the intervention (i.e., can treatment of the impairment improve functioning or prevent functional loss)?
- Are there any possible negative effects of the treatment (contraindications)?
- What is the cost-benefit ratio?

If it is determined that no treatment can be justified, the physical therapist should consider other options such as the following:

- Discussing the decision to decline intervention with the patient to ensure patient agreement and understanding of the decision
- Referring the patient to an appropriate practitioner or resource
- Assisting in modifying the environment in which the individual lives, goes to school, or works to ensure maximal performance despite the impairment, activity limitation, or participation restriction
- Teaching the individual to appropriately compensate for the impairment during activities or participation in more complex social roles.

If the impairment is amenable to treatment, decide whether to treat the impairment, activity limitation, or both. Building Block 2-1 illustrates this point.

Selecting and Justifying Treatment Interventions

After a decision has been made to treat a specific impairment or activity limitation, the next step is to select an appropriate intervention or combination of interventions with the proper sequencing (e.g., moist heat before joint mobilization, which

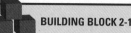

BUILDING BLOCK 2-1

Consider a 72-year-old man 4 weeks s/p total knee replacement. He presents with weakness of the quadriceps and reduced flexion ROM of the knee. Would you choose to treat the impairments with specific exercise instruction to increase quadriceps muscle performance and tibiofemoral joint mobility or teach the patient the functional task of sit to stand? Please defend your answer.

is followed by stretching and ends with a functional task that employs the new mobility).

Physical therapists may select an intervention from among the following possibilities[1]:

- Therapeutic exercise
- Functional training in self-care and home management (including basic ADLs and instrumental ADLs)
- Functional training in community or work reintegration (including instrumental ADLs, work hardening, and work conditioning)
- Manual therapy techniques (including mobilization and manipulation)
- Prescription, fabrication, and application of assistive, adaptive, supportive, and protective devices and equipment
- Airway clearance techniques
- Integumentary repair and protection techniques
- Physical agents and mechanical modalities
- Electrotherapeutic modalities

Numerous patient factors must be taken into consideration to determine which of the described interventions are appropriate. This information is obtained from the history and systems review (see Displays 2-1 and 2-2). An awareness of the patient's physical environment for living and/or working, or the recreational activities to which the patient wishes to return is important in developing patient-centered interventions and achieving functional outcomes. For example, a successful outcome may not be reflected in increased strength in the physical therapy office by a hand-held dynamometer, but may be observed in the use of that strength in a functional manner in the patient's environment, such as walking up a flight of stairs with 20 lb of groceries.

The process of selecting and justifying treatment intervention must be based on the integration of research evidence, clinical expertise, and patient values, called "evidence-based medicine (EBM)."[56] EBM aims to improve health care outcomes by balancing findings from research with clinical experience and patient/family preferences. The internet has greatly increased the ease with which many clinicians can access and rapidly sort current information. Of the numerous databases available for information, a few are particularly relevant to physical therapy. PubMed is probably the best known database. It is maintained by the National Library of Medicine and is free to the public at www.ncbi.nlm.nih.gov/PubMed. The American Physical Therapy Association's (APTA) Hooked on Evidence Initiative is a new and exciting grassroots effort to systematically find and evaluate research with relevance to physical therapy practice. More information about the process involved is available on their website, which can be accessed from the APTA website or at www.apta.org/hookedonevidence/index.cfm.

Patient-Related Instruction

Patient-related instruction is the process of imparting information and developing skills to promote independence and to allow care to continue after discharge.[1] It must be an integral part of any physical therapy intervention (Fig. 2-3) and will be featured in this text to enhance the therapeutic exercise intervention.

When patient education is not possible (e.g., the patient is an infant, comatose, there is a cognitive deficit or language barrier), educating family members, significant others, friends, or other caregivers is essential. Patient-related instruction offered to a support person, even when educating the patient is possible, can promote compliance by teaching the support person to intervene in an appropriate manner and encouraging the display of appropriate attitudes toward the patient's activity limitations and disabilities.

Patient-related instruction is critical to enhance compliance in following through with interventions and preventing future limitations in activity or restrictions in participation. Imparting your knowledge of the patient's function/disability process enables the patient to gain confidence in your skills, which further enhances compliance. Patient-related instruction may include the following:

- Education pertaining to the
  - pathologic process and impairments contributing to activity limitation and participation restriction
  - the prognosis
  - and the purposes and potential complications of the intervention

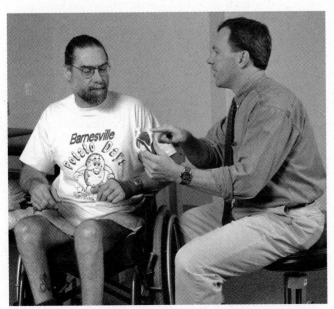

FIGURE 2-3. Patient-related instruction is an integral part of physical therapy intervention. By helping the patient understand his impairment and activity limitations, the clinician promotes patient compliance with the therapeutic intervention program. In addition, patient satisfaction is promoted by taking the time to educate the patient regarding the cause(s) of his condition, self-management techniques, and prevention.

- Instruction and assistance in making appropriate decisions about management of the condition during the ADLs (e.g., work station ergonomic modifications, altered movement patterns and body mechanics, and altered sleep postures)
- Instruction and assistance in implementing interventions under the direction of the physical therapist (e.g., training a support person in techniques of therapeutic exercise in the event that cognitive, physical, or resource status of the patient requires assistance to perform a home management program)

Patient-related instruction confers several benefits:

- Increased patient, significant other, family, and caregiver knowledge about the patient's condition, prognosis, and management
- Acquisition of behaviors that foster healthy habits, wellness, and prevention
- Improved levels of performance in employment, recreational, and sports activities
- Improved physical function, health status, and sense of well-being
- Improved safety for the patient, significant others, family, and caregivers
- Reduced participation restriction, secondary conditions, and recurrence
- Enhanced decision making about the use of health care resources by the patient, significant others, family, or caregivers
- Decreased service use and improved cost containment

Patient-related instruction represents the first and most important step toward directing responsibility for treatment outcome from the physical therapist to the patient. A thorough understanding of the individual's disablement process and the factors that may impede improved functional outcome are necessary to provide comprehensive and personalized patient-related instruction. The successful practitioner is one who is skillful in the delivery of an active treatment approach based on treatment specific to the individual's disablement profile and on education that places the patient (or caregiver) in the position of taking responsibility for the outcome.

Outcome

As the patient/client reaches the termination of physical therapy services and the end of the episode of care, the physical therapist measures the global outcomes of the physical therapy services by characterizing or quantifying the impact of the physical therapy interventions on the following domains[1]:

- Health condition (disorder or disease)
- Body functions/structures
- Activities
- Participation
- Risk reduction/prevention
- Health, wellness, and fitness
- Personal/environmental factors
- Patient/client satisfaction

An outcome is considered successful when the following conditions are met:

- Activity and participation is improved or maintained whenever possible.

- Activity limitation or participation restriction is minimized or slowed when the status quo cannot be maintained.
- The patient is satisfied.

At each step of the patient management process, the physical therapist considers the possible patient outcomes. This ongoing measurement of patient outcomes is based on the examination and evaluation of impairments, functional status, and level of participation restriction. To evaluate the effectiveness of the intervention, the physical therapist must select criteria to be tested (e.g., impairments and activity limitations) and interpret the results of the examination. Outcomes can be measured through outcome analysis. This is a systematic examination of patient outcomes in relation to selected patient variables (e.g., age, sex, diagnosis, interventions, and patient satisfaction). It can be part of a quality assurance program, used for economic analysis of a practice, or used to demonstrate efficacy of intervention.

Modification

Although positive outcomes are not synonymous with improved impairment measures, measurement of impairments and functional status should be performed to determine the efficacy of the intervention plan. By measuring both variables, the therapist can determine whether changes in the impairment are associated with changes in functional status.[55] If functional status has not changed, consider modifying the intervention plan. Modification of intervention is based on the status relative to the expected outcome and the rate of progress. Display 2-5 illustrates additional factors to consider with respect to modification of an intervention.

Prudent clinical reasoning assists the clinician in determining the need for modification and the best adjustments

---

> **DISPLAY 2-5**
> ## Factors to Consider When Modifying an Intervention
>
> - Medical safety
> - Patient comfort
> - Patient's level of independence with the intervention (especially related to therapeutic exercise intervention)
> - Effect of the intervention on the impairments and functional outcome
> - New or altered symptoms due to intervention by other health care providers
> - Patient finances, environment, and schedule constraints
>
> The intervention may be modified by one of the following actions
>
> - Increasing or decreasing the dosage of the intervention, especially in the case of therapeutic exercise intervention (see the section on "Exercise Modification" in this chapter)
> - Treating different impairments
> - Changing the focus to activity limitations
> - Consulting or referring to a physical therapist with advanced training or certification in a content area
> - Referring the patient to another health care provider specializing in a system that is beyond the PT scope of practice
> - Improving physical therapy techniques, verbal cues, and teaching skills

---

> **DISPLAY 2-6**
> ## Patient Management Concepts
>
> - Develop an examination or evaluation schema pertinent to the patient.
> - Diagnose the patient's impairments, activity limitations, and disabilities.
> - Develop a prognosis based on the patient's individual disablement process.
> - Develop a plan of care designed to improve function (i.e., the right things).
> - Apply appropriate judgment and motor skills to provide the appropriate intervention.
> - Continually use clinical reasoning to modify the intervention as needed for a positive outcome.

to implement. In determining and implementing revised goals and interventions, the clinician uses the additional data gathered from the reevaluation. This reevaluation and modification process continues until the decision to stop treatment is reached.

Physical therapists have a responsibility to demonstrate to patients and third-party payers that physical therapy is efficient and cost-effective and provides patient satisfaction. In daily practice, physical therapists should adhere to the same principles of measurement used in research. Changes should be carefully documented in an effort to demonstrate that physical therapy intervention is related to successful outcomes in an efficient and cost-effective manner.

In the current health care environment, physical therapists are faced with the challenge of practicing in an increasingly competitive marketplace. As marketplace competition continues to grow, patient satisfaction with physical therapy is emerging as an outcome variable of critical importance. The results of one study show that patient satisfaction with care is most strongly correlated with the quality of patient-care provider interactions.[57] This includes the care provider spending adequate time with the patient, demonstrating strong listening and communication skills, and offering a clear explanation of treatment and prevention strategies.

In today's healthcare market, complex reimbursement models, greater public scrutiny, and disclosure of clinical quality and patient safety performance standards are demanding a new, more equitable, and effective reimbursement model for hospitals and physician services. Pay-for-performance is an emerging payment model that links quality of care with the level of payment for healthcare services. While still in its infancy, a new model that bases reimbursement on high-quality clinical performance should sweep health care within 5 to 20 years.

Now more than ever, successful patient management is vital to the growth of our profession. As discussed in detail, successful patient management entails many aspects of clinician and patient/client interaction. Display 2-6 succinctly summarizes patient management concepts.

CLINICAL DECISION MAKING

At each juncture in the patient management model, clinical decisions are made. Appropriate decisions are crucial for a successful outcome. However, the clinical reasoning process involved in patient management presents the greatest challenge to the physical therapist. The following aspects are found to be most difficult in the clinical decision-making process:

- Organization of evaluation findings into a diagnosis
- Development of a prognosis based on the patient's activity limitations and disabilities
- Development of realistic patient-based goals
- Development and implementation of an intervention that is effective and efficient

Display 2-7 summarizes clinical decision-making tips in relation to patient management to help the physical therapist address some of these challenges. The effectiveness of clinical decision making is based on obtaining pertinent data. The physical therapist must possess

- Knowledge about what is pertinent
- The skill to obtain the data
- The ability to store, record, evaluate, relate, and interpret the data

These actions require knowledge of the function/disability process; clinical experience and skill in treating impairments and activity limitations; and disciplined, systematic thought processes. Common to those who strive to excel in clinical decision making are the following characteristics:

- Wide range of knowledge
- Ongoing acquisition of knowledge
- Need for order or a plan of action
- Questioning unproven conventional solutions
- Self-discipline and persistence in work

Information regarding clinical decision making and the process involved warrant their own text. However, this text strives to include theoretic information and pertinent issues related to clinical decision making. This information empowers the physical therapist with some of the necessary tools to make appropriate clinical decisions regarding the design and application of treatment plans.

THERAPEUTIC EXERCISE INTERVENTION

Of the three components of physical therapy intervention (see Display 2-4), this text presents information regarding the direct intervention of therapeutic exercise and patient-related instruction associated with therapeutic exercise intervention.

After a thorough examination and evaluation has been performed; a diagnosis and prognosis have been developed; and the clinician understands the relationships between the pathology, impairments, activity limitations, and participation restrictions, a plan of care is determined through the clinical decision-making process. Therapeutic exercise may be the basis of the intervention or may be one component of the intervention, but it should be included to some extent in all patient care plans. Therapeutic exercise includes activities and techniques to improve physical function and health status resulting from impairments by identifying specific performance goals that allow a patient to achieve a higher functional level in the home, school, workplace, or community or in recreational or sports endeavors. It also incorporates activities to allow well clients to improve or maintain their health or performance status for work, recreation, or sports and prevent or minimize future potential functional loss or health problems.

To develop an efficient, effective therapeutic exercise intervention, consider these variables:

- Which elements/components of the movement system (defined subsequently) need to be addressed to restore function?
- Which activities or techniques are chosen to achieve a functional outcome, including the sequence within a given exercise session and the sequence of gradation in the total plan of care?
- What is the purpose of each specific activity or technique chosen?
- What are the posture, mode, and movement for each activity or technique?
- What are the dosage parameters for each activity or technique?

The following section presents a therapeutic exercise intervention model to assist in organizing all the details necessary to prescribe an effective, efficient exercise prescription.

Therapeutic Exercise Intervention Model

A three-dimensional model has been developed to assist the clinician in the clinical decision-making process regarding exercise prescription (Fig. 2-4). Three axes are used to visualize three components of exercise prescription and their relationships:

1. Elements of the movement system as they relate to the purpose of each activity or technique
2. The specific activity or technique chosen
3. The specific dosage

DISPLAY 2-7
Clinical Decision-Making Tips for Patient Management

Examination: Prioritize the problems to be assessed and the tests and measures to be implemented.

Evaluation: Consider and analyze all examination findings for relationships, including the progression and stages of the symptoms, diagnostic findings by other health care professionals, comorbidities, medical history, and treatment or medications received.

Diagnosis: Segregate findings into clusters of symptoms and signs by common causes, mechanisms, and effects.

Prognosis and Plan of Care: Develop long-term and short-term goals based on patient safety, needs, and goals and on information regarding the natural history and expected clinical courses of the pathology, impairment, or diagnosis.

Intervention: Determine whether impairments correlate with an activity limitation or disability and are amenable to physical therapy treatment. Select and justify a method of intervention. The most credible source of justification is based on relevant research literature.

Outcome: Measure the success of the intervention plan according to functional gain and make appropriate modifications when necessary.

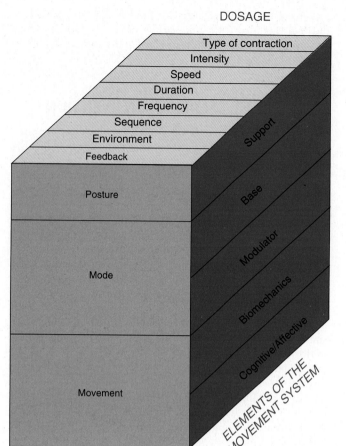

DOSAGE

ACTIVITY

FIGURE 2-4. Therapeutic exercise intervention model. Note the three-dimensional model indicating the relationship between elements of the movement system, activity, and dosage.

Elements of the Movement System

To prescribe the appropriate exercise, factors regarding the patient's activity limitation(s) and participation restriction(s) must be considered. The most critical factor is the patient's functional status. Each exercise prescription has two common goals: (a) to restore functional movement as best as possible and (b) prevent or minimize functional loss in the future.

Sahrmann[58] describes movement as a system that is made up of several elements, each of which has a unique basic function necessary for the production and regulation of movement. The optimal actions and interactions of the multiple anatomic, physiologic, and psychologic systems involved in movement must be considered. Ideal movement can be thought of as the result of a complex interaction of several elements of the movement system as defined by Sahrmann[58] and modified for the purposes of this model:

- *Support element*: The functional status of the cardiac, pulmonary, and metabolic systems. These systems play an indirect role in that they do not produce motion of the segments, but provide substrates and metabolic support required to maintain the viability of the other systems. Examples of components included in this element would be cardiopulmonary status (including breathing patterns) and hormonal factors.

- *Base element*: The functional status of the neuromusculoskeletal systems. This element provides the basis for movement, including components such as ROM, extensibility/stiffness properties of nervous tissue, muscle, fascia, and periarticular tissues; joint mobility and integrity, muscle performance, and the overall health of the neuromusculoskeletal tissue (e.g., irritability level, level of injury, and postsurgical status).

- *Modulator element*: The physiologic status of the neuromuscular system. This element is particularly related to motor function, including components such as patterns and timing of muscle recruitment, muscle cessation patterns, and feed-forward and feedback systems.

- *Biomechanical element*: The functional status of static and dynamic kinetics and kinematics. The biomechanical element is an interface between motor control and musculoskeletal function, thereby affecting the pattern of muscle use and the shape/integrity of bones and joints. Components of the biomechanical element include static forces affecting alignment and muscle torque capability, and dynamic forces affecting arthro/osteokinematics.

- *Cognitive or affective element*: The functional status of the psychologic system as it is related to movement. Components of this element include learning ability, compliance, motivation, and emotional status.

(*Note*: The cognitive element is not an original element of the movement system as defined by Sahrmann.[58])

The elements of the movement system are along the horizontal axis of the therapeutic exercise intervention model (see Fig. 2-4). The diagnostic process can determine the impairments that are related to the patient's activity limitations and participation restriction. To begin planning the therapeutic exercise intervention, the impairments should first be related to the elements of the movement system. This process not only illustrates the complex interaction of the elements of the movement system, but also guides the clinician toward the most appropriate activities or techniques, the sequence of exercise, and the specific dosage to treat the impairments related to the activity limitations and participation restriction. For example, a person with knee pain with a posture impairment of genu valgus may require orthotic intervention to correct the biomechanical element before muscle performance (base element) or motor control (modulator element) training. Changing the alignment at the knee is prerequisite to effective base or modulator element training. It may then be decided that muscle performance training is prerequisite to motor control training due to the fact that the patient's strength, power, or endurance are below functional levels. Muscle performance dosage parameters are different from motor control dosage parameters (see "Dosage" in a subsequent section of this chapter). Understanding the sequence of intervention based on a prioritization of the elements of the movement system, and that dosage parameters are different for the different elements/components of the movement system, can assist in organizing the complex data collected during the examination.

After evaluating a patient, it may be apparent that one, a few, or all elements of the movement system are related to the activity limitation and participation restriction. Most often, the interaction of the elements is critical, but one or two elements usually are pivotal to effect change. After determining the activity limitation(s) and participation restriction(s), the

BUILDING BLOCK 2-2

History

A 42-year-old female graphic designer presents with a diagnosis of impingement syndrome of the shoulder. She spends a large part of her day at a monitor creating design documents. She has two children aged 1 and 3. She likes to garden and cook. Activity limitation is an inability to raise the arm to groom her hair.

Evaluation

A pivotal impairment is determined to be a thoracic kyphosis that results in the scapula resting in an excessive

anterior tilt (Fig. 1). The scapula, resting in anterior tilt, fails to adequately posterior tilt during upper extremity flexion (Fig. 2). As a result, the glenohumeral joint mechanically impinges under the acromion process, and tissues in the subacromial space (e.g., bursa, biceps tendon, rotator cuff tendons) undergo microtrauma resulting in pain (i.e., impairment), inflammation (i.e., pathology), and the inability to raise the arm without pain (i.e., activity limitation). List examples of activity limitations and participation restrictions that result from this movement impairment.

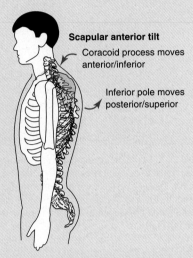

Scapular anterior tilt
Coracoid process moves anterior/inferior

Inferior pole moves posterior/superior

FIGURE 1. Thoracic kyphosis with excessive scapular anterior tilt. With anterior tilt of the scapula, the inferior pole moves posterior/superior and the coracoid process moves anterior/inferior.

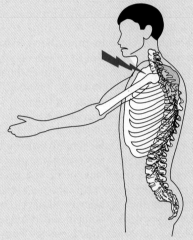

FIGURE 2. Lack of scapular posterior tilt leads to glenohumeral impingement.

next step is to determine which element(s) is/are involved. Determining which elements are involved will guide you in choosing the appropriate activity or technique, the proper dosage related to the element for which the exercise is prescribed, and in the sequence in which the exercises should be prescribed to be most efficient at restoring normal movement. Building Block 2-2 is provided for a clinical example of this clinical decision-making process.

Display 2-8 lists the impairments related to the case in Building Block 2-2 as they relate to the elements of the movement system.

As can be seen from this example, different impairments are correlated with each element of the movement system. A specific exercise can be prescribed to address each impairment associated with an element of the movement system (e.g., stretching the pectoralis minor to address the base element). Most often, the interaction of elements is critical; therefore, one exercise may address numerous elements of the movement system (see Building Block 2-3).

When instructing a patient in the performance of any exercise, provide verbal, visual, or tactile feedback to focus on the correlating element of the movement system, or provide instruction to the patient regarding the interaction

 DISPLAY 2-8
Elements of the Movement System Related to Impairments

- **Support element impairment:** Using accessory muscles of inspiration (pectoralis minor) versus diaphragm for breathing, potentially leading to overuse and shortening of pectoralis minor
- **Base element impairment:** Short pectoralis minor and short head of biceps pulling coracoid process anterior and inferior, lengthened and weak lower trapezius not providing sufficient counterforce leading to scapular anterior tilt.
- **Modulator element impairment:** Reduced recruitment of lower trapezius and serratus anterior not counterbalancing the anterior scapular tilt
- **Biomechanical element impairment:** Thoracic kyphosis contributing to the anterior tilt of scapula
- **Cognitive and affective element impairment:** Patient is clinically depressed, and the physical manifestation is a slumped posture contributing to the thoracic kyphosis.

BUILDING BLOCK 2-3

Wall slides (Fig. 2-7) is a good choice of exercise for the patient described in Building Block 2-2. This exercise can simultaneously address several impairments. List three impairments that this exercise addresses and indicate the correlating element of the movement system.

of elements. For example, tactile feedback or surface electromyography on the lower trapezius during a specific exercise (see Self-Management 25-2: Facelying Arm Lifts in Chapter 25) can assist in recruitment (modulator element). The sequence in which each exercise is prescribed is based on prioritizing which elements are pivotal to restoring function and which elements must be improved for other elements to follow (see Building Block 2-4).

Attempts should be made to prescribe exercise that will address the complex interaction of the elements of the movement system. For example, to restore normal shoulder girdle movement, instruction in diaphragmatic breathing (i.e., support element) may be pivotal to reduce the activity (modulator element) of the pectoralis minor (accessory muscle of respiration), improve thoracic spine alignment (biomechanical element), and increase thoracic spine and rib cage mobility (base element). Another example is to design an exercise that will concurrently stretch the pectoralis minor and strengthen (in the shortened range) the lower trapezius (i.e., base element) (Fig. 2-5). Optimizing the recruitment strategy (i.e., modulator element) during specific exercise and during functional movement is always necessary to achieve the best functional outcome.

Display 2-9 summarizes the factors to consider before determining the relevant and prioritized list of the elements of the movement system.

Activity or Technique

Along the vertical axis is the activity or technique chosen to ultimately achieve the functional goal. To be successful in choosing the proper activity or technique, first determine the element of the movement system associated with the impairment or activity limitation. Each element is associated with specific therapeutic exercise interventions. Table 2-2 cross-references the elements of the movement system with the most common therapeutic exercise activities or techniques. Though an argument can be made to prescribe a specific therapeutic activity or technique to address nearly any element of the movement system, this table refers the most common relationships between therapeutic activities/techniques and the elements of the movement system.

BUILDING BLOCK 2-4

Given the example of the women with impingement, is there another pivotal element of the movement system that might need to be addressed, prior to any other, for her to achieve a successful outcome? Explain your answer.

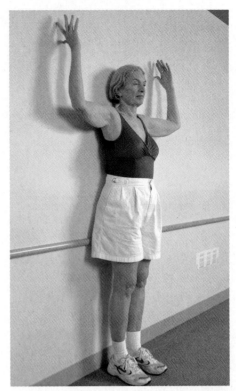

FIGURE 2-5. This exercise illustrates a patient performing a wall slide. The patient moves from the position shown here to the end position of the shoulders in full elevation. Note the arms are positioned in the scapular plane (slightly forward of the wall with thumbs touching the wall), the spine and pelvis are in neutral, and the feet are only a few inches away from the wall.

After identifying the elements of the movement system, the physiologic status of the body function or structure must be considered. This information assists in determining the activity or technique, posture, movement, and mode parameters. For example, if muscle performance (i.e., base element) is pivotal to return to an activity or participation, the chosen activity or technique may depend on the force or torque capability of the affected muscle(s). If the force or torque capability is less than fair muscle strength, as determined by Kendall,[59] a gravity-lessened position active ROM activity or an against-gravity active assisted technique may be chosen. Another related impairment may be related to reduced muscle recruitment from prolonged immobilization (i.e., modulator element) or muscle amnesia. If the ability to recruit is poor, a gravity-lessened active ROM activity may be chosen with tactile feedback or against-gravity active ROM

DISPLAY 2-9
Considerations in Clinical Decision Making Relevant to the Elements of the Movement System

- Identify the activity limitations and related impairments to be treated.
- Relate activity limitations and impairments to be treated with the appropriate elements of the movement system.
- Prioritize elements of the movement system.

TABLE 2-2 Therapeutic Activities Cross-Referenced With Elements of the Movement System

ACTIVITES	SUPPORT	BASE	MODULATOR	BIOMECHANICAL
Stretching (active and passive)		✓		
ROM (passive, active assisted, active)		✓		
Strengthening[a]		✓		
Neuromuscular reeducation			✓	
Developmental activities		✓	✓	
Breathing	✓			
Gait training	✓		✓	✓
Aquatic	✓	✓		
Balance and coordination training			✓	✓
Body mechanics and ergonomics training				✓
Movement training			✓	✓
Posture awareness training			✓	✓
Aerobic or muscular endurance[b]	✓	✓		

[a]Strengthening activities include active assistive, active, and resistive exercise using manual resistance, pulleys, weights, hydraulics, elastics, robotics, mechanical, or electromechanical devices.

[b]Aerobic or muscular endurance activities include use of cycles, treadmills, steppers, pools, manual resistance, pulleys, weights, hydraulics, elastics, robotics, mechanical, or electromechanical devices.

with neuromuscular electrical stimulation as an adjunctive intervention (discussed later in this chapter), both of which are chosen to augment muscle reeducation.

Stage of Movement Control   Another factor to consider in choosing an activity is the stage of movement control (Display 2-10). Mobility is defined as the presence of a functional range through which to move and the ability to initiate and sustain active movement through the range.[60] A person with musculoskeletal dysfunction may exhibit impairments in either or both parameters of mobility. For example, after total knee arthroplasty, a person may experience passive mobility restrictions caused by pain, swelling, and soft-tissue stiffness or shortness and have decreased ability to initiate knee motion as a result of reduced muscle force/torque production or reduced recruitment capability. The cause of the mobility restriction must be determined on a case-by-case basis to determine the most appropriate exercise intervention (see Chapter 7).

Stability in the construct of stages of movement control is defined as the ability to provide a stable foundation from which to move.[60] A precursor to achieving the stability necessary for movement, or dynamic stability, is optimal posture. The individual must be able to maintain optimal posture without a load before optimal posture can be maintained during movement of a limb. Mobility and stability are not mutually exclusive. Achieving mobility before addressing stability is unnecessary; the two stages of movement control can occur concurrently.

For example, as mobility after total knee arthroplasty is achieved passively, active motion must be prescribed. For optimal active motion, the knee requires a stable proximal base from which to move (i.e., pelvis and trunk) and distal base for weight bearing (i.e., foot and ankle). Stability must be achieved at these regions for optimal active motion to take place.

Controlled mobility is defined as the ability to move within joints and between limbs,[60] following the optimal path of instant center of rotation (PICR) (see Chapter 9 for clarity on the definition of the PICR). This requires proper recruitment of synergists that perform movement and proper length and recruitment, if necessary, of muscles providing a stable foundation for movement. The previous example would progress from exercises improving knee mobility, as well as pelvic-trunk and foot-ankle stability, to functional movement patterns. To walk, the knee must flex and extend at proper stages in the gait cycle. The trunk, pelvis, ankle, and foot must move into proper position at each stage of the gait cycle and provide proximal and distal stability for optimal knee function. The activity may involve the swing phase of gait, which requires a stable pelvis from which to swing the lower limb (Fig. 2-6A), or the stance phase of gait (Fig. 2-6B), which requires a stable foot for optimal knee loading.

DISPLAY 2-10
Stages of Movement Control

Mobility: A functional range through which to move and the ability to sustain active movement through the range

Stability: The ability to provide a stable foundation from which to move

Controlled mobility: The ability to move within joints and between limbs following the optimal PICR

Skill: The ability to maintain consistency in performing functional tasks with economy of effort

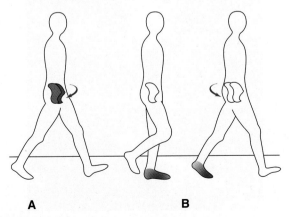

A   **B**

FIGURE 2-6. (A) Swing phase of gait requires a stable pelvis. (B) Stance phase of gait requires a stable foot.

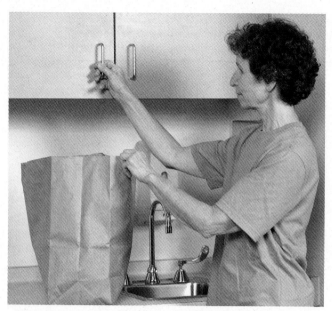

FIGURE 2-7. Grasping a cabinet door requires freedom of movement in space in a coordinated manner within and between the joints of the upper extremity, trunk, and pelvis.

The final progression in the stages of movement control is skill. Skill implies consistency in performing functional tasks with economy of effort.[61] Skill in the upper extremities most often requires freedom of movement in space in a coordinated manner within and between the hand, wrist, forearm, elbow, shoulder girdle, trunk, and pelvis (e.g., grasping a cabinet door) (Fig. 2-7). Occasionally, closed chain (weight-bearing) movements are required in the upper extremity (e.g., gymnast performing a handstand on the balance beam) (Fig. 2-8). Skill in the lower extremities requires coordination of open chain (nonweight-bearing) movements (e.g., swing leg in kicking a soccer ball) (Fig. 2-9) and closed chain movements (e.g., stance leg in kicking a soccer ball) within and between the foot, ankle, tibia, femur, pelvis, and trunk for movement on varied surfaces. For total body movement

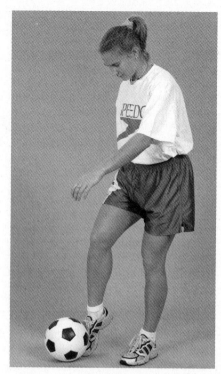

FIGURE 2-9. Skill in lower extremities requires coordination of open and closed chain movement. The swing leg performs an open chain movement as the stance leg performs a closed chain movement.

to be optimal, coordinated movement must occur within and between each segment involved in the movement (e.g., the tennis serve) (Fig. 2-10).

Commonly, patients are asked to perform skill-level activities without first developing proper foundations for functional

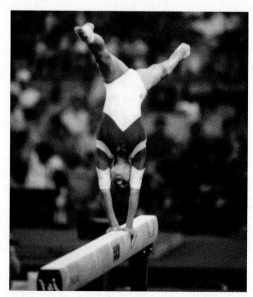

FIGURE 2-8. A gymnast performing on the balance beam represents an upper extremity closed chain movement.

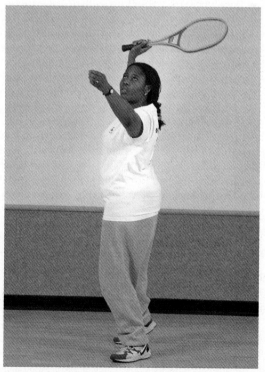

FIGURE 2-10. A tennis serve represents a total body movement, which is coordinated within and between each segment involved in the movement.

DISPLAY 2-11

Considerations Involved in Clinical Decision Making Related to Choice of Activity or Technique

- Determine the element of the movement system related to the impairment or activity limitation to be treated.
- Consider the physiologic status of the movement system.
- Determine the stage of movement control.

BUILDING BLOCK 2-5

A patient has sustained a grade 2 muscle strain to the hamstrings. It is in the intermediate stage of healing and repair (between 4 to 8 weeks poststrain). Describe two to three therapeutic activities to restore muscle strength with the mode, posture, and movement, specifically described.

How would you progress each of your choices as the patient moved toward 8–12 weeks of healing?

movement control. Conversely, patients may be prescribed exercises developing the other stages of movement control without finalizing the intervention with skill-level activities during functional movements. Skill is a necessary stage of movement control despite the prognosis of the patient (e.g., walk 10 ft with a walker versus run a marathon), which must be worked toward by achieving optimal function at each prior stage of movement control.

In summary, an activity can be as simple as performing a dynamic knee extension movement in sitting (i.e., mobility) or as difficult as an integrated movement pattern such as walking on an uneven surface (i.e., skill). An understanding of the level of involvement of the support, base, modulator, and cognitive/affective elements of the movement system help to determine the complexity of the task and the stage of movement control in which to intervene. Display 2-11 summarizes the factors to consider before determining the activity or technique.

Mode, Posture, and Movement After choosing the activity or technique, further breakdown of the activity is necessary for precise prescription. The mode, which is the method of performing the activity or technique, must be chosen. For example, if aerobic exercise is chosen, the mode can be cycling, swimming, walking, or a similar activity. If strengthening is chosen, the mode can be weights, manual resistance, or active assisted exercise. If balance and coordination training is chosen, the mode can be a balance board, balance beam, or computerized balance device. The initial and ending postures (e.g., standing, sitting, supine, prone, wide base of support, and narrow base of support) need to be determined. Included in this information is proper hand placement and angle of application of the force if the activity is performed manually. When using elastics, pulleys, mechanical, or electromechanical devices, proper equipment placement and angle of application of force must be determined. These descriptions must be included in the beginning and ending posture information. The movement needs to be specifically defined (e.g., partial squat through a 30-degree arc, unilateral arm raise through full-range, proprioceptive neuromuscular facilitation diagonal of the upper extremity to chest height).

The physiologic status of the body function or structure must be taken into consideration when determining the mode, posture, or movement of the exercise. Building Block 2-5 presents tissue injury as a cause of reduced muscle performance. You are challenged to consider the status of the tissue when determining the activity, posture, movement, and mode of exercise to address reduced muscle performance.

The quality of performance of the exercise is critical to the outcome (i.e., modulator element of the movement system). In relation to base or modulator elements, an obvious but often neglected concept is that a muscle cannot be strengthened if it is not recruited. Even if the correct activity is chosen, and the mode, posture, and movement are carefully selected, proper execution of the exercise is necessary to ensure a successful outcome. For example, hip abduction while sidelying can be performed with at least five different recruitment patterns (Fig. 2-11 and Display 2-12).[58] Attention to precision of movement and recruitment patterns is vital and must always be promoted to the best of the individual's capability.

Dosage

The third axis is related to dosage parameters (see Fig. 2-4). When determining dosage, physiologic status of the affected body functions/structures and the patient's learning capability must be considered. The anatomic site comprises the specific tissues involved (e.g., ligament, muscle, tendon, bone, cartilage, skin, and nerve). The physiologic status of the affected body functions/structures includes the severity of the tissue damage (e.g., partial versus complete tear), the irritability of the condition (e.g., easily provoked and difficult to resolve versus difficult to provoke and easy to resolve), the nature of the condition (e.g., chemical versus mechanical mediated pain), and the stage of the condition (e.g., acute, subacute, and chronic). For patients recovering from an injury, the dosage parameters are modified according to the tissues involved and the principles of tissue healing (Table 2-3). In the early stages of healing, tissues tolerate low-intensity passive or active activities, but in the later stages, tissues tolerate more aggressive resistive activities (see Chapter 10).

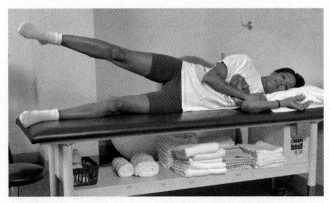

FIGURE 2-11. Hip abduction in the sidelying position. Optimal execution is with the pelvis and femur in the frontal plane and the movement of hip abduction occurring in the frontal plane with a stable pelvis. This requires recruitment of all of the hip abductors and proximal lumbopelvic muscles working in synergy.

DISPLAY 2-12
Variations in Performing Sidelying Hip Abduction

1. Sidelying with pelvis in frontal plane and abducting the hip with all of hip abductors in synergy (see Fig. 2-11)
2. Sidelying with pelvis rotated backward and femur rotated laterally, causing the movement to move toward the sagittal plane and resulting in recruitment of hip flexors
3. Sidelying with pelvis in frontal plane with femur rotated medially and flexed, resulting in recruitment of tensor fascia lata
4. Sidelying with pelvis in frontal plane, but movement is at the pelvis (hip hike), resulting in recruitment of lateral trunk muscles
5. Sidelying with pelvis in frontal plane, but movement is abduction of opposite hip, resulting in recruitment of opposite hip abductors

DISPLAY 2-13
Considerations Involved in Clinical Decision Making Related to Choice of Dosage Parameters

- Determine the anatomic sites involved in the current condition.
- Determine the physiologic status of the tissue(s) involved.
- Consider the patient's learning capability.

The patient's ability to learn, or learning capability, influences the schedule and the amount of reinforcement, feedback, or sensory input needed to perform the activity successfully. If a patient has difficulty learning a motor task, the dosage may be altered according to the principles of learning (see Chapter 3). For example, various forms of feedback (e.g., verbal, visual, and tactile) combined with numerous, low-intensity repetitions may be required initially for optimal performance of an activity. As skill is acquired, feedback and repetitions may be reduced and a more complex activity eventually may be prescribed.

After the anatomic and physiologic elements and the learning capabilities are understood, specific dosage parameters can be determined. Display 2-13 summarizes the factors to consider before determining dosage parameters. Parameters related to dosage include

- Type of contraction (i.e., eccentric, concentric, isometric, dynamic, or isokinetic)
- Intensity (i.e., amount of assistance or resistance required)
- Speed of the activity or technique
- Duration tolerated (i.e., number of repetitions or number of sets, particularly related to endurance and stretching activities)
- Frequency of exercise (i.e., number of exercise sessions in a given period)
- Sequencing of the exercise prescription (i.e., stretch before strengthen, low intensity warm-up before moderate or intense aerobic activity, or single joint

uniplanar movement before multijoint multiplanar movement)
- Environment in which the exercise is performed (i.e., quiet, controlled environment of a private room in a physical therapy clinic versus a loud, chaotic, uncontrolled, and outside environment)
- Amount of feedback necessary for optimal performance of the activity

SUMMARY

In summary, numerous variables in this model must be considered in prescribing an exercise, and variables often overlap (e.g., learning capabilities under dosage is similar to stages of movement control under activity, which is similar to modulator and cognitive/affective elements for the movement system). The task of organizing this data can be overwhelming. This three-dimensional model may help to visualize the relationships among the components of exercise prescription. It is the goal of this text that this model assists in organizing the data necessary to develop an effective, efficient therapeutic exercise intervention.

Exercise Modification

When the desired patient outcome is not met in a reasonable time frame, modification is based on evaluating how the following possibilities affect the lack of progress achieved with the therapeutic exercise intervention:

- The physical therapist may choose the wrong activity, dosage of exercise, or both.
- The physical therapist may not be able to effectively implement or teach the exercise.
- The patient may not be able to learn the exercise well enough or misunderstand or forget the instructions or dosage.
- The patient may not follow through with the prescription.

TABLE 2-3 Body Function/Structure Impairment Categories			
STAGE OF RECOVERY	**STAGE 1**	**STAGE 2**	**STAGE 3**
Onset of injury	Recent		Remote
Symptoms	↑ Severity ↑ Irritability		↓ Severity ↓ Irritability
Activity level	Decreased use of segment/ limb in function	Segment/limb used—not optimal	Near normal use of segment/ limb in function
Precautions/restrictions	Yes	Guarded	No
Outcome scores	High participation restriction		Low participation restriction

To be most effective and efficient with exercise prescription, constant reexamination and reevaluation of changes in impairments, activity levels, and participations are required. The exercises must be continually modified to increase or decrease the difficulty to ensure continual progress is being made with minimal setbacks. Numerous parameters can be modified to render an exercise more or less difficult. Four general parameters can be varied in an exercise prescription: biomechanical, physiologic, neuromuscular, and cognitive/affective. Display 2-14 outlines parameters that can be varied and provides examples for various types of exercise. The reader is strongly encouraged to review Display 2-13 before continuing further in the text.

If you've paid careful attention to these basic methods and principles, but the patient is not responding to the intervention, you must realize that all has been done within the scope of your therapeutic knowledge, expertise, and experience and that the patient should be discharged if you feel maximum improvement has been attained. If not, the patient should be referred to another practitioner for further treatment.

DISPLAY 2-14
Exercise Modification Parameters

Biomechanical

Stability
- Size of base of support
    Example: It is more difficult to balance with feet close together or in tandem than feet wide apart, and in sidelying rather than supine.
- Height of center of mass
    Example: Sit-ups may be done first with hands at the sides, progressed to forearms folded across the chest, progressed to hands clasped behind the neck. This upward shift of arm weight moves the center of mass toward the head by stages, progressively increasing the difficulty of the exercise.
- Support surface
    Example: The stability of the support surface can be progressed from a static or stable surface to a mobile base, such as foam, a balance board, or a trampoline.

External Load
- Magnitude
    Example: Increased magnitude of resistance alters the weight of the segment and thereby increases the difficulty of movement; however, it may also increase feedback from muscle and joint receptors and enhance the response.
- Gravitational forces
    Example: The force of gravity on a segment is maximal when the part is horizontal and diminishes as it moves toward the vertical. Knee flexion in prone is more difficult at the beginning of the movement and becomes easier as the motion progresses. Hip abduction is gravity reduced in prone or standing and against gravity in sidelying.
- Speed (see Chapter 5)
    Example: A medium rate is usually easier than very rapid or very slow.
- Length of lever arm
    Example: In prone exercises for scapular adductors (middle and lower trapezius), raising the arms with the elbows flexed gives less resistance than if the arms are nearly or completely straight.
- Point and angle of application of manual or mechanical resistance
    Example: A muscle pulling at or near a right angle to the long axis of the segment exerts its force more effectively than when its angle of pull is very small.

Number of Segments Involved
- Fewer segments may not always be easier than more segments, especially as in fine motor control.

Length of Muscle
- A muscle is better able to exert active tension when it is in a lengthened state than after it has undergone considerable shortening. When it is desirable to limit the participation of a given muscle in a movement, it is placed in a shortened position, or "put on slack." The active tension exerted by a muscle spanning more than one joint at a given joint depends on the position of the second joint over which it passes, because this determines the length of the muscle. For instance, the hamstrings are more effective as knee flexors when the hip is flexed and less effective when the hip is extended. Similarly, if the goal is to isolate the gluteus maximus during hip extension, the participation of the hamstrings is reduced if hip extension is done with the knee flexed compared with the knee extended.

Passive Tension of Two-Joint Muscles
- The hip can be flexed to only 70 to 90 degrees with the knee extended but considerably more if the hip and knee are flexed. Similarly, the ankle can dorsiflex more when the knee is flexed than when the knee is extended. These considerations are particularly important in planning effective stretching activities and in analyzing stabilization of body segments in all types of exercise. Altering joint positions or the use of external supports such as pillows can reduce or increase the tension of two-joint muscles based on the goal of the exercise.

Open Versus Closed Kinetic Chain
- The kinetic chain is related mostly to specificity of exercise. If the desired activity is in the closed kinetic chain, this position should be used for training whenever possible. However, the closed kinetic chain often cannot isolate muscle function as well as a specific open kinetic chain exercise.

Stabilization (External or Within)
- If stability is required for a movement, use of external straps or prepositioning a limb may assist stabilization if the patient is unable to stabilize with proper patterns internally. For example, in supine, the trunk can stabilize with greater ease if the hip and knee are flexed and held in place by the hands while the other limb slides down and back during an abdominal strengthening exercise (Fig. 1). This is an example of prepositioning to offer external stability.

Physiologic

Duration
- Duration of activity in seconds, minutes, or hours
- Number of repetitions or sets performed

Frequency
- Number of exercise sessions in a given time period

Speed
- Slower is not necessarily easier (see earlier)

Intensity of Contraction or External Load
- Percentage of maximum voluntary contraction

Type of Muscle Contraction
- Eccentric, isometric, concentric

(continued)

DISPLAY 2-14
Exercise Modification Parameters (Continued)

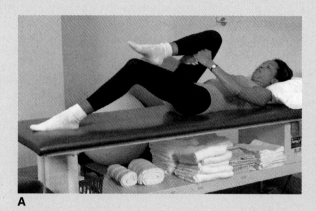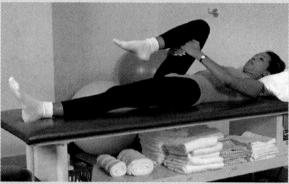

A   B

FIGURE 1. Leg slide movement for strengthening lumbopelvic stabilizing muscles. The hip and knee are flexed and held close to the chest as the other limb slides down and back. This modification reduces the stabilizing force needed by the trunk muscles due to the amount of hip flexion in the stationary limb. The more proximal the stationary limb is relative to the center of mass, the less difficult the exercise becomes, the more distal the stationary limb is relative to the center of mass, the more difficult the exercise becomes. This photograph illustrates the mid position of the exercise. (A) The patient should end with the extremity as close to full extension as the length of the hip flexors will allow (B).

Sequence of Exercise
- May require beginning with less complex tasks or less strenuous activity in early stages of learning or healing and progressing to less need for "warm-up" activities as skill is achieved and tissues are in more advanced stages of healing

Rest Between Repetitions and Sets
- As strength or endurance improves, less rest is necessary between repetitions and sets. Be cautious of overtraining, especially in presence of neuromuscular disease or injury.

Neuromuscular

Sensory input
- Visual, proprioceptive, and tactile inputs can be manipulated. If the eyes are closed, visual input is eliminated, leaving the vestibular, proprioceptive, and tactile receptors to detect any disturbance. The tactile input can be varied by standing on soft foam. The proprioceptive input can be varied with head movement.

Sensory Facilitation or Inhibition
- Techniques such as cutaneous and pressure input, approximation, and traction can alter muscle responses. Prolonged pressure on the long tendons such as the quadriceps, biceps, hamstrings, or finger flexors seems to inhibit responses. The placement of manual contacts is critical to facilitate the desired response. Contacts are placed in the direction toward which the segment is to move. Approximation or compression into or through a joint stimulates the joint receptors and may facilitate extensor muscles and stability around a joint. Traction separates the joint surface and is incorporated if increasing ROM around a joint is desired.

Number of Segments Involved
- In weight-bearing postures, joint involvement usually refers to the weight-bearing segments; for example, prone on elbows does not require participation of the forearm and hand or

the lower body compared with quadruped. The placement of manual contacts or other external forces also influences the number of segments involved. For example, contacts placed on the scapula and pelvis in sidelying involve the entire trunk, whereas contacts positioned on the lumbar spine and pelvis result in more isolated activity of the lower trunk.

Stage of Movement Control
- Mobility, stability, controlled mobility, skill (see Display 2-9 for the definitions of stages of Movement Control)

Cognitive or Affective

Frequency and Duration of the Activity
- Increased frequency and duration of the activity increases the practice schedule to enhance learning.

Initial Information Provided
- Care should be taken to provide enough information to perform the activity with the correct strategy, but not to give too much information, which may overwhelm the learner.

Accuracy Provided
- As skill is acquired, increased accuracy of cues is provided to "fine tune" a movement.

Variability of Environmental Conditions
- Initially reduced number of external distractions is provided with increasing external distractions toward a functional environment as skill is acquired.

Complexity of Activity
- Number of steps involved; as in breaking down components of gait into single tasks and then uniting them into the integrated complex motor task of gait with numerous steps

Anxiety Level
- Initially, greater focus on the activity is combined with the least emotional distractions to enhance early learning.

ADJUNCTIVE INTERVENTIONS

To complete this chapter on patient management, adjunctive interventions were chosen to be included in this section to provide insight into the complementary role they play in therapeutic exercise prescription. The interventions presented in this section are considered adjunctive to therapeutic exercise in that they are not regarded as essential to achieving a functional outcome.

When choosing to use an adjunctive intervention, a decision must be made regarding the benefit of its use in conjunction with therapeutic exercise. The clinician should be reasonably sure that combining the adjunctive intervention with the therapeutic exercise would produce more rapid or optimal functional recovery. Make it clear to the patient that the adjunctive intervention is being used to augment the exercise and that the exercise and modified posture and movement habits will ultimately change the impairments and activity limitations for long-term improvement. There are conditions for which physical agents, mechanical and electrotherapeutic modalities, and orthotics are imperative to achieve improved physical function and health status, in which case these interventions are not considered adjunctive (e.g., significant soft-tissue inflammation, severe pain disorders, skin conditions, nerve injury, impaired motor function, and structural abnormalities).

Physical agents, mechanical modalities, and electrotherapeutic modalities can play a vital role in the total plan of care for a patient and serve as important adjuncts to therapeutic exercise. Elaboration of the role of each of these therapies can be found on the website. Additional adjunctive interventions such as taping and orthotic prescription are presented in Units 5 and 6.

KEY POINTS

- The physical therapist integrates five elements of care—examination, evaluation, diagnosis, prognosis, and intervention—in a manner designed to maximize the patient's outcome.
- An understanding of each component of the patient management model assists the clinician in maximizing patient satisfaction and in delivering the most effective and efficient services possible.
- The clinician's knowledge, expertise, experience, and ongoing acquisition of knowledge and experience are the determinants for successful patient management.
- Critical clinical decisions are those involved in determining which impairments from the list generated from the examination are most closely related to activity limitation and participation limitation and therefore warrant intervention.
- Patient-related instruction must be an integral part of any physical therapy intervention.
- The three-dimensional therapeutic exercise intervention model is designed to help organize the data necessary to make clinical decisions regarding therapeutic exercise intervention.
- Exercises must be continually monitored to determine the need for modification to increase or decrease difficulty to ensure continual progress is being made with minimal setbacks. To be most effective with exercise modification, the clinician must possess thorough understanding of the parameters that can be modified.

- Therapeutic exercise can be complemented with adjunctive interventions if the additional intervention can lead to a higher level of functional outcome in a shorter period.

CRITICAL THINKING QUESTIONS

1. Read Case Study No. 2 in Unit 7.
   a. List the physiologic, anatomic, and psychologic impairments.
   b. List the activity limitations.
   c. Correlate the impairments to the activity limitations.
   d. Choose the impairments and activity limitations you feel warrant treatment.
   e. Correlate the impairments and activity limitations you have chosen to treat with the elements of the movement system.
   f. Prioritize the elements of the movement system.
2. Still using Case Study No. 2, you have decided to prescribe exercises to improve knee mobility, because you know the patient requires 70 degrees of knee flexion to perform simple ADLs. You would like to use a sit to stand movement to work on knee mobility. Recall that she requires moderate assistance with sit to stand transfers.
   a. Describe the posture, mode, and movement of the activity.
   b. Describe all pertinent parameters of dosage.
3. The patient has progressed to 70 degrees of flexion and no longer requires assistance with sit to stand transfers. How would you modify the mobility exercises to make them more difficult? Use the principles of exercise modification listed in Display 2-12.
4. The patient is having difficulty with recruitment of her quadriceps.
   a. What adjunctive intervention would you use?
   b. Describe the posture, mode, and movement of the activity.
   c. Describe all pertinent parameters of dosage.

REFERENCES

1. American Physical Therapy Association. Guide to physical therapist practice. 2nd Ed. American Physical Therapy Association; Phys Ther 2001;81:9–746.
2. Jette AM, Branch LG, Berlin J. Musculoskeletal impairments and physical disablement among the aged. J Gerontol 1990;45:M203–M208.
3. Bradley EM, Wagstaff S, Wood PHN. Measures of functional limitation (disability) in arthritis in relation to impairment of range of joint movement. Am Rheum Dis 1984;43:563–569.
4. Rothstein JM, Echternach JL. Hypothesis-oriented algorithm for clinicians. Phys Ther 1986;66:1388–1394.
5. Topp R, Wooley S, Khuder S, et al. Predictors of four functional tasks in patients with osteoarthritis of the knee. Orthop Nurs 2000;19:49–59.
6. World Health Organization. International Classification of Functioning, Disability and Health: ICF. Geneva, Switzerland: World Health Organization, 2001.
7. Guccione AA, Cullen KE, O'Sullivan SB. Functional assessment. In: Sullivan SB, Schmitz TJ, eds. Physical Rehabilitation: Assessment and Treatment. 2nd Ed. Philadelphia, PA: FA Davis, 1988.
8. Nagi S. Disability concepts revisited: implications for prevention. In: Pope AM, Tarlov AR, eds. Disability in America: Toward a National Agenda for Prevention. Washington, DC: National Academy Press, 1991.
9. Atlas SJ, Deyo RA, Van Den Ancker M, et al. The Maine-Seattle back questionnaire: a 12-item disability questionnaire for evaluating patients with lumbar sciatica or stenosis: results of a derivation and validation cohort analysis. Spine 2003;28:1869–1876.
10. Beaton DE, Schemitsch E. Measures of health-related quality of life and physical function. Clin Orthop 2003;413:90–105.
11. Takken T, van der Net J, Helders PJ. Relationship between functional limitation and physical fitness in juvenile idiopathic arthritis patients. Scand J Rheumatol 2003;32:174–178.

12. Hazes JM. Determinants of physical function in rheumatoid arthritis: association with the disease process. Rheumatology (Oxford) 2003;42:17–21.
13. Mason JH, Anderson JJ, Meenan RF, et al. The Rapid Assessment of Disease Activity in Rheumatology (RADAR) Questionnaire: validity and sensitivity to change of a patient self-report measure of joint count and clinical status. Arthritis Rheum 1992;35:156–162.
14. Meenan RF, Mason JH, Anderson JJ, et al. AIMS2: the content and properties of a revised and expanded Arthritis Impact Measurement Scales health status questionnaire. Arthritis Rheum 1992;35:1–10.
15. Jette AM, Davies AR, Cleary PD, et al. The functional status questionnaire: reliability and validity when used in primary care. J Gen Intern Med 1986;1:143–149.
16. Haley SM. Motor assessment tools for infant and young children: a focus on disability assessment. In: Forrsberg H, ed. Treatment of Children with Movement Disorders: Theory and Practice. Basel, Switzerland: S Karger, 1992.
17. Frey WD. Functional outcome: assessment and evaluation. In: Delisa JA, ed. Rehabilitation Medicine: Principle and Practice. Philadelphia, PA: JB Lippincott, 1988.
18. Haley SM, Coster WJ, Ludlow LH. Pediatric functional outcome measures. In: Jaffe KM, ed. Pediatric Rehabilitation. Philadelphia, PA: WB Saunders, 1991.
19. Law M. Evaluating activities of daily living: directions for the future. Am J Occup Ther 1993;47:233–237.
20. Heinemann AW, Linacre JM, Wright BD, et al. Relationships between impairment and physical disability as measured by the Functional Independence Measure. Arch Phys Med Rehabil 1993;74:566–573.
21. Mahoney FL, Barthel DW. Functional evaluation: the Barthel index. Md State Med J 1965;14:61–65.
22. Hamilton BB, Laughlin JA, Fiedler RC, et al. Interrater reliability of the 7-level functional independence measure (FIM). Scand J Rehabil Med 1994;26:115–119.
23. Berg K, Wood Dauphinee S, Williams JI, et al. Measuring balance in the elderly: validation of an instrument. Can J Public Health 1992;2:S7–S11.
24. Creel GL, Light KE, Thigpen MT. Concurrent and construct validity of scores on the Timed Movement Battery. Phys Ther 2001;81:789–798.
25. Granger CV, Cotter AC, Hamilton RB, et al. Functional assessment scales: a study of persons after stroke. Arch Phys Med Rehabil 1993;74:133–138.
26. Gresham GE, Labi ML. Functional assessment instruments currently available for documenting outcomes in rehabilitation medicine. In: Granger CV, Gresham GE, eds. Functional Assessment in Rehabilitation Medicine. Baltimore, MD: Williams & Wilkins, 1984.
27. Guccione AA. Arthritis and the process of disablement. Phys Ther 1994;74:408–414.
28. Bergner M, Babbitt RA, Carter WB, et al. The sickness impact profile: development and final revision of a health status measure. Med Care 1981;19:787–805.
29. Roland M, Morris RA. A study of the natural history of back pain, part I: the development of a reliable and sensitive measure of disability in low back pain. Spine 1983;8:141–144.
30. Fairbanks JCT, Couper J, Davies JB, et al. The Oswestry low back pain disability questionnaire. Physiotherapy 1980;66:271–273.
31. Waddell G, Main CJ, Morriss EW, et al. Chronic low back pain, psychological distress, and illness behavior. Spine 1984;9:209–213.
32. Keith RA, Granger CV. The functional independence measure: a new tool for rehabilitation. In: Eisenberg MG, Greysiak RC, eds. Advances in Clinical Rehabilitation. New York, NY: Springer Publishing, 1987.
33. Butland RJA, Pang J, Gross ER, et al. Two, six, and twelve minute walking test in respiratory disease. BMJ 1982;284:1604–1608.
34. Steffen TM, Hacker TA, Mollinger L. Age- and gender-related test performance in community-dwelling elderly people: six-minute walk test, Berg Balance Scale, Timed Up & Go Test, and gait speeds. Phys Ther 2002;82:128–137.

35. Shields RK, Enloe LJ, Evans RE, et al. Reliability, validity, and responsiveness of functional tests in patients with total joint replacement. Phys Ther 1995;75:169–176.
36. Stewart A, Ware JE, eds. Measuring Functioning and Well-Being: The Medical Outcomes Study Approach. Durham, NC: Duke University Press, 1992.
37. Lawliss GF, Cuencas R, Selby D, et al. The development of the Dallas pain questionnaire: an assessment of the impact of spinal pain on behavior. Spine 1989;14:512–515.
38. Ware JE, Sherbourne CD. The MOS 36-item short-form health survey (SF-36), I: conceptual framework and item selection. Med Care 1992;30:473–483.
39. Davidson M, Keating JL. A comparison of five low back disability questionnaires: reliability and responsiveness. Phys Ther 2002;82:512–515.
40. Sahrmann SA. Diagnosis by the physical therapist—prerequisite for treatment: a special communication. Phys Ther 1988;68:1703–1706.
41. Rose SJ. Physical therapy diagnosis: role and function. Phys Ther 1989;69:535–537.
42. Delitto A, Synder-Mackler L. The diagnostic process: examples in orthopedic physical therapy. Phys Ther 1995;75:203–210.
43. Van Dillen LR, Sahrmann SA, Norton BJ, et al. Movement system impairment-based categories for low back pain: stage 1 validation. J Orthop Sports Phys Ther 2003;33:126–142.
44. Coffin-Zadai CA. Disabling our diagnostic dilemmas. Phys Ther 2007;87:641–653.
45. Rose SJ. Description and classification: the cornerstone of pathokinesiological research. Phys Ther 1986;66:379–381.
46. Fritz JM, Wainner RS. Examining diagnostic tests: an evidence-based perspective. Phys Ther 2001;81:1546–1564.
47. Fosnaught M. A critical look at diagnosis. Phys Ther 1996;4:48–53.
48. Balla JL. The Diagnostic Process: A Model for Clinical Teachers. Cambridge, England: Cambridge University Press, 1985.
49. Guccione AA. Physical therapy diagnosis and the relationship between impairments and function. Phys Ther 1191;71:499–503.
50. Dekker J, Van Baar ME, Curfs EC, et al. Diagnosis and treatment in physical therapy: an investigation of their relationship. Phys Ther 1993;73:568–577.
51. Jette AM. Diagnosis and classification by physical therapists: a special communication. Phys Ther 1989;69:967–969.
52. Baker SM, Marshak HH, Rice GT, et al. Patient participation in physical therapy goal setting. Phys Ther 2001;81:1118–1126.
53. Straus SE, Sackett DL. Using research findings in clinical practice. BMJ 1998;317:339–342.
54. Kane R. Looking for physical therapy outcomes. Phys Ther 1995;74:425–429.
55. Rothstein JM. Outcome assessment of therapeutic exercise. In: Bajmajian JV, Wolf SL, eds. Therapeutic Exercise. 5th Ed. Baltimore, MD: Williams & Wilkins, 1990.
56. Sackett DL, Straus SE, Richardson WS, Rosenberg W, Haynes RB, Evidence-Based Medicine. How To Practice and Teach EBM. 2nd Ed. New York, NY: Churchill Livingstone, 2000.
57. Oermann MH, Templin T. Important attributes of quality health care: consumer perspectives. J Nurse Scholarsh 2000;32:167–172.
58. Sahrmann SA. Diagnosis and Treatment of Movement Impairment Syndromes. St. Louis, MD: Mosby, Inc., 2002.
59. Kendall FP, McCreary EK, Provance PG. Muscles Testing and Function. 4th Ed. Baltimore, MD: Williams & Wilkins, 1993.
60. Sullivan PE, Markos PD. Clinical Decision Making in Therapeutic Exercise. Norwalk, CT: Appleton & Lange, 1995.
61. Gentile AM. Skill acquisition: action, movement, and neuromotor processes. In: Carr JH, Shephard RB, eds. Movement Science: Foundations for Physical Therapy in Rehabilitation. 3rd Ed. New York, NY: Aspen Publishers, Inc., 2000

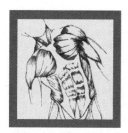

chapter 3

Principles of Self-Management and Exercise Instruction

LORI THEIN BRODY

Patient education is a critical component of patient care. Changes in the structure of the medical system, reimbursement issues, and an increase in the prevalence of chronic problems require educating patients about their conditions and teaching them self-management strategies. Patient-related or client-related instruction is defined as the "process of informing, educating, or training patients/clients, families, significant others, and caregivers with the intent to promote and optimize physical therapy services."[1] Instruction, education, and training of patients or clients include information on their current condition, the diagnosis, the prognosis and plan of care, health and wellness issues, and risk factors for pathology, impairments, activity limitations, and participation restrictions.

Teaching in the clinic can take many forms. Serving as a clinical mentor for a physical therapy intern and teaching parents how to assist their child in stretching exercises are obvious examples of teaching in the clinic. Clinicians also teach patients during the evaluation and treatment sessions. A study of the perceptions of physical therapists regarding their involvement in patient education showed that therapists educate 80% to 100% of their patients.[2] These therapists primarily recognized teaching range-of-motion (ROM) techniques, home exercise programs, and treatment rationales. Clinicians recognize but may underestimate the importance of educating their patients on important issues such as the relationship between symptoms and their patients' daily routines and the expected response to the exercise program. Patients' satisfaction with treatment and willingness to adhere are often based on the fulfillment of their expectations. The more time spent educating the patient on prognosis and expectations from the rehabilitation program, the more likely the patient is to adhere to and be satisfied with the treatment program. Gahimer and Domholdt[3] found that therapists educated their patients primarily in the areas of information about illness, home exercises, and advice and information. Moreover, the patients reported attitudinal or behavioral changes ranging from 83.8% to 86.5% as a result of this education. Health education and stress counseling were addressed less frequently during the treatment session.

PATIENT EDUCATION

Teaching in the clinic is a constant and ongoing process. As changes in health care occur, many clinicians are finding that their role has changed from full-time, hands-on providers of rehabilitation services to part-time educators, administrators, and clinicians.[3] In the past, patients were educated on a "need to know" basis. Patients were passive recipients of information deemed necessary by the clinician. This has changed and patient education is not optional but mandated. Informed consent requires that clinicians provide their patients with sufficient information to make an intelligent, well-informed choice about their health care. Informed consent does not mean just agreeing to the plan of care determined by the provider but also includes risks associated with the treatment, other treatment alternatives, and the potential consequences of not receiving the treatment.

Patient learning is categorized as cognitive, affective, and psychomotor.[4] In therapeutic exercise, all three domains are part of the patient education process. The cognitive domain includes information and facts about the patient's condition and the rehabilitation program. This might include descriptions of the anatomy, biomechanics, or pathomechanics of the condition. Educating patients about therapeutic exercise theory and the rationale behind the exercise choices also falls into the cognitive domain. A study of patients with a mean 10-year history of low back pain found that 51% of these patients had noticeable improvement in their pain 1 week after being provided with an individualized biomechanical treatment booklet. At both the 9- and the 18-month follow-up assessments, statistically and clinically significant improvements were reported in pain management, number of episodes of care, and perceived benefit.[5]

Affective domain education addresses the patient's attitude and motivation. This is also a critical component of the rehabilitation program. Possessing the cognitive information and the psychomotor skill to execute the exercise program is of little use when the patient is unmotivated to participate. The patients' attitudes toward their condition and their attitudes and beliefs about the likelihood of the therapeutic exercise program remediating their symptoms are essential for program adherence. This topic is explored further in the section on "Adherence and Motivation."

Finally, the psychomotor domain is of obvious import when considering therapeutic exercise. Learning the proper motor programs and exercise performance are critical for therapeutic exercise prescription. The nuances of muscle activation and control during therapeutic exercise distinguish this type of rehabilitative exercise from recreational exercise. The psychomotor domain is explored in further detail in the "Motor Learning" section.

Clinical teaching, particularly in the area of the home exercise program, is also important, because in-house supervised physical therapy services are often inadequate to achieve the patient's goals. For example, performing stretching exercises three times per week for 30 minutes under the clinician's supervision probably will be insufficient to produce a change. The development of a thorough, complementary home exercise program is essential. Exercise prescription for the home, workplace, or school can prove to be an interesting challenge for the clinician and patient. Helping the patient establish a daily exercise program as a routine can make a positive lifelong impact.

Improving Outcomes

Depending on the specific circumstances, the provision of rehabilitation services may be limited to a few visits. In this situation, the patient may be carrying out the rehabilitation program at home or at a local health club with intermittent rechecks for status and progression of the program. To ensure safety during exercise and improvement in the patient's symptoms, the exercise program must be executed properly. Frequently, the patient appears to understand proper performance of the exercises, but he or she subsequently forgets the instructions, resulting in improper technique. This problem can result in a lack of improvement and potentially in exacerbation, or worsening, of the symptoms. The patient should understand which signs and symptoms predict an exacerbation so that he or she can modify the exercise program appropriately. This education can prevent an exacerbation and potential reinjury (Building Block 3-1).

Self-Management

Self-management has become increasingly important today as people are living longer with chronic health conditions. Patients with chronic conditions such as arthritis, heart disease, stroke, and diabetes are living longer and must learn how to manage their symptoms and to prevent complications of the disease process. Similarly, greater longevity results in a larger population of older adults. These individuals require education to prevent a decline in their health status and to maintain their overall level of health and well-being. An individual seeing a physical therapist for knee osteoarthritis may have a poor understanding of the role of therapeutic exercise in maintaining knee and total body health. Extensive patient education may be necessary to help that patient achieve optimal function. Patients who are hospitalized for acute or

chronic conditions are being discharged earlier. This results in a greater demand for outpatient services and the need for patient and family/caregiver education to manage a more challenging situation.

When prescribing a rehabilitation program, educating the patient about the effects of the therapeutic exercise program on specific symptoms can empower him or her to self-manage the situation. The more clearly patients understand the relationships among various activities (including the exercise program) and their symptoms, the better able they will be to regulate their activity levels. This makes the patient a partner in the rehabilitation program. A recent study examined the impact of patient education and counseling regarding pain management, physical activity, and exercise in patients with low back pain and high levels of fear avoidance behavior.[6] While both groups improved with standard physical therapy intervention, those who received additional education and counseling had significantly fewer days off work than those without this education. This finding reinforces the importance of educating patients about their condition and strategies to effectively manage their symptoms. The patient still looks to the clinician for guidance and education regarding the physical problem, but the clinician gives the patient some responsibility in the decision-making process. This approach gently guides the patient in the self-management process.

Holmes et al.[7] successfully used a self-management approach in the treatment of a woman with impingement syndrome and adhesive capsulitis. She was seen for six visits over 10 weeks and followed up for 1 year. The authors felt that the intensive patient education allowed the patient to develop an internal sense of control and prevented the development of an external focus in which the patient depends on the therapist for the management of the condition. Motivation exhibited by patients may be a manifestation of their locus of control beliefs.[8]

CLINICIAN-PATIENT COMMUNICATION

Communication is a two-way conversation, not a one-way provision of factual information. It requires skill on the part of the provider as well as an understanding of the verbal and nonverbal components of communication. Communication has many facets and components, each requiring appropriate interpretation and responses. Body language and posture, eye contact, physical contact, tone of voice, type of questioning, and listening ability all impact rapport and trust. Clinicians must recognize their own verbal and nonverbal communication and recognize similar cues from the patient. They must then respond appropriately from these patient cues, reflecting back the patient's concerns and providing support.[4]

Communication is most effectively accomplished when the clinician has established rapport with the patient. Rapport is a quality of interaction that is difficult to define but is comprised of an ability to make patients feel cared for and respected.[4] The patient must trust the care provider, and the care provider must be able to accept and empathize with the patient's situation. This does not mean that the provider should support poor health behavior choices but should acknowledge the challenges the patient may be facing. This acknowledgement is followed by active problem solving to eliminate barriers to good choices and to design a support system that will facilitate and reward positive choices.

BUILDING BLOCK 3-1

Kathy is a 53-year-old high-level recreational tennis player. She sustained an acute rotator cuff tear during a fall 8 months ago and 2 months later underwent rotator cuff repair. Physical therapy was initiated 2 weeks post-op, and Kathy has been making steady progress on her ROM and strength. However, she is frustrated at the rate of her progress and feels as though she should be farther along in her recovery than she currently is. She has requested to add aquatic physical therapy in hopes of accelerating her progress. She belongs to a health club and has access to a pool there. She has been performing her land-based rehabilitation program faithfully.

Review of Kathy's land-based program reveals that she has been performing exercises correctly. However, in her zest to hasten her progress, she was overexercising, increasing her pain and slowing her progress. Given this information, what are key aspects of education for this patient?

Individual differences significantly affect the patient-clinician relationship. Fundamental personality differences, values, and teaching and learning styles influence communication and may ultimately affect adherence and outcome. Possessing important skills to assess the patient's willingness and style of communication and learning can enhance the rehabilitation program. These skills include the ability to actively listen to and reflect on the patient's reports and to provide appropriate feedback.[9,10] Sluijs et al.[11] found lack of positive feedback to be one of the primary factors related to lack of adherence to a rehabilitation exercise program. Cameron[8] suggests improving the quality of the interaction by showing sensitivity to the patient's verbal and nonverbal communications and understanding of and empathy with the patient's feelings.

Patient education implies a willingness to participate by the patient and the clinician. The patient's readiness to learn depends on many factors, including the relationship with the health care provider. The clinician must be able to assess the patient's readiness and willingness to learn. The relationship is based on how the patient is coping with the particular situation. Schwenk and Whitman[10] described a control scale in which the control level of the patient and that of the clinician were inversely related. As the clinician uses less controlling or assertive behaviors, the patient's control of the situation increases. The converse is also true; the active and assertive clinician is likely to push the patient into a more passive role. If the patient is unwilling to be in such a role, conflict will ensue or the clinician will become more passive, relinquishing some control to the patient.

The clinician's attention to the patient's needs can guide the appropriate communication style. In the initial visits, a more passive listener role gives the patient an opportunity to explain his or her needs. This gives the clinician an opportunity to hear the patient's concerns, expectations, and goals. Fundamental skills necessary for active listening include close observation of the patient's words, intonation, and body language. Eye contact, along with affirmation and reflection of the patient report, can clarify what the clinician heard and validate the patient report (Fig. 3-1). This gives the clinician an opportunity to discuss the recovery prognosis given the adherence to the treatment program, which, along with discussion of the clinician's expectations of the patient, can enhance communication and the rehabilitation process. Several studies have shown the "Pygmalion effect" in a variety of settings in which the instructors' expectations were matched by students' achievements.[12–15]

Although communicating the expectations of all involved participants is important, it is equally important to provide realistic expectations in the form of short-term and long-term goals. Setting reasonable and achievable goals can provide one form of positive feedback for the patient. Occasionally, the patient's motivation can be improved by education about reasonable goals. The ability to perform the same level of exercise or activity at a lower level of pain is a reasonable short-term goal. The patient may only see that he or she is performing at the same level and perceive this as a lack of progress. Clarification on how progress is defined and reasonable expectations regarding progress can improve patient adherence and satisfaction (see Building Block 3-2). Some advocate a contract approach in which the specific obligations of each party in the attainment of the therapy goals are set forth and a timeline is determined.[8]

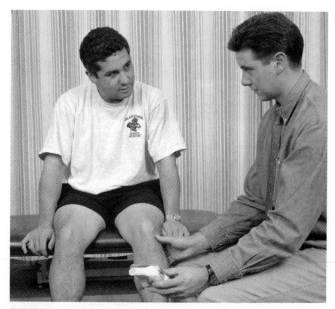

FIGURE 3-1. In appropriate cultural situations, eye contact can enhance communication.

ADHERENCE AND MOTIVATION

Patient compliance with a treatment regimen is a subject of a great deal of research. The terms *compliance*, *adherence*, and *therapeutic alliance* are often used to discuss the extent to which a patient's behavior coincides with medical advice.[8] Some feel that the term compliance is too dictatorial on the part of the caregiver and seems to neglect the philosophy of "patient as partner" in determining the plan of care. The term adherence is used throughout this chapter. The best-designed rehabilitation program achieves little if the patient is not compelled to participate. A study by Sluijs et al.[11] demonstrated a complete adherence rate of only 35%, with 76% of the patients "partly" compliant with their rehabilitation program. The factors related to nonadherence were barriers that patients perceived, lack of positive feedback, and the degree of helplessness. These are issues in the affective domain of patient education and learning.

Health Behavior Models

Clinicians spend a great deal of time designing what they believe to be the best plan of care for their patients. However, even the best intervention plans will fail in the absence of

 BUILDING BLOCK 3-2

Kathy returned to physical therapy for a follow-up visit. She is still worried that she will not be able to play again. She is currently 3 months post-op. Her physician performed an ultrasound to assess healing and felt that her rate of healing was as expected given her age and tissue quality. She remains frustrated at what she perceived to be a lack of progress despite improvement in impairments and increased functional use of the arm. How would you counsel the patient?

patient participation. The factors associated with compliance with medical professional recommendations have been well-studied. Some studies focus on eliminating unhealthy behaviors (smoking, excessive alcohol use), whereas others focus on initiating healthy behaviors (good eating habits, exercise, compliance with medication schedules).[8,11,16] A number of behavior change models have been put forth. For example, the Health Belief model stresses a reduction of environmental barriers to healthy behaviors including perceived barriers, benefits, self-efficacy, and severity.[17,18] Other models include the Health Locus of Control, Self-Efficacy and Transtheoretical, or stages of change model.[17,19] Of these models, the Transtheoretical model has been applied to many aspects of exercise behaviors.

The Transtheoretical model emphasizes the temporal aspect of a behavior change, underscoring the ability to change a behavior over a variable length of time. Individuals may spend varying lengths of time in different stages as they slowly make changes, or they may get stuck in one stage. Additionally, the patient may move through some of the stages several times before completing the behavior change.[19] The stages identified in this model include *precontemplation*, *contemplation*, *preparation*, *action*, and *maintenance*.

In the precontemplation stage, the individual has no intention of changing or does not see any need for change. Prochaska[20] quantifies this stage by a person stating he or she did not intend to change within the next 6 months. A person in this stage will be reluctant to begin any rehabilitation program and generally does not see the need or benefit of it. The individual may feel forced to come for rehabilitation by some outside party (physician, family member, employer), and no amount of explanation or information will improve adherence.

Individuals in the contemplation phase are seriously considering change but have not yet initiated it. Individuals in this stage state that they are planning to make a change within the next 6 months. Those in the preparation stage indicate that they are planning to change in the next month or had made some changes but had not fully achieved the change. Individuals in the action stage have reached some criterion level of change (such as quitting smoking or exercising three times per week) within the past 6 months. Those in the maintenance stage had reached the criterion level of behavioral change more than 6 months earlier.[20]

Applications

The patient will be more willing to adhere to a rehabilitation program if attention is given to the stage of readiness to begin such a program.[16,19,21] The first step is truly listening to the patient to identify clues as to their state of readiness for change. This can be done by using open-ended questions to explore issues related to adherence and to facilitate the patient's personal involvement. Help the patient identify potential barriers to participation and request input as to how these barriers can be removed or minimized. Patients need to believe that the pros of participation outweigh the cons and that they are capable of achieving the expected outcomes if they participate.[20,22,23] Help the patient in the precontemplation phase to identify personal goals that might be achieved by participation in the rehabilitation program. Build rapport through regular appointments and reflective conversation.[23] For the patient in the contemplation phase, build motivation through encouragement and the provision of information. Review the pros and cons of participation, reflecting the patient's own personal goals. Enhance adherence by educating the patient regarding the relationships among the injury or pathology, the exercise program, and the expected outcome. The clinician may purposefully link the exercise to the patient's specific problem or goals, but the patient may not understand this relationship. He or she should understand this relationship to ensure active participation in the treatment program. Friedrich et al.[24] found that compliance with physical exercise, energy conservation, and joint protection was increased by patient education in a group of patients with rheumatoid arthritis. For those in the action phase, actively engage them in plan of care formulation and provide support for the plan. Help identify barriers to implementation and address these in the treatment plan. Patients in the action and maintenance phases need positive reinforcement to continue participation and prevent relapses.

Motivation is a key factor in exercise adherence. Every person experiences various influences on motivation. What motivates one person is unlikely to motivate another. The clinician should attempt to determine which factors motivate the patient to adhere to the exercise program and use these as the "carrot" or reward. These factors vary tremendously and may include return to activities the patient enjoys (e.g., gardening, sports, leisure, recreational activities), return to work, return home (e.g., from hospital or intermediary care facility), ability to shop or carry out instrumental activities of daily living, or the ability to care for a child. After the motivators are identified, the exercise program should be tailored to those activities. Inability to participate in these activities is often one of the primary reasons the patient sought medical attention initially.

When designing the rehabilitation program with motivation and adherence in mind, use caution when using "exercise files." If the exercise program seems nonspecific or unrelated to the patient's functional needs, adherence could become a problem. In the early rehabilitation phases, some exercises may not seem particularly "functional" to the patient, but they are important aspects of the treatment program. Explaining the importance of the exercise educates the patient about the condition, assures the patient of the clinician's understanding of the problem and the potential solution, and treats the patient as an educated participant in the rehabilitation process. Further explanation of how the exercises will progress to more functional activities or how a specific exercise is related to the motivating activity validates the importance of that activity and verifies that this is important to the patient.

As the exercise program progresses, it should reflect more and more closely the activity to which the patient will be returning. The same physical therapy goals can be achieved while increasing motivation and function by using functional activities as the exercise program. For example, for the individual recovering from shoulder surgery who is unable to unload the dishwasher, transferring dishes of increasing weight from the counter to the shelf for progressively longer periods is more motivating and interesting than lifting a 1-lb weight (Fig. 3-2). This type of activity has the added benefit of requiring distal muscle function that more closely replicates the actual important activity than lifting a weight or using resistive tubing. Weights and tubing are useful adjuncts to the rehabilitation program and, when possible, should be used in a way that duplicates the functional activity. Rather

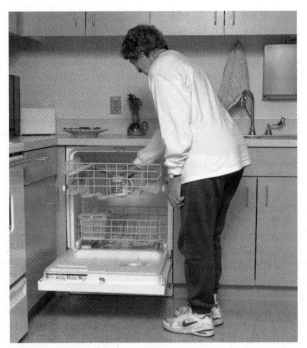

FIGURE 3-2. Choose home exercises reflective of the patient's usual activities.

than performing a series of cardinal plane shoulder exercises, mimicking activities such as a tennis swing, raking, sawing, or throwing a ball can increase strength and reinforce important motor programs (see Building Block 3-3).

A therapeutic exercise program requiring the fewest lifestyle changes increases the patient's adherence to it. Rather than trying to add more activities to the patient's day (often asking that exercise be performed several times per day), choose exercises that can be incorporated into his or her day. If an exercise program requires a 15- or 30-minute time block carved out of a person's busy day once or twice daily, adherence is difficult despite the patient's desire to participate. If the exercises can be blended into activities that the patient already does during the day, adherence becomes much easier. A study by Fields et al.[25] examined the relationships among self-motivation or apathy, perceived exertion, social support, scheduling concerns, clinical environment, and pain tolerance to adherence to sport injury rehabilitation in college-age recreational athletes. Of the variables under consideration, significant differences were seen between adherers and nonadherers in self-motivation,

BUILDING BLOCK 3-3

Kathy returns to physical therapy and is pleased with the progress but is anxious to return to tennis. She can see how she is getting stronger and her ROM is nearly full. She is concerned that she will not be able to make the arm movements necessary to play tennis. Her exercise program has focused on cardinal plane strengthening from 0 to 90 degrees on land and on overhead swimming strokes and diagonal patterns in the pool. How might you modify her exercise program to address her concerns?

 DISPLAY 3-1
Home Exercise Program for an Office Worker with Adhesive Capsulitis

Impairments
1. Decreased ROM in all directions in a capsular pattern
2. Decreased strength tested by manual muscle tests in all major shoulder muscle groups
3. Resting pain at 4 on 0–10 (0 = least; 10 = most pain); activity pain at 8 and 0–10.

Activity Limitations
1. Unable to use the arm for activities of daily living
2. Unable to lift weight with the arm held away from the body
3. Unable to get the arm over the head for work and daily activities

Participation Restrictions
1. Unable to fulfill all roles at work because of limitations
2. Unable to participate in leisure activities

Home Exercises
1. Stretching for shoulder elevation while in warm shower
2. Active use of the arm for personal hygiene, including showering, combing hair, dressing, eating, and pendulum exercises during dressing
3. Scapular retraction exercise with abduction in front of the mirror during grooming three times per day, looking in the mirror each time
4. Shoulder flexion or abduction stretch on the desk when talking on the phone
5. Passive shoulder external rotation stretch at the file cabinet every time
6. Isometric exercise while reading morning mail
7. Walk with large arm swings during lunch hour
8. Supine overhead stretches on the couch during the evening news
9. Use the arm as much as possible for cooking, dishwashing, housework, and yardwork
10. Resistive tubing exercises sometime during the day—patient's choice.

---

scheduling concerns, and pain tolerance; of these factors, scheduling concerns contributed most to the overall group difference. In another study, Sluijs et al.[11] found that the strongest factor in nonadherence was the barriers patients perceived. The most frequent complaint was that the exercise program required too much time and that the exercises did not fit into the patient's daily routine. An example of an exercise program for a patient with adhesive capsulitis can be found in Display 3-1.

Fitting exercise into the patient's daily routine establishes a conditioned response that may carry over after therapy is concluded. For example, if a patient needs to increase the length of the gastrocnemius-soleus complex by stretching several times each day, instructing that person to stretch for 20 to 30 seconds each time he or she ascends the stairs is less burdensome than doing this as part of an exercise routine at the day's end. For the individual needing to increase shoulder flexion ROM, leaning ahead with his or her arm forward and flexed on the desk or kitchen counter before making a phone call is a productive use of time. This may become a conditioned response, and whenever the phone rings, the individual associates that activity with stretching his or her shoulder, or whenever the patient climbs the stairs, he or she thinks of calf stretching. This technique works particularly well with postural reeducation exercises (Fig. 3-3).

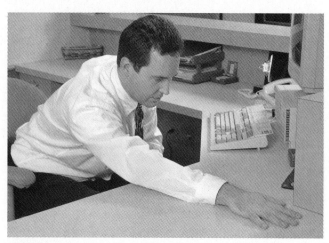

FIGURE 3-3. The clinician should prescribe exercises that can be performed during other home or work activities.

ISSUES IN HOME EXERCISE PROGRAM PRESCRIPTION

The home exercise program is an increasing component of the overall treatment program for most patients. In some cases, the patient performs the exercises independently, whereas, in other cases, a family member or other health care provider assists in the exercise program. In either situation, clarity in goals and exercise procedures is essential to ensure an optimal outcome.

Understanding Instructions

One of the fundamental steps in ensuring a positive outcome after initiation of a rehabilitation program is the patient's ability to understand the therapist's instructions. Many variables affect this aspect of patient care, including language or cultural barriers, reading or comprehension levels, hearing impairment, and clarity of instructions. The best-designed rehabilitation program may fail because it has not been carried out well. Do everything possible to ensure that your instructions are clear and easy to understand. While affective domain issues may be relevant here, much of the learning issues are related to the cognitive domain.

Cultural Barriers

Identify any cultural barriers to understanding early in the rehabilitation course. Language differences may hinder the use of even the simplest terminology. Although an individual may appear to understand many words in English, communicating thoughts about medically related issues is likely to be difficult. Use of an interpreter, whether a professional or a family member, can minimize communication difficulties in this area.

Other cultural barriers to adherence may exist and should be identified to the best of your ability. Religious or other cultural customs may prevent individuals from exercising on certain days or from wearing clothing that allows a body part to be visualized or palpated during exercise. In major metropolitan areas, a multitude of cultures exist. It is difficult to know all the intricacies of many cultures and customs. Do your best to know the times and meanings of your patient's ethnic or religious holidays. Seek information on cultural or religious customs related to eye and physical contact, including the appropriate type of greeting. This includes not only appropriate eye contact (avoiding eye contact is a sign of respect in some cultures) but also how the patient is addressed and if any physical contact (i.e., handshake) is appropriate.[26] Although these specific instances are difficult to know ahead of time, be alert to signs during the appointment that the patient is unwilling or hesitant to participate. Ask for permission to perform examination procedures in advance, or explain what needs to be done and determine what the patient needs to feel comfortable in the situation. In many cases, the patient feels most comfortable being examined by a therapist of the same sex. To the best of your ability, these issues should be addressed when scheduling the patient.

Clarity of Instruction

Simple aspects of the exercise program such as clear descriptions and legible writing are also important for adherence. Although written exercise programs may provide a personalized touch to the program, it may prove detrimental if the patient is unable to read your writing. Busy schedules and too little time contribute to hastily written patient instructions. Specific exercise descriptions may make perfect sense to the clinician but confuse the patient. Baseline knowledge assumed by the therapist may be too much for the patient and may result in incorrect exercise performance. Although the patient may be extremely bright and appears to grasp many aspects of medical care, clarity about which direction is "forward" or "up" is still necessary. Providers may find it useful to ask patients what they would name the exercise or how they would describe a certain movement. This simple act involves the patient in the exercise description and helps to personalize the home program. This contrasts an authoritarian position where the provider hands the patient a routine exercise handout that seems highly impersonal. Education around the home exercise program is another way to connect and develop rapport with the patient. Directions should be lengthy enough to be comprehensive without overburdening the patient with details. Full sentences are unnecessary, but key phrases or bulleted points can improve clarity.

Include pictures of the exercises and show the exercise in the start and finish positions. Communicating a three-dimensional movement on a single sheet of paper at a stationary point in time is difficult. Showing starting and ending positions or showing pictures from different angles helps clarify the three-dimensional nature of the movement. Arrows showing the direction of movement with marks clearly indicating the start and end positions are helpful. Often, exercise pictures show positions midway through the exercise, and the patient is unclear as to the full excursion of the movement. Throughout this book, Self-Management boxes present examples of exercise instructions.

Many clinics provide picture files or computer-generated exercises with pictures, descriptions, and exercise prescriptions included. These are helpful for the clinician, but use caution with these for the following reasons. First, the therapist frequently needs to modify the exercise in some way to adapt it to the specific patient needs. These modifications should be made on the patient's exercise record, not just verbalized. Do not assume that because an exercise is provided in one of these formats, it is the best or the only way to perform the exercise. Second, the exercise prescription should be individualized based on the patient's needs and ability to self-manage the problem, not necessarily prescribed as a certain number of sets and repetitions per day. This type of prescription may conflict with the goal of teaching the patient self-management skills. Exercises that appear to be "canned" or the standard sheet of exercises that is given to every patient with a certain diagnosis minimizes the individuality of the exercise program. Lack of individualization minimizes the skills of the therapist and may affect adherence if the patient feels his or her needs are not being met.

Communication with the patient regarding the exercise program should be written and verbal. Simply handing a patient the exercise program without having the patient perform each of the exercises increases the likelihood of non-adherence and incorrect performance. A study by Friedrich et al.[24] found that patients who received a brochure of exercises rather than a supervised instruction had a lower rating of "correctness" of exercise performance. A strong correlation between the quality of exercise performance and a decrease in pain was found.[27] Although patients may say they can remember their exercises, it is best to document the exercises with a written description that is reinforced with verbal cueing as the exercises are performed.

Organize the exercises to follow a logical sequence. An exercise program requiring frequent position changes is time-consuming and burdensome for the patient. Cluster exercises of a similar nature for ease of understanding and ease of performance. For example, cluster all exercises performed in a supine position to minimize position changes and group together shoulder rotation exercises because of their similar nature. Be sure to organize the exercises to simplify their performance and minimize the impact on the patient's lifestyle.

Psychomotor Aspects of Exercise Programs

Patient education and instruction in a home exercise program require more than the simple transfer of information from the provider to the client. While some aspects are clearly cognitive, many are psychomotor. Designing the home exercise program can impact the client's participation and eventual success. The program is designed to maximize learning a skill or concept and to facilitate carryover of that skill or concept to other environments, contexts, or situations. Important issues are not just cognitive or affective but also psychomotor. How the exercises are ordered and accomplished can affect the motor learning process. Thus, another important focus of home exercise program design and patient education is motor learning.

Motor Learning

Opportunities to enhance motor learning exist within the exercise program design. Motor learning is defined as the acquisition and/or modification of movement.[28] A number of strategies are available for promoting the acquisition of motor skills. Choices such as type of feedback, feedback schedule, open and closed loop response, and repetition and the organization of practice conditions impact the learning effect of training. These learning effects influence the patient's ability to learn, apply, and retain motor programs that can resolve or prevent decline or reinjury. For example, Herbert et al.[29] examined the effectiveness of different feedback schedules

on the performance and learning of a lumbar multifidus muscle activity. Those subjects who had a variable practice schedule performed better 3 to 4 months later than did those with a constant practice schedule.

Researchers and clinicians have attempted to characterize the process of learning a new motor skill. Visualize the last time you learned or watched someone else learn a new motor skill such as snowboarding, skating, or playing a musical instrument. Various theories related to the stages of motor learning exist and two three-stage theories will be summarized.

Fitts and Posner[30] call the first stage of their model the *cognitive*. In the cognitive stage, attention to the task is necessary to master the fundamental components of the skill. During this phase, gross motor strategies are developed. Overcorrection and exaggerated movements are typical in this phase. The second phase, or *associative* phase, is characterized by further refinement of these gross strategies. Movements are becoming more efficient with less overcorrection and more refined muscle activation. The third and final phase is the *autonomous* phase where the motor program is activated and implemented with little cognitive input.

Another model, the *systems three-stage model,* is based on controlling the movement and degrees of freedom as the central tenet of motor learning.[28] In the first phase, the learner uses muscle agonist-antagonist co-contraction to restrain movement and control the degrees of freedom. This stage of motor learning has been termed the *novice stage*.[31] Here, the learner simplifies movement by constraining or coupling some joints, thereby stabilizing or fixating these joints, decreasing the degrees of freedom to be managed. This is a relatively inflexible and inefficient movement pattern. The second phase is characterized by reducing constraint and increasing the degrees of freedom to be managed. This stage, the *advanced stage,* allows more coordinated movement without the constraint of agonist-antagonist co-contraction. Movement becomes more efficient and less rigid. The final phase, called the *expert phase,* sees the individual now releasing all degrees of freedom, and movement is allowed to proceed in the most efficient and coordinated manner. Movement is adaptable to multiple environments.

This type of learning process can be seen when teaching lumbar stabilization activities. In the early phase, the learner may overconstrain, tightening all muscles throughout the core at a maximum level in an attempt to stabilize the pelvis. As the patient progresses, learning appropriate pelvic control, the level of muscle activation in co-contraction is decreased. The patient contracts muscles in a coordinated fashion rather than in a mass recruitment manner. In the final phase, the patient activates core muscles in the right sequence and at the right level to match the task at hand.

Practice Conditions

Theories of motor learning have been tested using a variety of practice conditions. For example, using variable versus continuous practice conditions examines the carryover effect of a practiced skill to a new situation. A patient might perform an exercise at a continuous speed or a variable speed, followed by testing at a new speed. Supporters of variable practice strategies suggest that this program design is more likely to carry over to a new speed than practice at a single speed.

Other research in varying practice conditions examines the effects of mental and physical practice on performance.

Research into the effects of random and blocked task practice order has produced mixed results. The impact of cognitive problem-solving operations on motor skill acquisition has been termed *contextual interference*.[32,33] Contextual interference and its ability to enhance motor skill acquisition appear to be affected by many variables including practice schedule (random, blocked, combined) and the task difficulty. In general, it appears as though random practice conditions (where the patient practices several different tasks in random order) result in superior transfer skill performance compared with blocked practice conditions (practicing one task and then moving on to the next). However, blocked practice seems to be more effective in learning a new skill, with superior performance during the acquisition phase.[34] Thus, the stage of motor learning as well as the individual's capacity for learning must be considered when choosing random versus blocked practice conditions. It may be more appropriate to use a blocked practice schedule during the acquisition phase or with lower-skilled individuals, progressing to random practice conditions once the skill is acquired.

The generalization that random practice seems to be more effective in transfer and retention does not appear to be true in all populations. It does appear that children, perhaps because of less life experience and practice at many tasks, respond more robustly to a varied practice schedule than do adults.[28] Also, subjects with Parkinson disease performed better with a blocked order practice schedule.[35] However, while practicing at varied speeds may seem intuitively superior, the situation at hand must be considered. When training for tasks that will be performed in relatively fixed conditions or when the task being practiced can be enhanced by developing a unique response structure, the training should mimic that functional activity and trend toward a constant practice schedule.[36–38]

Attentional focus, or the act of directing attention to information sources or objects, is another variable impacting motor learning.[39] Attentional focus has been divided into external focus of attention, where the learner focuses on the action results, and internal focus of attention, where the learner attends to the body movements. For example, when learning to kick a ball, cues for an external focus asks the learner to attend to the movement of the ball and its position relative to the target. An internal focus would ask the learner to attend to the movements of the hip, knee, and foot while kicking. While numerous studies have found that groups trained with an external focus performed better, other studies suggest that preference for an external or an internal focus may be skill and/or age dependent.[40–43] A study of highly skilled and lesser-skilled golfers found that the highly skilled golfers performed better with an external focus of control, while the lesser-skilled golfers performed better with an internal focus.[42] Research into focus of control in children has found variable results.[39] In adults, it has been hypothesized that an internal focus constrains the motor system, altering the usual automatic control processes.[40,41] Therefore, in adults, particularly those of some skill level, an external focus of control will likely produce optimal results, while lesser-skilled adults may perform better with an internal focus of control. Children seem to have a preference for an internal focus of control, but this still requires further study.[39]

Finally, mental practice can have an impact on motor learning. Many high level athletes use mental practice to augment their physical training. Research has shown that the supplementary motor cortex, but not the primary motor cortex, is activated when mentally rehearsing a motion. Some research has shown improved performance when mental practice was combined with physical practice.[44] In general, mental rehearsal and imagery can be a useful adjunct to physical practice.[45–48] However, mental practice alone is not a sufficient substitute for physical practice.

Proper Exercise Execution

Although the patient may appear to follow the exercise instructions, he or she may still perform the exercise incorrectly. The patient may understand the instructions, but the instructions may be incomplete, the patient may read things into the instructions, or the patient may simply be unaware that he or she is not doing what the instructions call for. For example, the patient may think he or she is performing a trunk curl but rather is doing a full sit-up or is performing a straight leg raise without the necessary quadriceps set first.

Ensure proper performance by having the patient perform each of the exercises under your direction and guidance, with verbal and tactile cueing for proper performance. Encourage the patient to take notes during these sessions to enhance participation, responsibility, and understanding of the exercise program. Although written and verbal instructions help ensure proper performance, more instruction is occasionally necessary. Other options include having a family member observe the clinician instructing the patient, so that this individual may guide the patient's home exercise performance. Videotaping the exercise session allows the patient to see himself or herself performing the exercise, along with hearing the clinician's verbal cues and observing tactile cues for proper performance. The patient can replay this tape at home if a question regarding the exercise program exists.

When the patient returns for follow-up, ask him or her to demonstrate the home exercise program. In most cases, if the patient has been performing the exercises on a daily basis, the exercises should nearly be committed to memory. The ability of the patient to quickly recall the exercises with or without the assistance of the handout may provide a clue about adherence. Moreover, this shows precisely how the patient has been executing the exercise. Frequently, the exercise has been changed somewhat from the clinician's original intended performance, and this may affect the patient's progress since the last visit. Occasionally, the incorrect exercise performance can have negative consequences, such as increasing the patient's symptoms or hindering progress (Fig. 3-4).

Equipment and Environment

Along with determining what motivates the patient, determine the motivation derived from the use of exercise equipment. Performing exercises using body weight, objects at the home or office, or work tools may be more functional; however, the patient may feel like this is not really exercise if it does not involve weights or resistive bands. Patient education is necessary to ensure the patient knows the importance of these activities. However, preconceived ideas about exercise are frequently difficult to overcome, and adherence may be improved by use of some equipment. The financial cost of purchasing some equipment for home use may increase

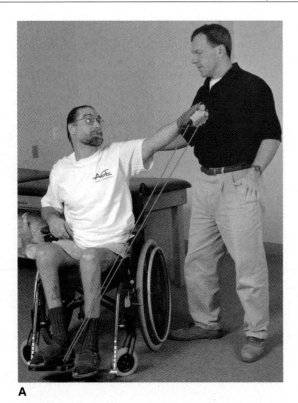
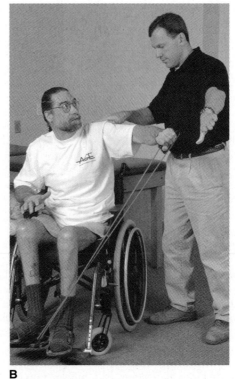

A   B

FIGURE 3-4. The exercise program must be reviewed at follow-up visits to ensure correct performance. (A) Incorrect position—substituting scapular movement for glenohumeral movement and incorrect degree of rotation. (B) Correct position—clinician corrects exercise performance.

or decrease adherence. If money must be spent to carry out the exercise program, the patient may decline participation. However, some patients feel obligated to use equipment that they have purchased. Assess the patient's position on this issue before issuing or recommending purchase of equipment.

When designing an exercise program with some specific equipment, ensure that the patient has a place to use the equipment (Fig. 3-5). Depending on the region of the country, homes may or may not have stairs. Other accommodations may be necessary if exercises require the use of a step. When prescribing exercises to be performed in a supine or prone position, a surface of the appropriate height and firmness must be available. Exercises often are easy to perform on the plinth in the clinic, but the quality or the ability to perform the exercise is negated at home because of the patient's environment. The patient must be able to comfortably transition positions to and from that surface. If the only available firm surface to carry out the exercise program is the floor, the patient must be able to easily get up and down from the floor. If not, the exercise program should be modified to increase the ease of participation in the program.

A final aspect of the environment that the clinician has little control over but should consider is the presence of a supportive family. Social support is an important factor in patient adherence to a treatment regimen. Social support includes both the medical community and the patient's family and immediate community. Social isolation has been determined to be a major factor in nonadherence to a medication regimen. Lack of social support has contributed to dropping out of treatment in a number of studies.[49] Social support is

particularly important when managing chronic disease, due to the ongoing nature of the problem.

Be sure to evaluate the role of the family and other support systems in the patient's immediate community. The family or work community can provide support or potentially have a negative effect. A supportive family can maximize the patient's opportunity to participate in medical care by being

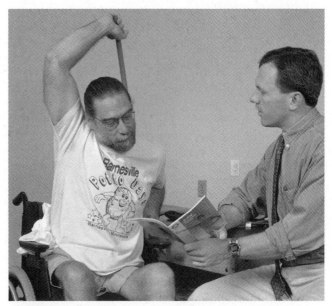

FIGURE 3-5. The clinician should choose equipment that can be easily used by the patient at home.

physically and emotionally supportive. Family members who take over duties normally carried out by the patient and advocate participation in the exercise program can enhance the patient's opportunity for improvement. Nonsupportive family members who criticize the patient for being injured or unable to carry out expected roles can create barriers to improvement.

If possible, involve the family members in the patient's care to ensure an understanding of the plan of care and prognosis. This will help them understand realistic goals and the plan to achieve them. If family members are nonsupportive, do your best to minimize their negative impact by providing additional support to your patient. Always be alert to signs of this situation and make referrals as necessary to ensure optimal participation in the rehabilitation program.

HOME EXERCISE PRESCRIPTION

Prescribing exercises for a home program is challenging. These exercises are performed without supervision, and patient education is critical to a successful home exercise program. Frequently, limited patient visit time further challenges the clinician to teach the patient all the necessary components of the self-management program. Providing a short, safe home exercise program is better than being too broad and overwhelming the patient with information on the first visit.

Considerations in Exercise Prescription

Exercise prescription can be difficult for several reasons. We know a great deal about exercise prescription in healthy individuals but less in those with impairment, injury, or disease. Determining the number of exercises and the quantity of repetitions, sets, bouts, and intensity within the context of the patient's daily activities is challenging. Too little exercise may not produce the desired result, but too much exercise may overwork the patient, resulting in a decline in progress. Many factors influence choices regarding the exercise prescription:

- Stage of healing
- Tissue irritability and symptom stability
- Daily activities
- Time between physical therapy visits
- Patient's time and willingness to participate

Stages of Healing

The acuity or chronicity of the injury affects the exercise prescription, including the regularity of supervised physical therapy and the time between visits. In the early stages, give the patient a few things to do at home between closely scheduled supervised visits. In the early phase, appointments may be more frequent because of the rapidity with which the patient's symptoms, impairments, and function are changing. The exercise program changes more frequently as goals are met and new goals established. In the early stage, the symptoms may be new to the patient, making determination of the appropriate exercise level difficult. Close follow-up of response to treatment is necessary to ensure forward progress. Conversely, in the intermediate to later stages, changes in the patient's symptoms and function occur more slowly, and the exercise program may be more extensive. The patient is often instructed in self-progression of activities.

DISPLAY 3-2
Questions Assessing Tissue Irritability

1. What activities or positions increase your symptoms?
2. How much time can you spend in that activity or position before your symptoms begin?
3. When you start feeling these symptoms, will they continue to progress despite discontinuing the activity or changing positions? Will changing the activity or position alleviate the symptoms?
4. After you begin experiencing your symptoms, how long do they last? How long until you return to "baseline"?
5. Is there anything you can do to relieve your symptoms?

Tissue Irritability and Symptom Stability

Tissue irritability has a significant effect on the rehabilitation program choices. This factor is somewhat subjective and is determined through a complete subjective examination. Questions regarding the patient's symptoms provide the clinician with the best information on this issue (Display 3-2).

Before deciding on the choice or intensity of the exercises, understand what kinds of activities or positions worsen the patient's symptoms. These activities or positions may or may not need to be avoided. If the patient can tolerate the activity or position for some time, is able to detect the prodromal signs that the symptoms are going to worsen, and understands that stopping the activity or changing position can alleviate the symptoms, use these activities or positions therapeutically. For example, if a patient with carpal tunnel syndrome enjoys knitting and this is one of the patient's functional goals, knitting may be used as part of the rehabilitation program. The patient must be able to recognize the onset of symptoms and be able to alleviate them by taking a rest period or discontinuing the knitting. Similarly, if a patient with back pain enjoys and is able to tolerate some walking, this activity can be a component of the exercise program. The patient must be able to detect the onset of symptoms and be able to relieve them by discontinuation, stretching, icing, or some other self-management intervention. Conversely, if the patient reports an unmanageable, inevitable worsening of symptoms once irritated, the exercise program should expressly avoid any position or activity that may exacerbate symptoms.

Be sure to consider the stability of the patient's symptoms as a component of tissue irritability. Individuals may have significant unpredictable fluctuations in their symptoms over the course of the day or week. If symptom changes cannot be associated with the time of day, position, or any specific activity, the exercise prescription can be difficult. If the patient is unable to determine what kinds of things make him or her better or worse, assessing the effects of the exercise program becomes yet another variable in the symptomatology. Deciding whether a specific exercise prescription is beneficial or deleterious is challenging if the patient's symptoms fluctuate randomly. When possible, it is best to proceed with fewer exercise interventions until a stable baseline of symptoms is achieved. This baseline then serves as a gauge of the effect of the exercise program.

Daily Activities

The patient's other daily activities affect the exercise prescription. Understanding the behavior of a patient's symptoms over a 24-hour period and how his or her normal daily routine affects the symptoms helps the clinician to gauge appropriate exercise levels. Frequently, the patient is unaware of the impact of certain routine activities on his or her problem, or the patient must perform some activities that worsen his or her symptoms (such as sitting or walking). For example, the individual with patellofemoral pain should be counseled about the importance of good shoes, particularly if standing for a large portion of the day. Despite the fact that standing behind a cash register for 8 hours may exacerbate the patient's symptoms, this work may be necessary to provide financial support for the family. The individual with back pain may need to lift a child out of a crib several times each day, despite the fact that this activity is painful. The clinician must educate the patient about the impact of these activities on symptoms and provide suggestions to minimize their negative effects. Moreover, the clinician must educate the patient regarding modification of the exercise program based on the symptoms related to participation in these activities. On days when the patient's symptoms may be increased because of excessive standing, working, or lifting, he or she may need to decrease the rehabilitation exercise level. Failure to recognize the impact of daily activities on symptoms may cause the clinician to erroneously assume that a change in the patient's symptoms was caused by the exercise program alone.

Time Between Physical Therapy Visits

The time between follow-up visits affects the exercise prescription. For the patient attending supervised physical therapy one or more times per week, the clinician may be more willing to give the patient more challenging exercises for the home program, knowing that the patient will be monitored more closely in the clinic. For those patients who live some distance away or who have longer intervals between supervised visits for other reasons, the clinician should provide exercises that are less likely to overwork the patients. This program is supplemented with instructions on how to progress exercises if they become too easy (e.g., increase time, repetitions, intensity) or an intermediate phone follow-up can take place. In many cases, interim contact with the patient via a phone call or e-mail can assess the patient's progress. The therapist can make suggestions on how to modify the home program until the patient's next clinic appointment.

Patient's Time and Willingness

The amount of time the patient has available to exercise is an important factor affecting exercise prescription. If the patient claims to have little time available for the home exercise program, be sure to respect the patient's position on this issue. The therapist should educate the patient about the importance of the program in a nonjudgmental fashion, followed by conscious choices about priority exercises. Make an effort to select exercises considered to be the most important for the exercise program. More is not always better, and giving thoughtful consideration to the core exercises is beneficial for the clinician and the patient. Choosing exercises that have the greatest impact for the least time commitment can minimize the time requirement and maximize the benefits. The patient will probably appreciate your concern and attention to his or her needs. Couple this approach with education regarding the importance of the home exercise program to achieve the determined goals in as expedient and efficient a time frame as possible. Emphasize your own and the patient's responsibilities in achieving those mutually defined goals.

Determining Exercise Levels

Determining the appropriate level of exercise can be difficult, particularly when the patient has had little or no experience with the specific problem previously or little previous experience with exercise. Although many individuals exercise regularly, many others have little experience with exercise. Knowing how to respond to different sensations felt during the rehabilitation exercises can prove frustrating to the patient. Many patients ask whether to continue exercising if the exercise produces pain. Despite the fact that pain is a subjective symptom, acknowledge this sensation. Consider pain in the context of change from the patient's baseline symptom level and how the symptoms behave over the subsequent 24-hour period.

Curwin and Stanish[50] provide guidelines originally designed to help determine readiness to return to a sport. However, these same guidelines are nicely adapted to evaluate patient's exercise program (Table 3-1). The column in Table 3-1 entitled "Description of Pain" refers to the level of pain during rehabilitation exercise performance, and the category "Level of Sports Performance or Activity" could be retitled "Level of Exercise Program Performance." Activity levels that keep the

TABLE 3-1 Curwin and Stanish Classification for Determining the Appropriate Level of Discomfort Associated with Home Exercise Prescription

LEVEL	DESCRIPTION OF PAIN	LEVEL OF SPORTS PERFORMANCE OR ACTIVITY
1	No pain	Normal
2	Pain only with extreme exertion	Normal
3	Pain with extreme exertion and 1–2 hours afterward	Normal or slightly decreased
4	Pain during and after any vigorous activities	Somewhat decreased
5	Pain during activity and forcing termination	Markedly decreased
6	Pain during daily activities	Unable to perform

From Curwin S, Stanish WD: Tendinitis: Its Etiology and Treatment. Lexington, MA: DC Heath and Co., 1984:64.

patient within his or her optimal loading zone are generally levels 1 through 3. Occasionally, some patients may be able to tolerate exercise at level 4 without any residual effects. In these cases, progress may need to be reassessed on a weekly basis rather than on an exercise-session-to-exercise-session or a daily basis. Patients with adhesive capsulitis often experience pain at level 4, but this level of pain does not interfere with their overall function or progress. These guidelines provide the patient and the clinician common criteria with which the exercise program prescription is evaluated.

Despite the clinician's best efforts, some patients experience an exacerbation of their symptoms, which may or may not be related to the exercise program. Although the first response of the clinician and the patient may be some level of distress, an exacerbation is not always a negative experience. An exacerbation can be a "teachable moment" with valuable lessons learned. At some point, whether days, weeks, months, or years later, most patients experience some type of symptoms related to the current problem. The patient with patellofemoral pain may experience a milder level of pain after a hiking vacation, or the individual with low back pain may notice some back discomfort after a long plane flight. Some patients experience a complete exacerbation of their symptoms at some future point. Patients must learn how to manage the exacerbation.

Frequently, several weeks have passed by the time the patient decides to seek medical attention and gets appointments with a physician and/or physical therapist. The optimal time for intervention has passed, and the patient may be struggling with secondary problems resulting from compensation or movement changes made because of pain or other impairments. One of the best services the clinician can offer the patient is instruction on how to manage the acute return of symptoms. Instruction may include the use of modalities such as ice, appropriate activity modifications or rest, changes in the maintenance exercise program, or education regarding when to seek medical attention.

In addition to possibly preventing reentry to the medical system through immediate, appropriate symptom management, self-management has the added benefit of enhancing patients' confidence in their ability to resolve the symptoms. The exacerbation experience coupled with instruction in appropriate management under the clinician's guidance can greatly decrease the patient's anxiety. Patients are often fearful

about participating in activities that may provoke their symptoms, afraid that they will be "back where they started" in the early stages of their injury. Learning that an exacerbation does not necessarily send them back to the initial phase and that they can successfully manage the problem empowers patients to make appropriate activity choices. Eventually, patients may choose to participate in activities they enjoy at the expense of getting a little sore, knowing that they can successfully manage the symptoms independently (see Building Block 3-4).

Formulating the Program

When possible, formulate the exercise program after the patient's baseline level of symptoms has stabilized and the previously mentioned factors (e.g., tissue irritability) have been determined. Ensuring the patient's understanding of what the "baseline" feels like allows better communication between the clinician and the patient regarding the behavior of his or her symptoms and the effects of the exercise program. Symptoms that are unstable or fluctuating without determinable cause make assessing the effects of intervention difficult. Ask the patient to articulate his or her "normal" level of symptoms to assist in determining the stability of symptoms. If patients have difficulty determining the stability of their symptoms, slow progression is necessary. When the patient is able to perform the same exercise program for three consecutive sessions without an increase in symptoms, progression is appropriate.

If intervention needs to be implemented before the establishment of a stable baseline, give the patient as few exercises as possible. This minimizes the impact of the exercise program, thereby lowering the possibility of exacerbating the symptoms. If the patient's symptoms do worsen, you will have an easier time determining the cause, and changes can be made more appropriately. As symptoms resolve and the baseline stabilizes, increase activities systematically and gradually. Do this by increasing the time and repetitions or by adding new exercises slowly.

How the exercise program is progressed depends on each person's stage of injury, specific goals, and stability of symptoms. For the individual who is in the intermediate to late healing stages and has demonstrated stable symptoms, several exercises can be progressed simultaneously. For those with unstable symptoms and frequent exacerbations, keep rehabilitation program changes to a minimum. In this way, any positive or negative response to the change can be more easily identified and remedied.

Teach patients how to modify their exercise program based on their activity level on any given day. Put exercises in the context of their daily routine. On days when the patient is more active (e.g., working overtime, child care, shopping, yard work), modify the home exercise program to prevent overload. On days when the patient is more sedentary (e.g., bad weather, day off from work), increase the exercise program. In this way, the patient begins to understand the impact of his or her overall activity level on his or her symptoms. This assists the patient in the self-management of symptoms in the future.

Choosing exercises that can be incorporated into activities already performed during the day should be a fundamental aspect of the exercise program. This type of exercise prescription results in short bouts of exercise performed several times

BUILDING BLOCK 3-4

Kathy had been performing racquet swings without a ball for 15 minutes/day as part of her rehabilitation program. On a warm sunny day, she decided that she wanted to start hitting a ball, so she joined her usual tennis partner for 40 minutes of light hitting on the court. She returned to physical therapy 3 days later with increased pain throughout the shoulder girdle. She reported that the pain was different from the pain she experienced when she injured her rotator cuff. She is again highly concerned that she will not be able to return to tennis. What are some possible educational strategies and recommendations?

throughout the day, thus improving motivation and adherence. In this case, the patient is unlikely to overwork in any single session, resulting in a lower chance of an exacerbation of symptoms. Moreover, the likelihood of exacerbation is decreased despite a greater volume of exercise than can be performed in any single session. For example, the individual with Achilles tendinitis may tolerate only two repetitions of 30 seconds of calf stretching at a time. If that individual performs those 2 repetitions 6 times spread out over the course of his or her day, the stretch has been performed 12 times. By contrast, if the patient tried to carry out the home exercise program in the evening after work and dinner, chances are that only two repetitions would be performed that day.

Finally, teach the patient that some exercise is better than none, and if time limitations exist, a couple of key exercises should be performed. Occasionally, other life events prevent completion of the full home exercise program despite the patient's willingness to adhere. Prioritize the exercises, highlighting those that are most important to complete if time does not permit completion of the entire program. Emphasize the importance of finishing all of the exercises when time permits, while suggesting that some exercise is better than none.

KEY POINTS

- Patient education and self-management have become increasingly important with greater life expectancy.
- Patient safety is the first consideration when designing a home exercise prescription.
- The best-designed treatment program is of little value if the patient does not adhere to the clinician's recommendations.
- The clinician must determine patient motivators to enhance likelihood of adherence.
- Exercises requiring the fewest lifestyle changes and imposing changes that mimic the patient's usual activities can increase adherence.
- Patient-clinician communication is enhanced by determining the patient's willingness to learn and listening actively to the patient's needs.
- Written and verbal instructions should be included in a home exercise program. Written exercises should include beginning and ending positions and any precautions.

- On subsequent visits, the patient should demonstrate the home exercise program to ensure correct performance of all exercises.
- Home exercise choices are affected by the acuity of the injury, tissue irritability, stability of symptoms, patient's daily activity level, time available for exercise, and factors affecting the length of follow-up.
- A symptom exacerbation can be a learning experience for the patient if educated properly and coached through the experience.
- Patients must be encouraged to take control of their exercise program and taught how to modify their home exercise program based on other activities and symptoms.
- Understanding the typical behavior of their symptoms allows patients to more easily recognize an exacerbation and be able to guide activity choice and intensity.
- Any cultural, language, education, visual, or hearing barriers should be identified early and appropriate accommodations made.
- Prioritize exercises so that the patient may perform at least some of his or her exercises on busy days.

CRITICAL THINKING QUESTIONS

1. How would your home exercise instruction differ for patients who are
   a. Visual learners
   b. Auditory learners
   c. Kinesthetic learners
2. Consider the patient in Lab Activities 1. How would you provide this patient with a home exercise program if he or she were blind?
3. A patient returns to see you and reports that the home exercise was not done because of a lack of time. How would you respond? What would be your strategy and rationale?
4. A patient returns to see you and reports that the home exercise program was not done because the exercises hurt. How would you respond? What would be your strategy and rationale?

LAB ACTIVITIES

1. Refer to Case Study 6 in Unit 7. Design a home program for this patient. Include written instructions and diagrams for all exercises. Teach your patient this home program while relaying the following emotions:
   a. Empathy
   b. Disinterest
   c. Hurry
   d. Insecurity
2. Using the exercises developed for the first question, modify each exercise to be performed throughout the day, incorporating the exercises into the patient's daily routine.

3. Using the exercises developed for the first question, prioritize the exercises for the patient and explain your rationale for the prioritization to the patient. Use language the patient can understand.
4. Your patient desires to return to several sporting activities. Choose two of the exercises you have given the patient, and modify them to mimic a sporting activity to which the patient would like to return.
5. Teach someone else in the class who does not know how to tie a necktie how to do this without looking at each other and without using the words *yes* or *no*.

REFERENCES

1. The American Physical Therapy Association. Guide to Physical Therapist Practice. 2nd Ed. Phys Ther 2001;81(1):S1–S738.
2. Chase L, Elkins JA, Readinger J, et al. Perceptions of physical therapists toward patient education. Phys Ther 1993;73:787–796.
3. Gahimer JE, Domholdt E. Amount of patient education in physical therapy practice and perceived effects. Phys Ther 1996;76:1089–1096.
4. Falvo DR. Effective Patient Education: A Guide to Increased Compliance. 3rd Ed. Sudbury, MA: Jones and Bartlett Publishers, Inc., 2004.
5. Udermann BE, Spratt KF, Donelson RG, et al. Can a patient educational booklet change behavior and reduce pain in chronic low back pain patients? Spine J 2004;4(4):425–435.
6. Godges JJ, Anger MA, Zimmerman G, et al. Effects of education on return-to-work status for people with fear-avoidance beliefs and acute low back pain. Phys Ther 2008;88:231–239.
7. Holmes CF, Fletcher JP, Blaschak MJ, et al. Management of shoulder dysfunction. J Orthop Sports Phys Ther 1997;26:347–354.
8. Cameron C. Patient compliance: recognition of factors involved and suggestions for promoting compliance with therapeutic regimens. J Adv Nurs 1996;24:244–250.
9. Gieck J. Psychological considerations for rehabilitation. In: Prentice W, ed. Rehabilitation Techniques in Sports Medicine. 2nd Ed. St. Louis, MO: Mosby-Year Book, 1994.
10. Schwenk TL, Whitman N. The Physician as Teacher. Baltimore: Williams & Wilkins, 1987.
11. Sluijs EM, Kok GJ, van der Zee J. Correlates of exercise compliance in physical therapy. Phys Ther 1993;73:771–787.
12. Brophy J. Research on the self-fulfilling prophecy and teacher expectations. J Educ Psychol 1983;75:631–661.
13. Fisher A. Adherence to sports injury rehabilitation programmes. Sports Med 1990;9:151–158.
14. Horn T. Expectancy effects in the interscholastic athletic setting: methodological concerns. J Sport Psychol 1984;6:60–76.
15. Wilder KC. Clinician's expectations and their impact on an athlete's compliance in rehabilitation. J Sport Rehabil 1994;3:168–175.
16. Marcus BH, Simkin LR. The stages of exercise behavior. J Sports Med Phys Fitness 1993;33:83–88.
17. Chen CY, Neufeld PS, Feely CA, et al. Factors influencing compliance with home exercise programs among patients with upper-extremity impairment. Am J Occup Ther 1999;53:171–180.
18. Elder JP, Ayala GX, Harris S. Theories and intervention approaches to health-behavior change in primary care. Am J Prev Med 1999;17:275–284.
19. Marcus BH, Simkin LR. The transtheoretical model: applications to exercise behavior. Med Sci Sports Exerc 1994;26:1400–1404.
20. Prochaska JO. Strong and weak principles for progressing from precontemplation to action on the basis of twelve problem behaviors. Health Psychol 1994;13:47–51.
21. Peterson TR, Aldana SG. Improving exercise behavior: an application of the stages of change model in a worksite setting. Am J Health Promot 1999;13:229–232.
22. Bandura A, Adams NE, Beyer J. Cognitive processes mediating behavioral change. J Pers Soc Psychol 1977;35:125–139.
23. Nolan RP. How can we help patients initiate change? Can J Cardiol 1995;11(Suppl A):16A–19A.
24. Friedrich M, Cermak T, Maderbacher P. The effect of brochure use versus therapist teaching on patients performing therapeutic exercise and on changes in impairment status. Phys Ther 1996;76:1082–1088.
25. Fields J, Murphey M, Horodyski MB, et al. Factors associated with adherence to sport injury rehabilitation in college-age recreational athletes. J Sport Rehabil 1995;9:172–180.
26. Spector RE. Cultural Diversity in Health and Illness. Upper Saddle River, NJ: Prentice-Hall, Inc., 2000.
27. Brus HL, van de Laar MA, Taal E, et al. Effects of patient education on compliance with basic treatment regimens and health in recent onset active rheumatoid arthritis. Ann Rheum Dis 1998;57:146–151.
28. Shumway-Cook A, Woollacott MH. Motor Control: Translating Research into Clinical Practice, 3rd Ed. Philadelphia, PA: Lippincott Williams & Wilkins, 2007.
29. Herbert WJ, Heiss DG, Basso DM. Influence of feedback schedule on motor performance and learning of a lumbar multifidus muscle activity using rehabilitative ultrasound imaging: a randomized clinical trial. Phys Ther 2008;88:261–269.
30. Fitts PM, Posner MI. Human Performance. Belmont, CA: Brooks/Cole, 1967.
31. Vereijken B, van Emmerik REA, Whiting HTA, et al. Freezing degrees of freedom in skill acquisition. J Mot Behav 1992;24:133–142.
32. Jarus T, Gutman T. Effects of cognitive processes and task complexity on acquisition, retention, and transfer of motor skills. Can J Occup Ther 2001;68(5):280–289.
33. Jarus T, Goverover Y. Effects of contextual interference and age on acquisition, retention and transfer of motor skill. Percept Mot Skills 1999;88(2):437–447.
34. Memmert D. Long-term effects of type of practice on the learning and transfer of a complex motor skill. Percept Mot Skills 2006;103(3):912–916.
35. Lin CH, Sullivan KJ, Wu AD, et al. Effect of task practice order on motor skill learning in adults with Parkinson disease: a pilot study. Phys Ther 2007;87(9):1120–1131.
36. Lee TD, Genovese ED. Distribution of practice in motor skill acquisition: different effects for discrete and continuous tasks. Res Q Exerc Sport 1989;60(1):59–65.
37. Heitman RJ, Pugh SF, Kovaleski JE, et al. Effects of specific versus variable practice on the retention and transfer of a continuous motor skill. Percept Mot Skills 2005;100(3 Pt 2):1107–1113.
38. Wilde H, Magnuson C, Shea CH. Random and blocked practice of movement sequences: differential effects on response structure and movement speed. Res Q Exerc Sport 2005;76(4):416–425.
39. Emanuel M, Jarus T, Bart O. Effect of focus of attention and age on motor acquisition, retention, and transfer: a randomized trial. Phys Ther 2008;88:251–260.
40. Wulf G, Shea CH, Park JH. Attention in motor leaning: preferences for the advantages of an external focus. Res Q Exerc Sport 2001;72:335–344.
41. Wulf G, McNevin NH, Shea CH. The automaticity of complex motor skill learning as a function of attention focus. Q J Exp Psychol 2001;54:1143–1154.
42. Perkins-Ceccato N, Passmore SR, Lee TD. Effects of focus of attention on golfers' skill. J Sports Sci 2003;21:593–600.
43. Vance J, Wulf G. Tollner T, et al. EMG activity as a function of the performer's focus of attention. J Motor Behav 2004;36:450–459.
44. Overdorf V, Page SJ, Schweighardt R, et al. Mental and physical practice schedules in acquisition and retention of novel timing skills. Percept Mot Skills 2004;99(1):51–62.
45. Allami N, Paulignan Y, Brovelli A, et al. Visuomotor learning with combination of different rates of motor imagery and physical practice. Exp Brain Res 2008;184(1):105–113.
46. Sanders CW, Sadoski M, Bramson R, et al. Comparing the effects of physical practice and mental imagery rehearsal on learning basic surgical skills by medical students. Am J Obstet Gynecol 2004;191(5):1811–1814.
47. Bucher L. The effects of imagery abilities and mental rehearsal on learning a nursing skill. J Nurs Educ 1993;32(7):318–324.
48. Creelman J. Influence of mental practice on development of voluntary control of a novel motor acquisition skill. Percept Mot Skills 2003;97(1):319–337.
49. Becker MH, Green LW. A family approach to compliance with medical treatment: a selective review of the literature. Int J Health Educ 1975;18:173–182.
50. Curwin S, Stanish WD. Tendinitis: Its Etiology and Treatment. Lexington, MA: DC Heath, 1984.

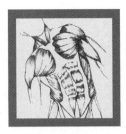

chapter 4

Prevention and the Promotion of Health, Wellness, and Fitness

JANET R. BEZNER

The function of protecting and developing health must rank even above that of restoring it when it is impaired.
                                                                —*Hippocrates*

Interventions aimed at preventing injury and illness are among the many tools physical therapists use on a daily basis to address the health needs of the patients we serve. Indeed, prevention, health promotion, fitness, and wellness efforts have recently garnered increased attention as the nation struggles to control escalating health care costs and to stop the progression of chronic diseases that have reached epidemic proportions.[1,2] It has been estimated that 50% of premature deaths in the United States are related to modifiable lifestyle factors,[3] so there is clearly a need for effective prevention programs and efforts aimed at reducing risk factors and improving health and wellness.

Traditionally the physical therapist's role in prevention and wellness has been narrowly focused on preventing a recurrence of the injury or illness a patient already has experienced or identifying risk factors and preventing escalation into disease. For example, when treating a patient recovering from an ankle sprain, some rehabilitation activities are directed toward preventing a recurrence of that injury. The approach may include direct interventions such as balance exercises or indirect interventions such as patient education. Some physical therapists perform biomechanical analyses such as running gait analysis or ergonomic workstation analysis to identify risk factors predisposing clients to injury. Although appropriate and worthwhile, these efforts do not produce the significant outcomes that primary prevention programs might, because they are applied after the onset of risk, illness, or injury. Contemporary physical therapist practice includes a role for the physical therapist in primary prevention—that is, interacting with clients to promote health and improve wellness before they become patients.

Physical therapists' efforts in health and wellness promotion require an expanded view of health beyond the biomedical or disablement models. Additionally, it is important to recognize that clients may not be motivated to participate in health-causing behaviors until they become symptomatic or ill. The purpose of this chapter is to explore the concepts of prevention, health promotion, fitness, and wellness. Because the remainder of this book discusses interventions aimed at injured or ill patients, this chapter focuses on primary prevention and the services that physical therapists can provide to clients before they become patients.

THE CONTEXT FOR PRIMARY PREVENTION

Numerous physical therapy professional references support a role for the physical therapist in health promotion and wellness. *The Guide to Physical Therapist Practice*, which defines the physical therapist's scope of practice, discusses the physical therapist's role in prevention and the promotion of health, wellness, and fitness.[4] The American Physical Therapy Association's (APTA) vision statement, goals, and objectives and several policy statements reference the role of the physical therapist in the provision of health and wellness services.[5] Numerous state licensing acts include within the definition of physical therapy a reference to promoting and maintaining fitness, health, or wellness in all age groups.[6] The accreditation criteria for physical therapist educational programs state that graduates of accredited programs are prepared to identify and assess health needs and provide appropriate prevention and wellness information and programs.[7]

Thus, the expectation that physical therapists participate actively in health and wellness practice exists in many professional documents. To provide such services, the physical therapist must first understand and differentiate the many terms used to describe these concepts.

Definitions

Prevention, Health Promotion, and Health Education

There are many terms used within the context of "prevention" within the US health care system. Differentiating these terms provides a valuable perspective for the delivery of appropriate services by physical therapists. Figure 4-1 illustrates the prevention to intervention continuum, ranging from health promotion services to rehabilitation. The associated pathologic state of the patient/client at each stage of prevention is shown across the top of the diagram. Prevention is divided into primary and secondary prevention services. Also referred to as public health, primary prevention includes health promotion, health protection, and preventive health services. Primary prevention takes place in the "prepathogenesis" period before the onset of disease. Secondary prevention services take place after the onset of illness or injury, in the presence of pathology, and include screening for the purpose of early diagnosis and treatment of disease, as well as disability limitation. Secondary prevention includes efforts to identify disease early by recognizing either the physiologic changes that precede illness or signs of subclinical illness. Examples include breast and prostate cancer screening, osteoporosis screening, medical preplacement evaluations, and accident reporting.[8] Also included within secondary prevention are efforts to limit disability for those with chronic diseases such as diabetes (i.e., a foot care educational program) or spinal cord injury (i.e., a program to prevent skin breakdown). Tertiary care, or rehabilitation, is the category that encompasses most of traditional physical

Prepathogenesis Period			Period of Pathogenesis		
Health Promotion	Health Protection	Preventive Health Services	Early Diagnosis and prompt treatment	Disability Limitation	Rehabilitation
Primary Prevention			Secondary Prevention		Tertiary

FIGURE 4-1. Differentiation of primary, secondary, and tertiary prevention.

therapist services. Although the physical therapist may use health education methods to provide information in the case of a secondary prevention effort, the health status of the patient/client determines whether this information falls under primary, secondary, or tertiary care. For example, providing information about how to be physically active for a client without injury or illness might be classified as primary prevention, whereas providing the same information to a client with diabetes would be considered secondary prevention, and including physical activity in an intervention plan for a diabetic client who is receiving rehabilitation for an amputation would be considered tertiary care.

In terms of primary prevention, health promotion is the most significant component for the physical therapist to understand. Health promotion can be defined as a combination of educational and environmental programs or actions that are conducive to health.[9] Three terms in this definition are worth exploring to fully understand the concept. They are combination, educational, and environmental. The term "combination" suggests that a variety of learning experiences are necessary to influence behavioral changes. It is rare that a single intervention can make a profound change. For example, when instituting an osteoporosis prevention program, it would be appropriate for the physical therapist to consider factors beyond the exercise program. Other health care providers on the program team might be enlisted to ensure that important factors such as nutrition and hormone status are addressed, which will reinforce the need to partake in physical activity, as well as provide valuable information about other useful interventions. The word "combination" also suggests that interventions should be matched to specific behaviors. In the case of the osteoporosis program, interventions should be planned to increase the quantity of weight-bearing activity the participants experience.

"Education" within the definition of health promotion refers to health education, which is "any combination of learning experiences designed to facilitate voluntary actions conducive to health."[9 (p.17)] Health education activities are planned out, rather than incidental experiences (e.g., designed), and facilitate behavioral changes without coercion (e.g., voluntary). Examples of health education initiatives include counseling a patient on the risks of smoking, providing an osteoporosis prevention class for a corporate wellness program, and teaching children how to carry and load their backpacks safely.

The word "environmental" in the definition is meant to encompass the myriad of social forces that influence health, including social, political, economic, organizational, policy, and regulatory issues.[9] It is critical to recognize that health promotion is broad and includes both individual and social/regulatory activities. For example, a physical therapist working for a large manufacturing company may want to begin a smoking cessation program to improve overall worker health. However, if the employer does not have a nonsmoking policy, efforts to stop smoking at the individual level will most likely be ineffective. Other illustrations of the broad net of health promotion include programs to increase the activity levels of youths or the elderly, corporate policies that provide release time to exercise, and funding to support or build public parks and trails.

Based on these definitions, it is apparent that the term health education falls under the umbrella of health promotion, and often the activities that would define each are overlapping.[9] More recently, it has been suggested that the terms health promotion and health education are not significantly different and, in fact, are often used interchangeably.[10] The bottom line is that both health promotion and health education refer to the "broad and varied set of strategies to influence both individuals and their social environments, to improve health behavior, and to enhance health and quality of life."[10]

The terms health promotion and health education are the most relevant aspects of primary prevention for the physical therapist. Health protection refers to strategies dealing with engineering the physical environment such as water fluoridation, whereas preventive health services refers to traditional medical system efforts to prevent injury and illness—for example, immunizations.

Physical Fitness, Exercise, and Physical Activity

Within the context of therapeutic exercise as discussed in this book, the physical therapist has a primary and important role in all types of prevention to keep people active. Several terms are used to describe what laypersons commonly refer to as "exercise." Physical activity has been defined as any bodily movement produced by skeletal muscles that results in energy expenditure.[11] Examples of physical activity include walking, performing yard or house work, and playing catch. Similarly, exercise is a type of physical activity that is planned, structured, repetitive, and is purposely aimed at improving physical fitness. Consistent with this definition, exercise is typically prescribed in terms of frequency, intensity, and duration in a dose adequate to improve physical fitness (discussed in greater detail in Chapter 6). Physical fitness is a set of attributes that people have or achieve and includes components of health-related (cardiorespiratory endurance, body composition, muscular endurance, muscular strength, flexibility) and athletic-related skills. Assessment of physical

CASE STUDY 4-1

A 36-year-old male (Derek Prager) has come to your practice following a left ACL repair performed 3 days ago. He tore his ACL 1 week ago sliding into second base during a company softball game. He had arthroscopic surgery to repair the ACL. He arrives to your office with his knee wrapped in an elastic bandage and using crutches. During your subjective history you obtain the following information from Derek.

- He is married and has two children; a 12-year-old daughter and a 10-year-old son. His wife works full-time outside of the home.
- He works approximately 60 hours per week as a construction foreman. He spends about 2 hours per day in his office and the rest of the day he is traveling between residential constructions sites supervising his crew. He tells you that his job has become much more stressful the past couple of years because of conflicts with his supervisor.
- Derek smokes a pack of cigarettes per day and has smoked for 16 years.
- He tells you that he was diagnosed with high cholesterol about a year ago. He is currently taking Lipitor (cholesterol lowering medication) once a day.
- His father died of a massive heart attack at age 60. He has an older brother who he describes as "a health nut." He participates in triathlons and eats "rabbit food."

- Derek's hobbies include watching sports on television, watching his children's sporting activities, and playing on the company softball team one night per week.
- Derek tells you that he has gained weight over the past 5 years but doesn't weigh himself and since his wife buys his clothes he doesn't pay much attention to changes in his clothing sizes.

In addition to the physical findings that you obtained regarding Mr. Prager's left ACL repair, you also obtain the following information.

- Height = 5'11"
- Weight = 208 lb
- Body mass index (BMI) = 29
- Relationship of BMI to weight status according to Centers for Disease Control and Prevention

  Below 18.5 = Underweight
  18.5–24.9 = Normal weight
  25.0–29.9 = Overweight
  30.0 and above = Obese

- Resting HR = 70 bpm
- Resting BP = 128/84

---

fitness is used to measure the impact of exercise or physical activity on the components of fitness, such as a 12-minute walk test to assess cardiorespiratory endurance. Based on decades of research on a wide variety of age groups, inclusive of both sexes and individuals with all types of chronic and acute disease, physical activity has been shown to be an extremely powerful resource to keep people healthy and to improve impairments, activity level, and participation level in those with health conditions.[12]

Wellness, Lifestyle, and Quality of Life

Wellness is defined in the *Guide to Physical Therapist Practice*, 2nd edition, as "concepts that embrace positive health behaviors and promote a state of physical and mental balance and fitness."[4] Since Dunn[13] conceptualized wellness in 1961 and offered the first formal definition of the term ("an integrated method of functioning which is oriented toward maximizing the potential of which the individual is capable."), wellness has been explained by various models and approaches.[14–21] Although the literature is full of definitions of, references to, and information about wellness, a universally accepted definition has failed to emerge. Several conclusions can be drawn, however, from the abundance of literature about wellness.

For many people, including the public, health and wellness are synonymous with physical health or well-being, and commonly consists of physical activity, efforts to eat nutritiously, and adequate sleep. Research has indicated that when the public is asked to rate their general health, they narrowly focus on their physical health status, and do not consider their emotional, social, or spiritual health.[22] Referring back to the definitions introduced earlier, it is obvious that wellness includes more than just physical parameters. Wellness and fitness are not synonyms; as indicated in Chapter 1, well-being or wellness is a broad term, like quality of life, that the ICF defines as encompassing the total universe of human life.

The common themes that emerge from the various models and definitions of wellness suggest that wellness is multidimensional,[13,15–21,23,24] salutogenic or health causing,[13,15,18,19,21,25,26] and consistent with a systems view of persons and their environments.[13,27–29] Each of these characteristics will be explored.

First, as a multidimensional concept, wellness is more than simply physical health. Among the dimensions included in wellness are physical, spiritual, intellectual, psychologic, social, emotional, occupational, and community or environmental.[30] Adams et al.[30] proposed six dimensions of wellness based on the strength and quality of the theoretical support

BUILDING BLOCK 4-1
Consider the patient in case study 4-1

1. Given the patient's history and examination findings, what health education and/or health promotion interventions might be indicated during the patient care episode?
2. Does Mr. Prager perform regular exercise?

TABLE 4-1	Definitions of the Dimensions of Wellness
Physical	Positive perceptions and expectancies of physical health
Psychologic	A general perception that one will experience positive outcomes to the events and circumstances of life
Social	The perception that family or friends are available in times of need, and the perception that one is a valued support provider
Emotional	The possession of a secure sense of self-identity and a positive sense of self-regard
Spiritual	A positive sense of meaning and purpose in life
Intellectual	The perception that one is internally energized by the appropriate amount of intellectually stimulating activity

Adams T, Bezner J, Steinhardt M. The conceptualization and measurement of perceived wellness: integrating balance across and within dimensions. Am J Health Promotion 1997;11:208–218.

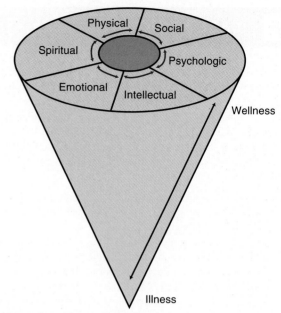

FIGURE 4-2. The Wellness model.

in the literature. The six dimensions and their corresponding definitions are shown in Table 4-1.

The second characteristic of wellness is that it has a salutogenic (e.g., health causing) focus in contrast to a pathogenic focus in an illness model.[26] Emphasizing that which causes health is consistent with Dunn's original definition.[13] It suggests that wellness involves maximizing an individual's potential, not just preventing an injury or maintaining the status quo. Wellness involves choices and behaviors that emphasize optimal health and well-being beyond the status quo.

Third, wellness approaches use a systems perspective. In systems theory each element of a system is independent and contains its own subelements, in addition to being a subelement of a larger system.[23,27,28] Further, the elements in a system are reciprocally interrelated, indicating that a disruption of homeostasis at any level of the system affects the entire system and all of its subelements.[27,28] Therefore, overall wellness is a reflection of the state of being within each dimension and a result of the interaction among and between the dimensions of wellness. Figure 4-2 illustrates a model of wellness reflecting this concept. Vertical movement in the model occurs between the wellness and illness poles as the magnitude of wellness in each dimension changes (see "black arrow" in Figure 4-2). The top of the model represents wellness because it is expanded maximally, whereas the bottom of the model represents illness.

The size of each dimension (a subelement in systems theory) represents how much wellness an individual possesses in that dimension. As wellness fluctuates in each dimension, an effect is generated on all of the other dimensions (reciprocal interrelation), see "red arrow" in Figure 4-2. According to systems theory, movement in every dimension influences and is influenced by movement in the other dimensions.[30] As an example, an individual who experiences a shoulder injury and undergoes surgery to repair the rotator cuff will probably experience at least short-term decreased physical wellness (the size of the physical dimension on the diagram

will decrease). Applying systems theory and according to the model, this individual may also experience a decrease in other dimensions, such as emotional, social or psychological wellness, in the postoperative period resulting from the connectedness or interrelatedness of all of the dimensions. The overall effect of the changes in these dimensions will be a decrease in overall wellness, which anecdotally we know occurs when patients experience a physical illness or injury. In other words, the individual also experiences a change in his or his emotional, social, or psychological states as a result of an unexpected injury that may significantly impact body image, self-confidence, energy level, comfort, personal finances, work, etc. Further applying the model in terms of an intervention plan, focus on a nonphysical state, such as the emotional or social dimension, can positively affect the physical dimension and result in improved wellness during recovery from a health condition.

The term health-related quality of life has already been defined in the context of the ICF model in Chapter 1. A similar term, quality of life, is "an individual's perception of their position in life in the context of the culture and value systems in which they live and in relation to their goals, expectations, standards and concerns. It is a broad concept affected in a complex way by the person's physical health, psychological state, level of independence, social relationships, personal beliefs and their relationship to salient features of their environment."[31]

The word lifestyle differs from wellness and thus is also important to consider, because many significant causes of disease, such as obesity and diabetes, involve lifestyle choices.[32] The simplest definition of lifestyle is perhaps "the consciously chosen, personal behavior of individuals as it may relate to health."[9] A more complex notion of lifestyle recognizes that personal behaviors are significantly influenced by social and cultural circumstances, indicating that behavioral choices may not be entirely under volitional control. For example, there is a great deal of controversy over tobacco advertising and its influence on certain populations. Consideration, therefore, of an individual's behaviors related to health and wellness, is most appropriately done within the context of social and cultural influences, and, more importantly, interventions designed to change behaviors should recognize the important influence of society and culture. This understanding of lifestyle is congruent with definitions of wellness, because it acknowledges that there are multiple influences on behavior.

In summary, the terms wellness and well-being can be used interchangeably and refer to an individual's perception of self in a broad sense. Quality of life is also a broad term that refers to an individual's perception of life in a broad sense. Finally, lifestyle is a term that describes personal behaviors that impact health.

Measurement of Wellness

As a result of the varied way that wellness has been defined and understood, a variety of wellness measures exist. A good wellness measure should reflect the multidimensionality and systems orientation of the concept and have a salutogenic focus. In the literature and in daily practice, clinical, physiologic, behavioral, and perceptual indicators are all touted as wellness measures. Clinical measures include blood lipid levels and blood pressure; physiologic indicators include skinfold measurements and maximum oxygen uptake; behavioral measures include smoking status and physical activity frequency; perceptual measures include patient/client self-assessment tools such as global indicators of health status ("compared to other people of your age, would you say your health is excellent, good, fair, or poor?")[33] and the SF-36 Health Status Questionnaire.[34]

Although clinical, physiologic, and behavioral variables are useful indicators of bodily wellness and are commonly used to plan individual and community interventions, they are incomplete measures of wellness.[35] Clinical and physiologic measures assess the status of a single system, most commonly within the physical domain of wellness. Overall, behavioral measures are a better reflection of multiple systems due to the influence of motivation and self-efficacy on the adoption of behaviors, but they do not describe the wellness of the mind. On the other hand, perceptual measures are capable of assessing all systems and have been shown to predict effectively a variety of health outcomes.[30,33,36–38] Perceptual measures can complement the information provided by body-centered measures.[35]

Although some perceptual measures assess only single system status (e.g., psychologic well-being, mental well-being), numerous multidimensional perceptual measures exist and can serve as wellness measures. Perceptual constructs that have been used as wellness measures include general health status,[34] subjective well-being,[39,40] general well-being,[41,42] morale,[43,44] happiness,[45,46] life satisfaction,[47–49] hardiness,[50,51] and perceived wellness.[30,52,53] Example questions from a few of these perceptual tools are listed in Table 4-2.

The influence of perceptions on health and wellness has been demonstrated repeatedly in a variety of patient/client populations and a variety of settings. Mossey and Shapiro[33] demonstrated more than 25 years ago that self-rated health was the second strongest predictor of mortality in the elderly, with age being the strongest predictor. Numerous other researchers have replicated these findings in other

TABLE 4-2 Sample Items from Perceptual Measurement Tools

INSTRUMENT	PERCEPTUAL CONSTRUCT	SAMPLE ITEMS (RESPONSES)
SF-36[31]	General health perceptions	"In general, would you say your health is" (excellent, very good, good, fair, or poor) "Compared to 1 year ago, how would you rate your health in general now?" (much better than 1 year ago, somewhat better, about the same, somewhat worse, much worse)
Satisfaction with Life Scale[44]	Life satisfaction	"In most ways my life is close to my ideal" "I am satisfied with my life" (7-point Likert scale from strongly disagree [1] to strongly agree [7])
Perceived Wellness Survey[28]	Perceived wellness	"I am always optimistic about my future" "I avoid activities that require me to concentrate" (6-point Likert scale from very strongly disagree [1] to very strongly agree [6])
NCHS General Well-Being Schedule[39]	General well-being	"How have you been feeling in general?" (In excellent spirits, In very good spirits, In good spirits mostly, I have been up and down in spirits a lot, In low spirits mostly, In very low spirits) "Has your daily life been full of things that were interesting to you?" (All the time, Most of the time, A good bit of the time, Some of the time, A little of the time, None of the time)
Philadelphia Geriatric Center Morale Scale[40]	Morale	"Things keep getting worse as I get older" "I am as happy now as when I was younger" (yes, no)
Memorial University of Newfoundland Scale of Happiness[43]	Happiness	"In the past months have you been feeling on top of the world?" "As I look back on my life, I am fairly well satisfied" (yes, no, don't know)

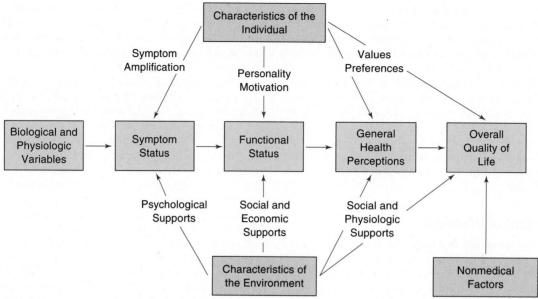

FIGURE 4-3. Health-related Quality of Life Conceptual model. (Reprinted with permission from Mokdad AH, Ford ES, Bowman BA, et al. Prevalence of obesity, diabetes, and obesity-related health risk factors, 2001. JAMA 2003;289:76–79.)

populations, lending support to the value of perceptions in understanding health and wellness and indicating that how well you think you are may be more important than how well you actually are. Patient's perceptions are critical in understanding and explaining quality of life.[35] Health perceptions provide an important link between the biomedical model with its focus on "etiological agents, pathological processes, and biological, physiological, and clinical outcomes" and the quality of life model, with its focus on "dimensions of functioning and overall well-being."[35] (Fig. 4-3). Health perceptions "are among the best predictors of general medical and mental health services as well as strong predictors of mortality, even after controlling clinical factors."[33,35]

Physical therapists assess perceptions as a part of the patient/client history, as recommended in the *Guide to Physical Therapist Practice*.[4] Some of the kinds of perceptions that can be assessed include perceptions of general health status, social support systems, role and social functioning, and functional status in self-care and home management activities, and work, community, and leisure activities. Although a few of these categories are included in overall wellness, such as general health status and social and role functioning, measuring wellness perceptions specifically can provide additional and more complete information about the patient that the physical therapist can use to formulate a plan and that can

be insightful to the patient/client. Therefore, perceptual tools should be included when measuring wellness within a primary prevention context and when examining patients/clients within a secondary or tertiary prevention context.

HEALTH PROMOTION AND WELLNESS-BASED PRACTICES

Establishing a wellness-based practice or offering health promotion and wellness services requires that the physical therapist or provider modify the traditional approach used to treat patients. Creating a successful wellness-based practice involves changing the focus from illness to wellness, being a role model of wellness, incorporating wellness measures into the examination, considering the client within his or her lifestyle or "system," and offering services beyond the traditional patient-provider relationship.

From Illness to Wellness

The types of services provided in a physical therapist wellness-based practice can be varied and are influenced by the population served, the skills and expertise of the physical therapist, and the setting in which the services are provided. Based on the definition and characteristics of wellness provided earlier in this chapter, wellness services can be provided in any setting and to any population—it just requires changing the approach to consider patients as clients who have the potential and opportunity to be more well.

The most common wellness-based practices are integrated within a traditional physical therapist practice in which patients convert to "members" after discharge for a specific diagnosis.[54] These patients/clients use the clinic or fitness facility to continue their exercise program. In this case, the client would have access to the facility to perform an individually or group prescribed exercise program and to the physical therapist who would be available to answer questions and progress the client's program. Additionally, to

---

BUILDING BLOCK 4-2
Consider the patient in case study 4-1

1. How do you think Mr. Prager's perceived wellness will be impacted by his knee injury?
2. How would you describe Mr. Prager's lifestyle?
3. What assessment tool would you use to measure perceptions?
4. Why use one of these perceptual instruments?

truly address "wellness," the provider must consider offering services beyond the physical domain. In other words, providing the "nonpatient" with the opportunity to continue an exercise program under the supervision of the physical therapist addresses the physical component of wellness, and while exercise can impact the other dimensions of wellness as described earlier, specific interventions aimed at the other dimensions of wellness would provide a holistic approach to wellness, as described below.

Establishing a wellness-based practice within an existing physical therapist practice requires several features. The facility should be available and staffed at convenient hours for clients and the staff should have expertise in exercise prescription as well as awareness and knowledge of wellness. For example, opportunities can be created to acknowledge the influence of social connections on wellness by offering group classes and group interaction among clients. The intellectual aspect of wellness can be tapped by providing educational resources and challenges for clients. For example, offering an educational class on topics such as progressing an exercise program or nutrition, followed by a test of understanding of the exercise prescription or the content of a class are activities that would use and challenge the intellectual dimension. Additional staff with expertise in mental and spiritual health can be retained as consultants to provide services in these dimensions when indicated or requested by clients. Some facilities provide an integrated experience, with mental and spiritual health as a component of the wellness program.

Establishing a wellness-based practice also requires that the provider assume the role of a facilitator or partner rather than that of an authority figure.[55] When a patient is ill it is often appropriate for the health care provider to act as the expert when the patient has limited ability to provide self-care and is relying on the provider for information and skills to recover and improve. In a wellness setting the best approach is to believe that the client knows best in terms of maximizing his or her potential; therefore, assuming a partner or facilitator role is more appropriate and will create a relationship in which the client feels empowered to take control. Rather than "making" the client well, the provider can view the client as a whole person within a biopsychosocial context and consider teaching the client how to achieve wellness. Being a role model and fulfilling the role of facilitator will establish a relationship and environment in which clients can attain greater wellness.

The Use of Screening as an Examination Tool within a Wellness-Based Practice

The Guide to Physical Therapist Practice defines screening as determining the need for further examination or consultation by a physical therapist or for referral to another health professional.[4] Screening is important and applicable in a health promotion context because it enables identification of the health status, personal goals, and available resources of the client. Within a physical therapist's scope of practice and a health promotion/wellness context, clients can be screened in numerous ways. Wellness programs routinely screen for osteoporosis, physical activity level, balance/risk for falls, muscle strength and endurance, flexibility, perceived wellness and quality of life, and motivation to change health-related

behaviors or adopt new behaviors. A number of tools have been developed and are available in the literature for use in screening clients. Example perceptual screening tools that can be used in a wellness or primary prevention context and their uses are listed in Table 4-3.

Screening tools can be used to identify whether or not a client has risks that should be investigated before participating in an intervention program. The physical therapist can also use the screening information to identify who should perform further examination and intervention, and the conditions under which the intervention should be performed (e.g., with or without supervision, the need for a medical diagnostic test). Screening tools can also identify a baseline from which progress can be assessed and documented. Depending on specific state law, screens may be performed on existing clients or can be used to identify those who would benefit from services.

Starting a Wellness-Based Practice

The mechanics of starting a specific wellness-based practice do not differ from starting or expanding any type of practice. The first step should include verifying that "wellness" or "health promotion" is included within the definition and description of physical therapy in the state practice act. Second, the liability policy should be checked to ensure coverage for wellness type activities. As with any new endeavor, physical therapists should spend time identifying and understanding the potential risks involved in the provision of wellness services.

Although great strides have been made in the area of insurance coverage for health promotion and wellness services, most insurers do not reimburse health care providers for these services. However, the public understands the value of these services and is becoming more and more willing to pay directly for them.[56] While there isn't a specific formula for determining the mechanics of charging for health promotion services and integrating these services into a physical therapist practice, following the same practice management and business principles used in creating any physical therapist practice, as well as knowing what other providers charge for health promoting services, will result in a service that will be competitive in the market as well as provide a valuable service for clients. A rich section of resources can be found on the APTA website (www.apta.org/Practice) in the Physical Fitness for Special Populations section of the Practice page. In the case of populations that are unable to afford these types of services, consider providing more affordable group and community programs, applying for state and federal grants to support programs, or providing pro bono services that offer recognition through positive public relations.

Other activities that should be well thought out and planned include marketing and advertising the program and evaluating program success. Although specifics of these activities are outside the scope of this chapter, they are key to overall program effectiveness. Whether you are starting a specific wellness-based practice or program or are adopting a wellness approach within an existing health care setting, shifting from a medical to a biopsychosocial focus, recognizing that, as important as they may be, there is more to wellness than physical parameters, and adding the assessment of perceptions to your examination toolbox are both approaches that will provide a strong basis for a wellness program.

TABLE 4-3 Perceptual Screening Tools

PERCEPTUAL SCREENING TOOL	USE	RESOURCE/REFERENCE	PHYSICAL THERAPY APPLICATION
Physical Activity Readiness Questionnaire	General activity screen for ages 15–69	Canadian Society for Exercise Physiology www.csep.ca	Indicates whether or not an individual should seek further medical consultation before beginning an aerobic exercise program.
Self-efficacy for Exercise Questionnaire	Assesses the beliefs one has regarding success with physical activity	Marcus et al.[61]	Provides the physical therapist with information about perceptions of success with physical activity, which can be a barrier to adopt an activity habit if not addressed.
Physical Activity Enjoyment Scale	Assesses how enjoyable a client finds exercise	Kendzierski and DeCarlo[62]	Provides information about how enjoyable a client finds exercise. Researchers have found that enjoyment is related to adherence to physical activity, so when enjoyment is low it should be addressed in the exercise prescription.
Motivational Readiness for Change Scale (Transtheoretical Model)	Assesses a client's readiness to change for any behavior (exercise, smoking, etc.)	Marcus and Simkim[63]; Prochaska and DiClemente[64]	Provides information from which the physical therapist can tailor the intervention for a specific behavior. For example, if a client is not ready to change, the intervention will be very different compared to a client who is ready to make a change.
Short Form 36 (SF-36)	General perceptual health status and outcomes questionnaire	Medical Outcomes Trust www.outcomes-trust.org	Provides information about perceptions in eight health concepts, including physical functioning, role limitations resulting from physical health problems, bodily pain, social functioning, general mental health, role limitations resulting from emotional problems, vitality (energy/fatigue), and general health perceptions. Can be used to determine the relative burden of an injury or illness and to document the relative benefits/outcomes of an intervention or interventions.
Perceived wellness survey	General perceptual wellness survey	Adams et al.[30]	Provides information about general wellness perceptions in six dimensions, including physical, emotional, social, psychologic, spiritual, and intellectual. Can be used to determine the relative burden of an injury or illness and to document the effect of an intervention on overall wellness.
Risk for falls	Assesses a client's risk for falling	Balance Self-Test www.balanceandmobility.com/patient_info/printout.aspx	Indicates an individual's risk for falling and thus the need for further examination and intervention.
Computer workstation checklist	Identifies clients at risk for injury as a result of computer use	www.osha.gov/SLTC/etools/computerworkstations/checklist.html	Identifies specific areas within a computer workstation where problems may exist that would benefit the worker to be addressed. Includes the areas of posture, seating, keyboard/input device, monitor, work area, accessories, and general issues.

PHYSICAL WELL-BEING: PHYSICAL ACTIVITY PROGRAMS

Transitioning a patient within a physical therapist practice from an intervention program addressing specific impairments to a general physical activity program addressing overall physical fitness and/or quality of life, and keeping in mind the impairments the physical therapist was addressing, is an approach physical therapists can and should consider. Physical therapists are uniquely qualified to create physical activity programs that enhance overall fitness and quality of life, while also addressing specific neuromusculoskeletal impairments that require the expertise of the physical therapist. Numerous government and research entities recommend that children and adults of all ages and health conditions partake in regular physical activity to improve overall health and well-being. The US Department of Health and Human Services, the Centers for Disease Control and Prevention, the National Center for Chronic Disease Prevention and Health Promotion, the President's Council on Physical Fitness and Sports, and the American College of Sports Medicine recommend that all adults should accumulate 30 minutes or more of moderate-intensity physical activity on most, and preferably all, days of the week.[12,57] Physical therapists within the context of primary prevention, can assist clients to achieve this goal safely and effectively by routinely inquiring about patient/client physical activity habits, conducting physical fitness assessments, prescribing physical activity to improve general health and well-being, and encouraging clients to adopt an active lifestyle.

Conducting Health-Related Physical Fitness Assessments

Clients who desire a physical activity program for improvement of overall physical fitness and/or quality of life should receive a physical therapist examination and evaluation similar to any other patient/client seen by a physical therapist. Parts of the examination may be abbreviated or taken from the patient/client existing medical record in the case of a patient/client who was treated by the physical therapist for a specific impairment or health condition in the recent past. Prior to engaging

in a physical activity or exercise program, clients should be screened to determine their readiness and appropriateness for exercise. For individuals who do not require medical evaluation as described in Chapter 6, preparticipation screening can be performed using a self-report questionnaire, such as the Physical Activity Readiness Questionnaire or PAR-Q[58-60] (see Appendix 3). Based on the answers to the seven questions on the PAR-Q, individuals between the ages of 15 and 69 can either appropriately participate in exercise or be referred to a physician for further evaluation before beginning an exercise program. All individuals who fall outside of the boundaries described should be referred to a physician for medical evaluation before participating in exercise training.

Depending on the client's goals for an exercise program, the five elements of physical fitness should be assessed to create a baseline and from which to prescribe exercise. Table 4-4 provides examples of the types of tests that can be

TABLE 4-4 Health-Related Physical Fitness Tests

PHYSICAL FITNESS PARAMETER	TEST NAMES	TEST DESCRIPTION	REFERENCE/ RESOURCE
Body composition	1. Body mass index 2. Waist to hip ratio 3. Skin fold measurements	1. Ratio of weight to height (weight in kg/height in ms) 2. Circumference of waist at smallest point/ circumference of hips at largest point 3. Uses skin fold calipers to assess amount of fat using standardized equations	58, 59
Cardiorespiratory endurance	1. Cooper 12-minute test 2. 1.5 mile test 3. 3-minute YMCA step test 4. Astrand-Rhyming cycle ergometer test	1. Participant walks or runs to cover the greatest distance in 12 minutes. 2. Participant runs or walks the distance in the shortest period of time. 3. Using a 12-in high step, the participant steps up and down at a rate of 24 steps/min for 3 minutes. Heart rate is measured immediately for 1 minute and used to estimate VO_2. 4. Participant cycles on a stationary cycle ergometer for 6 minutes at a standard resistance, pedaling at a rate of 50 rpm. Heart rate is taken twice and used to estimate VO_2.	59
Flexibility	1. Sit and reach test 2. Standard flexibility tests	1. Test to assess low back and hip joint flexibility; client in long sitting, reaches with both hands between outstretched legs as far as possible and tester measures distance reached. 2. Tests to determine joint range of motion specific to each joint.	58, 59
Muscular endurance	1. Total number of repetitions at a given amount of resistance 2. Total number of repetitions at a % of 1 repetition maximum (RM) 3. Curl up 4. Push up	1. Participant performs as many repetitions of a specific movement as possible at a submaximal level of resistance to fatigue. 2. Same as no. 1 using a percentage of 1 RM. 3. Participant is supine with knees at 90 degrees, arms at side, palms facing up. Client performs slow controlled curl-ups at a rate of 25 per minute. Tester counts the number per minute. 4. Male participants use standard "down" position and females "knee push up" position. Participant raises body by straightening elbows and returns to down position keeping back straight. Tester counts the number per minute.	58, 59
Muscular strength	1. Manual muscle testing 2. 1 RM	1. Manually applied resistance to specific muscle groups based on established norms and using standard scales. 2. The greatest resistance that can be moved through the full range of motion in a controlled manner with good posture.	59

used to assess each of the five elements of physical fitness. For example, for a client who desires to lose weight through physical activity and modification of eating habits, body composition and cardiorespiratory endurance should be assessed at a minimum to establish a baseline of weight, body fat, and cardiorespiratory fitness, and to establish goals and assess progress. If a general systems screen indicates impairments in musculoskeletal areas that might be impacted by physical activity, tests of muscular endurance and strength, and flexibility should also be performed. In general, a personalized physical activity prescription should be prescribed based on the patient/client's specific physical characteristics as often as possible, which will prevent injury, enhance comfort and participation, and promote overall physical fitness.

Establishing Physical Activity Interventions

Armed with the results of a patient/client history including goals for physical activity, systems review, and physical fitness testing, the physical therapist can establish a physical activity program for a client. Specific aspects of the history that may be useful when prescribing exercise include past experience with exercise or physical activity, dietary habits, social situation, and current medications. This information can be useful and necessary to ensure safety, enjoyment, compliance and effectiveness when creating an exercise program for a client.

There are numerous ways clients can become more physical active, including but not limited to walking, cycling, climbing stairs, doing yardwork and housework, and dancing. Clients who have been appropriately screened can engage in any type of physical activity that appeals to them and that they enjoy and will perform consistently. Setting a goal of 30 minutes per day of physical activity for an inactive client, consistent with government guidelines, provides great lattitude in terms of activity, and yet is achievable for most people. To achieve health-related benefits, physical activity can be performed in smaller bouts and does not need to be continuous or performed all at one time. For example, three 10-minute walks per day satisfy the goal of 30 minutes of moderate physical activity per day and perhaps can be incorporated more easily into the busy and demanding lifestyle of an individual who struggles to find time for physical activity.

Some clients may have specific goals that require more than the minimum amount of physical activity for health-related well-being, like running a marathon, playing recreational soccer, or losing weight. In these situations, specific exercise prescriptions should be established including well-defined and tailored doses of exercise in order to accomplish the specific client goal. The information in Chapter 6 is designed to assist in creating these types of exercise prescriptions.

KEY POINTS

- Prevention is classified as primary, secondary, or tertiary
- Health promotion and wellness fall into the realm of primary prevention, whereas most rehabilitation is secondary or tertiary prevention
- The terms health promotion and health education are often used interchangeably
- Physical activity is any bodily movement produced by skeletal muscles resulting in energy expenditure, whereas exercise is planned, structured, and repetitive and is a type of physical activity
- Wellness is multidimensional, salutogenic, and requires a systems perspective and can be used interchangeably with the term well-being
- Wellness extends beyond only the physical domain to include many other dimensions such as spiritual, intellectual, psychosocial, and emotional well-being
- Perceptual measures are often better predictors of general well-being than physiologic measures
- Wellness requires a vision beyond just the physical domain and the biomedical model
- Physical therapists should assess the physical activity level of their patients/clients and encourage patients/clients to become more physical active, including establishing physical activity programs to enhance health-related quality of life and well-being

REFERENCES

1. U.S. Department of Health and Human Services. Healthy People 2010. Washington, DC: U.S. Department of Health and Human Services, 2000.
2. Healthier US Initiative. Available at: http://www.healthypeople.gov/. Accessed March 17, 2008.
3. McGinnis JM, Foege WH. Actual causes of death in the United States. JAMA 1993;270:2207–2212.
4. Guide to physical therapist practice. 2nd Ed. Phys Ther 2001;81:471–593.
5. American Physical Therapy Association. Available at: http://www.apta.org/AM/Template.cfm?Section=About_APTA&Template=/TaggedPage/TaggedPageDisplay.cfm&TPLID=41&ContentID=23725. Accessed March 17, 2008.
6. Federation of State Board of Physical Therapy. The Model Practice Act for Physical Therapy. 4th Ed. Alexandria, VA: Federation of State Boards of Physical Therapy, 2006.
7. The Commission on Accreditation of Physical Therapy Education. Evaluative Criteria for Accreditation of Education Programs for the Preparation of Physical Therapists. Alexandria, VA, 2006.
8. Stave GM. The Glaxo Wellcome health promotion program: the contract for health and wellness. Am J Health Promotion 2001;15:359–360.
9. Green LW, Kreuter MW. Health promotion planning. An Educational and Environmental Approach. 2nd Ed. Mountain View, CA: Mayfield Publishing Company, 1991.
10. Glanz K, Rimer BK, Lewis FM. Health Behavior and Health Education. 3rd Ed. San Francisco: Jossey-Bass, 2002.
11. Caspersen CJ, Powell KE, Christenson GM. Physical activity, exercise, and physical fitness: definitions and distinctions for health-related research. Public Health Rep 1985;100:126–131.

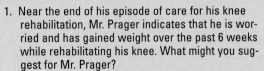

BUILDING BLOCK 4-3
Consider the patient in case study 4-1

1. Near the end of his episode of care for his knee rehabilitation, Mr. Prager indicates that he is worried and has gained weight over the past 6 weeks while rehabilitating his knee. What might you suggest for Mr. Prager?
2. You administer the PAR-Q to Mr. Prager. What does the PAR-Q indicate?
3. What assessment tool would you use to assess body composition?
4. How would you address stress with Mr. Prager?
5. Create a physical activity program involving walking that incorporates physical activity into Mr. Prager's lifestyle.

12. U.S. Department of Health and Human Services. Physical Activity and Health: A Report of the Surgeon General. Atlanta: U.S. Department of Health and Human Services, Centers for Disease Control and Prevention, National Center for Chronic Disease Prevention and Health Promotion, 1996.
13. Dunn HL. High Level Wellness. Washington, DC: Mt. Vernon, 1961.
14. Wu R. Behavior and Illness. New Jersey: Prentice-Hall, 1973.
15. Lafferty J. A credo for wellness. Health Ed 1979;10:10–11.
16. Hettler W. Wellness promotion on a university campus. J Health Promotion Maint 1980;3:77–95.
17. Hinds WC. Personal Paradigm Shift: A Lifestyle Intervention Approach to Health Care Management. East Lansing, MI: Michigan State, 1983.
18. Greenberg JS. Health and wellness: a conceptual differentiation. J School Health 1985;55:403–406.
19. Ardell DB. High Level Wellness. Berkeley, CA: Ten Speed Press, 1986.
20. Travis JW, Ryan RS. Wellness Workbook. 2nd Ed. Berkeley, CA: Ten Speed Press, 1988.
21. Depken D. Wellness through the lens of gender: a paradigm shift. Wellness Perspectives 1994;10:54–69.
22. Ratner PA, Johnson, JL, Jeffery B. Examining emotional, physical, social, and spiritual health as determinants of self-rated health status. Am J Health Promotion 1998;12:275–282.
23. Nicholas DR, Gobble DC, Crose RG, et al. A systems view of health, wellness and gender: implications for mental health counseling. J Ment Health Counsel 1992;14:8–19.
24. Whitmer JM, Sweeney TJ. A holistic model for wellness prevention over the life span. J Counsel Develop 1992;71:140–148.
25. World Health Organization. Basic Documents. 15th Ed. Geneva, Switzerland: WHO, 1964.
26. Antonovsky A. Unraveling the Mystery of Health: How People Manage Stress and Stay Well. San Francisco: Jossey-Bass, 1988.
27. Jasnoski ML, Schwartz GE. A synchronous systems model for health. Am Behav Scientist 1985;28:468–485.
28. Seeman J. Toward a model of positive health. Am Psychol 1989;44:1099–1109.
29. Crose R, Nicholas DR, Gobble DC, et al. Gender and wellness: a multidimensional systems model for counseling. J Counsel Develop 1992;71:149–156.
30. Adams T, Bezner J, Steinhardt M. The conceptualization and measurement of perceived wellness: integrating balance across and within dimensions. Am J Health Promotion 1997;11:208–218.
31. WHOQOL. Measuring Quality of Life. World Health Organization, Programme on Mental Health, Division of Mental Health and Prevention of Substance Abuse, 1997. Available at: http://www.who.int/mental_health/media/68.pdf. Accessed April 1, 2008.
32. Mokdad AH, Ford ES, Bowman BA, et al. Prevalence of obesity, diabetes, and obesity-related health risk factors, 2001. JAMA 2003;289:76–79.
33. Mossey JM, Shapiro E. Self-rated health: a predictor of mortality among the elderly. Am J Public Health 1982;72:800–808.
34. Ware JE, Sherbourne D. The MOS 36-item short-form health survey (SF-36). Med Care 1992;30:473–483.
35. Wilson IB, Cleary PD. Linking clinical variables with health-related quality of life. JAMA 1995;273:59–65.
36. Idler E, Kasl S. Health perceptions and survival, do global evaluations of health status really predict mortality? J Gerontol 1991;46:S55–S65.
37. Stewart A, Hays R, Ware J. Health perceptions, energy/fatigue, and health distress measures. Measuring functioning and well-being: the Medical Outcomes study approach. Durham, NC: Duke University, 1992.
38. Eysenck H. Prediction of cancer and coronary heart disease mortality by means of a personality inventory. Results of a 15-year follow-up study. Psychol Rep 1993;72:499–516.
39. Andrews F, Robinson J. Measures of subjective well-being. In: Robinson J, Shaver P, Wrightsman L, eds. Measures of Personality and Social Psychological Attitudes. Vol. 1. San Diego, CA: Academic Press, 1991.
40. Diener E. Subjective well-being. Psychol Bull 1984;95:542–575.
41. Campbell A, Converse P, Rodgers W. The Quality of American Life. New York: Russell Sage Foundation, 1976.
42. Fazio A. A concurrent validational study of the NCHS general well-being schedule. DHEW Publication Number (HRA) 1977;2:78–1347.
43. Lawton M. The Philadelphia geriatric center morale scale: a revision. J Gerontol 1975;30:85–89.
44. Morris J, Sherwood S. A retesting and modification of the PGC morale scale. J Gerontol 1975;30:77–84.
45. Fordyce M. The PSYCHAP inventory: a multi-scale to measure happiness and its concomitants. Soc Ind Res 1986;18:1–33.
46. Kozma A, Stones M. The measurement of happiness: development of the Memorial University of Newfoundland scale of happiness (MUNSH). J Gerontol 1980;35:906–912.
47. Diener E, Emmons R, Larsen R, et al. The satisfaction with life scale. J Pers Assess 1984;49:71–75.
48. Neugarten B, Havighurst R, Tobin S. The measurement of life satisfaction. J Gerontol 1961;16:134–143.
49. Wood V, Wylie M, Sheafor B. An analysis of a short self-report measure of life satisfaction: correlation with rater judgments. J Gerontol 1969;24:465–469.
50. Kobasa S. Stressful life events, personality, and health: an inquiry into hardiness. J Pers Soc Psychol 1979;37:1–11.
51. Williams P, Wiebe D, Smith T. Coping processes as mediators of the relationship between hardiness and health. J Behav Med 1992;15:237–255.
52. Adams TB, Bezner JR, Drabbs ME, et al. Conceptualization and measurement of the spiritual and psychological dimensions of wellness in a college population. J Am Coll Health 2000;48:165–173.
53. Bezner JR, Hunter DL. Wellness perceptions in persons with traumatic brain injury and its relation to functional independence. Arch Phys Med Rehabil 2001;82:787–792.
54. Ries E. In Sickness and in Wellness. PT Magazine 2003;11:44–51.
55. Ferguson T. Working with your doctor. In: Goleman D, Gurin J, eds. Mind Body Medicine. New York, NY: Consumer Reports Books, 1993.
56. Eisenberg DM, Davis RB, Ettner SL, et al. Trends in alternative medicine use in the United States, 1990–1997. JAMA 1998;280:1569–1575.
57. Pate RR, Pratt M, Blair SN, et al. Physical activity and public health. JAMA 1995;273:402–407.
58. American College of Sports Medicine. Resource Manual for Guidelines for Exercise Testing and Prescription. 3rd Ed. Baltimore, MD: Williams & Wilkins, 1998.
59. American College of Sports Medicine. ACSM's Guidelines for Exercise Testing and Prescription. 7th Ed. Philadelphia, PA: Lippincott Williams & Wilkins, 2006.
60. American Association of Cardiovascular and Pulmonary Rehabilitation. Guidelines for cardiac rehabilitation and secondary prevention programs. 3rd Ed. Champaign, IL: Human Kinetics, 1999.
61. Marcus BH, Selby VC, Niaura RS, et al. Self-efficacy and the stages of exercise behavior change. Res Q Exerc Sport 1992;63:60–66.
62. Kendzierski D, DeCarlo KJ. Physical activity enjoyment scale: two validation studies. J Sport Exerc Psychol 1991;13:50–64.
63. Marcus BH, Simkim LR. The stages of exercise behavior. J Sports Med Phys Fitness 1993;33:83–88.
64. Prochaska JO, DiClemente CC. The stages and processes of self-change in smoking: towards an integrative model of change. J Consult Clin Psychol 1983;51:390–395.

Impairments of Body Functions and Therapeutic Exercise

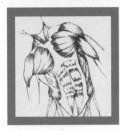

chapter 5

Impaired Muscle Performance

LORI THEIN BRODY AND CARRIE M. HALL

Muscular performance is an essential component of a person's life. Every human activity from breathing to walking to the bathroom to running a marathon requires muscle activity. Physiologic, anatomic, psychologic, and biomechanical factors affect muscle performance. Pathology and disease affecting the cardiovascular, endocrine, integumentary, musculoskeletal, neuromuscular, or pulmonary systems can also affect muscle performance and strength training can improve the function of these systems. Muscle performance impairments can be considered as impairments in muscle *strength, power,* or *endurance*. These impairments must be related to an activity limitation or participation restriction, or promote prevention, health, wellness, and fitness, to justify therapeutic exercise intervention. For example, an individual lacking the muscular ability to carry a bag of groceries into the house requires intervention to achieve this instrumental activity of daily living. A worker lacking the muscle endurance to maintain efficient posture and safe movement patterns throughout the workday requires intervention to prevent work disability. A person with osteoarthritis of the knee and poor quadriceps muscle performance requires quadriceps muscle training to prevent further knee joint deterioration.

Although not all scientific and clinical information on strength, power, and endurance production can be covered in this text, this chapter provides a strong foundation for this element of therapeutic exercise intervention. Fundamental terms and concepts are defined, the essential morphology and physiology of skeletal muscle relative to muscle performance are reviewed, and clinical applications are presented.

DEFINITIONS

Definitions of key terms vary from one researcher, text or profession to another. The following definitions are presented to clarify how these terms will be used throughout this text.

Strength

Impaired muscle performance is commonly treated by clinicians and is usually described as a strength deficit. However, strength is only one of three components of muscle performance (i.e., strength, power, and endurance). **Strength** is defined as the maximum force that a muscle can develop during a single contraction, and is the result of complex interactions of neurologic, muscular, biomechanical, and cognitive systems. Strength can be assessed in terms of force, torque, work, and power. If appropriate decisions are to be made regarding these impairments, operational definitions are necessary.

Force is an agent that produces or tends to produce a change in the state of rest or motion of an object.[1] For example, a ball sitting stationary on a playing field remains in that position unless it is acted on by a force. Force, described in metric units of newtons or British units of pounds, is displayed algebraically in the following equation:

$$\text{force} = \text{mass} \times \text{acceleration}$$

Kinetics is the study of forces applied to the body. Some of the factors influencing muscular force production include the neural input, mechanical arrangement of the muscle, cross-sectional area, fiber-type composition, age, and gender.[1]

All human motion involves rotation of body segments about their joint axes. These actions are produced by the interaction of forces from external loads and muscle activity. The ability of a force to produce rotation is **torque**. Torque represents the rotational effect of a force with respect to an axis:

$$\text{torque} = \text{force} \times \text{moment arm}$$

The **moment arm** is the perpendicular distance from the line of action of the force to the axis of rotation. The metric unit of torque is the newton-meter; the foot-pound is used in the older British system of units.

Clinically, the word strength is often used synonymously with torque. Large amounts of torque are produced by the musculoskeletal system during everyday functional activities such as walking, lifting, and getting out of bed. It is incorrect to conclude that a person is "strong" only because his muscles generate large forces. It would be just as erroneous to conclude that a person is strong only because he has large moment arms.

Torque can be altered in biomechanics through three strategies:

- Changing the force magnitude
- Changing the moment arm length
- Changing the angle between the direction of force and momentum

BUILDING BLOCK 5-1

A patient with thoracic spine and neck pain works at a research laboratory where the work stations are positioned such that it requires the patient to either (a) bend over a table top, or (b) to work with her arms extended well in front of her at shoulder height. Please apply the three principles of altering torque just discussed to minimize thoracic and cervical spine pain for this patient.

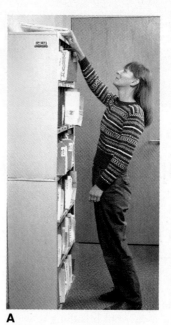
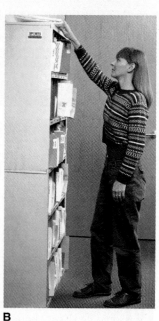

A   **B**

FIGURE 5-1. Individual standing at a work station using (A) poor posture or (B) good posture.

In the human musculoskeletal system, changing the force magnitude (i.e., tension-producing capability of muscle) can be altered by training, the moment arm can be decreased by positioning a load closer to the body, and the angle between the force and moment arm may be changed by altering joint alignment through postural education. See Building Block 5-1.

Power and Work

Power is the rate of performing work. **Work** is the magnitude of a force acting on an object multiplied by the distance through which the force acts. The unit used to describe work is the joule, which is equivalent to 1 N-m (the foot-pound unit is used in the British system). Work is algebraically expressed in this equation:

$$work = force \times distance$$

The unit of power in the metric system is the watt, which is equal to 1 J per second (foot-pound per second in the British system). Power can be determined for a single body movement, a series of movements, or for a large number of repetitive movements, as in the case of aerobic exercise. Power is algebraically expressed as:

$$power = work/time$$

For the simple movement of lifting or lowering a weight, the muscle must overcome the weight of the limb and the weight (force), acting some distance from the axis of rotation (torque) through a range of motion (work) during a specific time frame (power). This example summarizes the practical aspects of force, torque, work, and power in resistance training.

Endurance

Endurance is the ability of muscle to sustain forces repeatedly or to generate forces over a certain period. It is often measured as the ratio of the peak force that can be generated by a muscle at a given point in time, relative to the peak force that was possible during a single maximum contraction. Muscle endurance is the ability of a muscle group to perform repeated contractions against a load. This load can be externally applied or as a result of posture, such as when someone is working over a desk, counter, or work station all day (Fig. 5-1). Muscle endurance can be examined by isometric contractions, repeated dynamic contractions, or repeated contractions on an isokinetic dynamometer.

Muscle Actions

Poorly defined muscle actions can be a source of confusion and inaccuracy. Resistive exercise uses various types of muscle contraction to improve impaired muscle performance. Muscle actions can be divided into two general categories: static and dynamic. A static muscle action, traditionally referred to as **isometric**, is a contraction in which force is developed without any motion about an axis, so no work is performed. The amount of force generated by the muscle matches the external resistance applied.

All other muscle actions involve movement and are called dynamic or isotonic. An **isotonic exercise** suggests a uniform force throughout a dynamic muscle action. No dynamic muscle action uses constant force because of changes in mechanical advantage and muscle length. Isotonic is therefore an inappropriate term to describe human exercise performance, and the term **dynamic** is preferred.

Dynamic muscle action is further described as concentric or eccentric action. The term **concentric** describes a shortening muscle contraction, and the term **eccentric** describes a lengthening muscle contraction. A concentric contraction happens when the internal force generated by the muscle exceeds the external load, while an eccentric contraction occurs when the external resistance exceeds the muscle force and the muscle lengthens while still developing tension.[2] Eccentric contractions differ from concentric and isometric contractions in several important ways. Per contractile unit, more tension can be generated eccentrically than concentrically and at a lower metabolic cost (i.e., less use of ATP-derived energy).[3] Eccentric contractions are an important component of a functional movement pattern (e.g., required to decelerate limbs during movement), are the most energy-efficient form, and can develop the greatest tension of the various types of muscle actions.

The term **isokinetic** refers to a concentric or eccentric muscle contraction in which a constant velocity is maintained throughout the muscle action. A person can exert a continuous force by using an isokinetic device, which provides a resistive surface that restricts movement to a set, constant velocity. Some acceleration and deceleration occurs as the individual accelerates the limb from a resting position to the preset velocity and decelerates the limb to change directions. By constraining the speed of the isokinetic device, the limb moves at a constant velocity. Because the device cannot be accelerated beyond the preset speed, any unbalanced force exerted against it is resisted by an equal and opposite force. This muscular force may be measured, displayed, recorded, or used as concurrent visual feedback. Although the isokinetic device may be moving at a constant velocity, it does not guarantee that the user's muscle activation is at a constant velocity. Despite this inaccuracy, the terms isokinetic and isotonic to describe muscle action are likely to be employed for pragmatic reasons.

During functional movement patterns, combinations of static and dynamic contractions occur. Trunk muscles contract isometrically to stabilize the spine and pelvis during movements of the extremities such as reaching or walking. Lower extremity muscles are subjected to impact forces requiring combinations of concentric and eccentric contractions, sometimes within the same muscle acting at two different joints. Muscles commonly perform eccentric contractions against gravity, as in slowly lowering the arm from an overhead position.

Muscles often act eccentrically and then contract concentrically. The combination of eccentric and concentric actions forms a natural type of muscle action called a **stretch-shortening cycle** (SSC).[4,5] The SSC results in a final action (i.e., concentric phase) that is more powerful than a concentric action alone. This phenomenon is called **elastic potentiation**.[5] The SSC is discussed in more detail later in this chapter.

Exercise is described in terms of **dosage**. The components of the exercise dose include the exercise frequency, intensity, duration, volume, and rest interval. The exercise **frequency** is how often the exercise is performed, usually described as the number of days per week. The **intensity** is the amount of force necessary to achieve the activity, usually described as mass (in kilograms) or weight (in pounds). The intensity is often described as a percentage of a **repetition maximum (RM),** or the maximum amount of weight that can be lifted for a certain number of repetitions. For example, a 10 RM is the maximum amount of weight that can be lifted 10 times and a 1 RM is the maximum amount of weight that can be lifted once. The **duration** is the number of repetitions or time the exercise is performed. Often, a certain number of repetitions are performed in a **set,** and several sets of an exercise might be performed in a single session. The exercise **volume** is the total amount of exercise performed in a single session. Volume has been defined in different ways for different purposes. In weight training, volume is often defined as the product of the number of sets and repetitions and the weight. For example, the volume for 3 sets of 10 repetitions at 15 lb would be $3 \times 10 \times 15$ lb = 450 lb. It has also been defined as the total number of repetitions performed in a training session.[6] The **rest interval** is the amount of time between each set and/or between each exercise. The rest interval can be passive or active, where **passive rest** is simply resting before the next exercise bout, whereas **active rest** is rest where the person is performed a light activity such as walking or stretching between resistive exercise bouts. In order for resistive training to improve muscle performance the muscle must be overloaded. **Overload** means exercising or applying resistance above the loads currently or normally encountered.

FACTORS AFFECTING MUSCLE PERFORMANCE

The total force a muscle can produce is influenced by numerous factors. When prescribing therapeutic exercise intervention for muscle performance, knowledge of principles regarding muscle morphology, physiology, and biomechanics are critical. The following text discusses the primary factors influencing force production and, hence, muscle performance. For those needing a brief review of the structure of muscle and the physiology of muscle contraction, this material can be found on our website.

Fiber Type

Sedentary men and women and young children possess 45% to 55% slow-twitch fibers.[7] Persons who achieve high levels of sport proficiency have the fiber predominance and distributions characteristic of their sport. For example, those who train for endurance sports have a higher distribution of slow-twitch fibers in the significant muscles, and sprint athletes have a predominance of fast-twitch fibers. Other studies show that men and women who perform in middle-distance events have an approximately equal percentage of the two types of muscle fibers.[8] Any resistive rehabilitation program should be based on the probable distribution of fiber type of the individual.

Clear-cut distinctions between fiber type composition and athletic performance are true for elite athletes. A person's fiber composition is not the sole determinant of performance. Performance capacity is the end result of many physiologic, biochemical, and neurologic components, not simply the result of a single factor such as muscle fiber type.[9]

Fiber Diameter

Although the different fiber types show clear differences in contraction speed, the force developed in a maximal static action is independent of the fiber type but is related to the fiber's cross-sectional diameter. Because type I (slow) fibers tend to have smaller diameters than type II (fast) fibers, a high percentage of type I fibers is believed to be associated with a smaller muscle diameter and therefore lower force development capabilities.[10]

Muscle Size

When adult muscles are trained at intensities that exceed 60% to 70% of their maximum force-generating capacity, the muscle increases in cross-sectional area and force production capability. The increase in muscle size may result from increases in fiber size (i.e., hypertrophy), fiber number (i.e., hyperplasia), interstitial connective tissue, or some combination of these factors.[11,12]

Although the major mechanism for increased muscle size in adults is hypertrophy, ongoing controversy surrounds evidence of hyperplasia. Mammalian skeletal muscle does possess a population of reserve or satellite cells that, when activated, can replace damaged fibers with new fibers.[13,14] A mechanism exists for the generation of new fibers in the adult animal. Scientific models of exercise and stretch overload have shown significant increases in fiber number.[11] The mechanisms for fiber hyperplasia probably are the result of satellite cell proliferation and longitudinal fiber splitting.[11]

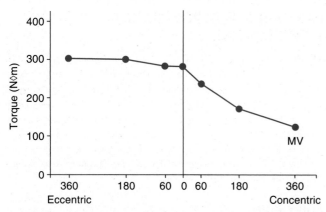

FIGURE 5-2. Relationship between the force and velocity of eccentric muscle contractions. (Adapted from Herzog W, Ait-Haddou R. Mechanical muscle models and their application for force and power production. In: Komi PV, ed. Strength and Power in Sport. 2nd Ed. Malden, MA: Blackwell Scientific Publications, 2003:176.)

Despite few investigations of the effect of strength training on interstitial connective tissue, it appears that, because interstitial connective tissue occupies a relatively small proportion of the total muscle volume, its potential to contribute substantial changes in muscle size is limited.[15]

Force-Velocity Relationship

Muscle can adjust its active force to precisely match the applied load. This property is based on the fact that active force continuously adjusts to the speed at which the contractile system moves. When the load is small, the active force can be made correspondingly small by increasing the speed of shortening appropriately. When the load is high, the muscle increases its active force to the same level by slowing the speed of shortening (Fig. 5-2).[16]

Slowing the speed of contraction allows a patient time to develop more tension during concentric contractions. This principle is evident during resistive exercise in the water, where the water's viscosity slows limb movement, allowing more time for tension development. However, during eccentric contractions, increased speed of lengthening produces more tension. This appears to provide a safety mechanism for limbs excessively loaded. Increasing the speed of a concentric contraction significantly lowers the amount of concentric torque developed. In contrast, increasing the speed of an eccentric contraction increases the amount of torque developed until a plateau speed is reached.

Length-Tension Relationship

A muscle's capacity to produce force depends on the length at which the muscle is held with maximum force delivered near the muscle's normal resting length (Fig. 5-3). The relationship between strength and length is called the length-tension property of muscle. The number of sarcomeres in series determines the distance through which the muscle can shorten and the length at which it produces maximum force. Sarcomere number is not fixed, and in adult muscle, this number can increase or decrease (Fig. 5-4).[17] Regulation of sarcomere number is an adaptation to changes in the functional length of a muscle.

Length-associated changes can be induced by postural malalignment or immobilization.[18,19] In muscles chronically

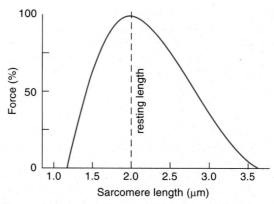

FIGURE 5-3. The length-tension curve depicts the relationship between muscle length and force development.

maintained in a shortened range because of faulty posture or immobilization, sarcomeres are lost, and the remaining sarcomeres adapt to a length that restores homeostasis; the new length enables maximum tension development at the new immobilized, shortened position.[20] For example, people who spend most of the day sitting can develop adaptive shortening of their hip flexor muscles. These muscles need to be stretched to avoid chronic shortening. In muscles immobilized or posturally held in a lengthened position, sarcomeres are added, and maximum tension is developed at the new increased length. This may be true of people at workstations where the scapular retractor muscles are lengthened due to thoracic kyphosis and a chronically protracted scapula. When a cast is removed or posture restored, the sarcomere number returns to normal. The stimulus for sarcomere length changes may be the amount of tension along the myofibril or the myotendon junction, with high tension leading to an addition of sarcomeres and low tension to a subtraction of sarcomeres.[21]

The clinical implication of the length-tension relationship is that the evaluation of muscle "strength" must be reconsidered. Muscles that tend to be shortened (e.g., hip flexors) may test as strong as normal-length muscles, because the manual muscle test position is a shortened position.[22] Conversely, the lengthened muscle (e.g., gluteus medius on the high iliac crest side) tests weak, because the manual

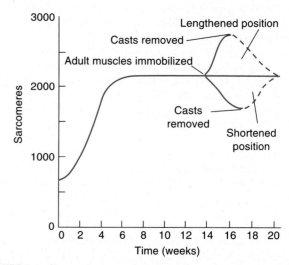

FIGURE 5-4. Changes in the number of sarcomeres in various conditions.

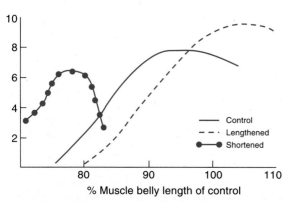

FIGURE 5-5. Changes in the length-tension relationship caused by length changes associated with immobilization. (Modified from Gossman, Sahrmann SA, Rose SJ. Review of length-associated changes in muscle. Experimental evidence and clinical implications. Phys Ther 1982;62:1799.)

muscle test occurs at a relatively shortened range, which is an insufficient position. According to animal studies,[26] the short muscles should develop the least peak tension, followed by the normal-length muscle and the lengthened muscle, which develops the greatest peak tension (Fig. 5-5). This finding reflects the number of sarcomeres in series. The lengthened muscle may be interpreted as weak although it is capable of producing substantial tension at the appropriate point in the range. This phenomena is called *positional strength*. A muscle should be tested at multiple points in the range to determine whether the muscle is positionally weak or weak throughout the range. See Building Block 5-2.

The emphasis of therapeutic exercise intervention should be on restoring normal length and tension development capability at the appropriate point in the range, rather than just strengthening the muscle. The positionally weak muscle should be strengthened in the shortened range, and the weak muscle should be strengthened dynamically throughout the range.

Muscle Architecture

The arrangement of the contractile components affects the contractile properties of the muscle dramatically. The more sarcomere lie in series, the longer the muscle will be, the more sarcomere lie in parallel, the larger the cross-sectional area of the muscle will be. These two basic architectural patterns affect the contractile properties of the muscles in the following ways:

- The force the muscle can produce is directly proportional to the cross-sectional area.
- The velocity and working excursion of the muscle are proportional to the length of the muscle.

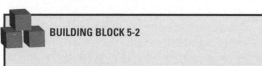

BUILDING BLOCK 5-2

Think of some other muscle groups that might not test "normal" when testing at mid-range position due to positional weakness (shortening or lengthening of the muscle).

BUILDING BLOCK 5-3

How might the rehabilitation of someone with a quadriceps muscle strain differ from someone with a hamstring muscle strain based upon the muscle architecture?

Generally, muscles with shorter fibers and a larger cross-sectional area are designed to produce force, whereas muscles with long fibers are designed to produce excursion and velocity.[24] For example, the quadriceps muscle contains shorter myofibrils and appears to be specialized for force production, whereas the sartorius muscle has longer fibers and a smaller cross-sectional area and is better suited for high excursion. See Building Block 5-3.

CLINICAL CONSIDERATIONS

Many factors impact the effectiveness of resistive exercise program. Issues such as medications and physical health, age, and program design can dramatically impact a person's ability to participate as well the physical response to the training stimulus.

Dosage

The exercise dosage can be altered in a variety of ways. Increasing the intensity or amount of weight is the most obvious means; changing the relationship to gravity, increasing the lever arm length, increasing sets and repetitions, decreasing the rest interval, and increasing the frequency are others. The dosage parameters of intensity, duration, and frequency are related and considered as training *volume*, and all must be considered when designing a resistive exercise program. The resistive exercise must be progressed to a functional activity to transition intervention at the impairment level to a functional situation (Fig. 5-6). Choose appropriate dosage

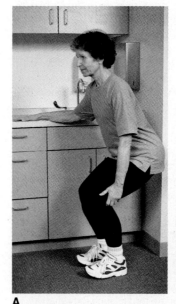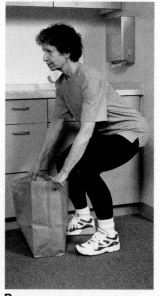

A   **B**

FIGURE 5-6. Progression of exercise. (A) Squat progressed to (B) squat with a bag of groceries.

DISPLAY 5-1
Dosage Variables for Individuals with Muscles of Various Strength Grades

Muscles Fair or Below Progressing to Muscles Above Fair
1. Gravity lessened or against gravity
2. Active assistive, active, or resisted
3. Range of motion
4. Lever arm length (bent elbow to straight arm)

Muscles Above Fair Strength Grade
1. Type of contraction (e.g., isometric, concentric, eccentric, isokinetic, plyometric)
2. Weight or resistance
3. Sets or repetitions
4. Frequency of training sessions (be cautious of overtraining)
5. Speed of movement (slower speed increases amount of force or torque generated during concentric exercise)
6. Distance (e.g., running, jumping, throwing)
7. Rest interval between sets

parameters based on the needs of the patient (Display 5-1). Determine whether the goal is to develop muscular strength, power, endurance, or some combination of these muscle performance parameters.

Patients with low levels of function often require resistive exercise prescriptions. Examination of many patients presenting with functional limitations reveals a less than fair grade of muscle strength. Patients with fair or lower muscle grades are unable to initiate resistive exercise against gravity with proper recruitment and movement patterns. When resistive exercise is prescribed against gravity, the patient is forced to train a faulty movement pattern. See Building Block 5-4.

Dosage parameters can be manipulated for maximum gains in strength, power, and endurance through a system of training called *periodization*. Periodization systematically varies the training dosage to prevent "plateaus" in training gains, to maintain interest, and to provide a well-balanced program. Varying the training program is essential to making long-term gains in training. Periodization breaks the training program down into cycles of a specific length and goals (i.e., hypertrophy, basic strength, power, and endurance). The cycles can vary from "minicycles" of 1 week to mesocycles of several months. Often a training program comprises a variety of cycles of variable lengths. Further discussion of periodization is presented later in this chapter in relation to training the advanced or elite athlete.

BUILDING BLOCK 5-4

A patient complains that she is unable to lift her arm overhead without pain. The patient is evaluated and is found to have a physiologic impairment of a muscle strength grade of fair for the lower trapezius and serratus anterior. How do these muscles function in arm elevation to an overhead position? Given their strength grade, what approach or approaches might be appropriate for initiating the rehabilitation program?

Intensity

Extensive strength training research has been performed on individuals without injury. Dosage parameters to increase strength began with DeLorme's classic paper in 1945.[25] He proposed a 10 RM, 10-set regimen. Later, DeLorme and Watkins[26] modified this regimen to a 10 RM, three-set regimen with loads increasing progressively for each set from one half to three fourths to a full 10 RM set. DeLorme called this regimen progressive resistance exercise (PRE), a term still used today (Table 5-1). DeLorme's three-set progressive resistance program has served as a control condition by which the effectiveness of other methods has been judged.

In 1951, an alternative to the DeLorme regimen was proposed by Zinovieff[27] at Oxford. He suggested adjusting the intensity of the load to allow for progressive fatigue. This was achieved by selecting an initial load that was just enough to permit each set to be completed. This regimen was called the Oxford technique. McMorris and Elkins[28] compared the DeLorme and Oxford techniques and found the Oxford technique to be slightly better, but the differences were not statistically significant.

The daily adjustable progressive resistive exercise (DAPRE) technique has been proposed as a more adaptable progressive exercise program than the Oxford or DeLorme approaches (see Table 5-1).[29] This program eliminates arbitrary decisions about the frequency and amount of weight increase. The DAPRE program can be used with free weights or with weight machines. A 6 RM is used to establish the initial working weight. Thereafter, weight increases are based on the performance during the previous training session.

These guidelines have been based on studies of uninjured subjects. When treating a patient with specific impairments, the resistive exercise dosage varies.[30] Exercise should be performed to substitution or form fatigue, the point at which substitution or alterations in form occur.

Duration/Volume

Duration or volume of resistive training can be considered the number of sets or repetitions of a specific exercise session. Most exercises are performed for a given number of repetitions and sets that can be considered the exercise duration or volume. In rehabilitation, resistive exercises might also be prescribed for a certain time interval such as 15, 30, or 60 seconds depending upon the goal.

In weight training for fitness, volume is often defined as the total number of repetitions performed during a training session multiplied by the resistance used. Intensity and volume are inversely related. The greater the intensity, the fewer repetitions are performed. When training at a low RM (near the 1 RM or maximum amount of weight that can be lifted), very few repetitions are performed, and strength gains are the chief goal. When training at 10 RM or higher, many repetitions are performed, and the goals are endurance and other aspects of muscle performance.

Very little stimulus is necessary to make strength gains in the beginner. In untrained individuals, one set of 10 RM, two to four times per week, may be adequate. In advanced or elite athletes, multiple set routines, three times per week, will be necessary to achieve strength and power gains. For this group, performing one set of an exercise is less effective for increasing strength than performing two or three sets, and there is

TABLE 5-1 Common Strength Training Dosages and DAPRE Program and Adjustments

TECHNIQUE	BASE REPETITION MAXIMUM (RM)	SETS	NUMBER OF REPETITIONS
DeLorme	10	1. 50% of 10 RM 2. 75% of 10 RM 3. 100% of 10 RM	10 10 10
Oxford	10	1. 100% of 10 RM 2. 75% of 10 RM 3. 50% of 10 RM	10 10 10
DAPRE	6	1. 50% of 6 RM 2. 75% of 6 RM 3. 100% of 6 RM 4. Adjusted weight based on number of reps performed in set 3[a]	10 6 As many as possible As many as possible, this number of reps is used to determine the working weight for the next day[a]

NUMBER OF REPETITIONS	ADJUSTED WORKING	ADJUSTED WORKING
Performed in set 3[a]	Weight for set 4[a]	Weight for next day[a]
0–2	Decrease 5–10 lb	Decrease 5–10 lb
3–4	Decrease 0–5 lb	Same weight
5–6	Keep weight the same	Increase 5–10 lb
7–10	Increase 5–10 lb	Increase 5–15 lb
11	Increase 10–15 lb	Increase 10–20 lb

[a]Adjustments for the DAPRE program.

evidence that three sets are more effective than two sets.[31] However, multiple sets pose higher risk for injury; therefore, careful technique must be employed to avoid injury.

For most individuals, a moderate training volume is sufficient to achieve strength gains and these gains can be made via any resistive training mode.[32] A review of meta-analyses concluded that a dosage of 60% of 1 RM, 3 days per week with a mean training volume of four sets per muscle group produced optimal strength gains in untrained subjects.[33] For recreationally trained nonathletes, an intensity of 80% of 1 RM, 2 days per week with a mean training volume of four sets per muscle group was best. Finally, for athletes, a training of 85% of 1 RM, 2 days per week with a mean training volume of eight sets per muscle group was necessary for optimal strength gains.

The rest interval between sets is another important variable to consider. Much research has been performed to determine the optimal rest interval to achieve different resistive training goals. Some controversy exists regarding single versus multiple sets and the length of the rest interval between sets.[34,35] Strength results might change when training at different rest intervals. Rest intervals will vary from <1 minute to 3 to 5 minutes depending on the intensity of the lift and the purpose of the training. The higher intensity required for strength training will necessitate longer rest intervals. For loads near 1 RM, a rest interval of 3 to 5 minutes allows for more recovery and the ability to train at a higher intensity for more repetitions.[34] For power training, a minimum of 3 minutes rest between activities such as plyometric jumps, will retain the necessary intensity. When training for muscle endurance, a circuit program with approximately 30 seconds between sets is sufficient. Muscles can be overloaded by decreasing the rest interval between sets.

Frequency

Training frequency depends on the rehabilitation goals. Isometric exercise is performed several times per day, and heavy dynamic exercise may be performed every other day. Frequency of one exercise is related to the exercise goal, intensity, duration, and other exercises in the patient's rehabilitation program. Individuals training for power lifting or body building lift daily or twice daily, whereas individuals in rehabilitation programs may perform resistive exercise 3 days per week and cardiovascular exercise on alternate days. Be sure to allow adequate time for recovery between training sessions. Shortening the recovery period between training sessions can produce persistent fatigue.[36]

Studies provide a variety of frequency recommendations, and these need to be balanced with intensity, duration, initial training status, and the goals of the training. Progressive resistive exercise training one time weekly with 1 RM for one set increases strength significantly after the first week of training and each week up to at least the sixth week.[31] Significant increases have occurred for beginners training 1 to 5 days per week.

Sequence

The sequence of training muscles can affect the development of strength. In general, multijoint exercises are advocated for strength and power gains. However, specific isolated muscle training is often necessary when rehabilitating individuals with impaired muscle performance. These exercises should be performed first before the patient gets fatigued. Follow these exercises with multijoint functional movement patterns. For training novice, intermediate, and advanced individuals wanting to increase strength, the American

College of Sports Medicine (ACSM) provides the following recommendations[37]:

- exercise large muscle groups before small and perform multijoint before single-joint activities
- when training all major muscle groups in one training session, rotate upper body and lower body activities
- when training upper body and lower body muscles on different days, alternate agonist and antagonist exercises
- when training individual muscle groups, perform higher intensity exercises before lower intensity exercises

Program Design

Program design simply means looking at the overall training session. This includes the activity sequence discussed in the previous section as well as overarching issues like interval training and circuit training. **Interval training** is a type of training that is used predominantly to build anaerobic metabolic systems, although depending upon the work:rest ratio, it can be used to train aerobic systems as well. Interval training prescription includes the exercise intensity and duration as well as the duration and activity for the relief interval.[2,6] The relief interval can be either passive (rest-relief) or active (active, or work-relief). The relationship of work:relief can vary from 1:1 or 1:1.5 when training the aerobic system to 1:12 to 1:20 when training the phosphagen system. The combination of high intensity and short duration places greater loads on the phosphagen system and requires a longer relief interval. A longer work interval (3 minutes or more) works the aerobic system, minimizing the necessity of a long relief interval. Interval training methods can be applied to resistance training by using weight equipment (free weights, variable resistance machines, elastic resistance) and training to obtain a certain number of repetitions within a given time frame. The relief interval can again be a passive rest interval or an active interval such as performing active movement without resistance, stretching, or another light activity. Interval training will be discussed in greater depth in Chapter 6 relative to the cardiopulmonary system.

Circuit training usually includes 8 to 15 exercise stations that are completed in a sequence or circuit. The stations can be general training for the major muscle groups, serving as a general fitness routine or a complement to a sports training program, or they can be specific. For example, a swimming team might perform circuit training 3 days per week with exercises focused on preventing injuries specific to swimmers. Exercises can be all one mode (i.e., variable resistance machines) or they can be a combination of stations such as variable resistance machines, free weights, elastic resistance and functional skills such as jumping. Participants complete two or three circuits at a given intensity depending upon goals with a prespecified relief interval of 15 to 30 seconds between stations. When designing the circuit, keep in mind the sequence considerations discussed previously.

Training Specificity

Training specificity suggests that "you get what you train for." The SAID principle (**S**pecific **A**daptations to **I**mposed **D**emands) embodies the notion of the idea first put forth in Wolff law. Wolff law states that bone will adapt to the loads placed upon it. The soft tissue corollary is called Davis law and states that soft tissues will remodel according to the loads placed upon them.[38] This specificity is particularly significant in terms of training range, mode, contraction type, and velocity.[39–41]

The greatest training effects are evident when the same exercise type is used for testing and training, although this principle varies by muscle contraction types. A muscle trained isometrically will show the greatest strength improvement when tested isometrically and a muscle trained dynamically will test stronger when evaluated dynamically. However, a study of concentric and eccentric quadriceps training found that specificity was related to eccentric training but not concentric training.[42] Concentric training showed increases only in concentric and isometric strength.[43] Studies have shown bilateral transfer; training one limb resulted in strength gains in the contralateral limb.[39,44] Further studies of bilateral versus unilateral training have shown improved bilateral scores when training bilaterally and improved unilateral scores when training unilaterally. These findings were consistent for upper extremity and lower extremity training.[45]

Range of motion (ROM) specificity also exists; strength improvements are greatest at the joint angles exercised.[40] A study of eccentric training showed isometric strength gains that were joint angle specific; a similar study of concentric training showed improvements throughout the range.[44]

The effects of posture on the specificity of training were assessed using squat and bench press lifts as the training tool. A variety of tests followed an 8-week training session that included skills such as vertical jump, 40-m sprint, isokinetic tests, and a 6-second bout on a power bicycle. The authors found results to support the concept of posture specificity, because the exercise postures similar to the training postures enabled the greatest improvements.[46]

The importance of training specificity is highlighted by the many variables affecting strength development. If the muscular system were the only system involved, then strength development would be predictable and linear. However, functional strength development is a complex relationship between the muscle tissue and the neural system dedicated to that tissue. This includes local and central nervous system mechanisms.

This specificity of exercise is evident to anyone who has trained for one activity (i.e., running) and subsequently discovered little transfer to another activity (i.e., tennis). Even resistive training, while providing a good strength base, does not transfer to other activities, even activities using the same muscle group. For example, a group of 12 men trained in a traditional isotonic strength program for knee flexor and extensor muscles.[47] They were tested isokinetically before and after the 12-week program. Their isotonic strength increased nearly 227% while their isokinetic strength at 60 degrees per second increased only 10%. Therefore it is important that resistive training serve as the training base upon which functional training is imposed.

Neurologic Adaptation

Muscle performance is determined by the type and size of the involved muscles and by the ability of the nervous system to appropriately activate muscles. The muscles responsible for producing the large force in the intended direction, called **agonists**, must be fully activated. Muscles that assist in coordinating the movement, called **synergists**, must be appropriately activated to ensure precision of rotating parts. Muscles producing force in the opposite direction of the agonists, called **antagonists**, must be appropriately activated or relaxed. The joint alignment and muscular recruitment patterns at the trunk, pelvis, hips, knees, ankles, and feet can alter which muscles are activated and when. For example, when performing a squat or step-up, the position of the center of gravity can determine whether or not the hamstring muscles are activated to co-contract and stabilize the knee. When an unfamiliar exercise is introduced into the resistive exercise program, the early increase in strength partially results from adaptive changes in the nervous system control. The clinician must ensure appropriate nervous system control over the movement pattern for the desired outcome. Inappropriate instruction or failure to monitor the exercise can render it ineffective or detrimental to the expected outcome.

DeLorme and Watkins[26] hypothesize that the initial increase in strength after PRE occurs at a rate greater than can be accounted for by muscle morphologic changes. The initial rapid increases in strength probably result from motor learning. When a new exercise is introduced, neural adaptation predominates in the first several weeks of training as the individual masters the coordination necessary to perform the exercise efficiently. Subsequently, hypertrophic factors gradually dominate over neural factors in the gain in muscle performance.[47] Although neurologic adaptations were once thought to dominate in the first few weeks of training, Staron et al.[48] found that morphologic changes begin to occur in the second week of training.

Other adaptations, such as the ability to fire motor units at very high rates to develop power, may require a longer period of training to attain and be lost more rapidly during detraining.[49] In the long term, further improvement in performance critically depends on the way the muscles are activated by the nervous system during training.[50]

Muscle Fatigue

Muscle fatigue may be defined as a reversible decrease in contractile strength that occurs after long-lasting or repeated muscular activity.[51] Human fatigue is a complex phenomenon that includes failure at more than one site along the chain of events that leads to muscle fiber stimulation. Fatigue involves a central component, which puts an upper limit to the number of command signals that are sent to the muscles, and a peripheral component. Peripheral changes in cross-bridge function associated with fatigue include a slight decrease in number of interacting cross-bridges, reduced force output of the individual cross-bridge, and reduced speed of cycling of the bridges during muscle shortening (Table 5-2).

When the patient is performing resistive training, be alert for signs of fatigue. Fatigue can lead to substitution or injury. The dosage for resistive exercise is often limited to *form fatigue*, the point at which the individual must discontinue the exercise or sacrifice technique.

Quality of motion usually is the most important factor in prescribing any exercise. Although this seems quite obvious, it is a concept that is often neglected. With resistive exercise, the patient cannot expect gains in force or torque production unless the muscle is recruited during the movement pattern. Because synergists can readily dominate a movement pattern, take care to ensure precision of motion during all exercise prescription. After the form is compromised (i.e., form fatigue), stop the exercise. Continuing to exercise with poor technique compromises the outcome and may be detrimental.

An example of the importance of technique is the traditional sit-up with and without holding the feet. Kendall et al.[22] provides a detailed analysis of muscle function during the sit-up. For this exercise, trunk muscle activation must be differentiated from hip flexor activation. For proper form, the trunk flexion phase must precede the hip flexion phase

---

TABLE 5-2 Chain of Events Leading to a Muscle Contraction

CHAIN OF EVENTS LEADING TO A MUSCLE CONTRACTION (ANATOMIC SITES OF FATIGUE)		MECHANISMS INVOLVED IN PROCESSING INFORMATION THROUGH THE CHAIN OF EVENTS (PHYSIOLOGIC PROCESSES RESPONSIBLE FOR FATIGUE)	
Central fatigue	Limbic, premotor, and association cortices ↓	Insufficient motivation or incentive	
	Sensorimotor cortex ↓	Insufficient cortical motoneuron activation	
	Spinal cord ↓	Depressed alpha motoneuron excitability	
Peripheral fatigue	Peripheral motoneurons ↓	Failure in neural transmission	Processes involved in delivery of sufficient electrical excitation from CNS to muscle
	Neuromuscular junction ↓	Failure in neuromuscular transmission	
	Sarcolemma ↓	Depressed muscle membrane excitability	
	Transverse tubules ↓	Failure of muscle action potential propagation	
	Sacroplasmic reticulum ↓	Insufficient release and/or reuptake of Ca^{3+}	Metabolic and enzymatic processes involved in providing sufficient energy for contraction
	Formation of actin-myosin cross-bridges ↓	Failure in excitation-contraction coupling, insufficient energy supplies, inadequate energy supply replenishment, metabolic accumulation	
	Muscle contraction		

From Currier DP, Nelson RM. Dynamics of Human Biologic Tissues. Philadelphia, PA: FA Davis, 1992:165.

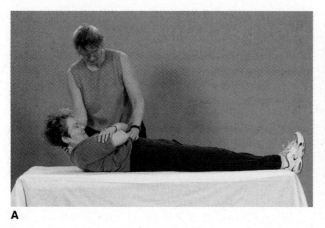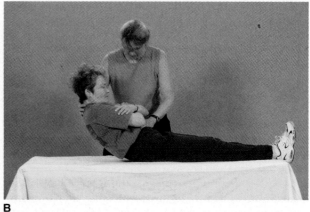

FIGURE 5-7. Two phases of a sit-up. (A) Trunk curl phase. (B) Hip flexion phase. Note: Refer to Chapter 17 for indications/contraindications for bent-knee versus straight-leg sit-up.

(Fig. 5-7). When the feet are free, the abdominal muscles tilt the pelvis posteriorly as the head and shoulders are raised. With the feet stabilized, the hip flexors are given distal fixation, and the trunk raising may become a hip flexor activity (Fig. 5-8). The trunk flexion phase is bypassed, and the motion is primarily hip flexion. Recruitment of the abdominal muscles is minimized, and recruitment of the hip flexors is maximized. When performing abdominal curls, the individual may exhibit proper technique for a few repetitions but then slip into faulty technique, or form fatigue, as the abdominal muscles fatigue. With the feet free, abdominal muscle fatigue results in an inability to complete the trunk curl and the feet will raise in an attempt to use the hip flexors. To ensure proper testing or training of the abdominal muscles, do not hold the feet during the trunk flexion phase.

As in the previous example, the proper exercise may be prescribed but performed incorrectly, therefore not achieving the desired result of increased abdominal strength. It is not good enough to perform the exercise; it must be performed correctly and with the appropriate recruitment pattern. *A person cannot strengthen a muscle that is not being recruited.*

Muscle Soreness

During resistive training, especially in an untrained state, minor lesions of the muscle structure and inflammation resulting in muscle soreness are common. Most people who

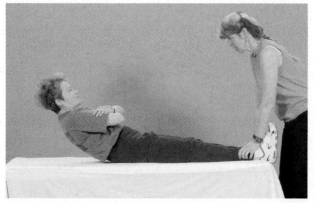

FIGURE 5-8. Improperly performed sit-up, with only a hip flexion phase. Note: Refer to Chapter 17 for indications/contraindications for bent-knee versus straight-leg sit-up.

initiate a resistive exercise program will feel some stiffness and soreness in the exercised muscles following activity. Soreness may be caused by myofibrillar damage localized to the Z band, membrane damage, or inflammatory processes. The serum or plasma level of creatine kinase is elevated and is an indicator of muscle damage, because the enzyme is found almost exclusively in muscle tissue.

A specific type of muscle soreness referred to as **delayed-onset muscle soreness** (DOMS) is common following exercises with a strong eccentric component. Delayed soreness, clearly linked to eccentric activity, usually peaks about 2 days after exertion and lasts for up to 7 days. Muscle function deteriorates, and muscle strength may be reduced for a week or more after intensive eccentric exercise. However, an adaptive process reduces the soreness after repeated training sessions.[52] The unaccustomed eccentric exercise and associated high muscle forces damage the sarcolemms causing a release of enzymes and myoglobin. Damage occurs to the muscle contractile and noncontractive structures, and abnormal metabolite accumulation in the muscle cell produces additional damage. Because eccentric contractions utilize a smaller number of motor units than concentric contractions, the excess stress on these motor units appears to be the source of tissue damage.[53] This results in the pain and inflammation associated with DOMS. The inflammation initiates the healing process, resulting in an adaptive process, protecting the muscle from similar damage in subsequent exercise bouts.[2]

Even during the soreness period, moderate activity is advised, because the adaptation response occurs before full recovery and restoration of muscle function. A single session of eccentric exercise provides a protective effect against DOMS in subsequent exercise bouts for up to 6 weeks.[2] Therefore when initiating a resistive training program that includes eccentrics, it is best to begin with a light exercise session to protect against significant DOMS.

Patients should be cautioned that eccentric training may lead to muscle soreness 24 to 48 hours after exercise, but that moderate exercise should continue during the recovery period. However, some research has shown attenuation of position sense and joint reaction angle following a bout of eccentric exercise.[54] Therefore, some caution is necessary in some populations such as female athletes, the elderly, and individuals performing work functions in at-risk environments (i.e., steel workers, roofers). A somewhat different type of soreness and reduced muscle function may occur during very long and intense exercise bouts. It is probably related to the total metabolic load, not muscle tension development.[52]

Lifespan Considerations

Prepuberty

Only about 20% of a newborn child's body mass is muscle tissue. The infant is weak, and muscular strengthening in the first months takes place by spontaneous movements. These movements should not be limited by tight clothes or constant bundling of the newborn. However, the infant and toddler should not be burdened with systematic resistive training; normal developmental progression provides an appropriate stimulus for the development of an optimal amount of muscular strength.

In the prepubertal phase, muscle mass increases parallel to body mass. Children are able to make strength gains above and beyond growth and maturation. Benefits of exercise in this age group include improved muscle performance, increased motor performance, improved body composition, an enhanced sense of well-being, and a positive attitude toward fitness. Moderate strength training is acceptable, but heavy resistance should be avoided because of the sensitivity of joint structures, especially at the epiphyses of bones. Resistive training at this age should focus on technique and the neurologic aspects of training. Maximum lifts are contraindicated, and submaximal resistive training focused on form is preferred (8 to 12 repetitions per set or more). During prepuberty, there are no differences between girls and boys with respect to trainability for strength. Boys have a small genetic advantage, which is completely compensated by the developmental advantage of girls.[55] There is no biologic basis for a sex-dependent difference in strength performance. Any difference in the strength between girls and boys, particularly in the shoulders and arms, appears to result from social expectations and gender roles in society. Muscle performance training should always be supervised by knowledgeable staff to avoid risk of injury. For improved strength gains, a frequency of 2 days per week is superior to 1 day per week in children beginning an introductory strength training program.[56]

Puberty

The ability to improve strength increases rapidly during puberty, particularly in boys. The increase in male sexual hormones is significant because of their anabolic (i.e., protein-incorporating) component. During maturation, the proportion of muscle in boys increases from 27% to 40% of body mass.[55] With the onset of puberty, the strengths of girls and boys diverge markedly. On average, the strength of girls is 90% that of boys at 11 to 12 years of age, 85% at 13 to 14 years, and 75% at 15 to 16 years.[55] Although this gender difference has a biologic basis, it does not completely account for the differences seen, suggesting continued societal influences.

General strength training is recommended during this phase. Optimal strength and muscular balance is critical for the quickly growing skeleton. Some precautions during strength exercise are still warranted. The epiphyses remain sensitive and liable to injury. Avoid heavy loads, unilateral burdens, or faulty techniques to prevent epiphyseal damage.

Early Adulthood

Strength potential is at its highest in the 18- to 30-year period.[56] The competent biologic structures show a state of good adaptability, the joints tolerate high loads, and the social situation makes specific use of strength necessary. Most individuals are actively involved in physical activity without the responsibility of working long hours. During this period, emphasis should be placed on a balanced fitness program for cardiopulmonary fitness, muscle performance, and flexibility.

Middle Age

The decrement of strength during this phase of life must be differentiated according to training activities, gender, and body area. Training for as little as 2 hours or more each week is sufficient to positively influence strength. A small amount of training increases the difference between active and inactive persons with increasing age. Persons from white-collar professions have the same or even more strength than persons from blue-collar professions; leisure time activities account more for existing strength than professional demands.[57]

Advanced Age

The body can adapt to strengthening exercise throughout the lifespan. It is possible to reverse existing muscular weakness in old age.[58] Strength increases result from relatively low stimuli because of the marked atrophy present at the onset of training in many elderly individuals. A study of older men (mean age, 70 years) demonstrated that the training-induced strength gains resulted from neural factors, as indicated by the increases in maximal integrated electromyography (EMG) in the absence of hypertrophy.[45] Neural factors are a significant mechanism by which older subjects increase strength in the absence of any significant evidence of hypertrophy. In general, fatigability increases with advancing age, and older muscles require a longer period of recovery after strenuous exertion. There is also a significant increase in the collagen content of muscle with advancing age. This is associated with thickening of the connective tissue and increased muscle stiffness.

The decrease in muscle performance with advancing age affects men and women differently. The absolute decline in strength is less steep in women than in men. Parts of the body are also affected differently. The arms are more affected than the trunk and legs, probably because of less use of the upper extremities in strength-related activities. Active elderly women surpass inactive men with respect to trunk muscle strength.

Adequate muscle strength helps to prevent or moderate the symptoms of degenerative changes of the joints. Resistive exercise by the elderly should be directed toward the muscles susceptible to atrophic changes.[60] Priority should be given to the deep neck flexors, scapular stabilizers, abdominal muscles, gluteal muscles, and quadriceps. Unjustifiably, little attention is paid to strength of the ventilatory muscles (i.e., diaphragm) and pelvic floor muscles. Training should include both multiple joint and single joint exercises, performed at moderate loads for one to three sets of 8 to 12 repetitions.

Additionally, the elderly should consider training for power, not just strength. Leg power has been shown to significantly influence the physical performance of mobility-limited elderly people.[61,62] In some cases, power training has been found to be more effective at improving physical function than traditional strength training[62–64] Fielding et al.[65] found high velocity resistance training to increase muscle power more effectively than low velocity training in older women. Power training in this group should include light to moderate loads performed for 6 to 10 repetitions with high velocity.

See Chapters 17 through 26 for resistive exercises for the spine, shoulder, arm, hip, knee, and pelvic floor.

With advancing age, the social needs and individual motivation for the use of strength lessen; the atrophy reflects the effects of disuse, not mere age-related changes. The voluntary and deliberate use of the motor system in daily life activities and intentional resistive training are able to counteract the loss of muscle mass with increasing age. The vigorous use of muscles, particularly among old persons, improves their health and sense of well-being.

Cognitive Aspects of Performance

The cognitive or mental aspects of strength and performance are most easily seen in elite athletes. The use of mental imagery techniques such as visualization and positive self-talk has been supported by sport psychologists and athletes alike. Positive cognitive strategies can enhance strength and performance, and negative strategies may have a negative or negligible impact. A study of different mental preparation techniques (i.e., arousal, attention, imagery, self-efficacy, and control-read conditions) showed that preparatory arousal and self-efficacy techniques produced greater posttest strength performance than in the control group.[66] A similar study showed no difference among the mental preparation conditions, but all performed significantly better than a control group.[67]

Some types of mental preparation can have a negligible or negative impact on strength performance. A study of relaxation-visualization training by non–strength-trained men showed poorer knee extensor measures for them than a control group. The investigators suggested that this training diverted their full concentration away from the exercise task.[68] A mental task requiring subjects to imagine situations making them angry or fearful produced increased levels of arousal but no change in strength performance.[69]

A study of the impact of imagery, preparatory arousal, and counting backward on hand grip strength found imagery to enhance grip strength in older and younger subjects.[70] Gould et al.[71] found that imagery and preparatory arousal improved strength performance. Different kinds of imagery and their impacts on power and endurance activities (i.e., seated shot-put and push-ups to exhaustion) have been studied. Results show that all imagery techniques have a positive impact and that using metaphors is particularly effective in improving power and endurance measures.[72]

The knowledge of results of isokinetic peak torque output (i.e., visual feedback) provides an important error-correction function. This type of training may help patients develop cognitive strategies that can be used to guide performance in clinical and nonclinical settings.[73] Studies suggest that mental preparation and the current mental state can affect strength performance. Consider this when performing and interpreting the results of resistive tests.

Effects of Alcohol

The deleterious effects of alcohol abuse on muscle have been well documented.[74] The myopathic changes seen in the alcoholic patient have at times been attributed to malnutrition or disuse. Experiments have demonstrated that, even with nutritional support and prophylactic exercise, normal subjects can develop alcoholic myopathy if they ingest large amounts of ethanol.[75]

Alcoholic myopathy has two clinical phases: an acutely painful presentation that follows "binges" and a chronic phase that consists of morphologic and functional alterations in muscle.[76] Acute alcoholic myopathy has morphologic features, such as fiber necrosis, intracellular edema, hemorrhage, and inflammatory changes, that can be seen under light microscope. Binges by chronic alcoholics can result in an acute myopathy characterized by muscle cramps, muscle weakness, tenderness, myoglobinuria, reduced muscle phosphorylase activity, and decreased lactate response to ischemic exercise. Exercise is contraindicated for persons with acute myopathy and those with myoglobinuria, because it may stress an already compromised system.

Changes seen in chronic alcoholic myopathy include intracellular edema, lipid droplets, excessive glycogen deposition, deranged elements of the sarcoplasmic reticulum, and abnormal mitochondria. Type II fiber atrophy has also been attributed to chronic alcohol abuse.[77] Type II atrophy suggests that alcoholic patients may exhibit specific deficits in muscle performance, such as an inability to generate tension rapidly and to produce power. For many patients, abstinence leads to full recovery of muscle function, but for others, the injury may be more severe and resistant to treatment, and this must be considered as a comorbidity when projecting the prognosis.

Effects of Corticosteroids

The widespread use of oral corticosteroid agents as anti-inflammatory and immunosuppressant agents has led to cases of steroid atrophy.[78] The primary biopsy finding in patients treated with prednisonelike steroids (e.g., prednisone, prednisolone, methylprednisolone) is type II fiber atrophy.[78] This reduction is thought to be most pronounced in type IIB fibers[79] and is believed to occur more often in women than men.[80] Corticosteroids are a potent catabolic stimuli, and the atrophy caused by prolonged corticosteroid use occurs as protein degradation exceeds protein synthesis. Goldberg and Goodman[81] believe that the constant use of the type I fibers during normal voluntary movement provides these fibers with a protective or sparing influence from the catabolic effects of steroids. Exercises recruiting type II muscle fibers may protect them from steroid-induced atrophy. Normal function can be expected to return within 1 year or, more often, within several months after steroid use has stopped.[80]

CAUSES OF DECREASE MUSCLE PERFORMANCE

Muscle performance can be impaired for a variety of reasons. Central or peripheral neurologic pathology decreases an individual's ability to effectively recruit and functionally use his muscles. Injury to the muscle from a strain or contusion decreases performance, as does disuse or deconditioning for any reason. The goal of examination/evaluation of muscle performance is to determine the *cause* of the impairment to develop the most efficient and comprehensive intervention plan. The following section discusses the potential factors that can cause impaired muscle performance, examination/evaluation results of each potential cause, and general intervention concepts for each specific cause.

Neurologic Pathology

Neurologic pathology can affect the contractile capacity of muscle as a result of pathology in the central or peripheral nervous system. The peripheral nervous system can be affected at the nerve root or peripheral nerve level.

Individuals with nerve root pathology may present with muscle performance impairments in the nerve root distribution. For example, nerve root compression at the L4–5 spinal level can produce quadriceps femoris weakness, while nerve root compression at the C5–6 spinal level can result in deltoid and biceps weakness. Therapeutic exercise intervention depends on the prognosis for the nerve root involvement. If the changes are relatively recent and resolution of the nerve root compression is expected through conservative or surgical management, preventive and protective measures are taken. The goal of therapeutic exercise intervention is not only to promote optimal muscle performance of the muscles innervated by the affected spinal segment (pending prognosis) but also promote spine stability and optimal movement patterns to alleviate any mechanical cause of nerve root pathology incurred by the spinal segment(s) (see Chapters 17 and 23). Peripherally, use resistive exercise to maintain/improve current strength levels, while training inner lumbar or cervical core and girdle muscles to provide proximal stability. Centrally, use resistive exercise to train inner core muscles (i.e., longus coli, transversus abdominis, lumbar multifidus, pelvic floor; see Chapters 18, 19, and 24 for detailed muscle performance training) to effectively stabilize the spine and relieve mechanical nerve root irritants. After the mechanical or chemical cause of nerve root injury is remediated, use specific, localized resistive exercise of the involved musculature to restore precise recruitment patterns.

Neurologic weakness may also result from a peripheral nerve injury. Compromise of the median nerve at the carpal tunnel, the radial nerve at the cubital tunnel, or the common peroneal nerve at the fibular head are examples of such injury. The pattern of sensory loss and weakness depends on which nerve and where along the nerve's course the damage occurs. Therapeutic exercise should be focused on remediating the mechanical cause of the peripheral nerve injury. For example, a depressed shoulder girdle may contribute to traction on the long thoracic nerve, causing motor changes in the serratus anterior. Exercise and posture education to elevate the shoulder girdles may alleviate the traction on the long thoracic nerve and ultimately restore normal innervation to the serratus anterior. Resistive exercise should also focus on maintaining and increasing the strength of the unaffected motor units in the involved musculature, and progressively strengthening motor units on reinnervation. Take care to avoid excessive strengthening of intact muscles for fear of creating significant muscle imbalance. Exercise should try to maintain muscle balance and efficient movement patterns without developing a dominant muscle group. Splinting, bracing, taping, or other supportive measures may be necessary to maintain balance.

Other neurologic conditions include neuromuscular disease such as multiple sclerosis, postpolio syndrome, and Guillain-Barré syndrome, and muscular paralysis or paresis resulting from spinal cord injury or cerebral vascular accident (CVA). Resistive exercise programs must consider the prognosis and tailor the exercises appropriately. In situations such as Guillain-Barré syndrome, certain cases of spinal cord injury and CVA, and progressive stages of multiple sclerosis, some recovery is expected. Exercise programs focus on maintaining strength in intact musculature and gently strengthening weakened muscles as recovery and remission advances. Avoid fatiguing weakened muscles during strengthening exercises. Dosage parameters generally include several short exercise sessions of a few repetitions interspersed throughout the day. During quiescent periods of diseases such as multiple sclerosis, a general conditioning program of balanced strengthening and mobility exercises is appropriate. When recovery is not expected, resistive exercise programs emphasize functional strength of remaining musculature. This includes strength for functional activities such as self-care, transfers, and mobility. Take care to avoid overworking these muscles. Unlike persons with full innervation who use their muscles efficiently, the individual with paralysis uses the few innervated muscles they have for nearly all their activities. The potential for overuse injuries is very high.

Muscle Strain

Muscle strain occurs along a continuum from acute macrotraumatic injury to chronic microtraumatic overuse injuries (see Chapter 11). Resistive exercise in the treatment of muscle strain injuries depends on where along this continuum the injury occurs. Resistive exercise that neither overloads nor underloads the tissue is optimal. Determining this resistance dosage is the challenge.

Acute traumatic injuries occur when a muscle is rapidly overloaded or overstretched and the tension generated exceeds the tensile capability of the musculotendinous unit.[82] The hamstring muscle is a common site of muscle strain injury. A combination of insufficient strength, reduced extensibility, inadequate warm-up, and fatigue has been implicated in hamstring injuries[83] (see Patient-Related Instruction 5-1: Preventing Muscle Strain). Strength, extensibility, and fatigue resistance protect a muscle from strain injury.

Eccentric loading is a common mechanism of muscle strain injury, and a muscle prepared for eccentric loading is less likely to sustain an injury. Eccentric loading should be an integral part of any resistance training program (see Selected Intervention 5-1: Lateral Kicks for an example of eccentric loading). A program to prevent muscle strain injuries should include dynamic resistive exercises with a strong eccentric component, flexibility exercises, an appropriate warm-up before activity, and attention to fatigue levels. The rehabilitation program after injury should also focus on these factors.

Patient-Related Instruction 5-1

Preventing Muscle Strain

Although some muscle strains are not preventable, precautions can reduce your risk of injury.

1. Warm-up before a vigorous activity; 5 to 7 minutes of a large muscle group activity such as walking, jogging, or cycling should suffice. This should be enough activity to break a sweat.
2. Stretch stiff and short muscles after your general warm-up. Stretch each muscle for 15 to 30 seconds for four repetitions.
3. Balance your sports or other leisure activities with strengthening exercises. Your clinician can help you focus on muscles susceptible to injury.
4. Avoid fatigue during the activity. Fatigue can increase your risk of injury.
5. Strengthen underused muscles to prevent overuse to susceptible muscles. Your clinician can help you determine which muscles these are and what specific exercises you need to perform to maintain muscle balance.

SELECTED INTERVENTION 5-1
Lateral Kicks

See Case Study No. 1

Although this patient requires comprehensive intervention as described in other chapters, only one exercise related to resistive training is described. This exercise would be used in the late phase of this patient's rehabilitation.

ACTIVITY: Resisted hip abduction and ankle eversion

PURPOSE: To increase the muscle performance of the ankle evertor and hip abductor muscles.

STAGE OF MOTOR CONTROL: Controlled mobility

MODE: Resistive band

POSTURE: Standing with one foot on the resistive band and the band around the other foot. A support should be readily available for balance as needed.

MOVEMENT: Standing on the uninjured leg, abduct the hip in the frontal plane, and evert (pronate) the ankle. Maintain good spinal posture throughout the exercise. Do not hike pelvis. Move only at the hip joint. Avoid moving out of the frontal plane. Moving toward flexion results in the motion performed by the flexor abductor group. Return to the start position.

DOSAGE: Two to three sets per day to form fatigue. If patient does not fatigue by 20 repetitions, increase the resistance of the band.

EXPLANATION OF PURPOSE OF EXERCISE: This exercise increases muscle performance in the hip abductors and ankle evertors in a synergistic fashion. Abductors are strengthened in both concentric and eccentric modes. It may be progressed to a higher speed to challenge stability.

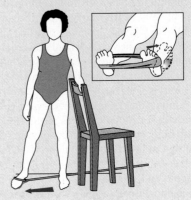

Muscles may also be strained from chronic overuse. For example, extensor digitorum longus (EDL) strain is common in workers performing continuous repetitive elbow, wrist, and hand activities as a result of using the EDL for wrist extension and elbow flexion. Training the individual to use the biceps for elbow flexion whenever possible (i.e., keep the hand supinated versus pronated during elbow flexion) can alleviate the overuse strain to the EDL. A thorough evaluation can determine the cause of the overuse problem. Ergonomic assessment and appropriate work site modification are also necessary to prevent a recurrence of the strain if ergonomics are at the root of undesirable posture or movement patterns. If left untreated, this impairment can quickly lead to disability.

Strain resulting from muscle dominance overuse is managed by reducing the loads imposed on the strained muscle. When the tensor fasciae latae dominates over the iliopsoas during hip flexion and gluteus medius during abduction, the tensor fasciae latae is at risk for an overuse strain. Improving the strength and recruitment patterns of the iliopsoas and gluteus medius can reduce the load on the tensor fasciae latae and allow it to recover. Postural habits (e.g., standing in medial rotation) and movement patterns (e.g., hip flexion or abduction with medial rotation) must also be modified to improve recruitment of the underused synergists.

A potential risk factor of muscle strain is gradual, continuous overstretching, which occurs when a muscle is continuously placed in a relatively lengthened, tension-producing position. For example, the lower trapezius in a person with forward shoulders is subjected to continuous tension and has adapted to a lengthened state. It may not take much force to produce a strain injury in a muscle that is already overstretched. This type of strain puts the muscle at risk for two forms of muscle weakness, one from length-tension changes and the other from overstretch strain.

Patient education is a key component of the rehabilitation program in the case of muscle strain associated with continuous overstretch. In the lower trapezius example, educate the patient about optimal postural habits to reduce tension on the lower trapezius. Improving postural habits and reducing tension on the lower trapezius with bracing or taping (see Chapter 26) will allow the muscle to heal more rapidly. In addition, it will promote adaptive shortening and therefore ultimately achieve a more optimal length-tension relationship and reduce the risk for future reinjury.

Disuse and Deconditioning

Muscle performance may be impaired because of disuse or deconditioning for a variety of reasons. Illness, surgery, specific physical conditions (e.g., pregnancy with twins), or injury may necessitate a period of decreased activity. Subtle muscle imbalances can lead to overuse of one muscle and to disuse and deconditioning of another.

Illness and injury are common causes of deconditioning. For example, illness such as pneumonia or an injury such as a herniated disk can result in a period of decreased activity and subsequent deconditioning. In these situations, total-body deconditioning occurs, and general conditioning is necessary. However, specific exercises also may be necessary to improve muscle performance and prevent secondary impairments. For example, an elderly individual may have relatively asymptomatic osteoarthritis until a bout with pneumonia produces general deconditioning. Subsequently, knee osteoarthritis becomes symptomatic because of impaired muscle performance in the lower extremity muscles involved in gait and other functional activities. Specific resistive exercises to recondition those muscles are necessary to restore proper biomechanics and prevent further disability.

Reduced activity levels can impair muscle performance in a similar manner. Multiparous pregnancies, exacerbation of a musculoskeletal injury, an episode of colitis, or social factors such as major life changes (e.g., job, school, divorce, family illness, death) can reduce activity levels and result in impaired muscle performance. For example, regular exercise may keep a woman's patellofemoral malalignment from becoming symptomatic. When her activity level decreases in the late stages of pregnancy, the combination of decreased activity, weight gain, and hormonal changes produces symptoms at the patellofemoral joint. Selective resistive exercises combined with patient education can prevent this exacerbation. Resistive exercises in the case of overall decreased activity must consider the muscles most likely to be affected, the patient's desired activity level and preference, and any underlying or residual medical conditions.

An overlooked source of deconditioning or disuse is a subtle muscle imbalance. When activating muscles for a functional movement, the body chooses the most efficient muscular and motor unit activation pattern. Certain motor units in a muscle may be preferentially recruited when a muscle is engaged in a particular task.[84] For example, motor units in the lateral portion of the long head of the biceps are preferentially activated when this muscle is engaged in elbow flexion, whereas motor units in the medial portion are preferentially activated in forearm supination. The recruitment thresholds of motor units in a muscle are also influenced by the type of muscle actions associated with a movement. In elbow flexion, biceps motor units have a lower threshold in slow concentric and eccentric actions than isometric actions; the reverse is true for the brachialis.[85] The recruitment thresholds of motor units of a muscle active in a movement may also be affected by changes in joint angle.[86] Some muscles or portions of a muscle may be overused while other muscles or portions are disused, and the resistive rehabilitation program must acknowledge this imbalance. In the previous example, instruction in general resisted elbow flexion may exacerbate the imbalance whereas specific training of the weaker recruitment pattern can restore muscle balance.

Length-Associated Changes

The principle of the length-tension curve affects muscle performance when a muscle is adaptively lengthened from prolonged posture and repetitive movement patterns of the muscle in the lengthened state. Examination of postural alignment controlled by the muscle suggests that the muscle is longer than ideal as in depressed shoulders or hip adduction and medial rotation. Muscles will test weak in the short range when compared with synergists, paired muscle of the other extremity, or other half of the axial skeleton (i.e., posterior gluteus and tensor fasciae latae, right and left posterior gluteus medius, or right and left external oblique muscles, respectively). As previously mentioned, this is referred to as positional weakness. Intervention should focus on strengthening the muscle in the shortened range, optimizing posture to reduce lengthening tension on the muscle, and altering movement patterns to recruit the muscle in the shortened range.

PHYSIOLOGIC ADAPTATIONS TO TRAINING

Strength and Power

The benefits of resistive exercise extend beyond the obvious improvements in muscle performance to include positive effects on the cardiovascular system, connective tissue, and bone. Moreover, these effects translate into function. Individuals perform their daily activities with more ease because they are functioning at a lower percentage of their maximum capacity. Improved functioning also enhances the patient's sense of well-being and independence. Additionally, strength training has shown crossover effects, where training one limb translates into muscle performance improvements in the contralateral limb.[39,87]

Muscle

The most obvious benefits of resistive training are for the muscular system. Regular resistive exercise is associated with several positive adaptations, most of which are dosage dependent (Table 5-3). The cross-sectional area of the muscle

TABLE 5-3 **Physiologic Adaptations to Resistance Training**	
VARIABLE	**RESULT AFTER RESISTANCE TRAINING**
Performance	
Muscle strength	Increases
Muscle endurance	Increases for high power output
Aerobic capacity	No change or increases slightly
Maximal rate of force production	Increases
Vertical jump	Increases
Anaerobic power	Increases
Sprint speed	Improves
Muscle Fibers	
Fiber size	Increases
Capillary density	No change or decreases
Mitochondrial density	Decreases
Enzyme Activity	
Creatine phosphokinase	Increases
Myokinase	Increases
Phosphofructokinase	Increases
Lactate dehydrogenase	No change or variable
Metabolic Energy Stores	
Stored ATP	Increases
Stored creatine phosphate	Increases
Stored glycogen	Increases
Stored triglycerides	May increase
Connective Tissue	
Ligament strength	May increase
Tendon strength	May increase
Collagen content	May increase
Bone density	Increase
Body Composition	
Percentage of body fat	Decreases
Fat-free mass	Increases

Adapted from Falkel JE, Cipriani DJ. Physiological principles of resistance training and rehabilitation. In: Zachazewski JE, Magee DJ, Quillen WS, eds. Athletic Injuries and Rehabilitation. Philadelphia, PA: WB Saunders, 1996.

increases as a result of an increase in the myofibril volume of individual muscle fibers, fiber splitting, and potentially an increase in the number of muscle fibers. This cross-sectional area increase primarily results from preferential hypertrophy of type II fibers. Changes in the muscle depend on fiber type and the stimulus. Hypertrophy of fast-twitch fibers occurs when all or most of the fibers are being recruited and is considered an adaptation for increased power output. Slow-twitch fibers hypertrophy in response to frequent recruitment. In repetitive, low-intensity activity, fast-twitch fibers are rarely recruited, and these fibers may atrophy while the slow-twitch fibers hypertrophy. A study by Staron et al.[48] examined the differences in the proportion of muscle fiber types in distance runners, weight lifters, and sedentary controls. The investigators found the weight lifters had a greater proportion of type IIA fibers and had a greater type IIA fiber area than the controls or distance runners.[88] Specificity of resistive training exists and must be considered when designing a training program.

Other changes occur on cellular and systemic levels. The capillary density is unchanged or decreases, and the mitochondrial density decreases. Some of these changes result from their number relative to total muscle volume. Although protein volume and cross-sectional area increase in response to resistive training, some of the cellular or systemic factors may remain unchanged, giving the perception of a decrease, although the decrease is only relative.

Energy sources necessary to fuel muscle contraction increase after resistive training. In general, levels of creatine phosphate, ATP, myokinase, and phosphofructokinase increase in response to a resistive exercise program.[89-92] Lactate dehydrogenase is variably changed.[90]

Neural adaptations occur with resistive training. Studies have shown increases in the muscle's ability to produce torque and increased neural activation, as measured by EMG.[49] Increases in muscle activity were also seen after resistive training that consisted of explosive jumping. Increased EMG values associated with greater power and maximal contraction were attributed to a combination of increased motor unit recruitment and increased firing rate of each unit.[93]

Connective Tissue

Although disuse and inactivity cause atrophy and weakening of connective tissues such as tendon and ligament, physical training can increase the maximum tensile strength and the amount of energy absorbed before failure.[94] Physical activity returns damaged tendons and ligaments to normal tensile strength values faster than complete rest.[95] Physical training, particularly resistive exercise, may alter tendon and ligament structures to make them larger, stronger, and more resistant to injury.

Bone

Weightlessness[96] and immobilization[97] can cause profound loss of bone density and mass. Weight-bearing activities that recruit antigravity muscles can maintain or enhance bone density and mass.[98] Weight training, particularly with a weight-bearing component, can substantially alter bone mineral density. Individuals in sports requiring repeated high-force movements such as weight lifting and throwing events have higher bone densities than distance runners or soccer players or swimmers.[99] Those who play tennis regularly have higher bone density in their dominant forearms, and professional pitchers have greater bone density in the dominant humerus.[100]

A 5-month study of weight training compared with jogging found that weight training produced significantly better increases in lumbar bone density than the aerobic exercise.[101]

These studies suggest that regular exercise, specifically exercise such as resistive training, can maintain or improve bone density. Resistive training to improve bone density is important for women of all ages. A study of adolescent female athletes found runners to have higher total body and site-specific bone mineral density than swimmers or cyclists, and that knee extension strength was an independent predictor of bone mineral density in this population.[102] Finally, a study of bone mass and exercise dosage found that daily loading regimens broken down into four sessions with recovery time in between improved bone mass significantly over a loading schedule that performed the training in a single, uninterrupted session.[103] Thus smaller exercise sessions separated by recovery periods may be a better prescription when increased bone mass is the goal.

Cardiovascular System

Resistive training benefits the cardiovascular system. The idea that strength training causes hypertension is erroneous. Most reports show that highly strength-trained athletes have average or lower than average systolic and diastolic blood pressures.[104] When performed properly and heeding the proper precautions, strength training can have a positive effect on the cardiovascular system.

Increased intrathoracic or intra-abdominal pressures may affect cardiac output and blood pressure during resistive exercise. In the classic model, increased intrathoracic pressures are thought to decrease venous return to the heart and decrease cardiac output. Intrathoracic pressure is inversely related to cardiac output and stroke volume and directly related to systolic and diastolic blood pressure during resistive exercise. Increased intrathoracic pressures may limit venous return and decrease cardiac output while causing an accumulation of blood in the systemic circulation that may increase blood pressure. Performing resistive exercises with a Valsalva maneuver, which elevates intrathoracic pressure, leads to a greater blood pressure response than performance of the exercise without a Valsalva maneuver.[105] Instructing the patient to breathe properly during exercise may reduce the increase in blood pressure sometimes seen during exercise.

Increased intramuscular pressure during resistive exercise may result in increased total peripheral resistance and increased blood pressure. Mechanically induced increases in peripheral resistance probably are the cause of higher blood pressures during isometric and concentric exercise compared with pressures during eccentric exercise.[106] Isometric or concentric exercise combined with a Valsalva maneuver can produce the greatest increase in blood pressure. This combination should be avoided, especially by individuals at risk for elevated blood pressure (see the section "Precautions and Contraindications").

Resistive exercise does result in a pressor response that affects the cardiovascular system by causing hypertension through exciting the vasoconstrictor center, which leads to increased peripheral resistance. If precautions are taken to ensure proper breathing and avoid isometric contractions in persons at risk for a pressor response, resistive exercise's benefits outweigh the risks. Long-term performance of resistive exercise can result in positive adaptations of the cardiovascular

DISPLAY 5-2
Benefits of Strength Training on the Cardiovascular System

- Decreased heart rate
- Decreased or unchanged systolic blood pressure
- Decreased or unchanged diastolic blood pressure
- Increased or unchanged cardiac output
- Increased or unchanged stroke volume
- Increased or unchanged maximal oxygen consumption
- Decreased or unchanged total cholesterol

system at rest and during work. Cardiovascular adaptations to resistive training are summarized in Display 5-2.

Endurance

The muscle's response to endurance training is different from its response to strength or power training. This response is expected because of the differences in training dosage. Muscular endurance depends on oxidative capacity, and training increases the muscle's metabolic capacity. Muscular endurance is often limited by a local accumulation of lactate, with glycolysis inhibition and a failure to regenerate ATP in the working muscle.[107] During prolonged activities, depletion of intramuscular glycogen reserves may contribute to impaired muscular endurance.

Muscles trained for endurance demonstrate cells with increased mitochondrial size, number, and enzymatic activity, as well as increased perfusion.[108] Increased enzymatic activity allows the muscle to better use the oxygen delivered, encouraging use of fats as a fuel and sparing glycogen. Muscles that are stronger use a smaller portion of the maximum voluntary contraction force with activity, thereby delaying the onset of muscular fatigue.

Muscles trained for endurance also demonstrate increased local fuel storage. Glycogen stores may be increased twofold, and when endurance training is combined with appropriate carbohydrate intake, stores may increase as much as threefold.[108] In addition to increasing fuel stores, the endurance-trained muscle also increases fatty acid use and decreases the use of glycogen as a fuel. This alteration allows more exercise before fatigue. Endurance muscle training improves the oxygen delivery system by increasing the local capillary network, producing more capillaries per muscle fiber.[108] Increased perfusion slows the accumulation of lactate in the working muscles.

EXAMINATION AND EVALUATION OF MUSCLE PERFORMANCE

Decreases in muscle performance may occur for a number of reasons. A thorough examination is necessary to determine the cause of impaired muscle performance and the link between impaired muscle performance and functional limitations or disabilities. After that relationship is established, the intervention must be matched to the cause of impaired muscle performance. The muscle test is only one small part of the examination process and must be used with additional information (e.g., range of motion, joint mobility, balance, sensory, and reflex integrity) to determine the specific cause of impaired muscle performance.

The tests and measures recommended by the *Guide to Physical Therapist Practice*[109] ensure comprehensive assessment of the patient's impairments, functional limitations, and disability. Within the examination is a subset of measures specific to the performance of the muscle. These tests include an analysis of functional muscle strength, power, or endurance; manual muscle tests; dynamometry; and electrophysiologic testing.

Manual muscle testing is the most fundamental of all strength tests. Length-tension relationships, muscle imbalance, and positional weakness must be considered when choosing manual muscle test positions. Close attention to substitution patterns and testing in a variety of positions minimizes the chance of erroneous results. When used reliably, hand-held dynamometers can provide muscle performance information that is more reliable than that of tests using the traditional criteria of 0 through 5.

Isokinetic dynamometers are commonly used to assess muscle performance. Computerized systems provide tremendous data reduction capabilities. Tests can be performed at a variety of speeds and comparisons made with antagonists, the contralateral limb, normative standards, or previous test results. These tools provide reliable data that can be used to assess progress, as a motivator, or as criteria for progression to more advanced rehabilitation phases. A variety of muscle actions can be assessed using this equipment.

Dynamic strength can also be determined using the RM method. For example, a 10 RM is the maximum amount of weight that can be lifted 10 times, and a 1 RM is the maximum amount of weight that can be lifted once. The amount of weight that can be lifted for a given number of repetitions can be determined and compared with that for the antagonist, the opposite limb, or to a previous test result.

The magnitude of measured increases in force or torque depends on how similar the test is to the training exercise.[110] For example, if athletes train their legs by doing the squat exercise, the increase in strength measured as maximal squatting is much greater than the strength increase measured in isometric leg press or knee extension tests. This specificity of movement pattern in strength training probably reflects the role of learning and coordination.[111] Improved coordination takes the form of the most efficient activation of all of the involved muscles and the most efficient activation of motor units within each muscle involved. Testing force production in the manner in which the muscle has been trained reflects the morphologic and neurologic adaptations.

CLASSIFICATION OF RESISTANCE EXERCISE

Resistive exercise can be broadly classified into categories comparing the force generated by a muscle or muscle group relative to an external load. This external load can be applied by numerous mechanisms such as a machine, a person (manual resistance), a stationary object or body weight. Exercises where the internal force generated matches the externally applied load are considered to be **isometric** exercises. In isometric exercise, no joint motion takes place, although muscle activation occurs. All other activities are **dynamic** involving joint motion. When the external load is less than the force generated by the muscle **concentric** contractions result, whereas when external loads exceed the internally generated force, **eccentric** contractions are produced. Resistance applied at a constant velocity is termed **isokinetic**.

Isometric Exercise

Isometric exercise is commonly used to increase muscle performance. Although no joint movement occurs and technically no work is performed (work = force × distance and distance = 0), isometric exercise is considered functional because it provides a strength base for dynamic exercise and because many postural muscles work primarily in an isometric fashion (see Self-Management 5-1: Cervical Spine Extension for an example of isometric exercise for postural muscles). Eccentric muscle contractions require that a concentric or an isometric contraction take place first, presetting tension in the muscle. For example, the quadriceps muscles preset tension to stabilize the knee in full extension at initial contact during the gait cycle. This allows a subsequent quadriceps eccentric contraction to decelerate the flexing knee to absorb shock. Therefore, isometric contractions are an essential component of many functional activities.

Indications

Isometric exercise is a valuable rehabilitation tool in many situations. It is a foundational exercise and isometric training often preceeds dynamic muscle training. Isometric exercise is preferred over dynamic exercise when joint motion is uncomfortable or contraindicated, such as postoperatively or with an unstable joint. Isometric exercise is essential to maintain muscle strength and prevent significant declines during immobilization.

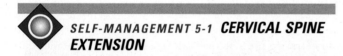

SELF-MANAGEMENT 5-1 *CERVICAL SPINE EXTENSION*

Purpose: To strengthen cervical extensors.
Position: Lying on your stomach with fists positioned under your forehead and a pillow under your trunk; a small towel roll under your chin may be necessary to keep your head in neutral.

Movement Technique: Remove your hands from your forehead and hold your head in a proper neutral position.

Hold for 10 seconds.

Dosage
 Repetitions: _____per set _____sets
 Frequency: _____sessions per day, _____ sessions
 per week

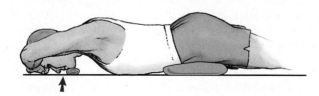

Isometric exercise is used for purposes other than muscle strength training. Isometric contractions are indicated when muscle reeducation is required. One of the benefits of isometric exercise is the ability to perform repetitive submaximal contractions as "reminder" or reeducation exercises. In contrast to isometric contractions to maintain strength during periods of immobilization or times when joint motion is contraindicated, isometric contractions for muscle reeducation can be submaximal. Following knee or hip injury or surgery, patients may have difficulty recruiting and activating the quadriceps muscles; following shoulder surgery or injury, patients may have difficulty recruiting and activating the rotator cuff musculature. Quadriceps setting and rotator cuff isometric exercises at a low, submaximal level can maintain connective tissue mobility (and at the knee, patellar mobility), and muscle mobility and function. These activities are typically initiated prior to dynamic resistive exercises. This prepares the patient for more advanced dynamic activities. Quadriceps and gluteal sets are also used to enhance circulation throughout the lower extremity during periods of bed rest.

These isometric setting exercises are also a prerequisite for more advanced dynamic exercises, particularly those requiring eccentric muscle contractions. This is a more complex neuromuscular activity than one might think. For example, if one were to catch an object being tossed at them, or to jump down from a given height, the brain must first signal the necessary muscles to preset isometric tension in order to decelerate the object upon catching, or the body upon landing, *respectively*. One of the significant challenges is teaching the patient *how* much tension to preset to accomplish a given task. In this case, isometric training at different percentages of maximal activation is useful.

Isometric exercise also functions as a component of dynamic exercise such as when weakness exists at a specific point in the ROM. Proprioceptive neuromuscular facilitation (PNF) techniques include isometrics as part of a dynamic program to enhance stability and strengthen muscles in a weak portion of the range (see Chapter 16). For example, while performing a diagonal pattern, the therapist may stop and apply an isometric contraction at a weaker portion of the range. Isometric contractions are also an important component of stabilization programs. **Stabilization** programs are a progressive series of exercises and activities designed to increase a patient's ability to dynamically control movement at a joint or series of joints. Stabilization exercises are an important component of treatment programs for shoulder, knee, and ankle instability, as well as the basis of treatment for many spinal problems. For example, PNF techniques such as alternating isometrics and rhythmic stabilization use isometric contractions as the basis for stability training.

This resistive mode is easy to understand and perform correctly, requires no equipment, and can be performed in almost any setting. Isometric exercise is most effective when individuals are in a low state of training, because the benefits of isometric exercise decrease as the state of training increases. Most gains are made within the first 5 weeks of the onset of training.[112]

Considerations in Isometric Training

Some factors are important in choosing isometric exercise for rehabilitation. Isometric strength is specific to the joint angle. Studies have demonstrated isometric joint angle specificity, noting that strength gained at one joint angle did not predictably carry over to other joint angles.[113] Neuromuscular changes accounted for the joint-angle–dependent effects, and obtaining generalized strength gains required multiple-angle training programs. Whitley[114] found significantly increased strength at all joint angles after 10 weeks of training at specific joint angles. Others have found this general transfer, although only after training was well advanced.[115] In the beginning training phase, the strength gains were transferred only when the muscle was at shorter than resting length.

Dosage

Like most resistive exercise programs, dosing the exercise is the most challenging aspect. Dosing for strength differs from dosing for muscle reeducation, and this differs from dosing for stabilization. Isometric exercise for these different therapeutic goals requires a specific approach for each.

Dosing for strength training has two important variables: intensity and range of motion. Because of the angle specificity, multiple-angle isometric training is recommended whenever possible. Muscle contraction should be maximal or nearly maximal and should be performed to fatigue. Exercise may be performed at a low frequency. Sample dosage parameters for isometric exercise prescription for strength are as follows

- Perform isometric contractions every 15 to 20 degrees throughout the ROM.
- Hold each contraction approximately 6 seconds (the first few seconds of the first maximum contraction appears to trigger the major training effect—after the first few seconds, the ability to maintain a maximal contraction drops off dramatically).[6]
- Hold the contraction long enough to fully activate all motor units, and repeat it frequently throughout the day.
- Isometric contractions have their greatest effect near maximal contraction, although this may not be possible in many clinical situations.

Dosing for muscle reeducation requires a different prescription. Contraction intensity is submaximal and can vary from very low intensity (<20% maximum voluntary contraction or MVC) to >50% MVC. Exercise at the lowest intensity immediately after injury or surgery to serve as a reminder how to contract the muscle. Following back surgery, the patient might perform abdominal muscle contractions at a very low level; following a patellar dislocation, a patient might perform low level quadriceps contractions. On the other hand, a patient who needs improved thoracic and cervical posture while at a workstation might perform scapular retraction isometrics at 50% or more of MVC throughout the day. Because intensity and volume are inversely related, isometric contractions for muscle reeducation are performed at a high volume. Activities that are performed for postural awareness may be put "on cue" asking the patient to perform a set of isometrics on cue, such as every time the phone rings, or every time a new email message arrives. Progression of these exercises is to dynamic strengthening, isometrics at a higher percentage of MVC, and/or isometric exercise with external resistance, such as holding a position against elastic resistance.

Isometric dosage for stabilization is somewhere between strengthening and muscle reeducation. Stabilization exercises are like muscle reeducation in that one of the goals is to train the muscles to dynamically maintain a joint or series of joints within a small range of postures that are the most optimal for the joint structures. An additional goal is to simultaneously strengthen the muscles required to do this. Thus the dosage is more flexible, and is specific to each patient situation. For stabilization activities, a common pattern would be initial training for muscle reeducation, where the emphasis is on contracting the right muscle group and avoiding the "overflow" phenomenon where the patient globally activates all muscles in the region. In the lower extremity, patients might activate quadriceps, hamstrings, and gluteal muscles while trying to perform a quadriceps set. In the core, the patient may activate all abdominal muscles when trying to activate only the deep trunk stabilizers. Once the correct activation has been achieved, the program might progress to program with strengthening emphasis, followed again by a muscle reeducation program to teach the patient to activate just enough motor units to accomplish the functional task safely.

Precautions

Use caution when prescribing isometric exercise for patients with hypertension or known cardiac disease. Isometric exercise can produce a pressor response, increasing blood pressure. Perform isometric exercise without breath holding or a Valsalva maneuver. Individuals with hypertension may benefit from simple, repeated contractions held only 1 to 2 seconds.

Dynamic Exercise

Dynamic resistive exercise can be performed in a variety of modes, postures, and dosages, as well as with a variety of contraction types (i.e., concentric, eccentric). Dynamic exercise implies joint motion and a shortening or lengthening contraction of the working muscle. Dynamic exercises have been called isotonic exercises in the past and the term is still in common usage today despite the technical shortcomings of the term.

Body weight, elastic bands, free weights, pulleys, manual resistance, and weight machines are a few modes of dynamic resistive exercise (see Patient-Related Instruction 5-2: Purchasing Resistive Equipment). Concentric and eccentric contractions can be used in different combinations depending on the mode of exercise chosen (i.e., most weight machines use concentric and eccentric contraction of the same muscle

---

◆ Patient-Related Instruction 5-2

Purchasing Resistive Equipment

Before purchasing resistive equipment for home use, the following information should be considered:

1. Is the equipment safe? Is it approved by a reputable organization?
2. How easy is the equipment to use? How long will it take to learn how to use it?
3. Is the equipment versatile? Can it be used to train a number of different muscle groups?
4. Will the equipment suit your needs as your training progresses?

Before purchasing equipment, consider joining a health club for a month or two to see:

1. Which equipment you tend to use regularly
2. What features you like about some equipment
3. What features you dislike or seem to be lacking

groups whereas manual resisted exercise can use concentric and/or eccentric contractions of opposing muscle groups). As with isometric exercise, each type of dynamic exercise has risks and benefits, and the training mode must be matched to the specific needs of the individual. The ACSM recommends that for novice and intermediate training, both free weights and machines be used, whereas the advanced and elite athletes' emphasis should be primarily with free weights.[37]

Although isokinetic exercise is a type of dynamic exercise, it is often considered in a different category from isotonic exercise. Although isotonic exercise can be performed at a constant velocity, it is performed against a constant load. Isokinetic exercise is performed at a constant velocity with accommodating resistance; that is, the isokinetic device "matches" the resistance applied by the subject. Specific indications and dosage for each type of dynamic exercise will be considered in the next section.

METHODS OF RESISTANCE TRAINING

The specific activities and dosage chosen to improve muscle performance depend on many factors, including the individual's age and medical condition, muscles involved, activity level, current level of training, goals (i.e., strength, power, and endurance), and cause of decreased muscle performance. The following sections describe the activities used to increase muscle performance and their relative risks and benefits. Be sure to match the appropriate training mode to the patient's goals.

Manual Resistance

Manual resistance can be applied by the clinician, the patient, or a family member. It is one of the most longstanding forms of resistance training in the rehabilitation profession. This is likely due to its ease of application and its versatility. Manual resistance can be applied at a variety of intensities, speeds, ranges, and contraction types. The speed, intensity, contraction type, and movement pattern can be varied during a given exercise. Several well-known techniques such as PNF are applied predominantly with manual resistance.

Indications

Manual resistance can be performed in almost any situation where resistance for rehabilitation is required. However, it becomes challenging in situations requiring high force levels, as in training for fitness, wellness, or sports. Manual resistance is especially effective in a number of situations. Manual resistance is quite effective when strength varies throughout the range of motion. A patient may have a portion of the ROM that is either weak or painful; the therapist can modulate the resistance more easily with manual techniques than with resistive equipment. The therapist can also apply specific tactile cues to facilitate recruitment at a weak portion of the range of motion. Similarly, manual techniques work well if a patient needs assistance through a portion of the ROM, followed by resistance at other positions. Manual techniques are quite useful when teaching proper movement patterns, as manual assistance/resistance can facilitate proper firing patterns. For example, a PNF technique called rhythmic initiation teaches proper movement patterns prior to the addition of resistance.

Manual resistance is indicated when manual contacts are necessary to ensure the proper muscle activation. For example, in some situations synergists may substitute for the desired primary muscle action. Palpation plus manual contacts and tactile cues can facilitate the proper muscle activation and stabilization. Manual cues with one hand can facilitate isometric stabilization contractions while the other hand facilitates and resists a dynamic contraction. PNF techniques are very effective for enhancing specific muscle activation patterns and intensities that can become resisted.

Manual resistance works well when needs a specialized technique such as alternating isometrics or rhythmic stabilization. These are techniques where agonist and antagonist are alternately activated within a small ROM and at progressively higher speeds until cocontraction provides stability. The alternating aspect of this activity makes manual techniques the optimal form of resistance. Additionally, when a variety of speeds is necessary, manual resistance offers the flexibility to change rapidly, enhancing motor learning opportunities.

Considerations

Manual resistance has the benefit of being readily available in the clinic and does not require specific positioning against gravity to achieve resistance. The amount of resistance can be modified as the exercise session progresses, with decreasing resistance as the patient fatigues. The resistance can be more finely adjusted through the range of motion and with every repetition to ensure maximum resistance through the exercise. The therapist is able to feel the change in force offered by the patient and can adjust the applied resistance appropriately. That way the patient can obtain the maximum resistance tolerated through the entire exercise set. The therapist's hand position is also easily modified to change the lever arm and resistance offered. Manual resistance also allows manual contact between the therapist and patient. For many patients, this tactile contact provides comfort and increases ease.

Another consideration is the labor intensive nature of manual resistance. Manual resistance requires the time, energy, and physical strength of a therapy provider. Depending upon the body part being exercised and the relative strengths, manual resistance can be physically taxing. Performing PNF diagonal patterns for the lower extremity can be physically difficult and could potentially result in injury to the therapist using poor body mechanics. Be sure to use proper body mechanics, maximizing hand positioning, base of support, and lever arms to minimize the stress and risk of injury.

Manual resistance is not practical for many home programs. Caregiver assistance is required and may place the caregiver at risk of injury. For all but the lightest of manual resistance applications (i.e., hand, wrist, foot) the resistance is too great and the body mechanics challenging. Few homes have sufficient tables or supports at the right height and firmness to allow the caregiver to use good body mechanics.

Measuring and defining manual resistance is difficult. Therapists use terms like "minimum," "moderate," and "maximal" but these are poorly defined and vary from one person to another. For situations where documentation needs to be precise, verifying the dosage of manual resistance can be difficult.

Techniques

Techniques for performing manual resistance require attention to patient positioning, therapist positions, manual contact, grading of resistance, and verbal cues. Attention to these details provides the safest experience for both the patient and therapist. Consider the following points, essential to manual resistance:

- Make sure that the patient's clothing allows you to see the muscles or joints associated with the exercise
- Position the patient so that full excursion of the movement is possible without restrictions
- Make sure that the patient is comfortable and as stable as necessary as dictated by the exercise goal
- Position yourself in the plane of the movement, using a wide base of support; shift your weight and step as necessary with the movement to maintain good body mechanics
- Use as wide a contact area as possible to prevent discomfort at the point of resistance or stabilization application
- Using a wide, gentle grip, take the patient's limb through the exercise ROM to teach them the movement pattern
- While continuing to move through the range, tell your patient that you will be gradually applying some resistance to the movement
- Be sure to gradually apply and slowly release the resistance to avoid sudden muscle contractions that might cause injury or pain

Video clips of some commonly-used manual resistance patterns can be found on the Web site.

Dosage

Dosing manual resistance can be challenging due to the inability to quantify the intensity of the exercise. The therapist is able to document sets and repetitions as well as a nominal description of the amount of resistance (i.e., minimum resistance, maximum resistance). Like all forms of resistance, manual resistance is applied with a specific goal in mind (i.e., strength, endurance, stabilization) and the sets, repetitions and relevant rest intervals are derived from the goal. The exercise should stop when form fatigue becomes evident. Exercises can be varied by speed, muscle contraction type (concentric, eccentric, isometric) ROM, and resistance. Manually resisted exercises can be performed in an open chain or a closed chain (see Fig. 5-9A and B).

Pulley System

Many pieces of exercise equipment are based on a pulley system where a weight plate is attached via a cable and pulley to a handle or lever that is controlled by the patient. In a standard pulley system, the cable attaches over a single or double round pulley. In other situations, the pulley or cam itself is elliptical, thereby providing variable resistance as they rotate through the cable's excursion. These are called **variable resistance** machines and will be considered in the next section. This section will focus on traditional pulley devices without an elliptical cam.

Most pulley systems consist of a simple cable and pulley attached to a weight stack of variable weight increments (i.e., 2.5, 5, or 10 lb). Most pulley systems are a single stack of weights that are freestanding or attached to a wall (Fig. 5-10). The other end of the pulley typically contains a clip or hook to which a number of different implements can be attached. These attachments may include a straight bar, cuff, handgrips, or various sizes and grips of implements designed to allow a wide range of exercises. Activities such as triceps pulls, biceps

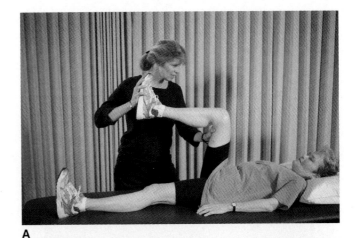

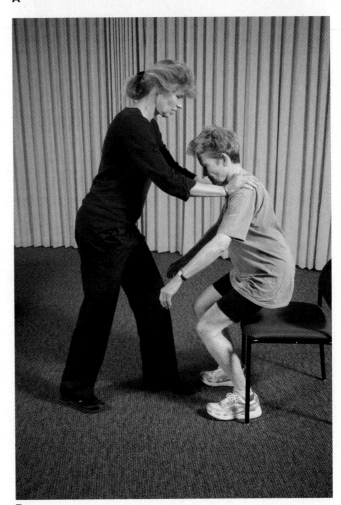

FIGURE 5-9. (A) Manually resisted open chain leg press and (B) manually resisted rise from a chair.

curls, latissimus pull-downs, rows, shoulder rotations, presses, leg lifts, and crunches are some of the many activities that can be performed with a pulley. Thus, a pulley is a versatile piece of equipment that allows someone to perform a large variety of activities with a single piece of equipment.

A pulley system is indicated any time resistive exercise through a range of motion is necessary. Pulleys are prescribed after baseline strength is established, as most pulley systems

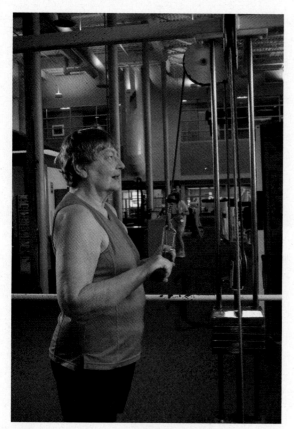

FIGURE 5-10. A standard pulley system.

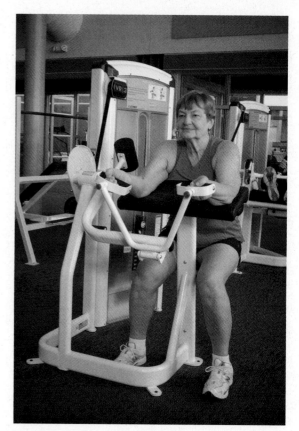

FIGURE 5-11. Variable resistance machine.

start with a minimum of 2.5 lb of resistance. Few pulley systems provide stabilization such as chairs or benches. Therefore most exercises require dynamic stabilization from the person performing the exercise. Chairs or benches can be set up to provide support or stabilization for specific exercises. For example, someone with limited standing tolerance or balance may be safer performing biceps curls seated rather than standing.

The most fundamental disadvantage of this type of system is the constant load provided by the equipment. When performing an exercise through a full ROM, the muscle will be maximally loaded only in the weakest portion of the range. The remaining portion of the ROM will be underloaded, failing to achieve the criteria necessary for strengthening. One technique to accommodate for this shortcoming is to train different portions of the ROM at different intensities. For example, the patient may train through the full range of motion at a lower intensity, then perform an additional set at a higher intensity in the mid-portion of the ROM, where the muscle requires higher resistance to overload.

Variable Resistance Machines

Resistive exercise machines are commonly found in rehabilitation clinics and health clubs. Most of these machines work in a similar fashion, although some differences exist. Historically, most weight machines were designed to isolate a specific muscle group such as the quadriceps femoris or biceps brachii. Some equipment trains multiple muscle groups in combination patterns such as a leg press or pull-up machine. Those machines using weight stacks have plates weighing 5 to 20 lb each. The weight stack configuration varies with the specific muscle action trained. A pin placed in the

weight stack selects the amount of weight to be lifted. The muscle contraction type is concentric during the lifting phase and eccentric during the lowering phase (Fig. 5-11).

The pulley or cam system is an important component of the weight machine. In contrast to a simple pulley system that provides a constant load through the ROM, a variable resistance machine contains an elliptical cam and pulley system that varies the resistance through the ROM. The kidney-shaped cam is an attempt to account for changes caused by varying length-tension relationships through the ROM. Variable resistance devices provide less resistance at the beginning and end of the ROM, and more resistance midrange.

Other machines use hydraulics to provide variable resistance through the range. Again, the machine is designed to provide more resistance in the mid-ROM, replicating "typical" length-tension ratios. Rather than alternating concentric-eccentric contractions of the same muscle groups, the hydraulic resistance machines typically provide reciprocal concentric contractions of opposing muscle groups (i.e., biceps-triceps).

Weight machines also differ in their adjustability. Lever arms and seat positions should be adjustable for a variety of body sizes. This ensures the ability to align the joint axis with the axis of the machine and prevent injury from poor posture or exercise mechanics. Stops and range-limiting devices should be available and easily adjustable.

An advantage of weight machines over other types of resistance is safety. Patients are stabilized effectively by the equipment, and the risk of falls or injury resulting from instability is minimized. It takes less time to learn weight machine exercises. After the adjustments are learned, the equipment is relatively easy to use, and novice weight lifters are less intimidated by the equipment. Weight machines are also relatively time-efficient because the machines are already set-up. Only a few simple adjustments are necessary, and the patient is ready to begin. These machines frequently isolate a specific muscle group to be trained, and the variable resistance accommodates for changing length-tension relationships better than other types of resistance.

One of the disadvantages of weight machines is their expense. They typically perform only a single exercise. For example, an expensive machine may train only biceps, whereas this could be done inexpensively with a couple of free weights and a bar. Another disadvantage is that weight increases are restricted to fixed increments (i.e., weight plates) on weight machines. Smaller changes of 1 or 2 lb are not possible on most machines. Despite the many size adjustments on weight machines, they still do not fit everyone. Most also have a fixed, two-dimensional movement pattern. Because the machine guides the patient through the ROM, little proprioception, balance, or coordination is learned from the experience. The stabilization helps with isolation but limits the patient from learning self-stabilization. Most machines are designed to perform bilateral exercise. In some cases, performing unilateral exercise is difficult, if not impossible.

Elastic Resistance

Elastic resistance in the form of elastic bands or tubing has improved greatly from its origins as "dental dam" used in dental procedures. Use of elastic resistance has increased significantly since its first appearance. It is relatively inexpensive, easy to use, small and light making it ideal for home and travel use, and can be used in an infinite variety of exercises. However, the trade-off for ease of use is the difficulty in quantifying and dosing an exercise program. Ongoing research is providing further information on forces generated with elastic resistance.[115–118]

Elastic resistance is a dynamic exercise but cannot be classified as isotonic or isokinetic. The variability in load through the range of motion does not allow it to be classified as isotonic and the variability in speed does not allow classification as isokinetic. It has unique characteristics that require it to be considered independent of other types of resistance. Elastic resistance is often compared with an isotonic pulley system. However, the unique characteristics of elastic do not allow a direct comparison with a pulley system.[119]

Unlike a pulley system which has a fixed load, the resistance provided by an elastic band varies with the thickness of the band and the elongation.[115,120,121] Any elastic material's resistance to stretch is proportional to its original cross-sectional area.[119] Therefore, doubling the cross-sectional area by folding (effectively doubling) the elastic doubles the resistance. Additionally, elastic resistance has unique force-elongation characteristics. The force increases as the elastic is stretched from 0% to 250% of its resting length. The force-elongation curve of Thera-Band (The Hygenic Corporation, Akron, OH, USA) elastic bands as well as the force in pounds can be found in Figure 5-12 and Table 5-4, *respectively*. The

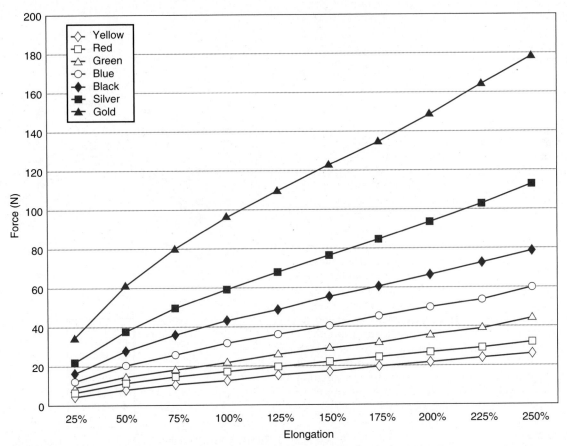

FIGURE 5-12. Force-elongation of Thera-Band elastic bands. (Used with permission of The Hygenic Corporation. Data from Page P, Labbe A, Topp R. Clinical force production of Thera-Band elastic bands. [Abstract]. J Orthop Sports Phys Ther 2000; 30(1):A47–A48.)

TABLE 5-4 Force-Elongation for Thera-Band Elastic Bands (Force in Pounds)							
ELONGATION (%)	YELLOW	RED	GREEN	BLUE	BLACK	SILVER	GOLD
25	1.1	1.5	2	2.8	3.6	5	7.9
50	1.8	2.6	3.2	4.6	6.3	8.5	13.9
75	2.4	3.3	4.2	5.9	8.1	11.1	18.1
100	2.9	3.9	5	7.1	9.7	13.2	21.6
125	3.4	4.4	5.7	8.1	11	15.2	24.6
150	3.9	4.9	6.5	9.1	12.3	17.1	27.5
175	4.3	5.4	7.2	10.1	13.5	18.9	30.3
200	4.8	5.9	7.9	11.1	14.8	21	33.4
225	5.3	6.4	8.8	12.1	16.2	23	36.6
250	5.8	7	9.6	13.3	17.6	25.3	40.1

(Used with permission of The Hygenic Corporation. Data from Page P, Labbe A, Topp R. Clinical force production of Thera-Band elastic bands. [Abstract]. J Orthop Sports Phys Ther 2000;30(1):A47–A48.)

percentage of elongation, or change in length of the elastic band, is calculated using the following formula:

$$\text{Percentage of elongation} = [(\text{final length}) - (\text{resting length}) / (\text{resting length})] \times 100$$

This force development is distinct from the torque created when functionally using elastic bands through a range of motion with changing moment arms. Like all elastic materials, the force developed when pulling that material in a linear fashion will increase as the material is lengthened until failure is reached. However, the actual amount of torque developed when using elastic bands through a range of motion (such as shoulder abduction) follows an ascending-descending pattern. That is, the torque increases from 0 to 90 degrees abduction as the moment arm increases, then decreases again as the moment arm decreases as the shoulder approaches 180 degrees. An example of strength curves can be found in Figure 5-13.

Indications

Elastic bands are indicated any time strengthening by an external resistance is required. Elastic resistance can be used in the clinic under a therapist's supervision. It also works well for home programs utilized on conjunction with in-house rehabilitation. Because it is light and easily transported, elastic resistance works well for those needing to perform exercise while at work or travelling. Resistive bands can be used for fitness or wellness training, providing challenges to muscle strength, power, endurance, as well as plyometric training, balance, and stabilization. They can be integrated into a practice or training session to provide additional activity-specific training. Resistive bands can be used for open chain or closed chain exercise, and core strength and stabilization. The tubing or bands can be attached to work or exercise equipment to provide functional resistance. It works well for individuals who have limited mobility, as the resistance can be applied in a variety of positions or postures. The resistance variation provides people with low physical capacity the opportunity to train and improve strength and function.[123-125]

Considerations

There are some issues to be considered when prescribing elastic band resistive exercises. First, although there is some data about the amount of resistance with different colors of elastic bands, patient implementation variables render it an inexact quantity. The amount of resistance varies with the elongation, so if the patient grasps the band at a different location, or initiates the exercise at a greater percent elongation, the torque may vary from one session to the next. The patient may not understand why the exercise seems easier one day and harder the next.

While the reproducibility of testing or exercise with elastic bands may be questioned due to issues of cross-sectional area, length and origin/stabilization, the reliability and validity of elastic band use has been established under controlled

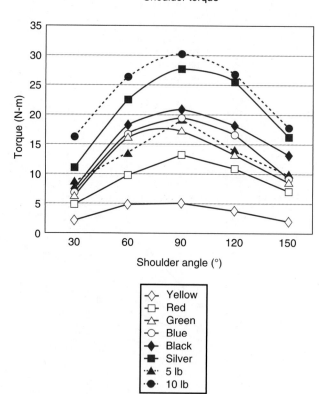

FIGURE 5-13. Strength curves of Thera-Band elastic tubing compare to free weights. (Used with permission of The Hygenic Corporation. Data from Page P, Labbe A, Topp R. Clinical force production of Thera-Band elastic bands. [Abstract]. J Orthop Sports Phys Ther 2000;30(1):A47–A48.)

conditions. Researchers found a 30-second elastic band elbow flexion test to be significantly correlated with a 30-second elbow flexion test using dumbbells (r = 0.62) and maximal isokinetic testing (r = 0.46). The test-retest reliability was high as well (ICC = 0.89).[120]

Another consideration is the impact of cyclic loading. Like any other elastic medium, loading the material results in changes such as creep. Additionally, cyclic loading (repeatedly stretching and relaxing the bands or tubing) can result in fatigue to the material. Over time, this fatigue can decrease the performance of the elastic and can eventually lead to failure. Research has shown that elastic bands stretch to 100% elongation for 500 cycles, resulting in a 5% to 12% decrease in force.[118] More importantly, the majority of the change occurred within the first 50 cycles. If patients are performing sets of 30 or more repetitions, the elastic can fatigue quickly. Therefore it is important to replace elastic bands frequently.

Like pulleys, elastic resistance exercises can be performed with or without external stabilization. If no stabilization is provided, be sure the patient is performing the exercise without substitution.

Dosage

Like any resistive exercise, the proper dosage is necessary to ensure achieving rehabilitation goals. Dosage is more difficult with elastic resistance because of the number of variables associated with this resistance mode. The length of the band, the percentage elongation, the color of band, and the origin of the elastic resistance all impact the torque developed.

Elastic resistance typically comes in a variety of colors and each color provides a different amount of resistance. Research on Thera-Band® elastic bands showed a 20% to 30% increase in force production between colors.[117] Increases in intensity should be accomplished by moving to the next higher level of resistance rather than doubling the elastic band. Doubling the elastic band will double the resistance, while increasing to the next higher level will provide only a 20% to 30% increase, a more moderate and safer intensity increase.

Another important variable in dosing elastic band exercise is the length of the band or tubing. The band should be elongated to no more than 250% of its original length.[119] To maintain the optimal ascending-descending torque curve, the length of the elastic should be equal to the length of the lever arm. In the case of exercise at the shoulder (i.e., abduction or flexion) the tubing should be equal to the length of the arm. This way the elongation through the full range of motion will be twice the length of the lever (a 200% elongation) resulting in an optimal torque curve for the shoulder musculature.

The angle of the origin of the tubing also impacts the torque curve and the subsequent resistance. An angle that is too acute will shift the torque curve to the left, increasing torque earlier in the range of motion. An angle that is too obtuse will shift the torque curve to the right, increasing torque later in the range of motion. This may be desirable in specific rehabilitation situations, but in general does not reproduce the torque curve of a normal muscle-joint interaction. The therapist should be aware of the impact of this angle on torque production. The origin of the elastic should be in the plane of the axis of rotation and in the direction of the desired motion.[119]

Finally, the resistance arm angle should be considered during exercise prescription. The resistance arm angle is the angle produced by the band or tubing and the lever arm (i.e., the hand and the band in the shoulder abduction example). The band and the limb should be aligned to ensure a normal physiological ascending-descending torque curve. If this alignment is incorrect, excessive torque may be produced at end range where the least amount is available. It is recommended that the band or tubing be aligned with the ending lever arm at a resistive arm angle of 15 degrees to 0 degree.[119] For example, in shoulder flexion, the band should be placed under the foot so that in the full 180 degrees overhead position, the band pulls nearly straight down, with the wrist:band angle at <15 degrees. A higher angle would place excessive load on the wrist extensor muscles.

Once the patient is properly positioned and the band or tubing color (resistance) and length determined, the number of sets and repetitions should be determined. The patient should start with slight tension on the band (approximately 25% elongation) and perform the exercise through the desired range of motion. Depending upon the patient's goals (strength, power, endurance, etc.) an increase or decrease in the band color might be indicated. Like free weights or weight machines, the resistance and number of repetitions depend upon the goal. For traditional strength or endurance training, repetitions at approximately 6 to 10 RM would be appropriate. For those doing power training, the intensity would be greater, with intensity at 90% of a 3 RM.[119]

As with any resistive exercise, substitution, form fatigue and stabilization are factors to be considered. Do not sacrifice form for additional resistance or repetitions. Training programs can be designed similar to those with traditional weights. As the patient fatigues, consider performing additional sets at a lower elastic band resistance, just as one might to a decreasing training schedule with free weights.

Free Weights

Free-weight training is the resistive exercise technique of choice for body builders and power lifters. Free weights and cuff weights are also commonly used in rehabilitation. Free-weight training is usually performed with hand-held weights that range from 0.5 up to 75 or more pounds. Free weights can also be combined on a bar with weight plates. Cuff weights typically range from 0.5 to 25 lb.

Free-weight training allows more discrete increases in resistance, and resistance can differ from one side to the other (see Self-Management 5-2: Standing Biceps Curls). For example, reciprocal biceps curls can be performed with 10 lb on the injured side and 15 lb on the uninjured side. Incremental increases of 1 to 2 lb or less are available, allowing a more gradual overload. The free-weight equipment is affordable, and a multitude of exercises can be performed with the same free weights. These exercises can include simple strengthening and endurance activities or power training techniques.

Free weight exercises can be performed in a multitude of different ways that meet the needs of individual patients or clients. For example, a variety of positions are available and and are not restricted by the design of the machine. Biceps curls can be performed in standing, sitting, supine or even prone. They can be performed symmetrically or reciprocally and the patient may have different weights in each hand.

SELF-MANAGEMENT 5-2 *STANDING BICEPS CURLS*

Purpose: To strengthen the biceps muscles

Position: Standing position, with shoulder girdles, spine, and pelvis in neutral. Hold a weight in each hand, palms facing sideway toward your thighs.

Movement Technique:

Level 1: Alternately bend your elbows, turning your palms upward as the weights clear your hips; and straighten your elbows, turning your palms sideways again as you move toward your hips. Do not alter your neutral shoulder, spine, or pelvic position as you lift and lower the weight.

Level 2: Bend and straighten your elbows simultaneously.

Hold _____ pounds in each hand

Dosage

Repetitions: _____ per set, _____ sets
Frequency: _____ sessions per day, _____ sessions per week

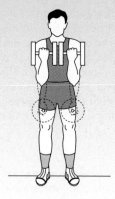

Level 2

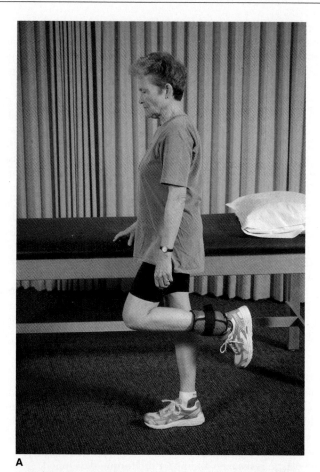

A

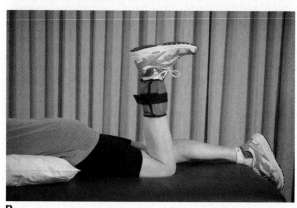

B

FIGURE 5-14. (A) Hamstring curl in standing and (B) hamstring curl in prone.

The exercise can be performed at a variety of different speeds and the working range of motion can be altered. Changing the position and/or range of motion can alter the relationship with gravity, affecting the working muscle group and contraction type. For example, a hamstring curl performed in standing provides concentric resistance during shortening and eccentric resistance while lengthening, both to the hamstring muscle group. This same exercise performed in prone provides concentric resistance with a decreasing moment arm against gravity until the knee approaches the 90-degree angle. At this position, there is no moment arm against gravity and no significant resistance. Continuing into further flexion produces and eccentric contraction of the quadriceps as they are lengthened while trying to slow the flexing knee (Fig. 5-14A and B). Free weight exercises provide a multitude of possibilities to match the exercise with the patient's goals.

One of the biggest advantages of free-weight training is the neural component of balance. Compared with the external

stabilization provided by a weight machine, the free weight usually has little external stabilization. These exercises require postural muscle stabilization beyond the work required to move the weight. The individual lifting with free weights must understand proper posture and spinal stabilization to prevent injury to the back. If balance is a rehabilitation goal, free weight exercise may be indicated.

The neural demands of free-weight exercise are a disadvantage for some. It takes longer to learn free-weight exercise, because the free-weight tasks usually are more complex than those with weight machines. Novice lifters may be at greater risk for injury because of poor technique (Fig. 5-15). Spotters are necessary for many of the free-weight lifts, increasing the

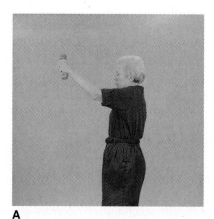

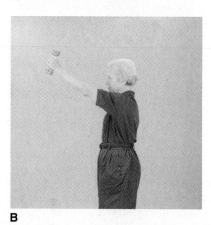

FIGURE 5-15. (A) Front arm raise performed with poor technique with excessive scapula elevation and (B) front arm raise performed with improved scapula stability.

personnel demands of this resistive technique. Because of the time required to load and unload bars, free-weight training can be less time efficient. However, for those using smaller hand-held weights, these can be more time efficient than weight machines due to the lack of setup time.

Safety tips for individuals training with free weights include working with a knowledgeable partner who can spot safely. Collars should always be used to lock the weights on the bar and prevent movement of the plates on the bar. Proper form and technique should be acquired before lifting with any weight.

Elastic bands, tubing, and pulleys are used in a similar fashion to free weights. One benefit of bands and pulleys over free weights is the ability to position the patient without regard to gravity (see Self-Management 5-3: Supine Shoulder Flexion). Free weights, resistive bands, and pulleys have the advantage of movement in a variety of three-dimensional patterns without fixed movement patterns. This allows highly specific training that matches individual needs. For example, resisted lunging patterns forward, backward, laterally, or diagonally can be performed with elastic bands, pulleys, or free weights. These movement patterns can be performed in whatever range is necessary for the individual, rather than in ranges dictated by a weight machine.

Isokinetic Devices

Isokinetic dynamometers are designed to provide maximum resistance through the entire ROM. The resistance provided

SELF-MANAGEMENT 5-3 *SUPINE SHOULDER FLEXION*

Purpose: To increase the strength of the shoulder muscles, especially serratus anterior.

Position: Lying on your back with the band tied around your foot. Hold the band in the ipsilateral hand with the arm next to your side and elbow bent to 90 degrees.

Movement Technique:

Level 1: Keeping your elbow bent, punch your hand toward the ceiling until your elbow is straight, then move your straight arm upward toward your head. Press backward into the surface you are lying on or pillow(s) as needed to support you at the end of your range of motion. Push back with an isometric contraction for 10 seconds. Return arm in reverse movement pattern. Repeat as prescribed.

Level 2: Perform level one with a straight arm.

Dosage

Repetitions: _____per set _____sets
Frequency: _____sessions per day, _____ sessions per week

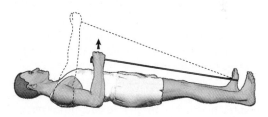

by these devices is termed "accommodating" because once the preset speed is achieved, the dynamometer "matches" the force applied by the patient. The dynamometer provides a counterforce equal to the force applied by the patient. Therefore the patient can obtain the maximum amount of resistance they can tolerate throughout the ROM. If a patient has pain or weakness in a specific portion of the ROM, the remaining portion can still be fully challenged. Additionally, patients can train at a variety of speeds.

The first isokinetic dynamometers performed resisted reciprocal concentric contractions at speeds fixed by the clinician. The dynamometer was passive in that the machine was unable to move independently; the patient was required to move the dynamometer arm. The new isokinetic devices are active computerized training and testing devices that are capable of actively moving the patient's limb for him or her. These dynamometers provide reciprocal concentric resistance at fixed speeds, and they provide multiangle isometric resistance, fixed resistance concentric and eccentric contractions, passive motion, and fixed speed concentric and eccentric contractions. Because these dynamometers now function in a variety of modes that the dynamometers are capable of performing, they have become multipurpose testing and training devices. While many dynamometers are capable of providing isometric and isotonic resistance, most providers still refer to these devices as isokinetic dynamometers, and emphasize the isokinetic capabilities of these devices.

Indications

The isokinetic mode is used most frequently for muscle performance testing and training. The dynamometers are capable of testing and training muscle groups around most major joints of the body. Muscles around the shoulder, elbow, forearm, and wrist in the upper extremity and the hip, knee, and ankle in the lower extremity are all readily tested and trained using an isokinetic dynamometer. Adaptive attachments allow training for pediatric patients, industrial medicine (i.e., lifting and work simulation attachments) and closed chain exercise and testing. Isokinetic testing is frequently performed as an alternative to 1 RM testing due to the computerize capabilities of the devices and safety issues. The dynamometer matches the patient's force output, thereby minimizing the chance of injury that is found when performing 1 RM testing, particularly in the presence of an injury. Tests can be performed in a limited range of motion and at a fixed speed to assess muscle strength or endurance. Test results are stored in the computer and can be compared with the results of future tests or to population-based norms.

Isokinetic testing is performed to assess muscle performance against some standard. The standard may be the contralateral side, a population norm or a percentage of the antagonist muscle performance. Testing is performed to assess progress after injury or surgery and to determine readiness to advance the rehabilitation program or to return to activity. In some situations testing is performed pre-season to provide guidance for the training program or to provide a baseline measure in the case of a future injury.

Testing is typically performed at two or three different speeds to capture speed-specific muscle impairments. Each dynamometer maker has specific testing protocols and standards to follow to ensure validity and test-retest reliability. The data is captured in a computer file and can be examined and manipulated in a variety of different ways (Fig. 5-16). Several important terms are used to describe isokinetic data results. **Peak torque** is the most common variable measured and is the maximum torque generated regardless of where in the ROM it is achieved. **Work** is the total amount of work performed under the torque curve, regardless of ROM, time, or speed. **Average power** is the amount of work (total work under the curve) performed per time unit (P = W/T). **Time to peak torque** is the amount of time it takes to achieve peak torque and the **peak torque angle** is the joint angle at which peak torque occurred. Other important and common comparisons are bilateral comparisons and agonist/antagonist ratios. In bilateral comparisons, one extremity is compared with the other to determine the absolute and/or relative difference from side-to-side. In agonist/antagonist ratios, the opposing muscles groups (i.e., quadriceps and hamstrings) are compared with the antagonist given as a proportion of the agonist (i.e., the hamstrings are 70% of the quadriceps). Normative standards for some agonist/antagonist ratios exist.

Isokinetic training is indicated any time the patient needs muscle activation throughout the range of motion. Isokinetics work well when there are fluctuations in torque production due to changes in the length-tension relationships or due to pain or pathology causing signification variation in torque production through the range. Unlike a fixed, constant load (i.e., isotonic) there is no minimum load to lift to complete the activity. If the patient is unable to continue the exercise, he or she can simply stop without worrying about dropping a weight. Isokinetic training also works well when a variety of speeds need to be trained. Velocity spectrum training (VSRP, velocity spectrum rehabilitation program), or training through a variety of speeds, is a commonly-used training regimen. Patients may start at a slow velocity (i.e., 60 degrees per second) and increase speed by 30 degrees per second up to a maximum velocity (i.e., 300 degrees per second) and then decrease speed incrementally until the starting speed is reached. A variety of training programs can be designed using this technique. The "slow velocity" VSRP generally ranges from 60 degrees per second to 180 degrees per second and back down, while the "medium velocity" VSRP ranges from 120 degrees per second to 240 degrees per second and the "high velocity" from 180 degrees per second to 300 degrees per second and back down.

The passive mode on an isokinetic dynamometer can be used to train isokinetically as well. The passive mode does precisely what the name implies: it passively moves the limb at a preselected velocity. The patient can use this mode in a variety of different ways. The patient might be instructed to relax and let the machine move and mobilize the joint. Alternatively, the patient might be asked to assist the machine in the direction it is moving (a concentric contraction) or to resist against it (an eccentric contraction). Why choose resisting against the passive movement rather than the active isokinetic or isotonic concentric and eccentric contractions? In the active modes, the patient must still generate enough torque to actively move the dynamometer arm and match the preset speed of the machine. In some cases, such as a postoperative surgery or an acute injury, this amount of force may still exceed the muscle's capacity. In the passive mode, the machine moves continuously, and the patient can provide resistance at the level and in the appropriate range of motion given the current injury status.

Considerations

The major advantage of isokinetic resistive training is its ability to fully activate more muscle fibers for longer periods. Because the machine matches the torque provided by the patient, it "accommodates" the patient's changing abilities throughout the ROM. In contrast, free weights (i.e., fixed resistance training) overload only the weakest portion of the range, but the stronger portion (usually the middle third) is not overloaded. For testing purposes, isokinetic dynamometers allow individuals to be tested at a variety of speeds, potentially identifying deficits at more functional speeds. Compared to a 1 RM strength measure, the isokinetic dynamometer produces a force curve through the ROM rather than a single measure. This allows more detailed evaluation of muscle function characteristics (i.e., time to peak torque, total work performed, etc.).

Isokinetic devices allow training at a variety of speeds. The positive effect of fast-speed training on performance is highlighted with isokinetic training. Training at faster speeds can assist the return to functional activities that require less muscle torque development but faster speeds of contraction. Speeds that more closely match the patient's function can be chosen to match functional velocities. Higher speeds can decrease joint compression forces in areas such as the

General Evaluation

Name:	
ID:	
Birth Date:	**(M/d/yyyy)**
Ht:	
Wt:	
Gender:	

Session:	
Involved:	**Left**
Clinician:	
Referral:	
Joint:	**Knee**
Diagnosis:	

Windowing:	**None**
Protocol:	**Isokinetic Bilateral**
Pattern:	**Extension/Flexion**
Mode:	**Isokinetic**
Contraction:	**CON/CON**
GET:	**18 FT-LBS at 30 Degrees**

		EXTENSION 60 DEG/SEC			FLEXION 60 DEG/SEC			EXTENSION 240 DEG/SEC			FLEXION 240 DEG/SEC		
# OF REPS (60/60): 5		UNINVOL	INVOLVED	DEFICIT	UNINVOL	INVOLVED	DEFICIT	UNINVOL	INVOLVED	DEFICIT	UNINVOL	INVOLVED	DEFICIT
# OF REPS (240/240): 15		RIGHT	LEFT		RIGHT	LEFT		RIGHT	LEFT		RIGHT	LEFT	
PEAK TORQUE	FT-LBS	92.0	81.8	11.1	68.0	68.9	-1.3	61.2	49.8	18.7	45.7	43.4	5.0
PEAK TQ/BW	5	38.3	34.1		28.3	28.7		25.5	20.7		19.0	18.1	
MAX REP TOT WORK	FT-LBS	113.1	76.4	32.4	69.5	69.8	-0.4	70.0	50.3	28.1	35.6	38.2	-7.2
COEFF. OF VAR.	%	6.6	6.8		5.5	6.2		9.6	12.5		16.0	7.9	
AVG. POWER	WATTS	83.5	60.0	28.1	52.6	56.0	-6.4	164.5	116.1	29.4	75.9	79.8	-5.2
TOTAL WORK	FT-LBS	496.8	346.5	30.3	304.4	317.2	-4.2	917.2	643.1	29.9	440.9	445.5	-1.0
ACCELERATION TIME	MSEC	30.0	30.0		40.0	40.0		50.0	50.0		80.0	80.0	
DECELERATION TIME	MSEC	40.0	100.0		80.0	90.0		80.0	90.0		100.0	80.0	
ROM	DEG	106.2	96.2		106.2	96.2		104.1	95.8		104.1	95.8	
AVG PEAK TQ	FT-LBS	84.0	76.8		64.9	64.6		54.7	41.3		37.1	35.9	
AGON/ANTAG RATION	%	74.0	84.3	G: 61.0				74.6	87.2	G: N/A			

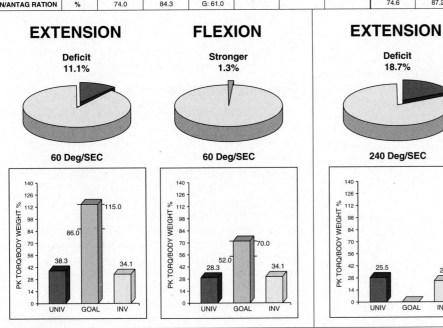

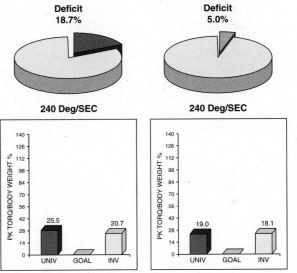

Comments:

PEAK TORQUE:	Highest muscular force output at any moment during a repetition. Indicative of a muscle's strength capabilities.
PEAK TQ/BW:	Represented as a percentage normalized to bodyweight and compared to an established goal
MAX REP TOT WORK:	Total muscular force output for the repetition with greatest amount of work. Work is indicative of a muscle's capability to produce force throughout the range of motion.
AVG POWER:	Total work divided by time. Power represents how quickly a muscle can produce force.
ACCELERATION TIME:	Total time to reach Isokinetic speed. Indicative of a muscle's neuromuscular capabilities to move the limb at the beginning of the range of motion.
DECELERATION TIME:	Total time to go from Isokinetic speed to zero speed. Indicative of a muscle's neuromuscular capability to eccentrically control the limb at the end of the range of motion.
AGON/ANTAG RATIO:	The Reciprocol muscle group ratio. Excessive imbalances may predispose a joint to injury.
DEFICITS:	1 to 10% No significant difference between extremities.
	11 to 25% Rehabilitation recommended to improve muscle performance balance.

Biodex   Rev 4.18b Sep 25 2006

FIGURE 5-16. Isokinetic test data analysis.

patellofemoral joint, decreasing the pain and discomfort often seen with heavy resistance exercises. Although less torque is generated at high speeds, the decrease in pain and more functional speeds may produce better results.

Studies assessing the speed variable favor slow-speed isokinetic training over fast-speed training for the development of strength.[126] High muscular tension is necessary for generating strength gains and is achieved when the isokinetic speed is slow enough to allow full recruitment and generation of a high resisting force.

The newer isokinetic dynamometers with computer interface also provides feedback for training purposes. This feedback can take many forms, such as visual when trying to reproduce a torque curve or produce enough force to raise a bar to a preset level. Feedback can be auditory with bells when a preset goal is met. Isokinetics can also provide neuromuscular training by requiring the patient to resist at a specific level that is submaximal, a relatively challenging task. While it may be easy for patients to push as hard as they can to achieve maximum torque production, it is often harder to regulate torque production at lower levels.

Isokinetic resistive training also has disadvantages. These devices are expensive to purchase and maintain. They require trained personnel for setting up patient training programs, testing, and data interpretation. From a biomechanical perspective, most training is done in a single plane, with a fixed axis at a constant velocity in an open kinetic chain. Testing and training in a single plane improve test reproducibility but do not necessarily carry over to function. We rarely move at a constant velocity in functional activities, although this feature provides for maximal loading through the ROM. Newer isokinetic devices have some closed-chain components, which have the advantage of testing a functional movement pattern but the disadvantage of being unable to tell where the muscle performance impairment lies.

Dosage

Isokinetic exercise is dosed similarly to other types of quantitative resistive training. Isokinetic devices have the advantage of computerized data reduction which helps to see and manage resistive exercise volume and intensity. The computerized system allows for storage of exercise training programs which can be programmed and executed with minimal setup. This data can then be tracked over time. Like any resistive exercise program, the volume of activity must be balanced with intensity and viewed within the context of the patient's daily activities.

Body Weight

Body weight can be effectively used as resistance. Resistive exercises for the lower extremity are the most obvious application of body weight as resistance, due to the high number of functional activities that require the lower extremity muscles to move body weight. Walking, running, sports, stair climbing, and transfers of all sorts are examples of activities requiring the movement of body weight. Upper extremity exercises using body weight are less common, but several examples exist. Push-ups, using the arms to push or pull oneself out of bed or a chair or sporting activities such as gymnastics are examples of upper extremity weightbearing activities. Many exercises using body weight as the primary resistance are classified as **closed chain**

exercises. Closed chain exercises are those activities where the distal segment is fixed on a rigid or semi-rigid surface. Squats, lunges, step-ups, or push-ups are considered closed chain exercises. **Open chain** exercises are those where the distal end is free, as in performing a straight leg raise, resistive knee extension, or biceps curl. Body weight can be minimized by altering the position of the body (i.e., push-ups from the knees rather than the feet), using a harness unweighting system, or using a pool. An advantage of using body weight as resistance is that it is always available and rarely requires equipment. A disadvantage is that it is difficult to isolate specific muscles that need strengthening, and the multijoint nature of closed chain exercises lends itself to subtle substitution. See more on closed and open chain exercise in Chapter 14.

THERAPEUTIC EXERCISE INTERVENTION FOR IMPAIRED MUSCLE PERFORMANCE

Therapeutic activities to enhance muscle performance are at the core of the intervention program for many patients. The clinician is faced with a multitude of variables to consider when designing this program. These variables are found in the intervention model in Chapter 2. Prioritizing and balancing all these variables to achieve the best patient outcome requires both knowledge and experience. The following sections will highlight the key variables to consider when designing a resistive exercise program for patients with impairments.

Program Initiation

One of the first variables to consider is the initial physical or training status of the patient. Realize that recommendations about the intervention model variables will change with the training status of the individual patient. Two patients with identical impairments may present with an inflammatory shoulder condition, one who is a regular exerciser, lifting weights 5 days per week and working construction, whereas the other is a sedentary individual, working at a desk job. The initial exercise prescription and progression plan will differ based on the difference in their initial physical condition and training status. The initial examination and evaluation is used to determine the starting point for the therapeutic exercise program. Once the starting point is determined, progress the rehabilitation program based upon the goals established and the gains made. Based upon the initial examination, the following questions should guide the therapist in determining the appropriate starting point for the program:

- What muscle or muscle group(s) need training? What type of muscle contraction does that muscle utilize to perform the functional activities that are limited?
- What type of training is required (i.e., strength, endurance, power, etc.) at this stage of the rehabilitation program? Should the muscle be isolated or worked as a synergist?
- What activity will best accomplish this goal? What range should be exercised?
- What is their current performance/training/strength status? Is strength above or below fair? Are the manual muscle tests normal? Approximately what resistance do you think they will tolerate and for how many repetitions?
- Given the patient's strength, what is the best mode to perform the exercise (i.e., manual resistance, free weights, body weight, isokinetics, etc.)?

- Are there any precautions necessary (i.e., blood pressure, diabetes, joint instability)?
- What is the stage of healing?

Answering these questions will provide the therapist with a starting place for the rehabilitation program (Table 5-5). If the patient reports increased symptoms or is unable to perform the exercise at the level chosen based upon the initial evaluation, a number of opportunities to decrease the exercise challenge exist. Many of these possibilities can be found in Chapter 2 and in Display 2-13. In general, decreasing the intensity, volume, complexity, or environment/stabilization can increase exercise tolerance. Once a set of exercises that do not exacerbate symptoms is developed, then the therapist can consider how to progress the exercise program.

Program Progression

Once the rehabilitation goals and the initial rehabilitation program are determined, the next step is determining the appropriate exercise progression. Exercises can be progressed a multitude of different ways ranging from the most obvious of increasing the exercise intensity, to changing the exercise to a more complex activity. It is possible to achieve continual advancement toward rehabilitation goals with the appropriate manipulation of program variables. Advancing an exercise program in a healthy individual training for health and wellness follows a more predictable pattern. However, progression in the presence of pathology or deficits is much more challenging.

The goal in patient progression is to narrow or eliminate the gap between the patient's current status and the desired functional status. How the therapist guides the patient to bridge that gap will likely vary from one individual to the next. The progression from program initiation to discharge requires a balance between exercise load and the loads applied with daily activities. The exercise load is the amount of stress and strain applied to the tissue of interest as a result of the rehabilitation program. The daily activity load is the stress and strain applied to the same tissue as a result of daily activities. The daily activity load may change from one day to the next depending upon the patient's activities on a given day. The therapist must teach the patient how to modify the rehabilitation program based upon that activity level. This will ensure that the total load placed on the tissue stays within the tissue tolerance. If not, then the likely result is an increase in symptoms.

Display 2-13 (Chapter 2) describes exercise modification parameters that can be used to increase or progress the program. Similarly, if a patient reports an increase in symptoms following program initiation, or the patient is not tolerating the activities at the level they were initiated, the display provides suggested modifications that can decrease the exercise challenge. The overarching goal is to continuously challenge the patient and to expand the training volume to bridge the gap between current and desired functional status. Figure 5-17 shows the relationship between progression variables/opportunities and expanding exercise volume. By systematically varying expanding volume and intensity, patients can continue progressing toward their goals.

TABLE 5-5	**Template for Determining Initial Therapeutic Exercise Prescription**	
EXAMINATION QUESTION	**THERAPEUTIC EXERCISE INTERVENTION MODEL DIMENSION**	**THERAEPUTIC EXERCISE PRESCRIPTION OBTAINED**
What muscle is impaired?	Muscle or muscle group	Muscle group to be trained
How does this muscle function primarily in this patient's activities? Is this the appropriate contraction type to begin with?	Movement	Type of muscle contraction for initial rehabilitation program, as well as contraction type to be progressed toward (if different)
In what range does the muscle function and does it need to be trained through that full range?	Movement	Working range of motion
What is the best mode for applying the resistance?	Mode	Exercise mode such as manual, pulley, elastic band, variable resistance equipment, etc.
What posture or position is this muscle used in functionally for this patient? Is this the best position to initiate training?	Posture	Beginning exercise posture as well as postural goal (if different)
At what speed does this muscle typically function? Is this the best speed to initiate training?	Speed	Beginning exercise speed as well as speed goal (if different)
What is the patient's baseline strength? What are the functional strength demands?	Intensity	Initial training resistance and resistance goals
What muscle function is the primary requirement? (i.e., power, strength, endurance) and at what frequency?	Frequency/duration	Initial training sets and repetitions and sets & repetitions goal
What other associated muscle or muscle groups need training? How do they work with the muscle group of interest? (i.e., synergist)	Sequence	Other supportive muscle groups to be trained and sequence for training
Are there any medical precautions or contraindications?	Overarching	Precautions and contraindications to exercise
What is the stage of healing?	Overarching	Volume and intensity limitations

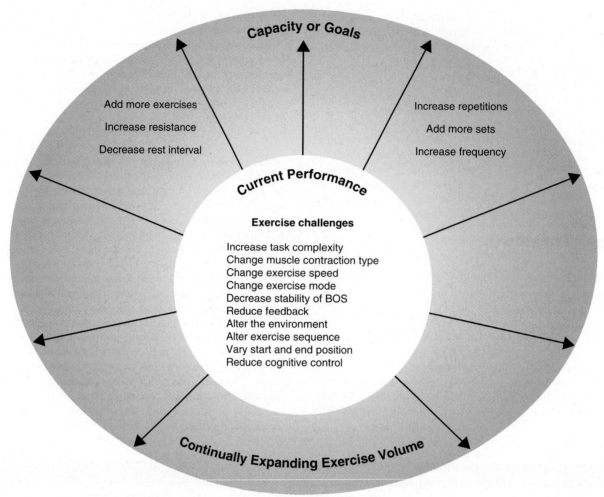

FIGURE 5-17. Exercise progression model.

How much the volume is increased depends upon the discrepancy between current and desired function. If a patient is functioning at a very low level due to injury, surgery, or pathology, then the increase in their total quantity of activity may be substantial. For others who may be very physically active but who still have pain, changing the exercise parameters within the same exercise volume may be preferable. For most patients trying to restore a previous or to obtain a higher level of function, program progression likely follows a variable course with volume increases balanced with exercise parameter changes. For example, a patient recovering from rotator cuff tendinosis may alternate exercise volume increases with changes from isometric or concentric contractions to eccentric, changes from slow speed to fast, and mode changes from free weights to elastic resistance and variable resistance machines (see Building Block 5-5). A variety of options exist depending upon patient goals and preferences.

Another consideration during program progression is the difference between current performance and current capacity. Although a higher capacity or level of function is the long-term goal, the program should be viewed in phases, each with a short-term goal. For example, a patient who sustained a second degree ankle sprain 2 weeks previously may desire to return to long-distance running. However, at this stage of healing, she is doing a series of rehabilitative exercises, deep water running and walking and standing intermittently as part of her job. She is experiencing some increased pain and swelling at the end of the day. It resolves by morning, and overall is making steady improvement. At this point she is likely performing close to her current physical capacity given the stage of healing. Therefore increasing her exercise volume might be inappropriate at this point as it may overwork the healing tissue. Rehabilitative exercise changes within the same working volume may be more appropriate at this stage of healing.

Options to increase the total volume are relatively clear; adding new exercises, resistance, sets, or repetitions are obvious ways to expand the exercise volume. Within a given volume,

---

BUILDING BLOCK 5-5

A 22-year-old marathon runner has had Achilles tendinitis for 6 weeks. She is currently able to run only 3 miles per day every other day before the symptoms prevent her from running any further. Describe how you might progress her strength program to prepare her to return to marathon training. The patient is unwilling to decrease her running at this point.

exercise parameter changes allow exercise progression toward a specific goal without (or with, if that is preferred) a change in total volume. Increasing task complexity can be accomplished a number of different ways. Increasing the number of body segments, the cognitive challenge, or the number of steps are examples of increasing task complexity. For example, increased coordination might be a patient goal. Rather than performing several exercises independently for several repetitions (blocked exercise), different exercises might be combined into a single task (i.e., rise out of a chair, walk across the room around a series of cones, reach up five times, then turn and sit down).

Changing muscle contraction type is another way to change and progress the exercise challenge. For someone recovering from knee surgery, changing from isometric quadriceps sets to straight leg raises and knee extension exercises is an exercise progression. For someone recovering from tendinosis, progressing from isometric contractions to eccentric contractions is another way to progress the exercise program without increasing the exercise volume. For general training purposes, it is important to train both concentric and eccentric muscle actions unless one type of action is preferred based on the pathology, impairments, or activity limitations. For example, patients who have difficulty descending stairs because of poor quadriceps control, but no trouble ascending stairs, should emphasize eccentric muscle actions.

Altering exercise speed can change the exercise impact. For many exercises, resistance varies with speed. For example, in the pool, increasing the speed increases resistance, while with isokinetic concentric exercise, decreasing the speed increases the resistance. When treating tendinosis, the rehabilitation program often progresses from exercises performed slowly to higher speeds.

Changing the exercise mode can alter the exercise challenge. Moving from isotonic resistance to isokinetic can provide more challenge through the range of motion. Changing from variable resistance machines to free weights can encourage more balance and stability. Likewise, decreasing stabilization in any way (with or without changing the mode) will place more challenge on the patient as they must provide internal stabilization to maintain balance and control in the exercise. Similarly, decreasing feedback requires the patient to rely on internal memory trace of correct motor performance rather than on external feedback provided by the therapist.

Changing the environment can provide numerous differing challenges to the patient. One important environmental change is moving from performing exercises in the pool in a minimally or unweighted environment to performing similar exercises on land, or vice versa. Another example is progressing from the structured environment of the clinic where the patient is used to focusing solely on the exercises at hand, to a community environment where there are many competing stimuli. Similarly, changing the exercise sequence can be a form of progression. Sequence preferences were discussed earlier in this chapter. A sample sequence progression might be performing two exercises training the same muscle group back-to-back rather than alternating the exercises with a different activity. For example, the patient might perform resisted knee extension immediately followed by resisted straight leg lifts rather than performing a hamstring curl or an upper body exercise in between.

For many individuals, changing the movement pattern or posture can significantly alter the activity. For example,

patients with spinal stenosis may need to perform exercises in slight flexion in the early stages. As symptoms improve, progression might include performing the same exercises closer to neutral or neutral towards an extended position. The movement for trunk stabilization exercises might progress from performing an exercise bilaterally (where the bilateral nature of the exercise provides balance and some stability) to performing the same movement unilaterally with the contralateral limb held close to the side. This asymmetric pattern would provide increase trunk stability challenge.

Finally, removing cognitive control asks the patient to progress the exercise from the cognitive motor control stage to the autonomous stage (see Chapter 3). This is simply done by engaging the patient cognitively while asking her to perform a motor skill. Thus the same task becomes more challenging as the patient is no longer allowed to cognitively focus on the exercise demands.

Finding the right balance of expanding volume and program changes within the same volume is no easy task. However, taking smaller incremental steps to progress the patient will minimize any significant regression should the program changes be too challenging. Ongoing communication and close monitoring either face-to-face or by other means can help ensure continuous forward progress toward goals. This communication should include patient education on the expected response to the exercise program and instructions for modification should symptoms increase.

THERAPEUTIC EXERCISE INTERVENTION FOR PREVENTION, HEALTH PROMOTION AND WELLNESS

Patients who successfully complete a rehabilitation program may want to continue a resistive exercise program to further the gains they have made and/or to prevent a recurrence of their injury. These individuals can transition into a fitness exercise program. The ACSM defines a *novice* as someone with no training experience, *intermediate* as someone with 6 months of consistent resistance training experience, and *advanced* as someone with years of resistive training experience.[37] *Elite* individuals are highly competitive athletes. Strength gains vary considerably among these training groups. You can expect muscle strength gains of approximately 40% in untrained individuals, 16% to 20% gains in intermediate, 10% in advanced, and 2% in elite athletes.[37] These gains can be expected over the course of 4 weeks to 2 years, with the majority of gains (especially in the untrained) occurring in the first 4 to 8 weeks. For untrained individuals, the responses to just about any training program will be profound, whereas making gains in intermediate, advanced, or elite athletes is much more difficult. Exercise prescription will need to be more creative and variable in these individuals.

While strength gains in the short term (4 to 8 weeks) can be encouraging for the participant, this rate of progress will level off after an initial period of training. At this point, program changes must be considered to continue progression toward exercise goals. The ACSM defines **progression** as the continued improvement in a desired variable (i.e., strength, power, endurance, muscle hypertrophy, etc.) over time until the individual goal has been achieved.[31] Continuing the initial training program for several months following program initiation is unlikely to sustain forward progress. Changes to the resistive training program are necessary to minimize training plateaus and to sustain forward progress. Like resistive training for rehabilitation, progressive overload can occur by increasing the exercise load, repetitions, or volume, or by changing the exercise speed, decreasing rest intervals, or by any combination of these variables. A periodized program to systematically vary exercise volume and intensity has been shown to be most effective for long-term progression.[37,127,128]

Dosage for Strength Training

For strength development, the ACSM recommends that novice and intermediate lifters train at an intensity of 60% to 70% of 1 RM for 8 to 12 repetitions.[37] All lifters should use both concentric and eccentric contractions. Untrained individuals require very little load to improve strength. Loads as little as 45% to 50% of 1 RM and less have been shown to increase strength in previously untrained individuals.[128,129] Novices should train the entire body 2 to 3 days per week whereas intermediate lifters should train similarly, unless desiring to progress to split workouts (upper body one day and lower another). In this case, the frequency should be 3 to 4 days per week, allowing training of each muscle group 1 to 2 days per week. The volume prescription should include either single or multiple sets initially (such as the DeLorme or DAPRE) and progressed to periodized training using multiple sets. Advanced lifters should train at 80% to 100% of 1 RM in a periodized plan.[37] Apply an approximately 2% to 10% increase in load when the individual can perform the current intensity for one to two repetitions over the desired number on two consecutive training sessions.[37] Base the intensity progression on the muscle group and activity.

The total training volume should be varied and progressed to continue strength gains. The training volume can be varied by changing the number of exercised performed in a session, by changing the number of repetitions performed in a set or the number of sets of exercise. Training volume dose-response recommendations for different populations have been made.[33] For untrained individuals, maximum strength gains were achieved at an intensity of 60% of 1 RM, 3 days per week with a mean training of four sets per muscle group. Recreationally trained athletes showed maximum strength gains at a dosage of 80% of one RM two days per week also training four sets per muscle group. For athletes, maximal strength gains were made when training at 85% of 1 RM, 2 days per week at a mean training volume of eight sets per muscle group.[33,130]

Some ongoing debate surrounds the question of single-versus multiple-set resistance training programs.[131–134] Many general strength training programs include a single exercise set of 8 to 12 repetitions.[135] For novice exercisers, either single- or multiple-set resistance programs will achieve strength gains, although multiple-sets produced superior gains in some research.[37,133,134] However, for trained individuals, multiple sets are more effective for strength building.[37,131,132]

Slow to moderate velocities are recommended for novice trainers unless the patient has difficulty generating torque or controlling movement at a specific functional speed. The ACSM recommends moderate velocities for intermediate training, and a spectrum of velocities from unintentionally slow to fast to maximize training gains in the advanced and elite athlete.[37] Unintentionally slow velocities are those where the load is so high that it requires the individual to lift slowly due to loading and/or fatigue. This type of training produces overload and a training response, whereas intentionally slow lifting, or submaximal lifting performed at a slow velocity (i.e., 5 to 10 second concentric, 5 second eccentric), do not produce sufficient overload.[136,137]

For novice, intermediate, or advanced training, the ACSM recommends rest intervals of 2 to 3 minutes for multijoint exercises using heavy loads.[37] For other exercises (including weight machines) they recommend a shorter rest interval of 1 to 2 minutes. This recommendation is the same for developing both strength and power.

Dosage for Power Training

Power requires a combination of strength, speed, and skill and the training program should reflect these variables. Effective use of power requires baseline strength at both fast and slow speeds, the ability to generate force quickly, efficient use of the SSC, and good neuromuscular coordination.

For power development, one to three sets of 30% to 60% of 1 RM for three to six repetitions should be incorporated into the intermediate training program.[37] Progression should use various loads planned in a periodized fashion. Advanced training should include a three to six set (one to six repetitions per set) power program incorporated into the strength program. Progression of power training requires both heavy loading (85% to 100% of 1 RM) for force development, and light to moderate loading (30% to 60% of 1 RM) performed at high velocity for increasing fast force production.[37] Focus only on heavy loading may actually decrease power output if not accompanied by quick, explosive-type exercises such as the loaded jump squat.[94] Rest period recommendations are the same as for strength training (see Building Block 5-6).

Plyometric Exercise

Functional activity seldom involves pure forms of isolated isometric, concentric, or eccentric actions, because the body is subjected to impact forces (Fig. 5-18), as in running or jumping, or because some external force, such as gravity, lengthens the muscle. In these movement patterns, the muscles are acting eccentrically and then concentrically. By definition of eccentric action, the muscle must be active during the lengthening phase. The SSC is the combination of an eccentric action followed by a concentric action. Training techniques that employ the SSC are called plyometrics. Examples of plyometric exercises include hopping, skipping, bounding and jumping drills for the lower extremity, and plyometric ball or elastic resistive exercises for the upper extremity. However,

 BUILDING BLOCK 5-6

A sprint athlete would like advice on how to increase performance for the 220-yard hurdles. Please provide some suggested strategies.

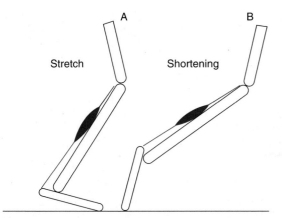

A   B

Stretch   Shortening

FIGURE 5-18. The SSC cycle in daily activities. At contact the muscle is stretched and contracts in a lengthening action (eccentric) (A). The stretch phase is followed by a shortening (concentric) action (B). The figure demonstrates the SSC, which is the natural form of the muscle function.

not all jumping or resistive band exercises are plyometric. Plyometrics are done with a specific goal in mind: to increase power and speed.

Plyometrics are quick, powerful movements that are used to increase the reactivity of the nervous system. Plyometrics enhance work performance by storing elastic energy in the muscle during the stretch phase and reusing it as mechanical work during the concentric phase. Bosco et al.[138] found that the amount of elastic energy stored in a muscle during eccentric work determines the recoil of elastic energy during positive work. Part of the developed tension during the stretching phase is taken up by the elastic elements arranged in series with sarcomeres (i.e., series elastic component or tendon). This mechanical work is stored in the sarcomere cross-bridges and can be reused during the following positive work if the muscle is contracted immediately after the stretch. The muscle's ability to use the stored energy is determined by the timing of the eccentric and concentric contractions and by the velocity and magnitude of stretch. A quick transition from eccentric to concentric (i.e., undamped landings) along with a high-velocity stretch of high magnitude produces the greatest benefits. The transition time between the eccentric and concentric contractions is called the amortization phase, and the distinction between plyometrics and other impact activities is the goal of decreasing this phase as much as possible.

Plyometrics are high-level activities. Because of the stored energy in the series elastic component, the tendon is susceptible to overuse injury when performing plyometric exercises. The individual should be in an advanced training stage before these techniques are employed. In an advanced exercise program, these techniques develop power and speed, the key muscle performance elements of athletics. Jumping from or to different heights, bounding (i.e., jumping for distance), progressive throwing programs, and throwing for speed or distance are methods of using SSC for enhancing speed or power performance. Before performing lower extremity plyometrics, the individual must be able to squat his or her body weight, perform a standing long jump equal to his or her height, and balance on a single leg with eyes closed. Programs should be well-planned and progressed slowly and appropriately for the individual and the goals. An example of a plyometric program can be found in Display 5-3. See Additional Reading for more plyometric materials.

DISPLAY 5-3
Sample Plyometric Activities

Easy
- Ankle bounces in place
- Ankle bounces side to side
- Ankle bounces with 90-degree turn
- Ankle bounces in stride
- Single leg push offs from box
- Lateral hopping over cones
- Forward hopping over cones

Intermediate
- Jump ups on box
- Side jumps on to box
- Tuck jump
- Multiple jumps forward
- Multiple jumps sideways
- Split squat jump
- Cone hops with turn
- Cone hops with land and sprint

Advanced
- Multiple box jumps with single leg land
- Squat jumps to multiple boxes
- Depth jumps with ball catch
- Standing long jump with 90-degree turn and sprint
- Depth jump with 90-degree turn and sprint
- Single leg bounding
- Bounding and vertical jump combination

Dosage for Endurance Training

Muscle endurance is necessary for a variety of activities and muscle groups. For example, postural muscles must provide sustained or repetitive contractions for long periods, such as during prolonged standing, walking, or work activities. Many lower extremity muscles need endurance for athletic endeavors such as distance running, tennis, or other sports and leisure activities. Repetitive work activities such as carpentry, factory work, or other manual labor require local muscle endurance to fulfill job requirements during 8- to 12-hour work shifts.

For development of muscular endurance in novice and intermediate training, the ACSM recommends relatively light loads with moderate to high volume (10 to 15 repetitions). For advanced training, various loading strategies should be used for multiple sets per exercise (10 to 25 repetitions) using a periodization scheme.[37]

Use shorter rest periods such as 1 to 2 minutes for high repetition (15 to 20 repetitions) and <1 minute for moderate (10 to 15 repetitions) sets.[37] The training frequency is the same as for strength training, and the training velocity should be slow when doing a moderate (10 to 15) number of repetitions, and moderate or fast velocities when performing higher numbers of repetitions (15 to 25 or more).

Dosage for the Advanced or Elite Athlete

The following techniques are used by those who train competitive athletes. These techniques can be used to provide variety, increase resistance, or maximize the workout time in daily workouts. These specific techniques are not well-studied, but do provide the recommended variability necessary for training the advanced or elite athlete. They are introduced to familiarize the therapist with the terminology used in training these athletes. Use good judgment based on scientific principles when using these techniques.

A superset consists of two sets of exercise involving opposing muscles that are performed in sequence without a rest between sets (e.g., a biceps curl followed by a triceps extension, without rest, proceeding to the remaining sets). Supersets can reduce workout time or allow more exercise to be performed during the same period.

A triset is a group of three exercises, each done after the other with little rest between muscle groups. Trisets can be used to exercise three different muscle groups or three angles of a complex muscle (e.g., flat, incline, decline bench press for the different fiber directions of the pectoralis major).

Pyramid training is a modification of the DeLorme training program. The regimen starts with a high number of repetitions and low weight (to warm-up), but instead of maintaining the repetitions constant and increasing the weight, the repetitions are reduced and weight is increased. After the series is completed, the individual works backward, taking off weight and adding repetitions. The number of repetitions and sets is arbitrarily established as long as the high-repetition, low-weight progression to a heavier-weight, low-repetition regimen is followed (Table 5-6).

A typical split routine consists of a series of exercises that usually emphasize two or three major muscle groups or body parts. This allows the individual to train on 2 consecutive days without overtraining muscle groups, because one muscle group is resting while the other is exercising. Body builders often follow a double-split routine, in which two sessions are performed on each day (Table 5-7).

Matveyev[139] described the basic ideas of periodized training programs for these athletes. A program is periodized when it is divided into phases, each of which has primary and secondary goals. The program is based on the premise that maximum strength gains are not made by constant heavy training but are made possible by different training cycles or periods. These cycles allow the athlete to reach maximum performance level at a predesignated time, usually the day of competition.

In his original model, Matveyev[139] suggested the initial phase of a strength-power program should contain a high volume (i.e., many repetitions) with lower intensity (i.e., low average weight lifted relative to maximum possible in each movement). Typical high-volume phases for weight lifters contain more training sessions per week (6 to 15),

TABLE 5-7 Example of a Split Routine for Total-Body Resistive Training

FOUR-DAY PROGRAM[a]	SIX-DAY, TWO SESSIONS PER DAY PROGRAM[a]
Monday: upper body	Monday AM: chest
Tuesday: lower body	Monday PM: back
Wednesday: rest	Tuesday AM: shoulders
Thursday: upper body	Tuesday AM: upper legs
Friday: lower body	Wednesday AM: triceps
Saturday: rest	Wednesday PM: biceps
Sunday: repeat sequence	Thursday AM: chest
	Thursday PM: back

[a]Abdominal and calf muscles are exercised each day.

more exercises per session (3 to 6), more sets per exercise (4 to 8), and more repetitions per set (4 to 6). As weeks pass, the volume decreases and intensity increases. The resulting higher intensity and lower volume represent the characteristics of a basic strength phase of training. Typical high-intensity phases for weight lifters contain fewer training sessions per week (5 to 12), fewer exercises per workout session (1 to 4), fewer sets per exercise (3 to 5), and fewer repetitions per set (1 to 3). A third, optional phase may include low volume (low repetitions) with high intensity (heavy weights) to work on power. The final phase is considered an active rest phase with very low volume and very low intensity.

Each phase may be several weeks to several months long. Two or more complete cycles may fit into a training year.

Stone et al.[140] proposed and successfully tested a periodized model of strength-power training with sequential phases that change rather drastically. An example is a phase to increase muscle size (five sets of 10 RM in core exercises), a phase to improve specific strength (three to five sets of 3 RM), and a phase to "peak" for competition (one to three sets of one to three repetitions). The use of 10 RM is higher than typically recommended in the early preparation phase but has proved to be successful in a number of studies.[140]

PRECAUTIONS AND CONTRAINDICATIONS

Be sure to consider certain precautions and contraindications when prescribing resistive exercise. Avoid using the Valsalva maneuver during resistive training, especially by patients with cardiopulmonary disease or after recent abdominal, intervertebral disk, or eye surgery. Educate patients to breathe properly during exercise, typically exhaling on exertion. Use isometric exercise with caution by persons at risk for pressor response effects (e.g., high blood pressure after an aneurysm).

Overwork phenomena may exist even at moderate training regimens over an extended period. Overtraining may lead to mood disturbances and reduce the effect of training by a decrease in performance. Avoid fatigue and overtraining by patients with metabolic diseases (e.g., diabetes, alcoholism), neurologic diseases, or severe degenerative joint diseases

TABLE 5-6 Sample Pyramid Training for a Squat Exercise for a Highly Trained Individual

SETS	REPETITIONS	WEIGHT
1	12	100
1	8	135
1	6	185
1	4	225
1	2	250
1	1	275

because of the risk of further joint damage. Overtraining may be the reason for a lack of progress, decreased performance, or development of joint pain and swelling.

Care should be taken when developing resistive exercise programs for prepubertal and pubertal children and adolescents. Minimize stress to epiphyseal sites and develop balanced exercise programs to avoid muscle imbalances.

An absolute contraindication to resistive exercise is acute or chronic myopathy, as occurs in some forms of neuromuscular disease or in acute alcohol myopathy. Resistive exercise in the presence of myopathy may stress and permanently damage an already compromised muscular system.

Scientific knowledge and common sense should be applied in prescribing resistive exercise. Caution should be taken with exercise in the presence of pain, inflammation, and infection. Although resistive exercise may be indicated, the mode and dosage should be carefully chosen.

KEY POINTS

- The term *muscle performance* includes strength, power, and endurance.
- The term *strength* should be clarified in terms of force, torque, and work.
- Muscle actions are static and dynamic. Static muscle actions are called *isometric*.
- A thorough knowledge of muscle morphology is necessary for effective/efficient therapeutic exercise prescription to improve muscle performance.
- Dynamic action is the preferred term over isotonic. Dynamic actions can be further divided into concentric and eccentric actions.
- The sliding filament theory describes the events that occur during muscle contraction.
- Basic muscle fiber types are slow oxidative, fast glycolytic, and fast oxidative glycolytic.
- Force gradation occurs by rate coding and the size principle.
- Overload training produces changes in the size of the muscle primarily through hypertrophy but also through hyperplasia.
- Muscle strength must be evaluated relative to the muscle's length because of length-tension relationships.
- Muscle architecture can significantly affect muscle force production.
- Specificity of training exists, especially relative to training velocity.
- Eccentric muscle contractions are the most energy-efficient contraction type and can develop the greatest tension of any muscle contraction type.
- Adaptations to resistive training are partially neurologic in that changes in performance often precede morphologic changes.
- *Form fatigue* is the point at which the individual must discontinue the exercise or sacrifice technique.
- Although dosage and goals differ, resistive training is beneficial from late childhood through old age.
- Impaired muscle performance can result from neurologic pathology, muscle strain, muscle disuse, or length associated changes.
- Adaptations to resistive training extend beyond the muscle to include connective tissues, the cardiovascular system, and bone.
- Activities to improve muscle performance include isometric, dynamic, plyometric, and isokinetic exercise.
- Dynamic exercise can be performed with a variety of modes, including free weight, resistive bands, pulleys, weight machines, or body weight; including various combinations of concentric and eccentric contractions.

◤ LAB ACTIVITIES

1. A series of musculoskeletal conditions is listed from i to viii. For each condition, perform the following
   a. Determine which muscles are involved. Include possible underused synergists that may lead to overuse of the muscle involved. List each muscle and describe its specific action.
   b. Design and perform one exercise for each muscle (group) given the manual muscle test grade of fair minus (3–/5). Include complete dosage parameters.
   c. Design and perform two exercises for each muscle (group) given the manual muscle test grade of good (4/5). Use an elastic band for one and a free weight for the other, and include complete dosage parameters.
   d. Progress the exercises in question 1c to two functional activities.

Musculoskeletal and neuromuscular conditions
   i. Achilles tendinitis
   ii. Iliotibial band fascitis
   iii. Patellar tendinitis
   iv. Hamstring strain
   v. Peroneal nerve palsy (i.e., common peroneal nerve; list muscles innervated)
   vi. Supraspinatus tendinitis
   vii. Middle trapezius strain resulting from overstretch
   viii. Lateral epicondylitis

2. Using free weights or a weight machine, determine the 1, 6, and 10 RM for a bench press and leg extension. Determine the dosage for Oxford, DeLorme, and DAPRE programs.

3. Pick three muscle groups throughout your body (one upper quarter, one lower quarter, and one trunk). Design two different resistive exercises for each muscle group using a variety of equipment, including elastic bands, free weights, and pulleys and weight machines if available. Determine the dosage for a DeLorme program.

- Plyometric activities use the SSC to enhance muscle performance.
- The dosage of exercise to improve muscle performance depends on the goal (i.e., strength, power, and endurance) as well as the initial fitness level of the individual (i.e., novice, intermediate, advanced, and elite).
- Precautions and contraindications to resistive exercise must be known to ensure safety to the patient/client.

CRITICAL THINKING QUESTIONS

1. Consider each of the questions in the Lab Activities in the next section. How would your dosage differ if you were training for
   a. strength
   b. power
   c. muscle endurance
2. Design a muscle performance program for a woman confined to bed rest for 3 weeks after an acute lumbar fracture without neurologic involvement. Include dosage parameters for strength and endurance.
3. Consider Case Study No. 5 in Unit 7. List muscles with impaired muscle performance. Determine whether the muscle requires strength, endurance, or power training. Decide on one activity for each muscle and determine the dosage relative to the goal (i.e., strength, power, and endurance) and initial fitness level for this patient. Develop the sequence of exercise for each session and include the frequency in the dosage parameters.

REFERENCES

1. Enoka RM. Force. In: Enoka RM, ed. Neuromechanical Basis of Kinesiology. Champaign, IL: Human Kinetics Books, 1988.
2. McArdle WD, Katch FI, Katch VL. Essentials of Exercise Physiology. 6th Ed. Baltimore, MD: Lippincott, Williams & Wilkins, 2007.
3. Abbott BC, Bigland B, Ritchie JM. The physiological cost of negative work. J Physiol (Lond) 1952;117:380–390.
4. Norman RW, Komi PV. Electromyographic delay in skeletal muscle under normal movement conditions. Acta Physiol Scand 1979;106:241.
5. Komi PV. Stretch-shortening cycle. In: Komi PV, ed. Strength and Power in Sport. Oxford: Blackwell Scientific Publications, 1992.
6. Baechle TR, Earle RW. Essentials of Strength Training and Conditioning. 2nd Ed. Champaign, IL: Human Kinetics, 2000.
7. Bell RD, MacDougall JD, Billeter R, et al. Muscle fiber types and morphometric analysis of skeletal muscle in six year old children. Med Sci Sports Exerc 1480;12:28–31.
8. Saltin B, Henriksson J, Nygaard E, et al. Fiber types and metabolic potentials of skeletal muscles in sedentary man and endurance runners. Ann N Y Acad Sci 1977;301:3–29.
9. Campbell CJ, Bonen A, Kirby RL, et al. Muscle fiber composition and performance capacities of women. Med Sci Sports 1979;11:260–265.
10. Billeter R, Hoppeler H. Muscular basis of strength. In: Komi PV, ed. Strength and Power in Sport. Oxford: Blackwell Scientific Publications, 1992.
11. Antonio J, Gonyea WJ. Skeletal muscle fiber hyperplasia. Med Sci Sports Exerc 1993;25:1333–1345.
12. MacDougall DJ. Hypertrophy or hyperplasia. In: Komi PV, ed. Strength and Power in Sport. Oxford: Blackwell Scientific Publications, 1992.
13. Bischof R. Analysis of muscle regeneration using single myofibers in culture. Med Sci Sports Exerc 1989;21(Suppl):S163–S172.
14. Schultz E, Jaryszak DL, Gibson MC, et al. Absence of exogenous satellite cell contribution to regeneration of frozen skeletal muscle. J Muscle Res Cell Motil 1986;7:361–367.
15. MacDougall JD, Sale DG, Alway SE, et al. Muscle fiber number in biceps brachii in body builders and control subjects. J Appl Physiol 1984;57:1399–1403.
16. Herzog W, Ait-Haddou R. Mechanical muscle models and their application for force and power production. In: Komi PV, ed. Strength and Power in Sport. 2nd Ed. Malden, MA: Blackwell Scientific Publications, 2003.
17. Tabary JC, Tabary C, Tardieu C, et al. Physiological and structural changes in the cat's soleus muscle due to immobilization at different lengths by plaster cast. J Physiol 1972;224:231–244.
18. Oudet CL, Petrovic AG. Regulation of the anatomical length of the lateral pterygoid muscle in the growing rat. Adv Physiol Sci 1981;24:115–121.
19. Kendall HO, Kendall FP, Boynton DA. Posture and Pain. Baltimore, MD: Williams & Wilkins, 1952.
20. Williams PE, Goldspink G. Longitudinal growth of striated muscle fibers. J Cell Sci 1971;9:751–767.
21. Herring SW, Grimm AF, Grimm BR. Regulation of sarcomere number in skeletal muscle: a comparison of hypotheses. Muscle Nerve 1984;7:161–173.
22. Kendall FP, McCreary KE, Provance PG. Muscles Testing and Function. 4th Ed. Baltimore, MD: Williams & Wilkins, 1993.
23. Williams PE, Goldspink G. Changes in sarcomere length and physiological properties in immobilized muscle. J Anat 1978;127:459–468.
24. Josephson RK. Extensive and intensive factors determining the performance of striated muscle. J Exp Zool 1975;194:135–154.
25. DeLorme TL. Restoration of muscle power by heavy resistance exercises. J Bone Joint Surg Am 1945;27:645–667.
26. Delorme TL, Watkins AL. Progressive Resistance Exercise. New York, NY: Appleton Century, 1951.
27. Zinovieff AN. Heavy resistance exercise: the Oxford technique. Br J Physiol 1951;14:129–132.
28. McMorris RO, Elkins EC. A study of production and evaluation of muscular hypertrophy. Arch Phys Med Rehabil 1954;35:420–426.
29. Knight KL. Knee rehabilitation by the daily adjustable progressive resistive exercise technique. Am J Sports Med 1979;7:336–337.
30. Krusen EM. Functional improvement produced by resistance exercise of the biceps muscles affected by polio-myelitis. Arch Phys Med 1949;30:271–278.
31. Clarke HH. Muscular Strength and Endurance in Man. Englewood Cliffs, NJ: Prentice-Hall, Inc., 1966.
32. Gonzalez-Bandillo JJ, Gorostiaga EM, Arellano R, et al. Moderate resistance training volume produces more favorable strength gains than high or low volumes during a short-term training cycle. J Strength Cond Res 2005;19(3):689–697.
33. Peterson MD, Rhea MR, Alvar BA. Applications of the dose-response for muscular strength development: a review of meta-analytic efficacy and reliability for designing training prescription. J Strength Cond Res 2005;19(4):950–958.
34. Willardson JM. A brief review: factors affecting the length of the rest interval between resistance exercise sets. J Strength Cond Res 2006;20(4):978–984.
35. Ahtiainen JP, Pakarinen A, Alen M, et al. Short vs. long rest period between the sets in hypertropic resistance training: influence on muscle strength, size and hormonal adaptations in trained men. J Strength Cond Res 2005;19(3):572–582.
36. Busso T, Benoit H, Bonnefoy R, et al. Effects of training frequency on the dynamics of performance response to a single training bout. J Appl Physiol 2002;92:572–580.
37. Kraemer WJ, Adams K, Cararelli E, et al. American College of Sports Medicine position stand. Progression models in resistance training for healthy adults. Med Sci Sports Exerc 2002;34:364–380.
38. Tippett SR, Voight ML. Functional Progression for Sport Rehabilitation. Champaigne, IL: Human Kinetics, 1995:4, ISBN 0–873–22660–7.
39. Seger JY, Thorstensson A. Effects of eccentric versus concentric training on thigh muscle strength and EMG. Int J Sports Med 2005;26(1):45–52.
40. Morrissey MC, Harman EA, Johnson MJ. Resistance training modes: specificity and effectiveness. Med Sci Sports Exerc 1995;27:648–660.
41. Kanehisa H, Miyashita M. Specificity of velocity in strength training. Eur J Appl Physiol 1983;52:104–106.
42. Higbie EJ. Effects of concentric and eccentric isokinetic heavy-resistance training on quadriceps muscle strength, cross-sectional area and neural activation in women. Doctoral Dissertation, University of Georgia, 1994.
43. Weir JP, Housh DJ, Housh TJ, et al. The effect of unilateral concentric weight training and detraining on joint angle specificity, cross-training, and the bilateral deficit. J Orthop Sports Phys Ther 1997;25:264–270.
44. Weir JP, Housh DJ, Housh TJ, et al. The effect of unilateral eccentric weight training and detraining on joint angle specificity, cross-training, and the bilateral deficit. J Orthop Sports Phys Ther 1995;22:207–215.
45. Taniguchi Y. Lateral specificity in resistance training: the effect of bilateral and unilateral training. Eur J Appl Physiol 1997;75:144–150.
46. Wilson GJ, Murphy AJ, Walshe A. The specificity of strength training: the effect of posture. Eur J Appl Physiol 1996;73:346–352.
47. Frontera WR, Meredith CN, O'Reilly KP, et al. Strength conditioning in older men: skeletal muscle hypertrophy and improved function. J Appl Physiol 1988;64(3):1038–1044.
48. Staron RS, Karapondo DL, Kraemer WJ, et al. Skeletal muscle adaptations during early phase of heavy-resistance training in men and women. J Appl Physiol 1994;76:1247–1255.
49. Hakkinen K, Komi PV. Electromyographic changes during strength training and detraining. Med Sci Sports Exerc 1983;15:455–460.
50. Sale D. Neural adaptation to strength training. In: Komi PV. Strength and Power in Sport. Oxford: Blackwell Scientific Publications, 1992.
51. Edman PK. Contractile performance of skeletal muscle fibers. In: Komi PV, ed. Strength and Power in Sport. Oxford: Blackwell Scientific Publications, 1992.
52. Friden J, Seger J, Sjostrom M, et al. Adaptive response in human skeletal muscle subjected to prolonged eccentric training. Int J Sports Med 1983;4:177–183.

53. McHugh MP, Connolly DA, Eston RG, et al. Electromyographic analysis of exercise resulting in symptoms of muscle damage. J Sports Sci 2000;18(3):163–172.

54. Paschalis V, Nikolaidis MG, Giakas G, et al. The effect of eccentric exercise on position sense and joint reaction angle of the lower limbs. Muscle Nerve 2007;35(4):496–503.

55. Crasselt W, Forchel I, Kroll M, et al. Zum Kinder- und Jugendsport—Realitaten, Wunshe und Tendenzen. [Sport of Children and Adolescents—Reality, Expectations, and Tendencies.] Leipzig: Deutsche Hochschule fur Korperkultur, 1990.

56. Hettinger TH. Isometrisches Muskeltraining. [Isometric Muscle Training.] Stuttgart: George Thieme Verlag, 1968.

57. Yokomizo YI. Measurement of ability of older workers. Ergonomics 1985;28:843–854.

58. Grimby G, Danneskiold-Samse W, Hvid K, et al. Morphology and enzymatic capacity in arm and leg muscles in 78–81-year-old men and women. Acta Physiol Scand 1982;115:125–134.

59. Moritani T. Training adaptations in the muscles of older men. In: Smith EL, Serfass RE, eds. Exercise and Aging: The Scientific Basis. New Jersey: Enslow Publishers, 1981.

60. Janda V. Muskelfunktionsdiagnostik. [Functional Diagnostic Tests for Muscles.] Berlin: Verlag Volk & Gesundheit, 1986.

61. Bean JF, Kiely SK, Herman S, et al. The relationship between leg power and physical performance in mobility-limited elderly people. J Am Ger Soc 2002;50:461–467.

62. Bottaro M, Machado SN, Nogueira W, et al. Effect of high versus low-velocity resistance training on muscular fitness and functional performance in older men. Eur J Appl Physiol 2007;99(3):257–264.

63. Miszko TA, Cress ME, Slade JM, et al. Effect of strength and power training on physical function in community-dwelling older adults. J Gerontol A Biol Sci Med Sci 2003;58(2):171–175.

64. de Vos NJ, Singh NA, Ross DA, et al. Optimal load for increasing muscle power during explosive resistance training in older adults. J Gerontol A Biol Sci Med Sci 2005;60(5):638–647.

65. Fielding RA, LeBrasseur NK, Cuoco A, et al. High-velocity resistance training increases skeletal muscle peak power in older women. J Am Ger Soc 2002;50:655–662.

66. Wilkes RL, Summers JJ. Cognitions, mediating variables, and strength performance. J Sport Psychol 1984;6:351–359.

67. Weinberg R, Jackson A, Seaboune T. The effects of specific vs. nonspecific mental preparation strategies on strength and endurance performance. J Sport Behav 1985;7:175–180.

68. Tenenbaum G, Bar-Eli M, Hoffman JR, et al. The effect of cognitive and somatic psyching-up techniques on isokinetic leg strength performance. J Strength Cond Res 1995;9:3–7.

69. Murphy SM, Woolfolk RL, Budney AJ. The effects of emotive imagery on strength performance. J Sport Exerc Psychol 1988;10:334–345.

70. Elko K, Ostrow AC. The effects of three mental preparation strategies on strength performance of young and older adults. J Sport Behav 1992;15:34–41.

71. Gould D, Weinberg R, Jackson A. Mental preparation strategies, cognition and strength performance. J Sport Psychol 1980;2:329–339.

72. Gassner GJ. Comparison of three different types of imagery on performance outcome in strength-related tasks with collegiate male athletes. Dissertation thesis, Temple University, 1997.

73. Hobbel SL, Rose DJ. The relative effectiveness of three forms of visual knowledge of results on peak torque output. J Orthop Sports Phys Ther 1993;18:601–608.

74. Rubin E. Alcoholic myopathy in heart and skeletal muscle. N Engl J Med 1979;301:28–33.

75. Song SK, Rubin E. Ethanol produces muscle damage in human volunteers. Science 1972;175:327–328.

76. Rubin E, Perkoff GT, Dioso NM, et al. A spectrum of myopathy associated with alcoholism. Ann Intern Med 1967;67:481–492.

77. Hanid A, Slavin G, Main, et al. Fiber type changes in striated muscle of alcoholics. J Clin Pathol 1981;34:991–995.

78. Mastaglia FL, Argov Z. Drug-induced neuromuscular disorders in man. In: Walton J, ed. Disorders of Voluntary Muscle. 4th Ed. Edinburgh: Churchill Livingstone, 1981.

79. Stern LZ, Fagan JM. The endocrine myopathies. In: Vinken PJ, Bruyn GW, Ringel SP, eds. Handbook of Clinical Neurological Disease of Muscle: Part 2. Amsterdam: North Holland Publishing, 1979.

80. Bunch TW, Worthingham JW, Combs JJ, et al. Azathioprine with prednisone for polymyositis: a controlled clinical trial. Ann Intern Med 1980;92:356–369.

81. Goldberg AL, Goodman HM. Relationship between cortisone and muscle work in determining muscle size. J Physiol (Lond) 1969;200:667–675.

82. Malone TR, Garrett E, Zachazewski JE. Muscle: deformation, injury, repair. In: Zachazewski JE, Magee DJ, Quillen WS, eds. Athletic Injuries and Rehabilitation. Philadelphia, PA: WB Saunders, 1996.

83. Worrell TW, Perrin DH. Hamstring muscle injury: the influence of strength, flexibility, warm-up and fatigue. J Orthop Sports Phys Ther 1992;16:12–18.

84. Desmedt JE, Godaux E. Spinal motoneuron recruitment in man: rank ordering with direction but not with speed of voluntary movement. Science 1981;214:933–936.

85. Tax AM, Denier van der Gon JJ, Gielen CAM, et al. Differences in central control of m. biceps brachii in movement tasks and force tasks. Exp Brain Res 1990;79:138–142.

86. Van Zuylen EJ, Gielen CAM, Denier van der Gon JJ. Coordination and homogenous activation of human arm muscles during isometric torques. J Neurophys 1988;60:1523–1548.

87. Munn J, Herbert RD, Hancock MJ, et al. Resistance training for strength: effect of number of sets and contraction speed. Med Sci Sports Exerc 2005;37(9):1622–1666.

88. Staron R, Hikida RS, Hagerman FC, et al. Human muscle skeletal muscle fiber type adaptability to various workloads. J Histochem Cytochem 1984;32:146–152.

89. Costill DC, Daniels J, Evans, et al. Skeletal muscle enzymes and fiber composition in male and female track athletes. J Appl Physiol 1976;40:149–154.

90. Tesch PA, Komi PV, Hakkinen K. Enzymatic adaptations consequent to long term strength training. Int J Sports Med 1987;8(Suppl):66–69.

91. MacDougall JD, Sale DG, Moroz JR, et al. Mitochondrial volume density in human skeletal muscle following heavy resistance training. Med Sci Sports 1979;11:164–166.

92. Thorstensson A, Spokin B, Karlsson J. Enzyme activities and muscle strength after "sprint training" in man. Acta Physiol Scand 1975;94:313–316.

93. Hakkinen K, Komi PV, Alen M. Effect of explosive type strength training on isometric force and relaxation time, electromyographic and muscle fibre characteristics of leg extensor muscles. Acta Physiol Scand 1985;125:587–600.

94. Stone MH. Implications for connective tissue and bone alterations resulting from resistance exercise training. Med Sci Sports Exerc 1988;20:S162–S168.

95. Tipton CM, Mattes RD, Maynard JA, et al. The influence of physical activity on ligaments and tendons. Med Sci Sports 1975;7:165–175.

96. Vogel JM, Whittle MW. Proceedings: bone mineral content changes in the Skylab astronauts. Am J Roentgenol 1976;126:1296–1297.

97. Hanson TH, Roos BO, Nachemson A. Development of osteopenia in the fourth lumbar vertebrae during prolonged bed rest after operation for scoliosis. Acta Orthop Scand 1975;46:621–630.

98. White MK, Martin RB, Yeater RA, et al. The effects of exercise on postmenopausal women. Int Orthop 1984;7:209–214.

99. Nilsson BE, Westlin NE. Bone density in athletes. Clin Orthop 1971;77:179–182.

100. Jones HH, Priest JS, Hayes WC, et al. Humeral hypertrophy in response to exercise. J Bone Joint Surg Am 1977;59:204–208.

101. Lane N, Bevier W, Bouxsein M, et al. Effect of exercise intensity on bone mineral. Med Sci Sports Exerc 1988;20:S51.

102. Duncan CS, Blimkie CJ, Cowell C, et al. Bone mineral density in adolescent female athletes: relationship to exercise type and muscle strength. Med Sci Sports Exerc 2002;34:286–294.

103. Robling AG, Hinant FM, Burr DB, et al. Shorter, more frequent mechanical loading sessions enhance bone mass. Med Sci Sports Exerc 2002;34:196–202.

104. Fleck SJ. Cardiovascular adaptations to resistance training. Med Sci Sports Exerc 1988;20:S146–S151.

105. Fleck SJ, Henke C, Wilson W. Cardiac MRI of elite junior Olympic weight lifters. Int J Sports Med 1989;10:329–333.

106. Miles DS, Gotshall RW. Impedance cardiography: noninvasive assessment of human central hemodynamics at rest and during exercise. Exerc Sports Sci Rev 1989;17:231–264.

107. Shephard RJ. Muscular endurance and blood lactate. In: Shephard RM, Astrand P-O, eds. Endurance in Sport. Oxford: Blackwell Scientific Publications, 1992.

108. Lash JM, Sherman WM. Skeletal muscle function and adaptations to training. In: American College of Sports Medicine: Resource Manual for Guidelines for Exercise Testing and Prescription. 2nd Ed. Philadelphia, PA: Lea & Febiger, 1993.

109. Interactive Guide to Physical Therapist Practice. Vol 1.0. Alexandria, VA: American Physical Therapy Association, 2002.

110. Sale DG, MacDougall D. Specificity in strength training: a review for the coach and athlete. Can J Appl Sports Sci 1981;6:87–92.

111. Rutherford OM, Jones DA. The role of learning and coordination in strength training. Eur J Appl Phys 1986;55:100–105.

112. Atha J. Strengthening muscle. Exerc Sport Sci Rev 1981;9:1–73.

113. Muller EA. Influence of training and of inactivity on muscle strength. Arch Phys Med Rehabil 1970;51:449–462.

114. Whitley JD. The influence of static and dynamic training on angular strength performance. Ergonomics 1967;10:305–310.

115. Patterson RM, Jansen SWS, Hogan HA, et al. Material properties of Thera-Band tubing. Phys Ther 2001;81(8):1437–1445.

116. Page P, Labbe A. Torque characteristics of elastic resistance and weight-and-pulley exercise. [Abstract]. Med Sci Sports Exerc 2000;32(5 Suppl):S151.

117. Page P, Labbe A, Topp R. Clinical force production of Thera-Band elastic bands. [Abstract]. J Orthop Sports Phys Ther 2000;30(1):A47–A48.

118. Simoneau GG, Bereda SM, Sobush DC, et al. Biomechanics of elastic resistance in therapeutic exercise program. J Orthop Sports Phys Ther 2001;31(1):16–24.

119. Page P, Ellenbecker TS. The Scientific and Clinical Application of Elastic Resistance. Champaign, IL: Human Kinetics, 2003, ISBN 0–7360–3688–1.

120. Manor B, Topp R, Page P. Validity and reliability of measurements of elbow flexion strength obtained from older adults using elastic bands. J Geriatr Phys Ther 2006;29(1):18–21.

121. Thomas M, Muller T, Busse MW. Quantification of tension in Thera-Band and Cando tubing at different strains and starting lengths. J Sports Med Phys Fitness 2005;45(2):188–198.

122. Hughes CJ, Hurd K, Jones A, et al. Resistance properties of Thera-Band tubing during shoulder abduction exercise. J Orthop Sports Phys Ther 1999;29(7):413–420.

123. Tafel JA, Thacker JG, Hagemann JM, et al. Mechanical performance of exer-tubing for isotonic hand exercise. J Burn Care Rehabil 1987;8(4):333–335.

124. Puls A, Gribble P. A comparison of two Thera-Band training rehabilitation protocols on postural control. J Sport Rehabil 2007;16(2):75–84.

125. Han SS, Her JJ, Kim YJ. Effects of muscle strengthening exercises using a Thera-Band on lower limb function of hemiplegic stroke patients. Taehan Kanho Hakhoe Chi 2007;37(6):844–854.

126. Gettman LR, Ayres J. Aerobic changes through 10 weeks of slow and fast-speed isokinetic training. [Abstract]. Med Sci Sports 1978;10:47.

127. Stone MH, Potteiger MA, Pierce KC, et al. Comparison of the effects of three different weight-training programs on the one repetition maximum squat. J Strength Cond Res 2000;14:332–337.

128. Stone WJ, Coulter SP. Strength/endurance effects from three resistance training protocols with women. J Strength Cond Res 1994;8:231–234.

129. Sale DG, Jacobs I, MacDougall JC, et al. Comparisons of two regimens of concurrent strength and endurance training. Med Sci Sports Exerc 1990;22: 348–356.

130. Rhea MR, Alvar BA, Burkett LN, et al. A meta-analysis to determine the dose response for strength development. Med Sci Sports Exerc 2003;35(3): 456–464.

131. Rhea MR, Alvar BA, Ball SD, et al. Three sets of weight training superior to 1 set with equal intensity for eliciting strength. J Strength Cond Res 2002;16(4):525–529.

132. Ronnestad BR, Egeland W, Kvamme NH, et al. Dissimilar effects of one- and three-set strength training on strength and muscle mass gains in upper and lower body in untrained subjects. J Strength Cond Res 2007;21(1): 157–163.

133. Wolfe BL, LeMura LM, Cole PJ. Quantitative analysis of single- vs. multiple-set programs in resistance training. J Strength Cond Res 2004;18(1):35–47.

134. Munn J, Herbert RD, Hancock MJ, et al. Training with unilateral resistance exercises increases contralateral strength. J Appl Physiol 2005;99(5): 1880–1884.

135. Hass CJ, Garzarella L, de Hoyos D, et al. Single versus multiple sets in long-term recreational weightlifters. Med Sci Sports Exerc 2000;32(1):235–242.

136. Westcott WL, Winett RA, Anderson ES, et al. Effects of regular and super slow speed resistance training on muscle strength. J Sports Med Phys Fitness 2001;41:154–158.

137. Neils CM, Udermann BE, Brice GA, et al. Influence of contraction velocity in untrained individuals over the initial early phase of resistance training. J Strength Cond Res 2005;19(4):883–887.

138. Bosco C, Tihany J, Komi PV, et al. Store and recoil of elastic energy in slow and fast types of human skeletal muscles. Acta Physiol Scand 1982;116: 343–349.

139. Matveyev LP. Periodisienang das Sportlichen Training. Berlin: Beles Wernitz, 1972.

140. Stone MH, O'Bryant H, Garhammer J. A hypothetical model for strength training. J Sports Med Phys Fitness 1981;21:342–351.

chapter 6

Impaired Aerobic Capacity/Endurance

JANET R. BEZNER

Cardiovascular endurance is the ability of the cardiovascular system (i.e., heart, lungs, and vascular system) to take in, extract, deliver, and use oxygen and to remove waste products. Cardiovascular endurance, or aerobic capacity, supports the performance of repetitive activities using large muscle groups for extended periods. Clients and patients who work at home or on the job, participate in athletic endeavors of all levels, skill, and type, and who perform physical activity for fun or leisure, require adequate aerobic capacity. Concurrently, these activities also improve impairments in aerobic capacity, and are thus useful therapeutically in a rehabilitation setting.

The literature contains convincing evidence that the regular performance of cardiorespiratory endurance activities reduces the risk of developing disease, such as coronary heart disease, and is associated with lower mortality rates in both older and younger adults.[1-3] Despite this evidence, surveys of exercise trends among inhabitants of the United States (US) in the 1990s illustrated that approximately 15% of US adults performed vigorous physical activity (three times per week for at least 20 minutes) during leisure time, approximately 22% participated in sustained physical activity (five times per week for at least 30 minutes) of any intensity during leisure time, and about 25% of adults perform no physical activity in leisure time.[1] Adolescents and young adults (ages 12 to 21) were found to be similarly inactive and approximately 50% regularly participated in vigorous physical activity.[1] Since the Surgeon General's report was published in 1996, numerous efforts have been undertaken to monitor the prevalence of physical activity in the population. Based on Behavioral Risk Factor Surveillance System data collected between 2001 to 2005, the prevalence of regular physical activity (either vigorous or sustained as defined above) increased significantly by 8.6% (from 43.0% to 46.7%) among women overall and by 3.5% (from 48.0% to 49.7%) among men. Except for women between the ages of 18 to 24 years, significant increases in regular activity were reported in all racial/ethnic, age, and education-level categories examined. For men, significant increases in regular physical activity were found among 45- to 64-year-old respondents, non-Hispanic white males, non-Hispanic black males, high school graduates, and college graduates.[4]

Because of the widespread prevalence of physical inactivity among the US population, the US Public Health Service has created goals for exercise participation in the *Healthy People 2000* and the *Healthy People 2010* documents, aimed at improving the quality and increasing the years of healthy life.[5,6] In the mid-1990s, the US Department of Health and Human Services, the Centers for Disease Control and Prevention, the National Center for Chronic Disease Prevention and Health Promotion, the President's Council

on Physical Fitness and Sports, and the American College of Sports Medicine (ACSM) recommend that all adults should accumulate 30 minutes or more of moderate-intensity physical activity on most, and preferably all, days of the week.[1,7] In 2007, the recommendation was updated by the ACSM and the American Heart Association (AHA) for adults between 18 and 65 years of age, including adults in this age range with chronic conditions not related to physical activity.[8] The recommendation for adults to promote and maintain health is to perform moderate-intensity aerobic physical activity for a minimum of 30 minutes on 5 days each week or vigorous-intensity aerobic activity for a minimum of 20 minutes on 3 days each week. Also, a combination of moderate and vigorous-intensity activity can be performed to achieve the recommendation.[8] Toward this end, health care professionals have an opportunity to contribute to the overall well-being of the patients and clients we serve by prescribing meaningful physical activity programs based on the most contemporary scientific evidence. In order to adequately address the plethora of chronic diseases that are prevalent in individuals we serve, it is our responsibility to ensure that every patient/client is assessed and educated about the importance and power of regular physical activity related to the treatment and prevention of disease. In this chapter, the scientific basis of aerobic training will be presented along with guidelines for prescribing and supervising aerobic exercise and physical activity.

AEROBIC CAPACITY AND ENDURANCE
Definitions

There are many terms used in relationship to aerobic capacity and exercise that require clarification. *Physical activity* has been defined as any bodily movement produced by skeletal muscles that results in energy expenditure.[9] Similarly, *exercise* is a type of physical activity that is planned, structured, repetitive, and is purposely aimed at improving physical fitness.[9] *Physical fitness* is a set of attributes that people have or achieve and includes components of health-related (cardiorespiratory endurance, body composition, muscular endurance, muscular strength, flexibility) and athletic-related skills.[9] Being physically fit thereby enables an individual to perform daily tasks without undue fatigue and with sufficient energy to enjoy leisure-time activities and to respond in an emergency situation, if one arises.

Cardiorespiratory endurance training, or repetitive movements of large muscle groups fueled by an adequate response from the circulatory and respiratory systems to sustain physical activity and eliminate fatigue, is designed to achieve physical fitness.[1] Said another way, cardiorespiratory endurance is the ability of the whole body to sustain prolonged exercise.[10] Another term for cardiorespiratory endurance training is aerobic training, indicating the role of oxygen in the performance of this type of exercise. Anaerobic training, on the other hand, involves exercise performed in short bursts that does not require an ongoing supply of oxygen, such as strength training.[10]

The highest rate of oxygen that the body can consume during maximal exercise is termed *aerobic capacity, maximal oxygen uptake,* or VO$_2$ max.[10] VO$_2$ max is considered the gold standard measurement of cardiorespiratory endurance and aerobic fitness and can be measured in absolute (L per minute) or relative (mL/kg/min) terms.[10]

Normal and Abnormal Responses to Acute Aerobic Exercise

The performance of aerobic exercise can be easily assessed using commonly measured parameters, such as heart rate (HR), blood pressure (BP), and respiratory rate (RR). It is important for the clinician to know and recognize the normal and abnormal response to acute aerobic exercise so that a judgment can be made about the patient/client's response and exercise stopped prior to the development of a situation that could put the patient/client in danger. Moreover, patient/clients typically have several comorbidities that may lead to abnormal responses and therefore a safe environment for exercising can be created with careful monitoring of responses and application of the knowledge about what the responses indicate.

Normal Responses to Acute Aerobic Exercise

To assess an individual's response to exercise, it is important to understand the normal physiologic changes that occur as a result of the performance of physical activity. The ability to sustain aerobic exercise depends on numerous cardiovascular and respiratory mechanisms aimed at delivering oxygen to the tissues. The following changes would be expected *during* aerobic exercise and would be considered normal responses.[10–14]

Heart Rate   There is a linear relationship between HR, measured in beats per minute, and intensity of exercise, indicating that as workload or intensity increases, HR increases proportionally. The magnitude of increase in HR is influenced by many factors, including age, fitness level, type of activity being performed, presence of disease, medications, blood volume, and environmental factors such as temperature and humidity.

Stroke Volume   The volume or amount of blood ejected from the left ventricle per heart beat is termed the stroke volume (SV), measured in mL/beat. As workload increases, SV increases linearly up to approximately 50% of aerobic capacity, after which it increases only slightly. Factors that influence the magnitude of change in SV include ventricular function, body position, and exercise intensity.

Cardiac Output   The product of HR and SV is cardiac output (Q), or the amount of blood ejected from the left ventricle per minute (L per minute), (Q = HR × SV). Cardiac output increases linearly with workload because of the increases in HR and SV in response to increasing exercise intensity. Changes in Q depend on age, posture, body size, presence of disease, and level of physical conditioning.

Arterial-Venous Oxygen Difference   The amount of oxygen extracted by the tissues from the blood represents the difference between arterial blood oxygen content and venous blood oxygen content and is referred to as the arterial-venous oxygen difference (a-vO$_2$ diff), measured in mL/dL. As exercise intensity increases, a-vO$_2$ diff increases linearly, indicating that the tissues are extracting more oxygen from the blood, decreasing venous oxygen content as exercise progresses.

Blood Flow   The distribution of blood flow (mL) to the body changes dramatically during acute exercise. Whereas at rest, approximately 15% to 20% of the cardiac output goes to muscle, during exercise approximately 80% to 85% is distributed to working muscle and shunted away from the viscera. During heavy exercise, or when the body starts to overheat, increased blood flow is delivered to the skin to conduct heat away from the body's core, leaving less blood for working muscles.

Blood Pressure   The two components of BP, systolic (SBP) and diastolic (DBP) pressure, respond differently during acute bouts of exercise. To facilitate blood and oxygen delivery to the tissues, SBP increases linearly with workload. Because DBP represents the pressure in the arteries when the heart is at rest, it changes little during aerobic exercise, regardless of intensity. A change in DBP of <15 mm Hg from the resting value is considered a normal response. Both SBP and DBP are higher during upper extremity aerobic activity, compared to lower extremity aerobic activity. This increase is thought to be due to increased resistance to blood flow and a resulting increase in BP to overcome the increased resistance as a result of the smaller muscle mass and vasculature of the upper extremities compared to the lower extremities.[10]

Pulmonary Ventilation   The respiratory system responds during exercise by increasing the rate and depth of breathing in order to increase the amount of air exchanged per minute (L per minute). An immediate increase in rate and depth occurs in response to exercise and is thought to be facilitated by the nervous system, initiated by the movement of the body. A second, more gradual, increase occurs in response to body temperature and blood chemical changes as a result of the increased oxygen use by the tissues. Thus both tidal volume, or the amount of air moved into and out of the lungs during regular breathing, and RR, the number of breaths per minute, increase in proportion to the intensity of exercise.

Abnormal Responses to Acute Aerobic Exercise

Individuals with suspected cardiovascular disease or any other type of disease that may produce an abnormal response to exercise should be appropriately screened and tested before the initiation of an exercise program. This topic will be discussed in greater detail later in this chapter. However, abnormal responses may occur in individuals without known or documented disease and thus routine monitoring of exercise response is important and can be used to evaluate the appropriateness of the exercise prescription and as an indication that further diagnostic testing may be indicated.

In general, responses that are inconsistent with the normal response guidelines described previously are considered abnormal responses. Of the parameters described, HR and BP are most commonly assessed during exercise. The failure of HR to rise in proportion to exercise intensity, a failure of

DISPLAY 6-1
Signs and Symptoms of Exercise Intolerance

- Angina, typically manifested as chest, left arm, jaw, back or lower neck pain or pressure
- Unusual or severe shortness of breath
- Abnormal diaphoresis
- Pallor, cyanosis, cold, and clammy skin
- Central nervous system symptoms such as vertigo, ataxia, gait problems, or confusion
- Leg cramps or intermittent claudication
- Physical or verbal manifestations of severe fatigue or shortness of breath

American College of Sports Medicine. Resource Manual for Guidelines for Exercise Testing and Prescription. 3rd Ed. Baltimore, MD: Williams & Wilkins, 1998.

DISPLAY 6-2
Physiologic Adaptations to Cardiorespiratory Endurance Training

- Increased heart weight and volume
- Increased left ventricle size
- Increased SV
- Increased plasma blood volume
- Decreased resting and submaximal HRs
- Decreased time required for HR to return to resting after exercise
- Increased maximum cardiac output
- Increased total hemoglobin
- Decreased SBP and DBP in hypertensive clients
- Increased peripheral capillary formation
- More efficient blood distribution to active muscles
- Increased tidal volume during maximal exercise
- Decreased resting and submaximal RRs
- Increased RR during maximal exercise
- Increased pulmonary ventilation during maximal exercise
- Increased pulmonary diffusion during maximal exercise
- Increased a-vO_2 diff during maximal exercise
- Increase in VO_2 max
- Decreased body fat

SBP to rise or a decrease in SBP $\geq$ 20 mm Hg during exercise, and an increase in DBP $\geq$ 15 mm Hg would all be examples of abnormal responses to aerobic exercise.[13]

Signs and symptoms of exercise intolerance should also be recognized and include those listed in Display 6-1. Abnormal exercise responses, such as failure of HR to rise, often occur with exercise intolerance, defined as patient-related signs and symptoms; however, they can occur independently, so the clinician should be familiar with both. Knowledge of the normal and abnormal physiologic and symptom responses to exercise will enable the clinician to prescribe and monitor exercise safely and confidently and to minimize the occurrence of untoward events during exercise. Regular exposure to aerobic exercise results in changes to the cardiovascular and respiratory systems that can also be assessed by monitoring basic physiologic variables during rest and exercise. These adaptations will be discussed next.[14]

Physiologic and Psychologic Adaptations to Cardiorespiratory Endurance Training

In healthy individuals, cardiovascular training produces profound changes throughout the cardiorespiratory and vascular systems. The documented benefits of aerobic exercise are a result of the adaptations the oxygen delivery system undergoes secondary to the performance of regular activity. These adaptations, considered chronic changes, enable more efficient performance of exercise and thus affect cardiorespiratory endurance and fitness level. These chronic adaptations occur in the cardiovascular and respiratory systems and affect the values of both VO_2 max and body composition (see Display 6-2).

Cardiovascular Adaptations
Factors involving the heart that adapt in response to a regular exercise stimulus include heart size, HR, SV, and cardiac output (CO). The weight and volume of the heart and the thickness and chamber size of the left ventricle increase in trained individuals. As a result, the heart pumps more blood out per beat (SV) and the force of each contraction is stronger. SV is thus increased at rest, as well as during submaximal and maximal exercise, because of more complete filling of the left

ventricle during diastole compared with an untrained heart and an increase in plasma blood volume, discussed in the following section. Changes to HR include a decreased resting HR and a decreased HR at submaximal exercise levels, indicating that the individual can perform the same amount of work with less effort after training. Maximal HR typically does not change as a result of training. The amount of time it takes for HR to return to resting after exercise decreases as a result of training and is a useful indicator of progress toward better fitness. Because Q is the product of HR and SV (Q = HR × SV), it does not change much at rest or during submaximal exercise because HR decreases and SV increases. However, because of the increase in maximal SV, maximal Q increases considerably.[10,13,14]

Adaptations also occur in the vascular system and include blood volume, BP, and blood flow changes. Aerobic training increases overall blood volume, primarily because of an increase in plasma volume. The increase in blood plasma results from an increased release of hormones (antidiuretic and aldosterone) that promote water retention by the kidney and an increase in the amount of plasma proteins, namely albumin. A small increase in the number of red blood cells may also contribute to the increase in blood volume. The net effect of greater blood volume is the delivery of more oxygen to the tissues. Resting BP changes with training are most noteworthy in hypertensive or borderline hypertensive individuals, in whom aerobic training can decrease both SBP and DBP up to 10 mm Hg. During the performance of submaximal and maximal exercise, there is little change, if any, in BP as a result of training. Several adaptations are responsible for the increase in blood flow to muscle in a trained individual, including greater capillarization in the trained muscle(s), greater opening of existing capillaries in trained muscle(s), and more efficient distribution of blood flow to active muscles.[10,13,14]

Respiratory Adaptations

The capacity of the respiratory system to deliver oxygen to the body typically surpasses the ability of the body to use oxygen, thus the respiratory component of performance is not a limiting factor in the development of cardiorespiratory endurance. Nevertheless, adaptations in the respiratory system do occur in response to aerobic training. The amount of air in the lungs, represented by lung volume measures, is unchanged at rest and during submaximal exercise in trained individuals. However, tidal volume, the amount of air breathed in and out during normal respiration, increases during maximal exercise. RR is lower at rest and during submaximal exercise and increases at maximal levels of exercise. The combined increases in tidal volume and RR during maximal exercise of trained individuals produce a substantial increase in pulmonary ventilation, or the process of movement of air into and out of the lungs. Pulmonary ventilation at rest is either unchanged or slightly reduced and during submaximal exercise is slightly reduced following training. The process of gas exchange in the alveoli, or pulmonary diffusion, is unchanged at rest and at submaximal exercise levels, but increases during maximal exercise because of the increased blood flow to the lungs and the increased ventilation as discussed previously. These two factors create a situation that enables more alveoli to participate in gas exchange, and thus the perfusion of oxygen into the arterial system is enhanced during maximal exercise. Finally, a-vO_2 diff increases at maximal exercise in response to training as a result of increased oxygen distraction by the tissues and greater blood flow to the tissues because of more effective blood distribution. [10,13,14]

One net effect of these cardiovascular and respiratory adaptations on aerobic capacity is an increased VO_2 max after endurance training. A typical training program consisting of three times per week, 30 minutes per session exercise at 75% of VO_2 max, as discussed in a later section of this chapter, over the course of 6 months can improve VO_2 max 5% to 30% in a previously sedentary individual. Resting VO_2 max is either unchanged or slightly increased following training, and submaximal VO_2 is either unchanged or slightly reduced, representing greater efficiency. [10] The second net effect relates to body composition changes that have been documented as a result of aerobic exercise training. Whether caloric intake stays the same during training or is decreased, individuals lose fat mass as a result of training. Several mechanisms have been postulated to produce a loss of body fat secondary to training, including appetite suppression, an increase in the resting metabolic rate, and an increase in lipid mobilization from adipose tissue and thus the burning of fat for energy. [10]

Psychologic Benefits of Training

In addition to the myriad of cardiovascular, respiratory, and metabolic improvements that occur after aerobic training, *psychologic* benefits have also been documented, although are less well understood. An overall assessment of the literature in this area indicates that depression, mood, anxiety, psychologic well-being, and perceptions of physical function and overall well-being improve in response to the performance of physical activity. [1,15] The finding that exercise can decrease symptoms of depression and anxiety is consistent with the fact that individuals who are inactive are more likely to have depressive symptoms compared to active persons. Improvements in depression and mood have been found in populations with and without clinically diagnosed psychologic impairment, as well as in those with good psychologic health, although the literature is less conclusive in this specific area.

A number of factors have been postulated to explain the beneficial effects of aerobic training on psychologic function, including changes in neurotransmitter concentrations, body temperature, hormones, cardiorespiratory function, and metabolic processes, as well as improvements in psychosocial factors such as social support, self-efficacy, and stress relief. Further research is needed to verify the potential contribution of changes in these factors resulting from aerobic training to improvement in psychologic function. [1]

Despite the inability to explain why psychologic parameters improve in response to training, the effect on overall quality of life is positive. [16,17] Improvement in quality of life as a result of physical activity has been demonstrated in individuals without [18–22] and with disease, including coronary heart disease patients who are obese, [23] coronary heart disease patients who are elderly, [24] patients with chronic heart failure, [25,26] patients after coronary bypass graft surgery, [27] and patients with multiple sclerosis [28] and cancer. [29]

Dose-Response Relationship

The amount of physical activity associated with decreased risk for cardiovascular disease and death has been the topic of numerous studies. [30–34] Authors agree that an inverse linear dose response exists between the amount of physical activity performed and all-cause mortality. [30–32] Although the minimal effective dose of physical activity is unclear, expenditure of 1,000 kcal per week is associated with a significant reduction in all-cause mortality. [30,32] It is less clear whether additional benefits are achieved from the performance of vigorous physical activity compared with moderate intensity activity, such as the current guidelines to accumulate 30 minutes of moderate intensity activity daily. [30–32] Until additional research is performed clarifying this association, it appears that an exercise prescription based on an individual client's motivations and desires is the best approach to follow, with the aim of performing consistent with current recommendations to accumulate 30 minutes or more of moderate-intensity physical activity on 5 days each week. [1,8]

The dose-response relationship relative to improvements in quality of life has also been examined. The observed improvement in quality of life in individuals who participate in regular exercise is achieved from quantities of exercise considered to produce health-related (versus fitness-related) benefits. Fitness-related benefits include those resulting in significant changes in physical fitness level, as measured by cardiorespiratory endurance and body composition changes. Specific recommendations for fitness-related changes usually include vigorous, continuous activities with a focus on the specific parameters of exercise (intensity, mode, duration, frequency). Health-related benefits can be achieved through the performance of moderate intensity, intermittent activity wherein the focus is on the accumulated amount of activity performed. [7] The documented health-related benefits from the performance of regular exercise are shown in Display 6-3.

Although improvement in fitness level is a worthwhile goal and also results in the health-related benefits listed previously, exercise to achieve health-related benefits appears to be easier for most people to incorporate into their lifestyle

DISPLAY 6-3
Health-related Benefits from the Performance of Regular Exercise

- Decreased fatigue
- Improved performance in work- and sports-related activities
- Improved blood lipid profile
- Enhanced immune function
- Improved glucose tolerance and insulin sensitivity
- Improved body composition
- Enhanced sense of well-being
- Decreased risk of CAD, cancer of the colon and breast, hypertension, noninsulin-dependent diabetes mellitus, osteoporosis, anxiety, and depression

and thus provides a valuable exercise option.[35–37] The specific parameters necessary to achieve both fitness-related and health-related benefits of aerobic exercise are presented later in this chapter.

CAUSES OF IMPAIRED AEROBIC CAPACITY/REHABILITATION INDICATIONS

The ability of the body to use oxygen can be limited by disease and is affected by aging and inactivity. A systems review, conducted as a part of the examination, discussed in the next section, can identify the presence of or risk for pathology/pathophysiology, impairments, functional limitations, or disabilities that impact aerobic capacity.[38] Although injury to or diseases of the heart, lungs, and vascular system—the primary tissues involved in cardiovascular endurance—are the most obvious causes of impairment or functional limitation, diseases and conditions of other body systems also affect aerobic capacity.

There are three categories of diseases that directly affect the heart, including conditions of the heart muscle, diseases affecting the heart valves, and cardiac nervous system conditions.[39] Heart muscle conditions include coronary artery disease (CAD), myocardial infarction, pericarditis, congestive heart failure, and aneurysms.[39] The pathologic processes involved in the impairment of aerobic capacity in these heart muscle conditions involve obstruction or restriction of blood flow, inflammation, or dilation or distension of one or more heart chambers.[39] Aerobic capacity is impaired because the heart is weakened as a result of the disease or condition or blood flow is impaired, resulting in ischemia and necrosis of heart muscle and an inability to pump enough blood in response to increased demand from activity.

The heart valves can become diseased by rheumatic fever, endocarditis, mitral valve prolapse, and various congenital deformities. Valve defects increase the workload of the heart, as the heart must work harder to pump blood through a malfunctioning valve, resulting in impaired aerobic capacity.[39] The nervous system that controls cardiac muscle contraction, when diseased, produces arrhythmias such as tachycardia and bradycardia. Arrhythmias impair aerobic capacity by causing changes in circulatory dynamics because the heart is beating too slow or too fast, or skipping beats.[39]

There are numerous types of peripheral vascular disease, including arterial, venous, and lymphatic disorders, such as atherosclerosis, embolism, Buerger disease, Raynaud disease, deep venous thrombosis, venous stasis, and lymphedema.[39] Because aerobic capacity is determined by the condition and capacity of both the heart and the peripheral circulation, these conditions also produce impairments. The vascular system is used to transport oxygen to exercising muscles so that diseases of the peripheral vascular system disrupt circulation to peripheral muscles, producing a loss of function at rest and during exercise, impairing aerobic capacity. The most common disease of the vascular system is hypertension, considered a major risk factor for myocardial infarction, stroke, and cardiovascular death.

Conditions affecting the pulmonary system influence the ability of the lungs to bring in and absorb oxygen and expel carbon dioxide from cells in the body. These processes are of primary importance to cardiorespiratory endurance; therefore, diseases affecting ventilation and respiration impact aerobic capacity. Diseases affecting the lungs include lung tumors, chronic obstructive pulmonary disease (COPD; including bronchitis, bronchiectasis, emphysema), asthma, pneumonia, tuberculosis, cystic fibrosis, and various occupational lung diseases (pneumoconiosis).[39]

Disease of the neurologic, musculoskeletal, endocrine/metabolic, and integumentary systems may also negatively affect aerobic capacity. Conditions such as cancer, neuromuscular disease, cerebrovascular attacks, traumatic brain injury, spinal cord injury, osteoporosis, arthritis, and AIDS either directly or indirectly impair aerobic capacity and thus limit cardiovascular endurance.

Any medical condition necessitating hospitalization or bed rest can result in deconditioning of the cardiovascular system. Surgical procedures for the gallbladder, appendix, uterus, or other internal organs require a period of decreased activity. Accidents resulting in multiple system injuries can limit activity for long periods of time, resulting in deconditioning.

The effects of aging on the cardiovascular and respiratory systems are numerous, resulting in an overall decrease in aerobic capacity. Some of the factors that have been attributed to the decline in aerobic capacity documented with age include decrements in central and peripheral circulation including a decrease in maximal HR, SV, and a-vO$_2$ diff; increases in body fat and decreases in lean body mass; and lung function decline including a decrease in vital capacity and forced expiratory volume, an increase in residual volume, and a loss of elasticity in the lung tissue and chest wall.[10] Because the elderly respond to cardiovascular training with impressive improvements in aerobic capacity, it is difficult to differentiate between biologic aging and physical inactivity as the primary cause of the decline in aerobic capacity that occurs with age.

A sedentary lifestyle, or physical inactivity, impairs aerobic capacity and is considered a modifiable risk factor for cardiovascular disease (Display 6-4). Considering that more than 25% of the US adult population is sedentary, physical inactivity is more prevalent than the diseases discussed previously that cause impairment in aerobic capacity, and thus is a major public health concern.[6] On the positive side, as a modifiable risk factor, physical inactivity is mutable and can and should be addressed when identified during the examination of a patient.

DISPLAY 6-4
Risk Factors for Coronary Heart Disease

Major Risk Factors—Nonmodifiable
Increasing age
Male gender
Family history
Race
Postmenopausal (female)

Major Risk Factors—Modifiable
Physical inactivity
Cigarette smoking
Elevated serum cholesterol
High BP

Contributing Factors
Obesity
Response to stress
Personality
Peripheral vascular disease
Hormonal status
Alcohol consumption

Goodman CC, Snyder TEK. Differential Diagnosis for Physical Therapists. 4th Ed. St. Louis, MO: Saunders Elsevier, 2007.

EXAMINATION/EVALUATION OF AEROBIC CAPACITY

With the exception of clients with cardiovascular and pulmonary diseases, most clients who are referred to physical therapy do not have as their primary diagnosis impaired aerobic capacity. Because aerobic capacity influences any exercise a client may perform as a part of an intervention, and thus the outcomes that client will achieve, it is important that examination and evaluation of the cardiovascular and respiratory systems be included as a part of the examination and evaluation of all clients. The tests and measures described in this section are aimed at identifying the presence of disease, describing baseline aerobic capacity, and measuring change in aerobic capacity as a result of intervention(s). The clinician is assumed to have the knowledge and skill to perform the *basic* tests necessary to diagnose impairments and functional limitations in aerobic capacity; however, detailed information will be provided for the more *advanced* tests of aerobic capacity because many clinicians may not have experience performing these tests on a regular basis. Additional information may be obtained from the ACSM text[40] on exercise testing and prescription.

Patient/Client History

Specific portions of the general data generated from a patient/client history as defined in Chapter 2 are important to note when attempting to identify the presence of an impairment in aerobic capacity that either should be directly addressed in the intervention or that may influence the clinician's ability to set and achieve goals related to other impairments. Knowledge of the risk factors for coronary heart disease provides a basis for collecting the most relevant information regarding impaired aerobic capacity. As shown in Display 6-4, general demographic information such as age, gender, and ethnicity is very important to consider. Social/health habits

such as smoking and physical activity are important behaviors to inquire about during the history. Assessment of general health status in terms of physical, role, and social functioning as well as functional status and activity level can provide additional indication of limitations in cardiovascular endurance. Clinical tests of blood cholesterol are useful to identify clients at risk for coronary heart disease. Other factors that should be noted from the history include personality/behavior, pregnancy, and breast-feeding status, factors that also may modify the exercise prescription.[13]

Medication history is of primary importance to review, especially for clients with documented cardiovascular and pulmonary disease, but also for those with risk factors for disease. Many cardiac and pulmonary system drugs affect aerobic capacity, and thus clients using these drugs should be carefully monitored during any intervention that affects the cardiovascular and pulmonary systems, including therapeutic exercise, functional training, airway clearance techniques, integumentary repair techniques, electrotherapeutic modalities, and physical agents and mechanical modalities.

Specific questions that should be posed during the patient/client history to identify the presence of cardiovascular and pulmonary disease and the relevant aspects of the client's overall status that may affect aerobic capacity as discussed above can be found in Goodman and Snyder's text[39] on differential diagnosis.

Systems Review

After, and based on, the patient/client history, a systems review is conducted as a brief or limited examination of the status of the other major body systems (integumentary, musculoskeletal, neuromuscular), and the communication ability, affect, cognition, language, and learning style of the patient.[38] The systems review helps to identify impairments in other areas that may affect the performance of an activity or task within the plan of care. Further, the systems review may identify potential problems that require referral to another provider.

Because the primary intervention used to address aerobic capacity impairments, therapeutic exercise, requires adequate musculoskeletal, neuromuscular, and integumentary function, it is especially important to perform a thorough systems review in clients with cardiovascular and pulmonary impairments. Failure to do so could result in prescribing an intervention that the patient either cannot perform or that compromises the safety of the patient. At a minimum, skin integrity, muscle strength, joint range of motion, balance, gait function, and assessment of the ability to make needs known should be assessed.

Screening Examination

Before the initiation of an exercise program, individuals should be assessed to ensure safety and minimize risks.[13] Preparticipation screening can be performed using a self-report questionnaire, such as the Physical Activity Readiness Questionnaire or PAR-Q[13,40,41] (see Appendix 3). Based on the answers to the seven questions on the PAR-Q, individuals between the ages of 15 and 69 can either appropriately participate in exercise or be referred to a physician for further evaluation before beginning an exercise program. All individuals who fall outside of the boundaries described should

DISPLAY 6-5
ACSM Risk Stratification Categories

Low risk = men < 45 years of age and women < 55 years of age who are asymptomatic and meet no more than one risk factor threshold from Display 6-6

Moderate risk = Men ≥ 45 years and women ≥ 55 years or those who meet the threshold for two or more risk factors from Display 6-6

High risk = Individuals with one or more signs and symptoms listed in Display 6-7 or known cardiovascular (cardiac, peripheral vascular, or cerebrovascular), pulmonary (COPD, asthma, interstitial lung disease, or cystic fibrosis), or metabolic (diabetes mellitus, thyroid disorders, renal, or liver disease) disease.

American College of Sports Medicine. ACSM's Guidelines for Exercise Testing and Prescription. 7th Ed. Philadelphia, PA: Lippincott Williams & Wilkins, 2006.

DISPLAY 6-7
Major Signs or Symptoms Suggestive of Cardiovascular, Pulmonary, or Metabolic Disease

Sign or Symptom
- Pain, discomfort (or other anginal equivalent) in the chest, neck, jaw, arms, or other areas that may result from ischemia
- Shortness of breath at rest or with mild exertion
- Dizziness or syncope
- Orthopnea or paroxysmal nocturnal dyspnea
- Ankle edema
- Palpitations or tachycardia
- Intermittant claudication
- Known heart murmur
- Unusual fatigue or shortness of breath with usual activities

American College of Sports Medicine. ACSM's Guidelines for Exercise Testing and Prescription. 7th Ed. Philadelphia, PA: Lippincott Williams & Wilkins, 2006. (Put clarification/significance information on web site.)

be referred to a physician for medical evaluation before participating in exercise training.

The ACSM[40] has created guidelines delineating who should be medically evaluated, including maximal or submaximal exercise testing, before participation in vigorous exercise (defined as intensity > 60% VO_2 max). Those who do not require medical evaluation include those who meet the definition of low risk as per the ACSM Risk Stratification Categories (Display 6-5).[40]

DISPLAY 6-6
CAD Risk Factor Thresholds for Use with ACSM Risk Stratification

Positive Risk Factors and Defining Criteria
1. Family history—Myocardial infarction, coronary revascularization, or sudden death before 55 years of age in father or other male first-degree relative, or before 65 years of age in mother or other female first-degree relative
2. Cigarette smoking—current cigarette smoker or those who quit within the previous 6 months
3. Hypertension—SBP ≥ 140 mm Hg or DBP ≥ 90 mm Hg, confirmed by measurements on at least two separate occasions, or on antihypertensive medication
4. Dyslipidemia—Low-density lipoprotein (LDL) cholesterol > 130 mg/dL or HDL < 40 mg/dL, or on lipid-lowering medication. If total serum cholesterol is all that is available use > 200 mg/dL rather than LDL > 130 mg/dL
5. Impaired fasting glucose—Fasting blood glucose ≥ 100 mg/dL confirmed by measurements on at least two separate occasions
6. Obesity—BMI > 30 kg.m² or waist girth > 102 cm for men and > 88 cm for women or waist/hip ratio: ≥ 0.95 for men and ≥ 0.86 for women
7. Sedentary lifestyle—Persons not participating in a regular exercise program or not meeting the minimal physical activity recommendations (accumulating 30 minutes or more of moderate physical activity on most days of the week) from the US Surgeon General's Report

Negative Risk Factor and Defining Criteria
1. High-serum HDL cholesterol > 60 mg/dL

American College of Sports Medicine. ACSM's Guidelines for Exercise Testing and Prescription. 7th Ed. Philadelphia, PA: Lippincott Williams & Wilkins, 2006.

For those meeting the criteria for moderate risk in Display 6-5, it is recommended that medical examination and exercise testing be performed prior to the initiation of vigorous exercise training. In addition, for those in the moderate risk category, it is recommended that medical supervision (a physician should be in proximity and readily available should there be an emergent need) occur for maximal exercise testing.

Finally, for those in the high risk category, medical examination prior to moderate or vigorous exercise and medical supervision for maximal or submaximal exercise testing is recommended.

Tests and Measures

The examination categories directly relevant for the client with aerobic capacity impairment include tests and measures

BUILDING BLOCK 6-1
Patient/Client History and General Information

Susan is a 47-year-old nurse who consulted a physical therapist for primary complaints of posterolateral right (R) thigh pain. Past medical history was unremarkable. The pain was worse with weight bearing first thing in the morning, got better with limited activity, but worsened by the end of the day—especially if she had been on her feet quite a bit during the day. Secondary complaints included intermittent, dull low back pain, and occasional bouts of sharp pain in the arch of her R foot. She was diagnosed and treated by the physical therapist for iliotibial band fascitis and intermittent plantar fasciitis. The short- and long-term goals set for her were aimed at decreasing disability and returning the patient to a pain-free level of functioning. Susan met the goals established with regular treatment and requested that the physical therapist assist her with establishing a regular physical activity habit.

Based on the information provided, does the patient/client require medical evaluation prior to participating in aerobic exercise?

of aerobic capacity/endurance, anthropometric characteristics, and circulation. There are numerous tests and measures in each of these categories and often the most difficult task for the clinician is selecting the most appropriate test. Tests and measures should be selected based on data collected from the history, systems review, and screening, the means the client has available for following through with a program of aerobic exercise, client goals, and the equipment and monitoring equipment available.

Aerobic Capacity/Endurance

The development of an appropriate and useful exercise prescription for cardiorespiratory endurance depends on an accurate assessment of VO_2 max, which is most commonly achieved through the performance of a graded exercise test (GXT). Exercise tests can be maximal, in which an individual performs to his or her physiologic or symptom limit, or submaximal, in which an arbitrary stopping or limiting criterion is used.

Maximal Graded Exercise Tests   The most important characteristics of a maximal GXT are that it has a variable or graded workload that increases gradually and that the total test time equal approximately 8 to 12 minutes.[40] In addition, individuals undergoing maximal GXT testing are usually electrocardiogram (ECG)-monitored. The direct measurement of VO_2 max requires the analysis of expired gases, which requires special equipment and personnel and is thus costly and time-consuming.[40] VO_2 max can be estimated from prediction equations after the individual exercises to the point of volitional fatigue, or it can be estimated from submaximal tests. For most clinicians, maximal exercise testing is not feasible because of the special equipment required and the ECG monitoring, although it is the most accurate test of aerobic capacity. Additionally, it is recommended that maximal graded exercise testing be reserved for research purposes, testing of diseased individuals, and athletic populations.[13] Thus submaximal testing is most commonly used, especially with low-risk, apparently healthy individuals, and will be further described in this section. Individuals who wish to conduct maximal graded exercise testing are referred to the ACSM Guidelines for Exercise Testing[40] or the ACSM Resource Manual[13] for more detailed information.

Submaximal Graded Exercise Tests   Submaximal exercise tests can be used to estimate VO_2 max because of the linear relationship between HR and VO_2, and HR and workload.[13] That is, as workload or VO_2 increases, HR increases in a linear, predictable fashion. Therefore, the clinician can estimate max VO_2 by plotting HR against workload for at least two exercise workloads and extrapolating to age-predicted maximal HR (220 – age) to estimate VO_2 max (Fig. 6-1).[40] Submaximal exercise testing is based on several assumptions, as shown in Display 6-8. Failure to meet these assumptions fully, which is usually the case, results in errors in the prediction of VO_2 max. Therefore, submaximal testing typically results in less accurate VO_2 max estimations. However, submaximal tests are appropriately used to document change over time in response to aerobic training and, given the time and money saved, are very useful clinically.

ACSM[40] provides recommendations for physician supervision during graded exercise testing. For women younger than

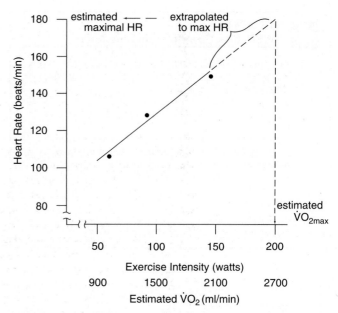

FIGURE 6-1. HR obtained from at least two (more are preferable) submaximal exercise intensities may be extrapolated to the age-predicted maximal HR. A vertical line to the intensity scale estimates maximal exercise intensity from which an estimated VO_2 max can be calculated. (From American College of Sports Medicine. ACSM's Guidelines for Exercise Testing and Prescription. 7th Ed. Philadelphia, PA: Lippincott Williams & Wilkins, 2006.)

age 55 and men younger than age 44 who are asymptomatic and have no more than one risk factor (Display 6-6), physician supervision is not deemed necessary during maximal or submaximal testing. Individuals in these age ranges who have two or more risk factors but no symptoms or disease can undergo submaximal testing without physician supervision. Physician supervision during submaximal and maximal testing is recommended for any individual with CAD or with symptoms of CAD. Last, during maximal testing for men older than age 45 and women older than age 55 with two or more risk factors but no symptoms, physician supervision is recommended.[40] Therefore, submaximal testing can be performed safely by physical therapists with any age individual who is symptom- or disease free, as defined by ACSM.[40]

Numerous testing protocols have been published and are available for submaximal exercise testing.[40] Because of the

---

  DISPLAY 6-8
Assumptions for Submaximal Exercise Testing

- A steady-state HR is obtained for each exercise work rate and is consistent each day.
- A linear relationship exists between HR and work rate.
- The maximal work load is indicative of the maximal VO_2.
- The maximal HR for a given age is uniform.
- Mechanical efficiency is the same for everyone (e.g., VO_2 at a given work rate).
- The subject is not on medications that alter HR.

Note: The most accurate estimate of VO_2 max is achieved if all of the preceding assumptions are met.

American College of Sports Medicine. ACSM's Guidelines for Exercise Testing and Prescription. 7th Ed. Philadelphia, PA: Lippincott Williams & Wilkins, 2006:68.

TABLE 6-1 YMCA Submaximal Bicycle Ergometer Test Protocol—Workload Settings

	HR < 80	HR 80–89	HR 90–100	HR > 100
Second Stage	750 kgm/min (2.5 kg) (125 Watts)	600 kgm/min (2.0 kg) (100 W)	450 kgm/min (1.5 kg) (75 W)	300 kgm/min (1.0 kg) (50 W)
Third Stage	900 kgm/min (3.0 kg) (150 W)	750 kgm/min (2.5 kg) (125 W)	600 kgm/min (2.0 kg) (100 W)	450 kgm/min (1.5 kg) (75 W)
Fourth Stage	1050 kgm/min (3.5 kg) (175 W)	900 kgm/min (3.0 kg) (150 W)	750 kgm/min (2.5 kg) (125 W)	600 kgm/min (2.0 kg) (100 W)

Resistance settings shown apply to ergometers with a 6 m/revolution flywheel.

requirement of reproducible workloads, treadmills, bicycle ergometers, and stepping protocols are most commonly used. Test selection should be based on safety concerns, familiarity with and knowledge of the testing protocol, equipment availability, and client/patient goals, abilities, and conditions (e.g., the presence of orthopedic limitations).

Bicycle Ergometer Tests. Two common bicycle ergometer tests are the YMCA protocol and the Astrand-Ryhming test.[40] In the YMCA protocol, the client performs two to four, 3-minute stages of continuous cycling, designed to elevate the HR to between 110 and 150 beats per minute during two consecutive stages. The client begins cycling at 50 revolutions per minute at a resistance of 150 kgm per minute or 0.5 kg and progresses to greater resistance in subsequent stages based on HR recorded during the last minute of the first stage according to Table 6-1. For example, if HR = 85 at the end of the first stage, the second stage workload would be 600 kgm per minute and the third stage workload would be 750 kgm per minute.

The test is terminated when two consecutive stages yield a HR reading between 110 and 150 beats per minute. The two HR measures and corresponding workloads are plotted on a graph and the line generated from the plotted points is extended to the age-predicted maximal HR and an estimation of VO$_2$ max is obtained.[40]

The Astrand-Ryhming test involves a single 6-minute stage, with workload based on sex and activity status:

- unconditioned females, 300 or 450 kgm per minute (50 or 75 W)
- conditioned females, 450 or 600 kgm per minute (75 or 100 W)
- unconditioned males, 300 or 600 kgm per minute (50 or 100 W)
- conditioned males, 600 or 900 kgm per minute (100 or 150 W).

Individuals pedal at 50 revolutions per minute and HR is measured during the fifth and sixth minutes. The two HR measures must be within 5 beats of one another and the HR between 130 and 170 beats per minute for the test to be completed. If the HR is <130 beats per minute, the resistance should be increased by 50 to 100 W and the test continued for another 6 minutes. The test may be terminated when the HR in the fifth and sixth minute differs by no more than 5 beats and is between 130 and 170 beats per minute. An average of the HRs is calculated and a nomogram is used to estimate

VO$_2$ max (Fig. 6-2).[40] The value determined from the nomogram is corrected for age by multiplication of a correction factor (Table 6-2).

Treadmill Tests. Submaximal treadmill tests are also used to estimate VO$_2$ max (Table 6-3). A single-stage submaximal treadmill test has been developed for assessing VO$_2$ max in low-risk individuals.[42] It involves beginning with a comfortable walking pace between 2.0 and 4.5 mph at 0% grade for a 2- to 4-minute warm-up, designed to increase HR to within 50% to 75% of age-predicted (220 − age) maximum HR, followed by 4 minutes at 5% grade at the same self-selected walking speed. HR is measured at the end of the 4-minute stage and VO$_2$ max is estimated using the following equation:

$$VO_2 \text{ max (mL/kg/min)} = 15.1 + 21.8 \times \text{speed (mph)} \\ - 0.327 \times \text{HR (bpm)} - 0.263 \times \text{speed} \\ \times \text{age (years)} + 0.00504 \times \text{HR} \times \text{age} \\ + 5.98 \times \text{sex (0 = F, 1 = M)}$$

Step Tests. Step tests were developed based on a need to test large numbers of individuals expeditiously and represent another mode of submaximal exercise testing. Several protocols have been developed,[43] but only one will be presented. The Queens College Step Test requires a 16.25-in step (similar to the height of a bleacher step).[43,44] Individuals step up and down to a 4-count rhythm (on Count 1 subject places one foot on step, on Count 2 subject places the other foot on the step, on Count 3 the first foot is brought back to the ground, on Count 4 the second foot is brought down). A metronome is useful to maintain the prescribed stepping beat. Females step for 3 minutes at a rate of 22 steps per minute, whereas males step at a rate of 24 steps per minute. At the end of the 3 minutes, a recovery 15-second pulse is measured, starting at 5 seconds into recovery while the individual remains standing. The pulse rate is attained and is converted to beats per minute by multiplying by 4. This value is termed the recovery HR. The following equations are used to estimate VO$_2$ max.

Females: VO$_2$ max (mL/kg/min) = 65.81 − [0.1847 × recovery HR (beats/min)]
Males: VO$_2$ max (mL/kg/min) = 111.33 − [0.42 × recovery HR (beats/min)]

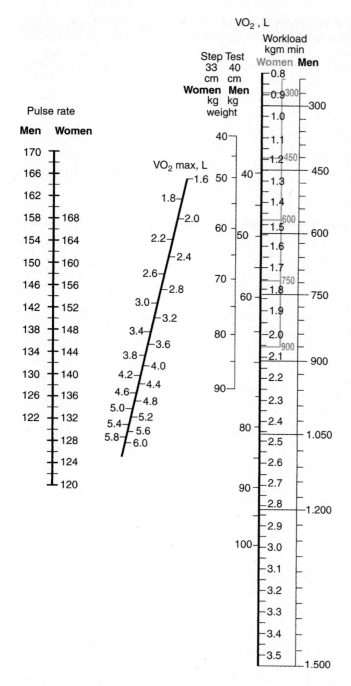

Males: $\dot{V}O_2max$ (mL/kg/min) =
111.33 − [0.42 × recovery HR (beats/min)]

FIGURE 6-2. The Astrand-Rhyming nomogram. A nomogram used to calculate aerobic capacity (VO_2 max) from pulse rate during submaximal work. The clinician must know the pulse rate, sex, and work load from the bicycle ergometer test performed on the client to determine absolute VO_2 max. VO_2 max values obtained from the nomogram should be adjusted for age by a correction factor (Table 6-2). (Reprinted from Astrand PO, Ryhming I. A nomogram for calculation of aerobic capacity [physical fitness] from pulse rate during submaximal work. J Appl Physiol 1954;7:218–221, with permission.)

Field Tests. Field tests refer to exercise testing protocols derived from events performed outside, or in the "field." They are also submaximal tests and, as with the step test, are more practical for testing large groups of people, appropriate when

TABLE 6-2 Correction Factor for Age for Astrand-Rhyming Nomogram

AGE	CORRECTION FACTOR
15	1.10
25	1.00
35	0.87
40	0.83
45	0.78
50	0.75
55	0.71
60	0.68
65	0.65

From p. 223 Bandy and Sanders, which was reprinted from American College of Sports Medicine, Guidelines for Exercise Testing and Prescription, 7th Ed. Baltimore, MD: Lippincott Williams & Wilkins, 2006:72.

time or equipment is limited, and when assessing individuals older than age 40.[43] A variety of field tests exist[43]; the Cooper 12-minute test and the 1-mi walk test will be discussed. In the Cooper 12-minute test, individuals are instructed to cover the most distance possible in 12 minutes, preferably by running, although walking is acceptable. The distance covered in the 12 minutes is recorded and VO_2 max estimated according to the following equation[43]:

$$VO_2 \text{ max (mL/kg/min)} = 35.97 \text{ (mi)} - s\ 11.29$$

A 1-mi walk test is another option in the field test category.[45] Individuals walk 1 mi as fast as possible without running and the average HR for the last two complete minutes of the walk is recorded. A HR monitor is necessary to record and average the HR over the last 2 minutes. If a HR monitor is not available, a 15-second pulse can be measured immediately on test completion. VO_2 max is estimated from the following equation[45]:

$$\begin{aligned} VO_2 \text{ max (mL/kg/min)} = {} & 132.85 - 0.077 \times \text{body weight} \\ & \text{(pounds)} - 0.39 \times \text{age (years)} \\ & + 6.32 \times \text{sex } (0 = F, 1 = M) - 3.26 \\ & \times \text{elapsed time (min)} - 0.16 \times HR \\ & \text{(beats/min)} \end{aligned}$$

All clients should be closely monitored during exercise test performance. Vital signs should be assessed before, during each stage or workload of the test, and after the test for 4 to 8 minutes of recovery.[13] In addition, the rating of perceived exertion (RPE) is commonly used to monitor exercise tolerance.[46] RPE refers to the "degree of heaviness and strain experienced in physical work as estimated according to a specific rating method"[46,p.9] and is an indicator of overall perceived exertion. The Borg RPE scale and instructions for use are shown in Figure 6-3.

Anthropometric Characteristics

Body composition is important to assess in individuals partaking in an aerobic exercise program because of the changes experienced in fat mass as a result of chronic training discussed earlier in this chapter. In addition, body composition is an important examination tool in the

TABLE 6-3 Submaximal Treadmill Exercise Test Results

STAGE	TREADMILL SETTINGS	DURATION	HEART RATE	BLOOD PRESSURE	SIGNS AND SYMPTOMS
Rest	N/A	N/A	85	132/86	None
Warm-up	3.0 mph 0% grade	3 minutes 15 seconds	102	140/84	None
Main	3.0 mph 5% grade	4 minutes	135	145/80	None
Cool down	2.0 mph 0% grade	4 minutes	90	130/80	None

RATING	DESCRIPTION
6	None at all
7	Extremely light
8	
9	Light
10	
11	Light
12	
13	Somewhat hard
14	
15	Hard (heavy)
16	
17	Very hard
18	
19	Extremely hard
20	Maximal

FIGURE 6-3. The rating of perceived exertion scale. (From Bezner J. Principles of aerobic conditioning. In: Bandy WD, Sanders B, eds. Therapeutic Exercise. Techniques for Intervention. Baltimore, MD: Lippincott Williams & Wilkins, 2001. Data from American College of Sports Medicine. The recommended quantity and quality of exercise for developing and maintaining cardiorespiratory and muscular fitness in healthy adults. Med Sci Sports Exerc 1990;22:265–274.)

presence of obesity and is considered superior to simple measures of height and weight. The gold standard measure of body composition is hydrostatic or underwater weighing that requires specialized equipment and the patient to tolerate total body immersion. Because of these limitations, several reliable measures of body composition estimation have been developed and are used widely, including body mass index (BMI), bioelectric impedance, near-infrared interactance, skinfold measurements, and waist to hip ratio. Bioelectric impedance, near-infrared interactance, and

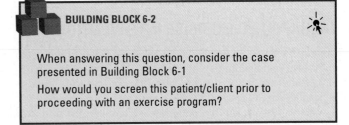

BUILDING BLOCK 6-2

When answering this question, consider the case presented in Building Block 6-1

How would you screen this patient/client prior to proceeding with an exercise program?

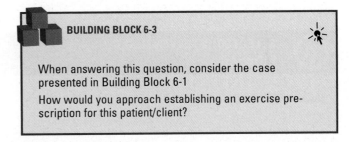

BUILDING BLOCK 6-3

When answering this question, consider the case presented in Building Block 6-1

How would you approach establishing an exercise prescription for this patient/client?

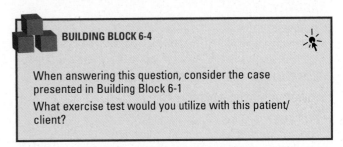

BUILDING BLOCK 6-4

When answering this question, consider the case presented in Building Block 6-1

What exercise test would you utilize with this patient/client?

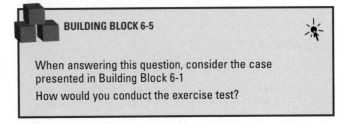

BUILDING BLOCK 6-5

When answering this question, consider the case presented in Building Block 6-1

How would you conduct the exercise test?

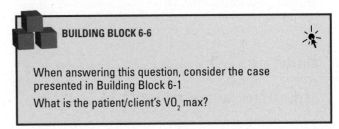

BUILDING BLOCK 6-6

When answering this question, consider the case presented in Building Block 6-1

What is the patient/client's VO_2 max?

skinfolds require specialized equipment and, in the case of skinfolds, specialized training; whereas the BMI and waist-to-hip ratio can be measured using height, weight, and circumferential measurements. The clinician is referred to ACSM's Guidelines for Exercise Testing and Prescription[40] for additional information about performing these tests.

Circulation

Assessment of BP; HR, rhythm, and sounds; and RR, rhythm, and pattern is important to establish a baseline and to determine impairments. In addition, these measures can be assessed over time to determine the effect of aerobic training on the cardiovascular and pulmonary systems and to document improvement.

THERAPEUTIC EXERCISE INTERVENTION

Impaired aerobic capacity/endurance involves the support element of the movement system, and as such is the underlying impairment for numerous functional limitations and disabilities and is thus a priority to address with the intervention plan. A wide variety of aerobic endurance activities exist and are the most efficient techniques to achieve the goal of improved aerobic capacity. The modes and dosage specifics used when establishing an aerobic endurance exercise prescription will be presented. A primary objective of the exercise prescription is to assist in the adoption of regular physical activity as a lifestyle habit and thus should take into consideration the behavioral characteristics, personal goals, and exercise preferences of the individual.[40] Given the critical epidemic of obesity and physical inactivity in the United States and the strength of the association between regular physical activity and reduction in mortality and morbidity, physical therapists should ensure that they include exercise testing and exercise prescription with all patients/clients with whom they interact.

Mode

Several modes of cardiovascular endurance training are available. Any activity that uses large muscle groups and is repetitive is capable of producing the desired changes. Such activities include walking, jogging, cross-country skiing, bicycling, rope jumping, rowing, swimming, or aerobic dance (see Selected Intervention 6-1). Although lap swimming is the most common aquatic cardiovascular exercise, water jogging, cross-country skiing, and water aerobics are

SELECTED INTERVENTION 6-1
Elliptical

Refer to Case Study No. 10

Although this patient requires comprehensive intervention, only one exercise is described:

ACTIVITY: Elliptical

PURPOSE: To increase cardiovascular endurance and musculoskeletal muscle endurance of quadriceps, gluteals, hamstrings, calf, trunk and upper extremity muscle groups

ELEMENTS OF THE MOVEMENT SYSTEM: Base, support

STAGE OF MOTOR CONTROL: Skill

POSTURE: Shoulders should be back, head up and slightly forward, chin up level and abdominals tight. Look forward, not down at your feet. Do not grip the handrails too tightly. Or "maintain a light grip on the handrails." Make sure that your weight is evenly distributed and that your lower body supports the majority of your weight.

MOVEMENT: Alternate hip flexion and extension in a walking pattern. Transfer weight completely from leg to leg during the activity, rather than shuffling or sliding the feet while bearing weight bilaterally. Move your arms in an alternate fashion with the legs (range of motion may be limited by individual needs).

SPECIAL CONSIDERATIONS: (a) All precautions to cardiovascular endurance exercise must be considered. (b) Individuals with balance and coordination difficulty should be assessed for ability to perform the activity safely.

DOSAGE: Ten minutes, adding 5 minutes every three sessions

RATIONALE FOR EXERCISE CHOICE: The elliptical is a total body exercise. Aerobic conditioning can be achieved,

along with shoulder, trunk, hip, and leg extensor muscle endurance training.

EXERCISE GRADATION: This exercise can be progressed by increasing the frequency, intensity, or duration of activity.

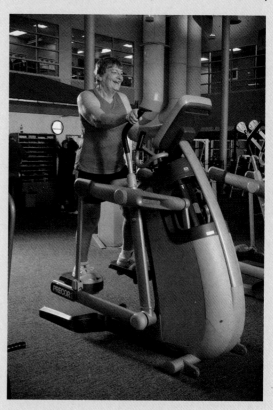

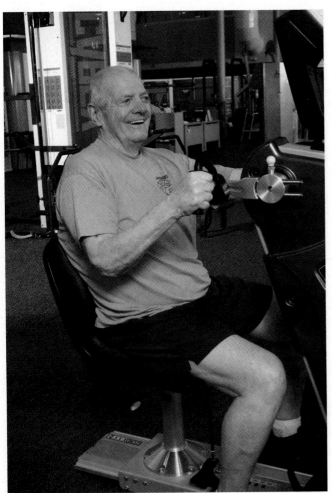

FIGURE 6-4. Upper body ergometer. An upper body ergometer is an exercise mode that provides an aerobic exercise alternative for those with significant lower extremity impairments or to provide variety in an exercise prescription. Because the smaller upper extremity muscles perform the exercise, lower HRs are experienced. In addition, it is difficult to monitor vital signs during activity. The seat on the device should be adjusted to allow slight elbow flexion in the outstretched position of the arm while the back maintains contact with the seat, and the seat height position should ensure that the shoulder is even with the axis of the crank arm. (From Bezner J. Principles of aerobic conditioning. In: Bandy WD, Sanders B, eds. Therapeutic Exercise: Techniques for Intervention. Baltimore, MD: Lippincott Williams & Wilkins, 2001. Courtesy of Henley Healthcare, Sugar Land.)

Patient-Related Instruction 6-1

Return to Impact Activity

Any return to impact activities such as jogging, impact aerobics, or sports requiring running or jumping should be preceded by impact progression. This approach ensures readiness to return to the activity and decreases the likelihood of setback. Prerequisites for impact progression include the following:

1. Adequate muscle strength and endurance
2. Full range of motion in the joints
3. No swelling

A suggested progression is as follows:

1. Two-footed hopping
2. Alternate-footed hopping
3. Single-footed hopping (optional)
4. Skill drills (optional)

This progression should be implemented as follows:

1. Begin on a low-impact surface (e.g., pool, minitramp, shock-absorptive floor).
2. Subsequently progress to the terrain you will be using.
3. Begin with 5 minutes, and increase by 2- to 5-minute increments when you are able to complete three consecutive sessions without pain, swelling, or technique compromise.
4. Return to your full activity is determined by the criteria set by your clinician. Remember that returning to activity is different from performing sport drills. During practice drills, mental attention is often given to awareness and protection of a recovering injury. When returning to the game, the majority of mental attention is given to the game. Therefore, practicing skills while mentally engaging in that sport activity is an important component of return to sport.

---

also effective aquatic training methods. An upper body ergometer is a good cardiovascular training tool and is especially well suited for individuals unable to use their legs (see Fig. 6-4).

The choice of exercise mode depends on the patient's goals and specific physical condition. Performing an activity that is convenient, comfortable, and enjoyable increases the likelihood of adherence. The amount of impact is also an important consideration when choosing the exercise mode. For the individual with lower extremity degenerative joint disease or the overweight individual, impact activities should be minimized. The pool is a better choice for those who need to minimize weight bearing or impact. Weight bearing can be completely negated by exercising in the deep end of the pool. For those desiring to return to impact activities, gradual impact progression can prepare the body for the demands of this type of loading (see Patient-Related Instruction 6-1: Return to Impact Activity).

Variety and cross-training in the cardiovascular endurance program are imperative. Alternating modes of activity can alleviate boredom and prevent overuse injuries resulting from repetitive activity. Individuals who have such low muscular endurance that they are incapable of performing the same repetitive activity for more than a few minutes can alternate activities within the training session and among sessions. Whereas one individual may bicycle 2 days per week, swim 2 days, and walk 2 days, another may bike, walk, and stair step for 10 minutes each daily.

Within one mode of exercise, several postures or equipment types are available. For example, during bicycling, the trunk posture selected depends on the goals. Bicycling may be performed on a recumbent bike (Fig. 6-5A), with the hips flexed 90 degrees or more and the low back supported, or it may be performed in a upright position with the arms moving (Fig. 6-5C), or in a forward leaning position (Fig. 6-5B). The optimal posture for maximal exercise benefit should be emphasized (see Patient-Related Instruction 6-2: Bicycling Guidelines).

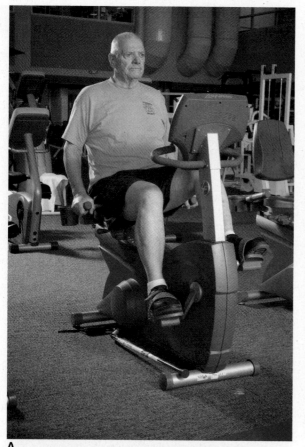

A

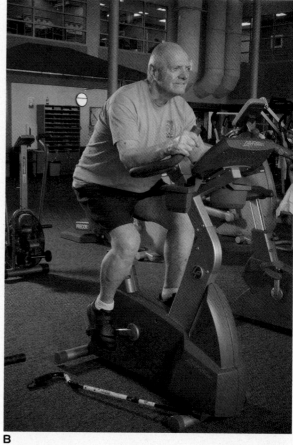

B

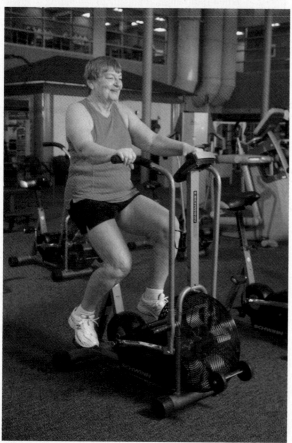

C

FIGURE 6-5. (A) Exercise on a semirecumbent bike positions the individual differently from exercise on a traditional bike. (B) Bicycling in a traditional position places more weight on the upper extremities, challenging the postural muscles more than in a recumbent position. (C) Exercise on an upright bike with moving arms places different loads on the patient.

> ### Patient-Related Instruction 6-2
> #### *Bicycling Guidelines*
>
> The following guidelines will keep your bicycling experience healthy and safe:
> 1. Seat height: The seat should be set so that your knee is slightly bent in the down-most position. If you place your heel on the pedal in the down position, your knee should be perfectly straight. When you place the ball of your foot on the pedal, your knee should be bent at the correct angle (15 to 20 degrees of knee flexion with the ankle in 90 degrees of dorsiflexion).
> 2. Cadence: Your pedal cadence should be high, at least 60 rpm or more. Your clinician may have other recommendations, depending on your specific situation.
> 3. Resistance: The resistance should be low enough to allow a higher cadence. Resistance too high can place extra stress on the knee. Keeping the resistance low and the cadence high produces the desired benefits without hurting your knees.
> 4. Safety: If riding outside, always wear a helmet, and obey your local bicycle laws.

> ### Patient-Related Instruction 6-3
> #### *Setting Up a Circuit*
>
> Your regular exercise routine can be enhanced and made more enjoyable by breaking up a continuous activity with stations of alternative activities. A circuit can be created outside along a normal walking or running route, or at your indoor exercise location. For example, a walking or jogging program through the neighborhood or on the treadmill can be broken up with the following activities performed at certain intervals throughout the session:
> 1. Calf raises
> 2. Abdominal curls or trunk plank
> 3. Push-ups
> 4. Squats
> 5. Dips
> 6. Lunge walks
> 7. Quadriceps, hamstring, and calf stretches

Dosage

Type

The training session itself may be performed using a variety of training techniques, from continuous activity to interval training. Continuous training relies on the aerobic energy system to supply energy for the exercise session and can be carried out for prolonged periods (see web site for review of energy systems). The individual exercises continuously, without rest, at a steady exercise rate. Although continuous in nature, several different activities can be combined within the same session, such as treadmill and bicycle or swimming and deep-water running.

Interval training incorporates rest sessions between bouts of exercise. This technique is useful for clients who are unable to maintain continuous exercise for the optimal length of time (e.g., 30 minutes) and for those recuperating from an orthopedic injury or who are deconditioned. When prescribing interval training, the ratio of the rest period to the training period determines the activity intensity and the energy system used. The aerobic energy system is used to a greater extent with longer training intervals and shorter rest periods. For example, performance of three bouts (intervals) of activity at an intensity of 50% of VO_2 max or greater for 10 minutes with a 2-minute rest period in between each bout would use the aerobic energy system.

The rest periods can be true rest (i.e., no activity) or a work-relief interval, during which light activity such as walking may be performed. High-intensity activity usually is combined with longer complete-rest intervals, and low to medium intensities are combined with shorter rest intervals or work-relief intervals. For example, a training session might include a set of ten 100-m sprints, in which each sprint may only take 10 to 20 seconds to complete, with a 10-minute complete rest interval between each sprint. Because high-intensity exercise of short duration uses the ATP-PCr and glycolysis systems for the provision of ATP, a longer rest period is required to allow muscle energy stores to be replenished (see Physiology Information on Web site). Less intense exercise, concomitantly, relying on the aerobic oxidative pathway, can be performed adequately from an energy availability standpoint for longer periods of time with shorter rest intervals that may consist of complete-rest or work-relief intervals.

Circuit training can be continuous or interval. Circuit training is a training technique in which the individual rotates through a series of exercise stations. A variety of upper extremity, lower extremity, core, and cardiovascular training exercises typically are included. The individual performs the activity at each station for a specified time (i.e., 30 seconds) and then moves on to the next station. The activity choices, activity intensity, and rest between stations determine the energy system used and whether the activity is interval or continuous. This type of training provides the opportunity for a well-balanced exercise program with variety. Multiple individuals can be trained simultaneously if there are adequate stations (see Patient-Related Instruction 6-3: Setting Up a Circuit).

Sequence

Cardiovascular endurance training may be performed as part of a comprehensive rehabilitation program that includes mobility, stretching, and strengthening activities. General warm-up activities should be performed initially, followed by stretching and the cardiovascular training session. The warm-up period should last 5 to 10 minutes to prepare the body for exercise. Large muscle group activity such as walking, calisthenics, or bicycling should be performed with gradually increasing intensity. The warm-up session may be a lower-intensity version of the cardiovascular training activity. Walking at a slower speed for 5 minutes may be used as a warm-up activity for faster walking or jogging. The warm-up activities increase muscle blood-flow, muscle temperature, and neural conduction. These changes, along with mental preparedness, can decrease the risk of muscle injury during exercise. After the warm-up, stretching exercises are performed, followed by the more vigorous cardiovascular endurance session.

The exercise session should be concluded with a cool-down period of 5 to 10 minutes to allow redistribution of blood flow that has changed with exercise, including prevention of lower extremity pooling of blood by enhancing venous return to the heart. Active muscle contraction by continued walking, cycling, or low-level calisthenics assists with blood flow redistribution. Stretching should conclude the session to ensure maintenance of the working muscle's optimal length.

Frequency

The frequency of cardiovascular training should be determined through consideration of the patient/client's goals, the intensity and duration of exercise, and the patient/client's baseline fitness level. The optimal frequency to achieve fitness-related benefits for most individuals is three to five times per week,[10,40] with those initiating a program beginning at three to four times per week and progressing to five. The optimal frequency to attain health-related benefits is 5 days per week of moderate-intensity activity and 3 days per week of vigorous-intensity activity.[8] The overload principle in terms of the interaction among intensity, duration, and frequency is important to consider when prescribing exercise. Individuals with very low functional capacities can perform daily or twice daily exercise because the total amount of exercise, considering intensity, duration, and frequency, is low.[40] In a highly trained individual, exercise at a greater frequency may be necessary to produce overload, depending on the exercise intensity.

Intensity

As with frequency and duration, setting the intensity of exercise should be based on the overload principle and consideration should be given to the functional limitations, goals, and fitness level of the individual. Exercise intensity indicates how much exercise should be performed or how hard one must exercise and is typically prescribed on the basis of HR max, HR reserve, VO_2 max, RPE, or METS (metabolic equivalents). Prescribing exercise intensity using HR is considered the preferred method because of the correlation between HR and the stress on the heart and because it is readily accessible for monitoring during exercise.[10] Several methods involving HR can be used.

When prescribing exercise as a percentage of maximum HR, either directly measured or on the basis of age-predicted maximum HR, the training range should be between 55% and 65% to 90% of HR max.[40] A second method involves the use of the HR reserve or Karvonen formula:

$$\text{Target HR range} = [(\text{HRmax} - \text{HRrest}) \times 0.60 \text{ and } 0.80] + \text{HRrest}^{40}$$

To obtain a HR range, two intensity levels are calculated in the formula, one equivalent to 0.60 of VO_2 max and one equivalent to 0.80 of VO_2 max. If exercise is prescribed using VO_2 max, 55% to 75% is also used as a training range and VO_2 max should be stated in relative terms (mL/kg/min), which accounts for the individual's body weight. The RPE can also be used to prescribe exercise intensity, within the range of 12 to 16 on the RPE scale shown in

Figure 6-3. RPE is especially useful for prescribing intensity for individuals who are unable to palpate pulse or when HR is altered because of the influence of medication and should be considered an adjunct to monitoring HR in all other individuals.[40]

METS may also be used to prescribe activity intensity. METS are used to estimate the metabolic cost of physical activity relative to the resting state. One MET is equal to 3.5 mL of oxygen consumed per kilogram of body weight per minute (mL/kg/min).[40] Therefore, when VO_2 is known, the intensity can be prescribed in METS by dividing relative VO_2 by 3.5 mL/kg/min. In general, walking at 2 mi per hour is the equivalent of approximately 2.0 METS, and walking at 4 mi per hour is the equivalent of approximately 4.6 METS.

Selection of an appropriate training range versus a specific training value has been recommended to provide greater flexibility in the exercise prescription, yet ensure that a training response will be achieved.[10] For example, an individual who is starting an exercise program might be given a target HR range between 60% and 70% of HR max instead of being told to keep target HR at a value equivalent to 60% of HR max.

Intensities between 70% and 85% HR max or 60% and 80% HR reserve are recommended for most people to experience improvements in cardiorespiratory endurance.[40] Health-related benefits can be realized at lower intensities, and thus lower intensities may be appropriate if the goal of exercise is to improve health rather than fitness.[47]

In the pool, the HR is decreased when exercising while immersed to the neck because of the Starling reflex and is therefore a poor gauge of workload. The HR of deep-water exercise is 17 to 20 beats per minute less than that of the comparable land-based activity.[48]

Increase exercise intensity by adding resistance, increasing speed, changing terrain (e.g., up hills), removing stabilization, or adding upper extremity activity. The method for increasing intensity is goal-specific and may be limited by other medical or physical conditions (e.g., rotator cuff tendinitis limiting the use of upper extremities). The intensity necessary to achieve a workload in the target training zone varies among individuals and usually correlates with the previously determined conditioning level.

Duration

Exercise duration can be manipulated to produce overload and a resultant cardiovascular training effect. Duration depends on the frequency, intensity, and the conditioning level of the patient. In general, exercise of greater intensity is performed for a shorter duration and exercise of lower intensity can be performed for a longer duration. Manipulation of these variables is goal-dependent. If the patient is required to perform an activity for a long duration (i.e., continuous walking as part of a job or recreation), progression of the activity program should focus more on increasing the duration and less on increasing the intensity.

The optimal duration recommended for aerobic training is between 20 and 30 minutes per session of exercise.[10,40] For individuals who are unable to perform 20 minutes of continuous exercise, discontinuous exercise can be prescribed.

Patient-Related Instruction 6-4
Frequency, Intensity, and Duration

Determining how often (frequency), how hard (intensity), and how long (duration) to exercise can be difficult. These parameters are related and must be balanced to find the right quantity of exercise for you. The following broad guidelines can be refined by your clinician:

1. Frequency: Generally, if you exercise more frequently (more times per day or days per week), the intensity and duration of those sessions should be lower. This recommendation allows adequate recovery before the next session. If the intensity and duration are high, you may not be fully recovered before the next session.
2. Intensity: The more intense the exercise, the shorter is the duration. Intense exercise cannot be sustained very long by most people.
3. Duration: Exercise that is lower in intensity can be sustained for longer periods. For example, sprinting can be sustained for seconds, but jogging can be sustained for up to several hours. The intensity and duration are inversely related; as one increases, the other must decrease.

That is, several 10-minute bouts can be performed, for example, until eventually exercise can be tolerated for 20 to 30 minutes continually. Duration can be progressed up to 60 minutes of continual activity.[40] The same activity or different activities may be performed in each of these sessions (see Patient-Related Instruction 6-4: Frequency, Intensity, and Duration).

PRECAUTIONS AND CONTRAINDICATIONS

In addition to the signs and symptoms of exercise intolerance described in the physiology of aerobic capacity and endurance section and Display 6-1, clinicians should be aware of the risks associated with exercise, as well as monitoring and supervision

BUILDING BLOCK 6-7

When answering this question, consider the case presented in Building Block 6-1

How would you create an exercise prescription for the patient/client?

BUILDING BLOCK 6-8

When answering this question, consider the case presented in Building Block 6-1

What normal cardiovascular changes would you expect during exercise?

guidelines. The incidence of cardiovascular complications during exercise has been documented to be extremely low for individuals without significant cardiac disease.[40] For persons with cardiovascular disease, the incidence of cardiovascular complications during exercise is considerably greater; however, the overall absolute risk of cardiovascular complications during exercise is low when considered in light of the health benefits associated with chronic exercise.

A profile has developed of individuals at greatest risk for cardiovascular complications during exercise.[40] The profile includes those with a history of multiple myocardial infarctions, impaired left ventricular function with an ejection fraction of <30%, rest or unstable angina pectoris, serious arrhythmias at rest, significant multivessel atherosclerosis on angiography, and low serum potassium. High-risk patients also show disregard for appropriate warm-up and cool-down, consistently exceed prescribed training HR, are more likely to be male, and to smoke cigarettes. Although this profile is helpful, it is important to note that a significant number of patients with one or more of these characteristics will never experience an exercise-related cardiovascular complication, and others without any of these characteristics may experience a complication. Therefore, the wise clinician will follow the recommendations in Display 6-9 when prescribing and monitoring aerobic exercise to reduce the incidence and severity of complications during exercise.

Endurance exercise places a significant load on the cardiovascular and musculoskeletal systems. Consideration should be given to any injury or disease affecting either of these systems. Individuals with degenerative joint disease

DISPLAY 6-9
Recommendations to Reduce the Incidence and Severity of Complications During Exercise

- Ensure medical clearance and follow-up
- Query patients/clients as to their reasons for initiating exercise, as some patients with new symptoms of cardiovascular disease initiate exercise programs in an attempt to reassure themselves that they are well
- Provide on-site medical supervision, if necessary
- Ensure medical personnel have training in cardiac life support when supervising vigorous exercise or testing
- Establish an emergency plan and procedures that are reviewed and practiced several times a year
- Educate patients/clients regarding the symptoms of cardiovascular disease
- Encourage patients/clients to start slowly and progress gradually
- Emphasize appropriate warm-up and cool-down procedures before and after vigorous exercise, including stretching
- Modify recreational game rules to minimize competition
- Maintain supervision during the recovery period
- Take precautions in the cold
- Consider added cardiac demands in the heat
- Seek full evaluation by a physician after patients/clients experience exercise-induced symptoms such as chest discomfort, unexpected dyspnea, or syncope, prior to returning to vigorous activity

American College of Sports Medicine. ACSM's Guidelines for Exercise Testing and Prescription. 7th Ed. Philadelphia, PA: Lippincott Williams & Wilkins, 2006:15.

should be encouraged to participate in non–weight-bearing exercises such as bicycling and water exercise, and those with low back pain should participate in activities that support or safely strengthen the back (e.g., semirecumbent biking, water activities). Individuals with osteoporosis should be encouraged to participate in weight-bearing activities. Positions and postures should be chosen that minimize the risk of fracture.

Graded Exercise Testing Contraindications and Supervision Guidelines

There are numerous contraindications to exercise testing, and guidelines for supervision of GXTs. Display 6-10 lists the absolute and relative contraindications to exercise testing. The relative contraindications should be considered in light of the potential benefits of exercise and a less vigorous prescription created for individuals in this category.

All clients should be closely monitored during exercise test performance. Vital signs should be assessed before, during each stage or workload of the test, and after the test for 4 to 8 minutes of recovery.[13] In addition, the RPE is commonly used to monitor exercise tolerance (Fig. 6-3).[46] Finally, individuals should be monitored for signs and symptoms of exercise intolerance. The guidelines for stopping an exercise test are presented in Display 6-11.

DISPLAY 6-10
Contraindications to Exercise Testing

Absolute
A recent significant change in the resting ECG suggesting significant ischemia, recent myocardial infarction (within 2 days) or other acute cardiac event
Unstable angina
Uncontrolled cardiac arrhythmias causing symptoms or hemodynamic compromise
Severe symptomatic aortic stenosis
Uncontrolled symptomatic heart failure
Acute pulmonary embolus or pulmonary infarction
Acute myocarditis or pericarditis
Suspected or known dissecting aneurysm
Acute infections

Relative
Left main coronary stenosis
Moderate stenotic valvular heart disease
Electrolyte abnormalities (e.g., hypokalemia, hypomagnesemia)
Severe arterial hypertension (i.e., SBP > 200 mm Hg and/or a DBP > 110 mm Hg) at rest
Tachyarrhythmias or bradyarrhythmias
Hypertrophic cardiomyopathy and other forms of outflow tract obstruction
Neuromuscular, musculoskeletal, or rheumatoid disorders that are exacerbated by exercise
High-degree atrioventricular block
Ventricular aneurysm
Uncontrolled metabolic disease (e.g., diabetes)
Chronic infectious disease (e.g., mononucleosis, hepatitis, and AIDS)

American College of Sports Medicine. ACSM's Guidelines for Exercise Testing and Prescription. 7th Ed. Philadelphia, PA: Lippincott Williams & Wilkins, 2006.

DISPLAY 6-11
Indications for Cessation of Graded Exercise Testing

- Onset of angina or angina-like symptoms
- Drop in SBP > 10 mm Hg from baseline BP despite an increase in workload
- Excessive rise in SBP > 250 mm Hg or DBP > 115 mm Hg
- Shortness of breath, wheezing, leg cramps, or claudication
- Signs of poor perfusion (lightheadedness, confusion, ataxia, pallor, cyanosis, nausea, or cold or clammy skin)
- Moderately severe angina (defined as 3 on standard scale)
- Increasing nervous system symptoms (ataxia, dizziness, or near syncope)
- Failure of HR to increase with increased exercise intensity
- Noticeable change in heart rhythm (sustained ventricular tachycardia and other indicates of ischemia on the ECG)
- Patient/client requests to stop
- Physical or verbal manifestations of severe fatigue
- Failure of the testing equipment or technical difficulties with ECG or BP monitoring

American College of Sports Medicine. ACSM's Guidelines for Exercise Testing and Prescription. 7th Ed. Philadelphia, PA: Lippincott Williams & Wilkins, 2006:78,106.

DISPLAY 6-12
General Guidelines for Exercise Program Supervision

Unsupervised = Low risk individuals from Display 6-5 with a functional capacity > 7 METs
Supervised = Low risk individuals from Display 6-5 with a functional capacity < 7 METs and Moderate and High risk individuals from Display 6-5

Modified from American College of Sports Medicine. ACSM's Guidelines for Exercise Testing and Prescription. 7th Ed. Philadelphia, PA: Lippincott Williams & Wilkins, 2006.

Supervision During Exercise

The screening or medical evaluation discussed in the screening examination section of this chapter provides information for determining which individuals may require supervision during exercise.[40] Referring to Displays 6-5 and 6-12, the clinician can determine whether a patient/client can exercise unsupervised or requires supervision. Notably, individuals with symptoms and cardiorespiratory disease who are considered by their physician to be clinically stable and who have been medically cleared for participation in an exercise program should be supervised during exercise.[40] Supervision means that the clinician is present during the exercise program and can monitor the patient/client response to exercise and provide support in the event that the patient/client develops symptoms during exercise.

PATIENT-RELATED INSTRUCTION/ EDUCATION AND ADJUNCTIVE INTERVENTIONS

Patient education regarding cardiovascular endurance training and its effects is a critical component of a physical activity or exercise program. Clinicians should recall the recent recommendation of the ACSM and the AHA that adults should perform moderate-intensity aerobic physical activity for a minimum of 30 minutes on 5 days each week or vigorous-intensity aerobic activity for a minimum of 20 minutes on 3 days each week to promote and maintain health. A combination of moderate and vigorous-intensity activity can be performed to achieve the recommendation.[8]

Patient education should include the "why" and the "how to" of the warm-up, training session, and cool-down phases. The patient should be alerted to signs or symptoms necessitating early cessation of the activity (including those in Display 6-1). These symptoms may be musculoskeletal (e.g., joint pain, muscle pain, cramps) or cardiovascular (e.g., shortness of breath, chest pain, lightheadedness), or they may be specific to the patient's particular diagnosis (i.e., reproducing the patient's original symptoms). The patient should be counseled regarding modifications in the exercise program based on fatigue level and other activities performed that day.

As the patient is prepared for discharge, education regarding a maintenance program is critical to continued adherence with the exercise program. Progression through a conditioning program should be individualized and is dependent on the client's functional capacity, premorbid state, health status, age, and individual preferences, goals, and tolerance of the training.[40] The client's objective and subjective training responses should most heavily influence training progression.[13] Signs and symptoms of overtraining include exercise and nonexercise fatigue, reduction in maximum performance, decreased interest in training compared with normal, decreased HR and RPE values at the same workload, and increased complaints of aches and pains.[49]

Emphasizing the importance of continued physical activity in long-term health maintenance can assist the patient in making exercise a lifelong commitment. Information about safe progression, exercise dosage, and signs and symptoms of overload can assist the patient in making appropriate exercise choices.

The documented success of programs designed to encourage the adoption of a regular exercise habit is similar to the success of changing other health-related behaviors such as smoking and weight reduction, in that approximately 50% of those who initiate the behavior will develop a lifelong habit.[50] Factors that have been found to be most predictive of exercise dropout or noncompliance include personal, program, and other characteristics. Personal characteristics that predict dropout include being a smoker, being sedentary during leisure time, having a sedentary occupation, possessing a Type A personality, being employed in a blue-collar occupation, being overweight or overfat, possessing a poor self-image, being depressed or anxious, and having a poor credit rating.[51] Program factors predicting dropout include inconvenient time or location, excessive costs, the prescription of high-intensity exercise, lack of exercise variety, exercising alone, lack of positive feedback, inflexible exercise goals, and poor exercise leadership.[51] Additional factors that have been identified to predict dropout are lack of spouse support, inclement weather, excessive job travel, injury, medical problems, and job change or move.[51] These factors in sum indicate that programs and individuals prescribing exercise can and should adopt specific strategies to enhance compliance with exercise prescription. Examples of these strategies are shown in Display 6-13.

DISPLAY 6-13
Strategies to Enhance Compliance with Cardiovascular Endurance Training Programs

- Minimize musculoskeletal injuries by adhering to the principles of exercise prescription
- Encourage group participation or exercising with a partner
- Emphasize mode variety and enjoyment in the program
- Incorporate behavioral techniques and base prescription on theories of behavior change
- Use periodic testing to document progress
- Give immediate feedback to reinforce behavior change
- Recognize accomplishments
- Invite spouse or significant other involvement and support of the training program
- Ensure that the exercise leaders are qualified and enthusiastic

Reprinted from Franklin BA. Program factors that influence exercise adherence: practical adherence skills for the clinical staff. In: Dishman RK, ed. Exercise Adherence. Champaign, IL: Human Kinetics, 1988:242–249, by permission.

The use of behavior change theories to enhance the adoption of exercise has received increased attention recently in the literature, specifically the application of the stages of change model, as discussed in Chapter 3. After identifying the stage the patient is currently in, the intervention can be tailored to enhance compliance and movement toward a lifelong habit. For example, an individual in contemplation is not quite ready for an exercise prescription. Efforts in this stage should focus on the provision of information about the costs and benefits of exercise, strategies to increase activity within the present lifestyle, and the social benefits of activity, for example.[52] Those in the preparation stage would benefit most from a thorough examination and exercise prescription. Whereas, those in the action or maintenance stage would benefit from learning about strategies to prevent relapse, making exercise enjoyable, and diversifying the exercise prescription to include more variety. Given the difficulty most people encounter when changing health-related behaviors, it seems prudent to use documented behavior change theories when possible, such as the stages of change model.

BUILDING BLOCK 6-9

When answering this question, consider the case presented in Building Block 6-1

How would you recommend the patient/client progress the exercise program:

BUILDING BLOCK 6-10

When answering this question, consider the case presented in Building Block 6-1

What education would you provide for the patient/client?

BUILDING BLOCK 6-11

When answering this question, consider the case presented in Building Block 6-1

What physiologic adaptations to the exercise program would you expect after 6 months?

BUILDING BLOCK 6-12

When answering this question, consider the case presented in Building Block 6-1

What psychologic adaptations to the exercise program would you expect after 6 months?

LIFESPAN ISSUES
Guidelines for Cardiovascular Endurance Training in the Young

Adolescents and children receive health-related benefits from regular exercise and should be encouraged to participate in regular activity because adopting an active lifestyle early in life may increase the likelihood of participating in physical activity in adulthood.[6] There are several key physiologic differences between children and adolescents compared with adults that the clinician should be aware of when prescribing aerobic exercise in young people. Resting and exercise BP values are lower in children than in adults, with a progressive increase with age seen until late adolescence when the values are similar to that of adults.[7] Children have smaller hearts and less total blood volume compared with adults, so SV is lower at rest and during exercise. To maintain cardiac output, HR is higher in children compared with adults. Overall cardiac output in children is lower than adults for the same absolute rate of work, so a-vO$_2$ difference increases to compensate for the lower SV.[10] Aerobic capacity, when expressed in L/min, is lower in children because of a lower maximal cardiac output capacity. However, as children develop and their pulmonary and cardiovascular function improves, aerobic capacity improves as well.[10]

Children lose more energy during exercise compared with adults when performing the same activity at the same intensity. In addition, children are less efficient at dissipating heat during exercise because they generate more metabolic heat per unit body size, sweat at a lower rate, and begin sweating at a higher core body temperature compared with adults.[40] Taken together, these factors indicate that children exercising in hot environments should do so at a lower intensity and they will need more time to acclimatize compared with adults.

Exercise testing in children is typically reserved for those with specific conditions in which cardiopulmonary capacity is necessary to be assessed.[40] Exercise testing in children can be performed for the same reasons the clinician would test adults—to assess symptoms, tolerance, and cardiopulmonary response to exercise in a monitored setting.[40] There are both treadmill and bicycle protocols and norms for children that can be referenced for use when exercise testing children.[40] Further, equipment that is safe and sized correctly for children is necessary for accurate testing and may not be available in all testing laboratory settings. More commonly, physical fitness testing is performed with children, which are more similar to the field tests discussed in the adult exercise testing section of this chapter. A popular physical fitness testing program is the President's Challenge Test[53] consisting of curl-ups or partial curl-ups, shuttle run, endurance run/walk, pull-ups or right angle push-ups, and V-sit or sit and reach. This program offers educational materials, tools, criterion-referenced standards and interpretation of results for schools and communities to apply in group or individual programs.

Regular participation in physical activity during childhood will result in gains in strength, endurance, bone formation, self-esteem and self-efficacy, and skill development.[40] A program of activity will also minimize risk factors for cardiovascular disease, manage weight, reduce anxiety and stress, provide social interaction, and can be a great source of fun and enjoyment.[40] The National Association for Sport and Physical Education developed a position statement for children aged 5 to 12 with the following useful recommendations:

- Children should accumulate at least 60 minutes, and up to several hours, of age-appropriate physical activity on all, or most days of the week. This daily accumulation should include moderate and vigorous physical activity with the majority of the time being spent in activity that is intermittent in nature.
- Children should participate in several bouts of physical activity lasting 15 minutes or more each day.
- Children should participate each day in a variety of age-appropriate physical activities designed to achieve optimal health, wellness, fitness, and performance benefits.
- Extended periods (periods of 2 hours or more) of inactivity are discouraged for children, especially during daytime hours.[54]

Children are at low risk for cardiovascular disease and are able to adjust exercise intensity to tolerance, so do not need a HR prescription.[40] No one program, activity, or methodology has been demonstrated to best improve physical activity in children.[40] Increasing children's physical activity participation on a regular basis and decreasing the amount of sedentary time spent are basic goals for a physical activity program for children. Fitness-based games and lifestyle activities should be used when addressing physical activity participation in children because they are fun and children are more likely to participate in activities that are fun versus highly structured. As children age, they can progress to league and team sports. Adolescents can benefit from league sports as well as cardiovascular exercise such as swimming, bicycling, and jogging. If desired, prescribing exercise using the parameters recommended for adults is safe for adolescents.

Children and adolescents are susceptible to overuse injuries; therefore, clinicians and parents should be aware of the signs and symptoms of overtraining. It is also important to recognize that children and adolescents should balance cardiovascular training with muscle strength and endurance training and activities to address flexibility, to address all of the elements of physical fitness.

Guidelines for Cardiovascular Endurance Training in the Elderly

Several factors affect the decline in physiologic function and physical performance that has been documented to occur with age. Technologic advances that require humans to expend less physical effort, decreased motivation levels and less energy, and the effects of aging all may contribute to the changes seen in the elderly and are sometimes difficult to differentiate. Maximum oxygen consumption decreases approximately 10% per decade with aging, beginning in the middle of the third decade in men and toward the end of the second decade in women. Maximum HR, SV, cardiac output, and peripheral blood flow also decrease with age.[10] In the lungs, residual volume increases with age but total lung capacity remains unchanged, so less air can be exchanged with each breath. The lungs and chest wall also lose elasticity with aging.[10] Body composition changes seen with aging include an increase in relative body fat and a decline in fat-free mass.[10] All of these changes documented in the elderly can be slowed by participation in regular physical activity, making a physically active lifestyle a powerful age deterrent.

The same exercise testing principles presented earlier in this chapter apply to the elderly population. A wide variety of testing protocols exist that are appropriate for use with the elderly population and traditional protocols can be used with slight modification. Appropriate tests are those in which the initial workload is low (2 to 3 METs) and wordload increments small (0.5 to 1.0 METs), and the test accommodates for impaired balance, coordination, vision, gait patterns, and weight-bearing.[40] The 6-minute walk test is used often as a measure of aerobic capacity in elderly patients and in elderly clients without disease.[55,56] To perform the test, patients walk as quickly as they can along a level surface for 6 minutes. The outcome measure of interest is the distance walked in feet or miles. The 6-minute walk test is a practical alternative to other exercise testing means in the elderly because it is easy to perform, patients can stop and rest anytime during the test, assistive ambulation devices may be used to perform the test, and it has been shown to be a reliable indicator of functional ability.[55,57]

The exercise prescription guidelines discussed in this chapter can be safely and appropriately applied to the elderly population. The ACSM and AHA recently published a physical activity recommendation for adults 65 years and older and for adults aged 50 to 64 with clinically significant chronic conditions or functional limitations that affect movement ability, fitness, or physical activity.[58] The recommendation is to perform a minimum of 30 minutes of moderate-intensity aerobic physical activity on 5 days each week or vigorous-intensity aerobic activity for a minimum of 20 minutes on 3 days each week. A combination of moderate- and vigorous-intensity activity can be performed to meet the recommendation. "Moderate-intensity aerobic activity involves a moderate level of effort relative to the individual's aerobic fitness. On a 10-point scale, where sitting is 0 and all-out effort is 10, moderate-intensity activity is a 5 or 6 and produces noticeable increases in heart rate and breathing. Vigorous-intensity exercise is a 7 or 8 and produces large increases in heart rate and breathing."[58(p. 1098)] The physical activity recommendation is in addition to activities of daily living like self-care, shopping and cleaning, or activities that are <10 minutes duration, like short walking bouts in the home or office. The recommendation emphasizes the importance of gradually increasing physical activity in the elderly to minimize the risk of overuse injury, to enhance enjoyment of physical activity, and allow for positive reinforcement through the accomplishment of small steps that lead to the achievement of activity goals.[58]

The effects of cardiovascular endurance training in the elderly include decreased BP, increased high-density lipoprotein (HDL) cholesterol, improved cardiovascular mortality rates, increased bone density, and maintenance of oxygen consumption values.[58] Chosen activities should minimize impact on the joints, emphasizing activities such as water exercise, bicycling, or stair climbing. As is true for all ages, exercise need not be vigorous and continuous to be beneficial. Select activities that are accessible, convenient, enjoyable, and safe for the participant. Progress the prescription by increasing exercise duration rather than intensity.[40] To maintain muscle strength and endurance and to improve mobility, balance, and agility, the elderly should be encouraged to participate in strength training and activities to maintain flexibility, in addition to a program of aerobic exercise.[40,59]

KEY POINTS

- Physical fitness is defined as a set of attributes that people have or achieve and includes cardiovascular endurance, or the ability of the whole body to sustain prolonged exercise.
- Aerobic capacity or maximal oxygen uptake (VO_2 max) is the highest rate of oxygen the body can consume during maximal exercise.
- During acute exercise, HR, SV, Q, a-vO_2 diff, BP, and RR increase proportionally to the exercise workload.
- Benefits of cardiovascular endurance training include positive changes in the cardiovascular and respiratory systems that provide protection from disease, and improved psychologic well-being and quality of life.
- Impaired aerobic capacity can occur as a result of primary cardiovascular and pulmonary disease, diseases of other systems that limit mobility, prolonged bed rest, aging, and a sedentary lifestyle.
- Areas of the patient/client history to which the clinician should pay special attention during the examination of individuals with impaired aerobic capacity include risk factors for cardiovascular disease, social/health habits such as smoking and physical activity, functional ability, and medication history.
- Patients/clients should be appropriately screened prior to the initiation of a cardiovascular training program to ensure safety and minimize risks, thus the clinician should be aware of general screening guidelines.
- Tests and measures used to examine patients/clients with impaired aerobic capacity include GXTs, body composition, and tests and measures of circulation such as BP.
- Exercise prescription can be based on the results of an appropriate exercise test administered before the initiation of a cardiovascular training program.
- Physical activity can be performed to produce health- or fitness-related benefits depending on the patient/client's goals and motivations. Most importantly, individuals should be regularly active.
- Cardiovascular endurance training can be performed using a variety of exercise modes and training techniques.

- Exercise prescription should be based on the individual's needs and interests and should take into consideration comorbidities that may affect activity performance.
- Cardiovascular endurance training is one aspect of a well-balanced exercise program including muscle strengthening and endurance activities and flexibility exercises.
- The clinician should be aware of the signs and symptoms of exercise intolerance and should be able to identify the contraindications for graded exercise testing.
- Supervision requirements for graded exercise testing and for the performance of aerobic exercise are based on the patient/client's history, risk factors, and abilities and the clinician should be able to appropriately determine the level of supervision required.
- Education about the specifics of the exercise prescription, including progression, and the implementation of strategies to enhance compliance will increase the likelihood of the patient/client adopting cardiovascular exercise as a lifelong habit.

CRITICAL THINKING QUESTIONS

1. Consider Case Study No. 1 in Unit 7.
   a. What activities to maintain cardiovascular endurance would you recommend for Lisa as she recovers from her ankle sprain? Be sure to consider the demands of her sport.
   b. What activities would you recommend if she were a long-distance runner? A hockey player? A wrestler?
2. Consider Case Study No. 2 in Unit 7.
   a. Assuming the patient has met the short-term goals, to plan an intervention program to achieve the long-term goals, what test and measure would you select to assess aerobic capacity? What tests and measures to assess circulation would you monitor during the test of aerobic capacity?
   b. To design a long-term aerobic exercise program for Sarah, determine the best strategies to incorporate to enhance compliance and increase the likelihood that she will adopt exercise as a lifelong habit.
3. Consider Case Study No. 3 in Unit 7.
   a. Design an intervention program to improve this journalist's cardiovascular endurance, including techniques to enhance compliance.
   b. According to the Transtheoretical Model of Behavior Change, what stage of change would you place Cathy in and what strategies are appropriate to incorporate to move her to the next stage?
4. Consider Case Study No. 8 in Unit 7.
   a. Recommend a GXT for George, considering the examination findings and his premorbid condition.
   b. Make recommendations for a cardiovascular exercise program, considering George's examination findings and his job.
   c. How would your intervention plan be different if George worked as a long-distance truck driver?

REFERENCES

1. U.S. Department of Health and Human Services. Physical Activity and Health: A Report of the Surgeon General. Atlanta: U.S. Department of Health and Human Services, Centers for Disease Control and Prevention, National Center for Chronic Disease Prevention and Health Promotion, 1996.
2. Blair SN, Kohl HW, Paffenbarger RS, et al. Physical fitness and all-cause mortality. JAMA 1989;262:2395–2401.
3. Paffenbarger RS, Hyde RT, Wing AL. Physical activity and physical fitness as determinants of health and longevity. In: Bouchard C, Shephard RJ, Stephens T, eds. Physical Activity, Fitness, and Health: International Proceedings and Consensus Statement. Champaign, IL: Human Kinetics, 1994.
4. Prevalence of regular physical activity among adults—United States, 2001 and 2005. MMWR 2007;56(46):1209–1212. Accessed on May 16, 2008 from http://www.cdc.gov/mmwr/preview/mmwrhtml/mm5646a1.htm#tab
5. Public Health Service. Healthy People 2000: National Health Promotion and Disease Prevention Objectives. Washington, DC: U.S. Department of Health and Human Services, 1990; DHHS pub. no. (PHS) 91–50212.
6. U.S. Department of Health and Human Services. Healthy People 2010 (conference edition, in two volumes). Washington, DC, January 2000.
7. Pate RR, Pratt M, Blair SN, et al. Physical activity and public health. JAMA 1995;273:402–407.
8. Haskell WL, Lee IM, Pate RR, et al. Physical activity and public health. Updated recommendation for adults from the American College of Sports Medicine and the American Heart Association. Circulation 2007;116:1081–1093.
9. Caspersen CJ, Powell KE, Christenson GM. Physical activity, exercise, and physical fitness: definitions and distinctions for health-related research. Public Health Rep 1985;100:126–131.
10. Wilmore JH, Costill DL. Physiology of Sport and Exercise. 2nd Ed. Champaign, IL: Human Kinetics, 1999.
11. Hasson SM. Clinical Exercise Physiology. St. Louis, MO: Mosby, 1994.
12. Berne RM, Levy MN. Cardiovascular Physiology. 7th Ed. St. Louis, MO: Mosby, 1997.
13. American College of Sports Medicine. Resource Manual for Guidelines for Exercise Testing and Prescription. 3rd Ed. Baltimore, MD: Williams & Wilkins, 1998.
14. Bezner J. Principles of aerobic conditioning. In: Bandy WD, Sanders B, eds. Therapeutic Exercise: Techniques for Intervention. Baltimore, MD: Lippincott Williams & Wilkins, 2001.
15. McAuley E. Physical activity and psychosocial outcomes. In: Bouchard C, Shephard RJ, Stephens T, eds. Physical Activity, Fitness, and Health: International Proceedings and Consensus Statement. Champaign, IL: Human Kinetics, 1994.
16. Caspersen CJ, Powell KE, Merritt RK. Measurement of health status and well-being. In: Bouchard C, Shephard RJ, Stephens T, eds. Physical Activity, Fitness, and Health: International Proceedings and Consensus Statement. Champaign, IL: Human Kinetics, 1994.
17. Rejeski WJ, Brawley LR, Shumaker SA. Physical activity and health-related quality of life. Exerc Sport Sci Rev 1996;24:71–108.
18. McMurdo MET, Burnett L. Randomised controlled trial of exercise in the elderly. Gerontology 1992;38:292–298.
19. Ruuskanen JM, Ruoppila I. Physical activity and psychological well-being among people aged 65 to 84 years. Age Ageing 1995;24:292–296.
20. Woodruff SI, Conway TL. Impact of health and fitness-related behavior on quality of life. Soc Ind Res 1992;25:391–405.
21. Norris R, Carroll D, Cochrane R. The effects of aerobic and anaerobic training on fitness, blood pressure, and psychological stress and well-being. J Psychosomatic Res 1990;34:367–375.
22. Influence of a medium-impact aquaerobic program on health-related quality of life and fitness level in healthy adult females. J Sports Med Phys Fitness 2007;47(4):468–474.
23. Lavie CJ, Milani RV. Effects of cardiac rehabilitation, exercise training, and weight reduction on exercise capacity, coronary risk factors, behavioral characteristics, and quality of life in obese coronary patients. Am J Cardiol 1997;79:397–401.
24. Lavie CJ, Milani RV. Effects of cardiac rehabilitation and exercise training programs in patients ≥ 75 years of age. Am J Cardiol 1996;78:675–677.
25. Kavanagh T, Myers MG, Baigrie RS, et al. Quality of life and cardiorespiratory function in chronic heart failure: effects of 12 months' aerobic training. Heart 1996;76:42–49.
26. Parish TR, Kosma M, Welsch MA. Exercise training for the patient with heart failure: is your patient ready? Cardiopulm Phys Ther J 2007;18:12–20.
27. Kurlansky PA, Traad EA, Galbut DL, et al. Coronary bypass surgery in women: a long-term comparative study of quality of life after bilateral internal mammary artery grafting in men and women. Ann Thorac Surg 2002;74:1517–1525.
28. Motl RW, Gosney J. Effect of exercise training on quality of life in multiple sclerosis: a meta-analysis. Mult Scler 2008;14:129–135.
29. Smith SL. Physical exercise as an oncology nursing intervention to enhance quality of life. Oncol Nurs Forum 1996;23:771–778.
30. Haennel RG, Lemire F. Physical activity to prevent cardiovascular disease. How much is enough? Can Fam Physician 2002;48:65–71.
31. Lee IM, Sesso HD, Oguma Y, et al. Relative intensity of physical activity and risk of coronary heart disease. Circulation 2003;107:1110–1116.
32. Lee IM, Skerrett PJ. Physical activity and all-cause mortality: what is the dose-response relation? Med Sci Sports Exerc 2001;33:S459–S471.
33. Manson JE, Greenland P, LaCroix AZ, et al. Walking compared with vigorous exercise for the prevention of cardiovascular events in women. N Engl J Med 2002;347:716–725.
34. Yu S, Yarnell JW, Sweetnam PM, et al. What level of physical activity protects against premature cardiovascular death? The Caerphilly study. Heart 2003;89:502–506.

35. Manson JE, Hu FB, Rich-Edwards JW, et al. A prospective study of walking as compared with vigorous exercise in the prevention of coronary heart disease in women. N Engl J Med 1999;341:650–658.

36. Andersen RE, Wadden TA, Bartlett SJ, et al. Effects of lifestyle activity vs structured aerobic exercise in obese women. JAMA 1999;281:335–340.

37. Dunn AL, Marcus BH, Kampert JB, et al. Comparison of lifestyle and structured interventions to increase physical activity and cardiorespiratory fitness. JAMA 1999;281:327–334.

38. Guide to Physical Therapist Practice. 2nd Ed. Phys Ther 2001;81:471–593.

39. Goodman CC, Snyder TEK. Differential Diagnosis for Physical Therapists. 4th Ed. St. Louis, MD: Saunders Elsevier, 2007.

40. American College of Sports Medicine. ACSM's Guidelines for Exercise Testing and Prescription. 7th Ed. Philadelphia, PA: Lippincott Williams & Wilkins, 2006.

41. American Association of Cardiovascular and Pulmonary Rehabilitation. Guidelines for cardiac rehabilitation and secondary prevention programs. 4th Ed. Champaign, IL: Human Kinetics, 2004.

42. Ebbeling CB, Ward A, Puleo EM, et al. Development of a single-stage submaximal treadmill walking test. Med Sci Sports Exerc 1991;23:966–973.

43. Maud PJ, Foster C. Physiological Assessment of Human Fitness. Champaign, IL: Human Kinetics, 1995.

44. McArdle WD, Katch FI, Pechar GS, et al. Reliability and interrelationships between maximal oxygen intake, physical work capacity and step-test scores in college women. Med Sci Sports Exerc 1972;4:182–186.

45. Kline GM, Porcari JP, Hintermeister R, et al. Estimation of VO_{2max} from a one-mile track walk, gender, age, and body weight. Med Sci Sports Exerc 1987;19:253–259.

46. Borg G. Borg's Perceived Exertion and Pain Scales. Champaign, IL: Human Kinetics, 1998.

47. American College of Sports Medicine. The recommended quantity and quality of exercise for developing and maintaining cardiorespiratory and muscular fitness in healthy adults. Med Sci Sports Exerc 1990;22:265–274.

48. McArdle WD, Katch FI, Katch VL. Exercise Physiology: Energy, Nutrition and Human Performance. 3rd Ed. Philadelphia, PA: Lea & Febiger, 1991.

49. Lehmann M, Foster C, Keul J. Overtraining in endurance athletes: a brief review. Med Sci Sports Exerc 1993;25:854–862.

50. Dishman RK. Exercise Adherence. Champaign, IL: Human Kinetics, 1988.

51. Franklin BA. Program factors that influence exercise adherence: practical adherence skills for the clinical staff. In: Dishman RK, ed. Exercise Adherence. Champaign, IL: Human Kinetics, 1988.

52. Marcus BH, Banspach SW, Lefebvre RC, et al. Using the stages of change model to increase the adoption of physical activity among community participants. Am J Health Promot 1992;6:424–429.

53. The President's Challenge. Physical Fitness Test. Available at: http://www.presidentschallenge.org/educators/program_details/physical_fitness_test.aspx, Accessed June 20, 2008.

54. National Association for Sport and Physical Education. Physical Activity for Children: A Statement of Guidelines for Children Ages 5–12. 2nd Ed. Reston, VA: NASPE, 2004.

55. Bean JF, Kiely DK, Leveille SG, et al. The 6-minute walk test in mobility-limited elders: what is being measured? J Gerontol A Biol Sci Med Sci 2002;57:M751–M756.

56. Lord SR, Menz HB. Physiologic, psychologic, and health predictors of 6-minute walk performance in older people. Arch Phys Med Rehabil 2002;83:907–911.

57. Hamilton DM, Haennel RG. Validity and reliability of the 6-minute walk test in a cardiac rehabilitation population. J Cardiopulm Rehabil 2000;20:156–164.

58. Nelson ME, Rejeske J, Blair SN, et al. Physical activity and public health in older adults. Recommendation from the American College of Sports Medicine and the American Heart Association. Circulation 2007;116:1094–1105.

59. Pollock ML, Lowenthal DT, Graves JE, et al. The elderly and endurance training. In: Shephard RJ, Astrand PO, eds. Endurance in Sport. Boston, MA: Blackwell Scientific, 1992.

chapter 7

Impaired Range of Motion and Joint Mobility

LORI THEIN BRODY

Most patients with orthopaedic conditions need mobility activities during the rehabilitation program. The clinician must provide hands-on rehabilitation techniques and instructions for a home exercise program. The execution of mobility activities is not as difficult as choosing the appropriate level of assistance and ensuring that the patient is performing the exercise with the correct level of assistance. Clear instruction and supervised practice in the clinician's presence can prevent misunderstandings about exercise performance.

Mobility exercises may be initiated early in the rehabilitation program and done throughout the rehabilitation program on a maintenance basis. Some individuals need progressive mobility exercises throughout the rehabilitation course, progressing from passive (PROM) to active assisted (AAROM) to active range of motion (AROM). Others use specialized mobility activities or stretching exercises. The choice of mobility activities depends on the stage of healing, length of immobilization, number and kind of tissues affected, and the specific injury or surgery. Understanding of the effects of decreased mobility and remobilization is the key to making appropriate mobility exercise choices. The clinician must also realize that immobilization is relative; it can be externally imposed by a brace or cast, or the patient may "self-immobilize" by discontinuing the use of the limb.

When considering mobility, the terms *arthrokinematic* and *osteokinematic* motion must be differentiated. **Arthrokinematic motion** refers to movements of the joint surfaces. Roll, spin, and glide are terms used to describe arthrokinematic motion. Arthrokinematic motion is a necessary component of osteokinematic motion that refers to movement of the bones. **Osteokinematic motion** is described in terms of planes (e.g., elevation in the sagittal plane) or relative movements (e.g., flexion, abduction). Mobility can be impaired by alterations in arthrokinematic motion, osteokinematic motion, or both.

Although decreased mobility is the most obvious mobility impairment encountered, the concept of mobility is relative, with the degree of mobility occurring along a continuum. That continuum encompasses **hypomobility**, or decreased mobility, and **hypermobility**, or excessive mobility. Hypermobility should not be confused with instability. **Instability** is an excessive range of osteokinematic or arthrokinematic movement for which there is no protective muscular control.[1] For example, someone may have excessive arthrokinematic anterior, posterior, and inferior glide at the shoulder (i.e., hypermobility) that is asymptomatic. Loss of dynamic muscular control at the shoulder produces instability and symptoms.

At the hypomobility end of the continuum, the concepts of contracture and adaptive shortening are important for understanding hypomobility. A **contracture** is a condition of fixed high resistance to passive stretch of a tissue resulting from fibrosis or shortening of the soft tissues around a joint or of the muscles.[2] Contractures occur after injury, surgery, or immobilization and are the result of the remodeling of dense connective tissue. Immobilization of a tissue in a shortened position results in **adaptive shortening**, which is shortening of the tissue relative to its normal resting length. Adaptive shortening also can result from holding a limb in a posture that shortens the tissues on one side of the joint. For example, protracting the shoulders in a rounded posture results in adaptive shortening of the pectoral muscles. This shortening can be accompanied by **stiffness** or a resistance to passive movement.

Somewhere between the ideas of hypermobility and hypomobility lies the concept of relative flexibility. **Flexibility** is the ability to move a joint or a series of joints through a ROM. **Relative flexibility** considers the comparative mobility at adjacent joints. Movement in the human body takes the path of least resistance. If one segment of the spine is hypomobile because of injury or disease, the segment is stiffer and has more resistance to movement than adjacent joints. When flexion, extension, or rotation is necessary, the adjacent joints produce most of the movement because of the resistance to motion at the hypomobile joint. Likewise, stiffness in the hamstrings is often compensated by lumbar spine motion, placing more load on the spine. Lengthening the hamstrings minimizes the stress placed on the spine and is the basis for hamstring stretching, an approach used by some persons to remedy back pain.

Relative flexibility is not always an impairment. For example, because of its biomechanical and anatomic properties, L5 is more adapted to produce rotation than any other lumbar segment. It is *relatively more flexible* in the direction of rotation. This is a clinical problem (i.e., impairment) only if the motion becomes excessive and is not muscularly controlled. This problem may occur because of relative stiffness at other spinal segments (above or below L5) or at the hips. For example, golfing requires a significant amount of total body rotation. If the hips, knees, and feet are relatively more stiff in rotation than the spine, the discrepancy may impose excessive rotation in the spine. If the thoracic spine or upper lumbar segments are stiff in rotation, the difference may impose excessive rotation on the L5 segment. L5 is the site of relative flexibility in the direction of rotation.

MORPHOLOGY AND PHYSIOLOGY OF NORMAL MOBILITY

Normal mobility, in its broadest definition, includes osteokinematic motion (movement of bones), arthrokinematic motion (movement of joint surfaces), and neuromuscular coordination to achieve purposeful movement. Normal mobility requires adequate tissue length to allow full ROM (i.e., passive mobility) and the neuromuscular skill to accomplish movement (i.e., active mobility).

Structures involved in passive mobility include the joint's articular surfaces and interposed tissues (e.g., menisci, labrum, synovial lining), joint capsule, ligaments and tendons (including insertions sites), muscles, bursae, fascia, and skin. Joints must have normal arthrokinematic motion, or the ability of an articular surface to roll, spin, and glide across another. The ability to accomplish active mobility requires an intact, functioning nervous system in addition to the structures necessary to allow passive mobility. Mobility is maintained in most individuals by routine, daily use of their limbs and joints in normal daily activities. However, adaptive shortening can occur in those who spend long periods in single postures (e.g., sitting most of the day), and mobility can be lost.

Normal mobility includes adequate joint ROM and muscle ROM. **Joint ROM** is the quantity of motion available at a joint or series of joints in the case of the spine. In contrast, **muscle ROM** is the functional excursion of the muscle from its fully lengthened position to its fully shortened position. Examination and treatment techniques for joint ROM impairments and muscle ROM impairments differ. Joint ROM impairments are examined using accessory or "joint play" motions (arthrokinematic motions) and are treated with joint mobilization, whereas muscle or other soft-tissue ROM impairments are examined using flexibility tests and treated with ROM or stretching exercises.

IMMOBILITY, IMMOBILIZATION, AND REMOBILIZATION

Individuals can lose mobility at a joint for several reasons. Trauma to soft tissue, bone, or other joint structures can diminish mobility. Operations such as total joint replacements, reconstructions, debridements, arthroplasties, osteotomies, and tendon transfers can reduce mobility, as can surgery for nonorthopaedic conditions. Mastectomy or other chest procedures may result in shoulder immobility, and bed rest after cardiac, gynecologic, or other surgical procedures may result in immobility in many joints. Joint disease such as osteoarthritis or rheumatoid arthritis and prolonged immobilization or bed rest for any reason frequently produce immobility. The inability to move a joint because of neuromuscular disease or pain can also result in mobility loss, and pain that inhibits movement can significantly alter mobility.

Immobility at a joint produces a self-perpetuating cycle that can be interrupted by several physical therapy interventions, including ROM modalities, resistive exercises, or mobilizations. Progressive adaptive shortening of the soft tissues occurs as the body responds to decreased loading. This shortening limits mobility and function, reducing the patient's ability to carry out normal activities of daily living, work, or leisure activities. The patient accommodates these limitations by substituting other joints or limbs to achieve functional goals, thereby contributing to the disuse. Pain results from disuse and progressive shortening of the joint capsule (a highly pain-sensitive structure), adding to the disuse. Weakness ensues because of changes in the length-tension ratios, furthering the patient's disinclination to use the limb (Fig. 7-1).

Decreased mobility has profound effects on bone and soft tissues, reflecting the body's ability to adapt to various levels of loading. The plastic nature of these tissues works in positive and negative ways. The specific adaptation to imposed demands principle is based on Wolff's Law and asserts that tissues remodel in accordance to the stresses placed on them. The effects of overload or tissue load greater than its normal usage, and its resulting hypertrophy, the enlargement of a tissue because of an increase in the size of its constituent cells,

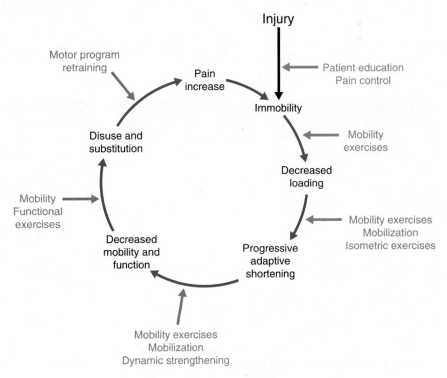

FIGURE 7-1. Self perpetuating cycle of immobility.

TABLE 7-1 Effects of Immobilization and Remobilization on Muscle and Tendon	
MUSCLE	**TENDON**
Position and composition specific muscle fiber atrophy	Decreased size and number of collagen fibers
Functional loss > muscle mass loss	Collagen fibers thinner and disorganized
Decreased electrical activity exceeding atrophy	Decreased load tolerance
Increased connective tissue	Decreased water and GAG[a] content
Increased subcutaneous fat deposition	Increased synthesis and degradation of collagen
Remobilization: lengthy rehabilitation necessary to restore muscle performance especially with longer immobilization	Decreased tensile strength, elastic stiffness and total tissue weight
	Remobilization: controlled mechanical stress increases tensile strength, and energy absorption capacity, facilitates normal gliding and soft tissue relationships, prevents excessive scar formation

[a] GAG, glycosaminoglycan
From References 4–53.

are well known, but the findings associated with underloading are less well known. Findings such as muscular atrophy, or wasting away of a tissue, and loss of joint motion are evident, but cellular changes, articular cartilage changes, and weakening of ligaments and their insertions are less obvious alterations. The clinician must prevent these effects when possible and consider them when implementing a rehabilitation program.

The following tables summarize the consequences of immobilization or decreased mobility on various tissues (Tables 7-1–7-4).[4–53] Further information can be found on the website. Generally, the effects reviewed are caused by immobilization of healthy, uninjured tissues (this is how most studies are done). This raises two important issues. First, immobilization usually is initiated in the presence of an injury (although tissue-lengthening procedures are exceptions), and the structural and mechanical properties of the injured tissues probably will be further compromised. The stages of healing can be found in Chapter 10 and should be considered in concert with the immobilization issues. Second, it is tempting to focus only on the injured tissue after immobilization. However, all surrounding tissues also are immobilized, and understanding the immobilization effects on these tissues ensures a safe and effective rehabilitation course.

Following immobilization, the patient typically goes through a course of structured remobilization.[3] The physiologic response to remobilization of previously immobilized tissues provides the scientific basis for many of the mobility interventions used. Be sure to consider the effects of remobilization on collagenous tissues prior to choosing any specific intervention techniques. The effects of remobilization on connective tissue vary with the type of connective tissue, the type of immobilization, and most importantly, the length of immobilization. Responses to the mobility activity are not necessarily linear and excessive exercise can disrupt the healing process. How the remobilization activity is dosed will impact the final quantity and quality of tissue. In-depth information on the specific tissue effects of remobilization on various tissues can be found on the website.

MOBILITY EXAMINATION AND EVALUATION

Perform a thorough examination before choosing a physical therapy intervention. This ensures appropriate indications and goal setting for the specific mobility technique chosen. Moreover, the evaluation, including subjective examination

TABLE 7-2 Effects of Immobilization and Remobilization on Ligament and Insertion Sites
EFFECTS OF IMMOBILIZATION AND REMOBILIZATION ON LIGAMENT AND INSERTION SITES
Decreased total collagen mass
Decreased strength and stiffness of ligament
Decreased load to failure
Shortening of ligament
Increased stiffness of associated joint
Disproportionate increase in young, immature collagen
Bony resorption and weakening at insertion sites
Increased avulsion rates
Remobilization: can restore structural and mechanical properties of ligaments but takes longer than the original immobilization period

From References 4–53.

TABLE 7-3 Effects of Immobilization and Remobilization on Articular Cartilage
EFFECTS OF IMMOBILIZATION AND REMOBILIZATION ON ARTICULAR CARTILAGE
Increased water content
Decreased proteoglycan content
Decreased chondrocyte population
Decreased articular cartilage thickness and stiffness
Articular cartilage softening
Collagen fiber splitting and fibrillation
Subchondral bone sclerosis
Osteophyte development
Remobilization: effects are time and load dependent; progressive joint deterioration may ensue with inappropriate loading post-immobilization

From References 4–53.

TABLE 7-4	**Effects of Immobilization and Remobilization on Bone**

EFFECTS OF IMMOBILIZATION AND REMOBILIZATION ON BONE

Decreased bone mass
Decreased bone synthesis
Decreased travecular bone volume
Weightbearing bone loss exceeds nonweightbearing bone loss
Remobilization: depends upon bone quality prior to immobilization; may return to normal faster or bone changes may not be reversed

and history taking, informs decisions about exercise dosage, activity type, and elements of the movement system specific to the individual.

The concepts of joint ROM and muscle ROM were clarified earlier. Examination procedures must identify the source of decreased mobility to effectively direct the treatment. Joint ROM is usually measured in the cardinal planes with a goniometer. Goniometric measurements are performed actively or passively, although the reliability of measurement is greater for active measures than for passive measures.[51] Isolated motions such as elbow flexion, knee extension, and ankle dorsiflexion are most commonly measured. Functional goniometric measurements with less stabilization and control can also be taken. Goniometric measurement of forward reach is a common functional assessment. Standards for normal goniometric mobility at each joint are published and provide a guideline for assessing mobility. When assessing joint ROM, the clinician must ensure proper patient positioning to avoid apparent joint motion limitations caused by poor muscle extensibility. For example, hip joint flexion ROM should be performed with the knee flexed to prevent limitations from hamstring excursion (Fig. 7-2).

Assessment of joint ROM with a goniometer does not identify the cause of limited motion. Joint ROM can be limited by capsular tightness, extrinsic soft-issue tightness, intrinsic joint blockage (i.e., knee meniscus tear blocking motion), or pain. Selective tissue tension testing assists the clinician in identifying the tissue at fault. Loss of joint motion in a capsular pattern or with a capsular end feel suggests that the joint capsule is the tissue at fault, and the treatment focus is joint mobilization. However, the clinician should remember that end-feel assessment is not a highly reliable measurement and that the pattern of capsular limitation does not always exist.[52]

Limitations in arthrokinematic motion decrease a patient's mobility, and increases in arthrokinematic mobility cause hypermobility. Arthrokinematic mobility is assessed through joint play maneuvers. Joint play is the movement of one articular surface on another and is not usually under voluntary control. Joint play is assessed by stabilizing one articular surface (by stabilizing the bone) and applying external pressure on the other to produce movement. For example, applying an anteroposterior glide at the proximal interphalangeal joint of the index finger requires stabilization of the proximal phalanx while the distal phalanx is moved in an anteroposterior direction. In some cases, stabilization of one segment is provided by the surrounding bony and soft-tissue structures and the supporting surface. For example, when performing posteroanterior unilateral vertebral pressure, the patient is stabilized in a prone position on the table while unilateral posteroanterior pressure is applied to the transverse process, producing rotation of the vertebral body that should be compared with the contralateral side.[1] Assessment of joint play can identify hypomobile, normal, or hypermobile conditions. These tests direct intervention for increasing capsular mobility, looking for other sources of mobility loss, or stabilization activities, respectively.

Unidirectional loss of motion suggests some other soft tissue (muscle-tendon unit, skin, fascia, neurologic tissue) is at fault, and other ROM techniques may be employed. Muscle ROM is generally assessed using flexibility tests, a few of which are quantified. For example, hamstring extensibility can be assessed goniometrically using the 90–90 straight-leg raise (Fig. 7-3).[1] The Thomas test for hip flexor extensibility and the Bunnel-Littler test for hand intrinsic or joint capsule extensibility are examples of flexibility tests. These tests, when performed correctly, can direct intervention for decreased musculotendinous extensibility as the cause of decreased mobility.

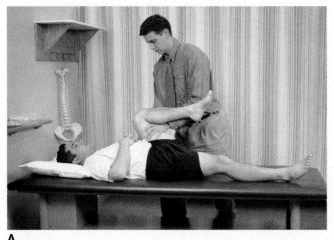
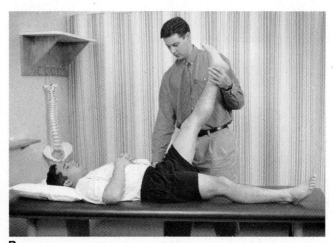

A   **B**

FIGURE 7-2. (A) Joint ROM at the hip. The knee is flexed to minimize effects of hamstring tension. (B) Muscle ROM for the hamstrings. The same hip flexion activity is done with the knee extended.

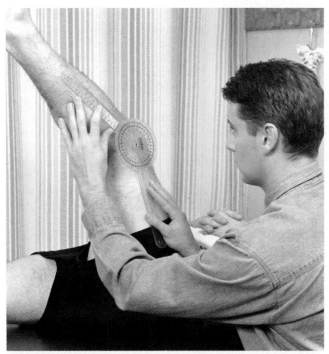

FIGURE 7-3. Assessment of hamstring flexibility goniometrically using the 90–90 straight-leg raise. The hip is flexed to 90 degrees, and the knee gradually extended from flexion to extension. The final angle of knee flexion is measured.

RANGE OF MOTION INTERVENTION FOR IMPAIRED MOBILITY

A variety of interventions are available to treat decreased mobility. After the tissues limiting mobility have been identified, appropriate ROM, stretching, or joint mobilization techniques should be applied. Adjunctive agents enhance the effectiveness of exercise interventions.

Elements of the Movement System

Although any of the elements of the movement system may contribute to decreased mobility, most problems with mobility arise from base elements or the extensibility and mobility of the soft tissues. For example, loss of normal hip extension ROM may contribute to low back pain by transferring the extension mobility requirement from the hip to the low back (i.e., relative flexibility). In this case, decreased mobility (i.e., impairment) in the hip contributes to low back pain (i.e., impairment). The pain arises from compression of the posterior elements of the spine and subsequent inflammation around the nerve roots (i.e., pathology) and an inability to sit for long periods (i.e., activity limitation). If left untreated, this condition may lead to participation restriction, such as the inability to work at a desk, participate in recreational activities, or sit in car.

In this example, the base elements are the shortened hip flexors and hip joint capsule pulling the pelvis into anterior tilt and the lengthened and weak abdominal muscles that are unable to provide sufficient counterforce. The biomechanical elements are the increased anterior pelvic tilt and increased lumbar lordosis contributing to posterior element compression in the spine. The modulator element is an inability to recruit the abdominal muscles to improve the

biomechanical elements. The cognitive or affective element is depression related to chronic low back pain.

The elements of the movement system involved must be prioritized and those elements amenable to physical therapy intervention determined. In this situation, intervention to increase the length of the hip flexors, decrease stiffness in the hip joint capsule, and improve the neuromuscular firing and muscular endurance of the abdominal muscles should be instituted.

Considerations in Choosing Mobility Activities

The clinician has many options for treating decreased mobility. Joint mobilization, ROM exercises, neuromobilization, and stretching are the more common interventions applied. ROM activities or joint mobilization can be used to increase joint ROM, and stretching techniques can be used to remedy limitations in muscle ROM. Joint mobilization is a technique that preserves or increases arthrokinematic motion. It is a necessary prerequisite for normal osteokinematic mobility. Attempting to perform ROM activities in the absence of normal arthrokinematic motion at the joint surface does not improve the impaired mobility and may increase the patient's symptoms. Self-mobilization activities such as lateral distraction at the glenohumeral joint or long-axis traction at the hip may precede ROM exercises.

When applying interventions to increase mobility, the clinician must consider the continuum of hypomobility to hypermobility and the concept of relative flexibility. Hypomobility can be mistreated if the possibility of adjacent hypermobility is ignored. For example, if a stiff segment exists at L4–5 and treatment is directed at decreasing stiffness there without stabilizing interventions directed at hypermobile segments above and below, symptoms of instability at these segments may increase. Treatment must include a comprehensive program to improve the mobility at the relatively more stiff segments or regions and to increase the stiffness at the relatively more mobile segment. Because motion always occurs along the path of least resistance, mobility occurs naturally at the stiff segment only if it is of equal mobility or more mobile than other segments. It is important to increase the stiffness at the site of relative flexibility. This is done by improving neuromuscular control, muscle performance capability, and length-tension relationships of the stabilizing muscles around the site of relative flexibility. These techniques are coupled with patient education, postural training, and movement patterns that improve the distribution of mobility.

The clinician must also consider the cause of decreased mobility and the prognosis for resolution of the mobility impairment. In some cases, such as idiopathic shoulder adhesive capsulitis, the specific cause of the problem is unknown, the rehabilitation program protracted and the prognosis and final outcome mixed. In this case, mobility interventions that the patient can perform independently will be an important component of the treatment program.

Range of Motion

Mobility activities at a joint or series of joints and articulations can offset some of the deleterious effects of immobilization. Movement about a joint, whether passive, active assisted, or active, produces a load in the soft tissues. This loading can

DISPLAY 7-1
Considerations When Performing ROM

- ensure patient comfort and safety
- ensure clinician safety by using good body mechanics
- support any areas at risk of injury resulting from hypermobility, fracture, etc.
- perform ROM slowly and rhythmically
- move through as full a range as possible
- avoid an excessively tight grip by grasping over as large a surface area as possible
- use cardinal plane motions, combined motions, or functional movement patterns

maintain the integrity of the tendon, ligament and bony attachments, articular cartilage, and muscle. The benefit is determined by the exercise and immobilization parameters and by the status of the tissues before immobilization. Mobility activities are specific exercises or functional activities performed to improve functional ROM about a joint. Mobility activities usually are performed through a joint ROM and can be performed in cardinal planes or in multiple planes using functional movement patterns (e.g., reaching, squatting). These activities can be performed actively, passively, or with active assistance (Display 7-1).

Passive Range of Motion

PROM exercises are mobility activities performed without any muscular activation (Fig. 7-4). These exercises are performed within the available ROM. Any overpressure at the end of the range would be categorized as stretching, not PROM. PROM and stretching can be combined to increase the ROM around a joint.[53]

Indications Noncontractile tissues potentially limiting passive mobility about a joint include the joint capsule, periarticular connective tissue, and overlying skin. Surgical incisions producing adhesions between the skin and underlying fascial layers limit their ability to glide during joint motion. Shortening, spasm, or contractures of the musculotendinous unit can also limit the

passive motion at a joint. Shortening of musculotendinous tissue should be differentiated from stiffness of the connective tissues. Stiffness in soft tissues is felt as an increased resistance to movement and can alter movement patterns passively and actively, resulting in musculoskeletal pain. Bone-on-bone approximation in the presence of degenerative joint disease, loose bodies, and pain can similarly limit passive mobility.

PROM is used when active movement may disrupt the healing process, when the patient is physically or cognitively unable to move actively, or when active movement is too painful to perform. Passive movements also are used to teach active or resistive exercises and to produce relaxation. Goals related to the prescription of PROM depend on the patient and the setting. In an orthopaedic setting, PROM is often used to prevent the deleterious effects of immobilization after an injury or surgery. Prevention of joint contractures and soft-tissue stiffness or adaptive shortening, maintenance of the normal mobile relationships between soft-tissue layers, decreased pain, and enhancement of vascular dynamics and synovial diffusion are goals of PROM.[53] These goals are difficult to measure and to document. The clinician must rely on his understanding of the pathologic process to provide the rationale for this intervention. Measurable outcomes related to PROM as prevention intervention may include decreased pain, expeditious restoration of motion and strength, and earlier return to function after activity is allowed (see Self-Management 7-1: Ankle Passive Range of Motion).

When the patient is comatose, paralyzed, on complete bed rest, wheelchair bound, or cognitively unable to maintain joint

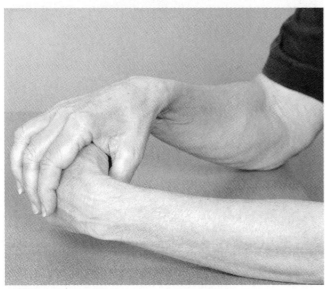

FIGURE 7-4. Self-range activity for wrist flexion.

SELF-MANAGEMENT 7-1 *Ankle Passive Range of Motion*

Purpose:	To increase ankle motion in all directions
Position:	In a sitting position with the ankle crossed across the knee, with a comfortable grip at the forefoot.
Movement Technique:	Move the ankle in upward and downward directions. Move the ankle in and out. Stay in a comfortable ROM. Hold briefly at the end of the range in each direction.

Dosage
   Repetitions: _____
   Frequency: _____

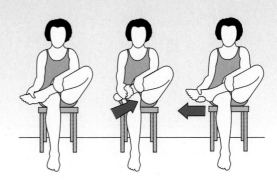

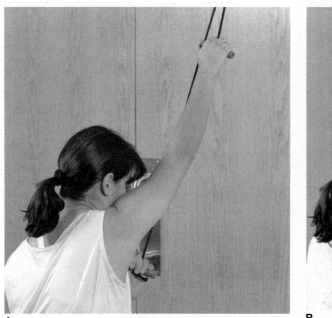
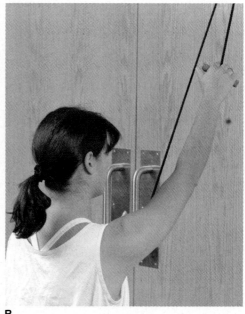

A   **B**

FIGURE 7-5. (A) Incorrect performance of shoulder flexion using pulleys. (B) Correct performance using proper posture and movement kinematics.

ROM, PROM is used to achieve the same goals as the orthopedic setting. Because of the long-standing nature of these problems and the profound effects of long-term immobility, prevention assumes even greater importance. The patient usually requires PROM exercise two or more times each day, necessitating provision of services by family members or other assistive personnel.

Modes   The exercise chosen should allow full available excursion. Several modes are available for the performance of PROM or stretching. Pulleys, continuous passive motion devices, family members, or various household objects such as the floor, counters, or chairs can be used to perform PROM. Holding the position at end range adds a stretching component to the PROM activity. Using pulleys to gain shoulder flexion can be helpful if performed properly without scapular or spinal substitution patterns (Fig. 7-5). The same can be said for self-mobilization activities such as stretching the arm forward on a counter (Fig. 7-6). Passive knee flexion can be easily performed using a towel and a smooth floor, by sitting on a chair, or while in a pool (see the section on ROM Self-Management).

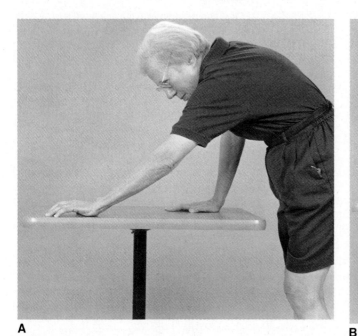
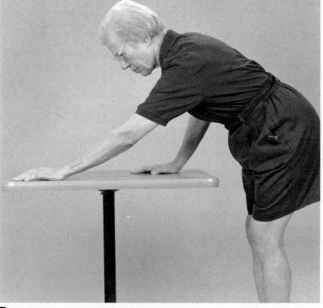

A   **B**

FIGURE 7-6. (A) Incorrect performance of passive shoulder flexion on a countertop. (B) Correct performance using proper posture and movement kinematics.

Techniques and Dosage The clinician's skill in performing PROM can significantly alter the response. The clinician's handling techniques can affect the patient's comfort and ability to relax during treatment. When active muscle contraction is contraindicated, positioning and handling should allow the patient to fully relax. Any apprehension could result in protective muscle contraction and possible injury. Proper positioning allows adequate stabilization while the clinician's hand control provides stabilization and command of the affected limb. The clinician should use a grip that provides control but considers the patient's condition. Avoiding painful areas or excessively tight grips that produce discomfort assures the patient of the clinician's control. ROM should be performed at a smooth and steady pace, avoiding abrupt movements or excessive speed that may cause protective muscle contraction. The clinician should always monitor the patient's response and be flexible enough to modify the technique when necessary. The hand position, ROM, and speed must be tailored for each patient.

The exercise dosage will vary with the purpose of the exercise. In general, the volume of exercise should be sufficient to achieve the physical therapy goals without overloading the tissues, particularly when performed during the healing process. It is best to perform fewer repetitions of an exercise, and return to that exercise performing additional set(s) of the exercise as the patient tolerates. For example, following cast removal for a colles fracture, the therapist might perform 5 to 10 repetitions of wrist flexion and extension, followed by a finger activity. If tolerated, add an additional set or two of the flexion/extension activity, with alternate activities between sets.

Active Assisted Range of Motion

AAROM can be defined as mobility activities in which some muscle activation takes place. In this situation, the patient is unable or not allowed to fully activate the muscle. AAROM is used when some muscle activation through the ROM is allowed or desired, but the patient requires some assistance to complete the ROM. AAROM is frequently used to initiate gentle muscle activity after musculotendinous surgical procedures such as rotator cuff or Achilles tendon repairs. The amount of assistance throughout the ROM may vary. Some individuals may require assistance throughout the entire range, but others may require minimal or no assistance in some ranges but nearly maximal assistance in other ranges. This variation may result from a painful arc, limitations imposed by the disease or injury, changing length-tension ratios, or synergist action.

Active assisted exercise is indicated for patients who are unable to complete the ROM actively because of weakness resulting from trauma, neurologic injury, muscular or neuromuscular disease, or pain. The weight of the limb may impede active movement using proper mechanics, and assistance may be provided to ensure proper exercise performance. Some injuries or operations necessitate limitations in active muscle contraction in the early phase of healing (see Self-Management 7-2: Knee-to-Chest Stretching).

The expected goals with AAROM intervention are the same as those accomplished with PROM. Prevention of the negative effects of immobilization, prevention of joint contractures and soft-tissue tightness, decreased pain, and enhancement of vascular dynamics and synovial diffusion can be accomplished with AAROM. The benefits of active muscle contraction extend beyond those of PROM. Active

SELF-MANAGEMENT 7-2 *Knee-to-Chest Stretching*

Purpose: To increase the mobility of the lumbar spine and hips in flexion

Position: Lying on your back, with your knees bent and feet flat on the floor

Movement Technique: Slowly bring one knee to your chest while grasping *behind your knee.* Bring the second knee to your chest. Hold for 15 to 30 seconds. Slowly lower one leg to the starting position, followed by the other leg.

Dosage
Repetitions: _____
Frequency: _____

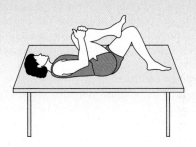

muscle contraction significantly enhances circulation. The pull of muscle on its bony attachments is a stimulus for bone activity while eliciting muscle activity. Active muscle contraction also assists in proprioception and kinesthesia, enhancing the individual's awareness of his position in space. Muscle contraction in this situation has little impact on true strength gains in most patients, but it teaches the patient how to actively fire the muscle. For example, individuals with rotator cuff injuries require assistance to activate these muscles after injury or surgery (Fig. 7-7). Moreover, active assisted exercise involves the patient in his rehabilitation, rather than acting as the recipient of a passive technique.

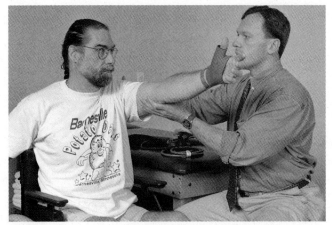

FIGURE 7-7. Active assisted shoulder flexion can be accomplished with assistance from the therapist.

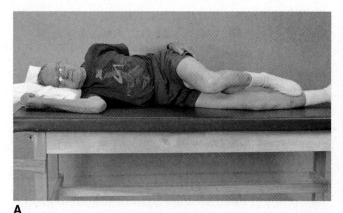 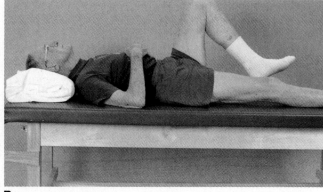

A   B

FIGURE 7-8. (A) Active hip flexion in a gravity minimized position. (B) Active hip flexion against gravity.

Hand placement and cueing during AAROM are important for optimal patient participation. When possible, tactile cueing should be on one side of the joint rather than using a grip on the flexor and extensor surfaces. This action cues the patient for the direction of assistance or resistance. This is particularly important when performing a technique such as AAROM when some ranges are assisted but others are not.

Active Range of Motion
AROM is defined as mobility activities performed by active muscle contraction. These activities can be performed against gravity or in a gravity-minimized position, depending on the individual's strength and the physical therapy goals (Fig. 7-8). Motions in cardinal planes, combination movement patterns, or functional activities such as reaching or combing one's hair are all examples of AROM. The expected goals or outcomes associated with AROM intervention include those associated with PROM plus the benefits of muscle contraction. These goals parallel those of AAROM, although the results are greater. In addition to the greater strength requirements, active exercise requires more muscle coordination because of the lack of assistance or guidance through the ROM. As with active assisted exercise, the strength gains are minimal in many patients. Only those with fair (3/5) strength or less can be expected to have their strength challenged. However, many patients can expect to be challenged proprioceptively and kinesthetically. For example, after knee injury or surgery, many individuals have difficulty activating the quadriceps femoris. Quadriceps setting exercises show patients how to activate the quadriceps, a prerequisite for functional activities. Although little or no tibiofemoral movement occurs, patellofemoral AROM occurs, with superior glide of the patella on the femur. An additional benefit of active exercise is independence in the rehabilitation program. Active exercise enhances the vascular

---

 SELECTED INTERVENTION 7-1
Active Range of Motion to Improve Mobility

See Case Study No. 4

ACTIVITY: Wand elevation exercise

PURPOSE: To increase shoulder mobility in abduction, scaption, and flexion

RISK FACTORS: Ensure appropriate stabilization and arthrokinematic motion to prevent substitution

ELEMENTS OF THE MOVEMENT SYSTEM: Biomechanical

STAGE OF MOTOR CONTROL: Mobility

POSTURE: The patient is standing in chest-deep water, with a wand in the hands.

MOVEMENT: The patient allows the buoyancy of the water and the assistance of the uninvolved arm to lift the arm in the frontal, scapular, or sagittal plane. Relaxation of the shoulder muscles allows passive stretch into abduction, scaption, or flexion.

DOSAGE: Sets of three to five repetitions with 30-second holding at the end of the range.

RATIONALE FOR EXERCISE CHOICE: This exercise passively assists motion into a functional, frequently limited range. The intensity of stretch is easily modified by changing water depth.

EXERCISE GRADATION: The patient should discontinue use of wand and progress to active then resisted movements.

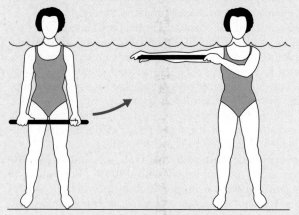

Wand shoulder abduction

benefits of ROM, with activities such as ankle pumps (i.e., repetitive dorsiflexion and plantarflexion) used postoperatively to prevent deep vein thromboses.

Indications   As with AAROM, active exercise is indicated when active muscle contraction is desired. Many exercise programs begin with a regimen of active exercise to ensure proper exercise performance before the addition of resistance. In some situations, the weight of the limb alone produces optimal loading and makes a good starting point for the rehabilitation program. After the patient learns the correct exercise technique, that exercise can be performed in a variety of modes that suit the patient's preferences (see Selected Intervention 7-1: Active Range of Motion to Improve Mobility).

Active mobility can be limited by the same noncontractile and contractile tissues that limit passive mobility. Shortening, stiffness, spasm, or contracture limit the joint's ability to move through a ROM. The strength and endurance of the muscle or muscle group can limit active motion. Strength below a fair (3/5) muscle grade implies an inability to complete the ROM against gravity. Poor neuromuscular coordination and balance, such as the inability to stand on a single leg, may limit active mobility. Strength in an agonist may be adequate to complete the ROM, but antagonist firing because of neurologic pathology or faulty neuromuscular control patterns may limit motion. The patient may lack adequate speed of movement or agonist or synergist coordination to achieve purposeful movement. Cardiovascular endurance limitations in patients with chronic obstructive pulmonary disease, emphysema, or other cardiovascular conditions can hinder the performance of active exercise. All these situations may necessitate AROM as a therapeutic intervention. See Building Block 7-1.

Technique   Prior to performing AROM, ensure that muscle activation is warranted and determine any precautions. Examples of precautions might be working only through a portion of the ROM, performing ROM in a gravity-minimized position only, or consideration of cardiac conditions. Once these are identified and the patient informed of these parameters, the therapist should demonstrate the exercise to be performed. The therapist can perform the exercise and then have the patient mirror the exercise, or the therapist may take the patient passively through the ROM and ask the patient to repeat this movement. Exercises can be performed through cardinal planes, diagonals, or functional movements. The speed, ROM, posture, and other important aspects of exercise performance should be monitored and explained to the patient.

Mirrors are useful so the patient receives both verbal and visual feedback about performance.

Dosage   Dosage for AROM depends upon the purpose of the activity. When using AROM to increase mobility, the exercise is typically dosed by the goal (i.e., continue repetitions until a ROM goal is achieved) or by the volume (i.e., number of repetitions × number of sets). For example, following shoulder surgery the patient might perform active shoulder flexion in sidelying until 100-degree flexion is achieved. Following knee surgery, the patient may be asked to perform 15 quadriceps set exercises every waking hour. When performing AROM as part of a strengthening routine, typical strengthening dosages should be implemented. The patient typically performs AROM exercise to fatigue, takes a rest interval, and performs additional sets. Patients performing AROM for position and kinesthetic sense should perform repetitions until form fatigue or muscle substitution. Again, this is followed by a rest interval and the exercise repeated or a different exercise initiated.

Active exercise should follow any passive technique to reinforce proper movement patterns and to overcome maladaptions to tissue stiffness. As new mobility is achieved, active exercise ensures the ability to use the new range effectively. For example, as hip flexion ROM improves from joint mobilization and stretching techniques, hand-knee rocking can be used to facilitate hip flexion ROM (see Fig. 17-26). As shoulder flexion mobility increases after stretching exercises, initiate active shoulder flexion exercises. Similarly, as knee flexion ROM increases after stretching, active knee flexion should follow (see Self-Management 7-3: Active Range of

SELF-MANAGEMENT 7-3 *Active Range of Motion for Shoulder Flexion*

Purpose: To increase active mobility in a forward and overhead direction

Position: In a sitting or standing position keeping your trunk in good alignment

Movement Technique: Reach your arm forward and up overhead. Reach as far overhead as is comfortable.

Dosage
Repetitions: _____
Frequency: _____

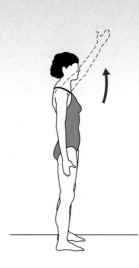

SELF-MANAGEMENT 7-4 *Active Knee Flexion*

Purpose: To increase active range of knee flexion and to initiate muscle activity

Position: Standing on your uninvolved leg on the floor or on a small step, with your involved leg hanging down next to the step, hold onto a stable object for support.

Movement Technique: Slowly bend your involved knee up behind you, then lower it slowly and in a controlled fashion. Be sure to keep your knees in line with one another.

Dosage
Repetitions: _____
Frequency: _____

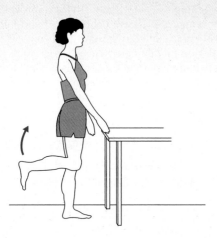

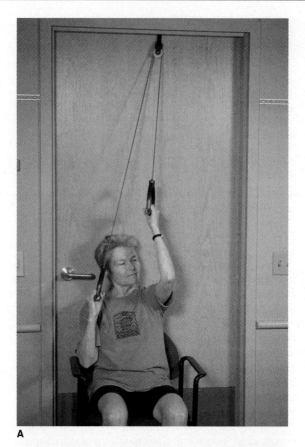

A

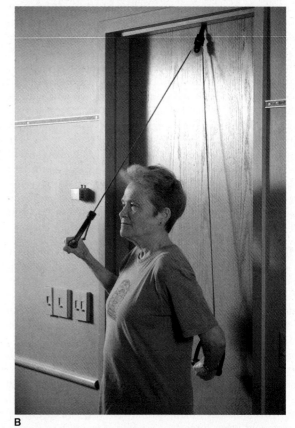

B

FIGURE 7-9. (A) Pulleys used for increasing shoulder flexion mobility. (B) Pulleys used to increase shoulder extension and internal rotation mobility.

Motion for Shoulder Flexion and Self-Management 7-4: Active Knee Flexion). A few repetitions to reinforce the new ROM and movement pattern are generally sufficient.

Independent ROM Activities
Most mobility conditions necessitating ROM intervention need these exercises daily. Therefore some exercises must be performed independently either by the patient or by a caregiver. For exercises provided by a caregiver, the therapist should instruct this individual in correct performance following the same guidelines utilized by the physical therapist. However, for the patient performing independent ROM activities, the therapist must provide tools, devices, or techniques that allow the patient to perform the ROM activity safely and effectively.

Pulleys ROM exercises can be implemented using a variety of different tools. Pulleys are one of the more common modes used for performing ROM exercises, particularly for the upper extremity. Pulleys are easily adjusted to increased shoulder ROM into cardinal planes such as flexion, abduction, and internal and external rotation (Fig. 7-9A and B). They can also be adjusted to increase mobility in diagonal or functional

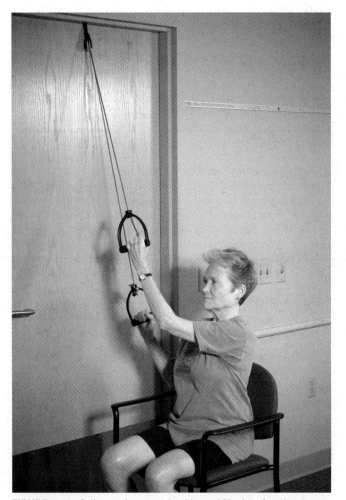

FIGURE 7-10. Pulleys to increase shoulder mobility in a functional diagonal pattern.

> **BUILDING BLOCK 7-2**
>
> A patient with adhesive capsulitis has been performing a home exercise program of pulleys working to increase independent active elevation of the shoulder. However, the patient is still unable to lift the arm against gravity above 90 degrees without scapular substitution. What are some changes to the exercise program that might make forward elevation easier?

For example, the patient might begin by performing PROM and progress (either in the same exercise session or over time as healing permits) to AAROM. As tolerated, the patient might include stretching at the end of the ROM. Dosage is typically the same as if the exercise were applied manually by a physical therapist. See Building Block 7-2.

The patient should be adjusted to that the pulley is directly in line with the axis of the joint being exercised. This facilitates normal biomechanics. If alignment is not correct, then altered joint mechanics follows and may produce pain. Monitor the patient closely for proper mechanics, avoiding excessive scapular elevation as substitution for glenohumeral motion. Educate the patient on the importance of proper mechanics and supervise the patient performing the exercise independently prior to initiating this exercise.

Cane Exercises   A cane, t-bar, dowel rod, or other similar device can be used to assist ROM exercises. Most of these exercises would be considered active-assisted as most of these exercises require muscle activation to complete the ROM or to return to the starting position. Depending upon how the exercise is performed, canes can be used effectively for stretching as well. Cane exercises are most frequently used for upper extremity ROM activities. In some cases, the uninvolved extremity guides the involved extremity while both are performing the same movement. Shoulder flexion and elbow flexion are good examples of this type of movement. In other cases, the uninvolved extremity guides the involved extremity in a unilateral movement pattern. Examples of this include shoulder external rotation and shoulder abduction (Fig. 7-11A and B). Combination activities such as extension and internal

patterns (Fig. 7-10). Pulleys are simple as long as the patient is able to grasp the pulley handle. For those lacking hand strength or control, mitts or other assistive devices are available.

ROM exercises using pulley can be passive or active assisted, and can incorporate stretching at the end of the ROM. Some combination of these activities is also possible.

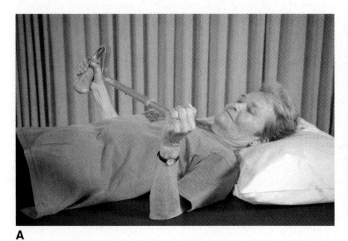

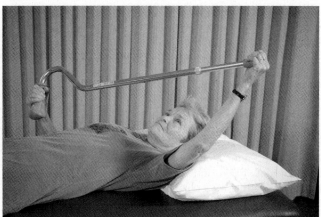

A   B

FIGURE 7-11. Cane exercise for shoulder (A) external rotation and (B) abduction.

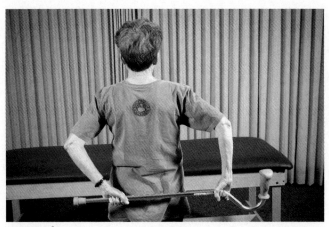

FIGURE 7-12. Cane used to increase shoulder extension and internal rotation mobility.

BUILDING BLOCK 7-3

The patient is a third grade teacher who was recently out of a cast following a left wrist colles fracture. He needs to increase his wrist AROM and PROM. Describe some activities he might do during his work day to increase ROM.

rotation can also be performed by grasping the end of the cane with the involved extremity while the uninvolved arm passively moves the arm into further internal rotation (Fig. 7-12).

Choosing cane exercises requires a good understanding of the limits of healing and confidence that the patient can perform the exercise competently without disrupting the healing process. Although the cane is held in both hands, patients sometimes mistakenly believe that the involved extremity is not working during the activity. In many cases, the muscles are actively working and the exercise more closely resembles a guided AROM activity than a PROM or AAROM activity. If the exercise is truly passive, ensure that the patient understands the ROM limits for the exercise. When starting the exercise program, demonstrate and then guide the patient through the exercise performance. Dose the exercise the same as if the activity was being performed manually. Be sure to allow sufficient rest periods between exercise sets or sessions.

Horizontal and Vertical Surfaces   Horizontal surfaces such as tabletops, desktops, floors and beds, and vertical surfaces such as walls, doors, and doorways provide ample opportunities for ROM exercises. Surfaces that allow the limb to slide easily (akin to a powder board or slide board) work best, although surface friction can be reduced by the addition of a towel, pillowcase, wax paper, or other similar material. Shoulder ROM in elevation can be performed by "walking" the fingers up a wall or doorway, or by walking the fingers out on a countertop, then forward bending at the hips to enhance the ROM. Similarly, sitting at a desk, the patient can reach the arm forward on the desktop, and then slide the chair back to achieve greater overhead elevation. External rotation ROM can be performed by placing the hand in a doorway and turning away from the involved shoulder.

Use the floor or a bed to increase hip and knee flexion ROM. Either sitting or supine on the floor, slide the heel toward the buttocks to perform AROM. Pull a pillowcase or towel placed under the foot to perform PROM or AAROM. Knee flexion ROM and ankle dorsiflexion ROM are easily performed sitting on a chair and sliding the foot back under the chair. A sock, pillowcase or wax paper will decrease friction between the foot and the floor. Similarly, these activities can be performed in supine with one foot on the wall. Slide the foot down the wall to increase hip, knee, and ankle flexion.

Crossing one ankle over the opposite knee and then sliding the foot down the wall will increase hip external rotation ROM.

These are only a few of the numerous examples of how horizontal and vertical surfaces can be used to perform self ROM. When choosing an exercise, determine the amount of muscle activation allowed to ensure picking an exercise that can be done safely. Then query the patient about surfaces available at home and at work. Design a program that will be easy to perform in their living and working environments. As best as possible, observe the patient performing the exercises. Dose the exercises the same as if they were being carried manually by the physical therapist. See Building Block 7-3.

Self-Range of Motion   In the absence of tools, equipment, or other means of independent ROM, the patient can use the arms or uninvolved upper extremity to perform self-ROM exercises. Self-ROM requires a baseline level of strength and coordination on the part of the patient, so the therapist should match patients with the appropriate level of activity. For example, a patient who has limited strength and mobility following a stroke may have insufficient strength or control to perform ROM on the involved arm or leg. Patients with multiple joint osteoarthritis or rheumatoid arthritis may not be able to use their arms to move other extremities due to pain.

Self-ROM can be performed in a variety of positions. The position chosen should consider the patient's strength and control, the desired working range, joint biomechanics (i.e., shoulder instability following a stroke, or hypomobility with impingement considerations) and the patient's ability to assume the preferred position(s). Modify the exercise as necessary to help the patient accomplish the activity. For example, when performing shoulder flexion ROM in supine, it may be necessary to flex the involved elbow to overcome gravity and lift the arm to the 90-degree position where gravity can begin to assist the exercise.

In the upper extremities, the supine position allows the final range of shoulder elevation to be assisted by gravity. If this same exercise were performed in sitting or standing, the biomechanics of the exercise would increase the physical challenge of achieving the full overhead position. In contrast, the same exercise performed in supine allows gravity to assist at the end of the ROM (Fig. 7-13A and B). Upper extremity ROM activities that work well in supine are shoulder elevation, horizontal abduction and adduction, and rotation. Elbow flexion and extension and forearm pronation and supination are performed either in supine or sitting. In sitting, these activities are performed with the arm supported in the tabletop. Wrist and hand activities can be performed in supine but may work better in a sitting position with the arm resting on a tabletop. This position allows easier visualization of the activity being performed. Finger activities can be performed in nearly any position as long as visualization and stabilization are sufficient. In any case, be sure to observe the patient performing these

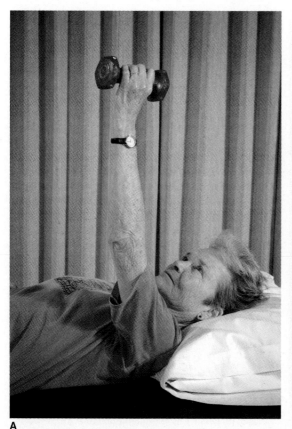 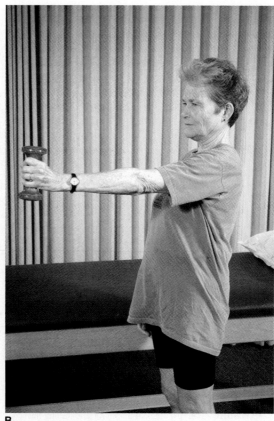

A   **B**

FIGURE 7-13. (A) Shoulder flexion in supine. Note that the moment arm length approaches zero at 90 degrees of forward flexion, and further flexion becomes assisted by gravity. (B) Shoulder flexion in standing. The resistance due to gravity increases as the arm approaches 90-degree flexion and continues to be resisted by gravity.

exercises in the clinic to ensure proper performance. The patient may begin ROM exercises in one position and progress to an alternative position as improvement is made.

Like the upper extremities, lower extremity ROM can be performed in supine or sitting. In supine, hip and knee flexion can be performed by grasping behind the thigh with a towel or hands and pulling the knee toward the chest. This exercise requires abdominal strength to initiate the lift, and arm strength to pull the thigh toward the chest. Hip abduction and adduction can also be performed in supine, sliding the leg in and out, while hip internal and external rotation is performed in the same position, rolling the leg in and out. Rolling the leg internally and externally on a bed is relatively easy, whereas sliding the leg in abduction and adduction can be challenging against the friction of the bed. Some alterations can make this exercise simpler. First, if sufficient strength and control exist, the patient can slide the uninvolved ankle under the involved ankle and use the uninvolved leg to assist the activity. Also, lower friction surfaces can be used. A powder board or slide board under the involved leg can decrease friction. Lastly, wearing clothing and utilizing bedding of fabric that is "more slippery" than higher friction materials such as flannel will improve the ease of this exercise.

Knee joint ROM exercises can be performed in supine by sliding the heel toward the buttocks, or in sitting. Sitting on the bed or floor, the patient slides the heel toward the buttocks. If ROM is to be passive, a pillowcase or towel under the foot can be pulled by the arms. In a chair, the patient can slide the foot forward and back, extending and flexing the knee, or if passive is preferred, the foot remains fixed on the floor and the patient slides his or her body forward and back over the fixed foot. Ankle PROM is easily performed passively by crossing the ankle over the opposite knee. Like the knee, PROM can also be performed with the foot fixed on the ground and moving the body anteriorly and posteriorly over it (Fig. 7-14A and B). Ankle AROM can be performed in nearly any position or posture. The same is true of the toes.

Trunk ROM exercises are more challenging because of the size and weight of the trunk. AROM exercises are performed in standing or sitting and involve trunk movements in cardinal, diagonal or functional movement patterns. However, on land, the effects of gravity may make these exercises uncomfortable. Many of these exercises are more comfortable in an aquatic environment. PROM is usually performed in prone or supine, with the exception of sidebending which is difficult to do passively independently. Passive extension is accomplished by a prone press-up while flexion is performed in supine in a knee-to-chest exercise. Passive trunk rotation can be performed in hooklying, rolling the knees from one side to the other.

Aquatic Environment   The pool is an ideal place to perform ROM exercises. The water's buoyancy makes performance of any upward movement easier than on land. The effects of gravity resisting elevation are minimized and the water's buoyancy assists movement. Thus, many ROM activities requiring upward movement become AAROM exercises. This attribute of buoyancy is particularly useful for movements

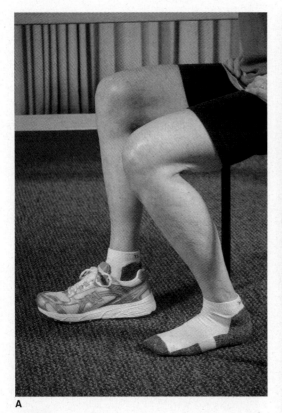
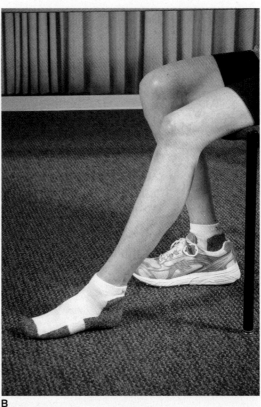

A   **B**

FIGURE 7-14. (A) Passive ankle dorsiflexion by moving chair forward. (B) Passive ankle plantarflexion by moving chair backward.

such as shoulder and arm elevation and hip flexion with knee extension during gait. The pool is particularly useful for individuals who lack the ability to perform self-ROM exercises on land. A few of the possible reasons for this include multiple joint involvement, generalized weakness, paraparesis or poor coordination.

Useful upper extremity movement patterns include cardinal plane flexion, extension, rotation, scaption, and abduction in a standing position. Combination patterns include functional diagonals, reaching and grasping, and pushing and pulling. Many of these combination patterns utilize all the joints throughout the upper quarter. Reaching behind the back also facilitates combination movements. These movements are generally supported or assisted by buoyancy.

Trunk movements are also easily performed in the water. Trunk rotation occurs passively by alternately flexing and extending the shoulder or actively by simply rotating the trunk. Sidebending and flexion and extension can be performed by actively moving the trunk on fixed lower extremities, or by moving the lower extremities on a fixed trunk, such as when performing a knee lift (Fig. 7-15). Normal walking or exaggerated walking facilitates trunk rotation as a component of normal gait.

Lower extremity movements are readily performed in isolation or in combination. Active hip flexion either with a straight leg or a bent knee is assisted by buoyancy. Similarly, active hip abduction is assisted by buoyancy. Marching in place or across the pool is a functional ROM activity facilitating hip flexion motion. Sidestepping facilitates hip abduction ROM. Lunging, lunge walking and squatting require multijoint movement in a functional pattern. Lifting the leg into

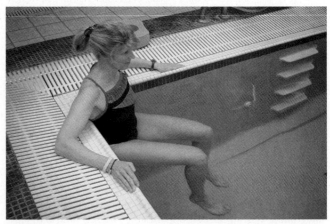

FIGURE 7-15. Knee lift, moving the lower extremities on a fixed trunk in the pool.

hip flexion, abduction and external rotation (i.e., Figure 4 lifts) facilitates the functional movement of crossing one ankle over the knee to don socks and shoes. Nearly any joint motion of the lower extremity can be performed actively or with assistance in the pool. See chapter 16 for more aquatic physical therapy suggestions.

STRETCHING

Stretching is one of the most common therapeutic exercise interventions applied by physical therapists. Although it is commonly prescribed and frequently utilized by rehabilitation experts, fitness experts, and the general public, proper applications and techniques are still not well-understood. New information about the indications, effects, and optimal dosage of therapeutic stretching is published regularly.[54,55] The therapist must stay abreast of new information regarding stretching intervention as it becomes available.

Indications

Stretching techniques are used to increase the extensibility of the muscle tendon unit and the periarticular connective tissue. Stretching is used to increase flexibility, which depends on joint ROM and soft tissue extensibility. Stretching techniques fall into four broad categories: static stretching, ballistic stretching, dynamic stretching, and proprioceptive neuromuscular facilitation (PNF) stretching. Specific stretching exercises and methods within these broad categories can increase muscle and connective tissue extensibility and joint ROM.[50,56–67] The clinician must determine which stretching methods and what sequence can best resolve the impairments and functional limitations of each patient.

Stretching can be used to increase the length and to decrease the resistance to elongation (decrease stiffness) in a muscle-tendon unit or other connective tissue. There are some cases where stiffness and resistance to elongation might be preferred. For example, patients with paralysis or paresis due to spinal cord injury might rely on stiffness to provide stability in various postures or tasks. Similarly, patients with joint instability need some tissue stiffness around the joint to provide stability. Functionally, athletes involved in jumping sports need a combination of flexibility and stiffness to maximize performance.[55] However, in many cases, patients need increased extensibility of soft tissues due to existing hypomobility. Tissues with poor flexibility can produce pain locally in the inflexible tissue, in adjacent joints due to faulty biomechanics or in opposing soft tissues as they become overworked attempting to overcome the resistance of the tight tissue.

Other tissues besides the musculotendinous unit may require stretching. Loose aerolar tissue, joint capsule, and supportive connective tissues may all benefit from stretching. Stretching can be combined with ROM exercises to maximize the impact of mobility activities. For example, a patient might perform ankle dorsiflexor and plantarflexor AROM followed by stretching of the Achilles tendon. Similarly, a patient might perform shoulder flexion PROM with a pulley followed by a prolonged stretch at end ROM.

Principles and Considerations in Stretching

Posture is a key aspect of any stretching activity performed. The starting and ending positions and the proper posture of associated joints are based on physiologic and kinesiologic factors. Physiologic factors such as the stage of healing affect the starting and ending positions for ROM and the position for stretching. For example, if a patient has just sustained an acute musculotendinous injury, ROM avoids the extreme position of the muscle range that would place too much stretch on the injured tissue.

Kinesiologic factors include the normal osteokinematics and arthrokinematics at the joint. For example, proper performance of shoulder flexion requires normal arthrokinematic motion at the glenohumeral, sternoclavicular, and acromioclavicular

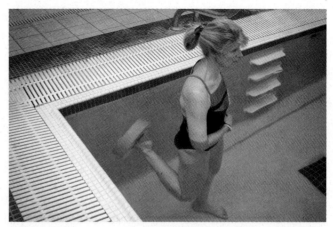

FIGURE 7-16. Knee flexion stretching performed in the pool using buoyant equipment.

joints and requires normal osteokinematic motion and associated arthrokinematic motion at the scapulothoracic articulation and thoracic spine. If motion is limited at any of these locations, substitution and faulty movement patterns occur. If an individual lacks glenohumeral arthrokinematic motion that limits glenohumeral flexion, scapulothoracic elevation or lumbar spine extension may substitute. Attempts to stretch the shoulder into further flexion can impinge subacromial soft tissues, cause substitution by adjacent joints, or both. The patient can learn an effective substitution pattern that prohibits normalization of movement patterns and the eventual progression to normal arthrokinematic and osteokinematic motion. Be sure to use joint mobilization techniques in this situation.

Another important kinesiologic factor is the stabilization of one attachment site of the muscle (usually proximal) or limb during stretching. For example, appropriately stretching the hamstring muscles requires proximal stabilization through proper lumbar and pelvic positions. Failure to stabilize proximally results in lumbar spine flexion, posterior pelvic tilt, and movement of the hamstring origin closer to the insertion, thereby minimizing the stretch. Maintaining correct posture that appropriately stabilizes is essential for effective stretching.

General procedures for stretching include a thorough examination to ensure stretching of the appropriate tissues. Before beginning the stretching perform a general warm-up to increase local blood flow and warm the tissue to be stretched. Active exercise for warm-up is preferable to local heat application, but hot packs can be used before stretching to warm local tissues. Use any relaxation techniques necessary to enhance the stretching procedure. As with ROM techniques, use a grip technique that is comfortable for the patient or use family members or equipment such as pulleys, towels, or bands, or the pool for stretching. Stretching can be performed using equipment or steps, walls, or bars in the pool (Fig. 7-16). The buoyant atmosphere and water's warmth often make stretching more comfortable (see Chapter 16). As always, listen to the patient and modify techniques as necessary to ensure optimal outcomes. Ensure that the patient is feeling a stretching sensation and not pain or any other sensation.

Neurophysiology of Stretching

In addition to the mechanical factors affecting stretching the neurophysiology of the gamma system must be considered in exercise prescription. The muscle spindle and Golgi tendon organ (GTO) play important roles in the modulation of stretching. The muscle spindle is a specialized sensory organ comprising intrafusal (nuclear bag and nuclear chain fibers) muscle fibers that lie in parallel with the extrafusal muscle fibers. Because they lie in parallel, stretching the extrafusal muscle fiber stretches and activates the intrafusal muscle fiber. The muscle spindle is sensitive to both changes in length and the velocity of these changes in the extrafusal muscle fiber. Type Ia and II afferent nerve fibers arise from the intrafusal fibers. The primary afferent nerve fiber from the nuclear bag intrafusal muscle fiber is principally sensitive to the rate of change of stretch.[68] If a muscle is stretched quickly, the type Ia fiber will facilitate contraction of the muscle being stretched. The type Ia receptor from the nuclear chain intrafusal muscle fiber responds to a maintained stretch and produces a maintained contraction. It is primarily affected by changes in muscle length, rather than velocity. Stimulation of type Ia fibers facilitates activation of the muscle being stretched. As with the type Ia fibers arising from the nuclear chain fibers, type II endings also arise primarily from the nuclear chain fibers and respond to maintained stretch with a maintained contraction.

The GTO (type Ib fiber) attaches to the muscle tendon in series with the extrafusal muscle fibers and is sensitive to tension in the muscle caused either by stretching or by active muscle contraction.[68] Its function is protective, to prevent overstretching or excessive contraction of the muscle. When stimulated, the GTO inhibits its own muscle and facilitates its antagonist. This decreases the tension in the muscle being stretched. Thus the GTO can override the stimulus from the muscle spindle, facilitating relaxation of the muscle being stretched rather than contraction. The GTO is primarily responsible for the autogenic inhibition mechanism.

Static Stretching

DeVries[57–59] is credited with the initial research on the use and efficacy of static stretching and ballistic stretching. Static stretching is a method of stretching in which the muscles and connective tissue being stretched are held in a stationary position at their greatest possible length for some period. Static stretching offers advantages of using less overall force, decreasing the danger of exceeding the tissue extensibility limits, lower energy requirements, and a lower likelihood of muscle soreness.[58] Static stretching also has less effect on the type Ia and II spindle afferent fibers than ballistic stretching, which would tend to increase a muscle's resistance to stretch and facilitate the GTO, thereby decreasing the contractile elements' resistance to deformation.

When performing static stretching, position the patient to allow complete relaxation of the muscle to be stretched. This position requires a comfortable, supportive surface, or other external stabilization. Take the limb to the point at which a gentle stretching sensation is felt, and hold the stretch for 15 to 60 seconds. Relax the stretch and then repeat. Proper limb alignment ensures that the proper tissues are being stretched without causing injury to adjacent structures (see Self-Management 7-5: Hip Stretching).

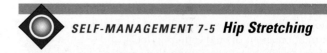

SELF-MANAGEMENT 7-5 *Hip Stretching*

Purpose: To increase the flexibility of the lateral hip and thigh muscles

Position: Standing with the involved leg out on the surface (e.g., table, step) in front of you

Movement Technique: Keeping your hips square (do not rotate your hips), bring your leg across in front of you a few inches; next, roll your entire leg in the same direction (across your body). Hold 30 to 60 seconds.

Dosage
Repetitions: _____
Frequency: _____

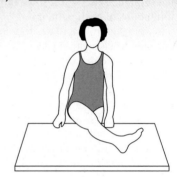

Ballistic Stretching

Ballistic stretching uses quick movements that impose a rapid change in the length of muscle or connective tissue. Initiated by active contraction of the muscles antagonistic to the muscles and connective tissue being stretched, these movements appear to be jerky in nature. Greater peak tension and greater energy absorption has been found with faster stretch rates, which is often the case with ballistic stretching.[69] Although ballistic stretching has been effective for increasing flexibility in athletes, there may be a greater chance of muscle soreness and injury.[58] Injury may result from excessive uncontrolled forces during ballistic stretching and proposed neurologic inhibitory influences (activation of type Ia afferent fibers) associated with rapid-type stretching.[61,70–75] For these reasons, ballistic stretching should be used only with selected patients, such as individuals preparing for plyometric activities. Research comparing ballistic stretching with static stretching has shown the two stretching techniques to produce different effects in the tissues.[76] Static stretching has been shown to decrease the passive resistive torque of the plantar flexors but have no effect on the Achilles tendon stiffness.[76,77] In contrast, the ballistic stretching had no significant effect on the plantarflexor passive resistive torque, but decreased the Achilles tendon stiffness.[76]

The patient performing ballistic stretching should be well stabilized and comfortable. Move the limb until a gentle stretch is felt, and then gently "bounce" at the end range. Take care to avoid ballistic stretching that is too vigorous, because it can produce muscle injury and pain.

Proprioceptive Neuromuscular Facilitation Stretching

PNF stretching techniques are widely used by the physical therapy community. These techniques seek to capitalize on the use of the neurophysiologic concept of stretch activation. PNF stretching techniques use a contract-relax (CR) sequence, an agonist contraction (AC), or a contract-relax–agonist contraction (CRAC) sequence.[78] It has been suggested that PNF stretching techniques increase muscle ROM by using reciprocal and autogenic inhibition to induce relaxation.[79–81] Others add that increases in mobility following PNF techniques may arise from an increased tolerance to stretch, or by changes to the viscoelastic properties of the stretched muscle.[79,82] This type of stretching has been shown to increase ROM, maximal isometric strength, rate of force development, and musculotendinous stiffness.[80,83] The ability to increase ROM while concurrently increasing stiffness would be a great benefit to athletes, particularly those in jumping sports.

CR stretching begins as does static stretching: support the patient and bring the limb to the end ROM until gentle stretching is felt. At that point, ask for and resist an isometric contraction of the muscle being stretched for approximately 2 to 5 seconds and then ask the patient to relax the muscle. Then increase the stretch and repeat the procedure two to four times.

AC stretching uses the principle of reciprocal inhibition. Take the limb to the position of gentle stretch and ask for a contraction of the muscle opposite the muscle being stretched. This facilitates the stretch and inhibits the muscle undergoing stretch. For example, when stretching the hamstring muscles, a simultaneous contraction of the quadriceps muscles can facilitate the stretch. Hold the muscle contraction for 2 to 5 seconds and repeat the technique two to four times.

CRAC is a technique that combines the CR and AC stretches. Take the limb to the point of gentle stretch, and perform a CR sequence (i.e., resistance applied against the muscle being stretched). After contracting the muscle being stretched, ask the patient to relax this muscle while contracting the opposing muscle group, thus facilitating the stretch. For example, when stretching the hamstring muscles, they are brought to a position of stretch. The hamstring muscles are contracted against resistance and then relaxed, and the quadriceps are contracted.

PNF stretching is indicated when muscle contraction in addition to stretching is appropriate. This type of stretching helps to improve strength and may help the patient better understand the continuum of contraction and relaxation. Some patients may find it easier to relax when contrasted with a muscle contraction. Each of these stretching techniques requires constant communication with the patient to ensure that neither overstretching nor excessive resistance produce muscle injury. These techniques can be performed independently with a family member or alone using a towel or other simple objects to provide resistance or assistance.

Dynamic Stretching

Dynamic stretching is a type of flexibility exercise where the limb is repeatedly taken through a ROM actively by the participant. The individual performs movements where the primary mover takes the limb through a ROM while the antagonist muscle relaxes and elongates.[84] For example, a reciprocal, dynamic knee extension with the hip at 90-degree flexion would be a dynamic flexibility stretch for the hamstring muscles (Fig. 7-17). The terms "dynamic stretching" and "dynamic warm-up" are often used interchangeably, as

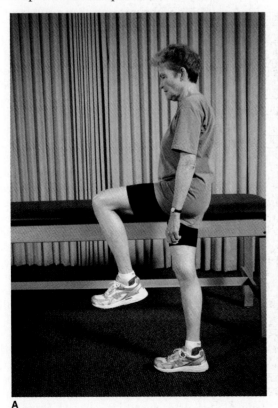 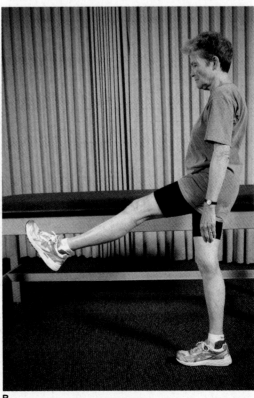

A   **B**

FIGURE 7-17. (A,B) Dynamic knee extension as a warm-up activity for the hamstring muscles.

BUILDING BLOCK 7-4

Denise is a 37-year-old mother of two who injured her right leg and hip in a motor vehicle accident (MVA) where she placed her foot against the floor of the car and sustained an impact injury up to her hip. She now has residual hip pain and limited mobility. She needs to increase hip external rotation ROM and hip strength. She is unable to tolerate a static stretch into hip external rotation. Please suggest alternatives.

the term "stretching" typically implies taking a structure to its end range and holding it for some period. Typically dynamic stretching takes the structure to the limits of the range but does not hold this position. Other examples of dynamic stretching include lunge walking forward and back, lunges or squats up to a toe raise, hamstring curls, hip extensions, and trunk activities. For those who cannot tolerate holding a static stretch, or who will be participating in activities requiring power or explosive speed, dynamic stretching is a good alternative to a traditional static stretching program. See Building Block 7-4.

Measures of performance are better following dynamic stretching compared with static stretching.[85–87] A 4-week dynamic stretching warm-up resulted in increases in quadriceps peak torque, broad jump, underhand medicine ball throw, sit-ups, and push-ups compared with static stretching.[85] Similarly, performance in the T-shuttle run, underhand medicine ball throw and the 5-step jump were improved immediately following a dynamic warm-up compared with a static warm-up.[86] Performance high-speed motor skills such as the 10-m sprint were also improved following dynamic warm-up compared with static stretching.[87]

Effects of Stretching

Stretching is one of the most accepted interventions in rehabilitation. Stretching has been studied to determine the effects of different stretching techniques and dosage.[88,89] The effects of stretching are divided into acute effects and chronic effects. Acute effects are the immediate, short-term results of stretching and are the result of elongating the elastic component of the musculotendinous unit (see Figs. 11-2 through 11-4). The effects of routine stretching exercises are acute in nature. Most research has been done on the acute effects of stretching.[81] It is clear that acute stretching can increase the ROM and mobility of the connective tissue. Research has consistently found increases in flexibility immediately following stretching.[88,90]

Less is known about the effects of long term stretching. Chronic effects are the long-term results of prolonged stretching and are the result of adding sarcomeres (usually because of immobilization in a lengthened position). Research has shown 30 minutes of daily stretching to increase the number of sarcomeres in series.[91] A study of immobilized soleus muscles found a 5% increase in length and a 4% increase in sarcomeres in series following a stretching dosage of 40 minutes per day, 3 days per week for 3 weeks.[92] Regular stretching appears to increase flexibility, although the research is not consistent.[54,88,93–96] Differences in results may be due to the subjects under study, or research design issues.

Stretching is used to lengthen shortened tissue and to decrease muscle stiffness. Contractile and noncontractile elements of muscle contribute to its resting tension and resistance to elongation.[75] Potential sources of stiffness are adhesions, epimysium, perimysium, endomysium, sarcolemma, contractile elements within the muscle fiber, and associated tendons and their insertions.[75] The relative contribution of the contractile elements to resistance to stretch appears to be velocity-related, with increased resistance to stretch occurring at higher velocities.[97] The farther the muscle is stretched, the greater is the relative contribution of noncontractile elements.[75]

The mechanism for short-term gains in flexibility after stretching techniques is unclear. Also, tissue compliance at rest is not necessarily related to tissue compliance during activity. It has been suggested that flexibility increases are not due to increased length or flexibility of the muscle, but rather due to an increased tolerance to the stretch.[98] Magnusson et al.[99] found that static and cyclic stretches both produce decreases in resistance to stretch, and that the increases in ROM were due to increased tolerance to the stretch, not to changes in the viscoelastic properties of the muscle. When comparing flexible versus inflexible individuals, the authors found that flexible subjects attained a greater angle of stretch with greater tensile stress and energy than inflexible individuals, apparently because of greater tolerance to the stretching sensation.[100] Additionally, strengthening exercises increased muscle stiffness that was unaltered by daily stretching.[101]

There is no agreement about which stretching technique is best.[50,56,60–64,66,67] According to some researchers, PNF techniques may be better than static or ballistic techniques for producing acute, short-term improvements in ROM.[102] These short-term improvements may result from contraction of antagonistic muscles while performing CRAC stretching, which is based on the principle of reciprocal inhibition.[70–74] Moreover, PNF techniques have been suggested to increase muscle performance as well, likely due to the isometric contraction component of the stretch.[96] Muscle stiffness has been decreased by performing a conditioning isometric or eccentric muscle action.[103] This muscle contraction causes a change in viscosity and resistance to molecular deformation, decreasing stiffness and resistance to stretch. Prestretch conditioning through active or passive movements (i.e., passive oscillations or active repetitive eccentric actions) may loosen actin-myosin bonds and increase stretching effectiveness.[78] However, in the absence of continued activity, the short-terms gains in flexibility may be lost. DePino et al.[104] found that improvements following four consecutive 30-second hamstring stretches were lost within 6 minutes of completing the last stretch.

Regardless of the type of stretching method used, flexibility gains made may be retained even after the individual has stopped stretching for some time. Zebas and Rivera[67] demonstrated retention of gains from 2 to 4 weeks after the cessation of a 6-week stretching program. Feland et al.[105] found retention of gains 4 weeks after cessation of a five times per week, 60-second hamstring stretching program in elderly individuals. Participating in a flexibility exercise program three to five times per week can produce gains. For individuals with significant flexibility deficits, stretching should be part of their daily routine. After the goal is achieved, stretching once each week may be sufficient to maintain gains.

Stretching has also been shown to improve muscle performance.[96] Research has shown stretching to increase hamstring torque production, bench press performance, trunk strength, power performance, and knee flexor and extensor strength and power.[96,106–108] The mechanism of improved muscle performance with stretching is unclear. However research has shown stretching to induce myoblast proliferation, increased muscle mass, and increased muscle fiber area.[92, 109] In some studies utilizing PNF stretching, the muscle contraction component may be responsible for increases in strength. Muscle activation in the contralateral leg working to stabilize the body while stretching has been suggested as another possible mechanism.[96] Regardless, a regular stretching program can improve muscle performance. There are limitations to the research and it is not being suggested that stretching can substitute for a well-designed resistive exercise program. However, in situations where resistive exercise is contraindicated or the patient is unable to perform these activities, a stretching program has been shown to provide strength benefits.

Stretching and Muscle Performance

The impact of stretching on muscle and functional performance has been the subject of ongoing research. The conventional wisdom that it is always necessary to stretch prior to an activity has been refuted. Again, the differences between the effects of a chronic stretching program and the acute effects immediately following a stretching session must be distinguished. Moreover, the therapist must consider the population under study prior to drawing any definitive conclusions about the relative merits of any particular stretching regimen. In many cases, this research is done on healthy athletes who have no impairments. Thus the applicability of this research to those patients with impairments of activity limitations due to hypomobility is limited.

It appears that chronic stretching can improve flexibility, muscle performance, and functional performance.[89,94,96,110–112] Research has shown that an 8-week program of regular stretching can increase active and passive flexibility and maximum torque and work.[81] A study of an intense stretching program (40 minutes per day; 3 days per week × 10 weeks) resulted in significant improvements in flexibility, standing long jump, vertical jump, 20-m sprint, knee flexion 1RM, knee extension 1RM, knee flexion endurance, and knee extension endurance.[96] However, other research has found no improvement in ROM, sprint time or vertical jump following a 6-week stretching program.[94] These differing results highlight the important issues in determining the efficacy of chronic stretching. Significant effects on performance were found when the subjects were inactive or only recreationally active and the stretching was intense (15 stretches per session).[96] No improvement in performance was found when the subjects were collegiate track athletes who performed only four stretches.[94] Therefore it is essential that the limitations of the evidence and the appropriateness of application in any patient situation be thoroughly considered prior to implementing a program.

In contrast to chronic stretching, acute static stretching of some lower extremity muscle groups has been shown to decrease muscle performance immediately after stretching.[84,113] Stretching, particularly slow static stretching has been shown to reduce maximum strength, rate of force development, power, and explosive performance.[114] This appears to be true regardless of the type of stretch (static or CR).[115] A bout of three 45-second stretches with 15-second rest periods to the hamstrings, quadriceps, and plantar flexors resulted in a decrease in balance scores, and in reaction and movement time.[116] Stretches held for as little as 15 seconds still produced declines in muscle performance immediately following stretching.[117] Muscle groups involved in performing a countermovement vertical jump such as the hamstrings, gluteals, trunk extensors, quadriceps, and hip flexors have been found to have decreased muscle performance immediately following static stretching.[113] Research has found that a general warm-up plus static stretching resulted in significantly lower gains in vertical jump height compared with a warm-up alone or a warm-up plus dynamic stretching.[84] The static stretching appeared to negate the positive effects of the warm-up. The magnitude of inhibitory effects following an acute bout of stretching seems to be affected by stretching duration. A study of isokinetic strength following a 30- or 60-second bout of quadriceps stretching found that peak torque decrements were greater with the 60-second stretch compared with the 30-second stretch.[113] In general, if the individual is participating in a sport that requires explosive power, a dynamic warm-up is preferable to static stretching to sufficiently warm the tissue without compromising explosive power.

Stretching and Joint Contractures

Joint contractures can occur following prolonged immobilization or surgery.[118] A joint contracture is an adaptive shortening of the connective tissue crossing and/or surrounding a joint that limits the ROM about that joint. The shortened tissues may be primarily the muscle-tendon unit or joint capsule.[118] However, following loss of joint ROM due to the primary soft tissue, other tissues secondarily shorten, lengthen, or are otherwise negatively affected. Depending upon the patient's history and the time interval between injury and physical therapy evaluation, it may be difficult to determine which tissue(s) are primarily at fault and which have secondarily adapted.

For those with joint contractures following prolonged immobilization, simple return to activity is insufficient in restoring joint ROM.[118] Stretching to the soft tissues and joint mobilization to the joint capsule are often employed to restore ROM.[119] Basic science research has shown that the tensile force produced by stretching, particularly long duration stretching, results in fibroblast proliferation.[120,121] Low-torque, long-duration stretching produced better outcomes than short-duration, high-torque activities.[122] This type of stretching can be applied manually but can prove tiring when applied by a therapist or family member. Other tools or devices can be utilized to provide this stretch. For some, just the weight of the limb is sufficient to provide this stretch. For example, a prone hang with or without an ankle weight will provide a prolonged stretch for someone with a knee flexion contracture (Fig. 7-18). A similar stretch can be performed in long sitting with distal traction provided by a weight stack or resistive band. This can be combined with weights on the top of the knee to provide additional force into extension (Fig. 7-19).

External devices are also useful for providing prolonged stretch.[123] A drop-out cast can be used to increase knee

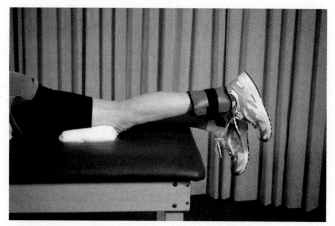

FIGURE 7-18. Prone hand to increase knee extension ROM.

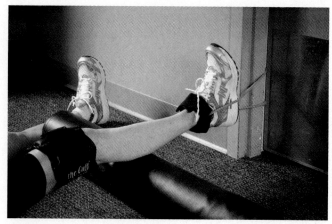

FIGURE 7-19. Prolonged passive knee extension with distal traction.

extension ROM. A study of four patients with knee flexion contractures found that this intervention can increase knee extension ROM without compromising knee flexion ROM.[124] Serial casting is another type of casting used to provide a low load long duration stretch. The limb is casted in a position that provides a slight stretch to the tissue. Once the tissue has accommodated to the new length, the cast is removed and a new cast applied, again, moving the limb into further stretch. Serial casting has the disadvantages associated with continuous immobilization. Significant atrophy and joint deterioration can occur from decreased loads on the tissues during immobilization. Because the immobilization is continuous, there is no opportunity for using the new range as it is acquired. Additionally, there is no opportunity to view the limb during immobilization. Atrophy, skin breakdown, or other complications can arise without the patient or clinician's ability to visualize the problem. Any suspected problem requires cast removal. Casting is also contraindicated in many patients due to such potential problems. Patients with diabetes, skin breakdown, hyperhidrosis, vascular disease, or sensory loss are not candidates for serial casting.

Commercial dynamic splinting systems such as Dynasplint (Severna Park, MD) are available to provide low load long duration stretching (Fig. 7-20A and B). These systems can be rented or purchased for home use by the patient. A variety of commercial systems exist (i.e., Dynasplint, Ultraflex, LMB Pro-glide, EMPI Advance, and SaeboFlex) and each has its own design and specifications. Most provide a three or four point tension to distribute loads across a larger surface area, decreasing the high stress region. Most importantly, these systems are designed to be used for only 6 to 8 hours per day. This allows visualization of the limb both during and following the stretching session. It also allows use of the limb between stretching sessions, negating many of the problems associated with prolonged immobilization.

These commercial systems are available for many different joints including the shoulder, elbow, forearm, wrist and hand, jaw, as well as the knee, ankle, and foot.[125] The splints are applied by a therapist and the patient or family member can learn how to don and doff the splint. The initial tension is set by the therapist and the patient is instructed in appropriate progression. Some splints, like the Dynasplint

have a preset load that remains constant during the stretching session. The tension should be at a low level that can be maintained for six to eight hours without pain. Other splints, like the Joint Active System allow the patient to set the tension at the beginning of the stretching session. The stretch is increased every few minutes up to s 30-minute session. The sessions are repeated throughout the day. The commercial systems are typically available for either rental or purchase. These systems are an adjunctive treatment to therapeutic exercise.

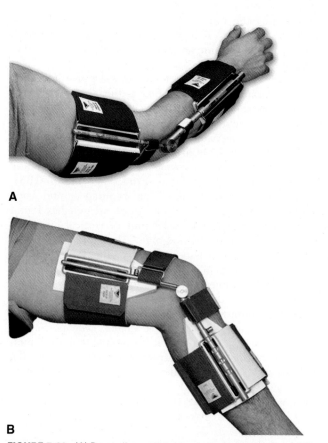

FIGURE 7-20. (A) Dynasplint used to increase upper extremity mobility. (B) Dynasplint used to increase lower extremity mobility.

JOINT MOBILIZATION TO INCREASE MOBILITY

Manual therapy techniques such as joint mobilization are used to improve the mobility of joints. The *Guide to Physical Therapist Practice*[126] defines mobilization/manipulation as a "continuum of skilled passive movements to the joints and/or related soft tissues that are applied at varying speeds and amplitudes, including small-amplitude/high velocity therapeutic movement." Manipulation is a type of mobilization that is generally performed at a high velocity through a small amplitude. Various models of manual therapy exist, each with its own definitions and classification of mobilization/manipulation. For example, Maitland[127] describes five levels of mobilization, whereas Kaltenborn[128] specifies only three (Fig. 7-21). Regardless of the classification system, these schools of thought all focus on increasing joint mobility by increasing the joint play, or motion between the joint surfaces. Use of mobilization/manipulation techniques requires an understanding of the normal joint architecture, arthrokinematics, and the specific pathology to determine which interventions are appropriate.

Researchers have examined the ability of joint mobilization techniques to increase joint ROM.[129,130] Hsu et al.[129] examined the effects of anterior and posterior translational mobilization performed in the resting position and at end abduction on shoulder rotation and abduction ROM in cadaver specimens. Both anterior and posterior glides at end range increased abduction ROM, whereas these same glides performed in the resting position were less effective. Small increases in lateral rotation were found after anterior glides in the resting position and in medial rotation after posterior glides at end range.

Roubal et al.[130] found that inferior and posterior mobilizations after a brachial plexus block in patients with adhesive capsulitis increased motion in flexion, abduction, internal rotation, and external rotation. Range increased in all four directions despite no anterior mobilization treatment, suggesting that mobility was limited more by capsular tension than joint geometry. In a series of case studies, Vermeulen et al.[131] found increased ROM in all directions, increased joint capsule volume, and increased function in a group of patients with adhesive capsulitis treated with end-range joint mobilization.

Biomechanics of Joint Mobilization

Movement occurs at a joint when one joint surface moves on another relatively fixed joint surface. Roll, spin, and glide (or slide) are the major categories of arthrokinematic motion found in human joints. Roll occurs when new points on one joint surface meet new points on the opposing joint surface. Spin is a pure rotational movement in which rotation occurs about a fixed axis. Motion of the radial head during pronation and supination is an example of spinning. Gliding or sliding occurs when one point on a moving surface continually comes in contact with new points on the opposing surface. Sliding is the predominant motion used in joint mobilization techniques. In most arthrokinematic motion, a combination of these movements occurs. In addition to roll, spine, and glide, compression and distraction of the joint can occur. Compression techniques are often used to facilitate muscular cocontraction and joint stabilization, whereas distraction is used in conjunction with joint mobilization to increase joint mobility or decrease pain.

Some joint play must exist for arthrokinematic motion to proceed normally as the limb moves through the ROM (osteokinematic motion). The type and direction of arthrokinematic motion is determined in part by the relative shape of the joint surfaces. Most joint surfaces are classified as either ovoid or sellar. In an ovoid joint, one joint surface is concave, whereas the other is convex. For example, at the glenohumeral joint, the glenoid fossa is concave, whereas the humeral head is convex. In a sellar joint, both surfaces are both concave and convex. The carpometacarpal joint of the thumb is an example of such a joint. The convex-concave rule dictates the direction of gliding of one joint surface on the other and forms the basis for joint mobilization techniques. When a convex surface is moving on a fixed concave surface (such as the humeral head moving on the stationary glenoid) the movement of the convex bone is in the direction opposite the convex articulating surface. In this case, the convex humeral head glides inferiorly as the humeral shaft moves superiorly. The opposite is true when a concave

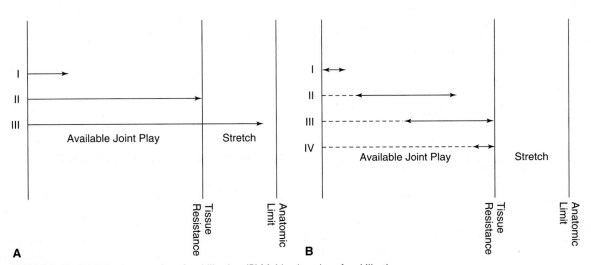

FIGURE 7-21. (A) Kaltenborn grades of mobilization. (B) Maitland grades of mobilization.

surface moves on a stationary convex surface. For example, movement of the concave tibial joint surface on the stationary concave femoral condyles is in the same direction as the tibial movement. Thus the tibial joint surface will move posteriorly as the tibia moves into flexion.

However, the human body does not always follow our rules, and the convex-concave rule is one of these. Following this rule at the shoulder would suggest that an anterior glide is used to increase mobility in external rotation, horizontal abduction, and extension, whereas a posterior glide is used to increase motion into internal rotation, horizontal adduction, and flexion. A study by Howell et al.[132] found that when the arm was placed in a maximally cocked position (abduction, extension, and lateral rotation) the humeral head was actually resting approximately 4-mm posteriorly. Additionally, Harryman et al.[133] found anterior humeral head translation with glenohumeral flexion and horizontal adduction and posterior translation with extension and lateral rotation. These apparent violations of the convex-concave rule may be the result of joint capsule tightening during rotation that is unique to the glenohumeral joint. Thus applying a single rule to all joints may mislead the clinician.

The primary indication for joint mobilization is a limitation in AROM and PROM at a joint. This is especially true in the case of a capsular end feel and loss of ROM in a capsular pattern. Remember that a number of structures can limit ROM at a joint; joint mobilization is most effective when the tissue limiting ROM is the joint capsule. This is generally assessed via joint play or joint accessory motion testing.

Small amplitude joint mobilization may be used for the reduction of pain. These oscillations stimulate joint receptors and decrease the perception of pain by the central nervous system. Joint traction or distraction is used to relieve the compression of painful joint surfaces and is used along with most mobilization techniques to separate joint surfaces during the mobilization procedure.

Joint mobilization is contraindicated in the case of joint infection, neoplasm, acute inflammation, or recent fracture. Caution must be used in cases of connective tissue disease, osteoporosis, hypermobility, or edema.

Mobilization Grades

Manual therapists use different mobilization grades depending upon their background and training. The two most commonly used grading systems are those developed by Kaltenborn and by Maitland.[127,128] They are distinguished by the number of grades and the criteria for each grade. Kaltenborn[128] defines three grades of mobilization by the amount of force applied, whereas Maitland[127] describes his grades by the amplitude and position in the range. Kaltenborn techniques are a sustained translation, whereas Maitland's are an oscillation. Kaltenborn[128] grades are

Grade I: a low level distraction force
Grade II: a greater force that takes up the available joint play
Grade III: a force that stretches the joint tissue after the available joint play has been taken up.

Maitland[127] grades are as follows:

Grade 1: small amplitude rhythmic movements near the beginning of the ROM

Grade 2: large amplitude rhythmic oscillations performed within the available range, but not reaching the limit
Grade 3: large amplitude rhythmic oscillations performed to the limit of the range and into the tissue resistance
Grade 4: small amplitude rhythmic movements performed at the limit of the range and into the tissue resistance
Grade 5: small amplitude, high-velocity thrust techniques performed at the end of the ROM for the purpose of breaking adhesions

Maitland[127] emphasizes not only the amplitude of the oscillations, but the rhythm and amount of pressure as well. He suggests that grade I oscillations for pain must be extremely gentle using a very light touch. The rhythm of oscillations can be varied from quick staccato movements into a stiff range, to smooth, rhythmic oscillations into and out of the painful or stiff region. When using grade II oscillations, the greater the pain, the slower and smoother should be the oscillations. Sustained stretch positions can be used as well, and the techniques should vary within the treatment session.

General Procedures

Be sure your patient is relaxed and positioned comfortably on the treatment table. Muscle guarding resulting from discomfort or apprehension will interfere with the treatment and place undue stress on both the patient and therapist. Position yourself to optimize body mechanics, making use of body weight and leverage to minimize your energy expenditure. Use external devices such as the table, positioning, belts, and wedges to stabilize and minimize therapist efforts. Be sure your grip is firm, using as large and wide a portion of your hand as possible. This will minimize painful pinching or a painful localized force application. Grasp as close to the joint line as possible with both the mobilizing and the stabilizing hand. Provide gentle traction to the joint while performing mobilizations. Understand the joint anatomy and arthrokinematics to minimize chances of painful joint compression forces. Oscillations are performed at a rate of 2 to 3 per second for approximately 1 minute. Reevaluate the joint and repeat, or choose another grade or direction as necessary.

Kaltenborn[128] suggests beginning the mobilization in the resting position if the purpose of the treatment is pain relief. The resting position varies from one individual to another. Find the position allowing the greatest ease of movement by trying gentle traction in a variety of positions. This position is the resting position. If the purpose of the mobilization is to stretch the tissue, then perform the mobilization nearer the limit of mobility. Performing the mobilization closer to the end range has proven more effective in increasing motion than performing mobilizations in mid-range.

Applications to Specific Joints

Selected mobilization techniques for the spine and extremities will be described. Realize that this is only an overview of techniques and is not comprehensive. Additionally, many modifications are available, and the specific positioning will vary with available resources and patient and therapist preferences. The descriptions can be found in Displays 7-2–7-8 and Figures 7-22–7-39.

DISPLAY 7-2
Shoulder Joint Mobilization

Glenohumeral Anterior Glide

Purpose: to increase shoulder external rotation and extension

Position: patient is prone with shoulder at edge of table and abducted to 90 degrees, elbow flexed to 90 degrees; mobilizing hand on posterior humeral head while stabilizing hand holds mid-humerus

Mobilization: anterior force applied by mobilizing hand to humeral head while stabilizing hand applies gentle traction

Glenohumeral Posterior Glide

Purpose: to increase shoulder flexion and internal rotation

Position: patient is supine with the shoulder at the edge of the table, scapula stabilized by the table or towel roll; abducted to 45 degrees and elbow slightly flexed; mobilizing hand on anterior humeral head and stabilizing hand supporting elbow

Mobilization: posterior force applied by mobilizing hand to humeral head while stabilizing hand applies gentle traction

Glenohumeral Inferior Glide

Purpose: to increase shoulder abduction and flexion

Position: patient is supine with the arm in 30- to 45-degree abduction; stabilizing hand supports scapula in axilla while mobilizing hand grasps distal humerus

Mobilization: inferior force applied by mobilizing hand while stabilizing hand holds scapula steady

Acromioclavicular Joint Anterior Glide

Purpose: to increase joint mobility

Position: patient is positioned sitting; stabilize the scapula with thumb along the scapular spine and fingers along acromion; mobilizing hand placed on posterior clavicle near joint line

Mobilization: mobilizing hand imposes an anterior force on the clavicle

Sternoclavicular Joint Superior/Inferior and Anterior/Posterior Glides

Purpose: superior glide increases depression, whereas inferior glide increases elevation; anterior glide increases protraction, whereas posterior glide increases retraction

Position: patient is supine with the stabilizing hand on the sternum and the mobilizing thumb or thumb and index finger on the proximal clavicle

Mobilization: superior glide—the index finger applies a superior force to clavicle; inferior glide—thumb applies an inferior force to clavicle; anterior glide—thumb and index finger lift the clavicle; posterior glide—thumb applies a posterior force to clavicle

Scapular Mobilization

Purpose: to increase mobility at the scapulothoracic articulation

Position: patient is in prone; superior hand is along scapular spine while inferior hand grasps inferior angle of the scapula

Mobilization: mobilize the scapula in elevation, depression, adduction, abduction, or rotation by pushing the appropriate direction

NEURAL MOBILITY

Pain perceived in various regions of the upper quarter (neck, upper back, chest, shoulder, and arm) or the lower quarter (low back, buttocks, hips and legs) can be the result of pathology in the spine and associated tissues, or from local structures. Neural tissues can be the source of pain, and vigorous stretching can exacerbate pain arising from these tissues.[134,135] A hallmark of neural tissue involvement in a pain syndrome if the response to provocation tests. Provocation tests are those examination procedures that selectively stress different neural tissues with functional positions.[134] These positions tension the neural tissues, and the area of tension or pathology can be identified by the results of these testing positions. For example, adding ankle dorsiflexion to a straight leg raise (SLR) maneuver increases the tension in the nervous system up to the cerebellum.[135] Adding hip movements to the SLR can help differentiate ankle symptoms arising from the neural structures versus local ankle structures.[136] In the upper extremity, components of shoulder abduction and

DISPLAY 7-3
Elbow Joint Mobilization

Elbow Humeroulnar Distraction

Purpose: to increase elbow joint mobility in flexion or extension

Position: patient is supine with the elbow flexed to approximately 70 degrees, wrist resting on the therapist's shoulder; both hands grasp proximal ulna

Mobilization: a distal force applied against the proximal ulna

Elbow Humeroradial Anterior or Posterior Glide

Purpose: anterior glide to increase flexion, posterior glide to increase extension

Position: supine with the elbow extended and supinated as far as possible; stabilizing hand grasping the medial distal humerus; proximal palm of stabilizing hand on anterior radial head with fingers on the posterior aspect

Mobilization: a posterior glide force provided by the palmar aspect of the hand, or an anterior force provided by the fingers

Elbow Radioulnar Anterior and Posterior Glide

Purpose: anterior glide to increase supination, posterior glide to increase pronation

Position: patient sitting or supine with the elbow in extension and supination for posterior glide or extension and pronation for anterior glide; stabilizing hand grasps proximal ulna with thenar eminence on anterior aspect and fingers on posterior aspect; mobilizing hand is in same position over the proximal radius

Mobilization: posterior force on radial head for posterior glide; anterior force on radial head for anterior glide, both while stabilizing hand holds ulna steady

DISPLAY 7-4
Wrist and Hand Mobilization

Interphalangeal or Metacarpal Palmar and Dorsal Glide

Purpose: palmar glide to increase flexion, dorsal glide to increase extension

Position: patient's palm faces down with joint in resting position; stabilizing hand holds proximal bony segment while mobilizing hand grasps distal bony segment

Mobilization: with mobilizing hand, move distal segment toward the palm to increase flexion or toward dorsum to increase extension while applying gentle traction

Thumb Metacarpal-Carpal Radial and Ulnar Glides

Purpose: ulnar glide to increase flexion; radial glide to increase extension

Position: patient's hand is positioned with the ulnar side down, joint in a resting position; stabilizing hand grasps distal forearm with grip around trapezium while mobilizing hand grasps first metacarpal

Mobilization: with mobilizing hand, glide metacarpal toward radius to increase extension, or toward ulna to increase flexion while applying gentle traction

Thumb Metacarpal-Carpal Dorsal and Palmar Glides

Purpose: palmar glide to increase adduction; dorsal glide to increase abduction

Position: patient's hand is positioned with the palm down, joint in a resting position; stabilizing hand grasps distal forearm with grip around trapezium while mobilizing hand grasps first metacarpal

Mobilization: with mobilizing hand, glide metacarpal toward palm to increase adduction, or toward dorsum to increase abduction while applying gentle traction

Wrist Palmar and Dorsal Glides

Purpose: palmar glide to increase extension, dorsal glide to increase flexion

Position: patient's forearm rests on table or wedge with the carpal joint at the edge; forearm is pronated for palmar glide and supinated for dorsal glide; stabilizing hand steadies the distal forearm against the table or wedge; mobilizing hand grasps the distal wrist

Mobilization: apply a downward force with mobilizing hand while applying gentle traction

DISPLAY 7-5
Hip Joint Mobilization

Hip Distraction/Distal Traction

Purpose: pain relief and general mobility

Position: patient is supine or prone on the table, with the pelvis stabilized with a belt; therapist grasps either the distal thigh or the distal calf, depending upon whether or not you want distraction through the knee joint; a belt can be used around your waist and hands to reinforce the grip and allow use of body weight

Mobilization: a distal traction force is applied to the leg by shifting your body weight backward

Hip Lateral Traction

Purpose: pain relief and general hypomobility

Position: patient is supine with pelvis stabilized with a belt; the hip may be in any degree of flexion to extension depending upon the direction of hypomobility; mobilizing belt is placed around your pelvis and the patient's proximal thigh

Mobilization: lean backward to apply a lateral traction force to the hip

Hip Anterior Glide

Purpose: increase extension and external rotation

Position: patient is prone with knee flexed to 90 degrees and a firm wedge or towel roll placed under the anterior pelvis; mobilizing hand just distal to posterior hip, and stabilizing hand grasps ankle to stabilize leg

Mobilization: anteriorly directed force through mobilizing hand via forward weight shift

Hip Posterior Glide

Purpose: increase flexion and internal rotation

Position: supine with hip near full flexion, knee flexed, pelvis stabilized on table or with additional wedges or support; mobilizing hands on patient's knee

Mobilization: a posteriorly directed force through the long axis of the femur

DISPLAY 7-6
Knee Joint Mobilization

Tibiofemoral Anterior Glide

Purpose: increase extension

Position: patient is prone with the knee at the edge of the table; mobilizing hand is just distal to knee joint and stabilizing hand supports anterior ankle

Mobilization: anteriorly directed force downward through mobilizing hand while stabilizing hand applies gentle distal traction

Tibiofemoral Posterior Glide

Purpose: increase flexion

Position: patient is supine or sitting with the knee at the edge of the table; mobilizing hand is just distal to the knee joint and stabilizing hand supports posterior ankle

Mobilization: a posteriorly directed force through mobilizing hand while the stabilizing hand applies gentle distal traction

Patellofemoral Joint Mobilization

Purpose: increased general patellar mobility; and superior glide for increased extension, inferior glide for increased flexion

Position: supine with knee supported by table, wedge, or towel roll; mobilizing thumb and index finger placed along patellar border oriented to direction of mobilization

Mobilization: apply a medially, laterally, superiorly, or inferiorly directed force to the patella

DISPLAY 7-7
Foot and Ankle Mobilization

Ankle Anterior Glide

Purpose: increase plantarflexion

Position: prone with foot hanging just over the edge of the table; stabilizing hand under the anterior distal tibiofibular joint; mobilizing hand on the posterior calcaneus, just distal to joint line

Mobilization: apply a downward, anteriorly directed force to the calcaneus while applying gentle traction

Ankle Posterior Glide

Purpose: increase dorsiflexion

Position: supine with foot just over the edge of the table; stabilizing hand under the posterior distal tibiofibular joint; mobilizing hand grasps anterior ankle just distal to joint line

Mobilization: apply a downward, posteriorly directed force to the ankle while applying gentle traction

Ankle Traction

Purpose: pain relief and general mobility

Position: supine with leg stabilized by a strap and foot just over the edge of the table; both hands grasp the foot, one posterior on the calcaneus and the other anteriorly over the midfoot

Mobilization: lean backward to produce a distal traction to the talocrural joint

Metatarsal and Phalanges Glide

Purpose: increase mobility of toes

Position: supine with foot over the edge of the table; stabilizing hand grasps metatarsal while mobilizing hand grasps phalanges

Mobilization: apply dorsal and ventral mobilizations while applying gentle traction

DISPLAY 7-8
Spine Mobilization

Cervical and Thoracic Spine Posterior to Anterior Glide

Purpose: increase segmental mobility and pain relief

Position: patient is prone with towel under forehead or on mobilization table; therapist's thumbs placed one on top of the other, directly over the spinous process to be treated; spread hands over the adjacent neck or back area, keeping shoulders directly above treatment area

Mobilization: apply a direct posterior to anterior force to the spinous process; this technique can also be performed with thumbs on the transverse processes unilaterally or bilaterally

Cervical and Thoracic Spine Lateral Glide

Purpose: increase general mobility and unilateral pain relief

Position: patient is prone; therapist's thumbs placed one on top of the other, directly over the lateral side (right or left) of the spinous process to be treated; spread hands over the adjacent neck or back area

Mobilization: apply gentle pressure to lateral border of spinous process

Lumbar Spine Posterior to Anterior Glide

Purpose: increase segmental mobility and pain relief

Position: patient is prone; therapist's ulnar border of the hand over the spinous process to be treated; the other hand reinforces the mobilizing hand by resting on top of it and grasping the radial border of the wrist with the fingers; keep your shoulders directly over your hands; this technique can be modified to provide unilateral pressure to the transverse process using your thumbs adjacent to one another

Mobilization: a gentle rocking motion provides an anteriorly directed force over the spinous process

Lumbar Lateral Glide

Purpose: increase segmental mobility and pain relief

Position: patient is prone with the therapist's thumbs (one on top of the other) on the lateral side of the spinous process to be mobilized

Mobilization: apply a horizontal pressure to the lateral border of the spinous process

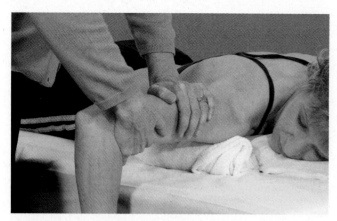

FIGURE 7-22. Glenohumeral anterior glide.

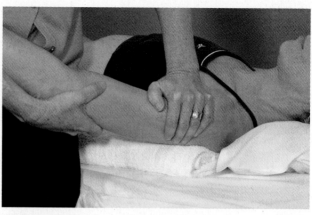

FIGURE 7-23. Glenohumeral posterior glide.

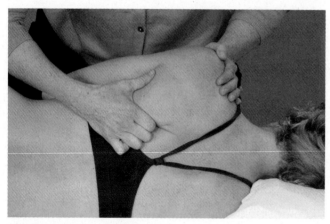

FIGURE 7-24. Scapular mobilization.

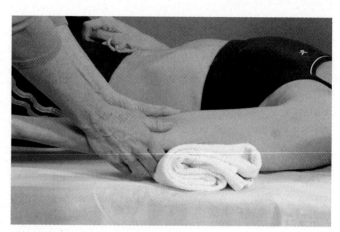

FIGURE 7-25. Humeroradial anterior glide.

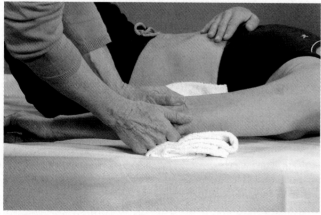

FIGURE 7-26. Radioulnar posterior glide.

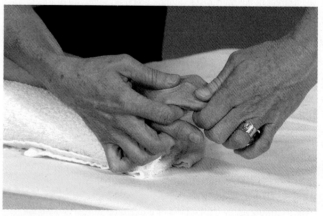

FIGURE 7-27. Interphalangeal palmar glide.

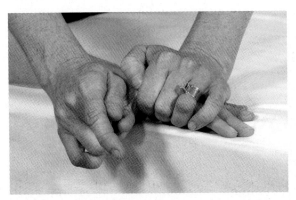

FIGURE 7-28. Thumb metacarpal-carpal dorsal glide.

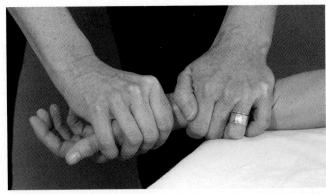

FIGURE 7-29. Wrist dorsal glide.

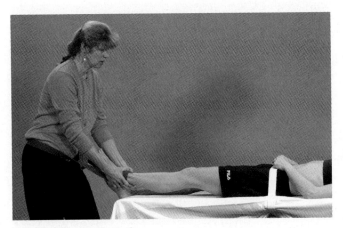

FIGURE 7-30. Hip distraction.

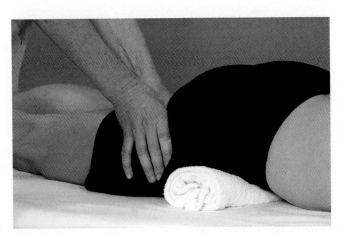

FIGURE 7-31. Hip anterior glide.

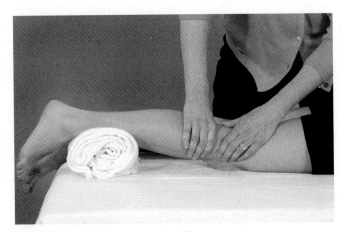

FIGURE 7-32. Tibiofemoral anterior glide.

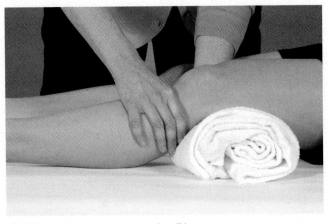

FIGURE 7-33. Tibiofemoral posterior glide.

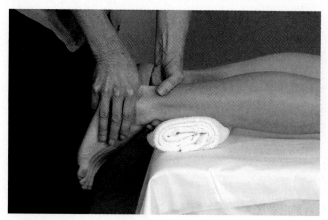

FIGURE 7-34. Ankle anterior glide.

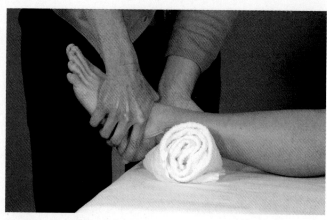

FIGURE 7-35. Ankle posterior glide.

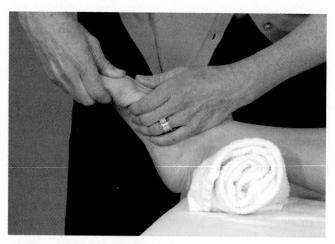

FIGURE 7-36. Metatarsal glide.

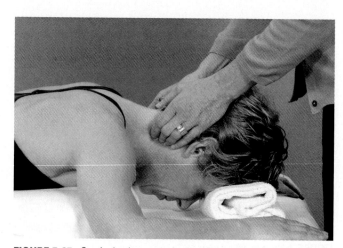

FIGURE 7-37. Cervical spine posterior to anterior glide.

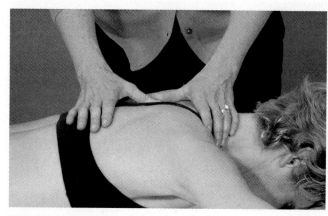

FIGURE 7-38. Thoracic spine lateral glide.

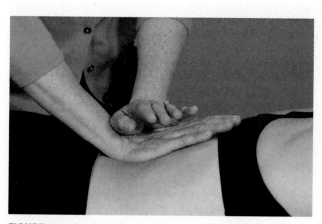

FIGURE 7-39. Lumbar spine posterior to anterior glide.

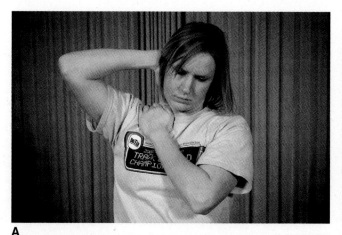
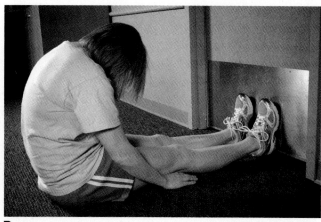

A   **B**

FIGURE 7-40. (A) Upper limb tension test 3 position. (B) Slump sit with ankle dorsiflexion.

lateral rotation, wrist and finger extension, forearm supination, elbow extension, and cervical lateral flexion can be used to determine involvement of median nerve structures.[136]

Mobilization of neural tissues is one part of an overall management strategy for patients with pain arising from these tissues. A thorough examination and evaluation is critical to ensure proper activity dosage. Mobilization can be passive, active, or some combination of both. Passive mobilization is rarely a treatment provided in isolation, but is generally combined with active movements, exercise, lifestyle modification, and education.[136] When performing, direct nerve mobilization, Butler[136] recommends starting the movements farther from the presumed site of pathology, and beginning with the rest of the body "unloaded" where there is less tension throughout the connective tissue system. If the patient has a number of positive tension tests, consider starting with the least provocative of these positions and examine the response to treatment before moving to the more acute or sensitive positions. With a successful response to the passive mobilization, the intervention can be progressed by adding active movements, increasing the repetitions, the intensity of the technique or moving techniques closer toward the presumed site of pathology. Additionally, an additional component can be added. For example, when tensioning a SLR, the patient can flex the cervical spine at the same time as dorsiflexing the ankle, thereby providing tension both from the proximal and distal ends.

Specific mobilization techniques have been described for problems in the extremities and trunk.[135,136] Mobilization begins with determining the starting position based upon examination results. Once a successful clinical program has been established, home exercises are incorporated to replicate the techniques used in the clinic (Fig. 7-40A and B). Further information on specific techniques can be found in Butler.[135,136]

Active movements following passive mobilizations should be functional. For example, when mobilizing the tissues associated with the median nerve, movements that place the wrist in extension with elbow extension are useful. A wall push-up, a chest-pass with a ball, or reaching overhead with the wrist extended are all examples of active movements, replicating the passive mobilization techniques. Once active movements are initiated and tolerated, progress the patient through AROM to resistive ROM following previously described guidelines.

TABLE 7-5 Precautions and Contraindications to Mobilizing Neural Tissues

PRECAUTIONS	CONTRAINDICATIONS
Potential of injury to other structures loaded during testing or treatment.	Recent onset of or worsening neurological symptoms; acute, unstable symptoms
Tissue irritability	Cauda equina lesions
Worsening symptoms, especially if a rapid worsening	Injury to the spinal cord
Unstable neurological signs or signs indicative of active disease process	
General health problems, especially those that involve connective or neural tissue	
Dizziness or circulatory problems	
Frank spinal cord injury with a minor secondary cord problem potentially amenable to treatment	

From Butler DS. Mobilisation of the Nervous System. St. Louis, MO: Churchill Livingstone, 1999.

A number of precautions and contraindications should be considered when examining and treating patients with mobilization directed at neural structures. These can be found in Table 7-5.

SELF-MOBILIZATION

Mobilization techniques performed only in the clinic may be of insufficient frequency to produce a significant change. Therefore, adding self-mobilization to therapist-provided interventions may provide a therapeutic dosage resulting in significant improvements. Mobilizations can be in the form of joint mobilizations performed with the use of assistive objects, or they can be soft tissue mobilizations or neural mobilizations designed to lengthen or relax associated soft tissues (Fig. 7-41).

Spine self-mobilization can be performed with the support of a chair or other rigid device that stabilizes the spine at a specific level. The patient can then extend or extend and

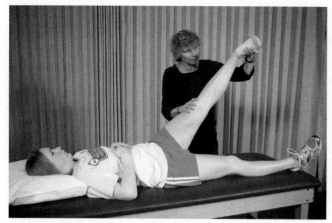

FIGURE 7-41. Neural flossing using a lateral hip stretch position with hip internal rotation.

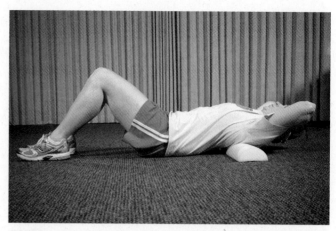

FIGURE 7-43. Half foam roll soft tissue mobilization for the spine.

rotate over the fixed chair (Fig. 7-42). This is most effectively done for the thoracic or lumbar spine. Alternatively, spine self-mobilization can be done using foam rollers or similar equipment. Foam rollers can be used in a variety of ways to provide mobilization. Half foam rollers can be placed flat side down with the patient lying on the curved part to mobilize the spine. Place a hypomobile segment at the end of the roll and relax the body over the edge to mobilize the segment (Fig. 7-43). The full foam roll can be used to mobilize soft tissue by rolling the stiff or shortened area over the roll (Fig. 7-44). Tennis balls taped together work well to mobilize soft tissues adjacent to the spine. Place the balls on either side of the spine while leaning against a wall. Slide up and down the wall to provide pressure and mobilization (Fig. 7-45).

Body rolling using a hollow 6- to 10-in diameter hollow ball provides additional opportunities for home programs

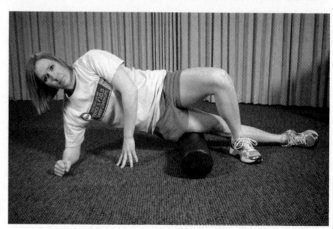

FIGURE 7-44. Foam roll for soft tissue mobilization of the iliotibial band.

utilizing mobilization techniques (Fig. 7-46).[137] Techniques to mobilize, stretch, and lengthen hypomobile tissues throughout the body are available for patients who have good general mobility. Many of these techniques require the ability to get up and down off the floor, to position the body and to move over the ball. This is not possible for some individuals with multiple joint involvement. However, for those who are mobile enough to utilize these techniques, self-mobilization with these assistive devices can be useful.

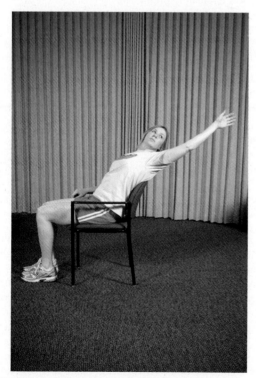

FIGURE 7-42. Thoracic spine mobilization using a chair.

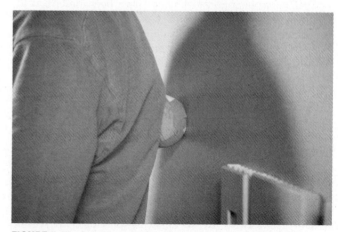

FIGURE 7-45. Soft tissue mobilization of spine using tennis balls.

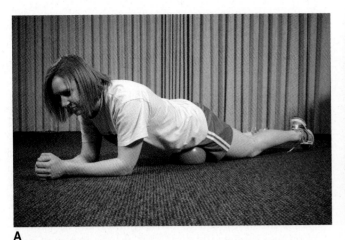

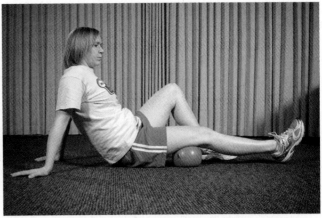

FIGURE 7-46. (A,B) Body rolling.

MOBILITY EXERCISE DOSAGE

The stage of healing (see Chapter 11) and the tissue response to loading relative to the patient's examination findings determine the dosage of mobility exercises. Each patient should be considered on an individual basis, with the dosage matched to the patient's needs. These needs extend beyond the physical impairments to include psychosocial and lifestyle issues.

Sequence

Mobility activities can be performed as part of warm-up exercises before aerobic or strengthening activities or as independent rehabilitative exercises. Use PROM or AAROM to teach AROM exercises, and use AROM as a teaching tool for resistive exercise. The sequence of exercise depends on the purpose of the ROM activity. ROM exercise as preparation for more difficult exercise should occur before that activity. When mobility exercises are being performed for the benefits of ROM increases, they should be performed in a sequence of easier to more difficult.

Most exercises performed passively can also be performed actively or with active assistance. This makes an easy progressive sequence for the patient to follow. For example, a single knee flexion exercise can be easily progressed by changing instructions. Progress knee flexion with a towel to active assisted by using some muscle activity and some passive assistance from the towel (Fig. 7-47). As the patient improves, the same exercise can be performed without assistance. The same is true for shoulder flexion exercises with a pulley or counter; the exercise can be performed with some level of assistance or completely actively.

The concept of active stretching is important when sequencing mobility activities. Active stretching is the use of active movement to stretch the agonist or to use the agonist in its new range. Stretching a short muscle should always be complemented with active stretching by strengthening the opposing muscle in the shortened range. Based on scientific studies of length-tension properties of skeletal muscle, it is hypothesized that a stiff or short soft-tissue structure cannot remain lengthened until opposing soft-tissue structures shorten.[138] The opposing muscle must be strengthened because its length-tension properties have been disrupted

because the short muscle is in need of stretch. It cannot generate sufficient tension in the short range to oppose the pull of the short muscle. By strengthening the lengthened muscle, particularly in the short range, its length-tension properties can improve, and it can provide a counterbalancing force to the short muscle. Stretching a short muscle can be done passively through a self-stretch or manual stretch, but it should always be accompanied with active stretching through strengthening the opposing muscle in the shortened range.

Active contraction of the antagonist in a shortened position is used to strengthen this muscle while simultaneously actively stretching the agonist. For example, after static stretching of the hamstrings, the patient can extend the knee in a sitting position while the paraspinal muscles stabilize the spine to prevent lumbar flexion. The quadriceps actively stretch the hamstrings into the new range. This repeated activity enhances mobility in the new range. This same sequence concept can be applied throughout the body, as in the treatment of low back and pelvic muscle imbalance. After static stretching of short hip flexor muscles, the patient should extend the hip in a walk stance position while the abdominal muscles stabilize the spine and pelvis (see Self-Management 7-6: Active Stretch for the Hip Flexor Muscles).

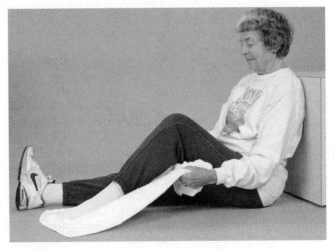

FIGURE 7-47. AROM at the knee using a towel for assistance as needed.

SELF-MANAGEMENT 7-6 *Active Stretch for the Hip Flexor Muscles*

Purpose: To stretch and use hip flexor muscles in the new range. This activity should follow hip-stretching exercises.

Position: In a stride position, with the leg to be stretched behind and with the opposite foot forward as in taking a step. Be sure to keep the back straight and abdominal muscles tightened.

Movement Technique: Shift your weight forward onto your front foot while maintaining proper hip and back position. Hold 30 to 60 seconds. Be sure that the hip of your back leg is being stretched as shown by the highlighted area in the illustration below.

Dosage
Repetitions: _____
Frequency: _____

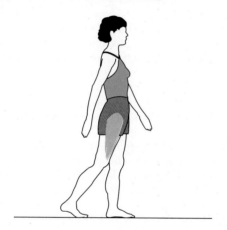

Frequency, Intensity, and Duration

As with resistive exercise, stretching dosage can be considered in terms of frequency, intensity and duration. Frequency is how often the stretch is performed, while duration is how long the stretch is held and intensity is how far into the end of the ROM the stretch is applied. The frequency of a therapeutic exercise program is often inversely related to the intensity and duration. Exercises of high intensity and duration are performed less frequently and vice versa. ROM activities, because of their purpose and goals, are generally a lower intensity exercise performed for a shorter duration. These exercises can be performed more frequently and usually take place in the home or work environment. Choose exercises that can easily and effectively be performed independently by the patient or with the assistance of a family member.

The exercise frequency is related to the purpose of the exercise, which can be considered relative to physiologic, kinesiologic, or learning factors. Physiologic purposes are those that enhance fluid dynamics, support articular cartilage nutrition, and maintain the integrity of the periarticular connective tissues. Kinesiologic purposes include maintenance of normal arthrokinematic motion and are closely tied to learning factors or choosing the correct motor program. Exercises

to teach postural set, appropriate sequencing, and patterning of muscle contraction or to teach a complex motor skill are examples of ROM as a tool for learning.

Exercises performed for physiologic or kinesiologic purposes are performed two to five or more times each day. The number of times depends on the environment and availability of exercise within that environment. If it is nearly impossible for an individual to perform exercises during the workday, asking him or her to carry out an exercise program five times each day is unreasonable. Similarly, if the ROM activities require the assistance of another, availability of that help dictates the frequency of the exercise program. As discussed in Chapter 3, an exercise prescription should fit within the context of the individual's day.

Exercises performed as learning tools are usually performed more frequently during the day. Examples of these exercises are postural reeducation activities such as scapular retraction and depression, chin tucks while sitting at a desk, and knee extension while driving without posterior pelvic tilt or lumbar flexion (Fig. 7-48). These kinds of exercises are often put "on cue" so that a specific stimulus can elicit the postural response, such as performing postural exercises every time the phone rings, every time a new page is started on a computer document, or every time an instructor poses a question. This type of programming places the exercise in the appropriate functional context, within the environment or situation where the exercise most needs to be performed. With time and repetition, individuals should find that, when the stimulus elicits the response, they are already in the appropriate posture. The intensity of this type of exercise is low, and the frequency is therefore increased.

The number of sets and repetitions depends on the frequency and the number of exercises performed. When several exercises are being performed to maintain ROM during a period of bed rest or in the early healing stages of an injury, the sets and repetitions may be fewer as multiple components of the joint and periarticular connective tissues are being mobilized. Conversely, when only a few exercises can be performed because of healing constraints or other medical conditions, more sets and repetitions of those exercises can be performed. When exercises are being performed frequently throughout the day, fewer sets and repetitions are performed during each session. When active exercise is being used to increase endurance, more repetitions and longer duration rather than greater frequency is the rule. The guiding principle in ROM prescription is understanding the physiologic, kinesiologic, and learning factors associated with each exercise in relation to the patient and exercise goals.

The length of time a stretch must be held to facilitate an increase in muscle flexibility remains a point of disagreement among clinicians. The clinical literature states that stretches should be held for a minimum of 30 seconds in young individuals and 60 seconds in older individuals. There does not appear to be any advantage to holding a stretch longer than those periods.[139-141] A study of individuals age 65 and older found that holding stretches for 60 seconds produced greater ROM gains that persisted longer than the gains for stretches held for 15 or 30 seconds.[105] A study of younger individuals found that holding stretches for 30 or 60 seconds produced greater benefits than stretches held 15 seconds, but there was no difference between the 30- and 60-second stretches.[139] Research into the viscoelastic tissue responses to stretching has shown little change

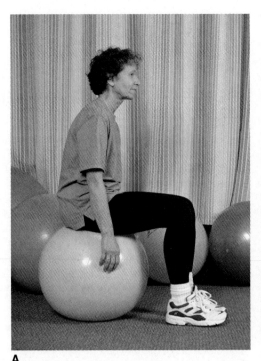
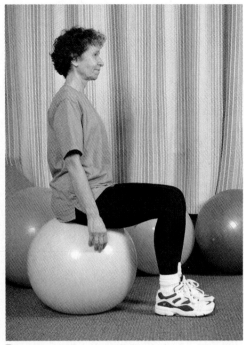

A   **B**

FIGURE 7-48. Chin tucks, pelvic tilts, and quadriceps setting can be performed while sitting on an unstable surface. (A) Poor posture. (B) Good posture with proper pelvic posture and chin tucks.

after four repetitions of stretching, suggesting that only a few repetitions are necessary to produce most of the elongation.[69] Other research suggests that it is the total time per day that the stretch is performed that is significant. A study comparing 10-second stretches with 30-second stretches performed for a total of 2 minutes per day found equivalent increases in hamstring flexibility.[142] If a patient is unable to hold a stretch for 30 seconds, then a shorter duration but higher repetition dosage may be equally effective.

However, the time that a patient or an athlete wants to hold a stretch may be based on the individual's perceived need or comfort level. When in doubt, a stretch should be held for a longer period rather than a shorter period. Although short-term flexibility improvements can be seen in one stretching session, studies on the length of stretching time necessary to effect long-term increases in muscle flexibility are still lacking. The intensity of stretching should be low to medium to prevent reflexive contraction. This contraction occurs in response to discomfort during stretching. The stretch should be comfortable enough to be easily held for 30 seconds.

HYPOMOBILITY EXERCISE PRECAUTIONS AND CONTRAINDICATIONS

PROM and stretching are not benign processes and are contraindicated when motion could disrupt the healing process. For example, passive motion into full shoulder external rotation may disrupt the healing process after a capsular shift procedure. Passive motion into hip adduction, flexion past 90 degrees, and internal rotation past neutral may result in dislocation of a recent total hip arthroplasty. Use caution to ensure that the activity is passive when active muscle contraction is

contraindicated, such as after a tendon transfer procedure. Ensure that the activity is producing *joint* ROM in the case of PROM and *muscle* ROM in the case of stretching. Moreover, control the speed and patient comfort to prevent inadvertent muscle contraction to oppose the passive exercise. Active muscle contraction in response to fear or pain could disrupt the healing process. Be aware of local anatomy, arthrokinematics, and the effects of PROM on these tissues. For example, passive shoulder ROM into full overhead flexion without adequate humeral head depression may compress a recent rotator cuff repair under the coracoacromial arch, producing pain and disrupting the healing process.

As with PROM, AAROM is contraindicated when motion or contraction may disrupt the healing process or affect the individual's health status. For example, individuals with unstable cardiac conditions are not candidates for active assisted exercise. When performing exercise with an active component, ensure that the type of muscle contraction performed (e.g., concentric, eccentric, isometric) is indicated and that the amount of tension generated is appropriate. The indications and contraindications for these contraction types are described in Chapter 5. Emphasize the importance of muscle relaxation between exercise repetitions to ensure adequate blood flow to the working muscles.

Contraindications and precautions for AROM are the same as those for active assisted exercise. Muscle contraction that may disrupt the healing process or affect the individual's health status are contraindications to AROM. The type of muscle contractions being performed should be safe for the specific situation, and the clinician should allow muscle relaxation between repetitions.

Stretching is contraindicated in the case of acute inflammation or infection in the tissues being stretched. Signs of inflammation or infection include increased warmth, tenderness, redness, or localized swelling. When stretching inflamed tissues, the patient will often report a sensation of pain prior to any sensation of stretching. This is an important reason to ask patients *what* they are feeling, not just *if* they are "feeling" the stretch. Some patients will assume that it is okay to feel pain. Use caution in patients with recent fracture, particularly if the fracture has been immobilized for some time, as the associated soft tissues will have weakened simultaneously. Additionally, the fracture site should be stabilized manually or by a supportive surface and the stretch should be designed to avoid torque directly over the fracture site.

Patient's osteoporosis should approach stretching cautiously as a quick muscle contraction in response to discomfort, as well as the force across the bone can produce a fracture. Similarly, the elderly are at risk of stretching injuries due to increased soft tissue stiffness. Those who have been in prolonged immobilization or those with very weak muscles will be at risk of stretch-related injuries or may lack sufficient strength to oppose a stretch applied too vigorously.

CAUSES AND EFFECTS OF HYPERMOBILITY

Although most clinicians are familiar with the treatment of persons with decreased mobility, many patients have problems related to excessive mobility. Most individuals do not seek medical attention primarily for possessing excessive mobility about a joint or throughout the body. More frequently, patients seek medical attention for pain, fatigue, or tendinitis. These pathologies, impairments, and functional limitations often result from the hypermobility.

Hypermobility should be differentiated from instability. Hypermobility is excessive laxity or length of a tissue, and instability is an excessive range of movement, osteokinematic, or arthrokinematic, for which there is no protective muscular control. Despite hypermobility, the individual may experience no symptoms of instability. For example, individuals with ACL-deficient knees may have measurable anterior laxity (i.e., hypermobility) at the tibiofemoral joint with no symptoms of instability. Conversely, individuals may have complaints of instability or "giving way" with no measurable laxity.

Hypermobility can be broadly categorized as excessive joint mobility resulting from trauma or a genetic predisposition or as excessive tissue length. Patients with traumatic or atraumatic hypermobility may seek medical attention for a number of complaints, which may or may not include frank instability.

Hypermobility at a joint caused by traumatic injury can lead to true instability, particularly at the glenohumeral joint, where a traumatic anterior inferior dislocation can result in recurrent dislocation. Similarly, sprains to the lateral ankle ligaments or medial knee ligaments can result in hypermobility and instability. Atraumatic hypermobility is common at the glenohumeral joint; persons with multidirectional instability often seek medical attention for symptoms of rotator cuff tendinitis. At the knee, hypermobility can result in secondary patellofemoral pain.

Hypermobility can develop in response to a relatively less mobile segment or region. In a multijoint system with common movement directions (e.g., spine), movement occurs at the segments providing the least resistance. Abnormal or excessive movement is imposed on segments with the least amount of stiffness. With repeated movements over time, the least stiff segments increase in mobility, and the stiffer segments decrease in mobility. A thorough examination, seeking to understand the impairment contributing to the hypermobility, is necessary.

THERAPEUTIC EXERCISE INTERVENTION FOR HYPERMOBILITY

Treatment techniques for hypermobility should be directed at the related impairments and functional limitations and at the underlying causes of hypermobility. For example, a patient with hypermobility at the spinal level probably has pain and decreased mobility at adjacent segments. These impairments must be treated along with the underlying hypermobile segment. Although it is important to address the patient's current complaints, failure to recognize hypermobility as the underlying cause ensures the return of symptoms. Hypermobility should be treated only if it is associated with instability or is producing symptoms elsewhere (i.e., hypomobile segment) because of relative flexibility.

Elements of the Movement System

The elements of the movement system are important in directing treatment of hypermobility. For example, a patient with spondylolysis at L4 (i.e., anatomic impairment) demonstrates faulty dynamic posture with increased lumbar lordosis during movement (i.e., impairment). This results in pain (i.e., impairment) and an inability to run and jump (i.e., functional limitation) and to participate in high school sports (i.e., disability).

In this situation, the spondylolysis is the base element, and the faulty dynamic posture is the biomechanical element. The spondylolysis is not amenable to physical therapy intervention, although the biomechanical element must be resolved to allow healing and prevent recurrence of the spondylolysis. The intervention should address the biomechanical element through stabilization exercises and postural exercises to be incorporated into daily activities.

Stabilization Exercises

The concept of stabilization exercises gained popularity in the treatment of conditions of the spine. Stabilization exercises are dynamic activities that attempt to limit and control excessive movement. These exercises do not imply a static position, but rather describe a range of movement (i.e., the neutral range) in which hypermobility is controlled. Stabilization activities include mobility exercises for stiff or hypomobile segments, strengthening exercises in the shortened range for hypermobile segments, postural training to ensure movement through a controlled range, and patient education. Supportive devices such as taping or bracing may be necessary initially to keep movement within a range where stability can be maintained. This range is different for every patient and condition. Patient education focuses on helping the patient find the limits of stability and work within those limits.

As mobility exercises to decrease hypomobility and stabilization exercises to increase stiffness improve symptoms, the stability limits increase, allowing the patient to work through a larger ROM. For example, a patient with an L4 spondylolysis may have short hip flexor and lumbar paraspinal muscles in combination with a hypermobile L4 segment. Stabilization focuses on increasing the length of the short muscles through static stretching, followed by active stretching through contraction of the abdominal muscles in a walk stance position. Initially, a stabilization brace may be used during exercise. As mobility of the short muscles and stiffness at the L4 segment improve, the brace can be discontinued and the walk stance position progressed to a lunge position.

Stabilization activities should be chosen based on the direction in which the segment is susceptible to excessive motion. In the previous example, the susceptible direction is extension; the spine tends to extend excessively, producing pain. Focus treatment on training the back to resist extension forces, rather than resisting motion in all directions. For the individual with anterior shoulder instability, the arthrokinematic motion of anterior glide is the symptom-producing hypermobility. Stabilization activities should focus on controlling anterior displacement and on treating the associated impairments.

Stabilization exercises can be performed in a variety of positions and using a range of equipment. When increasing the stability of a hypermobile segment, support (e.g., taping, bracing) and strengthening in the short range must be combined with mobility exercises for the hypomobile segment. This approach ensures balance in areas with variable relative flexibility. Gymnastic balls, foam rollers, balance boards, and proprioceptive exercises are effective ways to enhance stability.

Closed-Chain Exercise

Closed-chain exercise has been advocated for those with joint instability or hypermobility. For the lower extremity, exercises such as squats, lunges, or step-ups with the foot fixed are commonly used closed-chain activities. For the upper extremity, any weight-bearing exercise performed in the push-up or modified push-up position is considered to be closed-chain. Weight bearing with the hands against the wall or on a table or countertop is also an effective closed-chain position for the upper extremity. The rationale for this exercise is muscular cocontraction, decreased shear forces, and increased joint compression. Some of this theory is supported by scientific and clinical research.[143,144] Other studies dispute some aspects of this rationale, such as muscular cocontraction with a closed-chain position.[145,146] Particularly for the lower extremity when the foot spends a lot of time in contact with the floor, using closed-chain exercise for hypermobility makes good clinical sense. However, for the upper extremity, the closed-chain position is rarely the position of function. The closed-chain position remains an effective position for upper extremity training for individuals with hypermobility, but open-chain stabilization techniques should be incorporated as well. More information on the effects of closed-chain exercise can be found in Chapter 14.

Open-Chain Stabilization

Open-chain stabilization activities are available for the lower and the upper extremities. PNF techniques such as rhythmic stabilization and alternating isometrics can be used effectively to facilitate co-contraction about a joint (see Chapter 15). These techniques are particularly effective in the latter stages of rehabilitation when performed in the position of instability, such as abduction and external rotation for treating anterior glenohumeral instability (Fig. 7-49).

Stabilization exercises for the spine are difficult to categorize, because the spine is often fixed at one end and open at the other end. It is not a true closed or open system. Stabilization exercises for the spine are often initiated in a

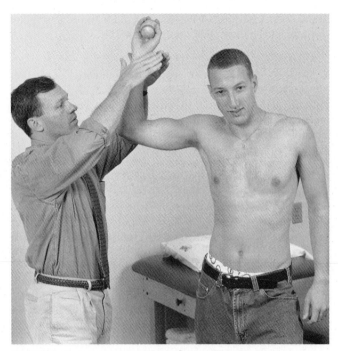

FIGURE 7-49. Rhythmic stabilization performed in a position of apprehension.

supine position with abdominal bracing exercises and progressed to sitting and standing positions. A variety of stabilization exercises can be performed on unstable surfaces such as a gymnastics ball or foam rollers to improve stability within a comfortable range. Sitting, prone, and supine activities combined with arm reaching and leg lifts can be used from early to advanced stages of stabilization training (Fig. 7-50).

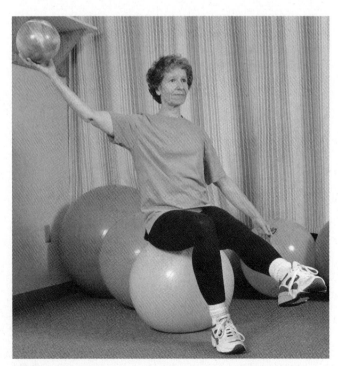

FIGURE 7-50. Sitting on a gymnastics ball while performing simultaneous arm and leg exercises is an example of an advanced spine stabilization exercise.

Many of these same activities can be used to improve stability throughout the upper and lower extremities.

Ballistic Exercises

Ballistic exercise has been shown to produce cocontraction about a joint through triphasic muscle activation. High-speed ballistic activities result in different patterns of agonist-antagonist muscle contractions from those of slower activities. Rapid ballistic movements result in synchronous activation of agonists and antagonists.[6,147,148] In contrast, the same movement pattern at a slow speed demonstrates only agonist muscle contraction, with braking provided by passive viscoelastic properties.[6] Although the viscoelastic properties also restrict movement at faster speeds, these properties are inadequate to halt fast movements.[147] These rapid ballistic movement patterns can be used with resistive tubing, balls, or inertial exercise equipment (Fig. 7-51).

The amount of antagonist activity needed to halt a movement is related to the velocity of the activity.[147] Subjects were asked to produce fast flexion movements of the thumb and fast extension movements of the elbow over three distances and at a variety of speeds. All movements resulted in biphasic or triphasic muscle contraction. A linear relationship was found between peak velocity and the amount of antagonist activation needed to halt the movement. Movements made through large angles (i.e., large amplitude) showed less antagonist activity than those made through small angles at the same speed, and fast, small-amplitude movements demonstrated an earlier onset of antagonist activity. The distance during fast movements is controlled primarily by the first agonist muscle contraction, and increasing antagonist torque is associated with decreasing distance, ultimately controlling the movement time.[148] Producing fast movements requires large agonist torque production, followed by an equally large or larger antagonist torque.

One study concluded that quick movements through small distances result in a large, quick antagonist burst and that slow movements over a long distance result in small and late antagonist bursts.[147] The antagonist burst timing is not specified solely by size; it is also a function of the movement amplitude. Timing and amplitude are regulated by the central nervous system. For example, flexing and extending the hip rapidly through a very small range elicits cocontraction of agonist and antagonist musculature, but flexing and extending slowly through a large range elicits reciprocal activation of the agonists and antagonists. If hip and pelvic stabilization is the goal, small-amplitude, fast movements are more likely to elicit cocontraction than slow, large-amplitude movements.

Another factor that affects antagonist activity is the subject's knowledge of the necessity for such a contraction. On study provided a mechanical stop for preventing further movement in some elbow flexion and extension tasks.[147] When the subjects knew that the stop was in place, the antagonist burst disappeared after two or three trials. This resulted in a faster movement, suggesting that the antagonist activity brakes and slows the motion. Some cognitive control over the braking mechanism exists.

This research supports the use of rapid, alternating movements, moving quickly through a short distance. Large-amplitude movement does not produce the same muscular coactivation as small-amplitude movement.

Exercise Dosage

Dosage parameters depend on the purpose of the exercise and the patient's tolerance for the activity. Any time rapid, alternating movements are used, fatigue can alter the proper performance and thus the outcome of treatment. Watch for signs of fatigue that result in substitution patterns or loss of the desired stabilization.

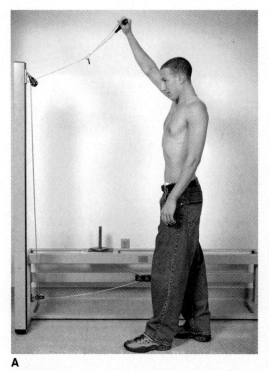
A

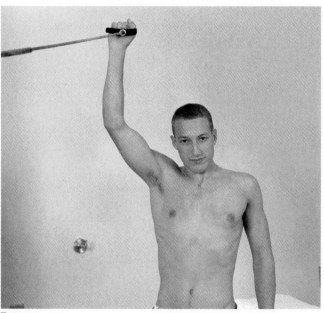
B

FIGURE 7-51. (A) Performance of rapid alternating shoulder flexion and extension at end ROM using impulse inertial exercise system. (B) Similar activity performed with tubing.

For rapid movements, sets for time often work better than a set number of repetitions. Patients can try to increase the number of repetitions of an exercise within the timed set.

As with all other exercise prescription, perform the exercise to fatigue without losing control. Monitor the time or number of repetitions, and, as the patient improves, change the exercise parameters to continue increasing the challenge. This may include increasing the resistance, repetitions, or speed, or decreasing the rest interval.

Hypermobility Exercise Precautions and Contraindications

An important precaution when treating areas of hypermobility is to ensure that areas of relative flexibility are identified. Stretching techniques to improve mobility in a hypomobile area may increase hypermobility in an adjacent area. Reinforce correct dynamic stabilization to ensure that intervention is isolated to the correct segment. For example, failure to stabilize the pelvis during hip flexor stretching increases lumbar extension, potentially increasing hypermobility in this area.

Any time dynamic stabilization activities are being performed at the limits of stability (e.g., resisted shoulder rotation at 90-degree abduction and full external rotation in a hypermobile shoulder), be sure that the individual has adequate control to prevent instability or dislocation. Progress activities according to the patient's ability to control the limits of stability. Fatigue of dynamic stabilizing musculature places the patient at risk for injury, and the fatigue level should be monitored throughout the exercise session.

Many stabilization exercises use eccentric muscle contraction to provide stability. Eccentric contractions are associated with delayed onset muscle soreness (see Chapter 5), fatigue, loss of control, and substitution. Consider this in the exercise dosage. Watch the patient closely for signs of fatigue and loss of control because the patient could be injured or develop excessive muscle soreness.

Any time activities are performed on a single limb, use caution to prevent falling and ensure that single-leg stance is indicated. Individuals with degenerative joint disease at the primary or adjacent joint may experience a symptom exacerbation due to excessive loads on the limb. A pool can minimize the quantity of weight bearing while performing single-leg stance activities (see Chapter 16).

LIFESPAN ISSUES

Be sure to consider that most studies on stretching and mobility exercises have been performed on young and middle-age adults, and few have been performed on children or the elderly. However, because of the aging of the population, more and more studies are being carried out on the elderly to determine how their responses to treatment differ from that of younger individuals. As noted in the section on "Stretching," the elderly benefit from holding their stretches for a longer time than do younger individuals.

As with many adults, children exhibit variable degrees of mobility, from shortened and tight muscles to hypermobility. In general, flexibility remains relatively stable through age 8, and then declines until about the ages of 11 to 15.[149] This decline is probably because of the adolescent growth spurt.

As with adults, flexibility in children can be improved by the stretching techniques outlined in this chapter. A study of elementary school children found that regular hamstring muscle stretching through the school year produced significant increases in SLR ROM.[150] Increases were greater for those stretching 4 days per week compared with those children stretching 2 days per week.

Joint mobilization techniques are not commonly used in children, although there may be special cases in which this technique is indicated. Joint mobilization has been considered for children with central nervous system disorders such as cerebral palsy.[151] As with adults, the primary indication for use in this population is joint hypomobility resulting from capsular tightness. However, use caution when using joint mobilization in any child. It may be contraindicated in some situations, such as Down syndrome in which joint hypermobility secondary to joint laxity is generally the case. Additionally, in any child with open epiphyses, the potential damage to the growth plate must be balanced against the potential benefits of joint mobilization. Alternative interventions to increase mobility may be safer choices.

Other issues exist at the older end of the lifespan. Joint mobility and muscular flexibility decline with aging.[105] Connective tissue changes occurring with aging impact the use of joint mobilization and stretching exercises. Aging muscle increases in stiffness as measured by passive length-tension plots, and the amount of muscle area occupied by connective tissue also increases.[152] Feland et al.[105] suggest using static stretching over PNF stretching because the muscles of the elderly are more susceptible to contraction-induced injury and have decreased capacity to recover from such injury. Older individuals have demonstrated greater muscle stiffness and a lower tolerance for stretching.[101]

Additionally, joint ROM decreases with aging. Declines of 20% in hip rotation and 10% in wrist and shoulder motion have been reported.[153] Walker et al.[154] showed declines in the lower extremity joint ROM of up to 57%. A 25% decrease in trunk side bending between the ages of 20 and 60 have also been reported.[153] Before performing joint mobilization in the elderly population, consider their decreased joint capsule tensile strength, diminished articular cartilage water content, and increased bone fragility. Joint mobilization should be approached cautiously because of all these connective tissue changes.

ADJUNCTIVE AGENTS

Clinicians often use various treatments or techniques to enhance the effects of another treatment. Forms of tissue heating are the most common adjunctive agents used in combination with ROM exercises to increase mobility. The ability of collagen to be easily and safely deformed or stretched is enhanced by increasing the temperature of the collagen. Because muscle is primarily composed of collagen, the ability of the muscle to be stretched may be enhanced by increasing the temperature of the muscle.[40] The critical temperature for beneficial effects appears to be approximately 39°C or 103°F.[10,155–158]

Intramuscular temperature may be increased by heating modalities or through exercise. The therapeutic temperature required may be efficiently achieved for the time necessary to complete a flexibility program using a deep-heating modality such as ultrasound.[159,160] Physiologically, the easiest and most appropriate way to increase intramuscular temperature is through the use of exercise. Active, submaximal resistive exercise of the muscle groups to be stretched should be performed before stretching. This type of exercise is capable of producing temperature increases to approximately 39°C after 10 to 15 minutes.

Heating techniques may prepare the tissue for mobility activities by increasing the tissue temperature, promoting relaxation and pain reduction, and increasing the local circulation. Forms of heat other than exercise can be categorized broadly as superficial-heating and deep-heating agents. Although heat can increase local circulation and temperature, it is not a substitute for warm-up exercises before a planned activity. A warm-up exercise such as walking, bicycling, upper body ergometry, or AROM exercise should take place before any therapeutic ROM activities. This approach increases core temperature and prepares surrounding tissues for the forthcoming activity.

Superficial Heat

The most common superficial heating agents include hot packs, paraffin, and warm whirlpools. These agents primarily increase skin temperature, with little penetration of heat to deeper tissues. Skin temperature increases are the greatest within the first 0.5 cm from the surface, with some increase in muscle temperature at 1 to 2 cm and less heating at 3 cm.[161] To achieve temperature elevations at increasing depths, a treatment time of 15 to 30 minutes is necessary.[161] The depth of penetration is significantly affected by the tissue composition. Areas with less soft tissue heat deeper than areas with greater subcutaneous fat. For example, superficial heat applied to the hands can increase tissue temperature to the joint, but heat applied to the thigh has only shallow penetration.

Hot packs are frequently used over larger surface areas such as the low back, thigh, and knee. Smaller areas such as the hand are more amenable to warm paraffin. The patient usually sits quietly while the treatment is applied. This produces relaxation but may leave the individual unprepared for vigorous exercise. In contrast, a warm whirlpool can provide superficial heating while simultaneously allowing exercise to be performed. AROM, PROM, or resistive ROM exercises can be performed while in a warm whirlpool, thereby extending the benefits of this heating modality.

Deep Heat

Ultrasound is the most common form of deep heat used in the clinic. The effects of ultrasound are mechanical and thermal, although in this context, the thermal effects are emphasized. The specific effects and depth of penetration are affected by the tissue type, the ultrasound wavelength or frequency, and the intensity. Ultrasound has the ability to elevate tissue temperatures to depths of 5 cm or more.[111] The temperature elevation in tissue has been associated with increases in collagen extensibility, changes in nerve conduction velocity, and increases in the pain threshold. Ultrasound intensities necessary to achieve tissue temperatures to a range of 40°C to 45°C range from 1.0 to 2.0 W/cm² delivered continuously for 5 to 10 minutes.[161]

The effects of ultrasound on tissue healing and tissue extensibility have been studied. Reed et al.[162] examined the effects of continuous ultrasound on knee medial collateral

ligament extensibility. The authors found that ultrasound did not increase extensibility beyond the effects of stretching. Although heating the tissue may not affect its extensibility, low-intensity ultrasound may facilitate healing. Enwemeka et al.[163] found that nine treatments of low-intensity ultrasound to the rabbit Achilles tendon resulted in significant increases in tensile strength, tensile stress, and energy absorption capacity compared with sham ultrasound. Ramirez et al.[164] expanded these results, showing that low-intensity ultrasound to rat Achilles tendons stimulated collagen synthesis in tendon fibroblasts. Additionally, ultrasound stimulated cell division during periods of subsequent rapid cell proliferation.

Superficial heat such as a hot pack commonly is used in combination with ultrasound to enhance the effects of treatment. The hot pack promotes relaxation and therefore increases the patient's tolerance for stretching, and the deep heat produces changes in the collagen elasticity, preparing it for subsequent stretching.

If extensibility gains are to be maintained after the heat and stretching session, stretching should be performed as the muscle cools to its preheated temperature. Ideally, this new length should be maintained for an extended period after the therapy session. This can be done by the use of splints or continuous passive motion devices.

KEY POINTS

- The effects of immobilization on the injured and uninjured soft tissues are profound. All tissues are affected, including insertion sites and bone.
- These effects are the result of the specific adaptations to imposed demands principle; tissue responds to loads placed on them. When underloaded, the tissue weakens.
- The period needed to restore normal structural, and mechanical properties to immobilized tissue can be two or more times the immobilization period.
- Joint ROM should be differentiated from muscle ROM. The specific goal dictates the type of mobility activity prescribed.
- A variety of contractile and noncontractile tissues can limit mobility at a joint.
- PROM exercise is a mobility activity performed without muscle contraction. AAROM is a mobility activity in which some muscle activity takes place, and AROM exercise uses active muscle contraction to perform the exercise.
- To increase flexibility, static, ballistic, and PNF stretching techniques can be used. The type of stretch chosen depends on the individual's impairments and lifestyle.
- Joint mobilization is an integral component of a comprehensive mobility program when capsular restriction is a key finding.
- Pulleys, machines, the pool, or objects found in the home or office can be used to perform mobility exercises.
- Mobility exercise prescription depends on the specific goal of the activity and the environment in which it will be performed.
- Hypermobility can be as disabling as hypomobility. Stabilization exercises such as closed-chain and rapidly alternating movements may be incorporated.
- Adjunctive agents such as heat can be used to enhance mobility activities.

LAB ACTIVITIES

Perform the following activities with your partner. Not all positions are optimal for performing each of the exercises, but the clinician occasionally is unable to change the patient's position. If not the optimal position, which position would be better and why?

1. With your patient in supine, perform the following:
   a. PROM shoulder flexion
   b. AAROM shoulder abduction
   c. PROM shoulder internal and external rotation
   d. CR stretching for pectoralis major
   e. PROM hip and knee flexion
   f. CR-contract stretching of the hamstring muscles
   g. PROM lumbar flexion
   h. PROM lumbar rotation
2. With your patient sitting, perform the following:
   a. PROM hip internal and external rotation
   b. AAROM knee extension
   c. CR stretching hip internal rotator muscles
   d. AAROM shoulder flexion
   e. AROM shoulder abduction
3. With your patient in a sidelying position, perform the following:
   a. PROM shoulder extension
   b. AAROM shoulder abduction
   c. CR stretching shoulder internal rotator muscles
   d. AROM shoulder flexion
4. With your patient in a prone position, perform the following:
   a. AAROM elbow extension
   b. PROM hip internal and external rotation
   c. AROM shoulder flexion

   d. CR stretching hip flexors
   e. CR-contract stretching for gastrocnemius
   f. CR-contract stretching for soleus
5. Decide how to best position your patient for the following:
   a. AROM shoulder external rotation in a gravity minimized position
   b. AROM scapular elevation
   c. AROM wrist extension in a gravity-minimized position
   d. CR stretching of hip adductor muscles
   e. AROM shoulder abduction in a gravity-minimized position
   f. PROM cervical rotation
   g. Static stretching of the triceps muscle
6. Choose five of the previous exercises and write a description of those exercises for a patient in a home exercise program. Include a picture of the exercise.
7. Consider Case Study No. 6 from Unit 7. Instruct your patient in the first phase of the exercise program. Explain and demonstrate.
8. The clinician is treating a postal worker with rotator cuff tendinitis resulting from hypermobility. This man sorts mail all day at eye level. The rotator cuff tendinitis has resolved with intervention. Instruct this patient in an exercise program to treat the instability. Explain and demonstrate.
9. Instruct a patient in a self-stretching program for the quadriceps, hamstrings, and iliotibial band. Explain and demonstrate three different stretches for each muscle group.

CRITICAL THINKING QUESTIONS

1. Consider Case Study No. 2 in Unit 7.
   a. Although the patient needs to increase knee ROM in both flexion and extension, which direction would you emphasize first and why?
   b. Discuss the advantages and disadvantages for various exercise modes to increase this patient's active knee ROM.
2. Consider Case Study No. 4 in Unit 7.
   a. How would your treatment differ if the patient were an elderly woman with severe osteoporosis?
   b. How would your treatment differ if the patient were 25 years of age and the joint accessory motion testing result indicated hypermobility?

REFERENCES

1. Magee D. Orthopedic Physical Assessment. 2nd Ed. Philadelphia, PA: WB Saunders, 1992.
2. Dorland's Illustrated Medical Dictionary. 26th Ed. Philadelphia, PA: WB Saunders, 1981.
3. Kannus P, Jozsa L, Renstrom P, et al. The effects of training, immobilization and remobilization on musculoskeletal tissue. I. Training and immobilization. Scand J Med Sci Sports 1992;2:100–118.
4. Kannus P, Jozsa L, Renstrom P, et al. The effects of training, immobilization and remobilization on musculoskeletal tissue. II. Remobilization and prevention of immobilization atrophy. Scand J Med Sci Sports 1992;2:164–176.
5. Hakkinen K, Komi PV. Electromyographic changes during strength training and detraining. Med Sci Sports Exerc 1983;15:455–460.
6. Lestienne F. Effects of inertial load and velocity on the braking process of voluntary limb movements. Exp Brain Res 1979;35:407–418.
7. Lieber RL, McKee-Woodburn T, Friden J, et al. Recovery of the dog quadriceps after ten weeks of immobilization followed by four weeks of remobilization. J Orthop Res. 1989; 7:408–412.
8. Appell HJ. Muscular atrophy following immobilisation: a review. Sports Med 1990;10:42–58.
9. Haggmark T, Eriksson E. Cylinder or mobile cast brace after knee ligament surgery: a clinical analysis and morphological and enzymatic study of changes in the quadriceps muscle. Am J Sports Med 1979;7:48–56.
10. Warren CG, Lehmann JF, Koblanski JM, et al. Heat and stretch procedures: an evaluation using rat tail tendon. Phys Med Rehabil 1976;57:122–126.
11. Lieber RL. Skeletal Muscle Structure and Function. Baltimore, MD: Williams & Wilkins, 1992.
12. Garrett W, Tidball J. Myotendinous junction: structure, function, and failure. In: Woo SL-Y, Buckwalter JA, eds. Injury and Repair of the Musculoskeletal Soft Tissues. Park Ridge, IL: American Academy of Orthopaedic Surgeons, 1988.
13. Tardieu C, Tabary J-C, Tabary C, et al. Adaptation of connective tissue length to immobilization in the lengthened and shortened positions in cat soleus muscle. J Physiol 1982;8:214–220.
14. Tipton CM, Vailas AC, Matthes RD. Experimental studies on the influences of physical activity on ligaments, tendons and joints: a brief review. Acta Med Scand Suppl 1986;711:157–168.
15. Enwemeka CS. Connective tissue plasticity: ultrastructural, biomechanical and morphometric effects of physical factors on intact and regenerating tendons. J Orthop Sports Phys Ther 1991;14:198–212.
16. Amiel D, Woo SL-Y, Harwood FL, et al. The effect of immobilization on collagen turnover in connective tissue: a biochemical-biomechanical correlation. Acta Orthop Scand 1982;53:325–332.
17. Andriacchi T, Sabiston P, DeHaven K, et al. Ligament: injury and repair. In: Woo SL-Y, Buckwalter JA, eds. Injury and Repair of the Musculoskeletal Soft Tissues. Park Ridge, IL: American Academy of Orthopaedic Surgeons, 1988.

18. Dahners LE. Ligament contraction: a correlation with cellularity and actin staining. Trans Orthop Res Soc 1986;11:56–66.

19. Laros GS, Tipton CM, Cooper RR. Influence of physical activity on ligament insertions in the knees of dogs. J Bone Joint Surg Am 1971;53:275–286.

20. Woo SL-Y, Inoue M, McGurk-Burleson E, et al. Treatment of the medial collateral ligament injury: II. Structure and function of canine knees in response to differing treatment regimens. Am J Sports Med 1987;15:22–29.

21. Noyes FR. Functional properties of knee ligaments and alterations induced by immobilization. Clin Orthop Relat Res 1977;123:210–242.

22. Amiel D, von Schroeder H, Akeson WH. The response of ligaments to stress deprivation and stress enhancement: biochemical studies. In: Daniel DD, Akeson WH, O'Conner JJ, eds. Knee Ligaments: Structure, Function, Injury and Repair. New York, NY: Raven Press, 1990.

23. Larsen NP, Forwood MR, Parker AW. Immobilization and retraining of cruciate ligaments in the rat. Acta Orthop Scand 1987;58:260–264.

24. Noyes FR, DeLucas JL, Torvik PJ. Biomechanics of anterior cruciate ligament failure: an analysis of strain-rate sensitivity and mechanisms of failure in primates. J Bone Joint Surg Am 1974;56:236–253.

25. Woo SL-Y, Gomez MA, Sites TJ, et al. The biomechanical and morphological changes in the medial collateral ligament of the rabbit after immobilization and remobilization. J Bone Joint Surg Am 1987;69:1200–1211.

26. Buckwalter JA. Mechanical injuries of articular cartilage. In: Finerman GA, Noyes FR, eds. Biology and Biomechanics of the Traumatized Synovial Joint: The Knee as Model. Rosemont, IL: American Academy of Orthopaedic Surgeons, 1992.

27. Troyer H. The effect of short-term immobilization on the rabbit knee joint cartilage. Clin Orthop 1975;107:249–257.

28. Videman T. Connective tissue and immobilization. Clin Orthop 1987;221:26–32.

29. Jozsa L, Jarvinen M, Kannus P, et al. Fine structural changes in the articular cartilage of the rat's knee following short-term immobilisation in various positions. Int Orthop 1987; 11:129–133.

30. Kiviranta I, Jurvelin J, Tammi M, et al. Weight bearing controls glycosaminoglycan concentration and articular cartilage thickness in the knee joints of young beagle dogs. Arthritis Rheum 1987;30:801–809.

31. Behrens F, Kraft EL, Oegema TR Jr. Biochemical changes in articular cartilage after joint immobilization by casting or external fixation. J Orthop Res 1989;7:335–343.

32. Burr DB, Frederickson RG, Pavlinch C, et al. Intracast muscle stimulation prevents bone and cartilage deterioration in cast-immobilized rabbits. Clin Orthop 1984;189:264–278.

33. Tammi M, Saamanen A-M, Jauhiainen A, et al. Proteoglycan alterations in rabbit knee articular cartilage following physical exercise and immobilization. Connect Tissue Res 1983;11:45–55.

34. Minaire P. Immobilization osteoporosis: a review. Rheumatology 1989;8(Suppl):95–103.

35. Schoutens A, Laurent E, Poortmans JR. Effects of inactivity and exercise on bone. Sports Med 1989;7:71–81.

36. Bailey DA, McCulloch RG. Bone tissue and physical activity. Can J Sport Sci 1990;15:229–239.

37. Evans EB, Eggers GWN, Butler JK, Blumel J. Experimental immobilization and remobilization of rat knee joint. J Bone Joint Surg Am 1960;42:737–758.

38. Whedon GS. Disuse osteoporosis: physiological aspects. Calcif Tissue Int 1984;36S:146–150.

39. Mazess RB, Whedon GD. Immobilization and bone. Calcif Tissue Int 1983;35:265–267.

40. Nishiyama S, Kuwahara T, Matsuda I. Decreased bone density in severely handicapped children and adults with reference to influence of limited mobility and anticonvulsant medication. Eur J Pediatr 1986;144:457–463.

41. Karpakka J, Vaananen K, Virtanen P, et al. The effects of remobilization and exercise on collagen biosynthesis in rat tendon. Acta Physiol Scand 1990;139:139–145.

42. Enwemeka CS, Spielholtz NI, Nelson AJ. The effects of early functional activities on experimentally tenotomized Achilles tendons in rats. Am J Phys Med Rehabil 1988;67:264–269.

43. Gelberman RH, Vande Berg JS, Lundborg GN, et al. Flexor tendon healing and restoration of the gliding surface: an ultrastructural study in dogs. J Bone Joint Surg Am 1983;65:70–80.

44. Gelberman RH, Woo SL-Y, Lothringer K, et al. Effects of early intermittent passive mobilization on healing canine flexor tendons. J Hand Surg 1982;7:170–175.

45. Gelberman RH, Botte MJ, Spiegelman JJ, et al. The excursion and deformation of repaired flexor tendons treated with protected early motion. J Hand Surg Am 1983;11:106–110.

46. Gelberman RH, Goldberg V, Kai-Nan A, et al. Tendon. In: Woo SL-Y, Buckwalter JA, eds. Injury and Repair of the Musculoskeletal Soft Tissues. Park Ridge, IL: American Academy of Orthopaedic Surgeons, 1988.

47. Woo SL-Y, Maynard J, Butler D, et al. Ligament, tendon and joint capsule insertions into bone. In: Woo SL-Y, Buckwalter JA, eds. Injury and Repair of the Musculoskeletal Soft Tissues. Park Ridge, IL: American Academy of Orthopaedic Surgeons, 1988.

48. Loitz BL, Frank CB. Biology and mechanics of ligament and ligament healing. Exerc Sports Sci Rev 1993;21:33–64.

49. Arnoszky S. Structure and Function of Articular Cartilage. Presented at the American Physical Therapy Association Annual Conference; June 12–16, 1993; Cincinnati, OH.

50. Markos PK. Ipsilateral and contralateral effects of proprioceptive neuromuscular facilitation techniques on hip motion and electromyographic activity. Phys Ther 1979;59:1366–1373.

51. Gajdosik RL, Bohannon RW. Clinical measurement of range of motion. Phys Ther 1987;67:1867–1872.

52. Hayes KW, Peterson C, Falconer J. An examination of Cyriax's passive motion tests with patients having osteoarthritis of the knee. Phys Ther 1994;74:697–709.

53. Frank C, Akeson WH, Woo SL-Y, et al. Physiology and therapeutic value of passive joint motion. Clin Orthop 1984;185:113–125.

54. Johnson E, Bradley B, Witkowski K, et al. Effect of a static calf muscle-tendon unit stretching program on ankle dorsiflexion range of motion of older women. J Geriatr Phys Ther 2007;30(2):49–52.

55. Ross MD. Effect of a 15-day pragmatic hamstring stretching program on hamstring flexibility and single hop for distance test peformance. Res Sports Med 2007;15(4):271–281.

56. Cornelius W, Jackson A. The effects of cryotherapy and PNF on hip extensor flexibility. J Athletic Training 1984;19:183–184.

57. deVries HA. Prevention of muscular distress after exercise. Res Q 1961;32:177–185.

58. deVries HA. Evaluation of static stretching procedures for improvement of flexibility. Res Q 1962;33:222–229.

59. deVries HA. The "looseness" factor in speed and oxygen consumption of an anaerobic 100 yard dash. Res Q 1963;34:305–313.

60. Loudon KL, Bolier CE, Allison KA, et al. Effects of two stretching methods on the flexibility and retention of flexibility at the ankle joint in runners. Phys Ther 1985;65:698.

61. Moore M, Hutton R. Electromyographic investigation of muscle stretching techniques. Med Sci Sports Exerc 1980;12:322–329.

62. Prentice WE. A comparison of static stretching and PNF stretching for improving hip joint flexibility. J Athletic Training 1983;18:56–59.

63. Sady SP, Wortman M, Blanke D. Flexibility training: ballistic, static or proprioceptive neuromuscular facilitation? Arch Phys Med Rehabil 1982;63:261–263.

64. Tanigawa MC. Comparison of the hold relax procedure and passive mobilization of increasing muscle length. Phys Ther 1972;52:725–735.

65. Voss DE, Ionta MK, Myers GJ. Proprioceptive Neuromuscular Facilitation: Patterns and Techniques. 3rd Ed. Philadelphia, PA: JB Lippincott, 1985.

66. Wallin D, Ekblom B, Grahm R, et al. Improvement of muscle flexibility: a comparison between two techniques. Am J Sports Med 1985;13:263–268.

67. Zebas CJ, Rivera ML. Retention of flexibility in selected joints after cessation of a stretching exercise program. In: Dotson CO, Humphrey JH, eds. Exercise Physiology: Current Selected Research Topics. New York, NY: AMS Press, 1985.

68. Crutchfield CA, Barnes MR. The Neurophysiological Basis of Patient Treatment. Vol I. The Muscle Spindle. 2nd Ed. West Virginia: Stokesville Publishing Co., 1972.

69. Taylor DC, Dalton JD Jr, Seaber AV, et al. Viscoelastic properties of muscle-tendon units. The biomechanical effects of stretching. Am J Sports Med 1990;18(3):300–309.

70. Entyre BR, Abraham LD. Antagonist muscle activity during stretching: a paradox reassessed. Med Sci Sports Exerc 1988;20:285–289.

71. Entyre BR, Abraham LD. Ache-reflex changes during static stretching and two variations of proprioceptive neuromuscular facilitation techniques. Electroencephalogr Clin Neurophysiol 1986;63:174–179.

72. Entyre BR, Lee EJ. Chronic and acute flexibility of men and women using three different stretching techniques. Res Q 1988;222:228.

73. Shindo M, Harayama H, Kondo K, et al. Changes in reciprocal Ia inhibition during voluntary contraction in man. Exp Brain Res 1984;53:400–408.

74. Zachazewski JE. Flexibility for sport. In: Sanders B, ed. Sports Physical Therapy. Norwalk, CT: Appleton & Lange, 1990.

75. Zachazewski JE. Improving flexibility. In: Scully RM, Barnes MR, eds. Physical Therapy. Philadelphia, PA: JB Lippincott, 1989.

76. Mahieu NN, McNair P, DeMuynck M, et al. Effect of static and ballistic stretchign on the muscle-tendon tissue properties. Med Sci Sports Exerc 2007;39(3):494–501.

77. Gajdosik RL, Allred JD, Gabbert HL, et al. A stretching program increases the dynamic passive length and passive resistive properties of the calf muscle-tendon unit of unconditioned younger women. Eur J Appl Physiol 2007;99(4):449–454.

78. Hutton RS. Neuromuscular basis of stretching exercises. In: Komi PV, ed. Strength and Power in Sports. Boston, MA: Blackwell Scientific, 1992:29–38.

79. Chalmers G. Re-examination of the possible role of Golgi tendon organ and muscle spindle reflexes in proprioceptive neuromuscular facilitation muscle stretching. Sports Biomech 2004;3(1):159–183.

80. Guissard N, Duchateau J. Neural aspects of muscle stretching. Exer Sports Sci Rev 2006;34(4):154–158.

81. Handel M, Horstmann T, Dickhuth HH, et al. Effects of contract-relax stretching training on muscle performance in athletes. Eur J Appl Physiol 1997;76:400–408.

82. Mitchell UH, Myrer JW, Hopkins JT, et al. Acute stretch perception alteration contributes to the success of the PNF "contract-relax" stretch. J Sport Rehabil 2007;16(2):85–92.

83. Rees SS, Murphy AJ, Watsford ML, et al. Effects of proprioceptive neuromuscular facilitation stretching on stiffness and force-producing characteristics of the ankle in active women. J Strength Cond Res 2007;21(2):572–577.

84. Holt BW, Lambourne K. The impact of different warm-up protocols on vertical jump performance in male collegiate athletes. J Strength Cond Res 2008;22(1):226–229.

85. Herman SL, Smith DT. Four-week dynamic stretching warm-up intervention elicits longer-term performance benefits. J Strength Cond Res 2008; June 9 [epub ahead of print].

86. McMillian DJ, Moore JH, Hatler BS, et al. Dynamic vs. static-stretching warm up: the effect on power and agility performance. J Strength Cond Res 2006;20(3):492–499.

87. Little T, Williams AG. Effects of differential stretching protocols during warm-ups on high-speed motor capacities in professional soccer players. J Strength Cond Res 2006;20(1):203–207.

88. Ford P, McChesney J. Duration of maintained hamstring ROM following termination of three stretching protocols. J Sport Rehabil 2007;16(1):18–27.

89. Bradley PS, Olsen PD. Portas MD. The effect of static, ballistic, and proprioceptive neuromuscular facilitation stretching on vertical jump performance. J Strength Cond Res 2007;21(1):223–226.

90. Decoster LC, Cleland J, Altieri C, et al. The effects of hamstring stretching on range of motion: a systematic literature review. J Orthop Sports Phys Ther 2005;35:377–387.

91. Williams PE. Use of intermittent stretch in the prevention of serial sarcomere loss in immobilized muscle. Ann Rheum Dis 1994;49:316–317.

92. Coutinho E, Gomes AR, Franca CN, et al. Effect of passive stretching on the immobilized soleus muscle fiber morphology. Braz J Med Biol Res 2004;37:1853–1861.

93. Beedle BB, Leydig SN, Carnucci JM. No differences in pre- and postexercise stretching on flexibility. J Strength Cond Res 2007;21(3):780–783.

94. Bazett-Jones DM, Gibson MH, McBride JM. Sprint and vertical jump performances are not affected by six weeks of static hamstring stretching. J Strength Cond Res 2008;22(1):25–31.

95. Woods K, Bishop P, Jones E. Warm-up and stretching in the prevention of muscular injury. Sports Med 2007;37(12):1089–1099.

96. Kokkonen J, Nelson AG, Eldredge C, Winchester JB. Chronic static stretching improves exercise performance. Med Sci Sports Exerc 2007;39(10):1825–1831.

97. Tillman LJ, Cummings GS. Biologic mechanisms of connective tissue mutability. In: Currier DP, Nelson RM, ed. Dynamics of Human Biologic Tissues. Philadelphia, PA: FA Davis, 1992.

98. Anderson B, Burke ER. Scientific, medical and practical aspects of stretching. Clin Sports Med 1991;10:63–86.

99. Magnusson SP, Aagard P, Simonson EB, et al. A biomechanical evaluation of cyclic and static stretch in human skeletal muscle. Int J Sports Med 1998;19:310–316.

100. Magnusson SP, Aagard P, Simonson EB, et al. Passive tensile stress and energy of the human hamstring muscles in vivo. Scan J Med Sci Sports Exerc 2000;10:351–359.

101. Magnusson SP. Passive properties of human skeletal muscle during stretch maneuvers. A review. Scan J Med Sci Sports Exerc 1998;8:65–77.

102. Stopka C, Morley K, Siders R, Schuette J, et al. Stretching techniques to improve flexibility in Special Olympics athletes and their coaches. J Sport Rehab 2002;11:22–34.

103. Hagbarth KE, Hagglund JV, Nordin M, et al. Thixotropic behavior of human finger flexor muscles with accompanying changes in spindle and reflex responses to stretch. J Physiol 1985;368:323–342.

104. DePino GM, Webright WG, Arnold BL. Duration of maintained hamstring flexibility after cessation of an acute static stretching protocol. J Athletic Train 2000;35:56–59.

105. Feland JB, Myrer JW, Schulthies SS, et al. The effect of duration of stretching of the hamstring muscle group for increasing range of motion in people aged 65 years or older. Phys Ther 2001;81:1110–1117.

106. Godges JJ, MacRae H, Longdon C, et al. The effects of two stretching procedures on hip range of motion and gait economy. J Orthop Sports Phys Ther 1989;10:350–357.

107. Worrell TW, Smith TL, Winegardner J. Effect of hamstring stretching on hamstring muscle performance. J Orthop Sports Phys Ther 1994;20:154–159.

108. Wilson GJ, Murphy AJ, Pryor JF. Musculotendinous stiffness: its relationship to eccentric, isometric, and concentric performance. J Appl Physiol 1994;76:2714–2719.

109. Stauber WT, Miller GR, Grimmett JG, et al. Adaptation of rat soleus muscles to 4 wk of intermittent strain. J Appl Physiol 1994;77:58–62.

110. Ferreira GN, Teixeira-Salmela LF, Guimaraes CQ. Gains in flexibility related to measures of muscular performance: impact of flexibility on muscular performance. Clin J Sport Med 2007;17(4):276–281.

111. Rubini EC, Costa AL, Gomes PS. The effects of stretching on strength performance. Sports Med 2007;37(3):213–224.

112. Fletcher IM, Anness R. The acute effects of combined static and dynamic stretch protocols on fifty-meter sprint performance in track-and-field athletes. J Strength Cond Res 2007 21(3):784–787.

113. Siatras TA, Mittas VP, Mameietzi SN, et al. The duration of the inhibitory effects with static stretching on quadriceps peak torque production. J Strength Cond Res 2008;22(1):40–46.

114. Kinser AM, Ramsey MW, O'Bryant HS, et al. Vibration and stretching effects on flexibility and explosive strength in young gymnasts. Med Sci Sports Exerc 2007;(40)1:133–140.

115. Wallmann HW, Gillis CB, Martinez NJ. The effects of different stretching techniques of the quadriceps muscles on agility performance in female collegiate soccer athletes: a pilot study. N Am J Sports Phys Ther 2008;3(1):41–47.

116. Behm DG, Bambury A, Cahill F, et al. Effect of acute static stretching on force, balance, reaction time and movement time. Med Sci Sports Exerc 2004;36(8):1397–1402.

117. Brandenburg JP. Duration of stretch does not influence the degree of force loss following static stretching. J Sports Med Phys Fitness 2006;46(4):526–534.

118. Trudel G, Zhou J, Uthoff HK, et al. Four weeks of mobility after 8 weeks of immobility fails to restore normal motion: a preliminary study. Clin Orthop Relat Res 2008;466(5):1239–1244.

119. Steffen TM, Mollinger LA. Low-load, prolonged stretch in the treatment of knee flexion contractures in nursing home residents. Phys Ther 1995;75:886–897.

120. Matsumoto F, Trudel G, Uhthoff HK, et al. Mechanical effects of immobilization on the Achilles tendon. Arch Phys Med Rehabil 2003;84:662–667.

121. Yasuda T, Kinoshita M, Shibayama Y. Unfavorable effect of knee immobilization on Achilles tendon healing in rabbits. Acta Orthop Scand 2000;71:69–73.

122. Usuba M, Akai M, Shirasaki Y, et al. Experimental joint contracture correction with low torque - long duration repeated stretching. Clin Orthop Rel Res 2007;456:70–78.

123. Branch TP, Karsch RE, Mills TJ, et al. Mechanical therapy for loss of knee flexion. Am J Orthop. 2003;32(4):195–200.

124. Logerstedt D, Sennett BJ. Case series utilizing drop-out casting for the treatment of knee joint extension motion loss following anterior cruciate ligament reconstruction. J Orthop Sports Phys Ther 2007;37(7):404–411.

125. McClure PW, Blackburn LG, Dusold C. The use of splints in the treatment of joint stiffness: biologic rationale and an algorithm for making clinical decisions. Phys Ther 1994;74(12):1101–1107.

126. Guide to Physical Therapist Practice. 2nd Ed. 2001;81:S680.

127. Maitland GD. Vertebral manipulation. 5th Ed. Boston, MA: Butterworth, 1986.

128. Kaltenborn FM. The spine: basic evaluation and mobilization techniques. Minneapolis, MN: Orthopedic Physical Therapy Products, 1993.

129. Hsu AT, Hedman T, Chang JH, et al. Changes in abduction and rotation range of motion in response to simulated dorsal and ventral translational mobilization of the glenohumeral joint. Phys Ther 2002;82:544–556.

130. Roubal PJ, Dobritt D, Placzek JD. Glenohumeral gliding manipulation following interscalene brachial plexus block in patients with adhesive capsulitis. J Orthop Sports Phys Ther 1996;24:66–77.

131. Vermeulen HM, Obermann WR, Burger BJ, et al. End-range mobilization techniques in adhesive capsulitis of the shoulder joint: a multiple-subject case report. Phys Ther 2000;80:1204–1213.

132. Howell SM, Glainat BJ, Renzi AJ, et al. Normal and abnormal mechanics of the glenohumeral joint in the horizontal plane. J Bone Joint Surg 1988;70A:227–232.

133. Harryman DT II, Sidles JA, Clark JA, et al. Translation of the humeral head on the glenoid with passive glenohumeral motion. J Bone Joint Surg 1990;72A:1334–1343.

134. Elvey RL, Hall T. Neural tissue evaluation and treatment. In: Donatelli RA, ed. Physical Therapy of the Shoulder. 4th Ed. St. Louis, MO: Churchill Livingstone, 2004.

135. Butler DS. Mobilisation of the Nervous System. St. Louis, MO: Churchill Livingstone, 1999.

136. Butler DS. The Sensitive Nervous System. Adelaide, Australia: Noigroup Publications, 2000.

137. Zane Y, Golden. The Ultimate Body Rolling Workout. New York, NY: Broadway Books, 2003.

138. Williams PE, Golkspink G. Changes in sarcomere length and physiological properties in immobilized muscle. J Anat 1978:127:459–468.

139. Bandy WD, Irion JM. The effect of time of static stretch on the flexibility of the hamstring muscles. Phys Ther 1994;74:845–852.

140. Lentell G, Hetherington T, Eagan J, et al. The use of thermal agents to influence the effectiveness of a low-load prolonged stretch. J Orthop Sports Phys Ther 1992;5:200–207.

141. Madding SW, Wong JG, Hallum A, et al. Effects of duration of passive stretching on hip abduction range of motion. J Orthop Sports Phys Ther 1987;8:409–416.

142. Cipriani D, Abel B, Pirrwitz D. A comparison of two stretching protocols on hip range of motion: implications for total daily stretch duration. J Strength Cond Res 2003;17(2):274–278.

143. Beynnon BD, Fleming BC, Johnson RJ, et al. Anterior cruciate ligament strain behavior during rehabilitation exercises in vivo. Am J Sports Med 1995;23:24–33.

144. Yack HJ, Collins CE, Whieldon TJ. Comparison of closed and open kinetic chain exercise in the anterior cruciate ligament-deficient knee. Am J Sports Med 1993;21:49–54.

145. Graham VL, Gehlsen GM, Edwards JA. Electromyographic evaluation of close and open kinetic chain knee rehabilitation exercises. J Athletic Training 1993;28:23–31.

146. Gryzlo SM, Patek RM, Pink M, et al. Electromyographic analysis of knee rehabilitation exercises. J Orthop Sports Phys Ther 1994;20:36–43.

147. Marsden CD, Obeso JA, Rothwell JC. The function of the antagonist muscle during fast limb movements in man. J Physiol 1983;335:1–13.

148. Wierzbicka MM, Wiegner AW, Shahani BT. The role of agonist and antagonist in fast arm movements in man. Exp Brain Res 1986;63:331–340.

149. Servedio FJ. Normal growth and development. Ortho Phys Ther Clin North Am 1997;6:417–437.

150. Santonja Medina FM, Sainz De Baranda Andujar P, Rodriguez Garcia PL, et al. Effects of frequency of static stretching on straight-leg raise in elementary school children. J Sports Med Phys Fitness 2007;47(3):304–308.
151. Harris SR, Lundgren BD. Joint mobilization for children with central nervous system disorders: indications and precautions. Phys Ther 1991;71:890–895.
152. Booth FW, Weeden SH. Structural aspects of aging human skeletal muscle. In: Buckwalter JA, Goldberg VM, Woo SL-Y, eds. Musculoskeletal Soft-Tissue Aging: Impact on Mobility. Rosemont, IL: American Academy of Orthopaedic Surgeons, 1993.
153. Schultz AB. Biomechanics of mobility impairment in the elderly. In: Buckwalter JA, Goldberg VM, Woo SL-Y, eds. Musculoskeletal Soft-Tissue Aging: Impact on Mobility. Rosemont, IL: American Academy of Orthopaedic Surgeons, 1993.
154. Walker JM, Sue D, Miles-Elkousy N, et al. Active mobility of the extremities in older subjects. Phys Ther 1984;64:919–923.
155. Lehmann JF, Masock AJ, Warren CG, et al. Effect of therapeutic temperatures on tendon extensibility. Arch Phys Med Rehabil 1970;51:481–487.
156. Rigby JF, Hirai N, Spikes JD, et al. The mechanical properties of rat tail tendon. J Gen Physiol 1959;43:265–283.
157. Rigby JF. The effect of mechanical extension upon the thermal stability of collagen. Biochem Biophys Acta 1964;79:334–363.
158. Warren CG, Lehmann JF, Koblanski JM, et al. Elongation of rat tail tendon: effect of load and temperature. Arch Phys Med Rehabil 1971;52:465–474.
159. Draper DO, Ricard MD. Rate of temperature decay in human muscle following 3 MHz ultrasound: the stretching window revealed. J Athletic Training 1996;30:304–307.
160. Rose S, Draper DO, Schulties SS, et al. The stretching window part two: rate of thermal decay in deep muscle following 1-MHz ultrasound. J Athletic Training 1996;31:139–143.
161. Michlovitz S, ed. Thermal Agents in Rehabilitation. 2nd Ed. Philadelphia, PA: FA Davis, 1990.
162. Reed BV, Ashikaga T, Fleming BC, et al. Effects of ultrasound and stretch on knee ligament extensibility. J Orthop Sports Phys Ther 2000;30:341–347.
163. Enwemeka CS, Rodriguez O, Mendosa S. The biomechanical effects of low-intensity ultrasound on healing tendons. Ultrasound Med Biol 1990;16:801–807.
164. Ramirez A, Schwane JA, McFarland C, et al. The effect of ultrasound on collagen synthesis and fibroblast proliferation in vitro. Med Sci Sports Exerc 1997;29:326–332.

chapter 8

Impaired Balance

COLIN GROVE, JUDITH DEWANE, AND LORI THEIN BRODY

Balance is an important consideration when rehabilitating patients with a variety of disorders, and balance training is increasingly being integrated into clinical practice.[1-4] Health conditions may result in or from impaired balance. For example, a patient who has undergone an anterior cruciate ligament reconstruction following a basketball injury may have residual impairments in single leg stance ability. Alternatively, a patient with impaired balance due to Parkinson disease may fall resulting in a hip fracture and increased mobility-related disability. The rehabilitation plan of care for each of these patients should include a balance component.

DEFINITIONS

Balance is the ability to maintain equilibrium or the ability to maintain the center of mass (COM) relative to the base of support (BOS).[5] Postural stability or sway is the normal, continuous shifting of the body's center of gravity (COG) over the BOS. Balance (postural stability) is maintained when a person is able to keep her sway within the limits of stability (LOS) or her maximum angle of displacement from vertical before losing equilibrium. Individuals rely on a variety of balance strategies (coordinated neuromuscular synergies) to maintain postural stability. When sway approaches the LOS, a corrective strategy is necessary to maintain stability. Thus, these limits represent the spatial area in which the individual can maintain equilibrium without changing her BOS. A certain amount of anteroposterior and lateral sway normally occur while maintaining balance. This sway envelope defines the LOS in anterior, posterior, and lateral directions. Normal anteroposterior sway in adults is 12 degrees from the most posterior to the most anterior position.[6] Lateral stability limits vary with foot spacing and height. An average-height adult with 4 in between the feet can sway approximately 16 degrees from side to side.[6] This stability limit is often characterized by a cone of stability (Fig. 8-1A and B). As long as the individual's sway envelope stays within the cone of stability, balance is maintained. When the COG is aligned in the middle of the sway envelope, the 12 degrees of anteroposterior sway and 16 degrees of lateral sway can easily occur.

The strategies that govern stability without causing a change in the BOS are known as in-place strategies. If sway exceeds the LOS, another type of corrective strategy must be employed to regain balance. These are referred to as change-in-support strategies and are used by the individual to establish a new BOS. Both types of strategies result from highly coordinated balance functions.

Coordination is defined as the ability to perform smooth, accurate, and controlled movements.[5,7] Coordination is necessary for the execution of fine motor skills such as writing, sewing, dressing, and the manipulation of small objects. Coordination is also necessary when performing gross motor skills such as walking, running, jumping, occupational tasks, and basic and instrumental activities of daily living. Coordinated movements are characterized by proper sequencing and timing of synergistic and reciprocal muscle activity. The proactive (preparatory) anticipatory postural adjustments and the reactive automatic postural response functions of the balance system that support all skilled movement share the characteristics of coordinated movements.

Skilled activities (throwing, kicking, hopping, and running) are not possible without appropriate balance function.[8] Thus, the concepts of coordination and balance are highly interrelated. However, despite their integrated relationship, balance and coordinated movements are felt to be controlled separately.[9] Evidence of the integration of these separately controlled functions is found in the observation of reprogramming of postural responses prior to measured changes in focal movement during a changing task or environmental context.[10]

Maintenance of balance requires that individuals have the ability to maintain a position of stability before, during, and immediately after voluntary activities, as well as the ability to react to external perturbations.[11,12] Balance functions also enable individuals to protect the body in the event of a fall[10] and allow for clear vision during head and/or body movements. A significant contributing factor to a person's ability to manage balance within her LOS is the position of the COG relative to the BOS. If an individual's COG is aligned more anterior, posterior, or lateral than center, a smaller sway envelop is tolerated before losing balance (see Fig. 8-1C).[6] For example, persons with Parkinson disease or with a significant thoracic kyphosis secondary to osteoporosis may have a static or dynamic anterior posture, decreasing tolerance for anterior sway. Alternatively, persons who have undergone right total knee arthroplasty or have sustained a left middle cerebral artery stroke may stand with their COG displaced toward the left and walk with a decreased ability to effectively load weight onto the right leg. This lateral postural displacement may increase this individual's risk for falling to the left.

Balance is far more complex than a simple relationship between the COG and the BOS. Effective and efficient performance and integration of multiple body systems is required for postural stability.[13] Specifically, stability is accomplished through the interaction of biomechanical (articular and muscular), sensory feedback (somatosensory, visual, and vestibular), self-perception (orientation in space, subjective postural, subjective visual vertical) dynamic control (control of walking and navigation), neuromuscular integration (neuromuscular synergies and adaptive and anticipatory action), cognitive processing (multitasking,

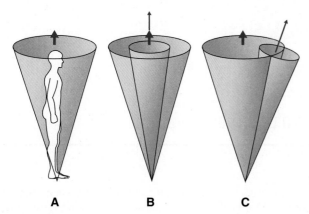

A   **B**   **C**

FIGURE 8-1. Relationships of the limits of stability, the sway envelope, and the center of gravity (COG) alignment. (A) The limits of stability are described by a cone-shaped sway envelope. (B) When the COG is aligned in the center, the sway envelope remains within the limits of stability. (C) When the COG is offset, as in a forward leaning posture, the sway envelope exceeds the limits of stability, and a balance restoration strategy must be implemented to regain balance.

information processing), affective (motivation and preferences), and cardiopulmonary (activity tolerance) systems. Figure 8-3 describes postural control and orientation from this perspective. Impairment in any of these systems can lead to altered balance and mobility function. A detailed examination enables the clinician to determine the system or systems at fault and drives treatment for impaired balance. Successful interventions also depend on the clinician's ability to prioritize interventions based on the relative impact of each underlying impairment in relationship to each other and the resulting activity limitations, participation restrictions, and mobility-related disability. See Building Block 8-1.

PHYSIOLOGY OF BALANCE

Identifying causes of and prescribing treatment for balance impairment requires an understanding of the various influences on balance control and their normal interactions. Again, biomechanical, sensory, self-perception, neural integrative, cognitive, and affective systems each directly influence balance control. The individual must effectively and efficiently process contributions from these systems within the central nervous system (CNS), then choose and execute an appropriate movement strategy. The actual movement or task performance, as well as the interaction with the environment must then be evaluated for accuracy and corrective action must be taken as necessary. An ecological model (Fig. 8-2) describes these interactions among the individual, the environment, and the functional task, with a circular network of domains demonstrating the integration of balance functions.[5,14] Any of these domains may dominate depending on the particular context.

Additionally, other individual body systems, such as the circulatory, respiratory, and integumentary systems, indirectly influence balance and mobility via the effects of disease, damage, or suboptimal function. For example, consider a patient with peripheral vascular disease who has swelling in the lower extremities and the subsequent impact of limitations in range of motion on balance reactions. Alternatively, consider the impact a venous stasis ulcer on the plantar surface of the foot has on weight acceptance a patient with diabetes mellitus.

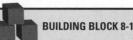

BUILDING BLOCK 8-1

A 75 year-old woman with multiple sclerosis (MS) presents to your clinic for evaluation and treatment of her gait instability following a recent fall. The patient fractured her right wrist as a result of the fall. The fracture was surgically repaired and she has recently been cleared for full weight bearing through her right hand. Prior to the fall, the patient had been using a front-wheeled walker for several years due to decreased stability while walking. In fact, she has fallen four times in the past year. You note that she stops walking whenever she tries to converse with you on the way to the exam room. Her past medical history is significant for the additional problems of depression, an anal cyst, and hypertension. She is taking multiple medications, including disease modifying agents, a benzodiazepine, prescription pain medication, a selective serotonin uptake inhibitor, and a calcium channel blocker. She lives alone in the home that she bought with her husband 40 years ago. There are three steps to enter the home that have a railing on the right side for ascending. Her three adult children live more than 2 hours away. The patient relies on volunteers for transportation since she is unable to drive. In fact, she rarely leaves her home. One of her regular companions spends 3 hours a day helping her with household chores and with completing her home exercise program for residual muscle weakness and adaptive shortening her right wrist and hand.

Give this woman's history, hypothesize impairments from each of the domains just discussed that you might find upon examination.

The primary systems that influence balance and mobility are depicted in Figure 8-3. Each of these systems is considered to be within the individual domain. The role of the integumentary system in balance typically occurs in select situations. Thus, this system will not be addressed further herein. Additionally, the influence of the cardiopulmonary

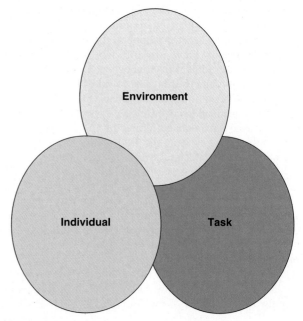

FIGURE 8-2. Ecological model of motor behavior.

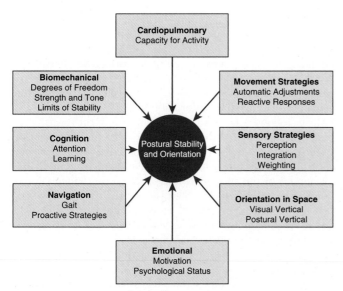

FIGURE 8-3. Systems model of postural stability and orientation.

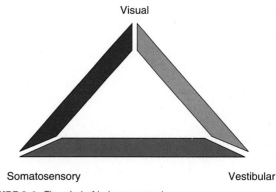

FIGURE 8-4. The triad of balance control.

system will not be considered further in this chapter. Refer to Chapter 6 for further information regarding examination and treatment of impaired aerobic capacity and endurance.

Biomechanical Contributions

An individual's LOS are largely a function of the size of the BOS and any impairments in biomechanical, sensory, or neural structure or function in the lower extremities. Individuals who are prone to falling tend to have smaller LOS.[15] The most important biomechanical constraint on balance is the size and quality of the BOS, the feet.[13] Any limitation in size, strength, range of motion, pain, or control of the feet will result in impaired balance.[16] Additionally, changes in lower extremity strength, range of motion, and flexibility can cause restrictions in moving the body on the BOS, and effect balance control. As previously stated, suboptimal postural alignment also affects balance control. In addition to primary biomechanical impairments, impairments in biomechanics may develop secondary to impairments iVn other systems, such as a patient with vestibular dysfunction who presents with complaints of pain and stiffness in the cervical region as a result of self-restriction of head movement.

Contributions of the Sensory Systems

Three sensory systems contribute to the maintenance of upright posture and orientation: somatosensory, visual, and vestibular. They are considered to be the sensory triad of postural control (Fig. 8-4). No single sense directly determines the position of the body's COG; the combined feedback from each system must be integrated. The somatosensory system gathers information from the individual (e.g., position of one body segment versus another or the position of the COG relative to the BOS), as well as the environment (e.g., various surface characteristics). The visual system provides information about task performance (e.g., orientation of the body relative to the task) and environmental cues (e.g., position relative to other objects, orientation to vertical, and environmental motion). The vestibular system provides an internal reference and final pathway, providing information about orientation of the head relative to gravity and movement of the head through space.[17]

Somatosensory Neurophysiology

The somatosensory system plays an important role in regulating posture and orientation. Information must be detected peripherally and transmitted centrally for processing. The peripheral receptors are an important source of that information. When a person steps onto a rug that slips beneath her foot, the acceleration of the slipping limb provides the first information to the balance system about impending peril. Information from the somatosensory system arises from peripheral sources such as the muscle, joint capsule, and other soft tissue structures. A variety of somatosensory receptors, each with unique functions and features, together provide information about movement and joint position. Information from these receptors is relayed to the medulla and brain stem through the dorsal column medial-lemniscal pathway.[17] This information assists in coordinating eye, head, and neck movements to stabilize the visual system and in maintaining postures and coordinated movement patterns.[18] The influence of each different form of somatosensory input varies. For example, joint afferent information does not contribute to a conscious sense of position.[18,19] This conclusion is based on studies in which local anesthetization of joint tissues failed to reduce joint position awareness and total joint replacement did not diminish joint position sense.[20] However, loss of proprioception function in the lower extremities has been associated with higher rates of falling.[21]

Visual Neurophysiology

The visual system contributes significant information about the body's position and movement in space. Vision plays a primary role in anticipatory postural control.[22] Incoming information from the visual system is used to preset the postural system for an anticipated change or perturbation.[22] The visual system provides information about the position of the head relative to the environment and orients the head to maintain level gaze. This system contributes significantly to head and neck posture. Vision can also function as visual proprioception when it gives information about the relationship of one body part to another.[22] The visual system also provides information about the movement of surrounding objects, thereby providing information about the speed of movement. Information entering the visual system travels through the optic nerve to the lateral geniculate nucleus (LGN) of the thalamus to the superior colliculus and through a few fibers to the inferior olivary nuclei. The LGN receives the largest projection and is the first center where information from the retina is represented.[22,23] From here, neurons project to the primary visual cortex in the occipital lobe (Brodmann area 17). As essential as vision is to anticipatory control, it is possible to balance without vision such as walking in the dark. In addition, visual inputs can be an inaccurate source of orientation information about self-motion. The visual system has been shown to have difficulty distinguishing between self-motion and object motion.[22]

Vestibular Neurophysiology

The vestibular system provides information on orientation of the head in space with respect to gravity and on acceleration. The vestibular system provides the gravito-inertial frame of reference for postural control.[22] Any movement of the head, including weight shifts to adjust posture, stimulate the vestibular receptors. There are two types of vestibular receptors, the semicircular canals and the otoliths of the macula. The semicircular canals function as angular accelerometers, and sense angular acceleration of the head.[22] The otoliths sense linear position and linear acceleration. The semicircular canals are particularly sensitive to fast head movements, while the otoliths respond mostly to slow head movements such as those movements during postural sway.[22] The vestibular nerve (cranial nerve VIII) projects to the vestibular nuclei and to the cerebellum. In fact, the vestibular system is the only sensory system that has direct, monosynaptic input to the cerebellum. The vestibular nuclei also receive input from other sensory systems, including the visual system. From the vestibular nuclei, two vestibulospinal tracts descend to the spinal cord for postural control.[23] Ascending projections include fibers to oculomotor nuclei to control eye movements and stabilize gaze via the vestibular ocular reflex. Ascending fibers also project via thalamic relays to the head of the caudate nucleus and to the parietal association area, where the information is integrated with other sensory information.

Interestingly, the vestibular system alone cannot provide the CNS a completely accurate picture of how the head and/or body is/are moving in space. The vestibular system is not able to distinguish between a simple head nod (head moving on a stable body) from a forward bend from the hips (head moving in concert with moving trunk).[22]

Neural Integration and Processing of Sensory Information

It is generally believed that the nervous system maintains an internal representation of the body in space. Balance control involves both postural and visual vertical orientation in space. Effective motor control depends on the accuracy of the internal maps of body and spatial orientation. Damage to the sensory systems or CNS may lead to impaired orientation in space. For example, the internal representation of visual, but not postural, vertical is tilted in individuals with unilateral vestibular loss.[24] However, the internal representation of postural, but not visual vertical, is tilted in individuals with hemi-neglect due to stroke.[24]

After information arrives from peripheral receptors, the information must be analyzed. Since no one sensory system can completely detail the body's position in space, the relative contributions from each system and integration of each system's information are critical. Integration and processing of incoming information occurs in the cerebellum, basal ganglia, and supplementary motor area.[25] The time required to process this information is important, particularly when a quick response is necessary. In adults, muscle response latencies to visual cues signaling perturbations to balance are slow, approximately 200 ms, compared to somatosensory responses that are activated in 80 to 100 ms.[22] Thus, the somatosensory system information is generally processed fastest, followed by the information from the visual and vestibular systems.[22,25] Researchers suggest that the nervous system preferentially relies on somatosensory inputs for controlling body sway when imbalance occurs from rapid displacement of the support surface.[22] However, balance function is also determined by the task and the context in which that task is being performed. Thus, the nervous system also needs information about the intended task and must resolve and ambiguity in sensory feedback from the environment in order to generate appropriate postural alignment, adjustments, and reactions.

Sensory organization is the process of resolving conflicting input; it is necessary because incoming information from a system may be inaccurate. For example, consider sitting stationary on a train in a station when an adjacent train begins moving forward. The visual system alone is unable to detect whether the adjacent train is moving forward or your train is moving backward. The brain must resolve inaccurate input from the visual system with the accurate information from the somatosensory and vestibular systems. Certain types of information from the visual system (e.g., moving visual fields) and the somatosensory system (e.g., moving sidewalks, compliant surfaces) are susceptible to error. Additionally, if an injury decreases the information processing rate, balance may be impaired. In fact, individuals with sensory loss from any sensory modality are limited in their ability to reweight (adjust the emphasis) sensory information as required by changes in environmental context, and, thus, are at increased risk for falling in certain situations.[15] If a single sensory system is impaired, other systems may adequately compensate for this impairment in most environmental contexts, and this concept is the basis for many treatment programs. However, balance may be significantly impaired if multiple sensory systems are damaged. See Building Block 8-2.

Generating Motor Output—Movement Strategies

After the sensory information is transmitted centrally, the information is processed, and a response is selected, the response output must be executed. This process is referred to as motor organization. The process of motor response organization involves the execution of coordinated and properly

BUILDING BLOCK 8-2

Consider the impact of impairments in specific sensory systems. Patients with impairment in the somatosensory system are more likely to demonstrate imbalance in which conditions? In which environmental contexts would you anticipate persons with vestibular impairments to show the greatest instability?

scaled neuromuscular synergies[26] to counteract either internal or external perturbations of the COM. Normal voluntary movement is dependent upon complex excitation and inhibition of muscular contractions, accurately controlled in force and extent, and appropriately organized in space and time, with a number of relevant postural adjustments[27] in the head and neck, trunk, and extremities.[8] Complex movements take longer to process and program than simple tasks. Motor processes develop early, resembling adult performance between ages 3 and 4 years.[26] Motor response programming is influenced by the movement and is the stage most often manipulated in treatment.[28]

The systems-level model of postural control proposed by Riach and Hayes[29] suggests that normal postural control is dependent on the parallel and integrated maturation of specific feedback and feedforward mechanisms. The feedback mechanisms of postural control are the automatic postural responses; these include the labyrinthine righting reflex, vestibulo-collic reflex, vestibulo-spinal reflex, and functional stretch reflexes. The feedforward mechanisms involve preparatory adjustments in body position that accompany a variety of activities.

Automatic Postural Responses

Although a multitude of postural responses are available when someone is destabilized, two broad classes of automatic responses are common. The automatic postural responses are classically referred to as the ankle, hip, protective extension, and stepping strategies and are characterized by stereotypical neuromuscular activation patterns. The ankle and hip strategies are in-place strategies since the BOS does not change. Alternatively, the protective extension and stepping strategies are change-in-support strategies. These responses are considered automatic due to their short response latencies. The earliest response latencies to surface perturbations are at 70 to 180 ms, much longer than stretch reflex latencies of 40 to 50 ms, but shorter than volitional reaction times of 180 to 250 ms.[14] This suggests that balance is learned and therefore trainable. These preprogrammed strategies (or synergies) are the fundamental movement unit engaged when balance is disturbed.[5,12,14]

Rather than determining which muscles to activate and when, the brain only needs to recognize which synergy to engage to meet the task demands in the particular environment, when to engage it, and at what intensity to respond. This is an example of synergistic neuromuscular control. These synergies have characteristics of feedforward (open loop) control, as the movement occurs too fast to rely solely on sensory feedback. Responses are also preprogrammed and automatic. These postural reactions are best described in terms of feedback control, or closed loop control. Selection of these movement patterns is triggered initially by sensory feedback. Sensory feedback experiences throughout development help the CNS learn the rules used to engage these strategies. Treatment procedures for reactive balance control impairments focus on eliciting these preprogrammed synergies to maintain postural control. However, remember that the motor output is situation dependent. The response to a stimulus will vary depending upon the environment in which it is elicited. Thus, be sure to vary the treatment environment; this allows the patient to develop movement strategies in a variety of situations.

The ankle strategy is the most commonly used, particularly when displacements are small. The ankle synergy displaces the

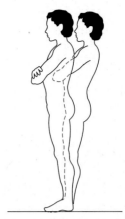

FIGURE 8-5. Ankle strategy in response to small perturbations.

COG primarily by rotation about the ankle joint (Fig. 8-5). This is accomplished as posterior displacement of the COG results in activation of the anterior tibialis, quadriceps, and abdominals to control the backward movement in typically developing children and healthy adults. Conversely, anterior displacement of the COG produces activation of the gastrocnemius, hamstring, and trunk extensors to slow the forward movement. Muscle activation on the stretched side of the body proceeds in a distal to proximal direction in both situations.[14,25]

The hip strategy is employed when ankle motion is limited, when the displacement is greater, or when standing on an unstable surface so that the ankle strategy is not effective. The hip strategy effectively produces rapid corrections making it the strategy of choice in situations where the perturbation is rapid and/or near the LOS. In this case, a posterior displacement of the COG (i.e., anterior translation of the surface) results in a backward sway with activation of the hamstring and paraspinal muscles (Fig. 8-6). Anterior displacement of the COG (i.e., posterior translation of the surface) produces forward sway with contraction of the abdominal and quadriceps muscles. In each case, the muscle activation on the unstretched side of the body proceeds from proximal to distal in an attempt to return the COG over the BOS. Little ankle activity occurs in this synergy.

If the displacement is great enough, the stepping strategy may be used to return the BOS under the COG. A forward, backward, or lateral step is elicited to regain postural control

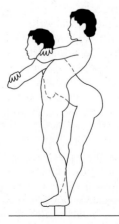

FIGURE 8-6. Hip strategy in response to larger perturbations.

in these circumstances. Most healthy individuals use the ankle strategy first, with the hip strategy employed in cases of limited ankle movement or greater displacement. However, factors such as age, risk for falling, and the presence of disease significantly influence which balance strategies are employed and may result in specific types of balance impairments. For example, elderly individuals who are at increased risk for falling tend to use hip, protective extension, and stepping strategies more frequently than those who are not at increased risk.[30]

Though early research identified three fundamental movement strategies to maintain equilibrium (ankle, hip, and the stepping strategies),[14,25] more recent studies suggest that these strategies rarely occur in isolation.[13] Additionally, the selection and execution of these strategies depends on the intensity of the disruption, the relative location of the COG to the LOS, the individual's awareness, and the individual's posture at the time of perturbation.[25]

In addition, underlying balance impairments may vary within a specific patient population. For example, individuals with Parkinson disease who demonstrate poorly coordinated automatic postural reactions show instability with external perturbations.[13] However, those with abnormalities in anticipatory postural adjustments show instability during self-initiated tasks.[13] Thus, knowledge of the individual's diagnosis is not sufficient to guide rehabilitation interventions. A careful and thorough examination encompassing each of the subsystems of balance control is needed.

Anticipatory Postural Adjustments

Volitional movements, such as reaching, stepping, or lifting objects cause displacements of the COM. A healthy individual is able to anticipate the postural requirements of tasks such as these and generate proactive movement strategies that prevent destabilization secondary to self-generated postural perturbations. These anticipatory postural adjustments represent feedforward mechanisms of postural control. Feedforward (or open loop) control characterizes actions that occur without sensory feedback. There are several examples of this type of postural adjustment. First, consider that the tibialis anterior on the contralateral limb fires just prior to step initiation of the ipsilateral limb in order to pull the COM forward and over the stance limb.[31] Second, electromyographic data shows that lower extremity muscles are the first to fire during reaching activities.[32] Third, during rising onto the toes, the gastrocnemius and soleus muscles are inhibited 150 ms prior to liftoff as the tibialis anterior pulls the COM forward over the anticipated new BOS.[33]

Persons with neurologic and orthopedic conditions may demonstrate poor feedforward postural control. Patients with Parkinson disease often have impaired anticipatory postural adjustments and will become unstable during lifting tasks. Similarly, pain and muscle weakness may interfere with anticipatory adjustments following total joint replacement. Some individuals, such as those with multifactorial dysequilibrium, may have difficulty with feedback and feedforward control mechanisms. It is often difficult to separate the feedforward and feedback aspects of postural control in a given task. Many tasks require both processes and these control mechanisms operate in parallel with each other. Careful analysis of postural control during task performance leads to a better understanding of impairments related to motor organization, and thus, more targeted treatment interventions.

Control of Walking—Navigation

Many of the concepts described thus far can also be applied to understanding adaptive control of walking. Patla[34] provides further insights into the requirements of adaptive gait. The nervous system must set up the body's initial posture and orientation necessary to initiate walking. Muscle activation patterns needed to propel the body in the intended direction must be determined, executed, and coordinated. The individual must be able to initiate and terminate walking as desired. Dynamic stability must be maintained as the body encounters both expected and unexpected destabilizing forces during movement. The individual must also be able to modulate locomotor patterns to accommodate for obstacles, changing terrain, and time constraints. The ability to navigate toward a point that is not seen is often required. Locomotor systems must also minimize fuel consumption and maximize structural integrity to promote longevity. The nervous system employs reactive, predictive, and proactive control strategies to accomplish these goals.[34] Reactive and predictive control of walking involves context-specific, neuromuscular synergies analogous to automatic postural responses and anticipatory postural adjustments involved during stance control. Proactive control strategies involve visually guided mechanisms used for obstacle avoidance or to alter global locomotor patterns in response to perceived or observed hazards in the environment.[34] For example, consider that walking characteristics change as one approaches a patch of ice on the sidewalk, even in advance of detecting any loss of traction under the feet.

Balance impairments related to any of the requirements for adaptive gait may arise related to a variety of health conditions. Persons with limited hip range of motion secondary to osteoarthritis may have difficulty setting up the posture required to initiate walking. An individual with cerebellar ataxia may demonstrate instability in waking due to problems coordinating muscle activation patterns or may have difficulty terminating walking at the appropriate time. Also consider the impact macular degeneration may have on an individual's ability to effectively recognize and avoid hazards in her path. The clinician can choose from a variety of tests developed to assist the understanding of balance impairments specific to the task of walking in order to drive clinical decision making regarding rehabilitation of balance and mobility. See Building Block 8-3.

Higher-level Influences

Information processing resources in the CNS are constrained. As a result, attention is both limited and selective. Attention has been shown to significantly influence balance control.[35–38]

BUILDING BLOCK 8-3

The use of an assistive device, such as a front-wheeled walker is an appropriate compensatory measure for individuals with variety of balance impairments (e.g., ineffective use of postural reactions). Why would you prescribe exercises to facilitate appropriate postural movement strategies for an individual who will continue to use an assistive device after the conclusion of rehabilitation?

The effect of attention is typically measured by the degree of interference between two tasks. The degree of interference is determined by several factors, including the relative task difficulty. This concept refers to the fact that specific personal (e.g., age, pathology, medications) and environmental (e.g., noise in the treatment area) factors influence attention capacity in highly individual ways. For example, increased age and a high number of comorbid health conditions tend to increase relative task difficulty. Therefore, when examining the effects of attention on balance control, care must be taken with regard to the types of tasks that are chosen for a given individual.

The individual's focus of attention also plays a significant role. Consider whether the individual should be encouraged to have an internal or an external frame of reference when completing a specific task. Research has shown that having an internal focus of attention is associated with greater performance errors, while successful functional outcome was associated with an external focus of attention.[39] For example, asking a patient to simply focus on clearing their foot as they attempt to step over an obstacle is more effective than instructing the patient to flex their knee 70 degrees at they try to clear the object.

The limbic system, emotional resources, and coping strategies also play important roles in determining balance control. Fear of falling significantly influences behavior on multiple levels. The selection of automatic postural responses is influenced by fear of falling.[40] Individuals make choices about the mobility based on the types of threats to postural instability encountered in their environment.[41] Confidence related to balance and perception of disability secondary to dizziness have also been shown to impact rehabilitation.[42,43]

Motor Learning

The ankle, hip, and stepping strategies are examples of feedback control; but these responses are controlled by motor programs that are preprogrammed collections of motor signals with a goal of achieving a specific task. In the case of balance, the goal is restoring the COG over the BOS. Each of the motor programs contains specific information about postural set and the sequencing and timing of muscle activation. If a movement is performed repeatedly with sufficient sensory feedback, motor learning occurs and a pattern is formed that guides future performance of the motor program.[14,22]

Several models of motor learning exist in the literature. Fitts and Posner[44] proposed that the learner passes through three stages when mastering a new skill. Consider learning a new task such as playing the piano or learning to swim from this perspective. The first phase is cognitive, in which full attention to instructions, the task, and performance feedback is necessary to develop gross problem-solving strategies. Performance during this phase is marked by a larger number of large errors, extreme variability, and little insight regarding how to improve.[45] The rehabilitation professional plays a critical role in this stage of learning balance control by working with the individual to select the appropriate tasks to be mastered, providing effective instruction, and guiding the individual with appropriate external feedback. The second phase is associative, in which further development and refinement of the movement strategies and acquisition of the ability to detect and identify one's own performance errors occur.[45] The movement patterns become more efficient, although still requiring attention to the task. The goal of training is to get

BUILDING BLOCK 8-4

Consider again your patient with MS and how her cognitive impairments may affect her rehabilitation. What strategies would you use to increase the likelihood of compliance with a home exercise program and a successful treatment outcome?

the learner to the autonomous (third) stage so that the movement can occur with little thought. The ability to balance while coordinating other physical and cognitive activities is an example of functioning at the autonomous stage and is the penultimate goal of rehabilitation.

Factors such as the quality of instruction and practice and the amount of practice influence whether or not a person reaches the autonomous stage of motor learning. Continued practice alone may not move the patient toward this stage. The early phase of training a new skill requires feedback. Learning relies on intrinsic and extrinsic cues to refine the movement program. As the process moves toward the autonomous level, more feedback should become intrinsic. Thus, the learner should be encouraged to develop her own internal problem-solving skills. Consider learning to drive from home to work in a new city. In the early stage, concentration on the task is required, and the individual can be overwhelmed with sensory information (e.g., other cars, signal lights, commercial signs). As driving this path is repeated, less attention to the task is required, until the drive eventually becomes automatic. Extraneous sensory information can be filtered out and only pertinent information processed. Repeating the pattern progresses it to the automatic stage. However, the patient must continue to learn and adapt to new situations. Continued exposure to new situations such as driving in unfamiliar areas teaches the nervous system how to learn or adapt quickly and effectively to new stimuli and situations.

The same learning process is applied to balance activities. As balancing on a single leg or on a balance board becomes easy, less attention is necessary, and the task becomes automatic. The nervous system must be challenged at a new level. This can be done by changing the surface, BOS, external perturbation, or visual or vestibular input (see Self-Management: Balance Activities in Chapter 21). Continued practice at grossly similar but continuously changing tasks can enhance the patient's ability to adapt to new situations. Exactly which tasks are practiced and which treatment variables are manipulated by the clinician depends on the unique balance impairments of the individual as they relate to her function in daily life. See Building Block 8-4.

EFFECTS OF TRAINING ON BALANCE

A variety of effects have been noted with training. Some training programs emphasize base elements such as strength, mobility, and cardiorespiratory exercise, while other programs use specific postural and balance training, or some combination of activities. Population-level-fall risk reduction programs have been implemented in countries around the globe in an attempt to proactively address risk factors on a community level as well.[46,47] In a systematic review by the Cochrane

Collaboration, McClure et al.[48] suggested that effective community-based intervention programs could be instrumental in driving public health policy as a result of their impact in terms of reducing falls and fall-related injuries.

Several community-level interventions have been developed and examined. The ancient art of T'ai Chi Chuan has been studied extensively for its effects on impairments in the elderly. Lan[49] studied the effects of Tai Chi on knee extensor muscle strength and endurance. They found increases in concentric and eccentric peak torque and the knee extensor endurance ratio in both men and women. Additionally, improvements in resting heart rate, 3-minute step test heart rate, modified sit and read, total body rotation testing, and single leg stance with eyes closed were found in a Tai Chi group compared with a control group.[50] The effects of Tai Chi directly on balance have been analyzed. Tai Chi was found to reduce the risk of multiple falls by 47.5%.[51] Yan[52] found that Tai Chi participants significantly reduced their vertical pressure variability compared to a walking or jogging group. Significant improvements have been found in self-reported physical functioning, general health status, arthritis symptoms, sensory organization testing, and the Dizziness Handicap Inventory (DHI) following Tai Chi training.[53–56] However, others have found computerized balance training to produce greater improvements in balance measures than Tai Chi, suggesting that Tai Chi may delay the onset to first or multiple falls by improving confidence without actually changing sway measures.[57] This is consistent with others who found significant self-reported benefits of Tai Chi training (improvements in daily activities) compared with individualized balance training.[58]

The Cochrane Collaboration found the following interventions to be effective in minimizing the effect of or exposure to risk factors for falling in the elderly on an individual level:[59]

- multidisciplinary, multifactorial, health/environmental risk factor screenin
- individualized muscle strengthening and balance retraining, prescribed at home by a trained health professional
- home hazard assessment and modification, professionally prescribe
- withdrawal of psychotropic medication
- cardiac pacing for appropriate patient
- Tai Chi group exercise intervention

The majority of patients with balance impairments will require skilled, individualized interventions that target the specific underlying impairments contributing to instability. The literature suggests that rehabilitation after lower extremity injuries that includes balance training results in improved static and dynamic balance[60] and contributes to greater success in return to play in athletes.[61] A three times per week program of balance and lower extremity strength training leads to improvements in balance measures equivalent to an individual 3 to 10 years younger, and increases in lower extremity strength.[62] According to Gardner et al.,[63] successful falls prevention programs include activities for strength, endurance, and balance training. Specifically, these authors recommend individually tailored exercises, criterion-based progression for strength and balance training conducted three times a week, use of a walking program to increase aerobic capacity, and follow-up with the exercise instructor over

several months to 1 year. Adherence to a program guided by these principles has resulted in reduced risk for falling for up to 2 years.[64]

EXAMINATION AND EVALUATION OF IMPAIRED BALANCE AND MOBILITY

Horak et al.[14] suggest the following keys to examination and designing a rehabilitation program including balance control: knowledge of the systems controlling equilibrium, knowledge of the systems likely disordered by aging and pathology, an understanding of the factors that are likely to influence recovery of function, attention to the environmental factors that influence balance and mobility, and adherence to the concepts of motor learning that govern task development. Additionally, a clinical framework, such as the systems model set within an ecological context, can facilitate our thinking about examination and intervention.[14] Given that balance- and mobility-related disability is both individually and contextually dependent, clinicians must also strive for a deep understanding of the lived-experience of the individual. Furthermore, clinicians must thoroughly understand the myriad of tests available for examining balance and gait. Perhaps most important, the clinician must work with the patient to develop meaningful and realistic goals for rehabilitation. Basing clinical decisions on knowledge from each of these domains can enhance the clinician's ability to choose the right measures for the right patient at the right time. Understanding the relative importance of specific impairments, activity limitations, and participation restrictions identified during the examination enhances the ability to prioritize the plan of care and select specific interventions.

The *Guide to Physical Therapist Practice*[65] describes three categories of balance assessments. They are

- Balance during functional activities with or without the use of assistive, adaptive, orthotic, protective, supportive, or prosthetic devices or equipment (i.e., ADL or IADL scales, observations)
- Balance (static or dynamic) with or without the use of assistive, adaptive, orthotic, protective, supportive, or prosthetic devices or equipment (i.e., balance scales, dizziness inventories, dynamic posturography, fall scales, motor impairment tests, mobility skill profiles)
- Safety during gait, locomotion, or balance (i.e., confidence scales, diaries, fall scales, and logs)

Thus, examination of balance impairment can range from the simple to the complex.[22,66] Simple, impairment level clinical measures, such as the ability to maintain a single-leg stance with the eyes closed or the Romberg test, are commonly used in the clinic. Measures of activity limitations, such as the Berg balance scale (BBS) and timed up and go are commonly used by certified clinical specialists.[67] Additionally, computerized balance testing systems are increasingly incorporated into clinical evaluation and treatment.[68–70]

As stated, balance impairment can arise from many sources. Thus, it is critical that the examination differentiate between biomechanical, motor, sensory, and other contributing causes of imbalance. This is the hallmark of a systems approach to examination. The systems model of postural control and orientation developed by Horak[71] provides the

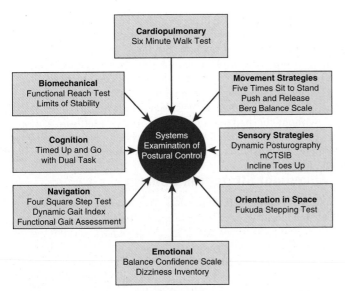

FIGURE 8-7. Examination of postural control from a systems model perspective.

foundation for this discussion regarding examination of balance (Fig 8-3).

It is also imperative that the clinician understand what is being testing. Consider the example of the sternal nudge test. The clinician attempts to disturb the patient's balance by trying to push the patient with instructions such as, "Don't let me push you over." The patient's response is to tighten all muscles in an attempt to resist the clinician's push. This tests the ability to tighten postural muscles, more so than balance reactions. Further, this test, like the single-leg stance and Romberg tests, is a static test, and tells little about the individual's ability to maintain balance while moving. However, this test may be a relevant indicator of balance control in crowd situations, where a patient may get pushed. Consider what is being tested, what determines a positive test, and how this test would subsequently direct treatment. This highlights the importance of an organized, thoughtful examination process designed to sequentially and specifically test the various systems involved in balance.

While most balance measures examine the performance of multiple body systems simultaneously, each assessment tool falls into a primary domain within the systems model (Fig. 8-7). The clinician should choose an evaluation battery that taps the multiple aspects of balance control, including musculoskeletal, sensory strategy, movement strategy, dynamic control, cognitive, and affective domains.

Biomechanical Domain

Evaluation of biomechanical causes of imbalance can be readily performed in the clinic. Crutchfield et al.[5] emphasizes the importance of distinguishing among a normal neurologic system working with an abnormal musculoskeletal system, an abnormal neurologic system working with a normal musculoskeletal system, or a combination of both. Joint range of motion, muscle length imbalance, impaired muscle performance, pain, or other postural abnormalities (e.g., kyphosis) can contribute to balance impairment. Loss of motion at a joint or series of joints (e.g., ankle, knee, and spine), decreased accessory motion, and muscle length imbalance alters posture

and movement strategies. Likewise, muscle impairments such as weakness or loss of endurance alter movement strategies. For example, gluteus medius weakness results in a predictable alteration in gait known as a gluteus medius limp. This weakness may prevent normal hip or stepping strategy use. Pain often produces changes in movement that, if continued, can produce secondary strength and mobility impairments. Limited ankle ROM prevents use of an ankle strategy, requiring the patient to use a hip strategy. This may be interpreted as faulty balance, although the hip strategy may be the best strategy available for that individual. Many of these impairments can be assessed using simple clinical measures such as goniometry and manual and functional muscle testing.

The functional reach test (FRT)[72] and tests of stability limits are examples of functional balance measures that can guide clinical decision making regarding potential biomechanical influences on postural stability. The FRT was originally developed as a performance-based assessment of unsupported dynamic standing balance impairment. This test is performed by observing how far forward an individual can reach while standing. Population-based normative data and/or data regarding risk for falling based on FRT scores is available for the elderly[72] and children.[73] Another version of the FRT provides information regarding the ability of the patient to reach in multiple directions.[74] The FRT requires minimal equipment and time to administer. An individual's stability limits can be quantified by performance-based scales, use of posture grids, or via computerized technologies utilizing force platforms.

Sensory Strategies Domain

Impairment of the sensory systems can result in balance impairment. Thus, each of the sensory systems contributing to balance control should be addressed. The somatosensory and visual systems may be tested directly. Basic, impairment level tests of the lower extremity sensations of light touch, vibration, proprioception, and kinesthesia should be considered. Screening for visual field defects, eye movement control, or sensitivity to visual motion may be pertinent depending on the specific case. The influence of the vestibular system must be tested indirectly and inferred through observing performance of vestibular outputs, such as the vestibular-ocular reflex and postural stability in sensory-deprived conditions.

Several components of sensory organization (functional utilization of sensory feedback for postural stability) can be tested readily in the clinic; however, a full examination of sensory contributions to postural sway requires more elaborate equipment such as a visual-conflict surround and rotating platform. The postural dyscontrol test or clinical test of sensory interaction in balance (CTSIB) combines and isolates information from the visual, vestibular, and somatosensory systems.[12,22] Systematically studying the contributions of each of these systems requires different testing situations, including standing with the eyes open on a fixed platform; standing blindfolded on a fixed platform; sway-referenced vision with fixed support; normal vision with sway-referenced support; absent vision with sway-referenced support; and sway-referenced vision and support[6] (Fig. 8-8).

Observation of performance while standing with the eyes open on a fixed surface provides a global view of stability when all sensory modalities are potentially available.

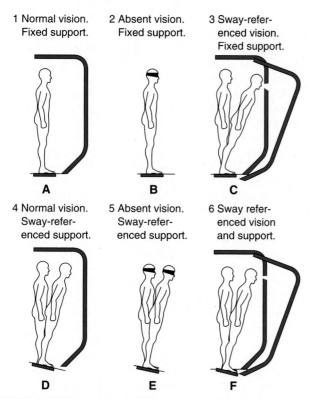

1 Normal vision. Fixed support.

2 Absent vision. Fixed support.

3 Sway-referenced vision. Fixed support.

A   B   C

4 Normal vision. Sway-referenced support.

5 Absent vision. Sway-referenced support.

6 Sway referenced vision and support.

D   E   F

FIGURE 8-8. The six balance testing situations: (A) standing quietly, eyes open; (B) standing quietly, with eyes closed; (C) standing with a visual box, and eyes open; (D) standing, and body rotates with body sway; (E) standing, rotating platform, with eyes closed; (F) standing on a rotating platform with a visual box.

Removing vision by closing or blindfolding the eyes provides information on the contribution of the somatosensory system. In the situation with sway-referenced vision with fixed support, the visual box moved as the subject swayed, presenting a sensory conflict: movement took place, but the eyes did not register movement. Joint receptors sensed the movement, but the eyes did not. The vestibular system provided the resolving information, indicating that movement had taken place. During this testing, normal subjects sway very little. The situation of normal vision with sway-referenced support presents a different conflict. In this case, the platform rotates in conjunction with the body sway. The visual system records movement, but the joint receptors do not. Once again, the vestibular system presents the resolving information. Greater sway occurs in this situation than in the previous three situations due to differences in sensory processing times between the somatosensory and other systems. The greatest sway is observed in situations of absent vision with sway-referenced support and of sway-referenced vision and support, for which inaccurate information is furnished from more than one source. Platform rotation provides inaccurate information to the visual and kinesthetic systems in the situation of absent vision with sway-referenced support. The rotating platform and visual box provides inaccurate visual and somatosensory information in the situation of sway-referenced vision and support. These tests suggest that individuals rely primarily on the somatosensory system for orientation and postural control and that, when somatosensory and visual information are removed or inaccurate, the vestibular system is left to provide postural control.[5]

Cohen and Blatchly[75] developed a streamlined version of the CTSIB. This modified version includes only the following four conditions: eyes open on a noncompliant, fixed surface; eyes closed on a noncompliant, fixed surface; eyes open on a compliant surface: and eyes closed on a compliant surface. This version has been used in adults,[75] children,[76] and patients with vestibular disorders.[77,78] The test may be performed with or without the patient standing on a force platform. Various ways of describing performance have been proposed, such as using an ordinal scale.[12]

Movement Strategies Domain

Assessing motor organization (movement strategies) in balance control can be conducted within the context of functional task performance inside or outside the context of standardized clinical assessment tools. Simple measures that provide insight regarding use of in-place anticipatory and reactive movement strategies include the FRT (described previously) and the Five-times-sit-to-stand Test (5× STS).[79] As a measure of upper extremity reaching ability, the FRT also assesses postural adjustments that anticipate upper extremity movement.[72,80] In addition to measuring functional lower extremity strength, the 5× STS also provides a basis for evaluating balance control during transitions when moving between sitting and standing. In this test, the individual is asked to rise to standing and sit back down (without use of the hands) as quickly and safely as possible five times consecutively while being timed.

Alternatively, the push and release test (PRT) provides information about corrective stepping (change-in-support) responses.[81] As opposed to the sternal nudge or "pull test" in which the individual knows the perturbation is coming, the PRT creates instability by having the patient attempt to maintain stability after being unexpectedly released from a position of gently leaning into the examiners hands. The reliability, sensitivity, and specificity regarding detecting balance impairments with the PRT have been found to be superior to other tests of perturbed stance, such as the sternal nudge.[81] Much information regarding movement strategies can also be gleaned from observing performance on test batteries such as the BBS.[82,11] The BBS rates performance from 0 (unable to perform) to 4 (normal) for 14 different tasks. Each task is performed without using the upper extremities for assistance.

Dynamic Control Domain

None of the measures introduced thus far provide the clinician with the necessary information required to drive clinical decision making regarding walking-related balance impairments. Insight into a patient's ability to step in multiple directions, a skill necessary for many functional tasks, including obstacle avoidance and navigation in crowed spaces, can be gleaned from the four square step test (4SST).[83] In the 4SST the patient is asked to step over four standard cones arranged on the floor in the shape of a "plus-sign." The test is timed and the patient must first step over each cone moving in a clockwise manner and then return to the starting position moving counter-clockwise. The timed up and go test (TUG) requires the patient to stand up from sitting in a chair, walk 3 m, turn around, return to the chair, and sit again.[22,84] The reliability of this test is high, and it correlates well with the BBS.[85] The dynamic gait index (DGI) is a measure of dynamic balance as it measures the patient's ability to modify gait in response to changing task demands.[86,22] The DGI has been shown to have good interrater and test-retest reliability.[18] Two major alternatives to the original DGI now exist. Wrisley et al.[87] expanded this test and created the functional gait assessment (FGA) in part in an attempt to capture information regarding balance control in patients with high-level problems. Preliminary normative data for the FGA now exists.[88] Alternatively, Marchetti and Whitney[89] found that a four-item version of the DGI could provide accurate information about faller status with comparable sensitivity and specificity to the original DGI.

Cognitive Domain

The timed up and go has been modified to include the simultaneous performance of a secondary cognitive task.[38] Repeating the TUG in this manner allows the clinician to gather information regarding the influence of divided attention on balance control during walking. Careful consideration should be given to which secondary cognitive task the patient is asked to perform. Patients should be allowed to practice a similar cognitive task prior to engaging in timed walking. The details of the task as well as the impact on walking performance and cognition should be documented clearly.

Affective Domain

Self confidence related to balance and perception of disability secondary to dizziness represent two important affective influences on balance and mobility. The activities-specific balance confidence (ABC) Scale consists of 16 questions for which patients are asked to rate their level of confidence that they will not lose their balance of fall while performing.[90] Average scores of <80% are considered abnormal and <50% have been correlated with a greater likelihood of being home bound.[90] The DHI is an assessment tool used to gauge self-perceived disability related to dizziness.[91] The DHI consists of 25 questions divided between physical, functional, and emotional subscales. Scores range from 0 to 100 with higher scores indicating greater disability. The degree of disability has been correlated with functional balance measures[43,92] and prognosis for recovery.[93] Each of these questionnaires also provides insight into the patient's lived experience of their health condition. See Building Block 8-5.

 BUILDING BLOCK 8-5

A 30-year-old previously healthy man is referred to physical therapy in the hospital 2 days after undergoing surgical resection of a vestibular schwannoma. The patient complains of vertigo, blurred vision, and feeling like he is intoxicated. He reports he has had difficulty walking to the bathroom with the nursing staff. What are two tests of postural control that you would prioritize to be completed during the initial evaluation that could be used subsequently in the outpatient setting as outcomes measures for this patient's rehabilitation? Why did you choose these tests?

Determining Risk for Falling

What is the likelihood that my patient will fall? This is one of the most important questions clinicians must answer. The ability to accurately answer this question has profound implications. Researchers and clinicians use each of the clinical tests of balance mentioned above to provide clues as to a person's risk for falling. The five-times-sit-to-stand test, PRT, FRT, four square step test, the BBS, Tinetti's balance and mobility assessment, the timed get up and go, and the DGI are used frequently in the clinic to stratify risk for falling.[11,22,72,82] The cut-off score associated with falls risk may vary by age. For example the cut-off score for the 5× STS was found to be 10 seconds for those under 60 years old and 14.2 seconds for those over age 60 years in a population of adults with balance disorders.[93] Cut-off scores may also vary by population. For example, a score of 15 seconds or longer on the 4SST identifies older adults with a history of multiple falls;[83]however, scores of 12 seconds or longer provide the same indication of prior falls status in persons with vestibular disorders.[94] Older adults who scored higher on the BBS were less likely to fall than those who scored below 45 of the 56 points.[22,95] Different cut-off scores for the BBS are applied to individuals with Parkinson disease[96] or those who are status-post traumatic brain injury[97] or stroke.[98] Like the BBS, the DGI can be used to determine falls status. Scores of <20 on the DGI indicate an increased association with previous falls, while scores of <17 are highly associated with prior falls status.[86] Likewise, individuals with vestibular disorders who score <19 on the DGI are 2.7 times more likely to have reported a fall in the previous 6 months.[99] Though performance indicators for the BBS and DGI have also been shown to vary by population and living arrangements, the BBS and DGI have been shown to agree 63% of the time for individuals with vestibular disorders.[100] It is critical that the clinician be mindful of who they are evaluating and how they are applying the information gathered. Further information regarding the psychometric properties, population-specific normative data, and/or cut-off scores related to falls risk for many of the assessment tools described in this text may be found online at www.thePoint.lww.com/BrodyHall3e.

Accurately diagnosing risk for falls is a complex and challenging task. This is due in part to the fact that most published indicators of falls risk only correlate with a person's recent history of falling. Predicting future falls requires careful analysis.[97,101,102] Currently, the best predictor of future falls is a history of previous falls.

TREATING IMPAIRED BALANCE
Diagnosis and Prioritization

The most important factor in treating balance and mobility impairments is diagnosing the underlying cause(s) and the factors contributing to these impairments. Remember that balance problems can result from biomechanical, neuromuscular, sensory, cognitive, or affective impairments. These impairments may be considered primary (a direct result of a health condition) or secondary (occurring in response to the development of primary impairments). Matching intervention strategies to underlying impairments is critical. Repetitive quadriceps strengthening exercises do little to improve balance if the primary underlying problem is a movement disorder. Conversely, the patient must have adequate strength to maintain balance. Many individuals are, in fact, lacking "core" strength, or strength in the trunk and pelvis, which provides a stable base for subsequent movement. Thus, a concurrent strength program is often necessary for treating balance impairment that result from a variety of primary causes.

Any musculoskeletal (base element) problem such as impaired muscle performance or mobility, or pain, should be emphasized early, with ongoing reevaluation and intervention for continued balance impairment as the fundamental musculoskeletal problems resolve. Chapters 5, 7, and 10 provide specific activities to treat these impairments. If the problem involves motor learning, then it would be considered a modulator element. Modulator elements are addressed throughout the plan of care. Additional modifying factors, such as the need for psychological interventions or cardiac rehabilitation, may need to be addressed early and incorporated into the plan of care as well. For example, consider those whose primary problem is a fear of falling. The impaired element of the movement system is within affective domain. A health psychologist or licensed counselor can assist the patient in developing the relaxation strategies needed in order for her to face her fear of falling and engage in the risks associated with balance rehabilitation.

There are many examples of how impairments in the primary systems supporting balance are incorporated into the treatment plan. For patients with discrepancies between actual stability limits and perceived stability limits, initiate postural sway activities within the actual stability limits. For those with sensory organization problems, design exercises requiring the patient to maintain balance during progressively more difficult static and dynamic activities within the appropriate environmental context; vary the sensory system emphasized with the different activities. Systematically eliminate, minimize, or alter the visual, vestibular, or somatosensory input, requiring the patient to reconcile input from the different systems based on the priorities identified while gathering subjective and objective data from your patient. For patients with impaired functional use of postural reactions, tasks designed to generate ankle, hip, and stepping responses may be prescribed. These examples demonstrate how accurate diagnosis leads to appropriate prioritization within the treatment plan.

Customization

There is strong evidence to support prescription of an individualized intervention program for balance retraining. Rehabilitation that includes balance training results in improved balance[60] and greater success in return to play in athletes.[61] Additionally, customized balance rehabilitation is more effective than generic exercise programs for reducing dizziness and improving balance in individuals with vestibular disorders.[103] Customized, multidimensional exercise programs also improve balance and mobility and reduce falls in geriatric populations.[104] The treatment suggestions described below must be matched to the underlying problem and patient.

Environmental Context

Rehabilitation takes place in an environmental context. There are three major factors to consider regarding the influence of the environment on balance rehabilitation; the physical location, appropriate safety measures, and the specific environmental features to be manipulated during task practice. The

physical location for balance training depends on the patient's situation. For the frail elderly or those with significant balance impairment, most of the training activity takes place in the clinic. Patients with higher baseline balance abilities and/or self-efficacy related to balance training or sufficient assistance at home will perform the majority of their training at home. Alternatively, patients who are ready to transition out of formal therapy or who desire to include more challenging, balance-specific activities (e.g., Tai Chi, yoga, and dance) into their routine health and wellness program may achieve their goals. Counseling individuals regarding identifying community-based programs that are appropriate for his/her needs and abilities may be a part of a successful plan of care. For athletes or other active individuals with musculoskeletal causes of balance impairments, balance activities may be carried out independently at home, at a local health club, or in a local pool.

Safety is a key factor when making choices about the exercise environment. A stable support should always be available for regaining lost balance. This support should be placed such that it does not interfere with the exercise and does not cause injury during an attempt to regain balance. Be alert for correct posture, avoidance of substitution, proper performance, and safety when providing direct interventions. Foster the patient's self-awareness and error correction. Simple activities such as postural awareness exercises may be performed safely at home by most patients. Realize that the clinic environment is designed for maximum patient safety, and may not reflect real world situations. Recommendations regarding exercising safely at home, including instructions to perform exercises in a corner, narrow hallway, nearby sturdy furniture, or with various forms of assistance may be appropriate.

The environment has a significant impact on patients and the choices they make regarding mobility. Factors such as distance, temporal demands, physical load, ambient conditions, attentional demands, terrain, frequency of postural transitions, and traffic density are examples of key environmental variables.[41] Distance refers to how far the individual must walk to complete each trip outside their home. Temporal demands include factors such as crowd speed, traffic lights, and amount of vehicular traffic. Precipitation, temperature, and available light are examples of factors related to the ambient conditions. Whether or not the individual must carry a load, such as a purse or grocery bags, relates to the required additional physical demands of each trip. Relevant features of the terrain may include the presence of grades, curbs, stairs, uneven surfaces (grass), shifting surfaces (gravel), and moving surfaces (elevators and escalators). The presence of distractions or being accompanied by a spouse, partner, or fried are examples of factors that alter the attentional demands of mobility. Even the occurrence of postural transitions such as the need to stop, start, turn, back up, and reach may influence choices about mobility. Individuals with mobility-related disability encounter fewer challenges and show avoidance behaviors with regard to temporal factors, physical load, terrain, and postural transitions.[41] The salience of these factors is individual;[105] thus, this is another aspect of rehabilitation that should be customized for each patient.

Whether exercising indoors or outdoors, surface characteristics, lighting, noise, cars, weather conditions, and a multitude of other external environmental conditions may overload the sensory systems, increasing the risk of a fall. Be sure to progress the patient to balance training in the types of environments they will encounter when they leave the clinic. This may require short "field trips" outside the clinic to reproduce these situations. If real world experience is not possible, consider the use of photographs, video tape, virtual reality, or gaming to facilitate discussion, mental rehearsal, or simulated practice of specific functional tasks within meaningful environmental contexts.

Mode

A variety of modes (e.g., supportive chair, therapeutic ball, firm floor, foam roll, foam pad, balance board, pool) can be used to treat balance impairment. The pool is an ideal place to train balance for some, because the water's movement causes perturbations, and the water's viscosity slows balance loss, giving individuals more time to respond (see Self-Management 16-3 in Chapter 16). A warm water pool may be an especially good mode for rehabilitating balance in persons with severe arthritis. More sophisticated, computerized balance testing devices can also be used for training. In fact, any mode used for testing balance can be used for training. One of the primary advantages of commercially available balance platforms is that they allow selective modulation of sensory systems and objective measures of progression.

SELF-MANAGEMENT 8-1 *Minitrampoline Balance*

Purpose:	To improve stability in single leg stance
Movement Technique:	Level I: While standing on the minitramp with a stable object at hand, practice standing on one leg. Make sure that your knee is slightly bent. Use the stable object for balance only if necessary.
	Level II: Close your eyes.
	Level III: Perform a minisquat.
	Level IV: Add resistance to the knee.
	Level V: Add movement to the arms.

Dosage
Repetitions: _____
Frequency: _____

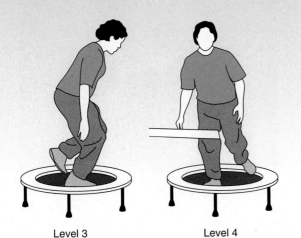

Level 3   Level 4

SELF-MANAGEMENT 8-2 *Sitting Balance on a Stable Surface*

Purpose:	To increase awareness of and expand stability limits
Movement Technique:	While sitting on a stable surface such as a chair, practice reaching forward, overhead, and to the side. You may look in the direction you are reaching or in a different direction, as recommended by your therapist.

Dosage
Repetitions: _____
Frequency: _____

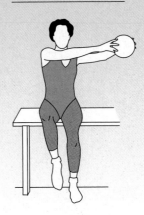

Intervention Strategies for Specific Systems—Examples

The sections that immediately follow contain specific examples of interventions categorized under the some of the primary subsystems supporting postural control. However, the same type of complexity represented in the model of normal balance function presented earlier also characterizes most if not all exercises prescribed as part of a balance rehabilitation program. Though a specific exercise (e.g., slow weight shifts on a noncompliant surface) may be prescribed for a primary purpose (e.g., retraining the ankle strategy), performance of this exercise requires the individual to draw on many other balance related resources. Therefore, it is important to bear in mind the various biomechanical, sensory, neuromuscular, cognitive, and affective requirements for each exercise prescribed. This type of task analysis allows the clinician to use exercises for more than one purpose or to make relatively simple modifications to alter the intent or level of difficulty of a given exercise.

Developing Orientation in Space

Since stability generally precedes mobility, some patients need to begin by working on maintenance of static postural alignment. Use a stable surface such as a hard floor or rigid chair for initiating sitting, kneeling, standing, and single leg standing. These body postures can be used to facilitate postural orientation and stabilization. Kinesiologic factors, such as achieving and maintaining proper COG alignment and control, as well as learning factors, such as internalization of balance strategies, provide the structural framework for the treatment postures chosen.

SELF-MANAGEMENT 8-3 *Sitting Balance on an Unstable Surface*

Purpose: To increase postural stability and trunk balance

Movement Technique: While sitting on the therapeutic ball, practice reaching forward, overhead, and to the side. You may look in the direction you are reaching or in a different direction, as recommended by your therapist.

Dosage
Repetitions: _____
Frequency: _____

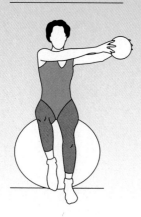

Utilize force platforms, scales, mirrors, or tape markings placed vertically on clothing while standing to train the patient to distribute weight equally on each lower extremity and/or align his/her body posture correctly. For those needing work on core trunk stability first, training may be initiated in a sitting position, which provides an opportunity to develop a sense of trunk posture and equity of weight bearing while sitting. Train sitting balance, trunk stability, and weight distribution on a chair, table, or therapeutic ball (see Self-Management, 8-1, 8-2, 8-3 and Fig. 8-9). Use a variety of arm positions, such as forward or lateral reaching, to change the postural challenge. Maintaining equitable weight distribution and trunk posture on an unstable surface such as a therapeutic ball creates an interesting and useful balance challenge. Static postures also may be used in combination with foam surfaces to alter the challenge to the patient. Keep in mind that unstable and foam surfaces will alter the sensory demands of this task.

More challenging static postures, such as standing heel to toe or a single-leg stance, should be included when the patient is ready. These postures minimize ankle strategy use and facilitate a hip synergy. For the athlete, postures encountered in sport should be duplicated and systematically challenged in the clinic. Lunge positions, single-leg stance with a variety of trunk postures, and squat positions are commonly encountered in sport. After stability and optimal posture are achieved in static positions, dynamic movement should be superimposed on the activity (see Selected Intervention 8-1). Adding dynamic movement increases use of automatic postural adjustments during the preparation for movement and reactive strategies to counteract perturbations of the COG. See Building Block 8-6.

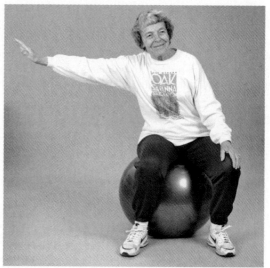

A

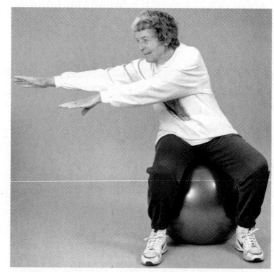

B

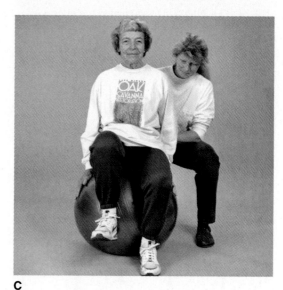

C

FIGURE 8-9. A variety of balance activities can be performed on a therapeutic ball: (A) single-arm lateral reach, (B) bilateral reaching, (C) assistance for balance while lifting one leg.

SELECTED INTERVENTION 8-1
Single Leg Balance on a Foam Roller

ACTIVITY: Single-leg balance on foam roller with added dynamic activity

PURPOSE: To increase stability limits and dynamic balance

PRECAUTIONS: Patient safety: ensure readiness for activity and safeguards in case of balance loss; adequate trunk control

POSTURE: Standing on a foam roller with dynamic control of head, spine, and lower extremity posture

MOVEMENT: Maintain balance while moving a ball into a variety of positions or while playing catch with ball

PROCEDURE: Isometric, concentric, and eccentric muscle contractions of the spine extensors, flexors, and abdominal oblique muscles. The closed-chain nature of the activity will produce cocontraction of lower extremity musculature including, but not limited to the gastroc-soleus, quadriceps, hamstrings, and gluteal muscles.

DOSAGE: Three to six sets of 30-second intervals

FUNCTIONAL MOVEMENT PATTERN TO REINFORCE GOAL OF EXERCISE: A variety of single leg instability situations are encountered in sports. The individual learns to control posture through core muscle contraction while performing a dynamic activity on an unstable surface.

BUILDING BLOCK 8-6

How might you conduct retraining of orientation to vertical posture in standing for an outpatient who has moderate left sided hemiparesis status-post right middle cerebral artery stroke and is not able to stand unsupported?

Retraining Movement Strategies

A variety of movement patterns superimposed on stable postures can increase the balance challenge and encourage development of proactive balance strategies. Adding anteroposterior and lateral sway assists the patient in determining and increasing her stability limits. Perform these in a variety of modes (e.g., supportive chair, therapeutic ball, firm floor, foam roll, foam pad, balance board, pool) and in a variety of postures (e.g., sitting, half kneeling, tall kneeling, standing, single-leg stance) using varying arm postures and/or movements. Trunk rotations with the arms in a variety of positions (e.g., abducted, forward flexed, arms across chest) with changes in head position (e.g., rotated, laterally flexed) to alter vestibular input can be combined in a multitude of ways. Proprioceptive neuromuscular facilitation (PNF) techniques in trunk rotation, called chops and lifts, are excellent dynamic movement patterns. These patterns include arm, trunk, and head rotation, flexion, and extension (see Chapter 15) (Fig. 8-10).

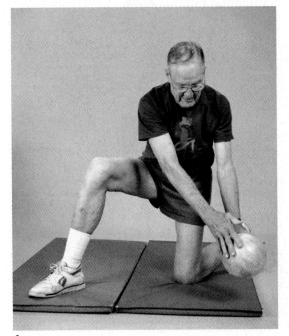
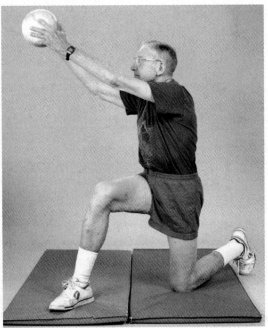

A　　　　　　　　　**B**

FIGURE 8-10. PNFs of chop and lift in half-kneeling position: (A) starting position and (B) ending position.

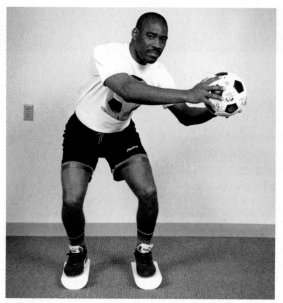

FIGURE 8-11. Foam rollers are used in bilateral stance when the person practices weight shifting while catching a ball.

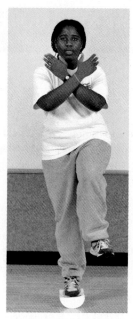

FIGURE 8-12. Tai Chi exercise to improve single leg balance.

For patients who need to train an ankle synergy, begin with weight shifts on a firm surface, with gradually increasing sway. As the patient improves, increase the compliance of the support surface. Training of the ankle strategy is encouraged when the individual is asked to maintain balance on any surface that is wide, noncompliant, or stable; when slow balance reactions are required; or when the COG is far from the LOS. Using rehabilitation balls, foam rollers, and foam surfaces provides uneven or unstable surfaces and encourages a shift toward use of proximal muscles for balance control (Figs. 8-11 and 8-12).

More challenging surfaces such as a minitrampoline can also provide a variety of balance experiences (see Self-Management 8-1). Modifying this simple task in these ways also alters the environmental demands and sensory feedback available for controlling balance and, therefore, prepares the individual to face these situations successfully in the real world.

Balance beams, lines drawn on the floor, and balance boards, are often used for balance training (Fig. 8-13). These intervention strategies are particularly useful for patients needing to train a hip synergy, as they prevent the use of an

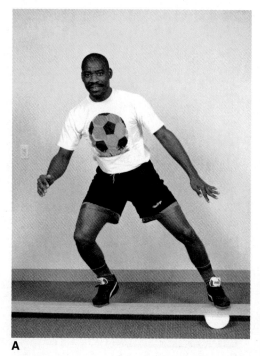

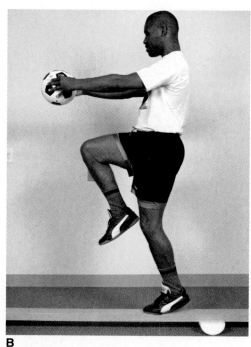

A   **B**

FIGURE 8-13. (A) Lateral movement on a balance beam on foam rollers.
(B) Adding a soccer ball to drill activities increases the challenge.

ankle synergy as a substitute. Training of the hip strategy is encouraged when the individual is asked to maintain balance on any surface that is narrow, compliant, or unstable; when rapid balance reactions are required; or when the COG is near the LOS.

Maki and McIlroy[106] suggests that training include mimicking the varied and unpredictable events that precipitate falls in the elderly, and that activities include not only COG displacements, but BOS compensatory movements. Thus, activities that require a change in BOS using stepping and reaching strategies should also be considered. Stepping exercises such as lunges provide an opportunity to control balance as the client first moves outside the stability limit and then restabilizes when her foot hits the ground. Starting with small steps and progressing to full lunges (Fig. 8-14) increasingly challenges the patient. Adding a concurrent arm activity can further challenge balance. For example, reciprocally swinging the arms during stepping can make the task easier, but performing a PNF chop or catching a ball can make it more difficult (Fig. 8-15). Completely eliminating the arms for balance by holding them across the chest or overhead can make the exercise extremely difficult for a person with poor trunk and hip stability.

More advanced balance exercises include hopping, skipping, carioka, slide board, and rope jumping (see Self-Management 8-4: Slide Board). Perform these exercises in a variety of patterns, with exaggerated step length or knee lift. Many can be performed backward, with a variety of step techniques incorporated. The "hop and stop" can be performed on a firm surface or a soft surface such as foam or minitramp (Fig. 8-16). The patient is asked to hop single or double footed and to "stick" the landing without losing balance. Exercise equipment such as a stepper can also challenge balance if performed without hand support, backward, or with the eyes closed. Closing the eyes assists in emphasizing the use of somatosensory and vestibular feedback control of balance. For athletes, reproducing movement patterns found in their sports can prepare them for the return to activity. Many traditional sports drills can be modified for use in a clinical setting. Changing the speed

of the stepping exercise to approximate functional speeds is essential to the movement strategy. These challenging tasks have elements of proactive and reactive dynamic balance. Consider which aspects to emphasize for each individual.

As mentioned previously, the pool provides an interesting and dynamic environment in which to challenge an array balance movement patterns. The viscosity and movement of the water constantly challenge posture and balance. Any arm or leg movement can potentially disrupt the patient's balance. For example, performing bilateral shoulder horizontal adduction and abduction results in posterior and anterior displacement of the body, respectively. Perform this exercise with the feet in stride, in normal stance, in a narrowed stance, or in single-leg stance for progressively increasing difficulty (see Self-Management 8-5: Shoulder Level Claps in the pool). The increased unpredictability experienced in the water may help prepare the individual for rapidly changing environmental conditions in the real world. See Building Block 8-7.

Facilitating Sensory Strategies

Awareness of posture and the position of the body in space are fundamental to balance training. Jeka[107] demonstrated that the use of light touch through a cane or balance aid enhances the use of somatosensory and can reduce postural sway. Compensatory strategies such as this can be used to increase spatial awareness, as well as facilitate performance and minimize the fear and anxiety sometimes associated with balance retraining.

There are many ways to facilitate relearning sensory strategies. As noted above, the environmental characteristics, such as the support surface, can be altered to change the mode of balance exercise. Understanding how to manipulate the surface or other environmental cues is critical to providing the appropriate sensory context in which patients practice. To that end, patients should be trained in situations that enhance the nervous system's ability to attend to specific types of feedback.

Patients who need to develop effective use of somatosensory feedback for balance control begin activities with the eyes closed on a stable surface. Attention to surface cues can

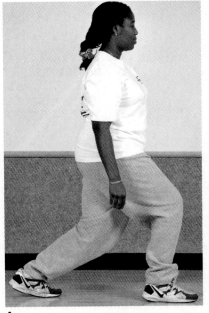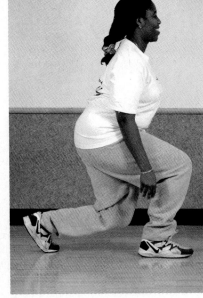

FIGURE 8-14. (A) Minilunges are progressed to (B) full lunges.

A

B

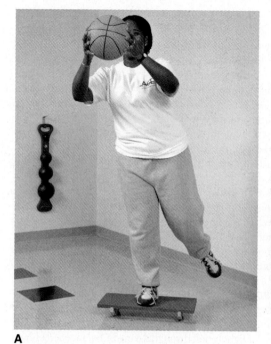

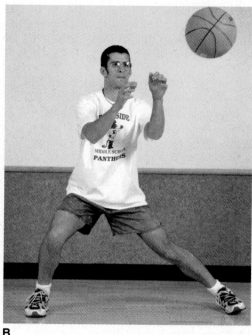

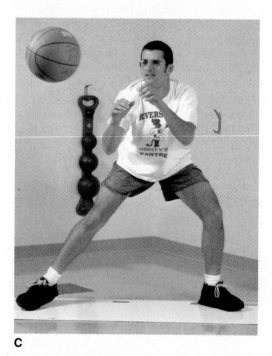

FIGURE 8-15. Catching a ball in a variety of situations increases task complexity: (A) on a balance board, (B) combined with lateral lunges, and (C) on a slide board.

be enhanced by having the individual perform exercises with her shoes off, while standing on a textured surface, or by using knobby insoles in the shoes. If the ability to use existing visual cues effectively for maintaining stability is compromised, training the patient on a compliant or unstable surface with the eyes open and fixed on or attending to visual references in the environment is appropriate. Attention to visual cues can be enhanced by asking the individual to fixate gaze on a stationary target <5 ft away or by performing the task near a doorway or other distinct cues of vertical alignment. Alternatively, patients with difficulty using vestibular feedback about head position and acceleration should be trained on compliant or

unstable surfaces with their eyes closed in order to force the nervous system to attend to vestibular inputs. The challenge to use vestibular cues for balance is increased by adding varied static head positions, active rotations, or tilts. Use caution with these activities for persons with vestibular disorders as these activities may cause dizziness. Real world environments often present patients with confusing and conflicting sensory information. Thus, patients also need training in how to resolve conflicting inputs. For example, patients may need to learn how to balance when standing still in an environment with overwhelming motion of the crowd, lighting, or displays. Partially distorting or obscuring vision may also help

SELF-MANAGEMENT 8-4 *Slide Board*

Purpose: To increase balance and coordination during a functional activity

Movement Technique: Level I: Laterally glide on a slide board.
Level II: Continuously catch and toss a ball.
Level III: Increase speed.
Level IV: Increase the number of balls tossed.

Dosage
Repetitions: _____
Frequency: _____

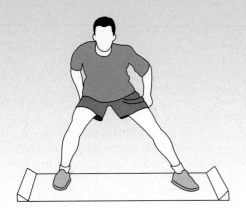

encourage patients to resolve sensory conflicts. Whether or not these specific sensory manipulations are included in the plan of care depends in large part on the underlying impairments and the patient's prognosis for functional recovery. Thus, understanding the expectations for recovery of function as they relate to the patient's health condition and their response to its influence on their life is critical to effective treatment planning. See Building Block 8-8.

Sequencing Considerations

Progression of exercise from simple to complex involves creating increasingly more challenging tasks for the individual to practice in meaningful environmental contexts. Variables related to the individual body systems contributing to balance control, characteristics of the environment, and task set-up can be sequentially and systematically manipulated to develop and progress a customized intervention program. Remember, there are complex relationships between each of these domains. Thus, manipulation of one variable in any given domain has broad implications.

Task Variables

Appropriate sequencing related to postural demands involves progression from stable postures (e.g., sitting) to more unstable postures (e.g., single-leg stance). Spatial characteristics such as the distance traveled with each step while side-stepping or the amplitude of arm movements produced while performing single limb stance should be considered. Generally, patients are progressed by increasing step length or the amount of reach. Temporal factors such as the velocity of movement and the time allowed to complete a series of movements can be used to influence performance. Patients may progress from

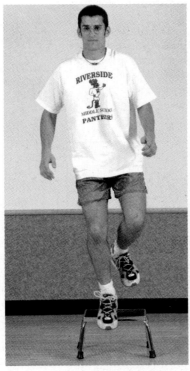

FIGURE 8-16. Hop and stop for dynamic balance. (A) The patient starts from a small stool, hops down, and (B) "sticks" the landing.

A

B

SELF-MANAGEMENT 8-5 *Shoulder Level Claps in the Pool*

Purpose: To increase upper back and chest strength and to challenge balance

Movement Technique: Level I: While standing in good postural alignment with your arms to the side at shoulder level, bring them forward and back to the starting position.

Level II: Bring your feet close together.

Level III: Stand on a single leg.

Level IV: Close your eyes

Level V: Add resistance to the hands.

Dosage
Repetitions: _____
Frequency: _____

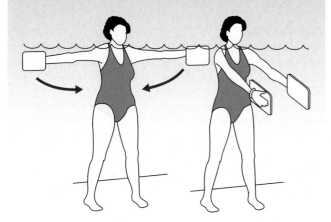

slow movement to attempting to control ballistic movements while maintaining a particular posture. Encouraging increased speed is easily accomplished by decreasing the time allowed to complete a block of practice. Whether or not the patient is asked to manage a physical load or simultaneously manipulate

BUILDING BLOCK 8-7

List several activities of daily life that require use of an ankle strategy that could be used as functional task practice in rehabilitation for a 52-year-old man who is in the chronic phase of recovery following an acute ankle sprain sustained while playing in a weekend basketball league. The patient is a ferry boat operator and must stand for long periods of time. Choose the ideal mode of exercise and several exercises for retraining the hip strategy for a 60-year-old, morbidly obese woman, status-post right total hip replacement. Explain your rationale. She is 2 months post-op and has minimal discomfort in the right hip. Her gait is antalgic and she continues to use cane and rates her osteoarthritic pain in the left hip and knee at 8/10 while walking.

BUILDING BLOCK 8-8

What parameters or variables would likely manipulate when retraining sensory strategies for a 57-year-old woman with diabetes mellitus and associated peripheral neuropathy (diminished vibratory sensation below the ankles bilaterally) and retinopathy (legally blind in both eyes)?

an object in the hand while maintaining stability is another consideration. The patient may begin by practicing walking on a level surface and eventually progress to walking while carrying a full glass of water or a large bag of groceries. Other task-related variables include the frequency, intensity, and schedule for practice. Patients progress from less to more frequent practice, fewer to greater repetitions, and blocked to random practice in order to address variables such as managing fatigue, encouraging motor learning, and developing greater motor control.

Individual Variables

The individual body systems that contribute to balance control can also be manipulated to create appropriate challenges and facilitate progress. As stated, base element problems related to the biomechanical system should be addressed early. Cognitive factors should be considered in all cases regardless of age or condition since many real world activities are performed under dual-task conditions. Training should begin with intense concentration and minimal cognitive distractions. Progression related to cognitive demands may involve having the individual perform a simultaneous cognitive task that requires listening, comprehension, mathematics, problem solving, etc. The patient's emotional engagement in training in terms of self-efficacy and their level of anxiety are additional considerations. Some individuals may need to practice deep breathing or other relaxation strategies in conjunction with task practice. As an indicator of self-efficacy, the patient should be encouraged to perform exercises that she is at least 70% to 80% confident in her ability to perform safely at home.

Facilitation of movement strategies as described earlier is often a critical component. The training plan should emphasize mastery of the appropriate use of in-place, automatic postural reactions for control of quiet stance before activities that involve executing change in BOS strategies, such as stepping correction responses. In terms of in-place responses, since the ankle strategy dominates stance control, this strategy should be addressed before impairments in the use of the hip strategy. While standing, start with simple sway activities that elicit an ankle strategy. Reinforce this strategy by verbal or tactile cuing and ensuring proper posture and firing patterns to prepare the patient for larger perturbations. Encourage the patient to gradually increase the stability limits by reaching or swaying farther. Progress the exercise by applying greater disruptions of the COG in order to elicit a hip strategy or a stepping strategy. After these responses are established, progress to more dynamic activities, unstable surfaces, and complex movement patterns. Additional critical variables involve the timing and scaling of these responses. Surface characteristics play a major role in movement strategy retraining. Progression is accomplished by increasing movement velocity and/or altering the surface.

Finally, sequencing training for appropriate use of sensory feedback for balance control described earlier should be considered. Generally, patients should be encouraged to perform exercises with all three major forms of sensory feedback available before progressing to practice in the environment's complex sensory conflicts. The use of somatosensory feedback should be encouraged by simply having the patient close her eyes while practicing on a stable surface. Once use of somatosensation is effective, retraining the use of vision can be facilitated by having the patient practice on an unstable surface with her eyes open while fixating their gaze on a stable target nearby. Eventually, practice emphasizing the use of vestibular feedback by balancing with the eyes closed on an unstable or compliant surface can be pursued. The dual sensory conflict created by practicing on an unstable surface while being exposed to visual feedback that is out of synch with their postural sway are the most challenging practice conditions. For example, retraining the ability to maintain dynamic stability while skating forward on one foot, while simultaneously trying to control a moving hockey puck, as teammates and defenders streak passed one's peripheral vision is a daunting task.

Environmental Variables

The terrain is one of the most commonly manipulated environmental variables. Not only can changing the terrain increase the level of difficulty, but, as we have seen, changing the surface can also be used to facilitate the use of specific sensory systems or postural reactions. Progression is best carried out from stable surfaces to unstable surfaces, noncompliant to compliant surfaces, flat surfaces to inclines, and stationary surfaces to surfaces that move. For example, performing postural sway in all directions with the arms folded across the chest while sitting on a firm chair is a good precursor to adding arm movements or for performing the same exercise on an unstable therapeutic ball. Ambient conditions play a major role and manipulating vision can serve to increase the challenge or determine whether the visual or vestibular system dominates balance control. Patients should exercise under good lighting conditions before progressing to practice in a dim room or in the dark. Closing the eyes is a simple and effective means to increase the difficulty of any exercise. Patients should demonstrate mastery in predictable environments prior to practicing under unpredictable conditions in order to minimize the effects of contextual variability. Vary displacements from those generated by the patient to an external force, and from an anticipated displacement to an unanticipated one to simulate balance control in crowds. Patients should be taught how to handle motion in the world around them (optokinetics) by first practicing in environments with no or very little environmental motion, such as a plain exam room on one end of the spectrum, and then progressing to more visually-busy environments, such as a crowded grocery store on the other end. Increasing the movement in the periphery during exercises will also challenge the balance system more.

Beginning with simple tasks on a stable surface and moving to progressively more unstable surfaces and complex tasks is the sequence plan, regardless of the age or condition of the patient. For an athlete, progression to a balance board, minitramp, slide board, or computerized balance training

BUILDING BLOCK 8-9

Describe an appropriate sequence for developing single leg stance for an otherwise healthy 22-year-old classical dancer recovering from left knee arthroscopy with resection of a medial meniscus tear.

system may occur rapidly. Although training the individual in postures or activities encountered in her sport can prepare her for those situations, many unpredictable situations occur, and unpredictable perturbations should be included in the training program to teach the nervous system how to respond to novel situations. See Building Block 8-9.

Feedback

Learning factors are essential in planning the activity mode for treating balance impairment. Early in the treatment program, simple balance challenges with external feedback are necessary. This allows the patient to develop gross strategies to manage the perturbation. As the patient learns and develops these gross strategies, increasing the balance challenge while decreasing the external feedback allows internal strategies to develop. Initially, ask the patient to describe what obstacles are in her path and what her strategies will be to negotiate through the room (enhanced use of cognition). Try to add distracters later in the rehabilitation process and look for more automatic postural presets. In the case of balance training, learning is the ultimate goal.

Mirrors and force platforms can provide visual postural biofeedback regardless of the position of exercise. This allows visual feedback (i.e., external feedback about position), which must be removed at some point to allow internalization of the balance strategies. Computerized force platforms allow for multiple variations of task practice with highly motivating performance feedback, and the ability to readily track progress.

EXPANDED ECOLOGICAL MODEL OF BALANCE REHABILITATION

As stated previously, the ecological model describes the interactions among the individuals, the environment, and the functional tasks.[5,14] The relationships between these domains are complex, dynamic, and lead to a highly individual experience of impaired balance and mobility. Figure 8-17 presents the variables available for manipulation by the clinician when developing interventions within the ecological framework discussed in this chapter. Systematic and skillful manipulation of specific variables related to the individual, environment, and the task provides the clinician with endless opportunities to customize a rehabilitation program for each person.

PRECAUTIONS AND CONTRAINDICATIONS

The most important precaution in balance training is the individual's safety. By definition, balance training challenges the patient's balance. Because the potential for falls is high, choose

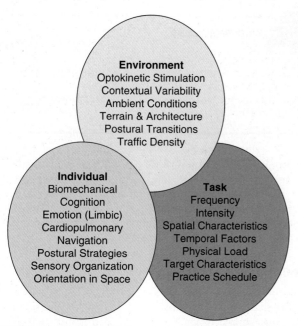

Environment
Optokinetic Stimulation
Contextual Variability
Ambient Conditions
Terrain & Architecture
Postural Transitions
Traffic Density

Individual
Biomechanical
Cognition
Emotion (Limbic)
Cardiopulmonary
Navigation
Postural Strategies
Sensory Organization
Orientation in Space

Task
Frequency
Intensity
Spatial Characteristics
Temporal Factors
Physical Load
Target Characteristics
Practice Schedule

FIGURE 8-17. Expanded ecological model of balance rehabilitation

activities that are appropriate for the patient's skill level. A well-performed evaluation and initiation of activities at a lower level than determined by the examination can ensure appropriate exercise choice. It is safer to start the patient with tasks that are simpler and safer and progress to more complex exercises than to misjudge and place the patient in an unsafe situation. Measuring the patient's self-efficacy regarding her ability to safely perform the prescribed exercise regime at home can also assist in selecting the appropriate level of challenge. Simply have the patient rate her level of confidence on a scale of 0% to 100% regarding their ability to perform each exercise. Select exercise which the patient has a high level of confidence performing.

The surrounding environment should have maximum safety as the principal design factor. Eliminate obstacles or unsafe objects from the exercise area and provide additional stabilization for the patient. A gait belt, hand contacts from the clinician, parallel bars, or other stable external objects for the patient to hold should be immediately available. Balance training is contraindicated for persons who are inherently unsafe in balance-challenged positions. For example, those with cognitive impairments may be unable to understand the purpose and mechanics of the activity.

PATIENT EDUCATION

Patient education is an ongoing process for the patient with balance impairment. Safety is the most important area of education. Counsel the individual with significant balance impairments regarding use of assistive devices to maintain stability. A walker, one or two crutches, or a cane can widen the BOS, thereby increasing the stability limits. Evaluate the home for potential balance hazards. Loose rugs, slippery floors or bathtubs, uneven doorway thresholds, and stairs without railings can be hazards. A recent systematic review by Lyons et al.[108] concluded that there is insufficient evidence to determine the overall effectiveness of these strategies in terms of risk reduction when used alone. However, these authors encourage the common sense use of home safety strategies given that there

is no evidence that these strategies do not work. Footwear can affect balance. Education regarding appropriate footwear is often essential. Shoes that slip on the foot or on the floor or shoes with rubber bottoms that stick on the floor can cause a fall. Additionally, consider the impact of eye conditions and surgical and optical vision correction strategies (glasses, mono-vision contact lenses, Lasik).

Educate the patient regarding the limits of her balance. Factors include time (e.g., walking more than 20 minutes), distance (e.g., after walking more than four blocks), time of day (e.g., better in the morning than in the evening), and environment (e.g., crowds, noise, lights). Anticipating and recognizing the situations that place her at risk can help her make appropriate, safe choices while still participating in desired activities.

The patient should be taught strategies to maximize balance in compromised situations. For reasons beyond their control, patients may find themselves in situations where their balance is at risk. For example, when coming out of a movie, a person may have difficulty adjusting to the light, noise, and crowds in the lobby. Patients should be counseled in strategies to optimize balance, which may include using an assistive device (when the patient normally does not use one), using a friend's arm for balance and escort through the lobby, sitting and planning a path where stable objects may provide some external assistance, or asking someone for assistance.

KEY POINTS

- Balance and coordination are separate concepts that are integral to each other and, together, support all skilled movement.
- Balance is a function of the interaction of multiple body systems including biomechanical, neuromuscular, sensory, perceptual, cognitive, emotional, and cardiopulmonary functions.
- Some musculoskeletal disorders or injuries are associated with balance impairment. Balance training should be incorporated into the treatment program.
- Aging is associated with balance impairment and places the elderly at risk for falls.
- Ankle strategies are used in response to small perturbations, and hip or stepping strategies are used to counter larger perturbations.
- Measurement of balance impairment should involve each of the assessment of each of the body systems contributing to postural control.
- Treatment should be aimed at the cause of the problem, whether biomechanical, sensory, motor, cognitive, affective, or a combination of impairments.

CRITICAL THINKING QUESTIONS

1. Consider Case Study No. 1 in Unit 7. Design a progressive balance program for this basketball player. How would your treatment program differ if she were a
   a. Gymnast
   b. Figure skater
   c. Wrestler
   d. Cross-country runner

LAB ACTIVITIES

1. With a partner, perform the following activities. Which balance strategy is elicited and why?
   a. With the patient's feet shoulder width apart, attempt to gently disrupt the patient's balance.
   b. With the patient's feet shoulder width apart, attempt a larger disruption of the patient's balance.
   c. With the patient standing heel to toe, attempt to gently disrupt the patient's balance.
   d. With the patient standing on a balance beam, attempt to gently disrupt the patient's balance.
   e. Restrict the patient's ankle mobility with a brace or tape. Attempt to gently disrupt the patient's balance.
   f. Repeat a to c on a soft foam surface.
2. Compare the amount of postural sway observed when standing with the feet together in the following conditions. Which activities are the most challenging and why?
   a. Eyes open on a stable surface.
   b. Eyes closed on a stable surface.
   c. Eyes open on a thick foam surface.
   d. Eyes closed on a thick foam surface.
   e. Eyes open on a rocker board.
   f. Eyes closed on a rocker board.
   g. Repeat tasks a to f while simultaneously rotating or tilting the head.
3. Compare the length of time balance that can be maintained in the following situations. Which muscles are working, and how are changes in COG compensated by postural changes? What do the arms attempt to do?
   a. Single-leg stance with eyes open (left and right)
   b. Single-leg stance with eyes closed (left and right)
   c. Single-leg stance, performing tubing-resisted shoulder horizontal abduction, unilateral and bilateral
   d. Single-leg stance, performing tubing-resisted shoulder flexion from 120 to 180 degrees of overhead flexion, unilateral and bilateral
   e. Single-leg stance, performing tubing-resisted hip extension
   f. Single-leg minisquats with the contralateral knee flexed
   g. Single-leg minisquats with the contralateral knee extended and hip flexed
   h. Single-leg minisquats on a minitramp
   i. Single-leg toe raises from a level surface
   j. Single-leg toe raises from the edge of a step
4. Compare muscle activity in the following situations:
   a. Single-leg minisquats on a minitramp, with tubing around the posterior knee pulling the knee into flexion
   b. Single-leg minisquats on a minitramp, with tubing around the medial knee pulling the hip into abduction
   c. Single-leg minisquats on a minitramp, with tubing around the anterior knee pulling the knee into extension
   d. Single-leg minisquats on a minitramp, with tubing around the lateral knee pulling the hip into adduction
5. Perform the following activities. Which activity is the most challenging to your balance?
   a. Repetitive single-leg hopping with arms free
   b. Repetitive single-leg hopping with arms across the chest
   c. Repetitive single-leg hopping with arms overhead
   d. Rope jumping on alternate feet
   e. Rope jumping on a single foot
   f. Single repetition of a single-leg hop, controlling and stopping the landing as quickly as possible (i.e., hop and stop)
   g. Hop and stop on a minitramp

2. Consider Case Study No. 5 in Unit 7. Design a progressive balance program for this woman. Include sitting, standing, and transitional postures and movements. What other interventions probably are necessary to improve her balance?
3. What aspects of home design can maximize an individual's independence if balance is impaired?

REFERENCES

1. Swanik CB, Lephart SM, Giannantonio FP, et al. Reestablishing proprioception and neuromuscular control in the ACL-injured athlete. J Sport Rehabil 1997;2:182–206.
2. Barrett DS, Cobb AG, Bentley G. Joint proprioception in normal, osteoarthritic, and replaced knees. J Bone Joint Surg Br 1991;73:53–56.
3. Corrigan JP, Cashmen WF, Brady MP. Proprioception in the cruciate deficient knee. J Bone Joint Surg Br 1992;74:247–250.
4. Lamb K, Miller J, Mernadez M. Falls in the elderly: causes and prevention. Orthop Nurs 1987;6:45–49.
5. Crutchfield CA, Shumway-Cook A, Horak FB. Balance and coordination training. In: Scully RM, Barnes MR, eds. Physical Therapy. Philadelphia, PA: JB Lippincott, 1989:825–843.
6. Nashner LM. Sensory, neuromuscular, and biomechanical contributions to human balance. In: Balance: Proceedings of the American Physical Therapy Association Forum; Nashville, TN, June 13–15, 1989.
7. Schmitz TJ. Coordination assessment. In: O'Sullivan SB, Schmitz TJ, eds. Physical Rehabilitation: Assessment and Treatment. Philadelphia, PA: FA Davis, 1994.
8. Williams HG, Fisher JM, Tritschler KA. Descriptive analysis of static postural control in 4, 6, and 8 year old normal and motorically awkward children. American J Phys Med 62(1):12–26.
9. Frank JS, Earl M. Coordination of posture and movement. Phys Ther 70(12):855–863.
10. Burleigh AL, Horak FB, Malouin F. Modification of postural responses and step initiation: evidence for goal-directed postural interactions. J Neurophysiol 72(6):2892–2902.
11. Berg KO, Maki BE, Williams JI, et al. Clinical and laboratory measures of postural balance in an elderly population. Arch Phys Med Rehabil 1992;73:1073–1080.
12. Shumway-Cook A, Horak RB. Assessing the influence of sensory interaction on balance. Phys Ther 1986;1548–1550.
13. Horak FB, Nashner LM. Central programming of postural movements: adaptation to altered support surface configurations. J Neurophysiol 1986;55(6):1369–1381.
14. Horak FB, Henry SM, Shumway-Cook A. Postural perturbations: new insights of treatment of balance disorders. Phys Ther 1997;77(5):517–533.
15. Horak FB. Postural orientation and equilibrium: What do we need to know about neural control of balance to prevent falls? Age Ageing 2006;35 (Suppl 2):ii7–ii11.
16. Tinetti ME, Speechley M, Ginter SF. Risk factors for falls among elderly persons living in the community. N Engl J Med 1988;319(26):1701–1707.
17. Stern EB. The somatosensory systems. In: Cohen H, ed. Neuroscience for Rehabilitation. Philadelphia, PA: JB Lippincott, 1993.

18. Rowinski MJ. Afferent neurobiology of the joint. In: Gould JA, Davies GJ, eds. Orthopaedic and Sports Physical Therapy. 2nd Ed. St. Louis, MO: CV Mosby, 1985.
19. Grigg P. Articular neurophysiology. In: Zachazewski JE, McGee DJ, Quillen WS, eds. Athletic Injury Rehabilitation. Philadelphia, PA: WB Saunders, 1996.
20. Grigg P, Finerman GA, Riley LH. Joint-position sense after total hip replacement. J Bone Joint Surg Am 1973;55:1016–1025.
21. Lord SR, Ward JA, Williams P, et al. Physiological factors associated with falls in older community-dwelling women. J Am Geriatr Soc 1994;42(10):1110–1117.
22. Shumway-Cook A, Woollacott MH. Motor Control Theory and Practical Applications. 2nd Ed. Philadelphia, PA: Lippincott Williams & Wilkins, 2001.
23. Fox CR, Cohen H. The visual and vestibular systems. In: Cohen H, ed. Neuroscience for Rehabilitation. Philadelphia, PA: JB Lippincott, 1993.
24. Karnath H O, Fetter M, Niemeier M. Disentangling gravitational environmental and egocentric reference frames in spatial neglect. J Cogn Neurosci. 1998;10(6):680–690.
25. Winstein C, Mitz AR. The motor system II: higher centers. In: Cohen H, ed. Neuroscience for Rehabilitation. Philadelphia, PA: JB Lippincott, 1993.
26. Nashner LM, Shuper CL, Horak FB, et al. Organization of posture controls: an analysis of sensory and mechanical constraints. Prog Brain Res 1989;80:411–418.
27. Garcin R. Coordination of voluntary movement. In: Visken PJ, Bruyun GW, eds. Handbook of Clinical Neurology. Amsterdam: South Holland Publishing Co., 1969.
28. Light KE. Information processing for motor performance in aging adults. Phys Ther 1990;70:820–826.
29. Riach CL, Hayes KC. Maturation of postural sway in young children. Dev Med Child Neur 1987;29:650–658.
30. Maki BE, Edmondstone MA, McIlroy WE. Age-related differences in laterally directed compensatory stepping behavior. J Gerontol A Biol Sci Med Sci 2000;55(5):M270–M277.
31. Halliday SE, Winter DA, Frank JS, et al. The initiation of gait in young, elderly, and Parkinson's disease subjects. Gait Posture 1998;8(1):8–14.
32. Bouisset S, Zattara M. Biomechanical study of the programming of anticipatory postural adjustments associated with voluntary movement. J Biomech 1987;20(8):735–742.
33. Horak FB, Macpherson JM. Postural orientation and equilibrium. In: Shepard J, Rowell L, eds. Handbook of Physiology: Section 12: Exercise, Regulation, and Integration of Multiple Systems. New York, NY: Oxford University Press, 1996.
34. Patla A. Adaptive human locomotion: influence of neural, biological, and mechanical factors on ctrol mechanisms. In: Bronstein AM, Brandt T, Woollacott MH, Nutt JO, eds. Clinical Disorders of Balance, Posture, and Gait. 2nd Ed. London: Arnold, 2004;Chap 2.
35. Stelmach GE, Zelaznik HN, Lowe D. The influence of ageing and attentional demands on recovery from postural instability. Aging (Milano) 1990;2(2):155–161.
36. Brown LA, Shumway-Cook A, Woollacott MH. Attentional demands and postural recovery: the effects of ageing. J Gerontol A Biol Med Sci 1999;54(4):M165–M171.
37. Rankin JK, Woollacott MH, Shumway-Cook A, et al. Cognitive influence on postural stability: a neuromuscular analysis in young and older adults. J Gerontol A Biol Sci Med Sci 2000;55(3):M112–M119.
38. Shumway-Cook A, Woollacott M. Attentional demands and postural control: the effect of sensory context. J Gerontol A Biol Sci Med Sci 2000;55(1):M10–M16.
39. Rotem-Lehrer N, Laufer Y. The effect of attention on transfer on a postural control task following an ankle sprain. J Orthop Sports Phys Ther 2007;37(9):564–569.
40. Adkin AL, Frank JS, Carpenter MG, et al. Postural control is scaled to level of postural threat. Gait Posture 2000;12(2):87–93.
41. Shumway-Cook A, Patla AE, Stewart A, et al. Environmental demands associated with community mobility in older adults with and without mobility disabilities. Phys Ther 2002;82(7):670–681.
42. Whitney SL, Wrisley DM, Brown KE, et al. Is perception of handicap related to functional performance in persons with vestibular dysfunction? Otol Neurotol 2004;25(2):139–143.
43. Brown KE, Whitney SL, Marchetti GF, et al. Physical therapy for central vestibular dysfunction. Arch Phys Med Rehabil 2006;87(1):76–81.
44. Fitts PM, Posner MI. Human Performance. Belmont, CA: Brooks/Cole, 1967.
45. Magill RA. Motor learning: concepts and applications. Boston, MA: McGraw-Hill, 1998.
46. Kempton A, van Beurden E, Sladden T, et al. Older people can stay on their fee: final results of a community-based falls prevention program. Health Promotion Int 2000;15:27–35.
47. Lindqvist K, Timpka T, Schelp L. Evaluation of an inter-organizational prevention program against injuries among the elderly in a WHO Safe Community. Public Health 2001;115(5):308–316.
48. McClure R, Turner C, Peel N, et al. Population-based interventions for the prevention of fall-related injuries in older people. Cochrane Database Syst Rev 2005;(1):CD004441.
49. Lan C, Lai JS, Chen SY, et al. Tai Chi Chuan to improve muscular strength and endurance in elderly individuals: a pilot study. Arch Phys Med Rehabil 2000;81(5):604–607.
50. Hong Y, LI JX, Robinson PD. Balance control, flexibility, and cardiorespiratory fitness among older Tai Chi practitioners. Br J Sports Med 2000;34(1):29–34.
51. Wolf SL, Barnhart HX, Kutner NG, et al. Reducing frailty and falls in older persons: an investigation of Tai/Chi and computerized balance training. Atlanta FICSIT Group. Frailty and Injuries: Cooperative Studies of Intervention Techniques. J Am Ger Soc 1996;44(5):489–497.
52. Yan JH. Tai chi practice reduces movement force variability for seniors. J Gerontol A Biol Sci Med Sci 1999;54(12):M629–M634.
53. Hain TC, Fuller L, Weil L, et al. Effects of T'ai Chi on balance. Arch Otolaryn Head Neck Surg 1999;125(11):1191–1195.
54. Wong AM, Lin YC, Chou SW, et al. Coordination exercise and postural stability in elderly people: effect of Tai Chi Chuan. Arch Phys Med Rehabil 2001;82(5):608–612.
55. Li F, Harmer P, McAuley E, et al. An evaluation of the effects of Tai Chi exercise on physical function among older persons: a randomized controlled trial. Ann Behav Med 2001;23(2):139–146.
56. Hartman CA, Manos TM, Winter C, et al. Effects of Tai Chi training on function and quality of life indicators in older adults with osteoarthritis. J Am Ger Soc 2000;48(12):1553–1559.
57. Wolf SL, Barnhart HX, Ellison GL, et al. The effect of Tai Chi Quan and computerized balance training on postural stability in older subjects. Atlanta FICSIT Group. Frailty and Injuries: Cooperative Studies on Intervention Techniques. Phys Ther 1997;77(4):371–381.
58. Kutner NG, Barnhart H, Wolf SL, et al. Self-report benefits of Tai Chi practice by older adults. J Gerontol B Psych Sci Soc Sci 1997;52(5):P242–P246.
59. Gillespie LD, Gillespie WJ, Robertson MC, et al. Interventions for preventing falls in elderly people. Cochrane Database Syst Rev 2003;3:CD000340.
60. Rozzi SL, Lephart SM, Sterner R, et al. Balance training for persons with functionally unstable ankles. J Orthop Sports Phys Ther 1999;29(8):478–486.
61. Fitzgerald GK, Axe MJ, Snyder-Mackler L. The efficacy of perturbation training in nonoperative anterior cruciate ligament rehabilitation programs for physical active individuals. Phys Ther 2000;80(2):128–140.
62. Wolfson L, Whipple R, Derby C, et al. Balance and strength training in older adults: intervention gains and Tai Chi maintenance. J Am Ger Soc 1996;44(5):599–600.
63. Gardner MM, Buchner DM, Robertson MC, Campbell AJ. Practical implementation of an exercise-based falls prevention programme. Age Ageing 2001;30(1):77–83.
64. Campbell AJ, Robertson MC, Gardner MM, et al. Falls prevention over 2 years: a randomized controlled trial in women 80 years and older. Age Ageing 1999;28(6):513–518.
65. Interactive Guide to Physical Therapist Practice, V. 1.0. American Physical Therapy Association, Alexandria, VA, 2002.
66. Russo SG. Clinical balance measures: literature resources. Neurol Rep 1997;21(1):29–36.
67. Andrews AW, Folger SE, Norbet SE, et al. Tests and measures used by specialist physical therapists when examining patients with stroke. J Neurol Phys Ther 2008;32(3):122–128.
68. Badke MB, Miedaner JA, Shea TA, et al. Effects of vestibular and balance rehabilitation on sensory organization and dizziness handicap. Ann Otol Rhinol Laryngol 2005;114(1 Pt 1):48–54.
69. Badke MB, Shea TA, Miedaner JA, et al. Outcomes after rehabilitation for adults with balance dysfunction. Arch Phys Med Rehabil 2004;85(2):227–233.
70. Badke MB, Pyle GM, Shea T, et al. Outcomes in vestibular ablative procedures. Otol Neurotol 2002;23(4):504–509.
71. Horak, F. Personal communication at: Advanced Competency in the Evaluation & Treatment of Complex Balance Disorders. North American Seminars, Indiana, 2002.
72. Duncan PW, Weiner DK, Chandler J, et al. Functional reach: a new clinical measure of balance. J Gerontol 1990;45:M192–M197.
73. Donahoe B, Turner D, Worrell T. The use of functional reach as a measurement of balance in boys and girls without disabilities ages 5 to 15 years. Pediatr Phys Ther 1994;6:189–193.
74. Newton RA. Validity of the multi-directional reach test: a practical measure for limits of stability in older adults. J Gerontol A Biol Sci Med Sci 2001;56(4):M248–M252.
75. Cohen H, Blatchly CA, Gombash LL. A study of the clinical test of sensory interaction and balance. Phys Ther 1993;73(6):346–351; discussion 351–354.
76. Westcott SL, Crowe TK, Deitz JC, et al. Test-retest reliability of the Pediatric Clinical Test of Sensory Interaction for Balance (P-CTSIB). Phys Occ Ther in Ped 1994;14:1–22.
77. Whitney SL, Wrisley DM. The influence of footwear on timed balance scores of the modified clinical test of sensory interaction and balance. Arch Phys Med Rehabil 2004;85(3):439–443.
78. Wrisley DM, Whitney SL. The effect of foot position on the modified clinical test of sensory interaction and balance. Arch Phys Med Rehabil 2004;85(2):335–338.
79. Cauka M, McCarty DJ. Simple method for measurement of lower extremity muscle strength. Am J Med 1985;78(1):77–81.
80. Fishman MN, Colby LA, Sachs LA, et al. Comparison of upper-extremity balance tasks and force platform testing in persons with hemiparesis. Phys Ther 1997;77:1052–1062.

81. Jacobs JV, Horak FB, Van Tran K, et al. An alternative clinical postural stability test for patients with Parkinson's disease. J Neurol 2006;253(11):1404–1413.

82. Berg KO, Wood-Dauphinee SL, Williams JT, et al. Measuring balance in the elderly: validation of an instrument. Can J Public Health 1992;83:S7–S11.

83. Dite W, Temple VA. A clinical test of stepping and change of direction to identify multiple falling older adults. Arch Phys Med Rehabil 2002;83(11):1566–1571.

84. Mathias S, Nayak USL, Isaacs B. Balance in elderly patients: the "get-up and go" test. Arch Phys Med Rehabil 1986;67:387–389.

85. DiFabio RP, Seay R. Use of the "fast evaluation of mobility, balance and fear" in elderly community dwellers: validity and reliability. Phys Ther 1997;77:904–917.

86. Shumway-cook A, Woollacott MH. Motor Control: Theory and Practical Applications. 1st Ed. Baltimore, MD: Williams and Wilkins, 1995.

87. Wrisley DM, Marchetti GF, Kuharsky DK, et al. Reliability, internal consistency, and validity of data obtained with the functional gait assessment. Phys Ther 2004;84(10):906–918.

88. Walker ML, Austin AG, Banke GM, et al. Reference group data for the functional gait assessment. Phys Ther 2007;87(11):1468–1477. Epub 2007 Sep 4.

89. Marchetti GF, Whitney SL. Construction and validation of the 4-item dynamic gait index. Phys Ther 2006;86(12):1651–1660. Epub 2006 Oct 24.

90. Powell LE, Myers AM. The Activities-specific Balance Confidence (ABC) Scale. J Gerontol A Biol Sci Med Sci 1995;50A(1):M28–M34.

91. Jacobson GP, Newman CW. The development of the Dizziness Handicap Inventory. Arch Otolaryngol Head Neck Surg 1990;116(4):424–427.

92. Vereeck L, Truijen S, Wuyts FL, et al. The dizziness handicap inventory and its relationship with functional balance performance. Otol Neurotol 2007;28(1):87–93.

93. Whitney SL, Wrisley DM, Marchetti GF, et al. Clinical measurement of sit-to-stand performance in people with balance disorders: validity of data for the Five-Times-Sit-to-Stand Test. Phys Ther 2005;85(10):1034–1045.

94. Whitney SL, Marchetti GF, Morris LO, et al. The reliability and validity of the Four Square Step Test for people with balance deficits secondary to a vestibular disorder. Arch Phys Med Rehabil 2007;88(1):99–104.

95. Bogle Thorbahn LD, Newton RA. Use of the Berg Balance Test to predict falls in the elderly. Phys Ther 1996;76:576–585.

96. Dibble LE, Lange M. Predicting falls in individuals with Parkinson disease: a reconsideration of clinical balance measures. J Neurol Phys Ther 2006;30(2):60–67.

97. Medley A, Thompson M, French J. Predicting the probability of falls in community dwelling persons with brain injury: a pilot study. Brain Inj 2006;20(13–14):1403–1408.

98. Mackintosh SF, Hill KD, Dodd KJ, et al. Balance score and a history of falls in hospital predict recurrent falls in the 6 months following stroke rehabilitation. Arch Phys Med Rehabil 2006;87(12):1583–1589.

99. Whitney SL, Marchetti GF, Schade A, et al. The sensitivity and specificity of the Timed "Up & Go" and the Dynamic Gait Index for self-reported falls in persons with vestibular disorders. J Vestib Res 2004;14(5):397–409.

100. Whitney S, Wrisley D, Furman J. Concurrent validity of the Berg Balance Scale and the Dynamic Gait Index in people with vestibular dysfunction. Physiother Res Int 2003;8(4):178–186.

101. Muir SW, Berg K, Chesworth B, et al. Use of the Berg Balance Scale for predicting multiple falls in community-dwelling elderly people: a prospective study. Phys Ther 2008;88(4):449–459; discussion 460–461. Epub 2008 Jan 24.

102. Dibble LE, Christensen J, Ballard DJ, et al. Diagnosis of fall risk in Parkinson disease: an analysis of individual and collective clinical balance test interpretation. Phys Ther 2008;88(3):323–332. Epub 2008 Jan 10.

103. Shepard NT, Telian SA. Programmatic vestibular rehabilitation. Otolaryngol Head Neck Surg 1995;112(1):173–182.

104. Shumway-Cook A, Gruber W, Baldwin M, et al. The effect of multidimensional exercises on balance, mobility, and fall risk in community-dwelling older adults. Phys Ther 1997;77(1):46–57.

105. Shumway-Cook A, Patla A, Stewart A, et al. Environmental components of mobility disability in community-living older persons. J Am Geriatr Soc 2003;51(3):393–398.

106. Maki BE, McIlroy WE. Postural control in the older adult. Clin Geriatr Med 1996;12(4):635–658.

107. Jeka JJ. Light touch contact as a balance aid. Phys Ther 1997;77(5):476–487.

108. Lyons RA, John A, Brophy S, et al. Modification of the home environment for the reduction of injuries. Cochrane Database Syst Rev 2006;(4):CD003600.

ADDITIONAL READING

Dietz V, Horstmann GA, Berger W. Significance of proprioceptive mechanisms in the regulation of stance. Prog Brain Res 1989;80:419–423.

Era P, Heikkinen E. Postural sway during standing and unexpected disturbance of balance in random samples of men different ages. J Gerontol 1985;40:287–295.

Hageman RA, Leibowitz JM, Blanke D. Age and gender effects on postural control measures. Arch Phys Med Rehabil 1995;76:961–965.

McCollum G, Leen T. Form and exploration of mechanical stability limits in erect stance. J Motor Behav 1989;21:225–238.

Nashner LM. Adaptation of human movement to altered environments. Trends Neurosci 1982;5:358–361.

Nashner L, McCollum G. The organization of human postural movements: a formal basis and experimental synthesis. Behav Brain Sci 1985;8:135–172.

Province MA, Hadley EC, Hornbrook MC, et al. The effects of exercise on falls in elderly patients. JAMA 1995;273:1341–1347.

chapter 9

Impaired Posture

CARRIE M. HALL

INTRODUCTION

Impairments in posture and movement are the basis of many regional musculoskeletal pain syndromes (MPS).[1] MPS are localized, painful conditions arising from irritation of myofascial, periarticular, or articular tissues.[1] Pain from trauma, such as strain, fracture, or dislocation, or pain caused by systemic disease, such as rheumatoid arthritis or cancer, does not fall into this category.

Regional MPS are often the result of cumulative microtrauma imposed on musculoskeletal tissue. Microtrauma can occur from overuse, which is defined as repetitive or prolonged, submaximal stress that exceeds the tissue's ability to adapt and repair.[2,3] Overuse can occur during a relatively short period, such as playing the first volleyball game of the season, or over a longer period, such as performing data entry tasks 8 hours a day, 5 days a week, for many years. Microtrauma can also be caused by movements repeated during activities of daily living with less than optimal starting alignment or faulty osteokinematic or arthrokinematic motion.

Pain indicates that a mechanical deformation or chemical process has stimulated the nociceptors in the symptomatic structures. However, describing the mechanisms that signal pain is not the same as identifying the cause of pain. The premise of this chapter is that mechanical stress related to sustained postural habits or repeated movement patterns

1. is the primary cause of pain
2. contributes to the recurrence of a painful condition
3. is associated with the failure of the condition to resolve

Intervention, therefore, focuses on correcting the factors predisposing or contributing to the sustained postures or repetitive movement. When correction is not possible (e.g., anatomic impairments, pathology, disease), modification of the posture or movement is indicated. Display 9-1 summarizes the factors influencing impairments of posture and movement.

It is generally accepted that impairments of posture and movement are related to the generation and perpetuation of MPS.[1,4–7] Although evidence exists that movement impairment is related to pain, there is still very little research to support a relationship between musculoskeletal pain and posture.[8]

Despite the lack of evidence, the inclusion of postural assessment in the Guide to Physical Therapist Practice[9] and the accreditation standards suggest that the profession considers postural alignment to have a role in patient care. Common knowledge would dictate that the emphasis of treatment for a patient with low back pain with a reduced lumbar extension curve would be different than a patient

with a lumbar lordosis. Sahrmann outlines a sound rationale for the discrepancy between the research data and the clinical experience of generations of physical therapists. In her 2002 commentary, she wrote:

> I believe some of the explanations are (1) a narrow definition of what constitutes posture; (2) attempts to find a linear correlation between pain and spinal curvature without identifying subgroups of extremes of increased or decreased curvature; (3) failure to consider alignment as only one of multiple factors causing pain; (4) attempts to relate postural faults and muscle weakness; and (5) limited research examining the relationship between alignment impairments and alterations in movement.[10]

She concluded that examination of alignment impairments has to be an important step in designing an appropriate treatment program for correcting mechanical impairments and that future studies need to better correlate relationships among specific alignment impairments, altered movement patterns, contributing muscle adaptations, patient modifiers, and mechanical pain problems.[10] Understanding these relationships will enhance our therapeutic intervention of these impairments.

This chapter defines the terms used in the evaluation and treatment of impairments of posture and movement, discusses factors influencing impairments of posture and movement, and outlines the principles of therapeutic exercise intervention for correction of posture and movement impairments.

DEFINITIONS

Posture

Posture is often considered to be a static function rather than being related to movement. However, posture should be considered not only a static function but also in the context of the position the body assumes in preparation for movement. Traditionally, posture is examined in standing and sitting positions, but posture should be examined in numerous positions, particularly postures in which the patient frequently assumes and positions related to frequently performed movements. For example, standing on one leg is 85% of the gait cycle and therefore should be considered an important posture to be examined.[11]

A useful definition of posture was provided by the Posture Committee of the American Academy of Orthopaedic Surgeons.[12]

> **Posture** is usually defined as the relative arrangement of the parts of the body. Good posture is the state of muscular and skeletal balance that protects the supporting structures of

the body against injury or progressive deformity irrespective of the attitude (e.g., erect, lying, squatting, and stooping) in which these structures are working or resting. Under such conditions, the muscles function most efficiently, and the optimum positions are afforded for the thoracic and abdominal organs. Poor posture is a faulty relationship of the various parts of the body, which produces increased strain on the supporting structures and in which there is less efficient balance of the body over its base of support.

Most physical therapists understand the relationship between posture and the musculoskeletal system, but an important message delivered by this definition is the interaction between posture, musculoskeletal tissues, and organ systems (e.g., lungs, abdominal organs, pelvic organs). This definition suggests that, without optimal support, organ systems may not function optimally. For example, respiratory insufficiency can result from kyphosis (increased thoracic flexion) or kyphoscoliosis (kyphosis superimposed lateral curve).[13] These postural faults can reduce mobility of the thorax and thereby increase the work of breathing.[14] Chronically altered respiratory mechanics have been cited as a contributing factor to cardiopulmonary pathology (e.g., pulmonary hypertension, right heart failure).[15]

Posture or carriage of the body describes the global relationships of body parts and should be considered differently than the orientation or alignment of one segment in relation to an immediately adjacent segment. For example, spino-pelvic balance in the sagittal plane can be considered as a global postural relationship linking the head to the pelvis whereas the shape and orientation (alignment) of each successive anatomic segment are closely related and influence the adjacent segment. Evidence in the literature demonstrates a relationship between the alignment of the sacrum, pelvis, femoral heads and developmental spondylolisthesis.[16] It is critical that the practitioner examine both posture orientation and segmental alignment to understand the relationship of individual segments to one another and to global posture orientation.

For the purposes of this chapter, the focus will be on examining and treating posture in the global sense. The reader is referred to regional chapters to understand segmental

alignment standards, the relationship of alignment faults to pathological conditions, and the treatment of existing segmental alignment faults.

Standard Posture

Although any posture a patient or client assumes for sustained periods on a daily basis should be evaluated and treated, this chapter considers only the upright standing posture. The **standard posture** refers to an ideal posture rather than an average or normal posture. This standard should be used as a basis for comparison; deviations from the standard are called *impairments of posture.*

An evaluation of postural faults necessitates a standard by which individual postures can be judged. The standing posture is used as the standard in this chapter and is illustrated from the back and side (Fig. 9-1). In the back view, a line of reference represents a plane that coincides with the midline of the body. It is illustrated as beginning midway between the heels and extending upward to midway between the lower extremities, through the midline of the pelvis, spine, and skull. The right and left halves of the skeletal structures are essentially symmetric. Hypothetically, the two halves of the body are in equilibrium.

In the side view, the vertical line of reference represents a plane that divides the body into front and back sections. Around this line of reference, the body is hypothetically in a position of equilibrium.

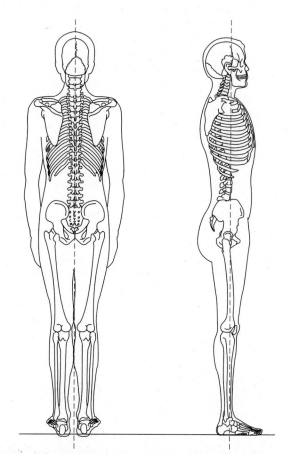

FIGURE 9-1. The back and side views of standard posture. The surface and anatomic landmarks that coincide with these views are listed in Table 9-1.

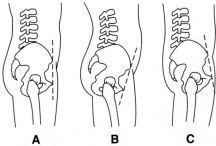

A   B   C

FIGURE 9-2. (A) The *neutral position* of the pelvis is one in which the anterosuperior iliac spines are in the same transverse plane and in which they and the symphysis are in the same vertical plane. (B) An *anterior pelvic tilt* is a position of the pelvis in which the vertical plane through the anterosuperior iliac spines is anterior to a vertical plane through the symphysis pubis. (C) A *posterior pelvic tilt* is a position of the pelvis in which the vertical plane through the anterosuperior iliac spines is posterior to a vertical plane through the symphysis pubis.

From a mechanical standpoint, it may be logical to assume that a line of gravity should pass through the centers of weight-bearing joints of the body. However, the on-center position is not considered stable, because it can be held only momentarily in the presence of normal external stresses.[17,18] For example, when the center of the knee joint coincides with the line of gravity, there are equal tendencies for the joint to flex and to hyperextend. The slightest force exerted in either direction causes it to move off center. If the body must call on muscular effort at all times to resist knee flexion, muscular effort is unnecessarily expended. To offset this necessity, the line of gravity is considered to be slightly anterior to the joint center. Ligamentous structures and ideal muscle length restrain the knee from moving freely posteriorly. At the hip joint, the same principles apply, but the hip is most stable when the line of gravity is slightly posterior to the center of the joint. The strong ligaments of the hip anteriorly prevent additional hip extension.

The pelvis is the link that transmits the weight of the head, arms, and trunk to the lower extremities, and it is considered key to the alignment of the entire lower body. Because of structural variations of the pelvis (i.e., women tend to have a shallow pelvis, with the anterior superior iliac spine [ASIS] inferior to the posterior superior iliac spine), it is not appropriate to use an anterior landmark in relation to a posterior landmark. The pelvis is considered to be in a neutral position when the ASIS and the symphysis pubis are in the same vertical plane (see Fig. 9-2A). The anatomic structures and surface landmarks that coincide with the line of reference for the side view are listed in Table 9-1. Specific alignment of the upper extremity is summarized in Display 9-2.[1]

Deviations in Posture

The following terms denote deviations in alignment with reference to segments of the body[19]:

- *Lordosis* is an increased anterior curve of the spine, usually of the lumbar spine, but it can affect the thoracic or cervical spine. If used without a modifying word, it refers to lumbar lordosis (Fig. 9-3).

TABLE 9-1 Anatomic Structures and Surface Landmarks that Coincide with the Line of Reference for the Side View of Posture

ANATOMIC STRUCTURES	SURFACE LANDMARKS
Through the calcaneocuboid joint	Slightly anterior to the lateral malleolus
Slightly anterior to the center of the knee joint	Slightly anterior to a midline through the knee
Slightly posterior to the center of the hip joint	Through the greater trochanter
Through the sacral promontory	Midway between the back and the abdomen
Through the bodies of the lumbar vertebrae	Midway between the front and back of the chest
Through the dens	Through lobe of the ear
Through the external auditory meatus	
Slightly posterior to the apex of the coronal sutures	

Kendall HO, Kendall FP, Boynton DA. Posture and Pain. Huntington, NY: Robert E. Krieger Publishing, 1970.

- *Kyphosis* is an increased posterior curve, usually of the thoracic spine but sometimes of the lumbar spine. If used without a modifying word, the term refers to the thoracic spine (Fig. 9-4).
- *Anterior pelvic tilt* refers to a position in which the vertical plane through the ASIS is anterior to a vertical plane through the symphysis pubis (Fig. 9-2B).
- *Posterior pelvic tilt* refers to a position in which the vertical plane through the ASIS is posterior to a vertical plane through the symphysis pubis (Fig. 9-2C).

DISPLAY 9-2
Alignment of the Upper Extremity

Side View
- Humerus
  No more than one third of the head of the humerus protrudes in front of the acromion.
  Proximal and distal humerus in line vertically
- Scapula
  The inferior pole is held flat against the thorax (if the thorax is in ideal alignment).
  30 degrees anterior to the frontal plane (i.e., scapular plane)

Back and Front View
- Humerus
  Antecubital crease faces anterior; olecranon faces posterior.
- Forearms
  Palms face the body
- Scapula
  The vertebral border of the scapula is parallel to the spine and is positioned approximately 3 in from the spine.
  The root of the scapula (where the spine of the scapula meets the vertebral border of the scapula) is at the level of T3.
  The vertebral border of the scapula is held against the thorax (if the thorax is in ideal alignment).

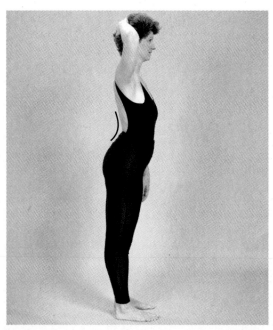

FIGURE 9-3. Marked anterior pelvic tilt and an exaggerated anterior curve of the lumbar spine. This curve is called a *lordosis.* Note that accompanying the anterior pelvic tilt and lordosis is flexion of the hip joint.

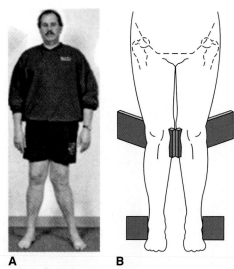

A   **B**

FIGURE 9-5. (A) This person has marked structural genu valgum or knock-knees. (B) Postural genu valgum results from a combination of lateral rotation of the femurs, supination of the feet, and hyperextension of the knees. With lateral rotation, the axis of the knee joint is oblique to the coronal plane, and hyperextension results in adduction at the knees.

- The normal angle between the tibia and femur in the frontal plane is about 170 to 175 degrees and is called the physiologic valgus angle of the knee.[20] If the valgus angle is <165 degrees, *genu valgum* (i.e., knock knees) exists.[20] Structural genu valgum can be associated with pronated feet, medially rotated femurs, anteverted hips, and coxa varum (Fig. 9-5A; see Chapter 20). Postural genu valgum results from a combination of lateral rotation of the femurs, supination of the feet, and hyperextension of the knees (see Fig. 9-5B).[19] Conversely, if the tibiofemoral angle approaches or exceeds 180 degrees, genu varum (i.e., bow legs) exists (Fig. 9-6A).[20] Structural genu varum can be associated with coxa valgum (see Chapter 20). Postural genu varum results from a combination of medial rotation of the femurs, pronation of the feet, and hyperextension of knees (see Fig. 9-6B).[19]
- In the sagittal plane, the tibiofemoral angle should be 180 degrees.[20] If the angle exceeds 180 degrees, *genu recurvatum* (i.e., hyperextension) exists (Fig. 9-7).[20]
- *Scapular adduction* is a rest position or movement in which the scapula is positioned or moving toward the

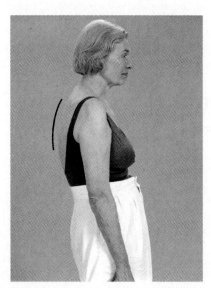

FIGURE 9-4. This person exhibits an exaggeration of the normal posterior curve of the thoracic spine. This is called a *kyphosis.*

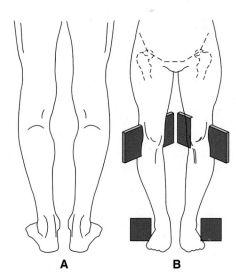

A   **B**

FIGURE 9-6. (A) Mild degree of structural genu varum, or bow legs. (B) Postural genu varum results from a combination of medial rotation of the femurs, pronation of the feet, and hyperextension of the knees. When femurs medially rotate, the axis of motion for flexion and extension is oblique to the coronal axis. From this axis, hyperextension occurs in a posterolateral direction, resulting in separation at the knees and apparent bowing of the legs.

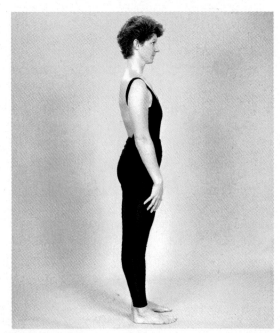

FIGURE 9-7. Moderate genu recurvatum or hyperextension of the knees.

vertebral column (see Fig. 9-8).[19] *Scapular abduction* is a rest position or movement in which the scapula is positioned or moving away from the vertebral column (Fig. 9-9).[19] The clinician should avoid using "retraction" for scapular adduction and "protraction" for scapular abduction.[19] The sternoclavicular joint moves into protraction and retraction. The scapula slides away from (abduction) or toward the spine (adduction) with protraction and rectraction at the SC joint, respectively.

- *Upward rotation of the scapula* is a position or movement about an axis perpendicular to scapular plane [21] in

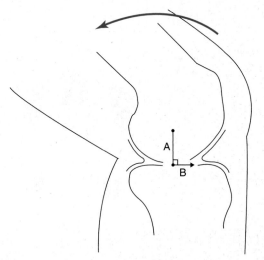

FIGURE 9-8. A normal knee with a line drawn from the instant center of the tibiofemoral joint to the tibiofemoral contact point (*line A*) forms a right angle with a line tangential to the tibial surface (*line B*). The *arrow* indicates the direction of displacement of the contact points. *Line B* is tangential to the tibial surface, indicating that the femur glides on the tibial condyles during flexion-extension motion.

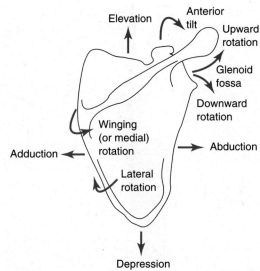

FIGURE 9-9. The positions and movements of the scapula.

which the inferior angle moves laterally and the glenoid fossa moves cranially (see Fig. 9-9).[19] *Downward rotation of the scapula* is a position or movement in which the inferior angle moves medially and the glenoid fossa moves caudally.[19]

- *Anterior tilt of the scapula* is a position or movement about a frontal axis parallel to the spine of the scapula[21] in which the coracoid process moves in an anterior direction.[19] *Posterior tilt of the scapula* is a position or movement in which the coracoid process moves in a posterior and cranial direction, whereas the inferior angle moves in an anterior and caudal direction (see Fig. 9-9).[19]
- *Elevation of the scapula* is a position or movement about a vertical axis in which the scapula moves cranially, and *depression of the scapula* is a position or movement in which the scapula moves caudally (see Fig. 9-9).[19]
- *Winging of the scapula* or *medial rotation* is a position or movement about a vertical axis perpendicular to the spine of the scapula[21] in which the vertebral border of the scapula moves posteriorly and laterally away from the rib cage and the glenoid fossa moves in an anterior and medial direction (see Fig. 9-9).[22] *Lateral rotation* of the scapula is the converse movement.[22]

MOVEMENT

Movement is the action of a physiologic system that produces motion of the whole body or of its component parts.[23] Evaluating active movement in the clinical setting requires precise observation and palpation skills and extensive knowledge of kinesiologic principles.

A useful criterion for assessing precise or balanced movement is knowledge of the *path of instantaneous center of rotation* (PICR) during active motion.[1,24–26] The instant center of rotation describes the relative uniplanar motion of two adjacent segments of a body and the direction of displacement of the contact points between these segments (Fig. 9-8).[24] The instant center of rotation changes over time because of altered joint configurations and external forces. The PICR is a trace of the sequential instant centers of rotation for a joint

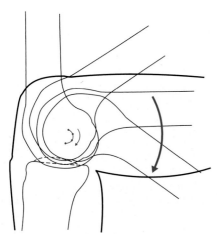

FIGURE 9-10. Semicircular PICR for the tibiofemoral joint in a normal knee.

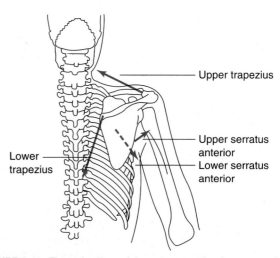

FIGURE 9-11. The action lines of the upper trapezius, lower trapezius, upper serratus anterior, and lower serratus anterior combine in a force-couple action to produce almost pure upward rotation of the scapula.

in different positions throughout the range of motion (ROM) in one plane (Fig. 9-10).

Efficiency and longevity of the biomechanical system requires maintenance of precise movement of rotating segments; the PICR must meet a kinesiologic standard.[1] Deviations in the PICR from the ideal for a given joint imply that the arthrokinematic joint motions have become altered, even if the osteokinematic motion is within the normal range. The quality or precision of the osteokinematic motion is affected. Various investigators have shown that PICR deviations provide a noninvasive means of identifying pathomechanics.[13,15,21] However, because the radiologic[27] or computational modeling methods[28] used to determine the PICR are not available to physical therapists, clinically reliable tools for measuring the PICR need to be established. Techniques used to qualitatively examine uniplanar, multiplanar, and total body movement patterns include precise observation, palpation of joint osteokinematics and arthrokinematics, and palpation or the use of surface electromyography to detect muscle activation patterns. The clinician relies on a thorough knowledge of kinesiologic principles to differentiate ideal from impaired movement patterns. A recommended reference to study clinical tools for assessing the PICR can be found in the recommended reading list at the end of this chapter.[1]

A major determinant of the PICR during active motion is the muscular force-couple action on the joint. **Force couple** is defined as two forces of equal magnitude but opposite direction with parallel lines of application.[18] The result of the forces is zero, meaning the body is not displaced (i.e., the body is in translatory equilibrium). The force couple causes the body to rotate around an axis perpendicular to the plane of the forces (Fig. 9-11).[18] In biomechanics, the instant center of rotation changes as the joint moves; consequently, the force-couple parameters change as the instant center of rotation changes.

Deviation of the PICR from the kinesiologic standard can be an indication of faulty muscle synergy in the force couple. **Muscle dominance** is defined as one muscle of a synergistic group of muscles that exceeds the action of its counterparts, causing a deviation of the PICR and potential disuse of the other synergists.[1] The factors that affect force-couple balance are discussed later in this chapter.

CONTRIBUTORS TO IMPAIRED POSTURE AND MOVEMENT

Pathokinesiology is defined as the study of anatomy and physiology as they relate to abnormal movement.[29] Pathokinesiology emphasizes abnormalities of movement as a result of pathologic conditions. For example, in hemiparesis, the abnormal movement is the result of pathology involving the nervous system.[1] However, the reverse can also occur—pathology can be the result of abnormal movement. This can be defined as **kinesiopathology**.[1] When movement deviates from the kinesiologic standard, the cumulative effect of repetitive movement can be pathology. Therefore, it is reasonable to assume that maintaining precise movement patterns can minimize abnormal stress. Kinesiopathology can also result from repetitive movements and sustained postures associated with activities of daily living including recreational, fitness, and sports activities. Clinicians use sustained postures and repetitive movements therapeutically to increase ROM and muscle length, improve joint mobility/stability, increase muscle performance, and improve balance and coordination. Most often, adaptations such as these are considered advantageous; however, they can also be detrimental and contribute to movement impairments. Everyday activities can change muscle performance, ROM/muscle length, joint mobility/stability, and motor control, which in turn can alter the relative participation of synergists and antagonists and eventually movement patterns.

The following sections describe the relationship between posture and movement and physiologic, anatomic, and psychologic impairments, lifespan considerations, and environmental factors.

Range of Motion

The normal limitation of joint motion in certain directions has postural significance in relation to the stability of the body, particularly in standing. For example, dorsiflexion ROM at the ankle with the knee straight is normally about

10 to 15 degrees. To prevent excessive hyperextension of the knees, when standing barefoot with the feet nearly parallel, the lower leg should not sway posteriorly beyond vertical alignment, nor should the hip move beyond its 10 degrees of extension. The combination of posterior sway of the tibia with hip extension in standing creates knee joint hyperextension. Excessive segmental joint ROM can allow proportional postural deviations in the corresponding directions.

Conversely, joint restriction also can affect postural alignment. Ankle, knee, or hip flexion contractures can cause deviations of posture in the corresponding directions.

With respect to movement, ROM impairment can contribute to movement dysfunction in that normal movement cannot occur at a joint with limited ROM and excessive ROM can allow extremes of movement that are detrimental to the joint, periarticular structures, and associated muscles. Typically, limited ROM at a joint encourages faulty movement at another segment. For example, a common faulty movement pattern seen associated with adhesive capsulitis of the shoulder is excessive scapula elevation. Normal ROM at a joint does not ensure accuracy of the PICR during active movement. Recall that precise active movement is dependent on balanced active force couples acting on the joint.

Muscle Length

Impairment of muscle length can both be the *result of* impaired posture and movement as well as *affect* posture and movement. Prolonged posture alterations can result in muscle length changes. The time a muscle spends in the shortened range and the amount a muscle is contracted in the shortened range determines whether it becomes shortened.[30–32] Conversely, the stimulus for lengthening a muscle is the amount of tension placed on the muscle over a prolonged period.[30–32]

Sustained postures, particularly those postures that are maintained in faulty alignments, can induce changes in the muscles and supporting tissues that can be injurious, especially when the joint is at the end of its range.[33]

A clinical example can provide a better understanding of these concepts. Consider a person with thoracic kyphosis with a scapula positioned in medial rotation (winging), downward rotation, and anterior tilt. The lower trapezius muscle can experience sustained tension, resulting in lengthening, from the 3D alignment faults coupled with gravity and the weight of a limb. In the case of the anterior tilt, the pectoralis minor experiences little to no counterbalancing tension from the lengthened lower trapezius and is assisted by gravity and the weight of the limb to remain in the shortened position. If the pectoralis minor contracts repeatedly in the shortened range (e.g., as an accessory muscle of respiration), it can develop adaptive shortening.

These alterations in the muscle length not only contribute to perpetuating the faulty posture but also contribute to altered length-tension properties and subsequent altered force couple action of the muscles, thereby ultimately affecting the PICR during active motion (see the section "Muscle Performance" for more details).[1] See Building Block 9-1.

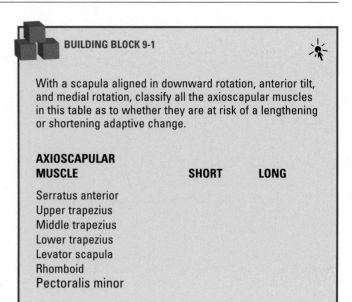

Joint Mobility

Joint mobility can be reduced or excessive. A joint can only move through a precise PICR if the joint has the available passive range in osteokinematic and arthrokinematic motions. However, normal passive joint mobility does not guarantee precise PICR during active motion.

Impairments in joint mobility rarely occur in isolation. Active motion is usually affected by a combination of factors such as muscle length, muscle performance, joint mobility, and motor control. For example, during active shoulder medial rotation in the prone position with the arm abducted to 90 degrees, the shoulder should be able to medially rotate 70 degrees without an associated anterior glide of the head of the humerus or anterior tilt or superior glide of the scapula.[34] The active ROM can be limited by stiff or short lateral rotators, stiff periarticular structures (particularly the posterior capsule), and/or weak or poorly recruited medial rotators.

In some cases, though the ROM may be normal, the *quality* of motion is affected. For example, during medial rotation, one deviation of the PICR that may be observed or palpated is an arthrokinetic motion of the head of the humerus gliding excessively anteriorly. This movement may result from one or a combination of factors, such as those previously mentioned, combined with specific weakness or poor control of the subscapularis; dominance of the pectoralis major, latissimus dorsi, and teres major muscles; and/or excessive extensibility of the anterior capsule. Joint mobility, whether limited or excessive, can affect active motion, particularly when combined with other impairments of body functions. See Building Block 9-2.

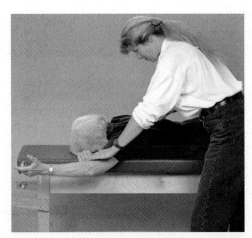

FIGURE 9-12. Manual muscle test position for the lower trapezius. Note that the arm is in elevation, positioning the scapula in upward rotation. The test position for the scapula is upward rotation, adduction, and depression. Failure to hold the test position indicates weakness.

Muscle Performance

A long-held belief is that deviations in posture reflect muscle weakness. However, the relationships between postural deviation and muscle strength have been questioned,[35,36] and the literature instead suggests that the relationship between muscle length and strength may contribute to postural deviation.[1]

Stretch weakness is a term used by Florence Kendall to describe the effect of muscles maintained in an elongated condition beyond neutral physiologic rest position.[19] This definition is based on the results of manual muscle strength testing, at which Kendall is an acknowledged expert.[19] For example, when the shoulders are maintained in a forward position and the scapulae are elevated and abducted, the lower and middle trapezius muscles are positioned in an elongated rest position. The manual muscle test would demonstrate weakness (Fig. 9-12). However, the apparent weakness of the posturally lengthened muscle may be an indication of altered length-tension properties such that the elongated muscle cannot produce tension in the shortened range (i.e., the manual muscle test position).[30–33] Length-tension properties of muscle are also discussed in Chapter 5.

If the elongated middle and lower trapezius muscles are tested in a relatively lengthened range, the force production capability is greater than in the traditional manual muscle test position. This phenomenon can be called a length-associated change.[33] For the muscle to become lengthened, it adds sarcomeres in series and, therefore, is capable of producing greater peak force than a normal-length or shortened muscle when tested at its optimal length. However, if the lengthened muscle is placed in a shortened position for manual muscle test, the filaments would overlap and be less efficient at producing force than a short or normal-length muscle. This is similar to flexing the knee to test the gluteus maximus in hip extension and thereby lessening the contribution of the hamstrings. When testing muscles in the shortened range, a more appropriate description may be *positional strength*, because it indicates only the torque the muscle can create in the short range.[1] One form of stretch weakness may be positional weakness. Testing the muscle at multiple points in the range and comparing findings with those for the opposite extremity (or half of the body when examining axial muscles)

can help to differentiate positional weakness from weakness resulting from strain, disuse, or neurologic involvement. The muscle with length-associated changes tests weak in the short range and strong in the lengthened range, whereas the other sources of weakness should test weak throughout the range.

The length-tension properties of the muscle correlate directly with the participation of the muscle in the force couple. The line of pull of its fibers determines the specific function of each muscle. No two muscles in the body have exactly the same line of pull. Whenever muscle weakness exists, the performance of some movement is affected or the stability of some part of the body is impaired. A muscle that becomes elongated over time exhibits positional weakness relative to the same point in the range of normal length or shortened synergists. Compared with its normal-length or shortened synergists, its participation in the force couple is lessened until it can achieve its optimal length-tension relationship. The result is a deviation of the PICR, which may contribute to microtrauma and eventually to macrotrauma, pathology, further impairment, and disability.

A clinical example may illustrate the relationship between length-tension properties and movement. In an individual with a functional limb length discrepancy with a high iliac crest on the right, the right hip is in postural adduction, which places the gluteus medius on stretch. During gait, the gluteus medius participates in the hip abduction force couple to decelerate hip adduction from the initial contact to midstance phase (see Selected Intervention 9-1). The tensor fascia lata (TFL) does not necessarily encounter the same stretch stimulus as the gluteus medius when the hip is in postural adduction (particularly the anteromedial fibers) and therefore can create better tension for abduction at initial contact when the hip is in more relative adduction. However, because the TFL is also a hip flexor and medial rotator, without strong counterbalance from the gluteus medius (particularly posterior gluteus medius), the PICR of the hip can deviate in the direction of flexion and medial rotation. The overstretched gluteus medius can generate greater counterbalancing tension only after the hip is adducted, flexed, or medially rotated, which places the muscle on stretch. The posturally lengthened muscle affects the force-couple action and ultimately affects active movement patterns. See Building Block 9-3.

The theory of "core strength" in the lumbopelvic and cervical regions is another key concept that certainly pertains to optimal posture and movement.[37–40] Chapter 17 discusses the theory of core strength in detail along with therapeutic exercise descriptions to develop core strength. The reader is referred to the section "Muscle Performance" in Chapter 17, The Lumbopelvic Region for the literature review, and detailed discussion of this topic.

With respect to the endurance component of muscle performance, the fatigability of a muscle affects its participation

BUILDING BLOCK 9-3

What kind of injury can the gluteus medius sustain if it chronically is activated in a stretched position? Could this be an explanation of lateral hip pain?

SELECTED INTERVENTION 9-1
Prone Hip Abduction

See Case Study No. 9

Although this patient requires comprehensive intervention, one critical exercise is described:

ACTIVITY: Prone hip abduction through full ROM

PURPOSE: Strengthen 2+/5 gluteus medius through full range (need to increase the muscle's ability to create tension through full range)

RISK FACTORS: No appreciable risk factors

EFFECT OF PREVIOUS INTERVENTIONS: None

ELEMENTS OF THE MOVEMENT SYSTEM: Base

STAGE OF MOTOR CONTROL: Mobility

MODE: Resisted exercise in a gravity-lessened position

POSTURE: Beginning and ending position—prone, with a pillow under stomach, hip slightly laterally rotated, elastic around the ankle (Fig. A)

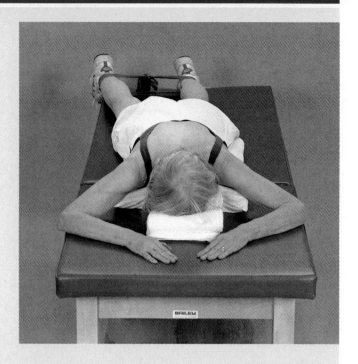

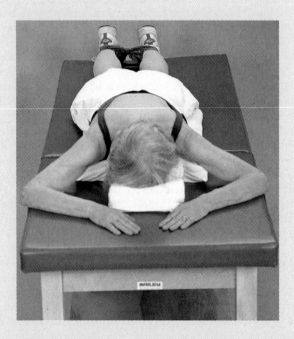

MOVEMENT: The hip extends just enough to clear from the supporting surface, abducts through the full available range (concentric), rests on the supporting surface, returns to a slightly extended position, and slowly adducts to the starting position (eccentric; Fig. B).

SPECIAL CONSIDERATIONS: Ensure that the gluteus medius is contracting throughout the entire activity (concentric and eccentric) and that the TFL is maximally relaxed. Ensure that full *end-range* motion is achieved and that the abdominal muscles are stabilizing the spine against extension and the pelvis against anterior tilt and side-bending forces imposed by motion of the hip. Be sure motion is isolated to the hip and that no motion occurs in the spine or pelvis.

DOSAGE

Special Considerations:
Anatomic: Gluteus medius
Physiologic: No strain, 2+/5 manual muscle test (MMT) grade
Learning Capability: Difficulty isolating gluteus medius over TFL may require tactile facilitation or surface electromyography with biofeedback on gluteus medius for better isolation.

Type of Contraction: Concentric during abduction motion and eccentric during adduction motion

Intensity: Light-resistance elastic tied around the ankle and taut in hip-neutral position

Speed of Activity: Moderate on concentric portions; slow on eccentric portion

Duration: To form fatigue for two sets (maximum of 30 repetitions)

Frequency: Daily

Environment: Home

Feedback: Initially tactile facilitation or surface electromyography with biofeedback, tapered after isolated contraction is achieved

(Continued)

Prone Hip Abduction (*Continued*)

RATIONALE FOR EXERCISE CHOICE: This exercise was chosen to increase the strength of the gluteus medius in isolation from the TFL. Because the MMT grade is 2+/5, a gravity-lessened position was chosen to allow full ROM. Light elastic was used to ensure concentric contraction of the gluteus medius during the abduction motion and eccentric contraction on the return from abduction in a gravity-lessened position. Full ROM is expected to work on length-tension properties of the gluteus medius (i.e., ability to create force throughout the range, including the shortened range).

EXERCISE MODIFICATION/GRADATION: As strength through a full range is developed, the exercise should be progressed to an against-gravity position (i.e., sidelying). After a 3+/5 MMT grade is achieved, standing functional activities should be introduced (i.e., stability and controlled mobility). After proximal stability and controlled mobility are achieved, the exercise can be progressed to functional gait activities (i.e., skill).

Within each activity level, specific dosage parameters can be manipulated to progress the exercise and prepare for gradation to the next level. At each level, care must be taken to ensure synergy between the gluteus medius and TFL in stabilizing the hip in the frontal plane by observing the pelvic and femur positions and preventing anterior pelvic tilt, Trendelenburg gait, or femur medial rotation. In closed chain positions, neutral pelvic, tibial, and foot alignment about all three axes complement the hip position.

FUNCTIONAL MOVEMENT PATTERN TO REINFORCE GOAL OF SPECIFIC EXERCISE:

Posture: Educate the patient about asymmetric postures that reinforce a weak, lengthened gluteus medius (i.e., standing with weight shifted to the involved side, resulting in a high iliac crest).

Movement: During gait, think of contracting gluteal musculature at heel strike to prevent a Trendelenburg gait.

---

in a force couple, particularly in repeated movements. Muscle fatigue affects movement, but muscle endurance often is not a factor in perpetuating optimal resting alignment; the length of the muscles and periarticular structures support optimal alignment. Little muscle activity is required to maintain a relaxed standing position.[41] However, in the presence of injury, even small demand on the musculature can be problematic.

Control of posture is a highly complex task in the human motor system. There is evidence that the postural control for stability and orientation requires proprioceptive input from numerous muscles in order to generate the appropriate torque in maintaining the body position.[42,43] The sensory organs involved in maintaining balance control and body orientation incorporates somatoafferent, vestibular, and visual input in order to assess the current body position, as well as external disturbances and feedback to previous control (efferent) strategies. Consequently, the motor process coordinates the trunk and lower limb muscles into combined postural strategies to decrease body sway and maintain it within the base of support. It has been suggested that the injury to the neck and/or the otolith structures that influence afferent feedback might contribute to loss of awareness and control of posture.[44] It could be hypothesized further that in a neck or ankle/foot injury the muscle-spindle inputs from a "proprioceptive chain," which functionally links the eye muscles to the foot muscles, are disturbed and therefore could contribute to faults in posture control and awareness. The practitioner needs to look at global strategies as well as local, segmental strategies, when it comes to examining and treating posture impairment. See Building Block 9-4.

Pain

Pain, posture, and movement are inextricably linked. Pain can induce abnormal movement, abnormal movement can induce pain, and it is often difficult to differentiate cause from effect. When a mechanical defect perpetuates the symptom or prevents resolution of the painful condition, the mechanical cause must be diagnosed and treated. Ultimately, the posture habits and movement patterns contributing to the mechanical cause of pain must be modified.

Pain may or may not alter a given posture or movement, depending on the severity of the symptom and the magnitude or intensity of stress imposed by the posture or movement. However, pain that is associated with posture and movement can lead the clinician to an understanding of the kinesiopathologic factors contributing to the pain. For example, if a patient has shoulder pain during swimming, it must be determined what movement impairments are associated with the pain experienced during the swim stroke and furthermore, what alterations to the movement pattern need to be made to reduce or eliminate the pain. For example, during movement testing of the shoulder, the patient is positioned prone with the arm abducted 90 degrees with the elbow flexed 90 degrees and the forearm hanging vertically off the side of the table (see Fig. 9-13). The patient is asked to actively medially rotate his shoulder. The examiner palpates and observes excessive

BUILDING BLOCK 9-4

Consider a 23-year-old that sustained a second degree ankle sprain. Provide an explanation as to why the physical therapist should consider closed chain balance drills in the plan of care.

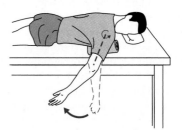

FIGURE 9-13. Illustration of movement test position for glenohumeral medial and lateral rotation.

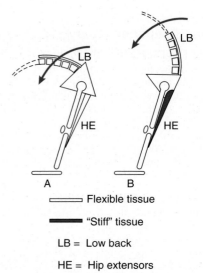

FIGURE 9-14. Figure A shows normal lumbopelvic rhythm. Figure B depicts faulty lumbopelvic rhythm with less movement of the pelvis relative to the hips. In men, this could result from the anthropometric characteristics of a heavy upper body relative to the lower body.

anterior translation of the humeral head during the movement and that this is associated with pain. When the humerus is manually prevented from moving anteriorly during the motion by the clinician, the pain is relieved. The anterior translation can be assumed to be contributing to the mechanical cause of the pain. The clinician must perform additional tests to determine the specific impairments that contribute to the anterior displacement of the head of the humerus such as a weak or overstretched subscapularis coupled with a dominant and short teres major or anterior deltoid.

Treatment is based on resolving the impairments associated with the kinesiopathologic pattern during specific exercises and eventually during functional movement patterns. By treating the movement impairment, the pain often resolves without necessarily requiring direct treatment of the tissue that is the source of pain. See Building Block 9-5.

Anatomic Impairments and Anthropometric Characteristics

Anatomic impairments can predispose persons to impairments of posture and movement that can result in MPS. Individuals with anatomic impairments (e.g., scoliosis, kyphosis from Scheuermann disease, hip anteversion) are predisposed to develop MPS because of altered posture habits and movement patterns. For example, an individual with Scheuermann disease typically has moderate to marked kyphosis. This patient is prone to even more exaggerated kyphosis beyond the anatomic impairment because of the effect of gravity and the weight of the upper extremities on the kyphotic posture. Increased thoracic kyphosis can give rise to thoracic, neck, shoulder, low back, or lower quadrant pain because of compensatory spinal, shoulder girdle, pelvic girdle, and lower extremity alignments.

The patient may adopt movement patterns that perpetuate the kyphotic posture. For example, during forward bending, instead of initiating the movement with concentric phasic activity from the rectus abdominis and controlling the lowering with eccentric spinal and hip extensors, the bending movement may be produced by tonic concentric rectus abdominis activity and phasic eccentric deceleration from the spinal and hip extensors. The latter movement pattern would

contribute to greater kyphotic forces on the thoracic spine than the former pattern.

Anthropometric characteristics can also contribute to impairments of posture and movement.[45,46] Consider a tall man with broad shoulders and a tall, narrow pelvis. Ideal lumbopelvic rhythm is such that motion at the lumbar spine should be accompanied by motion of the pelvis rotating over the hips.[47] The tall man with broad shoulders and a tall, narrow pelvis has a higher center of mass than an average-height woman with a relatively broader pelvis. When the man bends forward, the fulcrum point is more likely to be in the lumbar spine than at the hips because of the high center of mass. The man therefore has a greater tendency to bend with excessive lumbar flexion and limited pelvic rotation (Fig. 9-14). With repeated forward bending using this strategy over a lifetime, the hip joint is at risk for developing hypomobility in the direction of flexion, and the lumbar segments are at risk for becoming hypermobile in the direction of flexion. The hypermobility of the lumbar spine into flexion may be carried through other postures and movement patterns such as sitting, leaning forward in sitting, and the follow-through phase in serving the ball in tennis. Related impairments of muscle length and performance can result from impairments of movement and contribute to perpetuating and further exaggerating faulty movement. See Building Block 9-6.

Psychologic Impairments

Research points to a complex and dynamic interaction of biologic, psychologic, and social variables influencing movement and its relationship to pain and pain-related disability.[48] There is growing evidence that pain-related fear may be a particularly important mechanism in the onset and maintenance of pain-related disability.[49-54] Pain-related fear refers to the extent that an individual believes that certain movements or actions will result in either increases in pain levels or exacerbation of an injury that is associated with pain[49] and it is usually associated with avoidance of those movements or activities.[49,55-57] A reduction of activities on an ongoing basis can lead to the establishment of a cycle characterized by altered movement patterns, physical deconditioning, decreased self-efficacy, and negative affect[58] and can have a detrimental impact upon the musculoskeletal and cardiovascular systems,[59] further worsening the pain problem and leading to still greater avoidance of activities. Such a cycle, termed "fear-avoidance"[59] is thought to be maintained by both the reduction of anxiety that comes from the successful avoidance of feared activities[60] and the further entrenchment of pain-related fears as the individual allows themselves few opportunities to "challenge" their beliefs about the consequences of certain movements.

There is a considerable empirical support for the notion that pain-related fear is related to disability in patients with chronic pain.[51,61] Studies have shown that patients with high pain-related fear tend to overestimate their expected levels of pain in certain situations and to terminate activities earlier than those who predict less pain.[62] There are also indications that pain-related fear may be more strongly associated with disability than either pain severity or other biomedical characteristics of the patient's condition.[49,50,57,58,63] For example, Waddell et al.[64] found that fear-avoidance beliefs about pain were better predictors of self-reported disability in activities of daily living than were the anatomic pattern of pain, the time pattern of pain, or pain severity.

Though this research is compelling in presenting a biopsychosocial framework for the relationship between psychological and movement impairments, the physical therapist should not "throw the baby out with the bathwater." In other words, though we cannot underestimate the fear-avoidance component of movement impairment, we must also pay close attention to the quality of movement and teach the patient to move efficiently, safely, and with the least biomechanical stress to the affected tissues to address the impairments of body functions contributing to the pain.

It is beyond the scope of physical therapy practice to deal with the complexity of the biopsychosocial framework contributing to pain and movement impairment. A multidisciplinary approach toward complex chronic pain is warranted. If the physical therapist determines that the psychologic state of the patient is inhibiting recovery, referral to an appropriate mental health practitioner is indicated. Physical therapy intervention may need to pause until the psychologic condition improves, or it can proceed if it is determined that continued intervention is beneficial to psychologic recovery. As the psychological status improves, the PT's role is to reintroduce movements that have been avoided. As movement is restored, fear avoidance reduces—thus breaking the cycle of pain and fear avoidance of movement. See Building Block 9-7.

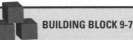

BUILDING BLOCK 9-7

Consider a 45-year-old female with a chronic history of hip and low back pain. She is able to perform a comprehensive self management program safely and has been able to control her pain 80% of the time. However, she is fearful to return to her health club which you feel is necessary for her to improve her global physical condition. How would you assist her in returning to her gym setting with a comprehensive gym-based program?

Lifespan Considerations

We all have observed the effect of age on posture and movement. Children are not expected to conform to an adult standard of posture and movement, primarily because the developing individual exhibits much greater mobility and flexibility than the adult.[65] Developmental deviations appear in many children at about the same age and improve or disappear without any corrective treatment, despite unfavorable environmental influences.[65] However, developmental deviations are perpetuated by habit in some children. Repeated observation (not a single examination) can determine whether a developmental deviation is being perpetuated by habit. If the condition remains static or if the deviation increases, corrective measures are indicated. A young child (younger than 5 years) is not likely to have habitual faults and can be harmed by corrective measures that are not needed. Any deviations considered severe require immediate attention, regardless of the age of the individual (Fig. 9-15). Developmental changes occur in the feet, knees, hips, pelvis, trunk, and shoulder girdle. Display 9-3 lists the common developmental deviations in children that should gradually diminish as the child reaches adolescence and adulthood.

One particular anatomic impairment that is not considered a normal developmental posture occurs during adolescence. Physical therapists working with preadolescent and adolescent populations should be routinely screening for the onset of scoliosis. After scoliosis is diagnosed, the adolescent can be referred to a physician specializing in the treatment

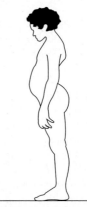

FIGURE 9-15. Severe developmental deviation. This amount of lordosis in an 8-year-old child is considered a severe developmental deviation necessitating intervention. A corset to support the abdomen is needed along with therapeutic exercises.

DISPLAY 9-3
Developmental Deviations in Posture

Feet
- Flat arches are normal in the small child.
- By age 6 or 7, expect good arch formation.

Knees
- Genu valgum is normal in a small child (about 2 in between ankles is normal for an average-height child).
- By age 6 or 7, genu valgum should be diminished or gone.
- Postural genu varum in the school-age child is not acceptable, and corrective measures should be taken, because it is difficult to change in the young adult.
- Genu varum may be compensatory for genu valgum by hyperextension of the knees.

Hips
- Femur medial rotation is the most common and often results from hip anteversion, foot pronation, knee hyperextension, postural genu varum, and less often, genu valgum. Check for structural sources and treat with the appropriate corrective measures.
- By adolescence, the femur should be in near-neutral alignment.
- Femur lateral rotation is more common in young boys.
- Persistent lateral rotation should be treated, because it can be detrimental in adulthood.

Lumbopelvic Region
- A protruding abdomen is normal for a child.
- By the age of 10 to 12, the abdomen should no longer be protruding.
- Lordosis peaks at age 9 to 10 and should gradually diminish thereafter.
- Handedness patterns emerge in school-age children, most commonly with the hip high and shoulder low on the dominant side. This should be monitored if it is borderline or excessive.

Shoulder Girdle
- Scapular tilting is normal in school-age children.
- The prominence should diminish as the child approaches adolescence.

From Kendall HO, Kendall FP, Boynton DA. Posture and Pain. Huntington, NY: Robert E. Krieger Publishing, 1970.

of scoliosis and a comprehensive management plan can be developed.

There is evidence that alterations in movement begin to occur in late middle age, probably because the functional abilities gradually decline.[66] In the broad sense, the execution of voluntary movements requires two goals to be achieved simultaneously: accurate performance of a goal-directed movement on the one hand, and maintenance of equilibrium and appropriate posture, or set of postures, on the other (for a review see Horak and Macpherson[67]; and Massion et al.[68]). Aging adds an additional problem with coordination between equilibrium and movement, causing progressive impairments at the CNS level as well as in the sensory motor system. According to Millanvoye,[69] decrements in performance are initially imperceptible, become detectable around the age of 40 to 45 and only become noticeable to the point that they cannot be ignored after the age of 60. Thus, the possibility of early detection of minor changes between young and aging adults in the coordination between equilibrium and movement may

provide a window into the evolution of fall risk as individuals age. Identification of these changes and their time course could provide the basis for preventive rehabilitation programs to diminish risk of traumatic falls and to enhance maximum autonomy.[70] Exciting research is on the horizon in this area, with a greater emphasis on prevention as we understand the effect of aging on equilibrium and movement.

Environmental Influences

The activities in which an individual participates and the surrounding environment may have favorable or adverse effects on posture and movement. The nature of the activities and the time spent doing them and whether the effect of habitual postures and movements during one activity are reinforced or counteracted by habitual positions or repeated movements in other activities determine the overall postural and movement effect. Stresses are put on the basic structures of the human body by increasingly specialized and limited or repetitive activity (e.g., working endless hours at a computer display terminal, going home exhausted, sitting most evenings in a recliner chair in front of a television).

The activities of an individual must be considered as a whole in gauging their postural or movement effects. Concentration on one type of activity can ensure muscle imbalance, but a combination of activities may be almost as unfavorable if each involves the same kind of movement or position. For example, a person working at a video display terminal who engages in piano playing in her leisure time has no real change in the type of activity.

Several environmental factors, such as workstations, beds, pillows, car seats, school chairs and desks, and footwear, influence posture and movement. These environmental influences should be made as favorable as possible. Patient-Related Instruction 9-1: Tips on Workstation Ergonomics outlines important tips for proper workstation ergonomics. This would be a useful handout to provide all your patients that spend time at a computer workstation. When major adjustments cannot be made, small adjustments often help considerably. A discussion of environmental influences is not complete without reference to body mechanics related to lifting and carrying. These strategies should be examined and favorably modified as much as possible for the individual's circumstances. A demonstration of proper lifting mechanics can be accessed on the website.

EXAMINATION AND EVALUATION

Posture

The lines and points of reference discussed under standard alignment are put to practical use in plumb line tests for postural alignment (Fig. 9-16). A plumb line test is used to determine if the points of reference of the individual being tested are in the same alignment as the corresponding points in the standard posture. The amount of deviation of the various points of reference from the plumb line reveals the extent to which the subject's alignment is faulty. When deviations from plumb alignment are evaluated, they are described as slight, moderate, or severe.[19] Additional alignment tests can be performed in several positions, such as sitting, recumbency, and single-limb stance. Deviations from acceptable standards can be noted.

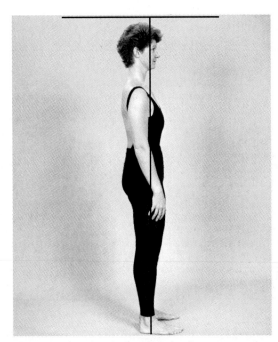

FIGURE 9-16. For the purpose of testing, the client steps up to a suspended plumb line. For the back or front view the subject stands with feet equidistant from the line; for side view, the point just in front of the lateral malleolus is in line with the plumb line. The base point should be the fixed reference point, because the base is the only stationary or fixed part of the standing posture.

DISPLAY 9-4
Definitions of Terms Regarding Muscle Length

- Tautness is defined as muscles or ligaments put on tension. It implies a state in which slack is taken up in the muscles or ligaments.
- A short muscle limits the ROM as it relates to the kinesiologic standard.
- An elongated muscle is longer than the kinesiologic standard; tautness appears after the motion has exceeded the normal joint range.
- The term tight is often used interchangeably with short or taut, but these terms do not have equivalent meanings. On palpation, a muscle that is short and drawn taut feels tight. A muscle that is elongated and drawn taut also feels tight on palpation. Because the word tight implies that a muscle should be stretched, the terms short and elongated are preferred to describe muscle length to ensure that stretching is applied only to short muscles.
- Stiffness is defined as the change in tension per unit change in length.[72] When passive motion of a joint is assessed, all the tissues crossing the joint contribute to the resistance, which can be referred to as joint stiffness.[1] For the purposes of this text, stiffness refers to the resistance present during the passive elongation of muscle and connective tissue, not during active muscle contraction or at the end of ROM.

In addition to standard posture assessment, the physical therapist must also examine specific segmental alignment of adjacent segments in a region. For example, the position of L5 relative to S1 may be relevant in a lumbar condition. If L5 is in a slight rotation, this may be a source of nociception due to the biomechanical stress on the tissues of the motion segment. Treatment of this specific segmental alignment fault may be vital to the reduction of symptoms and the overall recovery of the patient.

Posture can assist the clinician in generating hypotheses regarding muscle length. For example, anterior pelvic tilt can suggest short hip flexors and elongated abdominal muscles. Specific muscle length tests are necessary to determine actual muscle length. Definitions of terms regarding muscle length are outlined in Display 9-4.

Movement

Examination of movement in the clinical setting can be challenging, because sophisticated computerized movement analysis equipment is costly and is not user-friendly in the typical physical therapy setting. The clinician must therefore rely on the following test procedures for single-joint movement analysis:

- Palpation skills and precise observation of basic movement patterns at a single joint are used to determine how closely the movement pattern replicates the kinesiologic standard PICR for a given limb for that movement (e.g., observing or palpating the glenohumeral or scapulothoracic joints while raising the arm in flexion; or the spine, pelvis, knee, ankle, or foot during standing hip and knee flexion).

- Palpation or surface electromyography is used to determine the pattern and synchronization of muscle activity for a given movement, which is compared with known kinesiologic standards.

The clinician should rely on the following test procedures for anlalysis of multiple-segment movement:

- As in gait analysis, break the movement into phases, and look at each segment or component (i.e., group of segments) during each phase and relate the segmental movements to the process of movement. For example, the step-up can be broken into a swing and stance phase (Fig. 9-17). Each segment can be analyzed and relationships can be determined. For instance, a hip-hike strategy in the lumbopelvic region is related to insufficient hip and knee flexion and ankle dorsiflexion in the swing phase, and a Trendelenburg position (pelvis is dropped on the side opposite to the weak hip abductors) in the stance phase is related to similar abnormal movement patterns (i.e., hip adduction occurs in a hip-hike and Trendelenburg position).

- Similar movement pattern descriptions can be developed for each basic movement required for activities of daily living (e.g., rising from sit to stand, step-down, bed mobility, reaching). By describing movement pattern strategies, the variations in movement patterns and deviations from efficient and healthy patterns can be determined. The reader is referred to a more complete reference on this topic for specific regional movement impairment syndromes.[1]

Additional examination techniques can offer clues to expected outcomes. By compiling results of ROM, muscle length, joint mobility, and muscle performance tests, the clinician can

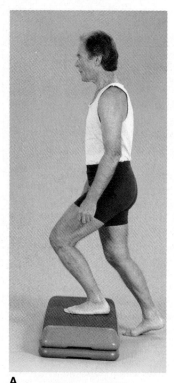
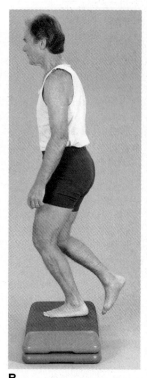

A   **B**

FIGURE 9-17. The step can be broken into two phases. (A) The swing phase in which the hip and knee are flexed to bring the foot to the surface of the step and (B) the stance phase in which the body is raised onto the step.

hypothesize about the quality of the PICR and the muscle recruitment patterns during active movement. The minimal essential tests of muscle length that should be included in any posture or movement examination of the lower and upper quadrant are listed in Display 9-5. The minimal essential tests of positional strength that should be included in any posture or movement examination for the trunk, upper quadrant, or

---

DISPLAY 9-5
Essential Muscle Length Tests

Lower Quadrant
- Hamstring: This test should distinguish between the medial and lateral hamstrings.
- Gastroc-soleus: This test should distinguish between the gastrocnemius and soleus.
- TFL and iliotibial band
- Hip flexors: This test should discriminate among the TFL, rectus femoris, and iliopsoas.
- Hip rotators: This test should distinguish between the medial and lateral rotators.

Upper Quadrant
- Teres major and latissimus dorsi
- Rhomboid major and minor and levator scapula
- Pectoralis major
- Pectoralis minor
- Shoulder rotators: This test should distinguish between the medial and lateral rotators.

DISPLAY 9-6
Essential Positional Strength Tests

Trunk
- Abdominal muscles: separate tests should be performed for the rectus abdominis and internal oblique,[10] external oblique,[1] and, if possible, transversus abdominis.[29]

Lower Quadrant
- Iliopsoas
- Gluteus medius
- Gluteus maximus
- Hamstrings
- Quadriceps
- TFL

Upper Quadrant
- Serratus anterior
- Upper, middle, and lower trapezius
- Infraspinatus and teres minor
- Subscapularis[1]

---

lower quadrant are listed in Display 9-6. Reexamination of the movement after additional tests have been performed can enable the clinician to better understand the complexity of movement.

INTERVENTION

Healthy, effective, and efficient posture, alignment, and movement are an integral part of general well-being. Efficiency and longevity of the human biomechanical system requires maintenance of precise movement of the rotating segments.[1] Good posture and movement are considered fundamental to health of the biomechanical system. Ideally, posture and movement instruction and training should become an integral part of any therapeutic intervention.

Although posture and movement alterations can each be considered as one type of impairment, they cannot be considered in the same way as impairment of muscle performance, ROM, muscle length, or joint mobility. Impairment in posture and movement can be the result of many factors, including physiologic, anatomic, and psychologic, and environmental factors. To develop an efficient, effective intervention for the treatment of posture and movement impairment, all the functional limitations and the related impairments resulting from and contributing to posture and movement impairment should be understood. The effect of predisposing risk factors, previous interventions, and environmental influences should also be taken into consideration.

This chapter has presented a foundation for developing therapeutic exercise interventions to treat posture and movement impairments. The remainder is devoted to describing therapeutic exercise intervention for posture and movement according to the intervention model described in Chapter 2.

Elements of the Movement System

Any or all elements of the movement system can be involved directly or indirectly in the development of posture and movement impairment and therefore should be dealt with in

DISPLAY 9-7

Elements of the Movement System and Factors Contributing to Impairment of Posture and Movement

Biomechanical Factors
- Impairments of body structures such as scoliosis or hip anteversion
- Impairments of body functions such as postural genu varum, thoracic kyphosis, or hip adduction as a result of chronically standing asymmetrically
- Anthropometric characteristics such as broad pelvis, tall pelvis, long legs, etc.

Base
- Overstretched gluteus medius, contributing to high iliac crest and functional limb length discrepancy
- Easily fatigued serratus anterior, contributing to reduced scapular upward rotation with repetitive overhead activities
- glutues medius strain, contributing to reduced activity level and altered movement patterns

Modulator Factors
- Reduced or loss of innervation of the gluteus maximus associated with hip hyperextension
- TFL dominance during hip flexion, contributing to hip flexion with medial rotation
- Latent timing of the vastus medialis oblique, contributing to patellofemoral movement impairment

Support Factors
- Inappropriate breathing patterns associated with abnormal rib cage alignment and with rib and thoracic spine movement patterns

Cognitive or Affective Factors
- Depression associated with slumped posture or shuffling gait
- Fear avoidance of movement
- Increased muscle tension associated with stress

treatment. Base and biomechanical elements usually require direct intervention for the correction of posture and movement impairments, whereas modulator elements are more critical to movement impairments than posture impairments. Impairments of the cognitive or affective element can limit the progress of an individual with posture or movement impairments. If this is the case, appropriate referral to a mental health practitioner may be required to reach the desired functional outcome. Impairments of the support element can affect posture and movement directly (i.e., faulty breathing patterns or reduced energy for movement) or indirectly through oxygen transport deficits in systemic disease that contributes to further faults in posture and movement.[15] Display 9-7 provides examples of impairments of the elements of the movement system associated with posture and movement.

Other bodily systems may be involved directly or indirectly and should be considered if necessary to improve posture or movement. For example, a patient presents with posture and movement impairments about the hip with the comorbidity of urinary incontinence caused by pelvic floor weakness and estrogen depletion.[71] Full correction of posture and movement impairments about the hip may not be achieved without attention to the pelvic floor dysfunction, which is caused by impairments of the movement,

urogenital, and endocrine systems. The link between the movement system and urinary incontinence is discussed in Chapter 18. In this case, without considering the associated urogenital problems and hormonal imbalances, the pelvic floor problem may not resolve, preventing optimal function of the pelvic floor muscles. Because two of the pelvic floor muscles are also used for hip function (i.e., obturator internus and piriformis), dysfunction of the pelvic floor may contribute to posture and movement impairment of the hip, which may contribute to further pelvic floor dysfunction, and so on as the cycle continues. All the systems involved must be addressed to resolve the posture and movement impairment at the hip.

Activity and Dosage

Numerous activities or techniques can be chosen to restore healthy and efficient posture and movement:

- Stretching short muscles and improving extensibility of stiff myofascial tissues
- Improving muscle performance in muscles exhibiting atrophy, weakness, strain, or poor endurance
- Supporting and strengthening elongated muscles
- Optimizing body mechanics, ergonomics, and posture awareness
- Normalizing segmental alignment
- Awareness training of preferred postural patterns
- Optimizing balance and coordination
- Training appropriate breathing exercises

This list is not conclusive in that essentially all therapeutic exercise interventions can affect posture and movement. Because posture and movement are components of the intervention model, every activity or technique should promote optimal posture and movement. No activity or technique should compromise kinesiologic standards of posture and movement unless modification is necessary as a result of the disease, pathology, or physiologic or anatomic impairment.

Identifying and prioritizing the elements of the movement system, combined with knowledge of the physiologic status of the component impairments, can help to determine the activities or techniques needed, including the posture, movement, and mode parameters. Dosage parameters depend on the component impairment (e.g., ROM, muscle length, joint mobility, muscle performance), stage of motor control, and physiologic status of the tissue being addressed.

To illustrate these points, consider a patient with a mild lower trapezius strain with thoracic kyphosis and abducted, anterior tilted, and downwardly rotated scapulae at rest (Fig. 9-18) and excessive scapular abduction, medial rotation, and anterior tilt during forward-reaching activities. Prevention of these impairments is preferable, and there should be careful scrutiny of any posture, activity, or technique that allows further stretching of the lower trapezius. The ideal length of periarticular structures and myofascial tissue helps to maintain ideal posture alignment with a minimum of muscular effort. When these tissues become overstretched, they fail to offer adequate support, the joint(s) deviate(s) from the neutral position, posture becomes faulty, and muscular effort is required to maintain ideal alignment. In this case, it is possible that the lower trapezius is strained

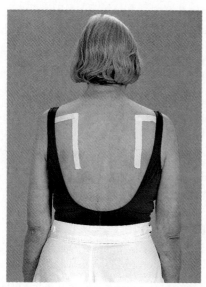

FIGURE 9-18. Although minimal, this figure illustrates abduction and downward rotation of the left scapula relative to the right.

by overstretching, and that the posture (thoracic kyphosis), scapula alignment (abducted and downwardly rotated), and movement patterns (scapula abduction, anterior tilt, and medial rotation) perpetuate this condition. Treatment of base (i.e., short range support [i.e., taping—see Chapter 25] and strengthening of the lower trapezius), biomechanical (i.e., reduced thoracic kyphosis, altered workstation ergonomics), and modulator elements (train reaching patterns without excessive scapula abduction, anterior tilt, or medial rotation) is indicated. Combining interventions to base, biomechanical, and modulator elements is more powerful than focusing on either element in isolation.

With respect to the base element, the goal is to improve muscle performance by altering length-tension properties of the lower trapezius. This component of muscle performance impairment is often overlooked but is critical to achieving muscle balance to restore healthy and efficient posture and movement. The tendency may be to stretch the opposing short pectoralis minor and major (also contributing to impairment of scapula posture and movement). However, if attention is focused *only* on stretching the short muscle without supporting and strengthening the lengthened muscle, equilibrium about the joint cannot be achieved. Another example of this principle is in the case of a person with an anterior pelvic tilt and lumbar lordosis. If the hip flexors are stretched without adaptive shortening of the abdominal muscles (see Chapter 17), the pelvis does not assume a neutral position in relaxed standing.

One activity that may be useful in this situation is to strengthen the adaptively lengthened muscles in the shortened range. The premise of this intervention strategy is to improve the strength of the lengthened muscle in the short range, where it has the greatest difficulty creating tension. If the focus of the exercise is on strengthening without attention to the ability to create tension in the shortened range, the exercise may reinforce the muscle imbalance by increasing the strength in the lengthened range. Careful

decisions must be made regarding the stage of motor control, posture, mode, movement, and dosage parameters to provide the optimal stimulus for strengthening without overloading the target muscle or promoting substitution of a dominant synergist (i.e., upper trapezius) or antagonist (i.e., pectoralis minor or major). The physiologic status of the tissue (i.e., length-associated changes or degree of strain) must be considered when determining each of these parameters.

Stability may be the starting point for the stage of motor control because strengthening is the chosen activity and specificity is critical so as not to strengthen in the lengthened range or the overused antagonist. Often, the lengthened muscle is unable to hold the limb against gravity when positioned in the short range as a result of the altered length-tension properties. Shortening the lever arm or exercising in a gravity-lessened position may be necessary for optimal strengthening (see Fig. 25-14 in Chapter 25). As the muscle becomes stronger in the shortened range, lengthening the lever arm and exercising against gravity can modify the exercise. Submaximal isometric contractions in the short range may be ideal initially, moving toward concentric–eccentric contractions throughout the range as the muscle performance and length tension improves and the tissues heal (if strain or tendiopathy is present). After stability and mobility are restored, the exercise can be progressed to controlled mobility and skill, with ultimate progression to functional movement patterns involving the total body as the final level of difficulty.

Dosage should follow the guidelines for strength training to improve muscle performance and generate hypertrophy of the lower trapezius to provide counterbalancing stiffness to the antagonists (pectoralis major and minor). Eventually, endurance dosage parameters can be applied as more functional movements are incorporated.

Simultaneous stretching of the pectoralis minor and major is not recommended due to the techniques that are often used for this type of stretching. The typical corner or doorway stretch (Figure 25-6) has a tendency to place excessive stress on the anterior capsule of the glenohumeral joint and thus is discouraged. Progressive strengthening of the trapezius has an elongating effect on the pectoralis minor and major and is a form of "active stretch" that is highly recommended (see Self-Management 25-2: Facelying Arm Lifts and Display 25-13: Activation Exercises for Trapezius and Serratus Anterior Based on EMG Analysis).

It may also be necessary to address breathing patterns if it is determined that the pectoralis minor is stiff because of overuse as an accessory muscle of respiration. Stretching addresses the base element, and breathing addresses the support element. Both of these interventions can begin at the mobility stage of motor control, progressing somewhat parallel to that for the lower trapezius toward controlled mobility and skill.

Ultimately, the isolated joint function of optimal movements of the scapula must be incorporated into total-body movement patterns (i.e., controlled mobility and skill). When this stage is appropriate, movement impairments of related areas may emerge. Perhaps the scapula abducts during forward-reaching movements because of a lack of hip flexion during reaching patterns or a lack of thoracic or hip rotation during cross-body

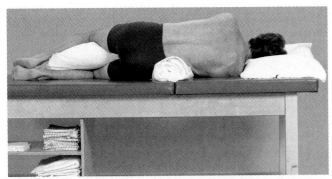

FIGURE 9-19. The use of pillows under the head, under the waist, and between the knees can position the spine in optimal alignment in sidelying.

reaching patterns. The related areas may require intervention to restore normal function to the shoulder girdle. A demonstration of the faulty movement pattern and corrected movement pattern can be viewed on the website.

Patient-Related Instruction and Adjunctive Interventions

Education regarding attention to postural alignment in frequently held or prolonged occupational or recreational positions is key to (a) optimizing joint position for rest and function, (b) reducing the tension placed on elongated muscles, and (c) increasing the tension placed on shortened muscles to restore muscle balance. Photographs of the patient in a typical rest posture and corrected posture can serve as powerful feedback for inducing change. Ergonomic modifications may be necessary to improve the patient's environment (see Patient-Related Instruction 9-1). If an on-site visit to the workplace is not feasible, a photograph of the workstation can be analyzed to provide suggestions for change. Other posture habits, including recumbent positions, can be analyzed and suggestions offered. Pillows under the head, under or between the knees, or under the waist in sidelying (Fig. 9-19) can be

suggested to offer optimal support to body regions while in recumbent positions. Footwear is another topic about which the physical therapist can provide recommendations (see Chapter 21).

Adjunctive interventions such as supportive devices (e.g., corsets, bracing, orthotics, taping) can be used temporarily to assist in creating length-associated and proprioceptive changes or used permanently to provide partial or complete correction of impairments of body structures. For example, taping can be used temporarily in the thoracic region to provide proprioceptive input for a patient about his or her kyphotic posture (Fig. 9-20). Every time the patient moves into excessive thoracic flexion, the tape serves as a reminder. Conversely, a permanent supportive device such as a corrective orthotic may be necessary to improve alignment throughout the kinetic chain and gait kinetics and kinematics in an individual with structural forefoot varus (see Chapter 21).

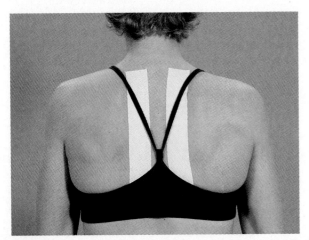

FIGURE 9-20. Taping along the thoracic spine can serve as biofeedback to discourage excessive thoracic flexion. The tape is best applied with the patient in a quadruped position, with the thoracic spine in a flat position.

KEY POINTS

- Many impairments in body functions can contribute to and perpetuate impairments in posture and movement.
- Evaluation of posture and movement impairment requires identification of deviations in posture and movement from acceptable standards and assessment of contributing factors such as impairments in body functions and environmental, structural, developmental, and emotional factors.
- Therapeutic exercise intervention for posture and movement impairment involves prioritization of the elements of the movement system and related impairments, careful determination of the appropriate activities or techniques and stage of motor control, and accurate prescription of dosage parameters for a successful outcome.
- Successful treatment of impaired posture and movement can directly affect the kinesiopathologic factors responsible for the development, perpetuation, or recurrence of MPS.

CRITICAL THINKING QUESTIONS

1. How are posture and movement impairments related to MPS?
2. Define ideal posture as it relates to surface landmarks from a side view.
3. Consider Case Study No. 9 in Unit 7.
   a. Given this patient's posture alignment, what muscles would you predict to be too long? What muscles would you predict to be too short?
   b. List the base, modulator, and biomechanical elements of the movement system that contribute to this patient's movement impairment.
   c. Develop an initial list of exercises, posture education, and movement retraining for this patient. Progress one of the listed exercises with respect to the stages of motor control.

LAB ACTIVITIES

1. Assess your laboratory partner's posture from the side and back views. Given your partner's alignment, which muscles would you predict to be too long or short?
2. Design an exercise program that stretches muscles that may be too short and strengthens muscles that are too long.
3. Assess your partner's strategy of rising from sit to stand. Break the movement into component parts. Assess the feet, ankles, knees, hips, pelvis, and lumbar, thoracic, and cervical spine about all three axes of motion during each component of the movement.

4. How would you provide feedback to change your partner's motor control strategy in rising from sit to stand? What verbal, tactile, and visual cues would you provide? What base element impairments may be contributing to the movement impairment?
5. Assess your partner's strategy of balancing on one limb. How does your partner move his or her center of mass over the base of support? What happens at the foot, knee, hip, pelvis, and spine? Do you think your partner uses a correct strategy? If not, what is faulty? Is one side different from the other? What contributing factors may be responsible for the faulty movement strategy?

CASE STUDY 9-1

See Case Study No. 9

Problem: Right hip pain with prolonged weightbearing

Short-term goal (4 to 6 weeks):
1. Patient has 3+/5 muscle grade in gluteus medius
2. Patient is able to walk 10 minutes with 2/10 pain and reduced Trendelenburg gait

Long-term goal (12 to 16 weeks)

• Patient has 4+/5 muscle grade in glutues medius
• Patient is able to walk miles with 1/10 pain

EXERCISE	EARLY PHASE	LATE PHASE
Hip abduction	Prone hip abduction (see Selected Intervention 9-1)	Sidelying hip abduction (Level V sidelying hip abduction—Self-Management 19-4)
Active stretch to Iliotibial Band (ITB)	Teach foam roll to self-mobilize Iliotibial Band (ITB) (Fig. 7-44)	Active stretch at the end of (Level V hip abduction—Self-Management 19-4: Performing Flexion and Extension Mobility Exercises During the *Day*)
Functional training	Squat (Figure 20-19)	Split squat (Level III walk stance progression—Self-Management 19-2: Patellar Mobilization Performed by the Patient)

REFERENCES

1. Sahrmann SA. Diagnosis and Treatment of Movement Impairment Syndromes. St. Louis, MO: Mosby, 2002.
2. Herring SA, Nilson KL. Introduction to overuse injuries. Clin Sports Med 1987; 6:225–239.
3. Leadbetter WB. Cell-matrix response in tendon injury. Clin Sports Med 1992; 11:533–578.
4. Bullock-Saxton J. Normal and abnormal postures in the sagittal plane and their relationship to low back pain. Physiother Prac 1988;4:94–104.
5. Raine S, Twomey LT. Attributes and qualities of human posture and their relationship to dysfunction or musculoskeletal pain. Crit Rev Phys Rehabil Med 1994;6:409–437.
6. Van Dillen LR, Gombatto SP, Collins DR, et al. Symmetry of timing of hip and lumbopelvic rotation motion in 2 different subgroups of people with low back pain. Arch Phys Med Rehabil 2007;88:351–360.
7. Van Dillen LR, Sahrmann SA, Caldwell CA, et al. Trunk rotation-related impairments in people with low back pain who participated in 2 different types of leisure activities: a secondary analysis. J Orthop Sports Phys Ther 2006;36:58–71.
8. Raine S, Twomey LT. Attributes and qualities of human posture and their relationship to dysfunction or musculoskeletal pain. Crit Rev Phys Rehabil Med 1994;6:409–437.
9. Guide to Physical Therapist Practice. 2nd Ed. Phys Ther 2001;81:9–746.
10. Sahrmann SA. Does postural assessment contribute to patient care? J Orthop Sports Phys Ther 2002;32:376–379.
11. Janda V. On the concept of postural muscles and posture in man. Aust J Physiother 1983;29:83–84.
12. Posture Committee of the American Academy of Orthopaedic Surgeons. Posture and its relationship to orthopedic disabilities: a report of the Posture Committee of the American Academy of Orthopedic Surgeons. Evanston, IL: American Academy of Orthopedic Surgeons, 1947:1.
13. Hobson L, Hammon WE. Chest assessment. In: Frownfelter D, ed. Chest Physical Therapy and Pulmonary Rehabilitation. St. Louis, MO: Mosby, 1987: 147–197.
14. Bates DV. Respiratory Function in Disease. 3rd Ed. Philadelphia, PA: WB Saunders, 1989.
15. Dean E. Oxygen transport deficits in systemic disease and implications for physical therapy. Phys Ther 1997;77:187–202.
16. Labelle H, Roussouly P, Berthonnaud E, Dimnet J, O'Brien M. The importance of spino-pelvic balance in L5-S1 developmental spondylolisthesis: a review of pertinent radiologic measurements. Spine 2005;30:S27–S34.
17. Johnson F, Leitl S, Waugh W. The distribution of the load across the knee: a comparison of static and dynamic measurements. J Bone Joint Surg Br 1980;62:346–349.

18. Nordin M, Frankel VH. Basic Biomechanics of the Musculo-skeletal System. Malvern, PA: Lea & Febiger, 1989.
19. Kendall FP, McCreary EK, Provance PG. Muscles Testing and Function. Baltimore, MD: Williams & Wilkins, 1993.
20. Norkin C, Levangie P. Joint Structure and Function. 2nd Ed. Philadelphia, PA: FA Davis, 1992.
21. Tsai N-T, McClure PW, Karduna AR. Effects of muscle fatigue on 3-dimensional scapular kinematics. Arch Phys Med Rehabil 2003;84:1000–1005.
22. Bagg SD, Forest WJ. A biomechanical analysis of scapular rotation during arm abduction in the scapular plane. Am J Phys Med Rehabil 1988;67:238–235.
23. Stedman's Concise Medical Dictionary. Baltimore, MD: Williams & Wilkins, 1998.
24. Frankel VH, Burstein AH, Brooks DB. Biomechanics of internal derangement of the knee. J Bone Joint Surg 1971;53:945–962.
25. Hollman JH, Deusinger RH. Videographic determination of instantaneous center of rotation using a hinge joint model. JOSPT 1999;29:463–469.
26. Smidt GL. Biomechanical analysis of knee flexion and extension. J Biomech 1973;6:79–92.
27. Penning L, Badoux DM. Radiological study of the movements of the cervical spine in the dog compared with those in man. Anat Histol Embryol 1987;16:1–20.
28. Liacouras PC, Wayne JS. Computational modeling to predict mechanical function of joints: application to the lower leg with simulation of two cadaver studies. J Biomech Eng 2007;129:811–817.
29. Hislop H. The not-so-impossible dream. Phys Ther 1975;55:1069–1080.
30. Williams PE, Goldspink G. Changes in sarcomere length and physiological properties in immobilized muscle. J Anat 1978;127:459–468.
31. Tabary JC, Tabury C, Taradiew C, et al. Physiological and structural changes in the cat's soleus muscle due to immobilization at different lengths by plaster casts. J Physiol 1972;224:231.
32. Goldspink G. Development of muscle. In: Goldspink G, ed. Growth of Cells in Vertebrate Tissues. London: Chapman & Hall, 1974;69–99.
33. Gossman MR, Sahrmann SA, Rose SJ. Review of length-associated changes in muscle, experimental and clinical implications. Phys Ther 1982;62:1799–1808.
34. Borich MR, Bright JM, Lorello DJ, et al. Scapular Angular Positioning at End Range Internal Rotation in Cases of Glenohumeral Internal Rotation Deficit. J Orthop Sports Phys Ther 2006;36:926–934.
35. Walker ML, Rothstein JM, Finucane SD, et al. Relationships between lumbar lordosis, pelvic tilt, and abdominal performance. Phys Ther 1987;67:512–516.
36. Diveta J, Walker M, Skibinski B. Relationship between performance of selected scapular muscles and scapular abduction in standing subjects. Phys Ther 1990;70:470–476.
37. Watanabe S, Eguchi A, Kobara K, et al. Influence of trunk muscle co-contraction on spinal curvature during sitting for desk work. Electromyogr Clin Neurophysiol 2007;47:273–278.
38. O'Sullivan PB, Dankaerts W, Burnett AF, et al. Effect of different upright sitting postures on spinal-pelvic curvature and trunk muscle activation in a pain-free population. Spine 2006;31:E707–E712.
39. Falla D, Jull G, Russell T, et al. Effect of neck exercise on sitting posture in patients with chronic neck pain. Phys Ther 2007;87:408–417.
40. Falla D, O'Leary S, Fagan A, et al. Recruitment of the deep cervical flexor muscles during a postural-correction exercise performed in sitting. Man Ther 2007;12:139–143.
41. Basmajian JV, DeLuca CJ. Muscles Alive. Baltimore, MD: Williams & Wilkins, 1985.
42. Panzer VP, Bandinelli S, Hallet M. Biomechanical assessment of quiet standing and changes associated with aging. Arch Phys Med Rehabil 1995;76:151–157.
43. Kavounoudias A, Gilhodes JC, Roll R, et al. From balance regulation to body orientation: two goals for muscle proprioceptive information processing? Exp Brain Res 1999;124:80–88.
44. Gosselin G, Rassoulian H, Brown I. Effects of neck extensor muscles fatigue on balance. Clin Biomech 2004;19:473–479.
45. Schache AG, Blanch PD, Rath DA, et al. Are anthropometric and kinematic parameters of the lumbo-pelvic-hip complex related to running injuries? Res Sports Med 2005;13:127–147.
46. Schache AG, Blanch P, Rath D, et al. Differences between the sexes in the three-dimensional angular rotations of the lumbo-pelvic-hip complex during treadmill running. J Sports Sci 2003;21:105–118.
47. Caillet R. Low Back Syndrome. Philadelphia, PA: FA Davis, 1981.
48. Turk DC, Monarch ES. Biopsychosocial perspective on chronic pain. In: Turk DC, Gatchel RJ, eds. Psychological Approaches to Pain Management. 2nd Ed. New York, NY: The Guilford Press, 2002:3–29.
49. Vlaeyen JS, Kole-Snijders AJ, Boeren RB, et al. Fear of movement/(re) injury in chronic low back pain and its relation to behavioural performance. Pain 1995;62:363–372.
50. Linton SJ. A review of psychological risk factors in back and neck pain. Spine 2000;25:1148–1156.
51. Fritz JM, George SZ, Delittlo A. The role of fear-avoidance beliefs in acute low back pain: relationships with current and future disability and work status. Pain 2001;94:7–15.
52. Vlaeyen JWS, de Jong J, Geilen M, et al. Graded exposure in vivo in the treatment of pain-related fear: a replicated single-case experimental design in four patients with chronic low back pain. Behav Res Ther 2001;39:151–166.
53. Vlaeyen JS, de Jong J, Geilen M, et al. The treatment of fear of movement/(re) injury in chronic low back pain: further evidence on the effectiveness of exposure in vivo. Clin J Pain 2002;18:251–261.
54. Peters ML, Vlaeyen JS, Weber WE. The joint contribution of physical pathology, pain-related fear and catastrophizing to chronic pain disability. Pain 2005;113:45–50.
55. Lethem J, Slade PD, Troup JDG, et al. Outline of fear-avoidance model of exaggerated pain perceptions. Behav Res Ther 1983;21:401–408.
56. Phillips HC. Avoidance behaviour and its role in sustaining chronic pain. Behav Res Ther 1987;25:273–279.
57. Asmundson GJG, Norton PJ, Norton GR. Beyond pain: the role of fear and avoidance in chronicity. Clin Psychol Rev 1999;19:97–119.
58. Crombez G, Vlaeyen JWS, Heuts PHTG, et al. Pain-related fear is more disabling than pain itself: evidence on the role of pain-related fear in chronic back pain disability. Pain 1999;80:329–339.
59. Bortz WM. The disuse syndrome. West J Med 1984;141:691–694.
60. Asmundson GJG, Norton GR, Allerdings MD. Fear and avoidance in dysfunctional chronic back pain patients. Pain 1997;69:231–236.
61. Woby SR, Watson PJ, Roach NK, et al. Are changes in fear-avoidance beliefs, catastrophizing, and appraisals of control, predictive of changes in chronic low back pain and disability? Eur J Pain 2004;8:201–210.
62. McCracken LM, Gross RT, Sorg PJ, et al. Prediction of pain in patients with chronic low back pain: effects of inaccurate prediction and pain-related anxiety. Behav Res Ther 1993;31:647–652.
63. Vlaeyen JS, Linton SJ. Fear-avoidance and its consequences in chronic musculoskeletal pain: a state of the art. Pain 2000;85:317–332.
64. Waddell G, Newton M, Henderson I, et al. A Fear-avoidance Beliefs Questionnaire (FABQ) and the role of fear-avoidance beliefs in chronic low back pain and disability. Pain 1993;52:157–168.
65. Kendall HO, Kendall FP, Boynton DA. Posture and Pain. Huntington, NY: Robert E. Krieger Publishing, 1970.
66. Vernazza-Martin S, Tricon V, Martin N, et al. Effect of aging on the coordination between equilibrium and movement: what changes? Exp Brain Res 2008;187:255–265.
67. Horak FB, Macpherson JM. Postural orientation and equilibrium. In: Towell LB, Shepherd JT, eds. Handbook on Integration of Motor Circulatory, Respiratory, and Metabolic Control During Exercise. Bethesda, MD: American Physiological Society, 1996:255–292.
68. Massion J, Alexandrov A, Frolov A. Why and how are posture and movement coordinated? Prog Brain Res 2004;143:13–27.
69. Millanvoye M. Le vieillissement de l'organisme avant 60 ans. Octare's (ed). Le travail au fil de l'âge, 2001:2–36.
70. Fletcher PC, Hirdes JP. Risk factors for falling among community-based seniors using home care services. J Gerontol A Biol Sci Med Sci 2002;57:492–495.
71. Sutherland SE, Goldman HB. Treatment options for female urinary incontinence. Med Clin North Am 2004;88:345–366.
72. Sternheim MM, Kane JW. Elastic properties of materials. General Physics. Toronto: John Wiley & Sons, 1986.
73. Woodley SJ, Nicholson HD, Livingstone V, et al. Lateral hip pain: findings from magnetic resonance imaging and clinical examination. J Orthop Sports Phys Ther 2008;38(6):313–328.

RECOMMENDED READING

Sahrmann SA. Diagnosis and Treatment of Movement Impairment Syndromes. St. Louis, MO: Mosby, 2002.

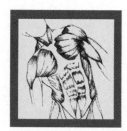

chapter 10

Pain

LORI THEIN BRODY AND KIMBERLY BENNETT

Pain is a psychosomatic experience that is affected by cultural, historic, environmental, and social factors. The prevalence of chronic pain increases from ages 18 to 70, and approximately 23% of patients in their seventh decade report chronic pain.[1] It is more common in women than in men. Unlike impairments such as motion or strength loss that can be observed and measured with tools such as goniometers and dynamometers, pain is elusive. Although limited motion produces observable activity limitations or participation restrictions, pain produces activity limitations and participation restrictions that are not always observable by the outsider. This situation produces anxiety for the patient and can be a source of conflict with spouses, family members, friends, and coworkers. The clinician must recognize the impact of pain on the patient and provide him or her with strategies to manage the pain.

DEFINITIONS

Pain is a component of most musculoskeletal conditions seen in the clinic. The International Association for the Study of Pain defines pain as "an unpleasant sensory and emotional experience associated with actual or potential tissue damage, or described in terms of such damage."[2] Acute pain is associated with muscle strains, tendinitis, contusions, surgery, or ligament injuries. Although it is important to acknowledge and treat acute pain, this pain is usually short-lived. Most individuals can tolerate this type of pain because they know that it is temporary. Acute pain is often successfully treated with nonnarcotic analgesics such as nonsteroidal anti-inflammatory drugs (NSAIDs) and agents such as ice.

Chronic pain is pain that persists after the noxious stimulus has been removed. It includes persistent pain after healing of an acute injury and pain with no known cause. It is not simply acute pain that has persisted too long. There may be no relationship between the extent of pathology and the intensity or anatomic location of the pain. Chronic pain is not short-lived and produces profound changes in the physical, psychologic, and social aspects of the patient's life. Chronic pain typically is a major component of problems such as fibromyalgia, chronic fatigue syndrome (CFS), myofascial pain syndrome, rheumatoid arthritis, and low back pain. Physical therapy focuses on treating the pain, the motion and muscle impairments, and the activity limitations and participation restrictions that result.

Referred pain is pain felt at a site far distant from the location of the injury or disease. Although the pain is felt elsewhere, the pain is still very real. Examination and evaluation can become difficult in the absence of understanding common pain referral patterns. Be sure to consider other distant sources of pain when examining the patient with acute or chronic pain.

PHYSIOLOGY OF PAIN

Pain is a complex sensory experience. The physiology of pain is far too complex to be covered in detail in this text. However, this brief overview provides an understanding of the physiology of pain and the scientific basis of interventions used to treat it.

Sources of Pain

Acute pain results from microtraumatic or macrotraumatic tissue injury. Microtrauma is defined as a long-standing or recurrent musculoskeletal problem that was not initiated by an acute injury. Microtrauma is exemplified by the overuse injury in which repetitive activity exceeds the tissue's ability to repair and remodel according to the imposed loads. The athlete playing in a weekend tennis tournament and the worker putting in overtime are prone to microtraumatic injuries. Macrotrauma is defined as an immediately noticeable injury involving sudden, direct, or indirect trauma.[3] Macrotrauma can produce pain through direct injury of tissues. Joint dislocations injure the joint capsule and periarticular connective tissue, and ligament or tendon injuries damage the respective collagenous tissues. Microtrauma and macrotrauma result in an inflammatory response that secondarily produces pain. Macrotrauma also produces pain directly through damage to the *nociceptors*, or pain receptors.

Chronic pain can arise suddenly or come on very gradually. It has strong psychologic, emotional, and sociologic effects. Individuals with chronic pain tend to have significant sleep disturbances, depressive symptoms, appetite changes, and decreased activity and socialization. Theories about the source of chronic pain suggest increased sensitization of nociceptors and spinal level changes that perpetuate positive feedback loops in the pain-spasm cycle.[4] Pain from inflammation in conditions such as osteoarthritis and rheumatoid arthritis sensitizes dorsal horn neurons to the inflammation. After inflammation of a joint or muscle, afferent input to the spinal cord increases the activity of the dorsal horn, spinothalamic tract, and thalamic neurons. The elevated activity increases the frequency of background firing of dorsal horn neurons and increases sensitivity to noxious and nonnoxious peripheral stimulation and joint motion. Repetitive stimulation with progressive build-up of the response in the dorsal horn neurons is termed "wind-up" and is a critical concept in understanding chronic pain.[5] When damage to the central

DISPLAY 10-1
Characteristics of NNP

1. Pain appears to be inappropriate compared with tissue pathology, or no tissue pathology may be evident
2. Hyperalgesia, where pain is greater than expected given the stimulus
3. Allodynia, where normally nonnoxious stimuli produces pain
4. Painful region extends beyond expected based on original tissue pathology

nociceptive system occurs, nonnociceptive afferent activity becomes capable of eliciting pain.[6] Stimuli that were previously innocuous become painful. This is referred to as nonnociceptive pain (NNP). These nonnociceptive afferents are not abnormal, but are working with a sensitized central nervous system (CNS). Bennett[5] describes four clinical features of NNP. They can be found in Display 10-1. The pathophysiology of NNP includes central sensitization of ongoing or past nociception, convergence of nociceptive and nonnociceptive inputs on the same secondary neuron in the dorsal horn, the experience of pain on wide dynamic range (WDR) neurons, and an expansion of the receptive fields, extending pain beyond the original boundaries.[5]

The peripheral receptive field of dorsal horn neurons increases in response to chronic pain.[7] The pain seems to spread from the originally painful area to adjacent areas. The basis for some of these changes may be an increased sensitization of WDR neurons from nociceptive input, causing them to respond more intensely to more nonnociceptive input and to afferent input from a larger area.[6] After being sensitized to nociceptive input from peripheral nerves, the WDR will respond to nonnoxious stimuli as intensely as they had to other stimuli before sensitization.[5] The increase in receptive field area, increased background firing, and increased sensitivity to mechanical stimuli after acute or chronic inflammation may set the stage for chronic pain that seems to spread along a limb or to adjacent areas.

Referred pain is considered to be an error in perception. For example, pain originating from deep visceral tissues may refer to the cutaneous region with the same segmental innervation. Pain originating from the genitourinary system may refer to the low back because of the common T11–L2 segmental origin. Cardiac pain refers to the shoulder because of the common T1–2 segments. As afferent input from the visceral receptors synapse in the dorsal horn, information is also incoming from skin afferents. Convergence of this incoming information in the dorsal horn results in the sense that the pain is originating from the skin. This same principle underlies the use of electrical stimulation at remote sites to decrease visceral pain.

Pain Pathways

Pain is transmitted from nociceptor and nonnociceptor afferents in the periphery. Nociceptors are defined as pain receptors that transfer impulses to the spinal cord and higher CNS levels. Nociceptors in the periphery are activated by mechanical stimuli such as strong pressure, irritants such as chemicals (e.g., bradykinin, substance P, histamine), or noxious elements such as heat and cold.

Nociceptors in peripheral tissues transmit pain information through A-delta and C fibers. A-delta fibers are small, myelinated fibers carrying information about pain and temperature. The information is carried to the spinal cord at an approximate speed of 15 m per second.[8] The A-delta fibers are most responsive to mechanical stimuli and probably are responsible for the sensation of pain in acute injuries. Type C fibers are slow, unmyelinated fibers carrying information about dull aching or burning pain from polymodal receptors. **Polymodal receptors** are receptors that respond to a variety of stimuli such as temperature and pressure. Type C polymodal fibers are found in the deeper layers of skin and in virtually all other tissues except the nervous system itself. They are also known as "free nerve endings" and are responsive to thermal, chemical, and mechanical stimuli. C fibers probably are responsible for the continued sensation of pain after the noxious stimulus has been removed. Transmission speed to the spinal cord is approximately 1 m per second.

At the spinal cord level, A-delta fibers enter the dorsal roots sending collateral that ascend and descend several segments before entering the gray matter. These fibers terminate on the cells of laminae I and V. The slower C fibers also enter the dorsal root and then enter the gray matter and synapse at the level of entry or ascend or descend a level or two before entering the substantia gelatinosa at laminae II and III. Some processing of information occurs in the spinal cord before the information is transmitted to higher levels. Important receptors at the termination of the primary nociceptive afferents in the dorsal horn have been found, in particular N-methyl-D-aspartate, which are activated and placed in a state ready for activation.[9] They are a primary mechanism in the development of windup, central sensitization, and changes in peripheral receptive fields.

Three types of interneurons found within the dorsal horn are categorized by their response to peripheral stimulation: low-threshold mechanosensitive, responding only to innocuous stimuli such as touching the skin; nociceptive-specific, responding only to high-threshold noxious stimuli; and WDR, responding to a wide variety of noxious and nonnoxious stimuli. Changes in the firing patterns of the WDR interneurons are suggested as an underlying cause of chronic pain, and convergence of stimuli from various receptors in the dorsal horn is the theoretic basis underlying the gate control theory. This convergence also may be the source of referred pain. Substance P is a neuromodulator shown to be responsible for the transmission of noxious information in the spinal cord.[7] It lowers the synaptic excitability threshold, sensitizing second-order spinal neurons. Substance P also facilitates the expansion of receptive fields and the activation of WDR interneurons by nonnociceptive afferent impulses.[5]

From the dorsal horn, these signals ascend through the contralateral spinothalamic tract in the ventrolateral white matter of the spinal cord to the ventral posterolateral nucleus of the thalamus. The spinothalamic tract transmits noxious and thermal information. The spinothalamic tract also sends collateral branches to the periaqueductal gray (PAG) nucleus of the brain stem. Synapses in this pathway are morphine-sensitive and are an important component of the pain-modulating system. Stimulation of the PAG nucleus has produced analgesia. The thalamus is capable of some conscious awareness of pain before this information reaches the postcentral gyrus of the cerebral cortex.[10] In addition to the spinothalamic tract, some noxious stimuli ascend in the ipsilateral dorsal column of the spinomedullary system.

Descending impulses also influence pain perception. The individual who continues to play sports despite a broken bone or the grandmother who lifts a car to save a child are examples of these descending influences at work. These systems are complex, and the relationships of the system components are being investigated. An overview is given to explain the rationale for some pain-control interventions.

Descending pain control occurs through opiate and nonopiate systems. Release of endogenous opiates from the brain stem related to exercise has achieved widespread publicity in the popular press. The "runner's high" that occurs with long-distance running has been attributed to the release of β-endorphin and methionine-enkephalin from CNS higher centers. Location of these opiates varies among the PAG, hypothalamus, thalamus, substantia gelatinosa, and midbrain structures.[4] Input to the enkephalinergic interneurons in the substantia gelatinosa comes from fibers descending from the midbrain (i.e., PAG) that use serotonin as the transmitter. Injection of opiates into the spinal cord inhibits noxious stimulus–elicited dorsal horn neuron activity.[4] Other neurons descending from the midbrain use noradrenaline as their transmitter and provide an analgesic action through direct inhibition of dorsal horn nociceptive neurons, rather than through the enkephalinergic interneurons.[8] Continued research in the area of descending influences may provide more effective pain control interventions in the future.

Pain Theory

Melzack and Wall proposed the gate theory of pain in 1965, with revisions added in 1982.[4] This theory replaced previously held pain theories such as the specificity and patterning theories.[4] The cornerstone of the gate theory is the convergence of first-order neurons and associated second-order neurons within the substantia gelatinosa (Fig. 10-1). The system has four components consisting of afferent neurons, internuncial neurons within the substantia gelatinosa, transmission cells (T cells), and descending control from higher centers.[11] The activity of T cells is regulated by the balance of large- and small-diameter fiber input from the periphery and by descending control from higher cells. This balance regulates the transmission of pain information.

The substantia gelatinosa modulates incoming information (i.e., regulates position of the gate) presynaptically, before information is passed to second-order neurons. When incoming information increases substantia gelatinosa activity, presynaptic inhibition occurs, closing the gate. Information is not passed from first- to second-order neurons for further transmission to higher centers. If peripheral receptors associ-

ated with large-diameter myelinated fibers are stimulated, activity in the substantia gelatinosa may close the gate to the slower C fiber pain information transmission.

This theory provides the rationale for interventions to "close the gate" to pain transmission. Several peripheral stimuli can close the gate to pain. Input from thermal modalities such as heat and cold can successfully decrease pain. When thermal impulses are transmitted, the input can "block" pain transmission from slower fibers at the substantia gelatinosa. Electrical impulses from transcutaneous electrical nerve stimulation (TENS) application can preferentially block pain impulse transmission (discussed in the "Adjunctive Therapies" section). Exercise can successfully decrease pain by stimulation of joint afferent receptors. These signals travel along A-beta fibers, which have larger diameters and carry information at higher speeds (30 to 70 m per second) than the slower pain fibers. This same mechanical stimulation of peripheral receptors can be achieved through tissue massage. Further revision of the gate theory of pain continues, because descending control from higher centers also influences the transmission of pain information.

EXAMINATION AND EVALUATION

A variety of tools helps the clinician assess and monitor the patient's pain level. Tools such as the McGill Pain Questionnaire (MPQ) assess affective qualities of pain, while the visual analog scale (VAS) is a nominal scale assessing pain intensity. Because of the multifaceted nature of pain, assessment should include information on the pain's intensity, location, and pattern over a 24-hour period (i.e., quantity of pain) and descriptors assessing the affective aspects (i.e., quality of pain). The impact of pain (i.e., activity limitations and participation restrictions) on the patient's life should be determined. Frequently tools such as the Beck depression and Beck anxiety questionnaires are used to assess the psychologic aspects of the patient's pain.

Clinicians perform examinations to determine the source of the patient's pain. This examination directs the subsequent treatment program to the source of pain. Structures within the musculoskeletal system have different levels of pain sensitivity. The periosteum of the bone is a highly pain-sensitive structure, whereas the joint capsule, ligaments, tendons, and muscle are less pain-sensitive. Interestingly, research has found that isometric muscle contraction normally increases the pain threshold, whereas in patients with fibromyalgia, the pain threshold actually decreases.[12] Additionally, compared with skin receptors, sensory input from muscle is a more potent catalyst of central sensitization.[5] Fibrocartilage and articular cartilage are not pain-sensitive structures, although injury or damage to these structures can produce a synovitis that results in pain. Perform a thorough evaluation to determine the source of the pain and to assess the characteristics of that pain. However, remember the pathophysiology of chronic pain and realize that the pain region and intensity may extend beyond discernible tissue pathology.

Pain Scales

The VAS and a 0 (least pain) to 10 (worst pain) scale are used to assess pain intensity. The simplest clinical tool consists of asking the patient to rate her pain on a 0 to 10 scale and recording this in the medical record. Follow-up visits ask the same question to determine the response to treatment. This

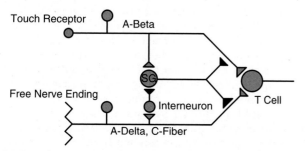

FIGURE 10-1. The gate control theory of pain. T cells, central transmission cells; SG, substantia gelatinosa.

type of scale has advantages and disadvantages. The clearest advantage is the ease of use. The patient is not burdened with forms to fill out or multiple questions to answer. Language and cultural barriers do not affect the use of this simple scale. The disadvantage is the minimal information acquired with such a tool. Only pain-intensity information is gathered. Information regarding the affective aspects of pain, pattern of pain, and the impact of the pain on the patient's life are absent. The patient is likely to remember the previous pain score, which reduces the reliability of this type of measurement. This type of scale presumes equal intervals between each level (i.e., the difference between a 1 and a 2 is equal to the difference between a 3 and a 4), and this may not be the case for the patient. Be sure to clarify the question being asked. Are you interested in the patient's current pain level or average pain level over the last 24, 48, or 72 hours? Are you interested in the worst pain and best pain in the last 24 hours or the last 7 days? Clarifying the question is critical due to the variable nature of patient's pain. Pain is often mediated by multiple factors such as time of day, activity level, and medication use. Consistency in collecting and interpreting this data is essential when using it to assess the efficacy of an intervention.

The VAS can be administered in several different forms (Fig. 10-2). A line with words placed at intervals along the line commonly is used. A single word may be used at each end, such as "no pain" and "worst pain," or several words

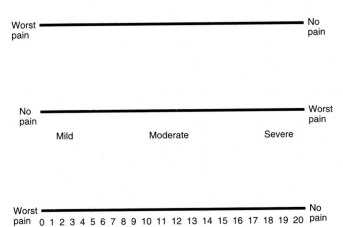

FIGURE 10-2. Variations of a VAS.

BUILDING BLOCK 10-1

A 36-year-old female with chronic neck pain and posttraumatic stress disorder has been coming to physical therapy weekly for soft tissue mobilization. The first week she reports her pain level at 8 on 0 to 10. On subsequent visits she reports her pain ranging from 5 to 9 on a 0 to 10 scale. Please provide recommendations on ways to gather pain information that would guide and inform her plan of care (primary goal: pain reduction).

may be placed along the continuum. The more words and lines dividing the continuum, the more the patient is likely to recall previous answers. Improve the reliability of a VAS by eliminating division marks and only marking both ends of the scale. The patient then places a mark along the scale corresponding to her current pain level. The distance from the left or right can be measured to assess progress. The direction of the scale should be altered occasionally. Reverse the "no pain" and "worst pain" sides of the scale or turn the scale from horizontal to vertical to minimize patient recall.[13] Combine these scales with other assessments, such as the location of pain (using a body diagram) and subjective descriptions of the quality of pain (see Fig. 10-2). See Building Block 10-1.

McGill Pain Questionnaire

The MPQ is one of the most widely used tests for the measurement of pain, and several forms of the questionnaire have been developed.[14–16] This pain questionnaire consists primarily of three classes of word descriptors to assess the subjective aspects of pain. The MPQ also contains an intensity score, a body diagram, and an assessment of pain relative to activities and pain patterns. The three major measures are the pain rating index (PRI), the number of words chosen (NWC), and the present pain intensity (PPI).

Part one contains word descriptors classified as three categories (i.e., sensory, affective, and evaluative) and 20 subcategories. Subcategories contain two to six words that are qualitatively similar but of increasing intensity. For example, one subcategory assesses the thermal aspects of pain through the descriptors "hot," "burning," "scalding," and "searing." Each word is assigned a numeric value. The patient is allowed to choose only one word from each subcategory and is not required to select an item from every category. The values are summed and the mean determined; the mean is the PRI score. The total number of subcategories selected is summed as the NWC score (Fig. 10-3).

The PPI is determined by use of a 5-point scale, asking about the current pain level and the level of pain when it is at its worst and at its best. The PPI is the current pain level. Part two categorizes the pattern of pain as constant, periodic, or brief and asks about activities that increase or relieve pain. A body diagram allows the patient to mark where the pain is located. The patient marks *E* for external pain and *I* for internal pain and then uses a VAS to document the quantity of pain.

The MPQ better assesses the many dimensions of pain with greater sensitivity than a VAS. The disadvantage is the

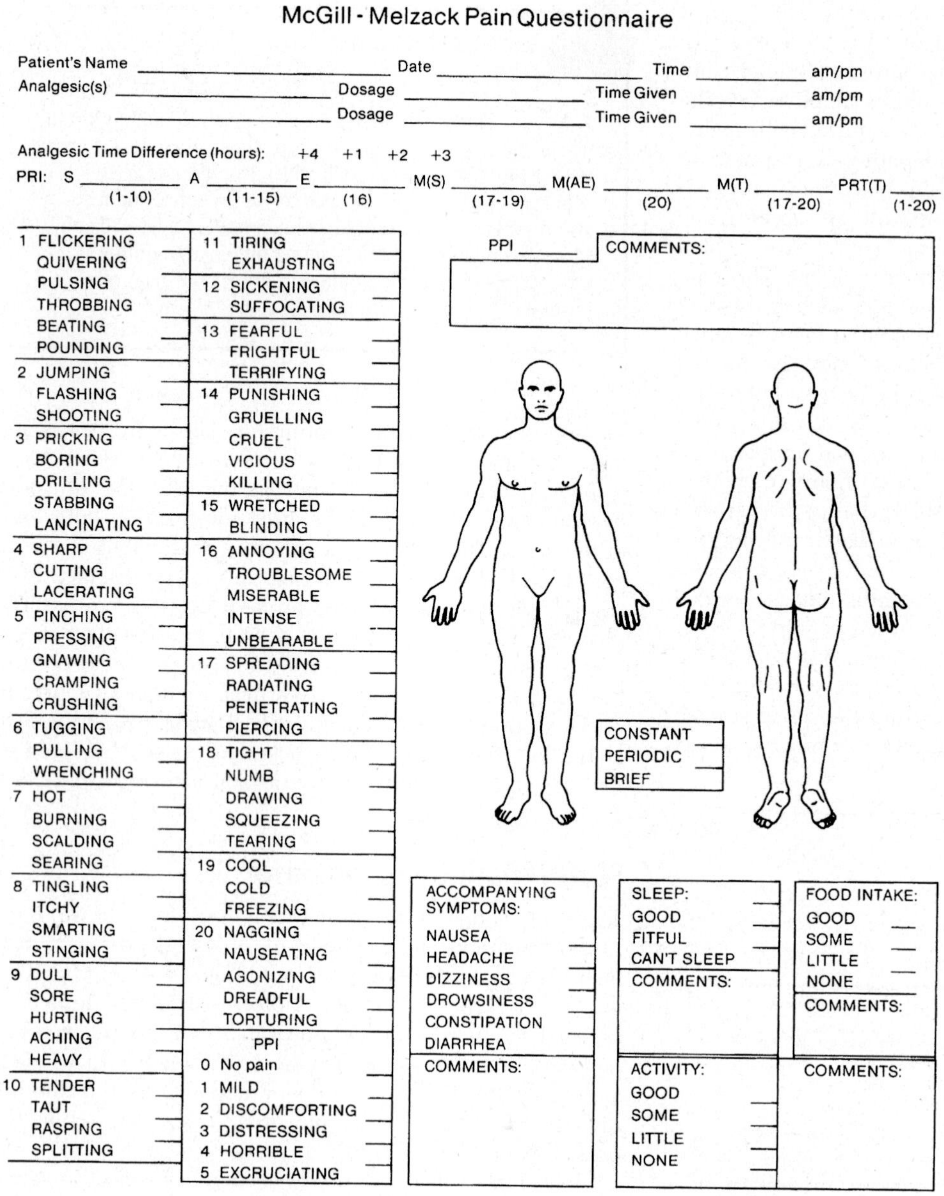

McGill - Melzack Pain Questionnaire

Patient's Name _____ Date _____ Time _____ am/pm

Analgesic(s) _____ Dosage _____ Time Given _____ am/pm

_____ Dosage _____ Time Given _____ am/pm

Analgesic Time Difference (hours):   +4   +1   +2   +3

PRI: S _____ A _____ E _____ M(S) _____ M(AE) _____ M(T) _____ PRT(T) _____
(1-10)   (11-15)   (16)   (17-19)   (20)   (17-20)   (1-20)

1 FLICKERING	11 TIRING
QUIVERING	EXHAUSTING
PULSING	12 SICKENING
THROBBING	SUFFOCATING
BEATING	13 FEARFUL
POUNDING	FRIGHTFUL
2 JUMPING	TERRIFYING
FLASHING	14 PUNISHING
SHOOTING	GRUELLING
3 PRICKING	CRUEL
BORING	VICIOUS
DRILLING	KILLING
STABBING	15 WRETCHED
LANCINATING	BLINDING
4 SHARP	16 ANNOYING
CUTTING	TROUBLESOME
LACERATING	MISERABLE
5 PINCHING	INTENSE
PRESSING	UNBEARABLE
GNAWING	17 SPREADING
CRAMPING	RADIATING
CRUSHING	PENETRATING
6 TUGGING	PIERCING
PULLING	18 TIGHT
WRENCHING	NUMB
7 HOT	DRAWING
BURNING	SQUEEZING
SCALDING	TEARING
SEARING	19 COOL
8 TINGLING	COLD
ITCHY	FREEZING
SMARTING	20 NAGGING
STINGING	NAUSEATING
9 DULL	AGONIZING
SORE	DREADFUL
HURTING	TORTURING
ACHING	PPI
HEAVY	0 No pain
10 TENDER	1 MILD
TAUT	2 DISCOMFORTING
RASPING	3 DISTRESSING
SPLITTING	4 HORRIBLE
	5 EXCRUCIATING

PPI _____ COMMENTS:

CONSTANT
PERIODIC
BRIEF

ACCOMPANYING SYMPTOMS:
NAUSEA
HEADACHE
DIZZINESS
DROWSINESS
CONSTIPATION
DIARRHEA
COMMENTS:

SLEEP:
GOOD
FITFUL
CAN'T SLEEP
COMMENTS:

FOOD INTAKE:
GOOD
SOME
LITTLE
NONE
COMMENTS:

ACTIVITY:
GOOD
SOME
LITTLE
NONE

COMMENTS:

FIGURE 10-3. The McGill-Melzack Pain Questionnaire. (From Melzack R. The McGill Pain Questionnaire: major properties and scoring methods. Pain 1975;1:277–299.)

time required to complete the questionnaire. A short form of the MPQ has been developed to address this issue.

Disability and Health-Related Quality of Life Scales

A variety of tools have been developed to assess pain and the impact of pain and resulting disability on patients' lives. Most tools broadly assess physical, social, and psychologic function. Some tools assess health perceptions, satisfaction, and various impairments. Each tool taps into these domains in a different way and at a different level. The tool must be matched to the population of interest.

The scales are classified in several ways but are broadly categorized into disease-specific and generic measures. Disease-specific scales are specific to a particular disease and are more responsive to issues of that population. Generic tools are applied across a variety of disease categories; the information has little relevance to a specific disease, and other important issues may not be tapped. However, use of these tools allows comparisons among disease or injury categories.

Commonly used generic tools are the Quality of Well-Being scale (QWB), the Sickness Impact Profile (SIP), the Duke Health Profile (DUKE), and the Short Form-36 (SF-36). The QWB taps five health concepts (i.e., physical functioning, mental health including psychologic distress, social or role functioning, mobility or travel, and physical or physiologic symptoms), and the SIP measures 12 concepts. Neither of these tools assesses pain directly. The DUKE measures seven health concepts, including self-esteem, health perceptions, and pain. The SF-36 is a derivative of the Medical Outcomes Study-149, a 149-item tool used as a generic assessment. The SF-36 is a 36-item tool measuring seven health concepts, including pain. Use caution when choosing a generic health assessment tool to ensure that critical parameters are being measured. The tool's range must allow for improvement or decline in the patient's status without exceeding the upper or lower limits of the measure (Fig. 10-4).

SF-36 HEALTH SURVEY

Instructions: This survey asks for your views about your health. This information will help keep track of how you feel and how well you are able to do your usual activities.

Answer every question by marking the answer as indicated. If you are unsure about how to answer a question, please give the best answer you can.

1. In general, would you say your health is:

(circle one)

Excellent	1
Very good	2
Good	3
Fair	4
Poor	5

2. <u>Compared to one week ago</u>, how would you rate your health in general <u>now</u>?

(circle one)

Much better now then one week ago	1
Somewhat better now than one week ago	2
About the same as one week ago	3
Somewhat worse now than one week ago	4
Much worse than one week ago	5

3. The following items are about activities you might do during a typical day. Does <u>your health now limit you</u> in these activities? If so, how much?

(circle one number on each line)

<u>ACTIVITIES</u>	Yes, Limited A Lot	Yes, Limited A Little	No, Not Limited At All
a. **Vigorous activities** such as running, lifting heavy objects, participating in strenuous sports	1	2	3
b. **Moderate activities**, such as moving a table, pushing a vacuum cleaner, bowling, or playing golf	1	2	3
c. Lifting or carrying groceries	1	2	3
d. Climbing **several** flights of stairs	1	2	3
e. Climbing **one** flight of stairs	1	2	3
f. Bending, kneeling, or stooping	1	2	3
g. Walking **more than a mile**	1	2	3
h. Walking **several blocks**	1	2	3
i. Walking **one block**	1	2	3
j. Bathing or dressing yourself	1	2	3

FIGURE 10-4. The SF-36 assessment tool. (From Medical Outcomes Trust; Boston, MA, 1992.) *(continued)*

4. During the <u>past week</u>, have you had any of the following problems with your work or other regular daily activities <u>as a result of your physical health?</u>

(circle one number on each line)

	Yes	No
a. Cut down on the **amount of time** you spent on work or other activities	1	2
b. **Accomplished less** than you would like	1	2
c. Were limited in the **kind** of work or other activities	1	2
d. Had **difficulty** performing the work or other activities (for example, it took extra effort)	1	2

5. During the <u>past week</u>, have you had the following problems with your work or other regular daily activities <u>as a result of any emotional problems</u> (such as feeling depressed or anxious)?

(circle one number on each line)

	Yes	No
a. Cut down on the **amount of time** you spent on work or other activities	1	2
b. **Accomplished less** than you would like	1	2
c. Didn't do work or other activities as **carefully** as usual	1	2

6. During the <u>past week,</u> to what extent has your physical health or emotional problems interfered with your normal social activities with family, friends, neighbors, or groups?

(circle one)

Not at all 1

Slightly 2

Moderately... 3

Quite a bit.. 4

Extremely..5

7. How much <u>bodily</u> pain have you had during the <u>past week</u>?

(circle one)

None 1

Very mild 2

Mild 3

Moderate 4

Severe 5

Very severe 6

8. During the <u>past week</u>, how much did <u>pain</u> interfere with your normal work (including both work outside the home and housework)?

(circle one)

Not at all 1

A little bit 2

Moderately... 3

Quite a bit.. 4

Extremely... 5

FIGURE 10-4. *(continued)*

9. These questions are about how you feel and how things have been with you <u>during the past week</u>. For each question, please give the one answer that comes closest to the way you have been feeling. How much of the time during the <u>past week</u>—

(circle one number on each line)

	All of the Time	Most of the Time	A Good Bit of Time	Some of the Time	Some of the Time	None of the Time
a. Did you feel full of pep?	1	2	3	4	5	6
b. Have you been a nervous person?	1	2	3	4	5	6
c. Have you ever felt so down in the dumps that nothing could cheer you up?	1	2	3	4	5	6
d. Have you felt calm and peaceful?	1	2	3	4	5	6
e. Did you have a lot of energy?	1	2	3	4	5	6
f. Have you felt downhearted and blue?	1	2	3	4	5	6
g. Did you feel worn out?	1	2	3	4	5	6
h. Have you been a happy person?	1	2	3	4	5	6
i. Did you feel tired?	1	2	3	4	5	6

10. During the <u>past week</u>, how much time has your <u>physical health or emotional problems</u> interfered with your social activities (like visiting with friends, relatives, etc.)?

(circle one)

All of the time... 1

Most of the time 2

Some of the time... 3

A little of the time... 4

None of the time.. 5

11.   How TRUE or FALSE is <u>each</u> of the following statements for you?

(circle one number on each line)

	Definitely True	Mostly True	Don't Know	Mostly False	Definitely False
a. I seem to get sick a little easier than other people?	1	2	3	4	5
b. I am as healthy as anybody I know	1	2	3	4	5
c. I expect my health to get worse	1	2	3	4	5
d. My health is excellent	1	2	3	4	5

FIGURE 10-4. *(continued)*

Health Concepts, Number of Items and Levels, and Summary of Content for Eight SF-36 Scales and the Health Transition Item

Concepts	No. of Items	No. of Levels	Summary of Content
Physical Functioning (PF)	10	21	Extent to which health limits physical activities such as self-care, walking, climbing stairs, bending, lifting, and moderate and vigorous exercises
Role Functioning Physical (RP)	4	5	Extent to which physical health interferes with work or other daily activities, including accomplishing less than wanted, limitations in the kind of activities, or difficulty in performing activities
Bodily Pain (BP)	2	11	Intensity of pain and effect of pain on normal work, both inside and outside the home
General Health (GH)	5	21	Personal evaluation of health, including current health, health outlook, and resistance to illness
Vitality (VT)	4	21	Feeling energetic and full of pep versus feeling tired and worn out
Social Functioning (SF)	2	9	Extent to which physical health or emotional problems interfere with normal social activities
Role Functioning Emotional (RE)	3	4	Extent to which emotional problems interfere with work or other daily activities, including decreased time spent on activities, accomplishing less, and not working as carefully as usual
Mental Health (MH)	5	26	General mental health, including depression, anxiety, behavioral-emotional control, general positive affect
Reported Health Transition (HT)	1	5	Evaluation of current health compared to one year ago

FIGURE 10-4. *(continued)*

One way to minimize some of the potential problems associated with generic tools is to use a disease-specific tool in combination with a generic measure. The Oswestry Low Back Disability Questionnaire, the Waddell Disability Index, and the Disability Questionnaire are used for individuals with back pain, and the McMaster-Toronto Arthritis Patient Reference Disability Questionnaire, the Arthritis Impact Measurement Scales (AIMS), the Health Assessment Questionnaire, and the Functional Capacity Questionnaire are used for individuals with arthritis. As with generic tools, disease-specific tools must match the population tested. Reliability of the tool must be determined for the population being evaluated. For example, if the AIMS reliability has been established for Caucasian women who are 65 or older, this tool may not be reliable or valid when applied to men between the ages of 40 and 60 (Fig. 10-5).

Other tools tap some of the psychosocial aspects of the pain experience. A large body of literature has developed around the issue of anxiety, fear and avoidance of pain in patients with chronic pain.[17–19] Fear-anxiety-avoidance models of pain and tools attempting to measure these constructs have been developed and tested.[20–28] The fear-anxiety-avoidance models were originally developed to explain the transition from acute to chronic pain. Now these models and measurement tools are used to formulate multidimensional treatment plans for patients with chronic pain, as well as to determine the efficacy of different interventions. Frequently, physical activity and rehabilitative exercises are a component of these intervention plans, as providers guide patients through structured activities to minimize their fear of movement.[29,30] The Fear-Avoidance Beliefs Questionnaire is commonly used to assess the patient's response and accommodations to the pain. Similar tools such as the Pain Anxiety Symptoms Scale (PASS), the Anxiety Sensitivity Profile, and the Fear of Pain Questionnaire attempt to determine how fear and anxiety impact a patient's function.[20,21,31–33]

INSTRUCTIONS

Check only one box in each section which best applies to you. We realize you may consider that two of the statements in any one section relate to you, but please just mark the box which most closely describes your problem.

SECTION I - PAIN INTENSITY

❏ I can tolerate the pain I have without having to use pain killers.
❏ The pain is bad but I can manage without taking pain killers.
❏ Pain killers give complete relief from pain.
❏ Pain killers give moderate relief from pain.
❏ Pain killers give very little relief from pain.
❏ Pain killers have no effect on the pain and I do not use them.

SECTION II - PERSONAL CARE (Washing, Dressing, Etc.)

❏ I can look after myself normally without causing extra pain.
❏ I can look after myself normally but it causes pain.
❏ It is painful to look after myself and I am slow and careful.
❏ I need some help but manage most of my personal care.
❏ I need help every day in most aspects of self care.
❏ I do not get dressed, wash with difficulty and stay in bed.

SECTION III - LIFTING

❏ I can lift heavy weights without extra pain.
❏ I can lift heavy weights but it gives extra pain.
❏ Pain prevents me from lifting heavy weights off the floor, but I can manage if they are conveniently positioned, e.g., on a table.
❏ Pain prevents me from lifting heavy weights, but I can manage light to medium weights if they are conveniently positioned.
❏ I can lift only very light weights.
❏ I cannot lift or carry anything at all.

SECTION IV - WALKING

❏ Pain does not prevent me from walking any distance.
❏ Pain prevents me from walking more than 1 mile.
❏ Pain prevents me from walking more than 1/2 mile.
❏ Pain prevents me from walking more than 1/4 mile.
❏ I can only walk using a stick or crutches.
❏ I am in bed most of the time and have to crawl to the toilet.

SECTION V - SITTING

❏ I can sit in any chair as long as I like.
❏ I can only sit in my favorite chair as long as I like.
❏ Pain prevents me from sitting for more than 1 hour.
❏ Pain prevents me from sitting for more than 30 minutes.
❏ Pain prevents me from sitting for more than 10 minutes.
❏ Pain prevents me from sitting at all.

FIGURE 10-5. The Oswestry Low Back Disability Questionnaire. (Adapted from Fairbank JCT, Davies JB, Couper J, et al. The Oswestry Low Back Pain Disability Questionnaire. Physiotherapy 1980;66:271–273.) *(continued)*

SECTION VI - STANDING

- ❏ I can stand as long as I want without extra pain.
- ❏ I can stand as long as I want but it gives me extra pain.
- ❏ Pain prevents me from standing for more than 1 hour.
- ❏ Pain prevents me from standing for more than 30 minutes.
- ❏ Pain prevents me from standing for more than 10 minutes.
- ❏ Pain prevents me from standing at all.

SECTION VII - SLEEPING

- ❏ Pain does not prevent me from sleeping well.
- ❏ I can sleep well only by using tablets.
- ❏ Even when I take tablets I have less than six hours sleep.
- ❏ Even when I take tablets I have less than four hours sleep.
- ❏ Even when I take tablets I have less than two hours sleep.
- ❏ Pain prevents me from sleeping at all.

SECTION VIII - SEX LIFE

- ❏ My sex life is normal and causes no extra pain.
- ❏ My sex life is normal but causes some extra pain.
- ❏ My sex life is nearly normal but is very painful.
- ❏ My sex life is severely restricted by pain.
- ❏ My sex life is nearly absent because of pain.
- ❏ Pain prevents any sex life at all.

SECTION IX - SOCIAL LIFE

- ❏ My social life is normal and gives me no extra pain.
- ❏ My social life is normal but increases the degree of pain.
- ❏ Pain has no significant effect on my social life apart from limiting my more energetic interests, e.g. dancing, etc.
- ❏ Pain has restricted my social life and I do not go out as often.
- ❏ Pain has restricted my social life to my home.
- ❏ I have no social life because of pain.

SECTION X - TRAVELING

- ❏ I can travel anywhere without extra pain.
- ❏ I can travel anywhere but it gives me extra pain.
- ❏ Pain is bad but I manage journeys over two hours.
- ❏ Pain restricts me to journeys of less than one hour.
- ❏ Pain restricts me to short necessary journeys under 30 minutes.
- ❏ Pain prevents me from traveling except to the doctor or hospital.

FOR OFFICE USE
Total Score

Therapist's Signature and Date	Patient's Signature and Date

FIGURE 10-5. *(continued)*

The literature on fear-anxiety-avoidance models suggests that anxiety and fear are separate cognitive constructs, with fear being a present-oriented emotive state associated with an imminent threat, while anxiety is a more general, future-oriented emotive state existing without an imminent threat.[20] It has been suggested that the pain-related fear is more disabling than the pain itself.[34] While this may be an oversimplification of the problem and true in only a small subsample of patients, the statement highlights the importance that the fear-avoidance-anxiety models have in patients with pain. The fear-avoidance beliefs can impact the transition from acute to chronic pain, and have been studied in patients with low back pain. Heightened focus on pain-related fear during the acute phase increased the risk of future chronic low back pain and disability.[22,28,35] Moreover, people with higher fear-avoidance beliefs who were currently pain-free had a greater risk of future low back pain.[36,37]

Fear-anxiety-avoidance behaviors can have a profound impact on a patient's physical, psychological, and social well-being. Avoidance behaviors are aimed at preventing a situation from occurring.[38] For patients with chronic pain, it is not possible to avoid pain, so these patients tend to avoid activities that they perceive will increase their pain. This may manifest as complete avoidance of some activities or decreased performance of activities. Pain-related fear has been associated with decreased walking speed,[39] decreased muscle performance,[40,41] and decreased physical task performance.[42] Patients may begin to avoid social situations that they fear will increase their pain. This can lead to increasing social isolation and decreased physical activity. The decreased physical activity associated with avoidance behaviors can also lead to further physical decline. Decreased aerobic fitness and decreased trunk mobility and muscle activation patterns have been found in patients with chronic low back pain.[43]

When treating patients with acute or chronic pain, give consideration to all components of pain. Although patients with acute pain may not exhibit all components of the fear-anxiety-avoidance models, researchers and clinicians are attempting to determine which factors in the acute pain situation might predict those patients who will go on to develop chronic pain.[22,26,27,44]

Generic, psychosocial, and disease-specific tools can be administered together to strengthen the information obtained. For example, the SF-36 may be combined with the Oswestry Low Back Disability Questionnaire for individuals with low back pain. A major concern about combination application is the burden placed on the patient who must fill-out a number of questionnaires.

THERAPEUTIC EXERCISE INTERVENTION FOR PAIN

Although many commonalities exist, the approaches to treating acute pain differ from the approaches to chronic pain. Application of acute pain interventions in the case of chronic pain will lead to frustration for the caregiver and the patient. Some combination of exercise and modalities are used; specific choices depend on the patient's circumstances. The treatment program should be tailored to each patient and be responsive to the pain pattern. For example, muscle stretching exercises are advocated for treating patients with myofascial pain resulting from shortening of sarcomeres found with sustained muscle fiber tension. However, resistive exercises are contraindicated in the early phases because of the early fatigue and lengthy recovery in muscle with active trigger points.[45]

Like many other medical conditions, the science of caring for people with acute or chronic pain is constantly growing. Clinicians must be aware of new research and literature that can provide strong evidence for interventions chosen. The American College of Occupational and Environmental Medicine regularly revises its recommendations for the treatment of various work-related disorders and includes a chapter on chronic pain (www.acoe.org). Progressive resistive exercise programs are the cornerstone of intervention programs for workers with chronic pain.

Acute Pain

The typical patient with acute pain has recently sustained an injury or undergone a surgical procedure. The pain is related to the acute trauma of an initial injury or an exacerbation of a preexisting injury. Pain medication may be taken for a short time after the injury or surgery. Acute pain is expected to resolve substantially over the course of a few days. Although some residual pain may continue for weeks after the injury or surgery, most pain is expected to resolve with only minimal discomfort remaining.

Acute pain of this type is treated with a combination of medication (i.e., prescription or over-the-counter drugs at the patient's discretion), gentle exercise, and ice. Ice is preferred over heat in the first 24 hours, and may be changed to heat thereafter depending upon the injury acuity and patient preference. Exercise is prescribed based on the specific injury or surgery and is directed at restoring the motion, strength, and function of the injured body part. Rehabilitation of the injured area is the prime focus and provides the framework for exercise prescription. Exercise in this phase is directed toward the primary joint and at prevention of injury at adjacent joints because of compensation. The clinician should include patient education about pain-relieving postures and skills to fulfill the activities of daily living and the instrumental activities of daily living (see Patient-Related Instruction 10-1: Management of Acute Pain). See Building Block 10-2.

Patient-Related Instruction 10-1

Management of Acute Pain

An increase in acute pain is a sign of doing too much. This may disrupt the healing process. In this situation, you should do the following:

1. Find a position of comfort that decreases or eliminates your pain. Your clinician can help you learn what these positions are.
2. Use a pain-relieving treatment such as ice for 10 to 15 minutes every hour.
3. Use an assistive device such as crutches, a cane, or a walker if your leg is involved, a sling or splint for your upper extremity, or a corset for your back. These devices reduce the stress on the injured area.
4. Take your medications as prescribed.

Chronic Pain

Treatment of chronic pain requires a team approach because of the multidimensional nature of the pain. Chronic pain is disabling and interferes with all aspects of the person's life. The clinician must work closely with the physician, psychologist, vocational counselor, alternative health-care providers, and the patient. In this way, a comprehensive treatment program can be established to ensure all aspects of the pain are being addressed. Therapeutic exercise is a major component of the treatment plan,[46–48] and has been shown to be effective in improving impairments and activity limitations in patients with chronic pain.[49–54] Different types of therapeutic exercise programs, including those focused on strength training, aerobic conditioning or flexibility appear to be successful in improving patient symptoms. Many adjunctive treatments and alternative therapies are often explored by the patient.[19,55] Herbal remedies, acupuncture, reflexology, and other therapies are often part of a patient's complete treatment program. An open dialogue with the patient ensures a thorough understanding of all therapies occurring simultaneously.

A critical component of chronic pain treatment is a realistic understanding of the goals of the treatment plan. Patient education is a key component; the clinician explains the likely source of pain, activity modifications or postures to minimize pain, and the expected outcomes of intervention. Ultimately, the goal is a return to the highest level of function while managing the pain.

Interventions to inhibit pain input or to facilitate non-nociceptive input are incorporated while simultaneously addressing associated impairments and activity limitations. Therapeutic exercise is used to affect the pain directly through endogenous opiates and indirectly through facilitation of non-nociceptive input and to treat the associated impairments and activity limitations. Exercises chosen may have very different goals. Exercise may be uncomfortable for the individual with chronic pain, and this discomfort may be necessary to achieve pain inhibition through endogenous opiates. This type of intervention requires extensive education regarding the purpose of the exercise and alternative options. It is essential to ensure communication and program adherence.

The goals of the therapeutic exercise program extend beyond treatment of impairments. Activity limitations and participation restrictions related to depression, sleep, and appetite are also of concern. Improvements in sleep patterns, mental state, and appetite may be the first markers of successful intervention, improving before any change in impairment measures (see Patient-Related Instruction 10-2: Why You Should Exercise When You Have Chronic Pain). See Building Block 10-3.

When designing the therapeutic exercise program, consider the current physical and psychologic status of the patient and take into account potential secondary problems

that must be prevented.[45] Direct the therapeutic exercise program toward the source of the pain, musculoskeletal impairments, or activity limitations and toward any secondary preventable problems identified during the evaluation process. Identify the elements of the movement system involved in the production of pain in order to facilitate prioritization of interventions.

Activity and Mode

The activity chosen to treat the individual with chronic pain depends on the source of the pain and results of the evaluation process. In addition to the specific interventions chosen to treat the source of the pain, other activities can help the patient.

The patient with chronic low back pain resulting from a herniated disk should receive treatment specific to the impairments and activity limitations associated with that injury, and several adjunctive measures can be used to treat the associated pain. Patients with chronic low back pain who were randomly assigned to active rehabilitation

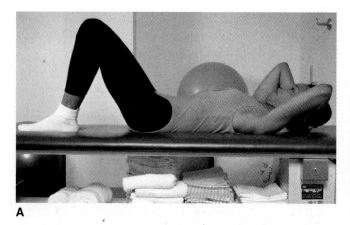

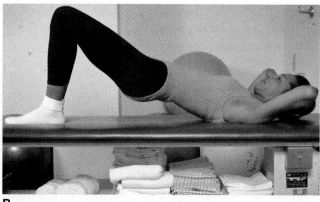

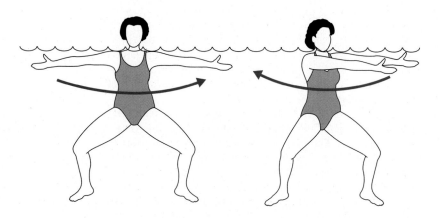

FIGURE 10-6. (A) A pelvic tilt exercise is a simple exercise for treating chronic low back pain. (B) Bridging is an advanced exercise for strengthening the abdominal and gluteal muscles. (C) Knee-to-chest stretching complements hip and low back strengthening.

compared with passive (massage and heat) treatment had significantly improved back pain intensity, functional disability, and lumbar endurance measured at a 1-year follow-up.[56] Individuals in pain, particularly those with chronic pain, are susceptible to changes in posture and movement patterns. These changes can perpetuate the original symptoms or cause secondary impairments or activity limitations. Regardless of the activity chosen, the therapeutic focus should be on awareness and use of proper posture and movement patterns.

Movement therapies such as Feldenkrais are helpful in restoring appropriate movement patterns. Total-body movement patterns are often more successful than isolated joint movement when treating individuals with chronic pain. Rhythmic activity of large muscle groups should be the activity of choice (Fig. 10-6). For those with mobility restrictions and pain due to

weightbearing Ai Chi exercise can be particularly useful. These activities should be balanced with specific exercises to address the impairments and activity limitations (Fig. 10-7).

Diagonal patterns used in proprioceptive neuromuscular facilitation (PNF) techniques (see Chapter 15) are useful for teaching the patient position and posture awareness while still using multisegmental movement. In addition to assisting in movement awareness, PNF patterns can increase mobility and muscle performance. These patterns can ensure proper muscle recruitment during movement. Substitution patterns often are difficult to observe but are easily palpated during PNF exercises. The posture and movements chosen for PNF should address the specific impairments and activity limitations determined during the evaluation. Bilateral, symmetric patterns are particularly helpful when one side is involved and needs retraining through the uninvolved side.

FIGURE 10-7. Ai Chi exercise as a form of mobility and strength exercise.

SELF-MANAGEMENT 10-1 *Proprioceptive Neuromuscular Facilitation Postural Technique*

Purpose: To improve postural control while moving the arms and sitting on an unstable surface

Position: Sitting on a therapeutic ball, with both feet flat on the floor, grasp wrist or a resistive band with both hands over one shoulder (Fig. A).

Movement technique: Level 1: Keeping your arms straight, and rotate your trunk and shoulders down past your opposite hip (Figs. B and C).

Level 2: Increase the resistance.

Level 3: Perform with one foot off the floor.

Dosage
Repetitions: _____
Frequency: _____

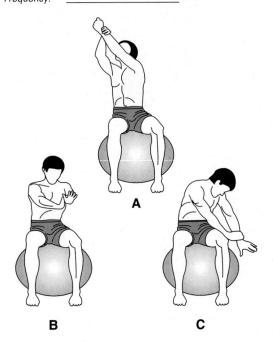

SELF-MANAGEMENT 10-2 *Supine Kicking with Optional Arm Movements*

Purpose: To increase strength and endurance of the neck, trunk, hip, and leg extensor muscles and to increase cardiovascular endurance

Position: Supine with arms in a comfortable position overhead or at the side

Movement technique: Level 1: Rhythmic, repetitive kicking, keeping knees relatively straight. and kicking from the hips; large or small fins may be used.

Level 2: Add arm movements in an underwater backstroke pattern. Bring arms up along the sides of your body to the shoulders, extend them straight out to the sides, then pull back down toward your sides.

Dosage
Repetitions: _____
Frequency: _____

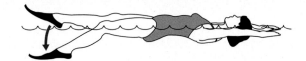

SELF-MANAGEMENT 10-3 *Jumping Jacks*

Purpose: Increase strength in shoulder and hip abductor muscles, initiate gentle impact, and initiate exercise using large muscle groups

Position: Start in chest-deep water, with feet together and arms at sides.

Movement technique: Bring both feet out to the sides while simultaneously bringing arms out to the side. Return to the starting position.

Dosage
Repetitions: _____
Frequency: _____

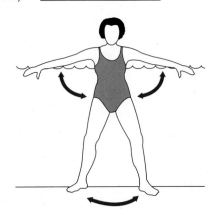

Bilateral patterns that emphasize trunk flexion and extension or rotation and sidebending are effective for normalizing specific movement patterns. The upper extremity diagonal patterns can be performed in a variety of postures and positions, depending on the patient's needs. Upper and lower extremity patterns can be combined for total-body movement patterns. These same patterns can be performed in a pool (see Self-Management 10-1: Proprioceptive Neuromuscular Facilitation Postural Technique).

Aerobic exercise is effective for treating chronic pain and is frequently recommended in the treatment of conditions such as fibromyalgia. The pool can be used for aerobic exercise, although consideration must be given to the water's resistance (see Self-Management 10-2: Supine Kicking With Optional Arm Movements and 10-3: Jumping Jacks). This resistance can produce muscle fatigue before reaching aerobic exercise

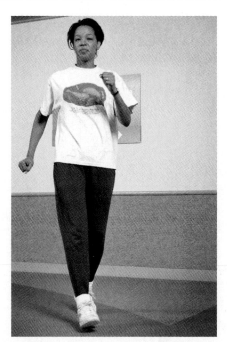

FIGURE 10-8. Walking on a track is a simple, continuous aerobic exercise available to most patients.

levels. Walking is a simple form of continuous exercise that can be performed by many persons (Fig. 10-8). Walking is particularly effective because it can be performed for several short bouts several times each day. A stationary bicycle such as a recumbent bike is also an effective tool, although less available. Other exercises enjoyed by the individual, such as aerobic dance, recreational dance, or traditional lap swimming, should be incorporated.

Activities such as yoga, Tai Chi, Ai Chi, or using a therapeutic ball allow a variety of large muscle group activities to be carried out while increasing posture awareness (Fig. 10-9). Many of these activities are done in a group setting or individually at home, providing flexibility to suit the needs of each patient (see Self-Management 10-4: Yoga Exercise). Group treatment of patients with fibromyalgia resulted in improved function and decreased tender points.[57]

The pool is a useful tool in the application of therapeutic exercise for those with chronic pain (see Chapter 16). The advantages include unweighting from the buoyancy and the warmth and contact of the water on the skin. Unweighting the sore limb or painful back allows movement with less pain and provides the opportunity for correct posture and movement patterns during activity or stretching (Fig. 10-10; see Self-Management 10-5: Hip External Rotation Stretch, 10-6: Deep Water March With Barbell, and 10-7: Elbow Flexion Extension). Movements that are too painful to perform on land are performed with greater ease and less pain in the water (Fig. 10-11). The water's warmth and skin contact may function to close the gate to pain at the spinal cord level. A disadvantage of pool use in treating chronic pain is the difficulty in determining proper muscle recruitment and movement patterns. The water's refraction causes distortion, and the clinician cannot observe movement and posture. Actual palpation and tactile cuing in the pool can overcome this problem. A second disadvantage for some individuals with conditions such as fibromyalgia or myofascial pain syndrome is the water's resistance. The viscosity of water provides enough resistance to exacerbate some chronic pain conditions. Choose positions and movement patterns to minimize resistance caused by turbulence (i.e., controlling the speed of movement) and viscosity (i.e., minimizing the

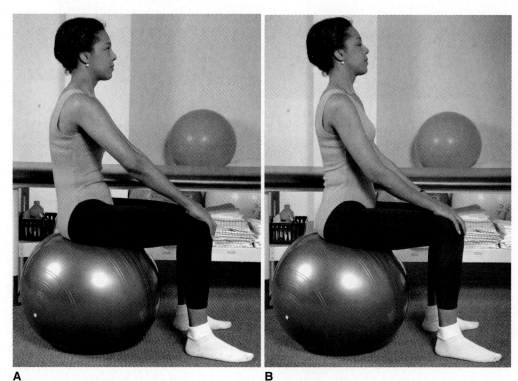

A **B**

FIGURE 10-9. Therapeutic ball exercises such as pelvic rocking can be performed at home and in the clinic. (A) Start position. (B) End position.

SELF-MANAGEMENT 10-4 *Yoga Exercise*

Purpose: To promote relaxation and pain relief and to increase mobility in the low back and hips

Position: Lying supine, with legs elevated on the wall (Fig. A).

Movement technique: Let the knees and hips bend, sliding the leg down the wall to a comfortable position (Fig. B). Hold 10 to 15 seconds, and return to the starting position.

Dosage
Repetitions: _____
Frequency: _____

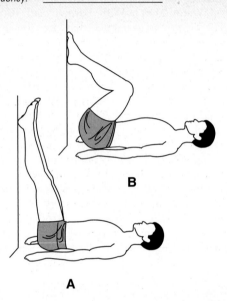

SELF-MANAGEMENT 10-5 *Hip External Rotation Stretch*

Purpose: To increase mobility of the hips

Position: While facing the ladder, set the foot of the hip to be stretched on a step of the ladder. Slide the foot across to the edge of the step. Keeping your foot there, let your knee roll out. Hold for 10 to 15 seconds.

Movement technique: Level 1: Assume the position described above until you feel a gentle stretch in your hip.

Level 2: Assume the position described above until you feel a gentle stretch in your hip. Use your hands to push your knee farther into rotation.

Dosage
Repetitions: _____
Frequency: _____

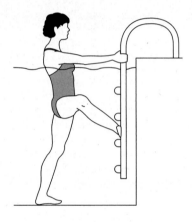

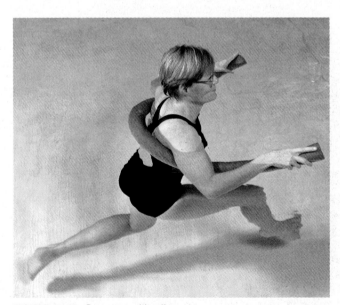

FIGURE 10-10. Deep water bicycling.

surface area; see Self-Management 10-8: Water Walking, Forward and Sideways). Dosing the therapeutic exercise in this situation can be challenging.

Dosage

As with the activity chosen, the dosage depends on the specific component of the movement system being treated and the purpose of the exercise, but some generalities about exercise and pain should be considered. The exercise dosage should not increase the pain. The chosen speed, repetitions, intensity, and duration should not increase pain within the exercise session, nor should symptoms increase after exercise.

If using aquatics as the exercise medium, the water's resistance can be a concern. Keep the first session brief (5 to 7 minutes) to assess the response to this intervention. As tolerance is demonstrated, the intensity or the duration may be increased (see Patient-Related Instruction 10-3: How Often and Hard Should You Exercise With Chronic Pain). The overarching goal is to increase the total volume of exercise (see Chapter 1). Initially, exercise volume might remain stable, while variables within the total volume (i.e., sequence,

SELF-MANAGEMENT 10-6 *Deep Water March with Barbell*

Purpose: To increase mobility through the low back, hips, and knees

Position: In water depth equal to your height or deeper, use a barbell or other buoyant equipment to support yourself.

Movement technique: Level 1: March in place through a comfortable range of motion at a comfortable speed.

Level 2: Add buoyant equipment to feet and ankles, increase the speed of marching, or do both.

Dosage

Repetitions: _____

Frequency: _____

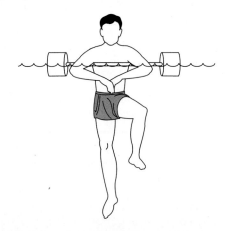

SELF-MANAGEMENT 10-7 *Elbow Flexion Extension*

Purpose: To increase mobility in the elbows, increase muscle strength and endurance in the upper extremities, and increase trunk stability

Position: Standing in shoulder-deep water, with your feet in a comfortable stance and arms at the sides

Movement technique: Level 1: Flex and extend the elbows with thumbs pointing up.

Level 2: Turn your palms up.

Level 3: Add gloves or other resistive equipment.

Dosage

Repetitions: _____

Frequency: _____

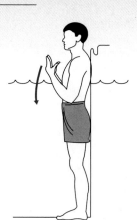

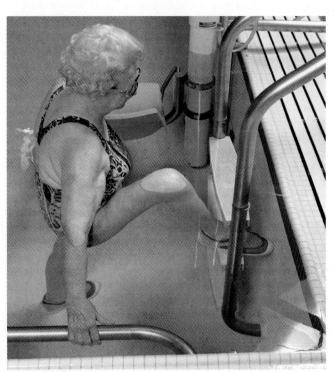

FIGURE 10-11. Knee-to-chest stretching can also be performed comfortably in the pool.

contraction type, etc.) are changed. When the optimum combination of variables is achieved, exercise volume can be slowly expanded. See Building Block 10-4.

The frequency is determined by the activity type and purpose and by the quantity of exercise performed before pain is experienced. For example, if only a few repetitions of activity at a low intensity for a short duration can be performed before experiencing pain, the exercises may be performed with greater frequency. Availability also affects frequency. A pool may not be available more than once each day or even less often. The frequency must be balanced against the intensity and duration of an activity. Some exercise should be performed daily, and matching a land-based exercise program to complement the pool program is necessary.

After the pain-free dosage is determined, progress the exercise parameters to those best suited to treat the patient's underlying pathology, impairment, or functional limitation. Advance the activity to a functional progression aimed at returning to previous activity levels.

ADJUNCTIVE AGENTS

Adjunctive agents are essential in the treatment of pain. In the case of chronic pain, more agents are used. The disabling nature of chronic pain leads individuals to seek out any

SELF-MANAGEMENT 10-8 *WaterWalking, Forward and Sideways*

Purpose: To increase mobility throughout the trunk, arms, and legs; increase trunk stability; and increase muscular strength and endurance in the arms, legs, and trunk

Position: Stand in water between waist and shoulder deep; deep water provides more resistance to walking.

Movement technique: Level 1: Step sideways, raising your arms out to the sides as you step and bringing back down to the sides as you bring your feet together.

Level 2: Walk forward with the opposite arm and leg reaching forward together. Be sure to walk normally using a heel-to-toe pattern.

Level 3: Add resistance gloves to hands.

Dosage
Repetitions: _____
Frequency: _____

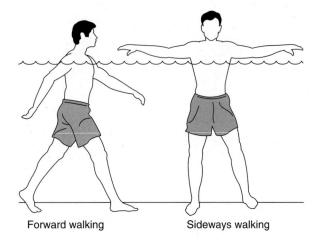

Forward walking   Sideways walking

other potentially pain-relieving therapy such as medications, chiropractic, massage therapy, relaxation techniques, acupuncture, biofeedback, and psychologic care.[45] Acupuncture, herbal remedies, dietary changes, and a host of other therapies may be employed. In particular, real acupuncture has proven better than sham acupuncture for relieving pain, improving global ratings, and decreasing morning stiffness.[45] It has been recommended as an adjunctive treatment in the management of fibromyalgia, chronic low back pain, myofascial pain, and osteoarthritis. Continuous communication with the patient ensures optimal team treatment and avoids conflicting interventions. Remain open-minded and supportive as the patient searches for solutions to his or her pain.

Transcutaneous Electrical Nerve Stimulation

TENS has been proven useful in the treatment of some types of pain.[58] Stimulation of the posterior tibial nerve and sciatic nerve was performed to see the effect on WDR neurons in the spinal cord. Results showed that electrical stimulation of peripheral nerves lead to inhibitory input to the pain pathways

Patient-Related Instruction 10-3

How Often and Hard Should You Exercise With Chronic Pain

1. Ideally, you should do something every day, at least once per day. Your clinician can give you further guidelines.
2. Many people do well by performing several short bouts of exercise spread throughout the day. These sessions may be only 5 to 10 minutes long.
3. Any aerobic activity should be continuous, working up to 10 to 20 minutes over time.
4. Stretches should be intense enough to feel a gentle pulling sensation.
5. Other exercises should be performed slowly until slight fatigue is felt or as otherwise instructed by your clinician.
6. If you feel any sharp, stabbing pain or numbness or tingling as a result of the exercise, discontinue the exercise. Use your pain-relieving measures, and tell your clinician.
7. You may feel some discomfort during or for a short time after exercise. This discomfort should not be confused with the pain that brought you to the clinic. Avoid exercises that increase this pain, but you may continue to exercise with some of the discomfort.
8. Ask your clinician if you are unsure about what to feel with your exercise program.

at the spinal cord.[59] One mechanism of pain relief with the application of an electric current is based on the gate theory of pain. Application of TENS selectively activates large A-alpha and A-beta fibers, which are stimulated at lower thresholds than the smaller C fibers. These impulses travel to the dorsal horn of the spinal cord, where facilitation of the small interneurons of the substantia gelatinosa inhibit pain transmission through presynaptic inhibition. Activation of these large-diameter fibers closes the gate to small-diameter fiber transmission.

Other theories suggest that TENS may function through antidromic (i.e., conducting impulses in a direction opposite to normal) stimulation of afferent neurons. Antidromic stimulation may decrease pain by blocking the nociceptive input to the spinal cord, and it may stimulate release of substance P, resulting in vasodilation. Vasodilation can decrease pain by increasing local circulation, which removes metabolic waste products and supplies oxygenated blood for healing. The increased local circulation may decrease local ischemia enough to decrease pain.[11]

BUILDING BLOCK 10-4

The patient in Building Block 10-3 has been performing a therapeutic aquatic exercise program of slow speed single plane shoulder movements, single plane hip movements, walking, and abdominal muscle isometrics. She exercises for 30 to 40 minutes and is tired at the end of the program, but has no increase in pain. She is doing the exercise program 4 days per week. How might her program be progressed?

TENS may effect the opiate pain-modulating system. Ascending projections from small-fiber afferents reach the PAG, which is rich with opiates. The PAG provides descending input to the dorsal horn, which probably is opiate-mediated. TENS may provide some analgesia through opiate-mediated activation of the brain stem.

The parameters for TENS application are varied. Consult any appropriate textbook for discussion of the benefits of different parameter settings.

Heat

Heat is commonly used as a primary or adjunctive agent to decrease pain. Trauma can produce a pain-spasm cycle that activates nociceptors. The nociceptors detect pain that produces reflex muscle activity that, if prolonged, results in muscle ischemia. The ischemia excites muscle nociceptors that perpetuate the muscle spasm. Chemical release at the time of injury or resulting from inflammation can also stimulate nociceptors. Vasoconstriction associated with a sympathetic response or vasoconstriction resulting from muscle spasm can produce pain. The application of heat can decrease pain from any of these sources.

According to the gate theory, heat application can decrease pain directly. Thermal sensations are carried to the dorsal horn of the spinal cord through large-diameter myelinated fibers. These impulses can close the gate, blocking the transmission of pain impulses through small-diameter fibers. The thermal sensations are transmitted to conscious levels preferentially over pain sensations. The increased circulation resulting from heat application decreases pain through two mechanisms. First, pain resulting from ischemia decreases as the local circulation is increased. The increased circulation may break the pain-spasm cycle as pain decreases and the muscle is provided with oxygenated blood. Second, the increased circulation may remove noxious chemicals associated with injury or inflammation, thereby decreasing pain.

Superficial heat in the form of hot packs is commonly used in the clinic and home to decrease pain and as a precursor to therapeutic exercise. Local heat application increases the extensibility of tissue, preparing it for subsequent exercise. Immersion in a warm pool or whirlpool can also decrease pain, although the water temperature is significantly lower than that of a hot pack because of the size of the area heated. The warmth and buoyancy effects of the water combine to decrease pain sensation. Ultrasound or diathermy can increase the heat's depth of penetration. Any of these modalities can provide valuable assistance in the reduction of pain.

Cold

Cold treatments are commonly used to decrease pain. Cold decreases pain through some of the same mechanisms as heat. Cold sensation is carried to the dorsal horn of the spinal cord through large-diameter afferent fibers and is capable of closing the gate to pain signals through smaller-diameter fibers. The drop in tissue temperature blocks synaptic transmission of any input, rendering the gate inactive. The decrease in pain may help to break the pain-spasm cycle. In acute injury, the vasoconstriction produced by cold may prevent edema that produces pain. Because the application of cold is somewhat noxious, the afferent input to the brain stem through the PAG could cause the release of endorphins at the spinal level; the decrease in pain would be modulated by higher centers.

Cold usually is applied by means of ice in the form of packs, bags, or ice massage. The length of application depends on the size of the area to be cooled, the area of the body to be cooled, the mode of application, local circulation, and patient sensitivity.

Medication

Drug therapy is commonly prescribed for individuals with acute or chronic pain. Many medications are available and act through different mechanisms and at different sites to relieve pain. Medications are administered orally, by intramuscular injection, by injection into other structures, or by intravenous infusion. The dosage necessary to produce analgesia varies among individuals and for various medications.

Acting peripherally, NSAIDs are commonly prescribed. Several chemical classes exist, all of which inhibit the synthesis or release of prostaglandins.[60] Analgesia generally occurs within 24 hours of NSAID administration, and antiinflammatory responses occur with continued administration. The major side effect of NSAIDs is gastrointestinal upset. Many NSAIDs are enteric-coated and long acting, decreasing the frequency of administration. Local injections of anesthetic agents can provide relief from pain in localized areas. Trigger-point injections with an anesthetic agent are commonly performed in individuals with chronic pain, particularly pain arising from myofascial tissues. Recently, botulinum toxin type A has been effective in reducing pain as measured by VAS, palpable muscle firmness, and pressure pain thresholds when compared with saline (placebo) injections.[45]

Cyclooxygenase (COX)-selective drugs are another classification of nonopioid analgesic medications. The COX-2 selective drugs (e.g., celecoxib, rofecoxib) work by inhibiting the synthesis of prostaglandins. These medications may decrease pain and inflammation with less gastric irritation.

At the spinal cord and higher levels, a variety of medications can be administered. When treating centrally-mediated pain, the preferred first line of medications includes the tricyclic antidepressants, serotonin-selective reuptake inhibitors (SSRIs) and the anticonvulsive medications, gabapentin and pregabalin. Antidepressant medications have analgesic effects, and administration may relieve pain at levels below those necessary to achieve antidepressant effects. These medications may be used at levels that have analgesic and antidepressant benefits. SSRIs typically cause less cardiovascular or anticholinergic side effects than tricyclics.[61] Side effects of the SSRIs include headache, nausean tinnitus, insomnia, and nervousness. Tricyclic antidepressants also have significant side effects, including orthostatic hypotension, potentially predisposing patients to falling. The tricyclics also have significant impact on the cardiovascular system, including altered heart rate, rhythm, and contractility, particularly in patients with existing cardiac disease.[61] Therefore, SSRIs are generally preferred to tricyclics in patients with known cardiac disease.

Anticonvulsive medications such as Gapabentin are used to treat neuropathic pain. Pregabalin has also been successfully used to treat neuropathic pain.[62] A recent study showed that the use of pregabalin (Lyrica) was cost neutral compared to "usual care" and resulted in a small but significant increase in the quality of life in patients with peripheral neuropathic pain.[63] Other medications such as muscle relaxants like the benzodiazepines also act as analgesics. Moreover, they help patients relax and sleep, which significantly improves their quality of life.

Narcotics acting at opioid receptors are also used to treat pain. Side effects of opioids include postural hypotension, sedation, and confusion. These effects may lead to a risk of falls, which should be considered in any rehabilitation program. Morphine and other strong narcotics are commonly used to relieve end-of-life pain and cancer pain. Bennett[5] suggests that opiates are the most effective medications for managing chronic pain and should not be withheld because of fear of addiction. Addiction is the use of medication for its mind-altering properties with manipulation of the medical system to acquire them. This is very different from the physical dependence seen in patients who need these medications to obtain pain relief.

Some patients receive inadequate pain control from traditional administration methods because of individual differences in absorption and metabolism of drugs or because of fluctuating plasma levels of the drugs or their metabolites. In this situation, patient-controlled analgesia (PCA) may be indicated. The PCA system infuses a drug in a desired location on demand or at a continuous rate.[64] Opioid analgesic drugs such as morphine, meperidine, and hydromorphone are commonly used.[64] In an on-demand system, a small button on the PCA system releases a preset dose of medication. The constant-rate infusion delivers a small but continuous dose to maintain steady plasma levels of the analgesic. A variety of safety features (i.e., the pump is programmed to prevent an overdose) are included in the system. Chronic pain from cancer, surgery, or labor and delivery is a common reason for the use of PCA.

FIBROMYALGIA AND CHRONIC FATIGUE SYNDROME

Significant impairments exist in patients with fibromyalgia syndrome (FMS), including widespread pain,[65] decreased joint range of motion,[66] and impaired respiratory[67] and cardiovascular status.[57] Patients frequently decrease work hours and change tasks[68–70] and they develop significant conflicts about life roles.[71] Twenty-five percent of patients with CFS are bedridden or unable to work.[72] These disabilities have negative economic and quality of life effects. Patients with FMS and CFS are being seen increasingly in the physical therapy clinic because carefully prescribed exercise has been shown to be of value in improved aerobic performance, tender point pain, well-being, pain levels, and self-efficacy.[73–79] Unfortunately, these conditions are poorly understood by the public and many health professionals. An understanding of the problems these patients encounter will provide a basis for a solid rehabilitation program.

Fibromyalgia Syndrome

The cause of fibromyalgia is uncertain. FMS is characterized by widespread body pain (in all four quadrants and the axial skeleton) and tenderness, fatigue, and morning stiffness.[1] These patients are highly sensitive to both painful and nonpainful stimuli, including touch, temperature, chemical, light, sounds, and smells.[80] FMS tends predominately to affect females (80% to 90% of patients). Patients typically are between 20 and 60 years of age,[81] though there have been

reports of children being affected.[82,83] The prevalence of fibromyalgia is about 2% of the general population, affecting approximately 5 million adults in 2005.[84] Persons with FMS are estimated to compose about 7% of the patients seen in general medical practices and up to 20% of the patients in general rheumatology practices.[81,85] Patients with fribromyalgia account for nearly 2.2 million ambulatory care visits at a total annual cost of approximately $6,000 per person.[86,87] Fibromyalgia has a significant impact on quality of life, with these patients scoring the lowest on 7 of 8 subscales of the SF-36 compared to patients with other chronic diseases, and having a 3.4 times greater likelihood of being diagnosed with major depression compared with age-matched peers without fibromyalgia.[88–90]

Etiology

One of the characteristics of FMS is the absence of consistent, positive laboratory findings.[65] Because its symptoms mimic those of other diseases (e.g., rheumatic diseases, multiple sclerosis, malignancies, hypothyroidism, anemia), a thorough medical evaluation is necessary to exclude other possible causes of the presenting complaints.[91] Onset of FMS can be insidious; it may occur after a viral infection[92–94] or trauma.[93–95] It also may be related to stress[96]; sleep disruption such as occurs in sleep apnea, sleep myoclonus, and alpha-delta sleep[97,98]; or be related to CNS mechanisms.[99] Increased excitability of spinal cord neurons after an injury, increased receptive field size of the neurons and reductions in pain threshold are examples of central sensitization.[80] It seems likely that multiple factors contribute over time until a threshold is reached such that a final event appears to be the precipitating factor.[100]

Many researchers have attempted to identify the causative factors of FMS, but the pathomechanics remain elusive. Historical references to FMS-like symptoms are found as far back as Hippocrates.[101,102] Straus[102] cites the treatise of an 18th century physician who describes such a disorder found predominately "among women... who are sedentary and studious," and that he felt was "precipitated by antecedent causes including grief and intense thoughts." In the 1800s and early 1900s, muscle inflammation (giving rise to the term *fibrositis*) was considered a cause. The term fibrositis has generally been disregarded based on the lack of histologic evidence of inflammation in the muscles of patients with FMS.[103,104] Later research on the possible causes of FMS has focused on peripheral (muscle physiology) and central (CNS function) phenomena.

Peripheral Origin   Aggressive exercise is not well tolerated by patients with FMS and often results in increased perception of pain and fatigue.[105–108] Muscle adaptation to decreased activity has been hypothesized to be at least partially responsible for the adverse reaction to overexertion, and muscle morphology and physiology in patients with FMS have been investigated.[109] No muscle morphologic changes specific to FMS have been found, but the muscles of patients with FMS have the appearance of inflammatory infiltrates, muscle pH changes related to ischemia, reduced oxidative capacity, and fiber changes.[80,104] In a very few muscle samples, evidence suggesting a mitochondrial disorder and possibly microcirculation compromise was documented, but these changes were not widespread in the muscle.[103,110–112] Neither muscle energy metabolism[113,114] nor enzyme levels[106] vary from those of controls, though a recent study showed decreased use of phosphorous metabolites at maximal work levels.[115] Reports of decreased exercise-induced muscle blood flow in patients with FMS[116] were not, however, accompanied by the expected decrease in capillary density that this finding suggested.[111] It is not clear whether localized metabolic or morphologic changes in muscle can account for the pain and fatigue associated with FMS. Peripheral changes may contribute to increased pain signals to the spinal cord, contributing to windup and central sensitization.[80] Even low levels of nociceptive input from the periphery can maintain the central sensitization.

Epidural blockade does reduce FMS tender points,[117] and there is evidence of increased nociceptor reactivity in patients with FMS,[118] which suggests that the pain may be of peripheral origin. Muscles of patients with FMS do not show a drop in surface electromyographic activity during short pauses between muscle contractions, which may be a response to perceived pain and fatigue.[119] Studies found that patients with FMS or CFS do not sustain repeated muscle contractions at the same intensity as controls.[120–122] Other studies show that they do.[123–124] However, when electrical stimulation of muscles accompanied repeated contractions, the contraction intensity and duration matched those of controls.[125] This finding suggests that the muscle itself is capable of normal work but that there may be a central mechanism limiting that work by producing symptoms of FMS and CFS, which the patient interprets as pain and fatigue.

Central Nervous System Origin Pain modulation may be disrupted in FMS at the spinal cord level or in higher CNS centers. Imaging studies are being utilized to obtain more information about the role of the brain in this disorder, as well as brain changes in response to interventions.[126] Although endorphin levels have been found to be normal,[127,128] lowered levels of serum tryptophan[129] and elevated levels of substance P[130] may amplify pain perception. Blunting of the hypothalamic-pituitary axis to stressors may also be a factor.[80]

Pituitary hormone secretion changes have been found in patients with FMS.[131–133] Growth hormone is adversely affected by sleep deprivation.[134] The production of an FMS-like state in healthy volunteers through alpha-delta sleep induction[135] may point to a role for abnormal growth hormone secretion in FMS symptom production.[111]

Another hypothesis in which CNS regulation is proposed to be aberrant suggests that the level where control is lost is the limbic system. This area affects sensory gating and processing of sensory input.[136] Autonomic nervous system dysfunction has also been suggested by the results of several studies.[106,137] An inverse relationship between sympathetic reactivity and pain sensitivity has been found. Stress and anxiety associated with FMS would be expected to increase sympathetic tone, but the expected commensurate increase in plasma and urinary catecholamines were not found.[138] A lowered level of sympathetic activation has been postulated, and may be a source of increased pain sensitivity in patients with FMS.[139]

Like other patients with chronic pain, central sensitization and temporal summation of pain, or "windup" occurs in patients with FMS.[80] The pain symptoms most frequently described by patients with chronic pain are those of a dull, aching, or burning pain, the symptoms transmitted by the unmyelinated C-fibers. When this type of pain is evoked, the perceived pain is greater for patients with FMS than for

controls, suggesting central sensitization in these patients.[80] In addition to windup, these patients experience expanding receptive field areas and spinal neurons taking on the properties of WDR neurons. Fibers that previously had no association with pain stimuli now begin transmitting pain, furthering the central sensitization phenomenon.[80]

The role of psychiatric and behavioral disorders in FMS is controversial. In one study, 20% to 40% of people with FMS in a tertiary care center were found to have current mood disorders and a lifetime incidence ranging from 40% to 70%. However this was felt to reflect health-care-seeking behavior in that population because lower lifetime incidences are noted to occur in patients with FMS in the general population.[100]

There may be a genetic predisposition to FMS because first-degree relatives of patients with FMS have a higher than expected frequency of FMS. It has been proposed[140,141] that FMS can occur with exposure of genetically susceptible individuals to any one or a combination of the triggers associated with FMS onset.[81–83,91,126]

The variety of triggers and variety of symptom, some of which predominate over others for given individuals, suggest there may be subgroups of patients with FMS. It may be that treatment must be tailored to individual patients.[142,143]

Signs and Symptoms

FMS is a chronic condition in which symptoms wax and wane but are typically unrelenting. In addition to pain and fatigue, this population experiences lowered respiratory function,[67] joint range, and muscle endurance and has strength impairments[57,144] and below average cardiovascular fitness levels.[57] FMS is listed in the American College of Rheumatology (ACR) classification of rheumatic disease as an extra-articular disorder. In a multicenter study,[65] which established the 1990 ACR criteria for definition of FMS, the most common symptoms of patients with FMS were fatigue, sleep disturbance, and morning stiffness (73% to 85% of patients). Pain all over, paresthesia, headache, and anxiety affected 45% to 69% of patients. Less common, but still significantly more frequent than in controls, were findings of irritable bowel syndrome, sicca syndrome (i.e., dry eyes and mouth), and Raynaud phenomenon (<35%). In this same study, factors found to affect the musculoskeletal symptoms of patients with FMS included cold, poor sleep, anxiety, humidity, stress, fatigue, weather changes, and warmth, as they did to a lesser degree in control subjects. These are still the accepted guidelines for the classification of fibromyalgia.[84]

The diagnostic criteria for FMS were developed from this study (Display 10-2). The diagnosis is based on finding at least 11 of 18 tender points (Fig. 10-12) in the presence of widespread pain (i.e., pain in all four quadrants of the body, including at least part of the axial skeleton) persisting for at least 3 months' duration. Tender points were defined as anatomically discrete and reproducible areas of heightened pain perception in patients with FMS. Diagnosis may also be made when the full 11 of 18 tender points are not present but other features commonly found in the study are.[100]

Activity Limitations

Several studies have examined the effect of FMS on everyday life. Fifty-five percent of working patients were found to have changed work tasks and to work shorter hours than before the illness. Motor tasks were reported as being more difficult

DISPLAY 10-2
Classification of Fibromyalgia*

1. **History of widespread pain.**
Definition: Pain is considered widespread when all of the following are present: pain in the left side of the body, pain in the right side of the body, pain above the waist, and pain below the waist. In addition, axial skeletal pain (cervical spine or anterior chest or thoracic spine or low back) must be present. In this definition, shoulder and buttock pain is considered as pain for each involved side. Low back pain is considered lower segment pain.
2. **Pain in 11 of 18 tender point sites on digital palpation.**
Definition: Pain on digital palpation must be present in at least 11 of the following 18 tender point sites:
Occiput: bilateral, at the suboccipital muscle insertions
Low cervical: bilateral, at the anterior aspects of the intertransverse spaces at C5–7
Trapezius: bilateral, at the midpoint of the upper border
Supraspinatus: bilateral, at origins, above the scapula spine near the medial border
Second rib: bilateral, at the second costochondral junction, just lateral to the junctions on upper surfaces
Lateral epicondyle: bilateral, 2 cm distal to the epicondyles
Gluteal: bilateral, in upper outer quadrants of buttocks in the anterior fold of muscle
Greater trochanter: bilateral, posterior to the trochanteric prominence
Knee: bilateral, at the medial fat pad proximal to the joint line

Digital palpation should be performed with an approximate force of 4 kg. For a tender point to be considered "positive," the subject must state that the palpation was painful. *Tender* is not to be considered *painful.*

For classification purposes, patients are said to have fibromyalgia if both criteria are satisfied. Widespread pain must have been present: for at least 3 months. A second clinical disorder does not exclude the diagnosis of fibromyalgia.

From Wolfe F, Smythe HA, Yunus MB, et al. The American College of Rheumatology 1990 criteria for the classification of fibromyalgia. Arthritis Rheum 1990;33:160–172.

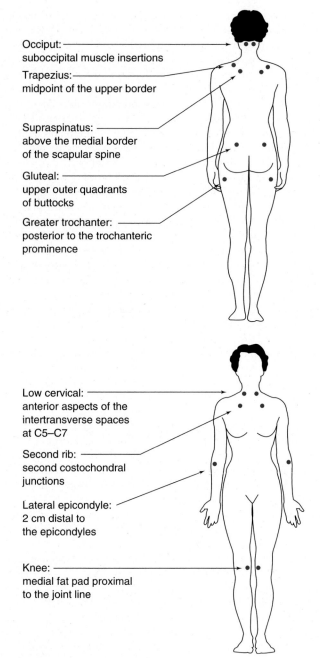

FIGURE 10-12. Location of 18 tender points.

to perform than before FMS onset, and 67% reported no or short pain-free periods.[68]

The lack of objective findings in light of the patients' perception of their illness is stressful and can lead to feelings of rejection and of being misunderstood or disbelieved. These feelings compromise the patient's ability to deal with the illness. Daily routines are disrupted, conflicts about life roles emerge and lead to further stress, and loss of physical fitness and loss of future opportunities occur. Patients need early and adequate information, along with acknowledgment of the conditions to minimize psychosocial consequences.[71]

Chronic Fatigue Syndrome

CFS is characterized by profound fatigue. Descriptions of similar illnesses are found throughout the medical literature.[101,102] These disorders include neurasthenia, myalgic encephalomyelitis, and chronic Epstein-Barr virus infection (i.e., "yuppie flu"). With an estimated incidence of 0.1%, CFS is much less prevalent than is FMS, and studies suggest that CFS affects both sexes and occurs across almost all races and ethnic groups.[145]

Etiology
Various studies have looked for the causes of CFS. Immune system changes have been reported in patients with CFS.

Early reports of viral markers have not been confirmed in later studies. The Epstein-Barr virus is not thought to be a causative agent in CFS onset, though some viral trigger may be involved.[146] Neuroendocrine changes, especially in hypothalamic hormone production or release of corticotrophin-releasing hormone, have been found.[147] CFS does not appear to be a form of depression, because neurohormonal and sleep-cycle findings characteristic of depression are not found in patients with CFS, though illness-related depression may occur, as it does in FMS.[145] Up to 70% of patients with CFS simultaneously present with FMS.[85]

New research has found a link between CFS and a retrovirus, the xenotropic murine leukemia virus-related virus (XMRV).[148] XMRV was first detected in patients with prostate cancer, and has subsequently been found in 67% of patients with CFS.[149] Further data analysis demonstrated evidence of the retrovirus in 95% of patients with CFS sampled.[150] The association between CFS and XMRV is unclear. It is unknown whether the virus is more prevalent in certain geographical areas, or if people with CFS are more susceptible to viruses and are therefore more likely to carry XMRV or its antibodies.[151] Patients with CFS also have a higher incidence of cancer, and it is unknown if XMRV is a factor in this increased incidence. The relationship between XMRV and other diseases like myalgic encephalomyelitis, atypical multiple sclerosis, and fibromyalgia is currently being investigated.[150] As new information becomes available, interventions and the role of therapeutic exercise may be modified and clinicians must continue to seek out current best evidence in the treatment of these conditions.

Signs and Symptoms

The onset of CSF is typically sudden, and the fatigue is profound. Twenty-five percent of patients with CFS are bedridden or unable to work, and 33% can work only part-time.[72] Patients with CFS may tolerate exertion at first, but 6 to 24 hours later, symptoms often increase. This must be considered by the clinician when designing and teaching an exercise program.

In 1994, the Centers for Disease Control and Prevention (CDC) published a working case definition of CFS[152] (Display 10-3). This definition is still curent.[153] Unexplained, debilitating fatigue of at least 6 months' duration that is unalleviated by rest and four of eight listed symptoms are required for case definition. Symptoms include impairment in memory or concentration, sore throat, tender cervical or axillary lymph nodes, muscular pain, multijoint noninflammatory arthralgia, new or different headaches, nonrefreshing sleep, and prolonged (at least 24 hours) generalized fatigue after previously tolerated exercise.

Among the eight symptoms detailed by the CDC, sleep disruption is reported by about 95% of patients with CFS. Other common complaints include neurocognitive difficulties, muscle weakness, frequent need for naps, dizziness, shortness of breath, and adverse responses to stress.[70] Comparison of the diagnostic criteria for FMS and CFS show a broad overlap, and their exact relationship is in question.[145]

THERAPEUTIC EXERCISE INTERVENTIONS FOR COMMON IMPAIRMENTS

Clinical manifestations of FMS and CFS include evidence of impairments that affect functioning. Studies carried out over the past 10 years[73–75,154–158] and reviews of treatment approaches for FMS and CFS[76,145,159] support the need for multidisciplinary intervention in the treatment of these impairments. Pharmacology, psychotherapy, education, and aerobic exercise are used successfully in many cases.[160–162]

Physical rehabilitation is an important part of treatment for patients with FMS or CFS. Evidence of deconditioning,[57] lowered respiratory function,[67] decreased joint range, depleted muscle endurance, and reduced muscle performance[66,144] has been found in these patients. Abnormal joint alignment and posture may contribute to peripheral stresses and amplify pain.[75,76,99] Deconditioning may make muscle more vulnerable to physiologic changes (hypothesized by some

DISPLAY 10-3

The Centers for Disease Control and Prevention Working Case Definition of Chronic Fatigue Syndrome

Fatigue criteria and four of eight symptom criteria must be present to fulfill the case definition.

Fatigue Criteria

1. Persistent or relapsing fatigue that
   a. Has been clinically evaluated
   b. Is of definite onset
   c. Is not the result of exertion
   d. Results in substantial reduction in activity
2. Other conditions that explain the fatigue have been excluded, including:
   a. Active medical conditions (e.g., untreated hypothyroidism)
   b. Previously diagnosed medical condition whose resolution has not been clinically documented (e.g., treated malignancies)
   c. Past or present psychotic or melancholic depression, bipolar disorder, schizophrenia, delusional disorders, dementia, anorexia nervosa, bulimia
   d. Alcohol or substance abuse within 2 years of the onset of fatigue or anytime thereafter

Symptom Criteria

Persistent or recurrent symptoms lasting more than six consecutive months:

1. Self-reported impairment in short-term memory or concentration, which causes substantial reduction of occupational, educational, social, or personal activities
2. Sore throat
3. Tender posterior cervical, anterior cervical, or axillary lymph node pain
4. Muscle pain
5. Multijoint noninflammatory arthralgias
6. New or different headaches
7. Unrefreshing sleep
8. Prolonged (at least 24 hours) generalized fatigue after previously tolerable levels of exercise

From Buchwald D. Fibromyalgia and chronic fatigue syndrome. Similarities and differences. Rheum Dis Clin North Am 1996;22:219–243.

researchers to underlie peripheral pain[80,96,102]) and affect neurohormonal regulation.[71,93] Stress is an exacerbating factor for some patients with these conditions. Careful prescription of an exercise program depends on significant findings during the initial evaluation. The clinician working with a patient with FMS or CFS should assess posture, strength, joint play, and cardiovascular conditioning to design a treatment program.

Therapeutic exercise can address six main areas of impairment:

1. Muscle power functions
2. Exercise tolerance functions (Impaired aerobic capacity)
3. Mobility of joint functions (Impaired ROM)
4. Muscle endurance functions (Impaired posture)
5. Emotional functions (Impaired response to emotional stress)
6. Pain

It is important to introduce exercise slowly, progressing intensity and duration as symptoms allow. The regimen

TABLE 10-1   **Exercise for Patients with Fibromyalgia**

Early Phase (Week 1-on)
Goal: stress and pain management
Relaxation
Progressie relaxation
Autogenic deep breathing
Visualization
Deep breathing
Stretch

Midphase (Week 2-on)
Goal: Musculoskeletal balance
Fluoromethane spray and stretch
Self-mobilizations
Neuromuscular techniques: hold and relax, contract and relax
Strain-counterstrain
Muscle system balance exercises (Sahrman)
Neutral spine (± tubing)
Closed chain eccentric exercise
Early aerobic exercise: supine bike, unloading equipment,
    easy exercises in water

Late Phase
Goal: Maintenance
Stretch, cont.
Musculoskeletal balance, cont.
General strength: resistance tubing, machines, closed chain
    eccentric exercise
Aerobic exercise: nonweight-bearing to weight-bearing and
    nonjarring actiities (ski machine, seated stationary bike,
    treadmill) and water exercises (aerobics, flotation belt)

depends on good communication between the clinician and patient. For consistency with the format being used in this textbook, exercises to address impairments are listed in the order used in other chapters, but this may not be the order in which they are introduced to the patient. The skillful therapist will choose interventions based on impairments found during evaluation and will structure them in a way that allows the patient to progress most smoothly toward functional goals.

There will be overlap in the impairments addressed within any given session but it is advisable to start with an emphasis on the less demanding regimens (e.g., relaxation and stretch) early in the course of treatment to build patient confidence in exercise and a greater acceptance of more aggressive exercise later. As treatment progresses increase the intensity and difficulty of the intervention, monitoring patient response and adjusting (and teaching the patient to monitor and adjust) appropriately, working toward functional goals. In general following the order outlined in Table 10-1 should help progress treatment with less likelihood of an adverse response to treatment and an increased confidence and willingness to participate on the patient's part.

Therapeutic intervention for a structured return to physical activity is suggested for patients with CFS because complete inactivity appears to promote fatigue.[145] Although little literature exists on the effect of exercise for CFS,[112] one study showed improvement in global self-assessment scores for patients with CSF after aerobic exercise training.[158] Treatment of FMS-like symptoms of CFS could follow the FMS protocols suggested in the next sections, and physical symptom exacerbation should guide progression of the program.

Impaired Muscle Power Functions

Muscle performance in patients with FMS declines compared with controls. Perception of pain and fatigue may limit production of muscle contraction force and eventually affect functional activities of the patient because of resulting deconditioning. When insignificant muscle imbalances are found or existing imbalances are being successfully addressed, patients can begin to direct their energy toward general strengthening routines for conditioning, especially if this goal is a priority for them. Strength training is initiated in the middle phase of treatment and for maintenance purposes. There is evidence that increasing general strength levels affects FMS symptoms positively.[79,161]

The same conditions apply to exercise prescription for general strengthening as apply to treatment of specific movement faults. The program should start with low-resistance and low-repetition work, avoid static holding, monitor symptoms, and progress slowly. Allowing the patient to choose the form of exercise may increase enjoyment and compliance. Exercise can be isometric or isotonic. If isometric activities are chosen, avoidance of prolonged static holding is important. Contractions should not be held longer than 3 to 5 seconds, with three to six repetitions of the exercise performed three times each week, a level that has been demonstrated to increase periarticular muscle strength.[163]

In dynamic exercise, slow movement through full range with return to the lengthened range allows a slight muscle stretch between contractions. Resistance tubing and, further into the program, resistance machines, which are designed to provide good body alignment and smooth resistance, seem preferable to free weights, perhaps because they allow more complete muscle relaxation between repetitions than free weights, which depend on static muscle contraction of the forearm and fi ngers. Aquatic therapy has been shown to be very effective for strengthening and aerobic exercise for patients with FMS.[162] Closed chain lengthening exercises of the Pilates type (a form of exercise developed and used with dancers, emphasizing strength and flexibility over bulking) are useful when the patient is ready for active movement. If no prior weight training has been done by the patient, calibrating the response by starting with three to five repetitions of three to five exercises at the lightest weight and monitoring the response over 24 to 48 hours can provide the baseline of the patient's tolerance. Patience is important in introducing exercise to decrease setbacks. Table 10-2 provides a sample program.

Exercise Tolerance Functions: Impaired Aerobic Capacity

Because aerobic exercise may have a positive effect on some of the impairments seen in patients with FMS, including endurance, pain, and flexibility, it should be introduced as soon as possible. Patients with FMS who participate in an aerobic exercise have been shown to improve overall well-being, improve ability to perform aerobic exercise, decrease tender point pressure pain, and reduce overall pain.[160] Exercise programs were performed for at least 20 minutes per day, 2 to 3 days per week and included strength training. The exercise should progress to being of moderate intensity.[161]

TABLE 10-2	Sample Strengthening Program

Water Program: 3 Days Per Week
- Warm-up: slow walking forward, backward, sideways: with or without arm movement depending upon upper extremity involvement (approximately 5 minutes)
- Slow-speed arm movements with short lever arm and decreased surface area (5–10 repetitions)
- Flexion/extension
- Horizontal abduction/adduction
- Abduction/adduction
- Rotation
- Slow speed leg kicks into flexion and abduction (5–10 repetitions)
- Squats or stepping exercise
- Bicycling with legs
- Gentle stretching and walk for cool down

Land Program: 3 Days Per Week
- Walking in home or around neighborhood
- Abdominal muscle strengthening (e.g., pelvic tilts, bridging, stabilization)
- Stepping exercise (such as wall slide, squat, stair step exercise)
- Upper extremity exercise with very light resistance (1–2 lb or less)
- Gentle stretching exercise

Initially, only a few minutes of the activity should be allowed (2 to 5 minutes, unless the patient is already active for longer periods without symptom flares). This allows the gradual build-up of tolerance. By the late phase of rehabilitation, the patient may be ready to work on elevation of the heart rate to 50% to 60% of the maximum heart rate. Monitoring techniques including the training index, pulse determination, and use of the perceived exertion scale[164] should be discussed so pacing and progress can be monitored. The patient should keep a record of exertion and symptoms to facilitate this assessment.

During the first session, it may be a good idea to make a contract with the patient to start preaerobic activities of daily walking, even if only one half of a block. For the patient who is able to walk more than one fourth of a mile, a high school track offers several advantages. Typically, it has a shock-absorbing surface; it is a safe place to use headphones without worrying about traffic, which may make it more enjoyable; accurate distance estimates are possible so progress in distance and rate can be tracked; and the patient who fatigues part way through can usually walk back to a car rather than all the way home or have to ask someone to come for him or her. It is important to consider the patient's interests and goals in designing a walking program and in suggesting a particular environment. Initially, the rate of walking should be slow and comfortable until tolerable levels, without a flare of symptoms, can be established.

Another approach to introducing exercise gently is to have the patient exercise on a recumbent bike or walking in a swimming pool. During the first session, the patient should walk or pedal about 2 to 3 minutes; 1 to 2 minutes can be added each session (at first not more than once a day) until, by the late phase of treatment, the patient may reach 15 minutes. After the patient is able to exercise on the bike or pool for 20 to 25 minutes, it should be possible to allow the patient to choose some other form of nonjarring aerobic exercise that is personally enjoyable.

SELECTED INTERVENTION 10-1
Treatment of the Patient with Fibromyalgia

See Case Study No. 7

Although this patient requires comprehensive intervention, as described in the patient management model, one exercise is described.

ACTIVITY: Hand to knee pushes

PURPOSE: To increase abdominal and hip flexor muscle strength; improve single-leg balance and trunk stability; and increase upper quarter strength through closed chain activity

RISK FACTORS: No appreciable risk factors

ELEMENTS OF THE MOVEMENT SYSTEM: Base

STAGE OF MOTOR CONTROL: Stability

POSTURE: Standing position on a single leg. The opposite hip and knee are flexed to 90 degrees. The opposite hand of the flexed leg pushes isometrically against the movement of hip flexion. A neutral spine is maintained, and concentration on abdominal muscle contraction is emphasized.

MOVEMENT: Isometric contraction of the abdominal, hip flexor, and contralateral upper quarter muscles.

SPECIAL CONSIDERATIONS: Ensure proper posture of the trunk, pelvis, and weight-bearing limb. Cue for an abdominal muscle contraction, using palpation as necessary. This exercise is contraindicated when an isometric muscle contraction is contraindicated.

DOSAGE: Hold contraction for 3 to 6 seconds at a comfortable intensity that does not cause hip flexor or shoulder fatigue. Repeat on the opposite side.

TYPE OF MUSCLE CONTRACTION: Isometric

Intensity: Submaximal
Duration: Hold for up to 6 seconds
Frequency: During each pool session

RATIONALE FOR EXERCISE CHOICE: This exercise addresses the many components of fibromyalgia, including trunk stability, single-leg stance stability, abdominal muscle endurance, and upper and lower quarter muscle endurance.

EXERCISE GRADATION: This exercise is progressed to greater intensity and more repetitions. More advanced stabilization exercises incorporating upper and lower extremity movements with resistance are then added.

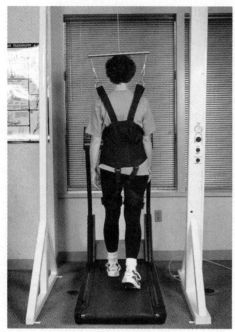

FIGURE 10-13. Unweighting equipment supports part of the patient's body weight. This decreases joint stress and body weight resistance, enabling the patient to do cardiovascular exercise with less physiologic stress.

In some clinics, unweighting equipment (e.g., harness) is available and has been used successfully in introducing patients to aerobic exercise[165] (Fig. 10-13). Water exercise is another form of reduced weight-bearing exercise. The patient can walk in the shallow end, move rhythmically, or participate in exercise classes. Community pool programs with classes for patients with fibromyalgia have the added benefit of social contact. For some patients with FMS, socializing has been markedly decreased because of fatigue and pain. Nonjarring sources of aerobic exercise for slightly more advanced patients may include a treadmill, ski machine, seated push-pull arm and leg machines, and minitramp.

In several studies of the effects of aerobic exercise on FMS, the first 10 to 12 weeks were problematic for musculoskeletal symptom flares and for adherence.[73,78] A systematic review of exercise in FMS[166] reports adherence to exercise and attrition in study subject numbers (25% average in the studies cited) was a problem. Some patients complained of a flare of pain or fatigue during and after exercise, and it is pointed out that positive findings reported with exercise in these studies might be due to attrition bias. Mengshoel,[78] however, maintains that patients can perform low-intensity dynamic exercise without a flare of symptoms.

More gradual introduction of aerobic exercise may solve some of this problem, and the knowledge that this is a common finding may help the clinician and the patient persevere beyond this point in conditioning.

In introducing aerobic exercise routines, the therapist should let the patient know that continuous monitoring and pacing are important. During periods of symptom flares, the patient should be encouraged to modify exercise intensity appropriately through trial and error of symptom response to exercise level over time. It is easy for patients to become discouraged and stop a program. Their records and the encouragement of the clinician may help them push through this

difficult time and allow them to comply with what appears to be one of a few treatment approaches with a positive impact on FMS.

Mobility of Joint Functions: Impaired Range of Motion

Restrictions in joint ROM may exist at any joint held for prolonged periods in abnormal alignment. Joints particularly affected by static poor posture can include craniovertebral, cervicothoracic, scapulothoracic, glenohumeral, radiohumeral, midthoracic, lumbopelvic and pelvofemoral, and subtalar joints. Intervention with soft-tissue and joint mobilization techniques where deemed appropriate should always be supported with exercises designed to balance muscles around the affected joints. Patient efficacy and responsibility with self treatment in this chronic condition is an important part of patient education for self management.

Where joint hypermobility or poor proximal stability is present, concurrent use of stabilization training (e.g., in craniovertebral flexion during self stretch of suboccipital muscles, uptraining of longus capitis and downtraining of scalenes and sternomastoid muscles) is necessary for the preservation of good joint alignment.

Flexibility exercises should be graded for exertion and time. The typical 20- to 30-second hold during stretching may be too long when effort is required to hold a limb. Passive support or decreased time may be necessary. Stretching should never be painful. Breathing instruction during training is important as breath holding can be a characteristic of patients with FMS.[67] (See Self-Management 10-9: Neuromuscular Relaxation of Suboccipital Muscles, 10-10: Neuromuscular Relaxation of a Second Set of Suboccipital Muscles, and 10-11: Neuromuscular Relaxation of a Third Set of Suboccipital Muscles.)

SELF-MANAGEMENT 10-9 *Neuromuscular Relaxation of Suboccipital Muscles*

Purpose:	To restore normal length to one group of suboccipital muscles and to decrease craniovertebral compression and possibly relieve headache
Position:	Lie on your back with your knees bent and neck supported on a small pillow or towel roll.
Movement technique:	Gently tuck your chin without lifting your head. Hold for 6 seconds. Relax.

Dosage
Repetitions: _____
Frequency: _____

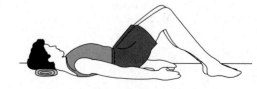

SELF-MANAGEMENT 10-10 *Neuromuscular Relaxation of a Second Set of Suboccipital Muscles*

Purpose: To restore normal length to a second set of suboccipital muscles and to decrease craniovertebral compression and possibly relieve headache

Position: Lie on your back with your knees bent and neck supported on a small pillow or towel roll.

Movement technique: Glide your head to the right without bending your neck.

With one finger tip on the bone behind your right ear, gently push your head to the right, but resist isometrically with your neck muscles.

Hold for 6 seconds.

Repeat on the opposite side.

Dosage
Repetitions: _____
Frequency: _____

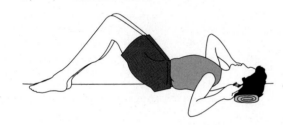

SELF-MANAGEMENT 10-11 *Neuromuscular Relaxation of a Third Set of Suboccipital Muscles*

Purpose: To restore normal length to a third set of suboccipital muscles and to decrease craniovertebral compression and possibly relieve headache

Position: Lie on your back with your knees bent and neck supported on a small pillow or towel roll.

Movement technique: Lift your chin about one-eighth of an inch, so your head tips back.

Bring your right ear toward your right shoulder one-eighth of an inch, so your head tips to the right.

Turn your head one-eighth of an inch to the right, so your heads rotates to the right.

With one fingertip on the right temple, gently push your head back to the left, but your neck muscles resist so no motion occurs.

Dosage
Repetitions: _____ times on each side (do not alternate)

Frequency: _____

Muscle Endurance Functions: Impaired Posture

The biomechanical faults resulting from poor postural alignment can contribute to FMS pain,[76,99] and poor postural alignment can play into the reduced respiratory capacity of patients. Postural assessment in all postures typical for the patient (standing, sitting, resting, and static or repetitive work postures) is important in this regard. Patient education regarding the importance of normal posture is often needed. Instruction regarding appropriate adaptation of standing, sitting, and lying surfaces with shock-absorbing pads, supports, and equipment realignment may be needed. And, often, help training for correct muscle recruitment and endurance to maintain good alignment is necessary.

Along with stretching, strengthening for muscle balance around affected joints is necessary. The Sahrman approach to muscle balance in joint or movement dysfunction (see Chapter 9) appears to be an especially effective and well-tolerated approach to treating patients with FMS. These exercises are specific and can be progressed slowly, allowing pacing and monitoring of symptoms, ideally short of causing overexertion flares. Most do not require resistance equipment and are easily related to functional tasks (e.g., reaching overhead without shoulder or back pain, standing without back or hip pain).

Static posture is a starting point for return to function where dynamic activity against gravity is required. Stabilization exercises for trunk and proximal limb girdle muscles are useful when muscle weakness or joint hypermobility impairments exist and proximal control during functional tasks with the limbs is compromised. This is especially true for spinal segmental dysfunction. An approach that has been nonstressful for patients is the use of graded-resistance tubing attached to the wall or door, with the performance of extremity PNF diagonals while neutral trunk alignment is maintained during resisted limb movements (Fig. 10-14). This exercise can be progressed in difficulty by adding movement of the entire body (e.g., lunging) against resistance while holding a neutral alignment.

Eccentric control is an important part of functional activity, introducing control and balance to movement patterns, and one that is frequently lost in deconditioned patients. Closed-chain activities and movement therapies, including Tai Chi Chuan, Feldenkrais, and low-level therapeutic ballet classes are exercise strategies that may help restore periarticular muscle balance and function and stimulate vestibular balance (Fig. 10-15). They may be more interesting and fun for patients, and the patient's desire to be involved with one or the other of these forms of exercise should guide the choice. Introduction of these strategies should be slow, probably after successful introduction of concentric forms of exercise, and

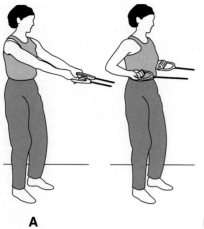

A   **B**

FIGURE 10-14. The use of graded-resistance tubing attached to the wall, with performance of upper extremity PNF diagonals provides a non-stressful stabilization exercise. (A) Holding onto the tubing, the patient crosses her wrists with her palms facing downward. (B) Maintaining her hand at waist level, the patient bends her elbows as she turns her palms upward.

always according to the patient's tolerance and carefully monitored for progression of intensity, duration, and frequency.

Emotional Functions: Impaired Response to Emotional Stress

If the evaluation indicates a need for stress management, it should be initiated in the early phase of treatment, probably within the first or second visit. Stress management may include an exercise program with relaxation, deep breathing, and stretch exercises. These are unlikely to be stressful to most patients and usually provide benefits that are

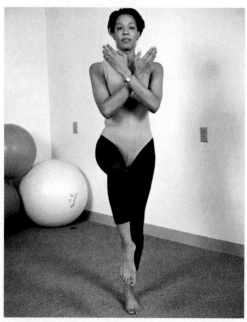

FIGURE 10-15. Tai Chi is an excellent exercise strategy to help restore control and balance to the movement patterns of deconditioned patients. The teacher should have experience working with patients with joint problems or chronic illness.

immediately obvious and typically pleasurable. This approach can provide a positive introduction to the benefits of exercise and offer an opportunity to demonstrate that exercise does not have to mean maximal exertion to be beneficial. Progressive relaxation, autogenic deep breathing, and visualization exercises (see Chapter 24) can be taught, or tapes can be made available to patients for use at home. In addition, patients may benefit from referral to an appropriate mental health professional for related services.

Instruction in diaphragmatic and lateral costal expansion breathing (see Chapters 22 and 24) can help respiratory function and is a good adjunct to any treatment requiring soft-tissue or joint mobilization of the thoracic cage. (See Self-Management 10-12: Neuromuscular Relaxation of Tight Rib Joints.) Relaxation in a warm pool along with diaphragmatic breathing while immersed provides resistance to the muscles

SELF-MANAGEMENT 10-12 *Neuromuscular Relaxation of Tight Rib Joints*

Purpose: To decrease tightness at the rib joints and decrease posterior costovertebral pain

Position: With help of your therapist or after you are experienced, push on the rib in the front that corresponds with the level of pain on the back.

Even though this might not have seemed painful to you until you touched it, it will almost feel like a red-hot type of pain if it is the correct level. The place you push in front is on the same side as the back pain and near where the rib attaches to the sternum.

After you have located the spot, place the fist of the same-side hand flat against the spot.

Press the opposite hand on top of your fist; your elbow on the side of the pain sticks out.

Movement technique: Stand next to a wall or have a partner gently resist that elbow as it starts to elevate from your side. Hold for a slow count of 6. *Be very gentle with resistance.*

Dosage

Repetitions: _____ times on each side (do not alternate)

Frequency: _____

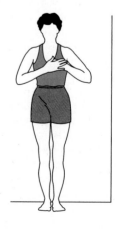

of inspiration. General stretching following accepted guidelines (see Chapter 7) can be prescribed if no joint instability has been found. It is often necessary to make the patient aware of the distinction between stretch and pain, which can be difficult when generalized pain and aching is chronic and patients have learned to disregard these signals. If static stretching is uncomfortable, consider gentle dynamic mobility to begin.

In introducing these exercises, it may be useful to suggest that the patient choose a pleasurable place at a time when interruptions are minimal. Enjoyable background music can be played. Defining this experience to the patient as a pleasurable and relaxing one that can have a positive impact on symptoms of FMS allows clinicians to reinforce success through an achievable task, builds patient confidence in the use of exercise therapeutically, and may help modify unrealistic beliefs about exercise.

Pain

The patient with fibromyalgia by definition has widespread pain and tenderness. During the intake evaluation the patient may also discuss isolated areas of joint pain. It is helpful to assess both the fibromyalgia and biomechanical aspects of the patient's symptoms and treat biomechanical faults (which may be postural, traumatic, or from some coexisting medical condition) as part of the whole approach. Elimination of pain of biomechanical origin (e.g., shoulder impingement resulting from abducted and downwardly rotated scapulae) by using hands-on or muscle balancing techniques will contribute to a decrease in emotional and physical stress, increase the sense of control, possibly eliminate a source of sleep disruption, and may better allow participation in an exercise routine aimed at the FMS symptoms without further exacerbating the fault.

Although aerobic and strengthening exercise have been shown effective in decreasing pain and tenderness in FMS, a systematic review of studies[166] has also shown that adherence and increased symptoms are problematic to some patients with FMS. Careful monitoring and adjusting of the exercise program for each patient, together with ongoing teaching about the rationale for exercise, may be useful in managing pain and apprehension, and maximizing adherence.

Transient relief of pain can be gotten from thermal and electrical modalities and patients can be taught self-application techniques. However, because pain may be central in origin, it is unlikely these will provide any long-term relief, but may offer the patient an increased sense of control over pain.

Cognitive behavioral therapy and neuropharmacologic approaches are useful in pain management, and the physical therapist who works with patients with FMS should be familiar with the outlines of these therapies in order to support efforts being made by other providers in conjunction with exercise therapy.[161,162]

PRECAUTIONS AND CONTRAINDICATIONS

Exercise can be a two-edged sword for patients with FMS or CFS. Overexertion can lead to a relapse or exacerbation of symptoms.[73,78,112,154,157] Because most persons with FMS or CFS have experienced this phenomenon, they may resist the idea of exercise, and adherence to an exercise program may be difficult.

Adherence

The patient's beliefs about the nature of the disease and the benefits of exercise play an important role in exercise adherence.[167] The process of negotiating for mutual therapeutic goals is an important part of treatment. Although the therapist may be modeling goals on a pathophysiologic concept of the disability, the patient's view is probably different. The patient's view is shaped by his or her perception of the disability and its effects, what he or she perceives to be helpful, and treatment goals and activities that are important personally. The therapist has the opportunity to influence these beliefs and positively affect treatment and adherence with the program through a process of mutual information sharing, listening, trust-building, and negotiation.

Adherence with exercise programs may be problematic. Patients with FMS and CFS may feel as if their energy reserves are nearly depleted and may want to avoid exercise. Patients may fear exercise based on past experience with exacerbations after overexertion. As more is being learned about the treatment of these conditions, patients may seek exercise prescription based on the encouragement of their physician or knowledge gained from support groups, literature, or word of mouth. Patients may hope for the clinician to reconcile the apparent discrepancy between their experiences and what they are told is helpful, making it easier for the clinician to convince the patient about the benefits of exercise.

One function of the initial assessment is to provide the opportunity for exchange of information. Another is to set mutual goals. During the assessment, the clinician should listen to and attempt to understand the patient's point of view. In this way, the patient can develop confidence in being part of a team. These are important processes in promoting the patient's adherence to an exercise program (see Chapter 3).

Pacing

Pacing is crucial for patients who are chronically fatigued.[168] For people who have been active exercisers before the onset of the disease, the inability to meet previous exercise goals may be a source of grief or frustration. Others may fear that exercise means lap swimming or jogging. The concept of therapeutic exercise and the importance of pacing needs to be carefully explained.

Most patients have experienced symptom flares with overexertion. Initiating an exercise routine requires starting slowly, with few repetitions (three to five may be enough the first time), light resistance (none to very minimal), and a limited number of exercises (usually, three is enough). Feedback 24 to 48 hours after exercise is necessary for pacing the progression of the program. Exacerbations of FMS were triggered in one study that looked at the effects of repetitive dynamic muscle contraction and sustained static muscle contractions in patients with FMS and in sedentary, healthy control subjects. It was found that, 24 hours after exercise, exercise-induced extremity pain had not returned to preexercise levels in patients with FMS.[108] Sometimes, a patient who is progressing the intensity and duration of an activity has a setback unrelated to exercise and needs to temporarily drop back to earlier levels of performance. Recognition and applause from the patient and the clinician for efforts to pace and avoid overexertion and avoid flares helps in redefining the value of exercise for the patient.

The training index is one form of monitoring that can be used to help the patient in pacing. The training index was originally introduced for use with cardiac patients by Hagberg[169] and modified by Clark[170] for use with patients with FMS. This is a quantitative measure of exertion based on simple calculations using pulse rate and the duration of exercise. The training index provides target values for basic cardiovascular fitness, which may be used by patients to track their progress toward these goals (see Patient-Related Instruction 12-1: Determining the Training Index to Track the Level of Exertion in Chapter 12). Some patients may find it helpful to keep a diary of daily activities to monitor possible correlations between symptoms and activity levels, and this may also be a useful pacing tool.

Pharmacologic and Psychologic Intervention

Pharmacologic therapy is based on findings of neurohormonal alterations and sleep disruption in CFS and FMS and on treating associated symptoms (e.g., fever in CFS, muscle pain, and gastrointestinal irritation in CFS and FMS). Low-dose tricyclic medications, which in much larger doses act as antidepressants, may be beneficial in addressing pain and sleep disruption. Selective serotonin-uptake inhibitors may help the fatigue component.[159] Buchwald[145] points to anecdotal reports of antiviral and immunomodulating drugs in the treatment of CFS. Simms[159] offers a complete review of the pharmacologic treatment of FMS.

The association of pain, fatigue, and disordered sleep of FMS and CFS with psychologic status is controversial.[101,171–173] This controversy is stressful for many patients.[71] As Hendriksson's studies point out, the effects of these chronic, long-term conditions can be profound.[68,71] Aside from the question of any possible causal relationship between psychopathology and CFS or FMS, various types of psychotherapeutic and educational interventions aimed at teaching coping strategies and at adjustment to lifestyle changes have been found to be beneficial.

One study[174] showed a 63% rate of return to work by patients with CFS after 1 year of cognitive behavioral therapy, and a study by Buckelew et al.[175] correlated higher self-efficacy with less pain and impairment in physical activities for patients with FMS. Self-efficacy can be defined as a belief that one can successfully do a thing. Self-efficacy has been shown to impact behavior, motivation, thoughts, and emotions.[175] A meditation-based stress-reduction program was also shown to be effective in improving physical symptoms.[176] Because CFS and FMS may be long-term, life-changing conditions, individual and group psychotherapy may be beneficial. In a review of programs using education for self-management of FMS, Burkhardt and Bjelle[177] concluded that self-efficacy and life quality can be enhanced for patients who undergo even short-term intensive treatment, with improvement lasting beyond the end of the program. Several organizations sponsor support groups and education classes throughout the United States and Canada (see Patient-Related Instruction 10-4: Organizations for Information About Fibromyalgia Syndrome and Chronic Fatigue Syndrome).

Patient-Related Instruction 10-4

Organizations for Information About Fibromyalgia Syndrome and Chronic Fatigue Syndrome

For information about fibromyalgia or chronic fatigue syndrome, contact one of these organizations:

- The Arthritis Foundation is an excellent source of information, has support groups, and provides leadership training. Phone numbers of local chapters can be found in phone books.
- Fibromyalgia Alliance of America provides patient information and support group resources (FMAA, PO Box 21990, Columbus, OH 43221-0990, (614) 457-4222).
- Chronic Fatigue Immune Deficiency Syndrome Association of America, Inc., provides patient information, support group resources, and data on research, treatment, and conferences (CFIDS Assoc., PO Box 220398, Charlotte, NC 28222-0398, (800) 848-7373)

KEY POINTS

- Pain impairment occurs with most musculoskeletal conditions and must be treated as a primary impairment along with any secondary limitations that may result.
- Nociceptors, or pain receptors, transmit impulses from the periphery to the dorsal horn of the spinal cord and higher CNS levels.
- Pain information is transmitted through A-delta and C fibers, which are small, unmyelinated neuronal fibers.
- Information is processed within the spinal cord and then ascends through the contralateral spinothalamic tract to the thalamus.
- The gate theory of pain states that incoming information from nonpain receptors (e.g., thermal, mechanical) can close the gate to pain information.
- Chronic pain may result from increased sensitization of nociceptors and spinal level changes that perpetuate positive feedback loops in the pain-spasm cycle.
- Descending impulses can influence pain perception through several mechanisms, including endogenous opiates.
- Pain can be assessed through direct measurement tools such as the VAS or MPQ questionnaires or through quality of life scales such as the SF-36.
- Fear-anxiety avoidance models help explain transitions from acute to chronic pain and can be measured with different tools.
- Therapeutic exercise is a cornerstone of treatment for chronic pain. It can remedy pain (through gating mechanisms and descending influences), secondary limitations caused by pain, and associated impairments and activity limitations.
- TENS, heat, cold, and medications are key components of a comprehensive pain treatment program.
- FMS and CFS are increasingly recognized in clinic patient populations, have widespread effects, and limit functioning.
- The cause of FMS is unclear; CFS may be viral in origin.

- Exercise appears to be one of a few effective treatments for FMS and possibly for CFS.
- Because of the fatigue and ease of symptom exacerbation with exertion, exercise prescription must be done carefully and thoughtfully, tracking responses continuously.
- Exercise for the treatment of FMS and CFS can be expected to address stress, posture, and mobility impairments; impaired muscle performance; and cardiovascular endurance.
- Exercise should be introduced slowly and progressed from exercises likely to lead to success to those that may be more stressful. Relaxation, breathing, stretching exercises, and gentle, limited walking exercises can progress to strengthening and to slowly progressing aerobic exercises.
- Physical therapy treatments should always attempt to model the concepts of pacing and limiting overexertion and overcommitment as they apply to daily activities of the patient and in therapeutic exercise.
- The physical therapist should attempt to encourage good communication and establish mutually acceptable goals in an attempt to contribute to the patient's adherence to the exercise program.
- Aerobic exercise should be progressed slowly, be nonjarring, and be pleasurable if possible.
- During physical therapy treatment, patients often are undergoing adjunctive treatments from other medical disciplines, which may stress them in terms of energy, time, and money. The therapist should be aware of the other commitments and help the patient prioritize realistically.
- The use of physical agents for pain control should be taught as self-treatment techniques, because using clinic time for their application may not be the best use of the patient's resources.
- Patients should be taught appropriate self-mobilization or neuromuscular techniques to cope with chronic biomechanical faults so that they have tools to manage their condition independently.

CRITICAL THINKING QUESTIONS

1. Consider Case Study No. 5 in Unit 7.
   a. This patient has pain with standing and walking. What interventions may improve this patient's ability to stand and walk without pain?
   b. This patient has pain with lumbar extension. How does your therapeutic exercise intervention address this problem?
   c. What suggestions can you give this patient to allow her to participate in social activities without pain?
2. Consider Case Study No. 7 in Unit 7.
   a. Design an exercise program to prevent further decline of her general deconditioning, with consideration of her overall fatigue and daily demands.
   b. Provide this patient with suggestions for energy-reducing measures to allow her to complete daily tasks without increasing pain or fatigue.
3. Outline the questions you would ask in the subjective portion of an evaluation of a patient with FMS. Be sure you cover the areas of their presentation that may affect development of the condition and that may contribute to its exacerbation.

4. What physical tests and measurements would you perform in the objective portion of the evaluation?
5. What forms of exercise would you need to introduce over time to the patient with FMS?
6. List the order in which you would probably introduce the various types of exercise over the course of treatment of the FMS patient.
7. Discuss special considerations for introducing exercise.
8. List the functional goals of physical therapy treatment that would be appropriate for this clinical population.

REFERENCES

1. Wolfe F, Ross K, Andreson J, et al. The prevalence and characteristics of fibromyalgia in the general population. Arthritis Rheum 1995;38:19–28.
2. Merskey H, Bogduk N, eds. Classification of Chronic Pain: Descriptions of Chronic Pain Syndromes and Definitions of Pain Terms. 2nd Ed. Seattle: IASP Press, 1994:210–211.
3. Quillen WS, Magee DJ, Zachazewski JE. The process of athletic injury and rehabilitation. In: Zachazewski JE, Magee DJ, Quillen WS, eds. Athletic Injuries and Rehabilitation. Philadelphia, PA: WB Saunders, 1996:3–8.
4. Newton RA. Contemporary views on pain and the role played by thermal agents in managing pain symptoms. In: Michlovitz S, ed. Thermal Agents in Rehabilitation. 2nd Ed. Philadelphia, PA: FA Davis, 1990.
5. Bennett RM. Emerging concepts in the neurobiology of chronic pain: evidence of abnormal sensory processing in fibromyalgia. Mayo Clin Proc 1999;74:385–398.
6. Kramis RC, Roberts WJ, Gillette RG. Non-nociceptive aspects of persistent musculoskeletal pain. J Orthop Sports Phys Ther 1996;24:255–267.
7. Sluka KA. Pain mechanisms involved in musculoskeletal disorders. J Orthop Sports Phys Ther 1996;24:240–254.
8. Bowsher D. Nociceptors and peripheral nerve fibers. In: Wells PE, Frampton V, Bowsher D, eds. Pain Management in Physical Therapy. Norwalk, CT: Appleton & Lange, 1988.
9. Siddall PJ, Cousins MJ. Spinal pain mechanisms. Spine 1997;22:98–104.
10. Werner JK. Neuroscience: A Clinical Perspective. Philadelphia, PA: WB Saunders, 1980.
11. Hanegan JL. Principles of nociception. In: Gersh MR, ed. Electrotherapy in Rehabilitation. Philadelphia, PA: FA Davis, 1992.
12. Kosek E, Ekholm J, Hansson P. Modulation of pressure pain thresholds during and following isometric contraction in patients with fibromyalgia and healthy controls. Pain 1996;64:415–423.
13. Scott J, Huskisson EC. Graphic representation of pain. Pain 1976;2:175–184.
14. Melzack R. The McGill Pain Questionnaire: major properties and scoring methods. Pain 1975;1:277–299.
15. Melzack R. The short-form McGill Pain Questionnaire. Pain 1987;30:191–197.
16. Melzack R, Katz J, Jeans ME. The role of compensation in chronic pain: analysis using a new method of scoring the McGill Pain Questionnaire. Pain 1985;23:101–112.
17. Martin AL, McGrath PA, Brown SC, et al. Anxiety sensitivity, fear of pain and pain-related disability in children and adolescents with chronic pain. Pain Res Manag 2007 Winter;12(4):267–272.
18. van den Hout JH, Vlaeyen JW, Houben RM, et al. The effects of failure feedback and pain-related fear on pain report, pain tolerance, and pain avoidance in chronic low back pain patients. Pain 2001;92(1–2):247–257.
19. Guzman J, Esmail R, Karjalainen K, et al. Multidisciplinary bio-psycho-social rehabilitation for chronic low back pain. Cochrane Database Syst Rev 2002;(1):CD000963.
20. Carleton RN, Asmundson GJ. The multidimensionality of Fear of Pain: construct independence for the Fear of Pain Questionnaire-Short Form and the Pain Anxiety Symptoms Scale-20. J Pain 2009;10(1):29–37.
21. Zvolensky MJ, Goodie JL, McNeil DW, et al. Anxiety sensitivity in the prediction of pain-related fear and anxiety in a heterogeneous chronic pain population. Behav Res Ther 2001;39(6):683–696.
22. Sieben JM, Portegijs PJ, Vlaeyen JW, et al. Pain-related fear at the start of a new low back pain episode. Eur J Pain 2005;9(6):635–641.
23. Olatunji BO, Sawchuk CN, Deacon BJ, et al. The Anxiety Sensitivity Profile revisited: factor structure and psychometric properties in two nonclinical samples. J Anxiety Disord 2005;19(6):603–625.
24. Roelofs J, Peters ML, Deutz J, et al. The Fear of Pain Questionnaire (FPQ): further psychometric examination in a non-clinical sample. Pain 2005;116(3):339–346.
25. Davidson MA, Tripp DA, Fabrigar LR, et al. Chronic pain assessment: A seven-factor model. Pain Res Manag 2008;13(4):299–308.
26. Vlaeyen JW, Linton SJ. Fear-avoidance and its consequences in chronic musculoskeletal pain: a state of the art. Pain 2000;85(3):317–332.
27. Swinkels-Meewisse IE, Roelofs J, Verbeek AL, et al. Fear-avoidance beliefs, disability, and participation in workers and non-workers with acute low back pain. Clin J Pain 2006;22(1):45–54.

28. George SZ, Fritz JM, Childs JD. Investigation of elevated fear-avoidance beliefs for patients with low back pain: a secondary analysis involving patients enrolled in physical therapy clinical trials. J Orthop Sports Phys Ther 2008;38(2):50–58.

29. Dehghani M, Sharpe L, Nicholas MK. Selective attention to pain-related information in chronic musculoskeletal pain patients. Pain 2003;105(1–2): 37–46.

30. Woods MP, Asmundson GJ. Evaluating the efficacy of graded in vivo exposure for the treatment of fear in patients with chronic back pain: a randomized controlled clinical trial. Pain 2008;136(3):271–280.

31. Coons MJ, Hadjistavropoulos HD, Asmundson GJ. Factor structure and psychometric properties of the Pain Anxiety Symptoms Scale-20 in a community physiotherapy clinic sample. Eur J Pain 2004;8(6):511–516.

32. Asmundson GJ, Bovell CV, Carleton RN, et al. The Fear of Pain Questionnaire-Short Form (FPQ-SF): factorial validity and psychometric properties. Pain 2008;134(1–2):51–58.

33. Roelofs J, McCracken L, Peters ML, et al. Psychometric evaluation of the Pain Anxiety Symptoms Scale (PASS) in chronic pain patients. J Behav Med 2004;27(2):167–183.

34. Crombez G, Vlaeyen JW, Heuts PH, et al. Pain-related fear is more disabling than pain itself: evidence on the role of pain-related fear in chronic back pain disability. Pain 1999;80(1–2):329–339.

35. Picavet HS, Vlaeyen JW, Schouten JS. Pain catastrophizing and kinesiophobia: predictors of chronic low back pain. Am J Epidemiol 2002;156:1028–1034.

36. Linton SJ, Buer N, Vlaeyen JWS, et al. Are fear-avoidance beliefs related to the inception of an episode of back pain? A prospective study. Psychol Health 1999;14:1051–1059.

37. Van Nieuwenhuyse A, Somville PR, Crombez G, et al. The role of physical workload and pain related fear in the development of low back pain in young workers: evidence from the BelCoBack Study; results after one year of follow up. Occup Environ Med 2006;63:45–52.

38. Leeuw M, Goossens ME, Linton SJ, et al. The fear-avoidance model of musculoskeletal pain: current state of scientific evidence. J Behav Med 2007;30(1):77–94.

39. Al-Obaidi SM, Beattie P, Al-Zoabi B, et al. The relationship of anticipated pain and fear avoidance beliefs to outcome in patients with chronic low back pain who are not receiving workers' compensation. Spine 2005;30:1051–1057.

40. Al-Obaidi SM, Nelson RM, Al-Awakhi S, et al. The role of anticipation and fear of pain in the persistence of avoidance behavior in patients with chronic low back pain. Spine 2000;25:1126–1131.

41. Goubert L, Crombez G, Lysens R. Effects of varied-stimulus exposure on overpredictions of pain and behavioural performance in low back pain patients. Behav Res Ther 2005b;43:1347–1361.

42. Vowles KW, Gross RT. Work-related beliefs about injury and physical capability for work in individuals with chronic pain. Pain 2003;10:291–298.

43. Geisser ME, Haig AJ, Wallbom AS, et al. Pain-related fear, lumbar flexion and dynamic EMG among persons with chronic musculoskeletal low back pain. Clin J Pain 2004;20:61–69.

44. Poiraudeau S, Rannou F, Baron G, et al. Fear-avoidance beliefs about back pain in patients with subacute low back pain. Pain 2006;124(3):305–311.

45. Borg-Stein J, Simons DG. Myofascial pain. Arch Phys Med Rehabil 2002;83: S40–S47.

46. Frost H, Klaber Moffett JA, Moser JS, et al. Randomised controlled trial for evaluation of fitness programme for patients with chronic low back pain. BMJ 1995;310:151–154.

47. Geiger G, Todd DD, Clark HB, et al. The effects of feedback and contingent reinforcement on the exercise behavior of chronic pain patients. Pain 1992;49:179–185.

48. Minor MA. Exercise in the management of osteoarthritis of the knee and hip. Arthritis Care Res 1994;7:198–204.

49. Busch AJ, Schachter CL, Overend TJ, et al. Exercise for fibromyalgia: a systematic review. J Rheumatol 2008;35(6):1130–1144.

50. Kay TM, Gross A, Goldsmith C, et al. Exercises for mechanical neck disorders. Cochrane Database Syst Rev 2005 Jul 20;(3):CD004250.

51. Pisters MF, Veenhof C, van Meeteren NL, et al. Long-term effectiveness of exercise therapy in patients with osteoarthritis of the hip or knee: a systematic review. Arthritis Rheum 2007;57(7):1245–1253.

52. Dagfinrud H, Kvien TK, Hagen KB. Physiotherapy interventions for ankylosing spondylitis. Cochrane Database Syst Rev 2008;23(1):CD002822.

53. Fransen M, McConnell S, Bell M. Exercise for osteoarthritis of the hip or knee. Cochrane Database Syst Rev 2003;(3):CD004286.

54. White CM, Pritchard J, Turner-Stokes L. Exercise for people with peripheral neuropathy. Cochrane Database Syst Rev 2004 Oct 18;(4):CS003904.

55. Rakel D, ed. Integrative Medicine. 2nd Ed. Philadelphia, PA: Saunders Elsevier, 2007.

56. Kankaanpaa M, Taimela S, Airaksinen O, et al. The efficacy of active rehabilitation in chronic low back pain. Effect on pain intensity, self-experienced disability, and lumbar fatigability. Spine 1999;24:1034–1042.

57. Bennett RM, Burckhardt CS, Clark SR, et al. Group treatment of fibromyalgia: a 6 month outpatient program. J Rheum 1996;23:521–528.

58. Robinson AJ. Transcutaneous electrical nerve stimulation for the control of pain in musculoskeletal disorders. J Orthop Sports Phys Ther 1996;24:208–226.

59. Hanai F. Effect of electrical stimulation of peripheral nerves on neuropathic pain. Spine 2000;25:1886–1892.

60. Baxter R. Drug control of pain. In: Wells PE, Frampton V, Bowsher D, eds. Pain Management in Physical Therapy. Norwalk, CT: Appleton & Lange, 1988.

61. Tierney LM, McPhee S, Papadakis MA. Current Medical Diagnosis and Treatment. New York, NY: Lange Medical Books/McGraw Hill, 2005.

62. Finnerup NB. A review of central neuropathic pain states. Curr Opin Anaesthesiol. 2008;21(5):586–589.

63. Annemans L, Caekelbergh K, Morlion B, et al. A cost-utility analysis of pregabalin in the management of peripheral neuropathic pain. Acta Clin Belg 2008;63(3):170–178.

64. Nolan MF, Wilson MCB. Patient-controlled analgesia: a method for the controlled self-administration of opioid pain medications. Phys Ther 1995;75:374–379.

65. Wolfe F, Smythe HA, Yunus MB, et al. The American College of Rheumatology 1990 criteria for the classification of fibromyalgia. Arthritis Rheum 1990;33: 160–172.

66. Mannerkorpi K, Burckhardt CS, Bjelle A. Physical performance characteristics of women with FM. Arthritis Care Res 1994;7:123–129.

67. Lurie M, Caidahl K, Johansson G, et al. Respiratory function in chronic primary fibromyalgia. Scand J Rehabil Med 1990;22:151–155.

68. Henriksson C, Gundmark I, Bengtsson A, et al. Living with fibromyalgia. Clin J Pain 1992;8:138–144.

69. Wolfe F, Anderson J, Harkness D, et al. Work and disability status of persons with fibromyalgia. J Rheumatol 1997;24:1171–1178.

70. Martinez JE, Ferraz MD, Sato EI, et al. Fibromyalgia versus rheumatoid arthritis: a longitudinal comparison of the quality of life. J Rheumatol 1995;22: 270–274.

71. Henriksson CM. Living with continuous muscular pain—patient perspectives. Scand J Caring Sci 1995;9:67–76.

72. Komaroff AL, Buchwald D. Symptoms and signs of CFS. Rev Infect Dis 1991;13(Suppl 1):S8–S11.

73. McCain GA, Bell DA, Mai FM, et al. A controlled study of the effects of a supervised cardiovascular fitness training program on the manifestations of primary fibromyalgia. Arthritis Rheum 1988;31:1135–1141.

74. Burkhardt CS, Mannerkorpi K, Hedenberg L, et al. A randomized controlled clinical trial of education and physical training for women with fibromyalgia. J Rheumatol 1994;21:714–720.

75. Goldman JA. Hypermobility and deconditioning: important links to fibromyalgia/fibrositis. South Med J 1991;84:1192–1196.

76. Rosen NB. Physical medicine and rehabilitation approaches to the management of myofascial pain and fibromyalgia syndromes. Baillieres Clin Rheumatol 1994;8:881–916.

77. Buckelew S, Conway P, Parker J, et al. Biofeedback/relaxation training and exercise interventions for fibromyalgia: a prospective trial. Arthritis Care Res 1998;11:196–209.

78. Mengshoel AM, Komnaes HB, Forre O. The effect of 20 weeks of physical fitness training in female patients with fibromyalgia. Clin Exp Rheumatol 1992;10:345–349.

79. Hakkinen A, Hakkinen K, Hannonen P, et al. Strength training induced adaptations in neuromuscular training in premenopausal women with fibromyalgia: comparison with healthy women. Ann Rheum Dis 2001;60:21–26.

80. Staud R. Biology and therapy of fibromyalgia: pain in fibromyalgia syndrome. Arthritis Res Ther 2008;10(6):208–215.

81. Wolfe F. Fibromyalgia: the clinical syndrome. Rheum Dis Clin North Am 1989;15:1–17.

82. Romano TJ. Fibromyalgia in children: diagnosis and treatment. W V Med J 1991; 87:112–114.

83. Gedalia A, Press J, Klein M, et al. Joint hypermobility and fibromyalgia in school children. Ann Rheum Dis 1993;52:494–496.

84. The Centers for Disease Control and Prevention. http://www.cdc.gov/arthritis/basics/fibromyalgia.htm. Accessed November 21, 2009. Last updated October 28, 2009.

85. Goldenberg DL, Simms RW, Geiger A, et al. High frequency of FM in patients with CF seen in a primary care practice. Arthritis Rheum 1990;33:381–387.

86. Hootman JM, Helmick CG, Schappert S. Magnitude and characteristics of arthritis and other rheumatic conditions on ambulatory medical care visits, United States, 1997. Arthritis Care Res 2002;47(6):571–581.

87. Robinson RL, Birnbaum HG, Morley MA, et al. Economic cost and epidemiological characteristics of patients with fibromyalgia claims. J Rheumatol 2003;30(6):1318–13125.

88. Picavet HSJ, Hoeymans N. Health related quality of life in multiple musculoskeletal diseases: SF-36 and EQ-5D in the DMC3 study. Ann Rheum Dis 2004;63:723–729.

89. Schlenk EA, Aelen JA, Dunbar-Jacob J, et al. Health-related quality of life in chronic disorders: a comparison across studies using the MOS SF-36. Qual Life Res 1998;7(1):57–65.

90. Patten SB, Beck CA, Kassam A, et al. Long-term medical conditions and major depression: strength of association for specific conditions in the general population. Can J Psychiatry 2005;50(4):195–202.

91. Freundlich B, Leventhal L. The fibromyalgia syndrome. In: Schumacher HR, ed. Primer on the Rheumatic Diseases. 10th Ed. Atlanta, GA: Arthritis Foundation, 1993.

92. Moldofsky H. Fibromyalgia, sleep disorder and chronic fatigue syndrome. Ciba Found Symp 1993;173:262–271.

93. Greenfield S, Fitzcharles MA, Esdaile JM. Reactive fibromyalgia syndrome. Arthritis Rheum 1992;35:678–681.

94. Buchwald D, Goldenberg DC, Sullivan JL, et al. The "chronic active Epstein-Barr virus infection" syndrome and primary fibromyalgia. Arthritis Rheum 1987;30;1132–1136.

95. Romano TJ. Clinical experiences with posttraumatic fibromyalgia syndrome. W V Med J 1990;86:198–202.
96. Dailey PA, Bishop GD, Russell IJ, et al. Psychological stress and the fibrositis/fibromyalgia syndrome. J Rheumatol 1990;17:1380–1385.
97. Moldofsky H. Sleep and fibrositis syndrome. Rheum Dis Clin North Am 1989;15:90–103.
98. Branco J, Atalaia A, Paiva T. Sleep cycles and alpha delta sleep in fibromyalgia syndrome. J Rheumatol 1994;21:1113–1117.
99. Yunus MB. Towards a model of pathophysiology of fibromyalgia: aberrant central pain mechanisms with peripheral modulation. J Rheumatol 1992;19:846–849.
100. Clauw DJ. Fibromyalgia and diffuse pain syndromes. Primer on the Rheumatic Diseases. 12th Ed. Atlanta, GA: The Arthritis Foundation, 2001.
101. Powers R. Fibromyalgia: an age-old malady begging for respect. J Intern Med 1993;8:93–105.
102. Straus SE. History of chronic fatigue syndrome. Rev Infect Dis 1991;13(Suppl 1):S2–S7.
103. Henriksson KG. Chronic muscular pain: aetiology and pathogenesis. Ballieres Clin Rheumatol 1994;8:703–719.
104. Yunus MB, Kalyan-Raman UP. Muscle biopsy findings in primary fibromyalgia and other forms of nonarticular rheumatism. Rheum Dis Clin North Am 1989;15:115–133.
105. Bengtsson A, Henriksson KG, Jorfeldt L, et al. Primary fibromyalgia: a clinical and laboratory study of 55 patients. Scand J Rheumatol 1986;15:340–147.
106. vanDenderen JC, Boersma JW, Zeinstra P, et al. Physiological effects of exhaustive physical exercise in primary fibromyalgia syndrome (PFS): is PFS a disorder of neuroendocrine reactivity? Scand J Rheumatol 1992;21:35–37.
107. Yunus M, Masi AT, Calabro JJ, et al. Primary fibromyalgia (fibrositis): clinical study of 50 patients with matched normal controls. Semin Arthritis Rheum 1981;11:151–171.
108. Mengshoel AM, Vollestadt NK, Forre O. Pain and fatigue induced by exercise in fibromyalgia patients and sedentary healthy subjects. Clin Exp Rheumatol 1995;13:477–482.
109. Bennett RM, Jacobsen S. Muscle function and origin of pain in fibromyalgia. Baillieres Clin Rheumatol 1994;8:721–746.
110. Henriksson KG, Bengtsson A, Larsson J. Muscle biopsy findings of possible diagnostic importance in primary fibromyalgia. Lancet 1982;2:1395.
111. Bengtsson A, Henriksson KG, Larsson J. Muscle biopsy in primary fibromyalgia: light microscopical and histochemical findings. Scand J Rheumatol 1986;15:1–6.
112. McCully K, Sisto SA, Natelson BH. Use of exercise for treatment of chronic fatigue syndrome. Sports Med 1996;21:35–48.
113. Jubrias SA, Bennett RM, Klug G. Increased incidence of a resonance in the phosphodiesterase region of ^{31}P nuclear magnetic resonance spectra in the skeletal muscle of fibromyalgia patients. Arthritis Rheum 1994;37:801–807.
114. Simms RW, Roy SH, Hrovat M, et al. Lack of association between fibromyalgia and abnormalities in muscle energy metabolism. Arthritis Rheum 1994;37:794–800.
115. Lund E, Kendall SA, Janerot-Sjoberg B, et al. Muscle metabolism in fibromyalgia studied by P-31 magnetic resonance spectroscopy during aerobic and anaerobic exercise. Scand J Rheumatol 2003;32:138–145.
116. Bennett RM, Clark SR, Goldberg, et al. Aerobic fitness in patients with fibrositis: a controlled study of respiratory gas exchange and 133 xenon clearance from exercising muscle. Arthritis Rheum 1989;32:454–460.
117. Bengtsson A, Bengtsson M, Jorfeldt L. Diagnostic epidural opioid blockade in primary fibromyalgia at rest and during exercise. Pain 1989;39:171–180.
118. Littlejohn GO, Weinstein L, Helme RD. Increased neurogenic inflammation in fibrositis syndrome. J Rheumatol 1987;14:1022–1025.
119. Elert J, Rantapaa-Dahlqvist SB, Henriksson-Larsen K, et al. Increased EMG activity during short pauses in patients with primary fibromyalgia. Scand J Rheumatol 1989;18:321–323.
120. Lindh M, Johansson G, Hedberg M, et al. Studies on maximal voluntary contraction in patients with fibromyalgia. Arch Phys Med Rehabil 1994;75:1217–1222.
121. Mengshoel AM, Forre O, Komnaes HB. Muscle strength and aerobic capacity in primary fibromyalgia. Clin Exp Rheumatol 1990;8:475–479.
122. Rutherford OM, White PD. Human quadriceps strength and fatigability in patients with post viral fatigue. J Neurol Neurosurg Psychiatry 1991;54:961–964.
123. Lloyd AP, Hales JP, Gandevia SL. Muscle strength, endurance and recovery in the post-infection fatigue syndrome. J Neurol Neurosurg Psychiatry 1988;51:1316–1322.
124. Stokes MJ, Cooper RG, Edwards RH. Normal muscle strength and fatigability in patients with effort syndromes. BMJ 1988;297:1014–1017.
125. Kent-Braun J, Sharma KR, Weiner MW, et al. Central basis of muscle fatigue in chronic fatigue syndrome. Neurology 1993;43:125–131.
126. Williams DA, Clauw DJ. Understanding fibromyalgia: lessons from the broader pain research community. J Pain 2009;10(8):777–791.
127. Yunus MB, Denko CW, Masi AT. Serum beta endorphin in primary fibromyalgia syndrome: a controlled study. J Rheumatol 1986;13:183–186.
128. Vaeroy H, Helle R, Forre O, et al. Cerebrospinal fluid levels of beta-endorphin in patients with fibromyalgia (fibrositis syndrome). J Rheumatol 1988;15:1804–1806.
129. Russell IJ, Michalek JE, Vipraio GA, et al. Platelet 3-H-imipramine uptake receptor density and serum serotonin levels in patients with fibromyalgia/fibrositis syndrome. J Rheumatol 1992;19:104–109.
130. Vaeroy H, Helle R, Forre O, et al. Elevated CSF levels of substance P and high incidence of Raynaud phenomenon in patients with fibromyalgia: new features for diagnosis. Pain 1988;32:21–26.
131. McCain GA, Tilbe KS. Diurnal hormone variations in fibromyalgia syndrome: a comparison with rheumatoid arthritis. J Rheumatol 1989;16(Suppl 19):154–157.
132. Neeck G, Riedel W. Thyroid function in patients with fibromyalgia syndrome. J Rheumatol 1992;19:1120–1122.
133. Bennett RM, Clark SR, Campbell SM, et al. Somatomedin-C levels in patients with fibromyalgia syndrome: a possible link between sleep and muscle pain. Arthritis Rheum 1992;35:1113–1116.
134. Davidson JR, Moldofsky H, Lue FA. Growth hormone and cortisol secretion in relation to sleep and wakefulness. J Psychiatry Neurosci 1991;16:96–102.
135. Moldofsky H, Scarisbrick P. Induction of neurasthenic musculoskeletal pain syndrome by selective sleep stage deprivation. Psychosom Med 1976;38:35–44.
136. Goldstein JA. Fibromyalgia syndrome: a pain modulation disorder related to altered limbic function? Ballieres Clin Rheumatol 1994;8:777–800.
137. Vaeroy H, Qiao ZG, Morkrid L, et al. Altered sympathetic nervous system response in patients with fibromyalgia (fibrositis syndrome). J Rheumatol 1989;16:1460–1465.
138. Yunus MB, Dailey JW, Aldag JC, et al. Plasma and urinary catecholamines in primary fibromyalgia: a controlled study. J Rheumatol 1992;19:95–97.
139. Okifuji A, Turk DC. Stress and psychophysiological dysregulation in patients with fibromyalgia syndrome. Appl Psychophysiol Biofeedback 2002;27:129–141.
140. Hudson JI, Goldenberg DL, Pope HG Jr, et al. Comorbidity of FMS with medical and psychiatric disorders. Am J Med 1992;92:363–367.
141. Buskila D, Neumann L, Vaisberg G, et al. Increased rates of fibromyalgia following cervical spine injury. A controlled study of 161 cases of traumatic injury. Arthrits Rheum 1997;40:446–452.
142. Raak R, Hurtig I, Wahren LK. Coping strategies and life satisfaction in subgrouped fibromyalgia patients. Biol Res Nurs 2003;4:193–202.
143. Drexler AR, Mur EJ, Gunther VC. Efficacy of an EMG-biofeedback therapy in fibromyalgia patients. A comparative study of patients with and without abnormality in (MMPI) psychological scales. Clin Exp Rheumatol 2002;20:677–682.
144. Jacobsen S, Danneskiold-Samsoe B. Inter-relationships between clinical parameters and muscle function in patients with primary fibromyalgia. Clin Exp Rheumatol 1989;7:493–498.
145. Buchwald D. Fibromyalgia and chronic fatigue syndrome. Similarities and differences. Rheum Dis Clin North Am 1996;22:219–243.
146. Buchwald D, Komaroff AL. Review of laboratory findings for patients with CFS. Rev Infect Dis 1991;13(Suppl 1):S12–S18.
147. Demitrak MA, Dale JK, Straus SE, et al. Evidence for impaired activation of the hypothalamic-pituitary-adrenal axis with chronic fatigue syndrome. J Clin Endocrinol Metab 1991;73:1224–1234.
148. Lombardi VC, Ruscetti FW, Gupta JD, et al. Detection of an infectious retrovirus, XMRV, in blood cells of patients with chronic fatigue syndrome. Science 2009;326(5952):585–589.
149. Schlaberg R, Choe DJ, Brown KR, et al. XMRV is present in malignant prostatic epithelium and is associated with prostate cancer, especially high-grade tumors. Proc Natl Acad Sci USA 2009 Sept 22;106(38):16351–16356.
150. The Whittemore Peterson Institute for Neuro-Immune Disease. http://www.wpinstitute.org/xmrv/xmrv. Accessed November 20, 2009.
151. Hohn O, Krause H, Barbarotto P, et al. Lack of evidence for xenotropic murine leukemia virus-related virus (XMRV) in German prostate cancer patients. Retrovirology 2009 Oct 16;6:92.
152. Fukuda K, International Chronic Fatigue Syndrome Study Group. The chronic fatigue syndrome: a comprehensive approach to its definition and study. Ann Intern Med 1994;121:953–958.
153. The Centers for Disease Control and Prevention. http://www.cdc.gov/cfs/cfsdefinitionHCP.htm. Accessed November 20, 2009. Last updated May 5, 2006.
154. Nichols DS, Glenn TM. Effects of aerobic exercise on pain perception, affect and level of disability in individuals with FM. Phys Ther 1994;74:327–332.
155. Isomeri R, Mikkelsson M, Latikka P. Effects of amitriptyline and cardiovascular fitness training on the pain of fibromyalgia patients. Scand J Rheumatol 1992;(Suppl 94):47.
156. Burckhardt CS, Clark SR, Campbell SM, et al. Multidisciplinary treatment of fibromyalgia. Scand J Rheumatol 1992;(Suppl 94):51.
157. Martin L, Nutting A, Macintosh BR, et al. An exercise program in the treatment of fibromyalgia. J Rheumatol 1996;23:1050–1053.
158. Fulcher KY, White PD. Randomised controlled trial of graded exercise in patients with the chronic fatigue syndrome. BMJ 1997;314:1647–1652.
159. Simms RW. Controlled trials of therapy in FMS. Baillieres Clin Rheumatol 1994;8:917–934.
160. Busch AJ, Barber KAR, Overend TJ, et al. Exercise for treating fibromyalgia syndrome. Cochrane Database Syst Rev 2007; Issue 4. Art. No.: CS003786. DOI:10.1002/14651858.CD003786.pub2.
161. Goldenberg DL, Burckhardt C, Crofford L. Management of fibromyalgia syndrome. JAMA 2004;292(19):2388–2395.
162. Hauser W, Arnold B, Eich W, et al. Management of fibromyalgia syndrome—an interdisciplinary evidence-based guideline. German Med Sci 2008;6:1–11.
163. Hicks JE. Exercise in patients with inflammatory arthritis and connective tissue disease. Rheum Dis Clin North Am 1990;16:845–870.
164. Borg GAV. Psychophysical basis of perceived exertion. Med Sci Sports Exerc 1980;14:377–381.
165. Essenberg VJ Jr, Tollan MF. Etiology and treatment of fibromyalgia syndrome. Orthop Phys Ther Clin North Am 1995;4:443–457.

166. Busch AJ Schachter CL, Peloso PM, Bombardier C. Exercise for treating fibromyalgia syndrome (Cochrane review). The Cochrane Library, 3. Oxford, Update software, 2002.

167. Jensen GM, Lorish CD. Promoting patient cooperation with exercise programs. Arthritis Care Res 1994;7:181–189.

168. Lorig K, Fries HF. The Arthritis Helpbook. 4th Ed. Reading, MA: Addison-Wesley, 1995.

169. Hagberg JM. Central and peripheral adaptations to training in patients with coronary artery disease. Biochem Exerc 1986;16:267–277.

170. Clark SR. Prescribing exercise for fibromyalgia patients. Arthritis Care Res 1994;7:221–225.

171. Goldenberg DL. Psychological symptoms and psychiatric diagnosis in patients with fibromyalgia. J Rheumatol 1989;16(Suppl 19):127–130.

172. Goldenberg DL. Psychologic studies in fibrositis. Am J Med 1986;81:67–70.

173. Yunus MB, Ahles TA, Aldag JC, et al. Relationship of clinical features with psychological status in primary fibromyalgia. Arthritis Rheum 1991;34:15–21.

174. Sharpe M, Hawton K, Simkin S, et al. Cognitive behaviour therapy for the CFS: a random controlled trial. BMJ 1996;312:22–26.

175. Buckelew SP, Murray SE, Hewett JE, et al. Self-efficacy, pain, and physical activity among FM subjects. Arthritis Care Res 1995;8:43–50.

176. Kaplan H, Goldenberg DL, Galvin-Nadeau M. The impact of a meditation-based stress reduction program on fibromyalgia. Gen Hosp Psychiatry 1993;15:284–289.

177. Burkhardt CS, Bjelle A. Education programs for fibromyalgia patients: description and evaluation. Baillieres Clin Rheumatol 1994;8:935–955.

Special Physiologic Considerations in Therapeutic Exercise

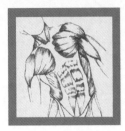

chapter 11

Soft-Tissue Injury and Postoperative Management

LORI THEIN BRODY

Most musculoskeletal problems resolve with conservative management. Patients who develop overuse injuries, or have mild sprains, strains, or contusions, can expect to return to full function within a matter of days or weeks. For example, most patients with acute low back pain recover within 12 weeks without surgery.[1] However, some musculoskeletal problems do not resolve with conservative management alone. In these cases, surgical intervention may be necessary to return the patient to optimal function. Understanding the fundamentals of connective tissue physiology and response to stress forms the basis for rehabilitation programs designed for both conservative and postoperative management. Be sure to consider this information in the context of interventions used to improve mobility and muscle performance, as discussed in Chapters 5 and 7.

PHYSIOLOGY OF CONNECTIVE TISSUE REPAIR

Soft tissues, including ligament, tendon, cartilage, and other connective tissues, respond to injury in a relatively predictable fashion. The repair process is similar in all connective tissues, although some variability between tissues (e.g., bone) exists. Healing is also affected by age, lifestyle, and systemic factors (e.g., alcohol abuse, smoking, diabetes mellitus, nutritional status, general health) and local factors (e.g., degree of injury, mechanical stress, blood supply, edema, infection).[2,3] An understanding of the healing phases helps the clinician choose treatment procedures that are appropriate at various points in the healing process.

Microstructure of Connective Tissues

Tendon, ligament, cartilage, bone, and muscle are some of the major connective tissues in the body. The three main components of connective tissue are fibers (i.e., collagen and elastin), ground substance with associated tissue fluids, solids (i.e., glycosaminoglycans such as proteoglycans), and cellular substances (i.e., fibroblasts, fibrocytes, and cells specific to each connective tissue).[3] The function of the various connective tissues is based on the relative proportions of intracellular and extracellular components such as collagen, elastin, proteoglycans, water, and contractile proteins. At least 15 types

of collagens (types I through XV) are known and differ fundamentally in the amino acid sequence of their constituent polypeptide chains (Table 11-1).[4,5]

Water makes up nearly two thirds of the weight of normal ligament, and collagen makes up 70% to 80% of the ligament's dry weight.[6] Nearly 90% of the collagen is type I, and 10% or less is type III collagen. Elastin is found in tiny quantities in ligaments, making up <1% to 2% of the total weight. Proteoglycans, another important solid found in ligaments, constitute <1% of the ligament's weight, but they are essential because of their water-binding properties.[2]

Tendon is a connective tissue attaching muscle to bone. Collagen forms 70% of the dry weight of tendon, and the overall proportions are 30% collagen, 2% elastin, and 68% water.[7] The low proportion of elastin accounts for the low elasticity of tendon. If tendon were more elastic, the tendon would elongate with muscle contraction, rather than transmitting the force to the bone. Muscle contraction would fail to move its insertion toward the origin, and no movement would take place. The structure provides some information about the function of this tissue.

Articular cartilage is composed of similar components, with nearly 80% of its weight from water. The high water content in articular cartilage, as in other viscoelastic tissues, is responsible for the mechanical properties of the tissue. The collagen makeup is primarily type II collagen, with small proportions of other collagen types.[5] Proteoglycans and their associated glycosaminoglycans are water-loving, or hydrophilic, molecules. Proteoglycans are responsible for the water-binding capabilities of articular cartilage, and proteoglycan loss results in a decreased water content and loss of the tissue's mechanical properties. Weight bearing causes tissue compression and fluid extrusion from the tissue, while unweighting pulls fluid back in because of the hydrophilic nature of the proteoglycans. This action provides nutrition and lubrication for the articular cartilage. Thus, weight bearing is critical for the health of articular cartilage. As proteoglycans are lost with degenerative joint disease, the ability to resorb fluid is impaired, decreasing the ability to absorb shock or transmit loads.

As with the other soft tissues of the body, bone is composed of solid and fluid components. Organic compounds

TABLE 11-1 Collagens of Connective Tissue

TYPE	DISTRIBUTION
I	Bone, ligament, tendon, fibrocartilage, capsule, synovial lining tissues, skin
II	Cartilage, fibrocartilage
III	Blood vessels, synovial lining tissues, skin
IV	Basement membranes
V	Pericellular region of articular cartilage when present,[a] bone, blood vessels
VI	Nucleus pulposus
VII	Anchoring fibers of various tissues
VIII	Endothelial cells
IX	Cartilage matrix[a]
X	Hypertrophic and ossified cartilage only
XI	Cartilage matrix[a]
XII	Tendon, ligament, perichondrium, periosteum
XIII	Skin, tendon

[a]Small amounts (<20%).
From Walker JM. Cartilage of human joints and related structures. In: Zachazewski JE, Magee DJ, Quillen WS, eds. Athletic Injuries and Rehabilitation. Philadelphia, PA: WB Saunders, 1996:123.

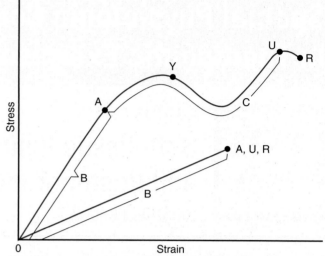

FIGURE 11-1. The stress-strain curve showing the elastic limit (A), elastic range (B), yield point (Y), plastic range (C), ultimate strength (U), and the rupture strength (R). (Adapted from Cornwall MW. Biomechanics of orthopaedic and sports therapy. In: Malone TR, McPoil T, Nitz AJ, eds. Orthopedic and Sports Physical Therapy. 3rd Ed. St. Louis, MO: Mosby, 1997:73; Rees JD, Wilson AM, Wolman. Current concepts in the management of tendon disorders. Rheumatology 2006;45:508–521.)

such as type I collagen and proteoglycans constitute approximately 39% of the total bone volume.[8] Minerals contribute nearly half of the total bone volume, and fluid fills the vascular and cellular spaces comprising the remaining volume. The primary minerals found in bone are calcium hydroxyapatite crystals. These minerals differentiate bone from other connective tissue and provide bone with its distinctive stiffness.

Response to Loading

When connective tissues are loaded, the *stress* can be plotted against the *strain* providing much information about the material properties of the tissue. The relative contributions of composite materials determine the mechanical properties of the specific tissue. However, some general concepts about connective tissue responses can be determined.

Tensile loads are resisted primarily by the collagen fibrils, which respond first by straightening from their resting crimped state. This straightening requires little force (Fig. 11-1). In the elastic portion of the curve, the collagen fibers respond to the load in a linear fashion up to 4% elongation.[7,9] After the load is removed, the tissue returns to its original length, a characteristic of the elastic range only up to the elastic limit. Beyond this point, removal of the stress does not result in a return to the tissue's original length. If the tissue is elongated beyond approximately 4%, plastic changes begin to occur (i.e., plastic range) as the cross-links begin to fail. Permanent deformation is the chief characteristic of the plastic range. After some fibers fail, the load on the remaining fibers is increased, accelerating tissue failure. The curve plateaus or even dips at the *yield point*. The *ultimate strength* is the greatest load the tissue can tolerate, and *rupture strength* is the point at which complete failure occurs.

The area under the curve represents the amount of strain energy stored in the tissue during loading. The viscoelastic nature of connective tissue results in an imperfect recovery after deformation, known as hysteresis. This difference between the loading curve and the unloading curve represents energy lost. This energy is lost primarily in the form of heat. A stretched tissue becomes warm in the process.

Other tissue qualities related to the load deformation curve are resilience and toughness. *Resilience* reflects a material's ability to absorb energy within the elastic range. As a resilient tissue is loaded quickly, work is performed, and energy is absorbed. When the load is removed, the tissue quickly releases energy and returns to its original shape. *Toughness* is the ability of a material to absorb energy within the plastic range. A critical quality of connective tissues is their ability to absorb energy without rupturing.

A relationship exists between stress and strain called the *elastic modulus*. The elastic modulus is the ratio of the stress divided by the strain and reflects the amount of stress needed to produce a given strain (i.e., deformation). The greater the stress necessary to deform the tissue, the stiffer is the material. For example, bone has a higher elastic modulus than meniscus and deforms less with a given load.

Cyclic loading alters the load deformation curve. Heat accumulates in the area of loading, disrupting the collagen cross-bridges. Cyclic loading produces microstructural damage that accumulates with each loading cycle. Damage accumulates faster at higher intensities of cyclic loading.[10] Failure as a result of cyclic loading, called fatigue failure, is the physiologic basis underlying stress fractures. Endurance limit or fatigue strength is the stress below which fatigue cracks do not begin to form.[10]

Connective tissues also demonstrate viscoelastic properties that provide these tissues with their uniquely mutable characteristics. These properties are creep and relaxation. When a tissue is held with a constant force, it begins to

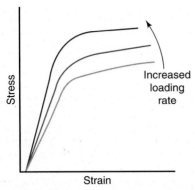

FIGURE 11-2. Three stress-strain curves for cortical bone tissues tested in tension at three different loading rates. As the testing rate increases, the slope (the elastic modulus) of the initial straight line portion increases. (Adapted from Burstein AH, Wright TM. Fundamentals of Orthopaedic Biomechanics. Baltimore, MD: Williams & Wilkins, 1994:120.)

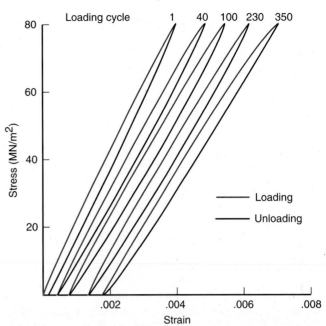

FIGURE 11-4. Effects of cyclic loading. When bone tissue is loaded cyclically to 90% of its tensile yield strength, nonreversible behavior (i.e., damage) is seen. By the 350th loading cycle, the elastic modulus has changed appreciably. (Adapted from Burstein AH, Wright TM. Fundamentals of Orthopaedic Biomechanics. Baltimore: Williams & Wilkins, 1994:125.)

lengthen until equilibrium is reached or until the tissue ruptures, depending on the magnitude of the force. This property is called *creep*. When a tissue is pulled to a fixed length, a certain force is required. As the tissue is held at this length, the amount of force necessary to maintain that length decreases. This property is called *relaxation*. These properties allow connective tissues to adapt to and function in a variety of loading conditions without being damaged. Tissues pulled into tension (i.e., stretched) lengthen and relax, which provides the rationale for stretching exercises to lengthen shortened soft tissues (Figs. 11-2–11-4).

Phases of Healing

The clinician must understand the phases of healing to formulate a plan of care matching the tissue's loading capabilities. The phases of healing provide a framework into which the rationale for physical therapy interventions fit. Understanding the healing process gives the clinician the tools to treat a variety of injury and surgical conditions.

Injury to the soft tissues arises from a number of sources. Physical traumas such as a sprain, strain, or contusion are most common, whereas injuries can also occur from bacterial or viral infections, heat, or chemical injury. Trauma causes direct damage to the cells in the immediate area of the injury, causing bleeding into the interstitial spaces. The bleeding initiates a cascade of events that promote healing of the injured tissue. The process can be considered in phases, although the continuum is an oversimplification of a very complex process.

Any of four outcomes may result from the inflammatory process: (a) resolution when the injury is mild and transitory, (b) replacement of the normal cell with fibrosis, (c) abscess formation in the presence of an infection, or (d) progression to chronic inflammation resulting from persistent injury or individual factors.[11] These factors include diabetes, corticosteroid use, and hematologic disease.[11] How the soft-tissue injury is managed is often responsible for the outcome of the injury.

Inflammatory Response

Healing of acute injuries passes through four major phases, beginning with the acute vascular-inflammatory response (Fig. 11-5). The purpose of the vascular changes is to mobilize and transport cells (white blood cells and leukocytes) to the area to initiate healing. When connective tissue is damaged,

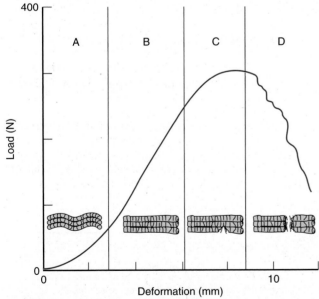

FIGURE 11-3. Stress-strain curve for ligament. As the ligament is distracted, fibers become progressively recruited into tension (A) until all the fibers are tight (B). The parts of the ligament that are tightened first are likely to be the first to fail (C) as the ligament reaches the yield point. Progressive fiber failures quickly result in ligament failure (D). (Adapted from Frank CB. Ligament injuries: pathophysiology and healing. In: Zachazewski JE, Magee DJ, Quillen WS, eds. Athletic Injuries and Rehabilitation. Philadelphia, PA: WB Saunders, 1996:15.)

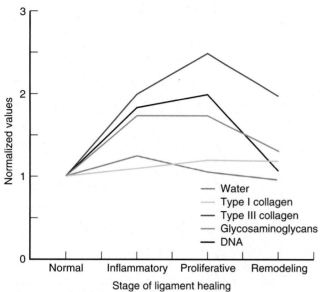

FIGURE 11-5. Changes in components of rabbit MCLs at various stages of healing. Values are normalized to that of uninjured ligament (normal = 1). (Adapted from Andriaacchi T, Sabiston P, DeHaven K, et al. Ligament: injury and repair. In: Woo SL-Y, Buckwalter JA, eds. Injury and Repair of the Musculoskeletal Soft Tissues. Park Ridge, IL: American Academy of Orthopaedic Surgeons, 1988:115.)

injured cells in the area release chemical substances (e.g., prostaglandins, bradykinin) that initiate the inflammatory response. The gap in the torn tissue is filled with erythrocytes and platelets.[1] The platelets form a plug to contain the bleeding and provide a scaffold for substances that will stabilize the clot. Local bleeding is a strong chemotactic stimulus, attracting white blood cells such as neutrophils and mononuclear leukocytes that help rid the site of bacteria and cellular debris through phagocytosis. Concurrently, in adjacent uninjured vessels, vasodilation occurs to increase local blood flow while capillary permeability is altered to allow greater exudation of plasma proteins and white blood cells. This produces swelling and edema in the area. In this phase, the damaged tissues and microorganisms are removed, fibroblasts are recruited, and some wound strength is provided by the weak hydrogen bonds of collagen fibers.[12] The inflammatory phase is essential in initiating the healing process. This phase is initiated immediately and lasts 3 to 5 days.[12]

Signs and symptoms observed in this phase are pain, warmth, palpable tenderness, and swelling. Pain and tenderness are caused by mechanical and chemical stimulation of nociceptors, and warmth and swelling are caused by acute inflammation. Limitations in joint or muscle range of motion (ROM) from pain or direct tissue damage are likely to occur. ROM testing usually reveals pain before the end of the ROM is reached.

Focus treatment procedures in this phase at decreasing pain and edema while preventing a progressive chronic inflammation. Ice is effective at reducing pain and edema. Compression also controls edema by forcing fluid to areas of lower hydrostatic pressure in the capillaries and lymph vessels.[11] Maintain the mobility and strength of adjacent joints and soft tissues while the acutely injured areas are rested (see Patient-Related Instruction 11-1: Acute Injury Management).

Patient-Related Instruction 11-1

Acute Injury Management

Take the following steps when an acute musculoskeletal injury or a flare-up of a preexisting injury occurs:

1. Ice the area for 10 to 15 minutes using cold packs or ice. Do this as often as possible throughout the day.
2. If possible, elevate the part to decrease swelling.
3. Apply compression in the form of an elastic sleeve or bandage. Remove the compression at night for sleeping.
4. Use a supportive or assistive device (e.g., sling, splint, cane, crutches, walker) to rest the injury.
5. Contact your clinician or physician regarding the need for further evaluation.
6. Resume previous program of care when instructed or able.

Proliferative/Fibroplasia Phase

The second phase, lasting from 48 hours to 6 to 8 weeks, is marked by the local presence of macrophages directing the cascade of events occurring in this proliferative phase. This phase may be referred to as the "repair-regeneration" phase, as there is a concurrent attempt at repair (replacement of the original tissue with scar tissue) and regeneration (replacement of the damaged tissue with the original tissue type).[13] Fibroblasts are actively resorbing collagen and synthesizing new collagen (primarily type III). The new collagen is characterized by small fibrils, disorganized in orientation and deficient in cross-linking.[12] Consequently, the tissue laid down in this phase is susceptible to disruption by overly aggressive activity. The greatest rate of collagen accumulation occurs between days 7 and 14.[13] As this phase progresses, a gradual decrease in tissue macrophages and fibroblasts occurs, and a grossly visible scar filling the gap can be seen.[14]

The warmth and edema resolves during this phase. Palpable tenderness decreases, and the tissue can withstand gentle loading. Pain is felt concurrent with tissue resistance or stretch of the tissue.

Treatment procedures in this phase include ROM exercises, joint mobilization, and scar mobilization to produce a mobile scar. These interventions are most effective during this stage of healing. Gentle resistance may be applied to maintain mobility and strength of the musculotendinous unit.

BUILDING BLOCK 11-1

A 72-year-old woman with a history of left knee osteoarthritis experienced an increase in symptoms after a day of walking for the Relay for Life 3 days ago. She reports pain averaging a 4 to 5 on a 0 to 10 scale during weight bearing, moderate swelling, and difficulty negotiating the stairs in her home. She is retired, but is an avid walker and enjoys weightlifting. Provide this patient with intervention strategies for this phase of treatment.

BUILDING BLOCK 11-2

Progress the 72-year-old patient from Building Block 11-1 to the next rehabilitation phase. Assume expected progress during the first phase.

In bone, this phase is referred to as the callus phase. Osteoclasts perform a function analogous to the macrophages in soft tissue. These cells debride the fracture ends and prepare the area for healing. The infrastructure for healing is assembled, including a capillary structure supporting callus formation. This callus bridges the gap between the fracture ends. The callus is an unorganized scaffold of cartilage that is easily deformed. Although the bone repair is relatively weak at this point, limited activity is allowed. This loading promotes remodeling and maturation.

Treatment goals focus on applying light loads that will provide a stimulus for the tissue to remodel. Keep these loads within the tolerance of the newly formed tissue by monitoring signs and symptoms closely. Any increase in pain, warmth, or edema is a signal that the loads are exceeding tissue capabilities. Loads can be in the form of stretching, joint mobilization, ROM activities, or weight bearing.

Remodeling and Maturation

As healing progresses to the third phase, the remodeling stage, a shift is made to the deposition of type I collagen. This phase is characterized by decreased synthetic activity and cellularity, with increased organization of extracellular matrix. The collagen continues to increase and begins to organize into randomly placed fibrils with stronger covalent bonds. At this point, tension becomes important in providing orientation guidance to the organizing collagen. The new collagen must orient and align along the lines of stress to best accommodate the functional loads required. This tension can be imposed by stretching, active contraction (in the case of the musculotendinous unit), resistive loads, or electrical stimulation. Active tissue remodeling occurs throughout this phase up until approximately 4 months postinjury. The final end point is unknown and the tissue will continue to remodel and mature for 1 to 2 years postinjury. Although patients are discharged from formal rehabilitation by the time they reach the maturation phase, it is important for them to continue their rehabilitation exercises. The tissue will continue to mature according to the stresses placed upon it, even following completion of formal rehabilitation.

As with the remodeling-maturation phase in soft tissues, loading is important in the final phase of bone healing. In this phase of bone healing, woven bone (i.e., immature bone) is replaced by well-organized lamellar bone.[3] Normal loading is necessary to remodel the bone in accordance to the stresses that it will bear (i.e., Wolff's Law). The linkage of electrical charges with mechanical loading is called the piezoelectric effect.[3] Piezoelectric effects in the calcium hydroxyapatite crystals resulting from loads orient the crystals along the lines of stress. In long, weight-bearing bones, activity differs on the concave and convex sides. On the concave side, osteoblasts lay down more bone where the bone is subject to compression (i.e., negative charge). On the convex side, osteoclasts digest bone that is subject to tension (i.e., positive charge). Imposition of normal functional loads is necessary for the final remodeling of bone. Electrical stimulation is used to enhance bone healing using the same piezoelectric effect.

PRINCIPLES OF TREATING CONNECTIVE TISSUE INJURIES

A variety of procedures are available to achieve physical therapy goals. Although detailing every situation the clinician may encounter is difficult, specific principles guide the decision-making process. These principles provide a framework and rationale for intervention choices.

Restoration of Normal Tissue Relationships

After connective tissue injury, the relationships of a variety of tissues are altered. After injury or immobilization, the tendon may fail to glide smoothly through the tendon sheath, the nerve may be adhered to surrounding tissues, folds of joint capsule may become adhered to one another, the skin may bind to underlying tissues, or fascial layers may fail to glide on one another. These normal relationships must be restored, or painful and restricted movement may result. Interventions such as active muscle contraction, passive joint motion or mobilization, modality use, or massage restore those relationships. Begin these preventive interventions as early as the healing process allows, often within the first 48 hours. Additionally, the normal length-tension relationship of the muscle must be recovered to ensure optimal function. Muscles damaged by contusion, disrupted by surgical procedures, or placed in a shortened position during immobilization are susceptible to these alterations. Use stretching techniques to restore the normal length-tension properties. For example, the Achilles tendon should be stretched regularly while a patient recovers from an ankle sprain or fracture.

Optimal Loading

After a connective tissue injury, a cascade of events facilitate the body's healing process. If this cascade is interrupted, healing is disrupted and chronic inflammation may ensue. During each of the healing phases, choose treatment procedures that aid the healing process without disrupting the normal chain of events. This requires optimal loading or choosing a level of loading that neither overloads nor underloads the healing tissue (Fig. 11-6). Effective application of optimal loads requires a thorough understanding of the mechanism of injured tissue loading, including which planes of movement place the greatest loads on the healing tissue.

BUILDING BLOCK 11-3

While it may be obvious that the mobility of tissues adjacent to the injured area should be mobilized, what about tissues more directly involved in the injury? For example, following a lateral ankle sprain, should the peroneal muscles be mobilized? Why or why not?

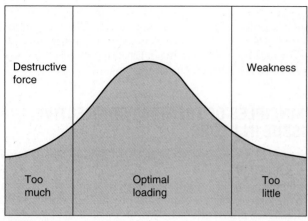

FIGURE 11-6. Optimal loading. Choose a load that neither overloads nor underloads the tissue of interest. (From Porterfield JA, DeRosa C. Mechanical Low Back Pain. Philadelphia, PA: WB Saunders, 1991:13.)

Consider the biomechanical effects of daily activities and therapeutic activities in the context of the stage of healing, and individual factors such as age, quality of the tissue, nutritional status, and fitness level. A stress that underloads a tissue in the remodeling phase probably overloads the tissue in the inflammatory phase. (Review Table 5-5 and Fig. 5-17.) An exercise that underloads a young athlete after an acute fracture would probably overload an elderly individual after a pathologic fracture. The medial collateral ligament (MCL) of the knee is loaded most in the frontal plane, with the knee near terminal extension. Avoid activities that load the knee in the frontal plane near full knee extension during the acute phase. However, in the late phases, when remodeling of the ligament is necessary, frontal plane loading is precisely the stimulus needed. Designing the treatment program requires consideration of all of the factors in the intervention model within the injury framework (see Patient-Related Instruction 11-2: Signs of Overload).

Specific Adaptations to Imposed Demands

Although the concept of optimal loading guides the *quantity* of activity (e.g., volume, intensity), the specific adaptations to imposed demands (SAID) principle expands to include the *type* of activity chosen. The SAID principle is an extension of Wolff's Law, which states that a bone remodels according to

Patient-Related Instruction 11-2
Signs of Overload

The following signs and symptoms suggest that exercise or activity is too much and should be decreased or modified:

1. Increased pain that does not resolve within the next 12 hours
2. Pain that is increased over the previous session or comes on earlier in the exercise session
3. Increased swelling, warmth, or redness in the injury area
4. Decreased ability to use the part

BUILDING BLOCK 11-4

A 26-year-old recreational soccer player sustained a second degree MCL sprain 8 weeks ago and is preparing to return to soccer. Design a late phase exercise program that would prepare this athlete to return to soccer. Assume full ROM and strength within 10% of the opposite leg.

the stresses that are placed on it. The SAID principle implies that soft tissues remodel according to the stresses imposed on them. Exercise is specific to the posture, mode, movement, exercise type, environment, and intensity used. For example, an exercise may be chosen to prepare the quadriceps muscle for weight bearing. The quadriceps muscle contracts eccentrically in a closed chain through the first 15 degrees of knee flexion during the loading response of gait. A closed chain eccentric quadriceps exercise such as a short-arc (0 to 15 degrees) leg press is a better choice than concentric isokinetic exercise. This is an example of the SAID principle guiding the activity choice.

The SAID principle also guides exercise prescription parameters. For example, in the late stage of healing, a patient returning to tennis should increase the speed and intensity of exercise, whereas the patient returning to marathon training should increase the exercise duration. When the stage of healing and optimal loading parameters allow, training should as closely as possible reflect the specific demands of the patient's functional task.

Prevention of Complications

Be sure to consider the effects of the connective tissue injury on surrounding tissues. For example, immobilization imposed while a fracture is healing is unhealthy for the joint's articular cartilage, ligaments, and surrounding musculature, although it is necessary for bone repair. Muscle atrophy and weakening of the immobilized ligaments ensue during the immobilization period. Use any available interventions that might minimize these effects. For example, electrical stimulation or isometric muscle contractions can be used to retard strength losses in the muscle, tendon, and tendon insertion sites. Active muscle contractions also prevent thrombus formation after surgery. ROM exercises at joints above and below injury sites may preserve some soft-tissue relationships and prevent loss of mobility. Weight bearing loads the articular cartilage and lessens degradation caused by immobilization.

MANAGEMENT OF IMPAIRMENTS ASSOCIATED WITH CONNECTIVE TISSUE DYSFUNCTION

Patients with acute soft-tissue injuries such as sprains and strains are commonly treated by physical therapy clinicians. Management of these injuries is discussed together because of the many similarities, and any differences are highlighted.

Sprain: Injury to Ligament and Capsule

A sprain can be defined as an acute injury to a ligament or joint capsule without dislocation. Sprains occur when a joint is extended beyond its normal limit, and the ligament or capsule tissues are stretched or torn beyond their limit. Sprains are common at the ankle (i.e., anterior talofibular and calcaneofibular ligaments), knee (i.e., medial and lateral collateral ligaments, anterior [ACL] and posterior cruciate ligaments [PCL]), wrist, and spine. A sprain may resolve with short-term immobilization, controlled activity, and rehabilitative exercises, but other sprains may require surgery to stabilize the joint.

Sprain Classification

Sprain severity occurs along a continuum from microscopic tearing and stretching of ligament or capsule fibers to complete disruption of the ligament. Sprains are classified by severity based on clinical examination or special testing (e.g., magnetic resonance imaging, arthrometer testing). Grade I sprains are mild sprains in which the ligament is stretched, but there is no discontinuity of the ligament. A grade II sprain is a moderate sprain in which some fibers are stretched and some fibers are torn. This produces some laxity at the joint. A grade III, or severe sprain, is a complete or nearly complete ligament disruption with resultant laxity (Table 11-2).

Examination and Evaluation Findings

Examination findings following a ligament sprain include ecchymosis and edema. Functional mobility losses include the mobility of a single joint (ICF b7100), the mobility of several joints (ICF b7101), or the loss of stability of a single (ICF b7150) or multiple (ICF b7151) joints. Additionally, muscle performance or power functions are typically decreased. When sprains occur in the lower extremity, gait pattern functions are impaired, and when the upper extremity is involved, functional reach and the ability to hold and manipulate objects may be impaired. Sprains of the spine can impact many aspects of functional mobility such as self-care, home and community mobility, and work. Joints proximal and distal to the primary joint injury may have associated injuries or compensation. Determine activity limitations and identify the relationship between impairments and those activity limitations.

TABLE 11-2	Classification of Sprain	
GRADE	**DESCRIPTION**	**CHARACTERISTICS**
I	Mild	Fibers are stretched without loss of continuity
II	Moderate	Some fibers are stretched and some are torn. Some laxity observed on examination
III	Severe	Ligament completely or nearly completely torn; laxity results.

From American Academy of Orthopaedic Surgeons. Athletic Training and Sports Medicine. Park Ridge, IL: American Academy of Orthopaedic Surgeons, 1991.

Strain: Musculotendinous Injury

A strain is an acute injury to the muscle or tendon from an abrupt or excessive muscle contraction. Strains are usually the result of a quick overload to the muscle-tendon unit in which the tension generated exceeds the tissue's capacity. Strains occur when a contracting muscle is excessively or abruptly stretched in the opposite direction. The person who reaches quickly to catch a falling object or the individual who suddenly stops or changes direction when walking or running is susceptible to a muscle strain. Overuse injuries are another type of muscle strain.

Strain injuries are difficult to classify and can be graded as mild, moderate, or severe based on clinical examination findings such as pain, edema, loss of motion, and tenderness. Muscle strains can be complete or incomplete, although complete tears are less common.

Most strain injuries occur at the myotendinous junction.[15] Structural features of the sarcomeres and connective tissues in this area suggest that load transmission occurs across the musculotendinous junction. As with many other structures in the body, transitions from one tissue type to another are areas of increased stress and risk of injury. In this case, the transition zone from contractile to noncontractile tissue creates an area of increased stress that is susceptible to injury. Factors that may contribute to muscle strain injuries include poor flexibility, inadequate warm-up exercise, insufficient strength or endurance, training errors, and poor coordination.[15]

Examination and Evaluation Findings

A history of an abrupt decelerating movement, change of direction, or quick stretch suggests a muscle strain injury. The musculotendinous junction or the muscle belly may be painful. Pain in the injured muscle is reproduced clinically by active or resistive contraction of the muscle and by stretching it. For example, a quadriceps strain is reproduced by stretching the knee into flexion and by resisting active knee extension. The muscle may need to be put on stretch during the active or resistive muscle contraction to stress the lesion. Occasionally, localized swelling and warmth may be observed.

Application of Treatment Principles

Although each intervention program should be directed toward the specific impairments, activity limitations, and goals for each patient, some general guidelines can help the clinician make informed choices that will maximize recovery and return to function.

Inflammatory Phase

Treatment principles in the early phase include optimal loading and prevention of secondary complications. As the inflammatory response initiates the healing response, an environment conducive to healing must be established. The appropriate balance of rest and loading ensures loads within the optimal loading zone for the patient's age, medical condition, and injury severity. Overload may perpetuate bleeding or the inflammatory response beyond its useful purpose, and underload may result in complications such as motion loss, scar tissue adhesions, or ectopic ossification.

Modality use in this phase usually includes cryotherapy and compression with elevation to decrease bleeding and

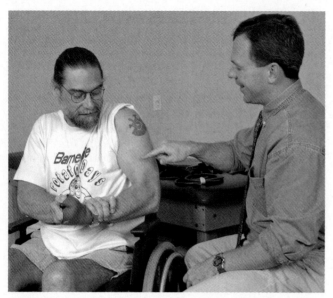

FIGURE 11-7. Clinician instructing patient on isometric biceps curl.

BUILDING BLOCK 11-5

A 63-year-old woman sprained her left knee 4 days ago when she slipped on the ice. She sustained first degree sprains of her MCL, joint capsule, and ACL. Due to underlying arthritis, her swelling and functional instability were significant. She has a 2+ effusion, is unable to fully bear weight on the left, has limited ROM and poor quadriceps function. Provide a list of goals and interventions for the first phase.

swelling. Most injuries allow passive or active ROM in a pain-free range, although exercise may be contraindicated in some severe cases. Isometric muscle contraction, in the absence of moderate or severe muscle strains, can lessen atrophy and serve as a learning activity, reminding the patient how to contract involved muscles (Fig. 11-7). Because the muscle is the primary tissue involved in a strain, active muscle contraction capability may be limited or reduced significantly. When treating lower extremity injuries, assistive devices, immobilizers, and weight-bearing restrictions can maintain tissue loading within the optimal loading zone. Treatments that impose rest or restriction must be balanced with activity that offsets the negative effects of immobility (see Selected Intervention 11-1: Isometric Ankle Eversion for the Patient After Ligament Reconstruction).

Getting the correct dosage is the greatest challenge. No standards exist to provide the clinician with precise frequency, intensity, and duration of exercise. This is one reason why the intensity of services is greater in the early phase of rehabilitation. More frequent contact with the clinician can ensure that the exercise dosage is appropriate for the patient's current physical condition. The rehabilitation program is modified as changes occur.

Proliferative/Fibroplasia Phase

As healing progresses to the proliferative phase, treatment principles focus on restoration of normal tissue relationships, optimal loading, and prevention of complications. Complications in this phase may result from changes in movement patterns to accommodate pain, weakness, or motion loss. These movement pattern changes can create excessive

---

SELECTED INTERVENTION 11-1
Isometric Ankle Eversion for the Patient After Ligament Reconstruction

See Case Study No. 1.

Although this patient requires comprehensive intervention as described in the patient management model, one specific exercise is described.

ACTIVITY: Isometric ankle eversion

PURPOSE: Increased ability to produce torque in the peroneal muscles without excessively loading the acutely injured tissue

RISK FACTORS: No appreciable risk factors

ELEMENTS OF THE MOVEMENT SYSTEM: Base

STAGE OF MOTOR CONTROL: Mobility

POSTURE: Any comfortable position such as sitting or supine. The lateral border of the foot is stabilized against a stationary object.

MOVEMENT: Patient performs an isometric ankle eversion contraction against a stationary object.

SPECIAL CONSIDERATIONS: Ensure that muscle contraction is at a submaximal level during the acute phase. Maximal muscle contraction can overload recently injured tissues. Be

sure eversion is not substituted with tibial external rotation, hip abduction, or external rotation.

DOSAGE

TYPE OF MUSCLE CONTRACTION: Isometric

Intensity: Submaximal
Duration: To fatigue, pain, or 20 repetitions
Frequency: Hourly or as frequently as possible during the day
Environment: Home

RATIONALE FOR EXERCISE CHOICE: This exercise was chosen to begin retraining the peroneal muscles. Isotonic exercises can overload the muscle in the acute phase, but submaximal isometric contraction maintains loading within the optimal loading zone. Gentle isometric activation "reminds" the muscle how to contract, providing a foundation for further strengthening in later phases.

EXERCISE MODIFICATION OR GRADATION: As healing progresses, isometric contractions may be performed at multiple angles. Isometric contractions should be progressed to isotonic exercise through a ROM. Closed chain exercise should be incorporated as weight bearing allows.

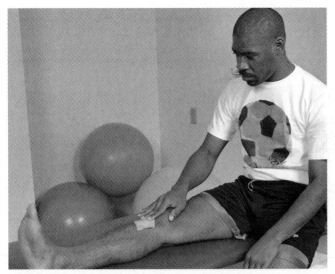

FIGURE 11-8. Scar mobilization performed by the patient.

loads on uninjured tissues that can become painful. These changes also become habitual and can be difficult to correct. Examples of these habits are hiking the shoulder (i.e., scapular elevation) during forward reaching and ambulating with a flexed knee. Faulty movement patterns are deleterious for the long-term health of the joint and should be corrected as quickly as possible.

Restoration of normal tissue relationships can prevent these faulty movement patterns by reestablishing joint ROM and muscle length. As healing occurs, connective tissue tends to shorten. Manual therapy, including joint mobilization techniques, stretching, and massage techniques, as well as postural education exercises, can facilitate restoration of these relationships. Connective tissue massage performed by the patient can increase scar tissue mobility (Fig. 11-8). This type of self-management increases the activity dosage to a level that can impact outcomes. Muscle contraction of the muscle opposing the short muscle is an active stretching technique that can restore normal tissue relationships (Fig. 11-9).

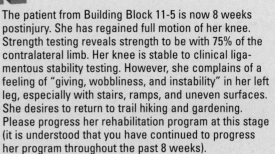

BUILDING BLOCK 11-6

The patient from Building Block 11-5 is now 8 weeks postinjury. She has regained full motion of her knee. Strength testing reveals strength to be with 75% of the contralateral limb. Her knee is stable to clinical ligamentous stability testing. However, she complains of a feeling of "giving, wobbliness, and instability" in her left leg, especially with stairs, ramps, and uneven surfaces. She desires to return to trail hiking and gardening. Please progress her rehabilitation program at this stage (it is understood that you have continued to progress her program throughout the past 8 weeks).

Optimal loading concepts provide the framework for exercise parameters. Understanding the effects of muscle contraction and the location and direction of loading on the healing tissue is fundamental to optimally loading the tissue. Loading is important in the repair-regeneration phase, because loads help orient newly forming collagen fibrils along the lines of stress. Excessive loading disrupts the healing process, and underloading results in randomly organized collagen. Weight bearing, active and resistive mobility activities, massage, and functional movement patterns can provide these loads. It is the clinician's charge, along with input from the patient, to prioritize these activities to close the gap between current and desired functional performance. By the end of this phase, mobility and a strength base should be established.

Remodeling and Maturation Phase

As the patient returns to activity, the guiding principles are optimal loading and SAID. The type and magnitude of loads encountered in the patient's daily routine, including work and leisure activities, determine the specific interventions chosen (Fig. 11-10). The goal in the final phase is to "fine-tune" or convert the baseline strength and mobility into functional movement patterns and activities that address the patient's activity limitations and participation restrictions. The exercises

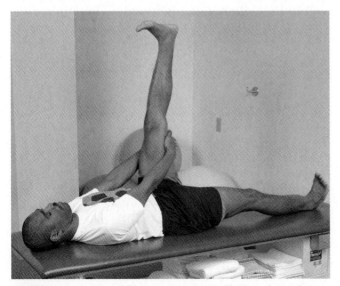

FIGURE 11-9. Active quadriceps contraction facilitating a hamstring stretch.

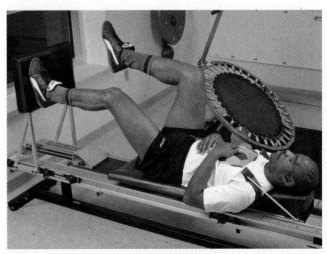

FIGURE 11-10. Example of impact loading in a horizontal position as a transitional activity between strengthening and impact loading in a vertical position.

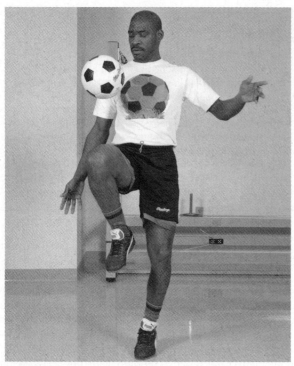

FIGURE 11-11. A soccer drill performed by a soccer coach is an example of a graded, progressive study.

generally consist of more whole-body patterns and functional activities related to the patient's lifestyle. At the same time, consider the status of healing tissue and the loads placed on it as you choose activities. For example, repeatedly throwing a fastball on a repaired elbow MCL excessively loads the repair at this point. A graded, progressive functional exercise is necessary to resume activities with such loads (Fig. 11-11). In the final phase, the patient should be instructed in a comprehensive home program to ensure continued maturation of the tissue according to the patient-specific loads.

Tendinopathy

Tendon failure can occur as a result of macrotrauma or microtrauma. Tendons are able to withstand high loads, but if these loads become repetitive, injury may result. Injury occurs on a microscopic or macroscopic level, with damage to the structural proteins and the blood supply. Adequate recovery and healing time must be allowed or tendinopathy will develop. As the understanding of tendon disorders has progressed, new classification schemes of tendon injury have been developed. In addition to the global categories of acute and chronic, tendon injuries have been subclassified as paratenonitis, tendinosis, tendinitis, and paratenonitis with tendinosis.[16] Each of these subcategories has treatment ramifications. Although tendon injuries are discussed in the context of connective tissue injuries, some of these injuries may be more suitably treated in a localized inflammation pattern. This will vary with classification. However, all tendon injuries will be discussed together for simplicity.

Classification of Tendon Injuries

Tendon injury can be classified by etiology (macrotrauma, microtrauma), by duration (acute, chronic), or by presumed histopathology (tendinitis, paratenonitis, tendinosis).

Tendinopathy is a global term for tendon disorders without presumptions about histopathology, duration, or etiology. Historically, the most common term for tendon injury was "tendinitis," implying inflammation.[17] (Rees) More recently, the term "tendinosis" is used as a histological description of degenerative tendon without inflammation. Examination of tissue with chronic tendinopathy has found little evidence of inflammation.

Tendon may be injured by acute macrotrama, such as landing from a jump, or microtrauma, such as the trauma associated with repetitive uphill walking. Acute macrotraumatic injuries occur as a result of a sudden contraction, often decelerating in nature, and they are followed by a lengthy but predictable outcome.[16] Loads during normal activities generally do not exceed 25% of the tendon's ultimate tensile strength.[18,19] However, loads during high-level activities, such as kicking, have been found to exceed this average level. For example, loads estimated in a weight lifter at the time of patellar tendon rupture were 17 times body weight.[20] Most acute injuries occur at the musculotendinous junction and result in a profound inflammatory reaction.[21] This reaction initiates the phases of healing outlined previously.

Microtrauma, or repetitive loads without adequate recovery time, can also result in injury to the tendon. Paratenonitis is an inflammation of the outer layer of the tendon (i.e., paratenon), whether lined with synovium or not.[16,22] Histologically, inflammatory cells are found in the paratenon or peritendinous areolar tissues, and, clinically, the cardinal signs of inflammation such as pain, crepitation, swelling, and palpable tenderness occur. Treatment procedures, including anti-inflammatory measures, are indicated.

Tendinosis is an intratendinous degeneration without an inflammatory response.[17,23,24] It is generally caused by atrophy from aging, microtrauma, or vascular trauma. Histologic findings include fiber disorientation, hypocellularity, scattered vascular ingrowth, and occasional necrosis or calcification.[16,22] Because there is no inflammatory response, none of the cardinal signs of inflammation are present, and anti-inflammatory measures are ineffective. A nodule may be palpable but nontender. Tendinosis may also occur with paratenonitis, in which paratenon inflammation accompanies intratendinous degeneration. Symptoms in this case may be confusing, combining signs of inflammation with a chronic degenerative tendon. Histologically, scattered vascular ingrowth may be present, although no true intratendinous inflammation exists. Areas of neovascularity are evident in both Doppler studies and ultrasound.[17,24] Degenerative Achilles tendons show high blood vessel density compared with healthy tendons.

The term *tendinitis* is used to describe an acute inflammatory process, usually the result of overuse in a young individual. Histologically, tendinitis is classified into three subgroups, each with different findings, from purely inflammation to inflammation superimposed on preexisting degeneration to calcification and tendinosis changes in chronic conditions. The symptoms in this group are proportional to the vascular disruption or atrophy and can be inflammatory, depending on the duration (Table 11-3).

Examination and Evaluation

History and subjective symptoms are of primary importance because of the differences in classification and treatment. The events leading up to the onset of pain in the chronic case are significant in that the predisposing factors may be identified and modified. Training errors, inappropriate equipment,

TABLE 11-3 **Classification Terminology of Tendon Injury**				
NEW	**OLD**	**DEFINITION**	**HISTOLOGIC FINDINGS**	**CLINICAL SIGNS AND SYMPTOMS**
Paratenonitis	Tenosynovitis, tenovaginitis, peritendinitis	An inflammation of only the paratenon, lined by synovium or not	Inflammatory cells in paratenon or peritendinous areolar tissue	Cardinal inflammatory signs: swelling, pain, crepitus, local tenderness, warmth, dysfunction
Paratenonitis with tendinosis	Tendinitis	Paratenon inflammation associated with intratendinosis degeneration	Same as above, with loss of tendon collagen, fiber disorientation, scattered vascular ingrowth, but no prominent intratendinous inflammation	Same as above, with often palpable tendon nodule, swelling, and inflammatory signs
Tendinosis	Tendinitis	Intratendinous degeneration resulting from atrophy (aging, microtrauma, vascular compromise)	Noninflammatory intratendinous collagen degeneration with fiber disorientation, hypocellularity, scattered vascular ingrowth, occasional local necrosis, or calcification	Often palpable tendon nodule that is asymptomatic; no swelling of tendon sheath
Tendinitis	Tendon strain or tear	Symptomatic degeneration of the tendon with vascular disruption and inflammatory repair response	Three recognized subgroups; each displays variable histology, from pure inflammation to inflammation superimposed on preexisting degeneration in chronic conditions: (1) acute, (2) subacute, (3) chronic	Symptoms are inflammatory and proportional to vascular disruption, hematoma, or atrophy-related cell necrosis. Symptom duration defines each group: (1) <2 weeks, (2) 4–6 weeks, (3) 6 weeks

From American Academy of Orthopaedic Surgeons. Athletic Training and Sports Medicine. Park Ridge, IL: American Academy of Orthopaedic, 1991.

environmental factors, excessive fatigue, or an apparently small injury without adequate recovery can precipitate tendon injury. Work or training restrictions or modification of the home or work environment may be necessary to give the body an adequate opportunity for recovery (Fig. 11-12).

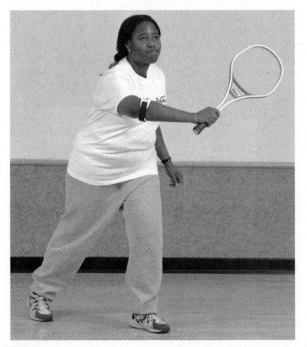

FIGURE 11-12. A tennis elbow strap can be used to decrease loads on the wrist extensor musculature during drills.

Treatment Principles and Procedures

Treatment of tendinopathies is based on the specific tendon injury, framed within the context of the tendon's role in function. Restoring the tendon to optimal length, cellularity, and ability to withstand loads is fundamental to complete rehabilitation. The optimal loading zone is the foundation principle for choosing loading techniques. Educate the patient about outside activities that maximize symptom resolution and minimize harmful effects. Rehabilitation should be of appropriate intensity, frequency, and duration such that, when combined with essential activities of daily living, it keeps loading within the optimal loading zone.

Anti-inflammatory measures are helpful when inflammation is a component of the tendinopathy. If you are treating inflammation as the primary problem, the injury may be treated in the localized inflammation practice pattern. Physical agents such as ultrasound and cold packs, as well as electrotherapeutic modalities such as electrical muscle stimulation and iontophoresis, can reduce inflammation. Use other physical agents or modalities as necessary to reduce the pain associated with inflammation, allowing greater participation in the therapeutic exercise program.

Incorporate stretching if muscle length is inadequate for the demands placed on the musculotendinous unit. In cases of recovery from an acute tendon injury, stretching is critical for restoring the normal length of the tissue. Moreover, in the early stages, stretching is a stimulus for the proper alignment of healing collagen. In healing tissue, gentle stretching to provide a stimulus for fiber orientation without disruption of the immature collagen facilitates the remodeling process. In the chronic tendon injury, stretching increases the tissue's resting length, allowing loading through a greater range and force dispersion over a larger surface area. Changes in resting length may affect the muscle spindle, altering its sensitivity and resultant muscle stiffness. As with resistive exercise, stretching should be prescribed according to intensity, frequency, and duration parameters. Too often, these prescriptive factors are neglected, leading to overload. For example, patients often believe that a strong stretching sensation is necessary to adequately stretch the muscle. However, a strong stretch can be just as damaging to an injured muscle-tendon unit as too much resistance. Patients should feel a "low" to "medium" stretching sensation during the stretch, without an increase in symptoms after the stretching session.

Progressive resistive exercises are a key component of the intervention program. Eccentric muscle contractions have been implicated in the development of tendinopathies.[25–28] Eccentric contractions allow the series elastic component (SEC) to contribute to force production. Tendon forms part of the SEC.[9] Other connective tissue proteins in parallel with the muscle fiber also contribute to force production. Eccentric contractions usually precede concentric contractions in activities such as jumping, allowing the SEC to contribute to force production. The force generated in the tissue during eccentric contractions depends on the velocity of the stretch, the distance moved, and the amount of load placed on the tissue (e.g., body weight, external loads). These parameters are used in the rehabilitation of tendon injuries.

Curwin and Stanish[9] outlined a progressive resistive exercise program in an attempt to strengthen the tendon tissue. Because eccentric muscle contractions allow the SEC to contribute to force production and because eccentric muscle contractions are frequently associated with the development of tendinopathies, this muscle contraction type is emphasized. Before an effective eccentric contraction can be performed, the individual must first be able to isometrically hold at the starting position. Thus, the first appropriate resistive exercise may be a submaximal isometric contraction. As the individual progresses, an eccentric program is initiated, with a progression of speed built into the program. The resistive eccentric program is performed slowly for the first 2 days, progressed to a moderate speed for 3 days, and then to a fast speed for 2 days. The resistance is then increased, and the speed progression instituted again. This program is easily performed at home, and intensity, frequency, and duration are clearly outlined to prevent overload (Fig. 11-13). Be sure to begin and end each session with stretching.

Others have advocated for a more aggressive eccentric training program.[25,27,29,30] This type of training has been studied in the Achilles and patellar tendons using high loads and decline boards. The subjects were asked to train at pain levels between 4 and 5 on a 0 to 10 scale (10 = highest pain imaginable).[25] Weight was added to the protocol when pain dropped below 3 on a 0 to 10 scale. This type of heavy load eccentric program has been successful in treating chronic Achilles and patellar tendinopathy, and has been more successful than programs using concentric contractions.[25,28–30] It is theorized that eccentric training interferes with the neovascularization apparent in chronic tendinosis, in a manner similar to that of sclerosing injections.[27,29,30] As with any soft-tissue injury, rehabilitation activities must mimic the demands placed on those tissues on return to activity. The prescription parameters are framed around the functional outcome. For the individual returning to a work, leisure, or

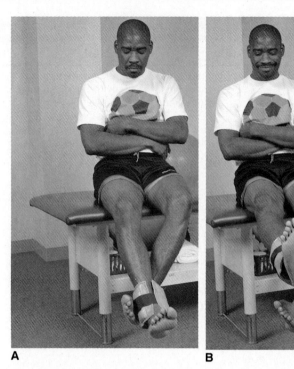

Figure 11-13. Eccentric quadriceps work with an ankle weight is performed by the patient. (A) Uninvolved leg lifts the relaxed involved leg. (B) Uninvolved leg is then lowered eccentrically by the involved leg.

home environment that places him or her at risk for reinjury, appropriate modifications to the environment or to the individual (e.g., technique, adaptive or supportive devices) must be made as part of the prevention and long-term care program.

Articular Cartilage Injury

Articular cartilage injury can lead to both short-term and long-term activity limitations and participation restrictions. The pain associated with damage to the articular cartilage can impact a person's ability to stand, sit, walk, or perform other important functional tasks necessary for self-care or employment. Damage to the articular cartilage can occur from mechanical injury or from other nonmechanical trauma. Nonmechanical traumas include infection, inflammatory conditions, or prolonged joint immobilization and can result in loss of proteoglycans. Proteoglycan degradation or suppression of synthesis from these conditions results in articular cartilage damage that may be irreversible. Mechanical damage to the articular cartilage (i.e., chondral injury) or to the articular cartilage and underlying bone (i.e., osteochondral injury) can happen as a result of blunt trauma, frictional abrasion, or excessive weight-bearing forces.[31] For example, knee hyperextension injuries or ankle rotational injuries can result in chondral or osteochondral injuries and ligamentous injuries. Excessive weight bearing and joint compression combined with rotation produce high shear forces on the articular cartilage, resulting in chondral or osteochondral injury.

In addition to the mechanism of injury, articular cartilage damage is also classified by size and depth. While more complex grading system exists, a simple classification describes whether it is partial or full thickness and the width of the lesion. Other important information includes the status of the joint surface and the location of the lesion. All of these factors (depth and diameter, articular surface and lesion location) have implications for prognosis and treatment.

Articular cartilage has a poor healing response. In adults, the tidemark prevents the underlying bony vascular supply from providing nutrition to the articular cartilage. The articular cartilage receives its nutrition by diffusion of synovial fluid. Therefore, chondral injuries that do not penetrate the underlying subchondral bone will lack sufficient blood supply to effect a healing response. While these injuries may not heal in adults, they may not worsen in the presence of loading that stays within the patient's optimal loading zone. This requires education and guidance through an appropriate rehabilitation program.

Examination and Evaluation

Important clinical information relative to rehabilitation includes the cause of the damage (i.e., mechanical or nonmechanical), area of damage (e.g., weight-bearing surface), classification of damage, and other factors that may affect health of the articular cartilage, such as general health, lifestyle factors, body weight, joint alignment, and stability. If surgery was performed, the status of the articular cartilage and the associated soft tissues should be available in the chart. Patient goals should be determined and a realistic prognosis determined based on available information. For example, an individual with an articular cartilage lesion on the weight-bearing surface of the medial femoral condyle in a varus-aligned ACL-deficient knee will have difficulty when returning to high-demand activities.

Other assessment procedures of merit include posture, ROM, muscle performance, and joint integrity and mobility examinations. Assessment of swelling and pain influences intervention choices and progression of the treatment program. A swollen and sore knee indicates that the joint is inflamed, which is unhealthy for the articular cartilage. Resolution of the swelling and inflammation as quickly as possible is imperative for the joint's health.

Treatment Principles

Minimum requirements for healthy articular cartilage are freedom of motion, equitable load distribution, and stability.[32] Beyond this, issues such as appropriate body weight, efficiency of movement to minimize joint loads, and avoiding overload are important in long-term joint health. Exercise is healthy for joints; joint motion and alternating joint loading and unloading (compressive forces) provide articular cartilage nutrition.[33] This nutrition is achieved by diffusion of synovial fluid across the joint surface. When joints are immobile or held in a single position for long periods of time (such as sleeping or riding in a car), stiffness and pain ensue due to lack of joint surface nutrition. Therefore, use a period of "preconditioning" or warm-up at the beginning of an exercise session or after periods of rest. Gentle muscle tightening exercises or ROM activities serve as good preconditioning exercises for people with articular cartilage injury.

Initiate treatment focused on restoration of motion as a primary goal. The aggressiveness of other interventions such as muscle performance exercises and progressive weight bearing is dictated by the other factors and the medical treatment. The articular cartilage has a better chance of recovery after injury or surgery when the loads across the recovering joint surface are controlled and progressed as healing occurs. Optimal recovery is more likely to take place in the presence of equal load distribution (i.e., medial and lateral compartments in the knee) and joint stability. For example, a knee with significant varus or valgus alignment excessively loads the medial and lateral compartments, respectively. This loading is the rationale for tibial osteotomy procedures, which attempt to balance load distribution medially and laterally. An unstable knee (anterior or posterior cruciate deficient) also places greater loads on the articular cartilage, and rehabilitation after articular cartilage injury or surgery in an unstable knee must proceed cautiously. A patient with Ehlers-Danlos syndrome will have more difficulty recovering from an acute facet joint injury than a patient without this connective tissue disease.

Restoration of motion in a compromised joint allows loads to be distributed across a greater joint surface area, decreasing peak focal loads. Mobility activities enhance fluid dynamics in the joint, assisting with lubrication and nutrition of the joint. Active and passive ROM activities are important for the recovery of articular cartilage lesions.

In addition to the restoration of motion, normalization of gait and increased muscle performance decrease loads on the articular cartilage.[34] Effective eccentric muscle forces during the loading response of gait can minimize articular cartilage and subchondral bone loads at the tibiofemoral joint. Strengthening activities play an important role in the protection of articular cartilage. Muscle performance exercises must be performed at a dosage that minimizes shear forces and maintains compressive forces within the tissue tolerance. Little empirical clinical evidence exists to provide guidance in program design.[34] Guidelines are generally a compilation of basic science, animal studies, biomechanics, and expert opinion.

Consider alternative exercise modes for patients with articular cartilage injuries of the lower extremity. Clinical research has shown the effectiveness of aquatic rehabilitation for persons with knee arthritis.[35] Water-based programs have shown significant reductions in pain and improvements in strength function in patients with knee and/or hip arthritis.[36–39] Compliance rates were 84% for water therapy and 75% for land therapy. Patients frequently report that pain is lower with exercise in the water compared with exercise on land.[38] Continued participation following the conclusion of formal rehabilitation is also common following aquatic therapy, theoretically maintaining gains achieved in therapy.[40,41] The results reinforce the notion that patients can improve strength and function effectively in either a land or aquatic environment. The key is the ability to provide a comprehensive program, whether on land, in the water, or some combination of both.

MANAGEMENT OF IMPAIRMENTS ASSOCIATED WITH LOCALIZED INFLAMMATION

Contusion

A contusion occurs as the result of a blow and can occur in any area of the body to a variety of tissues. No break in the skin occurs, although blood vessels below the skin may be injured, causing ecchymosis in the area. If the damage is more extensive and large blood vessels in the area are disrupted, a localized area of blood may accumulate in deeper tissues, forming a hematoma. When a deep-tissue hematoma occurs, ecchymosis may or may not be seen on the skin surface. For example, quadriceps femoris contusions frequently result in hematoma formation. This hematoma is easily palpable within the muscle, but it is rarely accompanied by ecchymosis. The severity of this type of injury can be deceptive, and if left untreated, may progress to myositis ossificans. Myositis ossificans is the formation of heterotopic bone within the muscle. Bleeding in the area of the contusion initiates the inflammatory response and healing process.

Examination and Evaluation

The history of a blow provides the best information for evaluation of a contusion. The size, location, and direction of the blow provide the clinician with valuable clues about the location and extent of soft-tissue injuries. After observation and palpation of the area for localized swelling or hematoma, assess joint mobility, muscle performance, and flexibility and function. A diagnosis and prognosis based on the evaluation guide treatment procedures. Muscle contusions at risk for ectopic bone formation (e.g., quadriceps femoris, biceps brachii) are treated more cautiously than simple subcutaneous tissue contusions, and the evaluation process must clarify the extent of tissue involvement.

Treatment Principles

Simple contusions generally resolve in a timely manner without secondary complications or long-term consequences. However, this will be determined by the extent and location of the contusion. Be sure to consider the many layers of soft tissue comprising most injured areas. Contusions that occur in areas of high loads or poor blood supply may eventually result in a chronic inflammation. For example, a blow to the Achilles tendon may result in secondary Achilles tendinitis. Also, deep muscle contusions are at a high risk for long-term complications. Quadriceps contusions left untreated may result in myositis ossificans or ectopic bone formation within the muscle. This bone results in significant impairments such as loss of motion and muscle performance, as well as activity limitations relative to gait. These impairments and activity limitations can result in participation restrictions in those who are physically active as part of their lifestyle.

Treatment principles are therefore grounded in an understanding of the consequences of the specific contusion. ROM must be restored as quickly as possible, although in the case of a deep muscle contusion, aggressive mobility early on can increase bleeding. Thus, a balance must be struck between treating the impairments and causing further damage. In the case of a quadriceps contusion where the risk of myositis ossificans is high, this balance can be difficult. Use ice to control swelling and local inflammation as necessary. Use measures of pain, muscle length, and muscle performance to guide the aggressiveness of treatment for this condition. When these measures decline, the pace of the program is too aggressive, potentially causing further damage. Muscle performance measures must be restored, and these activities progressed to functional skills such as walking, stair climbing, and upper extremity work tasks. Submaximal isometric contractions can be safely initiated in the early phases, and these exercises progressed to more challenging muscle performance activities as healing progresses.

MANAGEMENT OF IMPAIRMENTS ASSOCIATED WITH FRACTURES

A fracture can be defined as a break in the continuity of the bone.[42] Most fractures are the result of an acute injury (i.e., macrotrauma), although stress fractures can occur as the result of microtrauma. Fractures are categorized by whether the skin is broken (i.e., open or closed), the amount of disruption (i.e., displaced or nondisplaced), and the type of fracture (e.g., greenstick, comminuted). The type and degree of force required to fracture a bone usually injures the surrounding soft tissue as well. Most fractures are treated in the practice pattern of impairments associated with fracture. However, patients undergoing surgical stabilization may be more appropriately treated in the bony and soft-tissue surgical procedures pattern. All fractures are discussed together for clarity.

Classification of Fractures

Classification is first determined by whether the fractured bone is protruding through the skin. Fractures breaking the skin surface are considered open fractures; those that do not break the skin are classified as closed fractures. The continuity of the ends of the fracture is then considered. If the bone on all sides of the fracture remains in anatomic alignment, the fracture is considered nondisplaced. Nondisplaced fractures are more difficult to diagnose and require special studies such as radiography to verify. Fractures in which the ends of the bones are not in anatomic alignment with each other are considered displaced fractures.

Fractures are described by the type of break or disruption (Fig. 11-14). A greenstick fracture is an incomplete fracture that occurs in children. It is so named because of its resemblance to a green stick or twig that partially breaks when bent. Epiphyseal fractures also occur in children and are fractures through the growth plate. Salter and Harris[43] subclassified epiphyseal fractures into five different types depending on

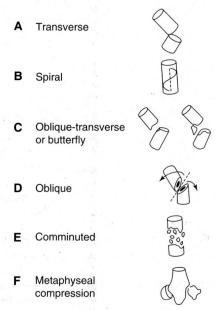

A Transverse

B Spiral

C Oblique-transverse or butterfly

D Oblique

E Comminuted

F Metaphyseal compression

FIGURE 11-14. Types of fractures. (A) Transverse, (B) Spiral, (C) Oblique-transverse or butterfly, (D) Oblique, (E) Comminuted, and (F) Metaphyseal fracture.

BUILDING BLOCK 11-7

A 65-old-female fell on the ice and sustained a proximal humeral fracture. She has mild osteoporosis. She was immobilized in a sling for 6 weeks and presents to physical therapy for a rehabilitation program. Which associated tissues should be considered and assessed at this point? Presume sufficient healing of the fracture.

the extent of fracture affecting the epiphysis and metaphysis. Children are also susceptible to avulsion fractures, in which a tendon or ligament is separated from its attachment by a small piece of bone. Because of the relative strength of the collagenous tissues compared with bone in this population, it is not uncommon to see young persons avulse structures such as ACLs or the proximal origin of the hamstring muscle from the bony attachments.

Comminuted fractures break into more than two fragments and are often the result of significant trauma, such as a fall or motor vehicle accident. Pathologic fractures occur in damaged or diseased bones, as in the elderly with osteoporosis. These fractures are produced with surprisingly minimal force. Stress fractures are overuse injuries in which the bone's ability to remodel is incapable of keeping up with the breakdown resulting from activity. Stress fractures occur in persons involved in repetitive activities such as running and jumping and in those with decreased bone density.

Application of Treatment Principles

When designing the rehabilitation program, consider associated soft tissues that have been injured and subsequently immobilized. Although the fracture may be of primary importance from the physician's perspective, rehabilitation of the associated soft tissues may be more challenging than the healing of the fracture. These soft tissues may have been injured at the time of fracture, they may be impaired because of the resultant immobilization, or both. Be sure to relay this information to the patient so realistic expectations after fracture treatment can be developed. Often patients believe that when the fracture is healed that the limb should be functional. Soft tissues can take longer to recover than bone, and ensuring that the patient understands this is important for prognosis and adherence.

Immobilized Fractures

The fracture site and joints above and below the fracture usually are immobilized for some time to allow healing. For patients with external fixation (e.g., cast, splint), physical therapy treatment focuses on rehabilitating the soft tissues that were damaged at the time of fracture and that were subsequently immobilized. The effects of immobilization on soft tissues are profound and consist of softening of the articular cartilage, shortening and atrophy of musculotendinous units, decreased mobility of the joint capsule and periarticular connective tissues, and decreased circulation. Consider these changes when initiating rehabilitation after immobilization. Optimal loading and restoration of normal tissue relationships are the goals when rehabilitating patients after fracture immobilization.

Initially, joint mobilization, stretching, and other gentle mobility activities can begin to restore ROM and normal soft-tissue relationships without overloading the tissues. Gentle strengthening in the form of isometrics or gentle isotonics stimulates increases in muscle performance. These same activities and controlled weight bearing load articular cartilage to reverse the changes resulting from immobilization. Electrical stimulation or biofeedback may be necessary in treating significant muscle atrophy. As impairments improve, initiate activities to alleviate any remaining activity limitations to facilitate the patient's return to work, leisure, and community activities.

Surgically Stabilized Fractures

Fractures of the hip and femur are examples of fractures that are frequently treated with surgical stabilization. The lengthy immobilization and significant lifestyle restrictions make conservative treatment of some fractures unrealistic. Open reduction and internal fixation (ORIF) provides immediate fixation of the fracture without the deleterious effects of immobilization.

When treating the individual who underwent surgical fixation of an acute fracture, treatment principles in the early phase focus on recovery from the traumas of the original injury and of surgery. The principles are the same as those for treating soft-tissue strains, sprains, and contusions when addressing postfracture and postoperative pain. When choosing exercises, be sure to consider the effects of the magnitude and direction of loading on the fracture site. The stability of the fracture and fixation guide exercise choice, and this information should be obtained from the chart or from the physician. For example, a patient with a fixated patellar fracture may avoid weight bearing to prevent distraction loads at the fixation site, but a patient with a fixated tibia fracture may be allowed to bear weight to compress the fracture. Activities that address impairments and activity limitations while keeping loads within the optimal loading zone can then be safely chosen.

Stress Fractures

Stress fractures are a type of overuse injury in which the osteoblastic activity cannot keep pace with osteoclastic activity. This occurs when repetitive loading without adequate recovery is imposed. The metatarsal bones, tibia, and spine are common sites of stress fractures.

The most important aspect of stress fracture care is decreasing loading to allow healing to occur. This may range from leisure activity limitation to short-term immobilization. During this phase, rehabilitation procedures include treating any impairment of mobility, muscle balance, or movement patterns that may have predisposed the individual to a stress fracture. If decreased bone mineral density is suspected as an

BUILDING BLOCK 11-8

Consider the patient in Building Block 11-7. She has active shoulder flexion from 0 to 85 degrees, abduction from 0 to 75 degrees, external rotation from 0 to 15 degrees, and internal rotation from 0 to 35 degrees. Passive ROM is slightly greater. Cervical spine ROM is decreased in all directions by ~25%. Provide a sample beginning rehabilitation program.

underlying problem, institute education or referral for proper evaluation and testing.

After loading at the fracture is allowed, determine the patient's optimal loading zone, or current capacity. The patient must learn which exercise or work parameters (e.g., intensity, repetitions, duration, and frequency) keep within that capacity. As tolerated, progress activities using the parameters described in Chapter 5 (Fig. 5-17). Progress parameters moving from patient's current status toward their desired performance or capacity. Choose activities that duplicate the activities to which the patient will be returning. If possible, the activity should be used as a component of the rehabilitation program. Use the functional activity, whether work, leisure, or recreational activities, as the measure of progress, and allow full return when the fracture has healed and is no longer painful to load.

MANAGEMENT OF IMPAIRMENTS ASSOCIATED WITH BONY AND SOFT-TISSUE SURGICAL PROCEDURES

Surgical procedures necessitating rehabilitation can be broadly categorized into soft-tissue procedures and bony procedures. Soft-tissue procedures are operations primarily directed at the soft tissues, such as tendons, ligaments, or joint capsules. In contrast, bony procedures are operations primarily directed at bone and adjacent tissues. These categories are not exclusive, because surgery often includes soft tissues and bone. However, the primary procedure may predominantly affect one or the other, and rehabilitation follows those guidelines. Not all surgical procedures can be discussed here, and as new surgical techniques are employed, the rehabilitation may change. The physical therapist should focus on the principles of treating patients with different categories of procedures, rather than on specific diagnosis-based protocols.

Frequently, a course of conservative management, including physical therapy, precedes surgery, and follow-up therapy is provided in the postoperative period. This gives the physical therapist the opportunity to participate in the patient's care in two critical perioperative periods. Many specific physical therapy outcomes can be achieved when the therapist has the opportunity for a preoperative visit. This visit allows positive interaction and development of a good rapport between the therapist and patient. Instruction in the postoperative exercise program occurs at a time when full attention can be given to the rehabilitation program, without the complications of postoperative pain and nausea. Teach the patient crutch training, wound care, bed mobility, precautions and contraindications to certain movements, and use of any immobilization or supportive equipment so that the patient is not overburdened with multiple instructions after surgery. Emphasize the importance of adhering to the prescribed exercises in the postoperative program. Consult with the patient about expected outcomes and return to function to reinforce realistic expectations after surgery.

Soft-Tissue Procedures

A multitude of soft-tissue procedures are routinely performed by surgeons and include transfer, reattachment or realignment of tendons, ligament reconstructions, capsular tightening,

debridement and synovectomy procedures, and stabilization techniques. Regardless of the specific procedure, consider the stages of healing and the effects of immobilization and remobilization on connective tissue. In addition to the specific tissues involved in the surgery, consider adjacent tissues that may be affected indirectly by the surgery. These tissues may include supporting musculature, tissues at adjacent joints, articular cartilage, and associated joint structures.

Some soft-tissue procedures often require a longer recovery period than bony procedures because of the difficulty in obtaining fixation in soft tissue. Capsular reefing or tightening surgeries in which soft tissue is sutured to soft tissue or tendon transfer or repair procedures in which soft tissue is attached to bone require adequate healing time to ensure fixation. Most important, be sure to understand the surgical procedure and communicate with the surgeon to ensure optimal rehabilitation for the patient.

The goals of therapeutic exercise in the perioperative period are to restore motion, strength, and function and to reduce pain. The principles of optimal loading and SAID provide the framework for intervention choices. Be sure to observe for and educate the patient about potential postoperative complications such as infection or deep vein thrombosis. Prevention of these complications by early detection minimizes the risk of and protracted course of care associated with these problems. The rehabilitation program should include exercises and modality treatments to be performed at home to reinforce self-management of the condition.

Ligament Reconstructions

The most common sites of ligament reconstructions are the ulnar collateral ligament at the elbow, the lateral ankle ligaments, and the ACL, PCL, and MCL of the knee. Ligament reconstruction should not be confused with a primary ligament repair. Ligament reconstructions generally use other tissues (e.g., tendon) to create a new ligament, rather than repairing the original ligament. Communication with the surgeon regarding the specifics of the procedure provides the clinician with information critical to proper patient care.

Not all individuals with ligament injuries are candidates for reconstructive procedures. Ample evidence exists supporting the conservative management of knee MCL injuries in the presence of an intact ACL. Many individuals are able to return to their previous activity levels after ACL injury without surgical reconstruction. Decisions regarding the appropriateness of reconstructive procedures are based on the patient's activity level, clinical signs and symptoms, and the natural history of the injury.

The postoperative rehabilitation course after ligament reconstructions depends on factors such as the graft material, fixation, quality of the tissue, status of the joint surfaces, comorbidities, and associated injuries. In the knee, bone-patellar and tendon-bone ACL reconstructions have solid, bone-to-bone fixation, whereas some other procedures may have soft-tissue fixation. Frequently, associated injuries or procedures affect the rehabilitation (e.g., meniscus injury or repair, ulnar nerve transposition). Comorbidities such as diabetes or degenerative joint disease may alter the typical postoperative procedures by accelerating some aspects (e.g., mobility), but in other cases, it may slow down elements of the rehabilitation program (e.g., weight bearing). Every individual should be considered in light of the specific situation.

SELECTED INTERVENTION 11-2
Quadriceps Setting for the Patient With a Knee Injury

See Case Study No. 10.

Although this patient requires comprehensive intervention as described in the patient management model, one specific exercise is described.

ACTIVITY: Quadriceps setting

PURPOSE: To increase superior glide of the patella, to teach activation of the quadriceps, and to maintain or increase strength in the quadriceps muscle

RISK FACTORS: No appreciable risk factors

ELEMENTS OF THE MOVEMENT SYSTEM: Biomechanical and neuromuscular

STAGE OF MOTOR CONTROL: Mobility

POSTURE: A variety of positions such as long sit, supine, or standing. The knee is fully extended.

MOVEMENT: Isometric contraction of the quadriceps muscle

SPECIAL CONSIDERATIONS: Ensure normal tracking of the patella. Avoid substitution with hip extensor musculature.

Check quadriceps muscle contraction by attempting to mobilize the patella. With an effective quadriceps set, the patella should not be mobile.

DOSAGE

TYPE OF MUSCLE CONTRACTION: Isometric

Intensity: Submaximal to maximal
Duration: Hold for up to 6 seconds for up to 30 repetitions
Frequency: Hourly or as frequently as possible

RATIONALE FOR EXERCISE CHOICE: Quadriceps setting is a key exercise to maintain the health of the extensor mechanism. This activity lubricates the patellofemoral joint, increases superior glide of the patella (necessary for full knee extension), and increases or maintains quadriceps muscle strength. Full knee extension with quadriceps activation is necessary for a normal gait.

EXERCISE GRADATION: Quadriceps setting is a foundation exercise that serves as a precursor to other exercises. This activity is progressed to more difficult exercises that require quadriceps muscle activation (i.e., any closed chain exercise).

Impairments after ligament reconstructive surgeries include pain, swelling, and loss of mobility and strength. Weight bearing and all weight-bearing activities are impaired after lower extremity procedures. These impairments may result in activity limitations, including inability to perform activities of daily living such as bathing, dressing, and household chores or an inability to participate in leisure activities. Associated participation restrictions may include an inability to fulfill expected roles as worker, student, or spouse (see Selected Intervention 11-2).

Tendon Surgery

Surgery to repair or transfer tendons is commonly performed in orthopedics. Whether a tendon has been torn acutely or has undergone a degenerative process over a protracted period, surgery to repair or debride the injury can maximize the outcome. Common areas of tendon surgery include the tendons of the hand and the rotator cuff, and Achilles and patellar tendons. As with ligament injuries, not all tendon ruptures need to be treated surgically. Many individuals return to a high level of function despite an unrepaired rotator cuff tear or conservative management of an Achilles tendon rupture.

The specific rehabilitation program depends to a great extent on the location and function of the musculotendinous unit, the location and extent of damage within the musculotendinous unit, the quality of the tissue, and the ability of the surgeon to effectively repair the damage. Areas of poor blood supply, inferior tissue quality, extensive damage, or comorbidities can deleteriously affect the surgical outcome. Communicate with the physician to ensure an understanding of the quality of the surgical repair to avoid overtreating or undertreating the patient.

Key issues after a tendon injury are the prevention of mobility impairment without overloading the tendon repair and prevention of excessive atrophy. Immobilization results in loss of normal tendon gliding within the tendon sheath and the associated soft-tissue and joint adhesions because of the restrictions placed on muscle-tendon stretch and contraction. Unlike ligament reconstruction surgery, after which strengthening exercises can be initiated early, these same exercises may overload the repaired tendon (Table 11-4).

Debridement

Surgical debridement is performed alone or combined with other procedures at a number at joints. Debridement refers to the removal of tissue from an area until healthy tissue is exposed. The purpose is to remove potential sources of pain or irritation and, in some cases, to stimulate a healing response. For example, in osteoarthritic knees, debridement may remove osteophytes and loose bodies, shave or trim areas of roughened articular cartilage, and trim or remove areas of torn meniscus. When performing a ligament reconstruction, the remains of the torn ligament are debrided before the reconstruction is performed, and the torn ends of a tendon are debrided before tendon repair.

Because of the variety of situations in which this procedure is used, rehabilitation is dictated by the primary procedure. Rehabilitation after debridement that accompanies tendon or ligament repair follows the repair guidelines. Debridement performed primarily (e.g., arthritis) is guided by the underlying pathology. Understanding the extent of debridement and the status of the joint (e.g., location, extent, and depth of articular cartilage changes, meniscus tears) ensures appropriate pacing of the rehabilitation program.

TABLE 11-4 **Sample Rehabilitation Program Following an Achilles Tendon Repair**

	PRECAUTIONS	ROM	THERAPEUTIC EXERCISE	PROGRESSION CRITERIA
Phase 1: Inflammatory phase to early proliferative phase surgery to 2 weeks	Boot locked in 20–30 degrees PF Touchdown WB using axillary crutches Avoid long periods of dependent positioning	NA for ankle; well limb and proximal joint mobility	Well limb training UBE or upper body circuit	Time-based; 2 weeks post-op
Phase 2: Proliferative fibroplasia phase 2–4 weeks post-op	Continue use of boot progressing to 10 degrees PF at week 2 and 0 degrees PF at week 3 WBAT using crutches and boot Watch for appropriate wound healing	AROM exercises in all ranges Joint mobilization	Isometric exercise of all muscle groups; submaximal for plantar flexion Hip and core strength UBE or upper body circuit	Time-based: 4 weeks post-op Pain-free active DF to neutral No wound complications
Phase 3: Late proliferative fibroplasia phase 4–8 weeks	Wean from boot Start with ¼–½ in heel lifts in tennis shoes for short distances on level surface Gradually reduce heel lift	Continue AROM, stretching, and joint mobilization	Progressive isotonic strengthening Static balance exercises Frontal and sagittal plane stepping drills Low-velocity functional movements Hip and core strength Pool exercise	Normal gait Squat to 30 degrees knee flexion with normal mechanics Stork stand with good control for 10 seconds. AROM from 5 degrees DF to 40 degrees PF
Phase 4: Remodeling phase ~8 weeks	Compensations Forceful impact	Continue ROM to 15 degrees DF and 50 degrees PF	Frontal and transverse plane agility drills, progressing from low to high velocity and to sagittal plane Progress hip and core exercise Multiplane single leg stance activities Bike, cross trainer, swimming	Squat and lunge to 70 degrees knee flexion with good mechanics AROM to 15 degrees DF and 50 degrees PF
Phase 5: Maturation phase ~4 months to discharge	Postactivity soreness should resolve within 24 hours. Avoid anything producing abnormal movement patterns	ROM as necessary	Impact control exercises progressing from 2 footed through alternate footed to single footed Movement control exercises Work- or sport-specific activities	Completion of functional progression or similar measure

DF, dorsiflexion; PF, plantarflexion; WB, weight bearing; UBE, upper body ergometer; WBAT, weight bearing as tolerated.

Synovectomy

Synovectomy, the removal of the synovial lining of the joint, is a procedure performed primarily in the case of rheumatoid arthritis and other diseases such as pigmented villonodular synovitis. The purpose of synovectomy in the case of rheumatoid arthritis is to remove the inflamed synovium and thereby relieve pain and swelling and perhaps retard the progressive joint destruction associated with chronic inflammation.[44,45] This procedure is performed only after conservative measures to control the pain and swelling have failed.

Rehabilitation after synovectomy is guided by the primary pathology, such as rheumatoid arthritis. Because this procedure has been performed as a last resort to control pain and swelling, every effort should be made during rehabilitation to restore motion and strength without increasing pain or swelling. These two factors guide the pace of the rehabilitation program and provide the clinician with the parameters for optimal loading.

Decompression

Decompression procedures are used to relieve pressure in an area and are commonly performed at the shoulder to reduce pressure on the subacromial soft tissues and in the spine to reduce pressure on the spinal cord. Surgery

TABLE 11-5	Sample Rehabilitation Guidelines Following Rotator Cuff Repair with Subacromial Decompression			
	PHASE 1: INFLAMMATORY PHASE TO EARLY PROLIFERATIVE PHASE	**PHASE 2: PROLIFERATIVE FIBROPLASIA PHASE**	**PHASE 3: EARLY REMODELING MATURATION PHASE**	**PHASE 4: REMODELING MATURATION PHASE**
Timeframe	Post-op to 2 weeks	Week 2 to week 5 or 6	Week 6 to Phase 3 goals met	Phase 3 goals to discharge
Immobilization	Sling continuously	Gradually wean out of sling; fully out of sling by week 6	NA	NA
Range of motion	Elbow, wrist, and neck AROM: up to 100 degrees elevation and 35 degrees external rotation	PROM progressing to AAROM for shoulder girdle in all cardinal planes Passive pendulum Neck and scapular mobility exercise; joint mobilization at cervical spine and scapulothoracic region as needed UBE within ROM limits and without resistance	AAROM progressed to AROM PROM to end range GH joint mobilization Cervical and thoracic mobility as needed	Mobilization as necessary for normal arthrokinematics
Neuromuscular exercise	Ball squeezes	Postural exercises Scapular retraction Core strengthening Submaximal multiple angle isometrics for shoulder rotation Manual resistance for secondary and distal musculature	Isotonic shoulder strength Scapular strength progressed to plyometrics Submaximal elastic resistance and isokinetic exercise	Total arm strength emphasizing patient's functional needs
Cardiorespiratory	Walking, stationary bike, or cross trainer with sling	Walking, stationary bike, or cross trainer with sling	May begin running if 5/5 strength in rotation	Sport- or work specific
Progression criteria	Time-based: 14 days post-op	Minimum 5 weeks post-op; pain controlled and mobility returning	Full AROM 5/5 strength Negative impingement signs	
Other	Ice or other modalities for pain			

AROM, active range of motion; GH, glenohumeral; AAROM, active assisted range of motion; UBE, upper body ergometer; PROM: passive range of motion

in the wrist to relieve pressure in the carpal tunnel and fasciotomies in the leg to reduce compartment pressures may be considered forms of decompression. The excessive pressure in these areas may result from bony or soft-tissue architecture, and decompression involves the release or removal of these soft tissues and shaving or removal of bony sources of pressure.

Rehabilitation after a decompression is guided by the primary pathology and the status of the tissues decompressed, which depends on the amount and duration of compression and on the type of tissue compressed. For example, if excessive pressure on a nerve has caused neurologic changes, rehabilitation focuses on recovery of nerve function. In the spine, a decrease in neurological symptoms in the arm (following cervical spine decompresssion) or the lower extremity (following lumbar decompression) is a sign that the decompression has been successful. As neurological symptoms decrease, progressive strengthening of the core and extremity musculature should increase. If pressure has caused poor muscle function (e.g., rotator cuff), rehabilitation focuses on recovery of muscle function. As rehabilitation progresses, avoid using activities or positions that may excessively compress the tissue just decompressed (Table 11-5).

Soft-Tissue Stabilization and Realignment Procedures

Soft-tissue stabilization procedures are performed in the case of joint instability resulting from capsular laxity. Capsular laxity can be the result of an acute injury such as a dislocation, or can be part of an overall pattern of hypermobility that has become symptomatic. Soft-tissue stabilization procedures are performed most frequently to correct an unstable shoulder and may be combined with other stabilization procedures (e.g., bony stabilization). A variety of surgical techniques can stabilize a joint with capsular laxity. Each technique has risks and benefits that should be evaluated on a case-by-case basis. Likewise, soft-tissue realignment procedures are performed to redirect the pull of soft tissues that may or may not be the result of instability. For example, proximal patellar realignment is used to enhance the effective pull of the vastus medialis obliques on the patella. Regardless of the procedure, the fixation usually is soft tissue to soft tissue, without bony stability.

Because of the lack of rigid fixation and length of time necessary for soft tissue to heal, the loads placed on the repair site are controlled for some time after stabilization. For example, when stabilizing the shoulder for anterior inferior glenohumeral instability, external rotation is limited for a

TABLE 11-6 Sample Rehabilitation Program Following an Anterior Shoulder Reconstruction with Bankart Repair

	PHASE 1: PROLIFERATIVE FIBROPLASIA PHASE	PHASE 3: PROLIFERATIVE AND EARLY REMODELING PHASE	PHASE 4: REMODELING PHASE	PHASE 5: REMODELING AND MATURATION
Timeframe	Weeks 2–6 postoperative	Weeks 6–10 postoperative	Weeks 10–15 postoperative	Weeks 18+
Range of motion	Sling immobilization for 3–4 weeks No external rotation with abduction for first 6 weeks PROM/AAROM for all ranges except external rotation only to neutral Begin AROM week 5	Continue AAROM and AROM Gentle joint mobilization as necessary Cervical spine and scapular AROM	Posterior glides if posterior capsule tightness present Stretching and joint mobilization for any motion limitations	As needed
Therapeutic exercise	Submaximal shoulder isometrics beginning week 3 Elbow, forearm, wrist, and hand exercise Cervical spine and scapular exercise Well limb activities	Core strengthening Postural exercise Rotator cuff strengthening in nonprovocative position Scapular strengthening and dynamic control Partial weight-bearing exercise	Progressive multiplane resistive exercise Stabilization exercises using PNF, rapid alternating, or closed chain techniques	Total arm/core functional exercise Dumbbell, resistive band, and medicine ball exercise Higher velocity strengthening and control exercise Inertial exercise Plyometric exercise Progress to functional program: throwing, swimming, and racquet sports
Cardiorespiratory fitness	Walking and stationary bike with sling	Walking, stationary bike, elliptical trainer	Walking, biking, elliptical trainer, and running	Sport- or work specific
Criteria for progression	Full AROM in all ranges except ER 5/5 IR/ER strength in neutral Negative apprehension and impingement signs	Full AROM 5/5 IR/ER strength at 45 degree abduction	Continued strength and function progress without apprehension or impingement	Discharge to sport/work when functional progression complete

IR/ER, internal rotation/external rotation; PNF, proprioceptive neuromuscular facilitation.

short time after surgery to allow the anterior capsule to heal. Because the repaired tissue is noncontractile, muscle activation is usually allowed early in rehabilitation, as long as ROM precautions are considered. As rehabilitation progresses into the range that stresses the repaired tissue, be alert for signs of progressive loosening of the repair, such as complaints of slipping or instability. Depending upon the specific procedure, mobility recovery should be full, without the return of instability symptoms.

Rehabilitation following stabilization procedures focuses on restoring mobility, strength, and function. The rate of progression of mobility activities may vary from one person to the next due to individual variations. Some patients are progressed slowly due to concern that the stabilization will "stretch out" or loosen. Differences in tissue quality, joint architecture, and surgical technique impact the progression of mobility activities (Table 11-6).

Meniscal and Labral Repairs

The meniscus of the knee and the labrum of the hip and shoulder are common sites of fibrocartilage repair. They tend to be less symptomatic because of the non–weight-bearing nature of the joint; therefore, surgery for repair is less common. When repairs are performed, they are often in the superior aspect of the joint where the superior labrum and long head of the biceps attachment meet. Repair of torn menisci of the knee is commonly performed alone or in combination with other procedures such as ACL reconstruction. In the knee in particular, the repair is of a soft tissue with an inferior blood supply. Healing may be enhanced by associated procedures to increase the blood supply to the area.

Important issues during rehabilitation include understanding the loads placed on the repair when the joint is in a variety of positions. These positions should be avoided in the early stages when the repair is still fragile. For example, full overhead positions may be avoided early after labral repairs in the superior zone. Full knee flexion in weight bearing is limited for several weeks after meniscal repair, because this position places high loads on the meniscus. Return to activities such as impact loading, jogging, deep knee flexion, and pivoting should be approached cautiously, particularly in the early postoperative phase.

Communicate with the surgeon regarding the location and extent of tissue repair. The type, location, and extent of tear provide important information about the rehabilitation protocol. At the knee, the margins of a longitudinal tear will be approximated with weight bearing, whereas the margins of a radial tear will be disrupted. Tears located in the peripheral one third, or vascular zone, have a better prognosis than those in the central one third, or avascular zone. However, surgical techniques have improved and meniscus tears in the avascular zone are repairable with good success.[46]

Meniscal allografts are being used in situations in which patients have undergone a complete meniscectomy, and are generally young and active (age 50 or less), have a varus alignment and mild to moderate tibiofemoral arthrosis. The goal is to perform the surgery early before extensive articular cartilage damage occurs.[47] In fact, meniscal allograft transplantation is contraindicated in patients with significant arthrosis.[48]

Rehabilitation following meniscal repair or transplantation focuses on limiting weight-bearing forces to control compressive and shear forces.[48] The rate of program progression will depend upon many individual factors, most importantly keeping joint loads within healing tissue tolerance. Appropriate progression requires attention to external factors (i.e. age, joint surface quality, body mass index, joint alignment, etc.) and internal factors (i.e. size and location of lesion, direction of tear, etc.) Maintain close communication with the surgeon to ensure progression that is consistent with surgical findings and procedures.

The rise of hip arthroscopy has expanded the understanding and treatment of hip pathology. Procedures such as debridement of loose bodies of removal of osteophytes that were previously performed as open techniques can now be done more efficiently arthroscopically. Additionally, arthroscopy has helped identify previously underrecognized problems such as labral tears and chondral injuries.[49] These injuries occur as acute traumatic episodes in athletic activities, such as landing directly on the greater trochanter. This impact can produce shearing of the articular cartilage on the acetabulum resulting in a chondral injury.[49]

Injuries to the acetabular labrum can occur acutely or as the result of aging and degeneration.[49–51] Femoral acetabular impingement can produce anterosuperior labral and chondral lesions.[51] Labral injuires have been classified in to four different types and occur in different locations.[51] Symptoms are similar to those of a meniscal or shoulder labral tear, where the patient experiences pain, clicking, catching, and instability. Hip arthroscopy can help to identify and correct the injury.[52] Like surgery for a torn meniscus, arthroscopy to debride the unstable labrum, maintaining as much of the tissue as possible will lead to the best outcomes. A sample rehabilitation program following hip arthroscopy can be found in Table 11-7.

Bony Procedures

Rehabilitation is often necessary after bony surgical procedures to restore motion at adjacent joints, strengthen related soft tissues, and increase general endurance. Most articular cartilage surgeries are a combination of soft tissue and bony

TABLE 11-7 Sample Rehabilitation Program Following Hip Arthroscopy for Labral Tears			
	PHASE 1: INFLAMMATORY AND EARLY PROLIFERATIVE PHASE	**PHASE 2: PROLIFERATIVE FIBROPLASIA PHASE**	**PHASE 3: REMODELING AND MATURATION PHASE**
Timeframe	Post-op to week 2–3	Completion of phase 1 to approximately week 6	Completion of phase 2 to discharge
Weight bearing	Crutches and limited weight bearing; normalize gait	Discontinue crutches when gait is normal without pain medication	Full weight bearing
Range of motion	AAROM, PROM all planes Gentle hip mobilization and distraction	Continue ROM and mobilization until full or desired ROM is achieved	Maintenance, patient-specific stretching
Neuromuscular exercise	Gait activities: marching, weight shifting, and normalizing gait (may use pool) Isometrics of all hip and knee musculature Short-arc dynamic hip exercises	Progressive gait activities including balance, direction changes, and functional movements (may use pool) Nonimpact hip and core muscle strengthening (resistive bands, swiss ball, etc.) Lower extremity strengthening (PNF, leg press, knee extensions, etc.)	Gentle impact on shock absorptive surfaces, 2 ft—2 ft progressing to single foot Progress to multiplane Dynamic control exercises reproducing functional activities Running program if returning to running sport Sport- and work-specific drills Progressive hip, leg, and core strengthening
Cardiorespiratory	UBE or pool without kick	Nonimpact: stationary bike, cross trainer, swimming, and deep water running	Sport- or work specific in neuromuscular and cardiorespiratory demands
Progression criteria	Normal gait without assistive device or pain medications on level surface Functional ROM without pain Good leg control during slow movements	Normal gait on all surfaces Completion of functional movement patterns without compensation Single leg balance ≥ 15 seconds	Return to work or sport when functional progression and/or work conditioning program is passed

procedures. The number of available procedures suggests that there is no one optimal treatment for those with articular cartilage injuries. Many individual parameters such as age, body mass, activity demands, status of the primary and adjacent joints, as well as specifics of the lesion itself weigh heavily in treatment planning.[53,54] The specific procedure, tissue damage, and the patient's general health, balanced with the optimal loading and SAID principles, guide intervention choices. The focus of these sections will be on the knee due to the volume of research and high utilization at this joint. However, use of many of these procedures is being extended to other joints.

Lavage/Debridement/Microfracture

Surgical procedures to remove loose fragments and other mechanical or chemical irritants may provide some temporary relief to joint pain in the degenerative joint. Simple arthroscopic irrigation (lavage) along with removal of loose bodies or other tissue fragments can produce improvement in many patients. The purpose of these procedures is to reduce inflammation and mechanical irritation by washing away fragments of cartilage and calcium phosphate crystals from the joint.[55] This procedure can decrease mechanical symptoms as well as night pain in the short term following surgery.[56] In some patients, lavage can decrease symptoms for up to 3 years. Additional debridement including smoothing of fibrillated joint surfaces, removal of osteophytes, or partial synovectomy may further reduce symptoms.[55] Patients with good joint space, a short duration of symptoms, good alignment, and a stable knee may do well with this procedure. However, neither lavage nor debridement addresses the underlying pathology, so improvements are short lived. As a result, the benefits of these procedures may be limited, and the improvements restricted to a small proportion of patients.

Others may require more aggressive treatment that attempts to stimulate healing. Microfracture is a procedure performed alone or in combination with other procedures in cases of articular cartilage lesions. This procedure is performed most commonly at the knee, where articular cartilage lesions may result from degenerative joint disease or acute injury. The microfracture technique can be used for isolated defects or for bipolar or "kissing" defects, where defects on opposing joint surfaces contact one another. These lesions produce impairments such as pain, swelling, and motion loss, as well as activity limitations such as the inability to walk distances, stand for long periods, or negotiate stairs.

The surgical procedure involves a diagnostic arthroscopy and correcting any associated intra-articular pathology. The zone of calcified cartilage is debrided, taking care to avoid abrading the subchondral bone. Subsequently, a surgical awl is used to make several small holes or "microfractures" that create a roughened surface to which a blood clot can adhere. This procedure stimulates a healing response and local fibrocartilage ingrowth. Unfortunately, the mechanical properties of the replacement fibrocartilage are significantly inferior to the original tissue.[55,56]

Rehabilitation after microfracture varies with the extent and location of the articular cartilage lesion. Large lesions on weight-bearing surfaces have a poorer prognosis than small lesions on non–weight-bearing surfaces. The joint with extra loads from excessive body weight, malalignment, or instability is likely to require a longer rehabilitation course, with

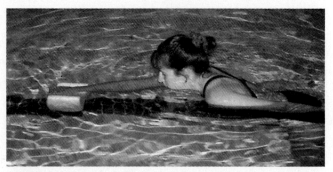

FIGURE 11-15. Using activities in a gravity-minimized environment can progressively load the lower extremity.

a greater likelihood of overloading the new fibrocartilage. These individuals may have weight-bearing and exercise limitations for up to 8 weeks after surgery. Depending upon the size and location of the lesion, weight-bearing (WB) can be progressed to partial weight bearing between weeks 2 and 4. The patient should be full weight bearing by week 8.

Restoration of motion and strength as quickly as possible without disrupting the healing process provides the best opportunity for healing of this fresh injury (Fig. 11-15). Many surgeons advocate the use of continuous passive motion with their patients for up to 6 weeks postoperatively.[56] Typically, PROM is performed immediately without restrictions in most cases.

Strengthening exercises in the early phase consist of multiangle isometrics and non–weight-bearing leg raise activities. The pool is an effective place for gait training, ROM and functional training and is initiated when incisions have healed. A stationary bike with light resistance can be used for mobility and strengthening as early as week 3 to 4. By week 4, with the progressive increase in weight bearing, balance and light weight bearing activities such as wall slides, mini-squats and lunges can be initiated or advanced. Hip and core strengthening are important as well. Strengthening exercises should continue and replicate functional activities by weeks 8 through 16, with gradual return to activities over the next 2 months.[57] High impact activities can be considered at 6 to 8 months postoperatively.

Osteochondral Autograft Transplantation

Several surgical techniques attempt to restore and preserve articular cartilage. More aggressive techniques are indicated in the case of full-thickness defects of the weight-bearing surface of a joint.[55,58] The osteochondral autograft transplantation (OAT) procedure transfers articular cartilage tissue from areas of low loading to areas of high loading. In addition to the knee, OAT procedures have been used with lesions on the talus, tibia, humeral capitellum, and femoral head.[58] Indications include focal chondral or osteochondral defects of weight-bearing surfaces or joint surfaces that are frequently loaded, age <50 years, concurrent treatment of instability, malalignment and meniscal injuries, and compliance with weight-bearing restrictions.[58] This procedure is performed most often at the knee, where bone plugs are removed from trochlea and intercondylar notch and placed on the articular surface lesions. When multiple plugs are used to fill a larger defect, the procedure is often termed a "mosaicplasty." Problems with this procedure are related to limitations in the graft size, obtaining good congruity of the graft and adjacent articular cartilage, and graft fixation. Additionally, few areas

TABLE 11-8 Rehabilitation Program Following OAT procedure

	PHASE I: INFLAMMATORY PHASE TO EARLY PROLIFERATIVE PHASE	PHASE 2: PROLIFERATIVE FIBROPLASIA PHASE	PHASE 3: REMODELING PHASE	PHASE 4: MATURATION PHASE
Timeframe	Weeks 0–6	Weeks 6–12	Weeks 12–26	Weeks 26+
Weight bearing	Brace locked in full extension Status will vary with location and size of lesion; follow physician guidelines *Generally* NWB for up to 4 weeks with progressive WB by 25% per week	Discontinue brace Progress WB based upon physician recommendations *Generally* full WB by 8–10 weeks	Full WB	NA
Range of motion	PROM as tolerated CPM for up to 8 hours per day Immediate full extension Stationary bike as tolerated Joint mobilization Flexion goal of 90 degrees by ~2 weeks	Continue PROM AROM in ranges that do not engage lesion Continue mobilization and stretching Knee flexion to ~130 degrees by week 8–10	Full ROM Continue stretching as needed	Continue maintenance stretching
Therapeutic exercise	Quadriceps sets Multiangle isometrics Leg raises Pool exercises Well limb exercise	Partial WB weight shifts Gentle leg press, wall slides, and lunges with resistive bands or weights through partial ROM Partial WB balance and proprioception drills Partial ROM resisted knee extension	Continue progressing strength exercises Increase resistance Leg press 0–90 degrees Squats 0–60 degrees Step-ups, Lunge walking, Elliptical trainer, Progressive walking, bicycling Functional activities that are nonimpact	Progress strengthening Progress balance and proprioception activities Functional progression Impact activities as determined by individual needs Return to work or sport

of a joint surface are truly "non–weight bearing," resulting in significant risk of donor site morbidity.[58]

Rehabilitation after an OAT procedure will vary with the size and location of the lesion and fixation stability. The general rules about rehabilitating any articular cartilage lesion apply here and are modified based on individual patient factors. General guidelines allow unloaded PROM as tolerated with emphasis on restoring full motion as quickly as possible, whereas AROM varies depending on the size, location, and fixation of the lesion. Typically, there is no period of strict immobilization. Particular attention should be paid to treatment of the underlying causes of the original articular cartilage lesion. Patients are generally non–weight bearing for 2 to 4 weeks, followed by a gradual progression of weight bearing over the next 3 to 4 weeks. This varies with the size and location of the lesion. Lesions that are found on a non–weight-bearing surface may be non–weight bearing for 1 week only. Muscle performance activities include isometric contractions in pain-free ranges and the non–weight-bearing leg raises immediately. Concentric active exercises in ranges that do not engage the lesion can begin as early as 1 week with light resistance as early as the second week after surgery.[58] Strength and functional activities progress and include balance and proprioception drills by 6 to 12 weeks postoperatively.[57] Low

impact activities are allowed at 6 to 8 months, while higher impact activities such as running and aerobics are no allowed until 8 to 10 months following surgery.[57] (See Table 11-8.)

Autologous Chondrocyte Implantation
The autologous chondrocyte implantation (ACI) procedure is indicated for cases of large, full thickness chondral lesions located on the femoral condyles or trochlear groove. Patients should be under 50 years of age and be willing to adhere to the postoperative protocol.[53] The lesion typically ranges in size from 2 to 10 cm² in diameter, but ACI has been successfully used in lesions up to 20 cm².[59] Other prerequisites include good alignment, ligamentous stability, and good ROM.[54] Any associated pathology must be corrected prior to or at the time of surgery. ACI procedures are considered when patients have failed other interventions such as marrow stimulation and osteochondral autograft techniques. While ACI can be used in joints with multiple chondral lesions, ACI is contraindicated for "kissing lesions" or significant bone loss.[55]

This procedure is performed in two stages. In the first stage, two to three full-thickness samples of healthy articular cartilage are harvested from the patient, typically from the superior peripheral edges of the lateral or medial femoral condyles.[53] These samples are cultivated and held until the second stage, performed anywhere from 6 weeks to 18 months after graft harvest.[53,55] The patient should obtain full motion and sufficient strength prior to the second procedure. In the second surgical procedure, the cartilage defect is debrided, avoiding disruption of the subchondral bone. Once the lesion is debrided and prepared, a periosteal flap is harvested from a different site (typically the superior medial tibia) and sutured over the lesion. The suture line is sealed with fibrin glue to ensure a watertight seal at the edges of the periosteal flap. The cultured chondrocytes are injected under the periosteal flap and the injected site closed with additional sutures and fibrin glue.

Rehabilitation after autologous chondrocytes implantation is similar to that of other articular cartilage procedures. A balance must be found between protection of the healing tissue and loading of the maturing tissue. The actual progression will vary with the size and location of the defect.[53,57] In general, full unloaded PROM is allowed early on, and the patient will be non–weight bearing or touch down weight bearing for the first 2 to 4 weeks, with progressive weight bearing over the next 2 to 4 weeks. Weight bearing is performed with axillary crutches and the knee locked in full extension. Full weight bearing without crutches is expected by 6 to 9 weeks. Full passive knee extension is expected immediately, with knee flexion to 90 degrees by week 2 and 130 degrees by week 8.[53,57] Isometrics that do not engage the lesion are initiated and progressed to short-arc isotonic exercises, again, in positions that do not engage the lesion. The pool is an ideal place to initiate and progress activities, particularly gait, weight bearing and balance activities. Return to activity is anywhere from 6 to 12 months depending upon the lesion, patient factors, and type of activity.

Open Reduction and Internal Fixation

ORIF of a fracture is commonly performed when closed reduction is impossible or when fracture healing would be protracted if treated without fixation. Goals of ORIF are to stabilize a fracture while allowing early motion and activity, to decrease the chances of nonunion, and to decrease the effects of immobilization on the limb. Surgical fixation may use plates, screws, wires, or other forms of hardware to stabilize the bone and fragments. In most situations, the hardware is left in permanently, although it may be removed if superficial location causes discomfort.

Rehabilitation after ORIF is directed at any impairments or activity limitations associated with the injury. Any force great enough to fracture a bone is likely to have produced some local soft-tissue damage, which must be treated as well. Restrictions (e.g., weight bearing, motion) are specific to the location and severity of the fracture and to the extent of associated soft-tissue injury. In general, surgical fixation stabilizes the fracture, and treatment focuses on associated soft-tissue damage and restoration of full function.

Fusion

Fusion is the operative formation of an ankylosis or arthrodesis.[60] Fusions are performed most commonly in the spine, although some joints in the extremities are fused. Spinal fusions are used to treat problems such as instability, facet pain, and disk disease. Glenohumeral joints are fused in cases of severe pain, especially in the presence of neurologic injury (e.g., axillary nerve, long thoracic nerve) that severely restricts

functional use of the arm. Knee joints are fused when severe arthritis produces pain and disability and total joint replacement is not a treatment option. Fusions about the ankle are used to treat hindfoot pain and arthritis.

The postoperative rehabilitation program must consider the mechanical changes that occur as a result of the fusion. Because mobility is limited at a joint (or series of joints in the spine), adjacent joints compensate to restore the presurgical mobility. How effectively these joints compensate or overcompensate has a profound impact on the result. If the hip and ankle are unable to adequately compensate for a fused knee, the patient has difficulty getting in and out of a car, a chair, and on and off the floor. Because the spine is a series of joints, adjacent segments can often compensate for fusion at one or more levels. However, adjacent segments may become hypermobile in response to the fusion, creating pain above or below the fusion. An important aspect of postoperative rehabilitation is focused on the adjacent joints and procedures necessary to ensure the long-term health of these joints. The muscles must be retrained to function in a new movement pattern.

Osteotomy

Osteotomy, the surgical cutting of a bone, is a procedure performed to correct bony alignment. This procedure is performed most commonly at the knee to correct excessive genu varus or valgus. Excessive varus or valgus places increased loads on the medial and lateral compartments of the knee, respectively. This may result in degeneration of the articular cartilage in that compartment. The purpose of performing an osteotomy is to redistribute weight off the compromised compartment and to disperse the load over a larger area. To correct for excessive varus, a high tibial osteotomy (or valgus osteotomy) is performed at the proximal tibia. To correct for excessive valgus, a distal femoral osteotomy is performed. These procedures remove a wedge of bone from the respective site, and the "fracture" is fixated with hardware.

Rehabilitation focuses on the precipitating issues that led to surgery (usually degenerative joint disease) and the preservation or restoration of motion and strength. An important consideration is the change in loading patterns on the articular cartilage. One compartment that has been excessively loaded will have decreased loading; the other compartment that has been underloaded will have increased loading. How well a compartment adapts to the increased load depends on many factors. The health of the articular cartilage in this compartment is probably the most important factor. Weight bearing and weight-bearing activities may have to be restricted until the joint can adapt to this change.

MANAGEMENT OF IMPAIRMENTS ASSOCIATED WITH JOINT ARTHROPLASTY

Joint replacement surgery is performed to remedy significant joint deterioration after other conservative or surgical measures have been exhausted. Joint replacement is performed in many joints, including the hip, knee, shoulder, elbow, wrist, and hand. The chief goal of joint arthroplasty is pain relief. Generally, the patient cannot expect increased joint motion, strength, or function other than that resulting from a decrease in pain.

Joint replacement is categorized by component design (i.e., constrained, unconstrained, or semiconstrained), fixation (i.e., cement or cementless), and materials (i.e., cobalt-chrome alloy, titanium alloy, or high-density polyethylene). A *constrained* design allows motion in only one plane; an *unconstrained* design allows motion in any axis. A *semiconstrained* allows full motion in one plane and some motion in other planes. Fixation is achieved with cement or with some type of biologic fixative. Biologic fixation may include a porous coat or similar surfaces that allow bony ingrowth into open areas on the surface. Recovery of components with this type of fixation is difficult in the patient in need of revision arthroplasty. Materials usually are a combination of metals and plastic.

In addition to total joint arthroplasty, joint resurfacing procedures are also available. Total surface arthroplasty (TSA) is being performed more routinely at the hip joint. While patients in the past underwent total joint arthroplasty for pain relief, more patients are requesting TSA to improve their quality of life and to remain active. TSA preserves more bone. In the hip procedure, the prosthesis is metal-on-metal, where the acetabulum is lined with a metal cup and the femoral head is capped with a metal prosthesis. Unlike a total hip arthroplasty, the femoral head is not removed in a TSA.

Rehabilitation issues are joint- and prosthesis specific. In general, restoration of motion, strength, and function and consideration of the underlying cause of the surgery constitute the rehabilitation framework. Consideration must also be given to the adjacent joints, which may be compromised by the same disease process and the excessive loads placed on them in the perioperative period. After recovery from the operation, the patient generally feels much better than before the surgery, with less pain in the affected joint. Education regarding the long-term health of the joint replacement and the adjacent joints is a large component of the patient care program.

KEY POINTS

- The composition and structure of connective tissues provide information about each tissue's mechanical properties and function.

- The unique viscoelastic characteristics of connective tissues are the result of their fluid and solid constituent materials.
- When connective tissues are loaded, the stress (i.e., force per unit area relative to the strain) or change in the length per unit length provides information about the tissue's ability to withstand loads.
- The viscoelastic properties of relaxation, creep, and hysteresis are the physiologic basis for changes seen with stretching.
- The stages of healing along with knowledge of the specific injury provide the clinician with guidelines for intervention selection throughout the episode of care.
- Restoration of normal tissue relationships, optimal loading, the SAID principle, and prevention of secondary complications are broad rehabilitation principles that guide treatment.
- Acute soft-tissue injuries such as sprains, strains, and contusions necessitate early intervention to avoid secondary complications.
- Management of tendon injuries and prognosis varies according to the injury classification.
- Interventions used in the treatment of bony or surgical procedures should have a solid foundation in basic science and require an understanding of the anatomy and kinesiology of the area.

CRITICAL THINKING QUESTIONS

1. Consider Case Study No. 2 in Unit 7, before her total knee replacement surgery. Presume that she came to your clinic 2 years earlier in an attempt to delay surgery. At that time, her motion was decreased by 15%, and her overall strength was decreased by 20%. Describe her exercise program. Provide the rationale for restoration of her joint motion and strength in the case of osteoarthritis of the knee.

2. a. The patient in the first question is given a home exercise program to carry out for 2 weeks, after which she returns to the clinic for reevaluation and progression. Explain to this patient how to differentiate the discomfort associated with some exercise from pain that may be related to harming her knee.

▼ LAB ACTIVITIES

1. A patient comes to the clinic Monday morning with acute Achilles tendinitis after a weekend tennis tournament.
   a. Instruct your patient in a home exercise program, including dosage, to be performed until he or she returns in 4 days.
   b. Explain to your patient about adjunctive agents and give any special instructions.
2. The patient returns 4 days later and is in a subacute phase of injury.
   a. Demonstrate five stretching techniques for the Achilles tendon.
   b. Instruct the patient in a home stretching program, including dosage.
   c. Demonstrate three ways to strengthen this muscle group, including dosage, using

   i. Concentric only
   ii. Isometric only
   iii. Eccentric only
3. This patient has improved with the exercise program and desires to return to basketball. Demonstrate the final phase of the rehabilitation program to prepare the patient for this activity.
4. Instruct each of the following patients on five exercises to increase knee flexion mobility:
   a. A 19-year-old student 2 weeks after a grade II MCL sprain of the right knee with a 0- to 90-degree ROM
   b. A 75-year-old woman who is unable to get up and down off the floor 2 weeks after a total right knee replacement with a 0- to 60-degree ROM

b. The patient in the first question is given a home exercise program to carry out for 2 weeks, after which she returns to the clinic for reevaluation and progression. Compared with her previous visit, her knee is more swollen and warm to the touch. She has lost 5 degrees of knee extension and 10 degrees of knee flexion. Her gait is significantly impaired. What are your recommendations at this time? When should you see her again and why?

3. Why are repeated eccentric muscle contractions associated with tendinitis?

4. If eccentric muscle contractions contribute to tendinitis, why are they used to treat tendinitis?

5. Consider Case Study No. 6 in Unit 7. How would your acute-phase mobility program differ if the patient
   a. Were generally hypermobile, demonstrating elbow hyperextension, knee recurvatum, and thumb to volar forearm?
   b. Were generally hypomobile, with a history of excessive scar formation?

REFERENCES

1. Andersson GB. Epidemiological features of chronic low-back pain. Lancet 1999; 354:581–585.
2. Frank C, Woo S-L, Andriacchi T, et al. Normal ligament: structure, function and composition. In: Woo SL-Y, Buckwalter JA, eds. Injury and Repair of the Musculoskeletal Soft Tissues. Park Ridge, IL: American Academy of Orthopaedic Surgeons, 1988:45–101.
3. Riegger-Krugh C. Bone. In: Malone TR, McPoil T, Nitz AJ, eds. Orthopaedic and Sports Physical Therapy. 3rd Ed. St. Louis, MO: Mosby, 1997.
4. Walter JB. Principles of Disease. 2nd Ed. Philadelphia, PA: WB Saunders, 1982.
5. Walker JM. Cartilage of human joints and related structures. In: Zachazewski JE, Magee DJ, Quillen WS, eds. Athletic Injuries and Rehabilitation. Philadelphia, PA: WB Saunders, 1996.
6. Woo SL-Y, Maynard J, Butler D, et al. Ligament, tendon and joint capsule insertions into bone. In: Woo SL-Y, Buckwalter JA, eds. Injury and Repair of the Musculoskeletal Soft Tissues. Park Ridge, IL: American Academy of Orthopaedic Surgeons, 1988:133–167.
7. O'Brien M. Functional anatomy and physiology of tendons. Clin Sports Med 1992;11:505–520.
8. Loitz-Ramage B, Zernicke RF. Bone biology and mechanics. In: Zachazewski JE, Magee DJ, Quillen WS, eds. Athletic Injuries and Rehabilitation. Philadelphia, PA: WB Saunders, 1996.
9. Curwin S, Stanish WD. Tendinitis: Its Etiology and Treatment. Lexington, MA: DC Heath, 1984.
10. Burstein AH, Wright TM. Fundamentals of Orthopaedic Biomechanics. Baltimore, MD: Williams & Wilkins, 1994.
11. English T, Wheeler ME, Hettinga DL. Inflammatory response of synovial joint structures. In: Malone TR, McPoil T, Nitz AJ, eds. Orthopaedic and Sports Physical Therapy. 3rd Ed. St. Louis, MO: Mosby, 1997.
12. Leadbetter WB. An introduction to sports-induced soft-tissue inflammation. In: Leadbetter WB, Buckwalter JA, Gordon SL, eds. Sports-Induced Inflammation. Park Ridge, IL: American Academy of Orthopaedic Surgeons, 1990:3–24.
13. Lee AC, Quillen WS, Magee DJ, et al. Injury, Inflammation, and Repair: Tissue Mechanics, the Healing Process, and Their Impact on the Musculoskeletal System. In: Magee DJ, Zachazewski JE, Quillen WS, eds. Scientific Foundations and Principles of Practice in Musculoskeletal Rehabilitation. St. Louis, MO: Saunders Elsevier, 2007:1–22.
14. Andriaacchi T, Sabiston P, DeHaven K, et al. Ligament: injury and repair. In: Woo SL-Y, Buckwalter JA, eds. Injury and Repair of the Musculoskeletal Soft Tissues. Park Ridge, IL: American Academy of Orthopaedic Surgeons, 1988:103–132.
15. Malone TR, Garrett WE, Zachazewski JE. Muscle: deformation, injury, repair. In: Zachazewski JE, Magee DJ, Quillen WS, eds. Athletic Injuries and Rehabilitation. Philadelphia, PA: WB Saunders, 1997:71–91.
16. Leadbetter WB. Cell-matrix response in tendon injury. Clin Sports Med 1992;11:533–578.
17. Rees JD, Wilson AM, Wolman RL. Current concepts in the management of tendon disorders. Rheumatology 2006;45(5):508–521.
18. Elliot DH. Structure and function of mammalian tendon. Biol Rev 1965;40:392–421.
19. Walker LB, Harris EH, Benedict JV. Stress-strain relationships in human plantaris tendon: a preliminary study. Med Elect Biol Eng 1964;2:31–38.
20. Zernicke RF, Garhammer J, Jobe FW. Human patellar tendon rupture. J Bone Joint Surg Am 1977;59:179–183.
21. Nicholas JA. Clinical observations on sports-induced soft-tissue injuries. In: Leadbetter WB, Buckwalter JA, Gordon SL, eds. Sports-Induced Inflammation. Park Ridge, IL: American Academy of Orthopaedic Surgeons, 1990: 129–148.
22. Clancy WJ. Tendon trauma and overuse injuries. In: Leadbetter WB, Buckwalter JA, Gordon SL, eds. Sports-Induced Inflammation. Park Ridge, IL: American Academy of Orthopaedic Surgeons, 1990:609–618.
23. Khan KM, Cook, JL, Bonar F, et al. Histopathology of common tendinopathies. Update and implications for clinical management. Sports Med 1999;27(6):393–408.
24. Pufe T, Petersen WJ, Mentlein R, et al. The role of vasculature and angiogenesis for the pathogenesis of degenerative tendons disease. Scand J Med Sci Sports 2005;15(4):211–222.
25. Bahr R, Fossan B, Loken S, et al. Surgical treatment compared with eccentric training for patellar tendinopathy (Jumper's knee). A randomized, controlled trial. J Bone Joint Surg Am 2006;88(8):1689–1698.
26. Jonsson P, Alfredson H. Superior results with eccentric compared to concentric quadriceps training in patients with jumper's knee: a prospective randomised study. Br J Sports Med 2005;39(11):847–850.
27. Ohberg L, Alfredson H. Effects on neovascularisation behind the good results with eccentric training in chronic mid-portion Achilles tendinosis? Knee Surg Sports Traumatol Arthrosc 2004;12(5):465–470.
28. Ohberg L, Lorentzon R, Alfredson H. Eccentric training in patients with chronic Achilles tendinosis: normalised tendon structure and decreased thickness at follow-up. Br J Sports Med 2004;38(1):8–11.
29. Mafi N, Lorentzon R, Alfredson H. Superior short-term results with eccentric calf muscle training compared to concentric training in a randomized prospective multicenter study on patients with chronic Achilles tendinosis. Knee Surg Sports Traumatol Arthrosc 2001;9(1):42–47.
30. Alfredson H, Pietila T, Jonsson P, et al. Heavy-load eccentric calf muscle training for the treatment of chronic Achilles tendinosis. Am J Sports Med 1998;26(3):360–366.
31. Buckwalter J, Rosenberg L, Coutts R, et al. Articular cartilage: injury and repair. In: Woo SL-Y, Buckwalter JA, eds. Injury and Repair of the Musculoskeletal Soft Tissues. Park Ridge, IL: American Academy of Orthopaedic Surgeons, 1988:465–482.
32. Arnoczky S, Adams M, DeHaven K, et al. Meniscus. In: Woo SL-Y, Buckwalter JA, eds. Injury and Repair of the Musculoskeletal Soft Tissues. Park Ridge, IL: American Academy of Orthopaedic Surgeons, 1988:465–482.
33. Ikenoue T, Trindade MC, Lee MS, et al. Mechanoregulation of human articular chondrocytes aggrecan and type II expression by intermittent hydrostatic pressure in vitro. J Orthop Res 2003;21:110–116.
34. Hambly K, Bobic V, Wondrasch B, et al. Autologous chondrocyte implantation postoperative care and rehabilitation: science and practice. Am J Sports Med 2006;34(6):1020–1038.
35. Bartels E, Lund, H, Hagen K et al. Aquatic exercise for the treatment of knee and hip osteoarthritis. (Protocol) Cochrane Database Syst 2007 Oct 17;14(4):CD005523.
36. Cochrane T, Davey R, Matthes Edwards, S.: Randomised controlled trial of the cost-effectiveness of water-based therapy for lower limb osteoarthritis. Health Technol Assess 2005;9(31):1–114.
37. Foley A, Halbert J, Hewitt, T, et al. Does hydrotherapy improve strength and physical function in patients with osteoarthritis: a randomised controlled trial comparing a gym based and a hydrotherapy based strengthening program. Ann Rheum Dis 2003;62:1162–1167.
38. Silva L, Valim V, Pessanha A, et al. Hydrotherapy versus conventional land-based exercise for the management of patients with osteoarthritis of the knee: a randomized clinical trial. Phys Ther 2008;88(1):12–21.
39. Wyatt F, Milam S, Manske R, et al. The effects of aquatic and traditional exercise programs on persons with knee osteoarthritis. J Strength Cond Res 2001;5:337–340.
40. Fransen M, Nairn, L, Winstanley, J, et al. Physical activity for osteoarthritis management: a randomized controlled clinical trial evaluating hydrotherapy or Tai Chi classes. Arthritis Rheum 2007;57(3):407–414.
41. Hinman R, Heywood S, Day A. Aquatic physical therapy for hip and knee ostearthritis: results of a single-blind randomized controlled trial. Phys Ther 2007;87(1):32–43.
42. American Academy of Orthopedic Surgeons. Athletic Training and Sports Medicine. Park Ridge, IL: American Academy of Orthopaedic Surgeons, 1991.
43. Salter RB. Textbook of Disorders and Injuries of the Musculoskeletal System. 2nd Ed. Baltimore, MD: Williams & Wilkins, 1983.
44. Insall JN. Surgery of the Knee. New York: Churchill Livingstone, 1984.
45. Rubman MH, Noyes FR, Barber-Westin SD. Arthroscopic repair of meniscal tears that extend into the avascular zone. Am J Sports Med 1998;26:87–95.
46. Noyes FR, Barber-Westin SD. Arthroscopic repair of meniscus tears extending into the avascular zone with or without anterior cruciate ligament reconstruction in patients 40 years of age and older. Arthroscopy 2000;16:822–829.
47. Stollsteimer GT, Shelton WR, Dukes A, et al. Meniscal allograft transplantation: a 1- to 5-year follow-up of 22 patients. Arthroscopy 2000;16:343–347.
48. Heckmann TP, Barber-Westin SD, Noyes FR. Meniscal repair and transplantation: indications, techniques, rehabilitation, and clinical outcome. J Orthop Sports Phys Ther 2006;36(10):795–814.

49. Byrd JWT. Hip arthroscopy in the athlete. N Am J Sports Phys Ther 2007;2(4): 217–230.
50. Narvani AA, Tsiridis E, Tai CC, et al. Acetabular labrum and its tears. Br J Sports Med 2003;37:207–211.
51. Martin RRL, Enseki KR, Draovitch P, et al. Acetabular labral tears of the hip: examination and diagnostic challenges. J Orthop Sports Phys Ther 2006; 36(7):503–515.
52. Enseki KR, Martin RRL, Draovitch P, et al. The hip joint: arthroscopic procedures and postoperative rehabilitation. J Orthop Sports Phys Ther 2006; 36(7):516–525.
53. Gillogly SD, Myers TH, Reinold MM. Treatment of full-thickness chondral defects in the knee with autologous chondrocyte implantation. J Orthop Sports Phys Ther 2006;36(10):751–764.
54. Gillogly SD, Voight M, Blackburn T. Treatment of articular cartilage defects of the knee with autologous chondrocytes implantation. J Orthop Sports Phys Ther 1998;28:241–251.
55. Lewis PB, McCarty LP, Kang RW, et al. Basic science and treatment options for articular cartilage injuries. J Orthop Sports Phys Ther 2006;36(10):717–727.
56. Gill TJ, Asnis PD, Berksom EM. The treatment of articular cartilage defects using the microfracture technique. J Orthop Sports Phys Ther 2006;36(10): 728–738.
57. Reinhold MM, Wilk KE, Macrina LC, et al. Current concepts in the rehabilitation following articular cartilage repair procedures in the knee. J Orthop Sports Phys Ther 2006;36(10):774–794.
58. Bartha L, Vajda A, Duska Z, et al. Autologous osteochondral mosaicplasty grafting. J Orthop Sports Phys Ther 2006;36(10):739–750.
59. Bentley G, Biant LC, Carrington RW, et al. A prospective, randomized comparison of autologous chondrocyte implantation versus mosaicplasty for osteochondral defects in the knee. J Bone Joint Surg Br 2003;85:223–230.
60. Dorland's Illustrated Medical Dictionary, 26th Ed. Philadelphia, PA: WB Saunders, 1981.

chapter 12
Therapeutic Exercise for Arthritis

KIMBERLY BENNETT

PATHOLOGY

An important principle of therapeutic intervention is that treatment should consider the underlying causes of disease as well as the resulting effects on body function and structure, activity and participation (see Chapter 1). This approach necessitates an understanding of the pathology and its relation to broader functional effects in order to guide treatment design, including the choice of intervention, understanding of precautions, and formulations of rational goals.

Arthritis literally means joint inflammation, but there are approximately 100 different forms of arthritis (inflammatory and noninflammatory, affecting not only joints but soft tissue as well). Osteoarthritis and rheumatoid arthritis, two of the most common forms of arthritis, are discussed in this chapter. Osteoarthritis represents a type of nonsystemic, mostly noninflammatory, localized pathology. Rheumatoid arthritis is a systemic, inflammatory disease that usually involves multiple joints and often affects organ systems. Because these two diseases have distinctly different pathologic mechanisms, and because of the widespread systemic effects of rheumatoid arthritis, some of the exercise design considerations vary.

Since many of the same principles of degenerative and inflammatory processes are encountered in the less common forms of inflammatory arthritis, similar thought processes can be applied to developing exercise approaches for patients with these diseases. Effects of the two diseases on joints and related structures are listed in Table 12-1.

Osteoarthritis

Etiology
Osteoarthritis is characterized by the breakdown of articular cartilage under load with resultant changes in bone and other soft tissue periarticular structures. The view that osteoarthritis is the result of passive wearing of cartilage with time is being replaced with an increased understanding of the interaction of biomechanical and molecular events which produce osteoarthritic changes,[1] though there is a highly positive correlation of incidence with age.[2]

Clinical Manifestations
Osteoarthritis typically affects weight-bearing joints and joints of the hand, is usually unilateral and often unicompartmental, and has no direct systemic effects.

The pathologic changes of osteoarthritis reflect damage to the articular cartilage and the joint's reaction to that damage. Cartilage damage diminishes the joint's ability to withstand loading forces which further stresses the articular cartilage,

leading to tissue damage that can result in low-grade synovial inflammation. If chronic, inflammation can lead to fibrosis of the joint capsule and resultant range restriction (see Chapter 20). Hypertrophic bone formation at joint margins (i.e., marginal spurring) leads to joint deformity and pain (Fig. 12-1).

Extra-articular soft tissue structures are affected by asymmetric joint deformity which in turn further affects joint function. A common example of this imbalance is seen in the osteoarthritic knee. Lateral compartment cartilage loss results in a valgus deformity of the knee, which stretches muscles and ligaments medially and shortens soft tissue structures laterally. In addition to affecting alignment of the knee and weight bearing through the joint, the deformity changes the mechanical advantage of medial and lateral muscle groups and the stability of the joint as stretched ligaments become lax. Joint pain and swelling, together with splinting and guarding, can lead to muscle disuse atrophy and loss of this important component of the shock-absorbing system. Significant functional deficits can develop as these clinical changes progress. In running, the tibiofemoral joint experiences forces 2.5 to 3.0 times body weight[3] and in deep knee bends, the patellofemoral joint is exposed to forces 10 times body weight.[2] Impairment of the joint elements responsible for efficient shock absorbing will in turn lead to further joint breakdown during activity.

Although cartilage failure may be the primary event in osteoarthritis, the overall effect of the disease is rarely confined to the involved joint.[4] Minor[4] cites studies of patients with osteoarthritis in the lower limb that showed joints adjacent to the affected joint can have limitations in range of motion (ROM) and strength and that contralateral joints can also be affected in ROM and in functional use. In attempting to improve overall function, the exercise program should focus on impairments at the affected joint and on secondary impairments and activity limitations at associated joints caused by the primary impairments and by inactivity. See Building Block 12-1.

Rheumatoid Arthritis

Etiology
Rheumatoid arthritis is a disease characterized by chronic, erosive synovitis in which an immune event triggers transformation of synovial cells causing them to proliferate. An invasive, fibroblast-like cell mass called pannus develops and erosion of cartilage and bone follows. Synovial fluid accumulates, and the joint swells, distending the capsule, pulling on its periosteal attachment, and causing pain and potential rupture. Ligaments and muscles around the inflamed joint are also subject to weakening and potential rupture.

TABLE 12-1	**Effects of Osteoarthritis and Rheumatoid Arthritis on Joint Structure and Function**		
STRUCTURE	**FUNCTION**	**EFFECTS OF OSTEOARTHRITIS**	**EFFECTS OF RHEUMATOID ARTHRITIS**
Cartilage	Shock absorption, joint congruence	Thickening to softening to thinning to loss	Erosion of cartilage
Synovium	Secretes synovial fluid for nutrition of cartilage, lubrication, and stability	Secondary involvement occasionally	Microvascular lining cells activated by inflammatory process, pannus formation
Ligaments	Stability, reinforce capsule and limit movement, guide movement	Abnormal joint alignment stresses	Erosion weakens
Muscles	Reinforce joint capsule, reflex joint protection, move joints	Immobility shortens pain, causes guarding and reflex inhibition, leading to weakness	Joint deformity interferes with peak torque generation; immobility shortens; myositis weakens; pain and effusion cause guarding and reflex inhibition leads to weakness
Bone	Structural support	Subchondral bone remodeling changes shock-absorbing properties, joint margin spurring leads to bony blockade and pain	Erosion leads to joint deformity, bony blockade, pain
Extra-articular system		Increased energy expenditure from abnormal movement patterns	Myositis, anemia, sleep disruption, fatigue, increased energy expenditure from abnormal movement patterns

Clinical Manifestations

Loss of cartilage and bone integrity, soft tissue disruption, and swelling lead to joint dysfunction as they do in osteoarthritis, but often the deformities are more severe, and usually the entire joint is affected rather than just one joint compartment (Fig. 12-2). As the disease becomes more chronic, contralateral joints are affected. The joint changes are usually reversible if the disease remits within 1 year and no structural deformity has occurred. Early intervention with an emphasis on education regarding joint protection strategies is important as irreversible changes usually occur between the first and the second year in more chronic forms of rheumatoid arthritis.[5]

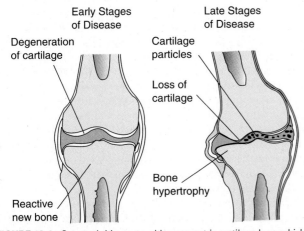

FIGURE 12-1. Osteoarthritis starts with asymmetric cartilage loss, which leads to abnormal forces on the joint. Soft-tissue imbalance, joint malalignment, and bony hypertrophy can result. Inflammation is not the major component of the osteoarthritis process. (Adapted from AHPA Arthritis Teaching Slide Collection. American College of Rheumatology, Atlanta, GA.)

BUILDING BLOCK 12-1

(OA)

A 65-year-old male is referred to you with complaints of left (L) knee pain. Since his recent retirement, he has spent three mornings a week at a driving range, and two times a week playing 18 holes of golf. He thinks his knee pain has gotten worse since his retirement when he was more sedentary. In addition to making it difficult for him to participate in his normal weekly golf game with friends (he is now limited to nine holes and that is getting painful enough that he is thinking of stopping altogether), he is finding it increasingly difficult to get up and down stairs, or to sit and get up from a low chair due to pain and a perception of weakness in his L leg.

He takes no medication, reporting to you that though his doctor has told him to take an over the counter anti-inflammatory, he has chosen not to as he doesn't believe in medicine and especially doesn't want to "get hooked" on pain medication.

Review of systems shows a moderately hypertensive individual, who is overweight. His radiology report states that there is marked cartilage degeneration in the left medial compartment of the tibiofemoral joint which is apparent in the varus angle of his L knee compared to right (R). When he has been on his feet a lot, his R knee can bother him a little in the last few weeks. His doctor has suggested increased activity for both weight and hypertension control.

1. Which joints should be examined in your initial evaluation of this patient?
2. What tests will you do in this examination?
3. Write a problem list based on the information in this case including at least two impairments of body structure or function, two for activity, and two for participation restrictions.

Early Inflammatory Response

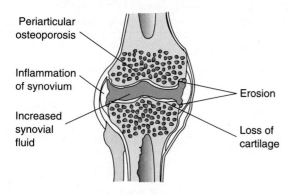

Post-Inflammatory Response

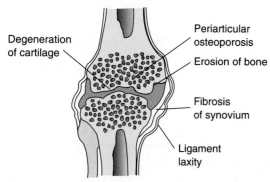

FIGURE 12-2. Early inflammatory joint response to rheumatoid arthritis includes pannus formation and erosion of cartilage and bone. Posinflammatory irreversible joint changes include destruction of cartilage, bone, and soft tissues and fibrosis of the joint capsule. Damage affects joint alignment, stability, and range of motion. (Adapted from AHPA Arthritis Teaching Slide Collection. American College of Rheumatology, Atlanta, GA.)

DISPLAY 12-1

Classification of Progression of Rheumatoid Arthritis

Stage I, Early

*1. No destructive changes on roentgenographic examination
2. Roentgenologic evidence of osteoporosis may be present

Stage II, Moderate

*1. Roentgenologic evidence of osteoporosis, with or without slight subchondral bone destruction; slight cartilage destruction may be present
*2. No joint deformities, although limitation of joint mobility may be present
3. Adjacent muscle atrophy
4. Extra-articular soft-tissue lesions, such as nodules and tenosynovitis, may be present

Stage III, Severe

*1. Roentgenologic evidence of cartilage and bone destruction in addition to osteoporosis
*2. Joint deformity, such as subluxation, ulnar deviation, or hyperextension, without fibrous or bony ankylosis
3. Extensive muscle atrophy
4. Extra-articular soft-tissue lesions, such as nodules and tenosynovitis, may be present

Stage IV, Terminal

*1. Fibrous or bony ankylosis
2. Criteria of stage III

*The criteria prefaced by an asterisk are those that must be present to permit classification of a patient in any particular stage or grade.

From Schumaker HR Jr, ed. Primer on the Rheumatic Diseases. 10th Ed. Atlanta: Arthritis Foundation, 1993:188–190.

Patients diagnosed with rheumatoid arthritis prior to the mid-1980s were typically treated with the least aggressive pharmacologic agents first, typically starting with nonsteroidal and then steroidal medications followed eventually by cytotoxic drugs like colloidal gold. As newer cytotoxic and biologic drugs aimed at interfering with immune system events leading to joint damage became available, this approach changed and patients diagnosed in the 1990s and later were more likely to be treated with steroidal and cytotoxic drugs immediately. The result of this is that you may see patients with more extreme joint deformities if the onset of their disease was prior to the 1980s and in some cases in patients from countries with limited access to these more expensive drugs as once joint deformities are present, they are not reversible. The newer approach is aimed at minimizing joint deformity in the patient with rheumatoid arthritis from the onset of the disease.

Display 12-1 summarizes the effects of rheumatoid arthritis on joint and extra-articular structures and function.

Unlike osteoarthritis, rheumatoid arthritis has systemic effects such as fatigue, malaise, anemia, and sleep disorders (i.e., pain and abnormal sleep cycles). Organ systems, including lungs and the cardiovascular system, may also be affected. Medications used to treat rheumatoid arthritis may contribute to myositis, gastrointestinal distress, and sleep disruption.

These systemic effects should be considered in designing exercise programs for the patient with rheumatoid arthritis.[5,6]

The course of rheumatoid arthritis is variable and characterized by exacerbations (i.e., flares) and remissions. During a flare, joints are hot and swollen, morning stiffness is present and often lasts longer than 60 minutes, and systemic effects may be more obvious. This is considered an acute phase of the disease. As the pain, swelling, systemic effects, and morning stiffness decrease, the disease state is considered to be subacute. Between exacerbations, the disease state is considered chronic.

The clinician needs to consider the phase of rheumatoid arthritis when designing an exercise program. After prolonged inflammation, synovial membranes fibrose, decreasing the vasculature such that joints may not appear hot and swollen. These are referred to as burned-out joints. Although it may appear that the disease has gone into remission (i.e., the subacute or chronic phase) and has ceased to damage the joint, the joint destruction and systemic effects continue,[5] and the disease state remains active.

Because symptoms wax and wane, the type and intensity of appropriate exercise also vary. *The clinician must consider the phase of rheumatoid arthritis when designing an exercise program, and the patient must be taught to modify the program to match the phase of their illness.* See Building Block 12-2.

In addition to the local pathologic changes caused by both rheumatoid and osteoarthritis, the resulting joint pain and effusion in both diseases trigger protective and reflex spasm

BUILDING BLOCK 12-2

1. List at least three characteristics of rheumatoid arthritis which distinguish it from osteoarthritis.
2. List three special considerations in designing an exercise program necessitated by the clinical manifestations of rheumatoid arthritis.

and immobility. Immobility leads to further muscle atrophy and loss of normal protective reflex responses.[3,7,8] Immobility combined with non–weight bearing has been shown in animal models to contribute to cartilage breakdown, aggravating the condition.[6,7] Diminished joint complex integrity can also lead to movement patterns that are energy inefficient, limiting activity. When a joint is abnormally aligned, muscles can no longer generate peak force, contributing to strength deficits. For these reasons and because of the effects of low-dose steroids on muscle[9] and the destructive effect of myositis in rheumatoid arthritis, muscles often atrophy significantly. Type II fiber deficits occur in patients with rheumatoid arthritis and osteoarthritis,[10,11] and isometric strength deficits have been reported for these patients compared with controls.[8,12–14] These impairments underlie the development of functional deficits as patients find it more difficult, painful, and less efficient to move. Exercise correctly prescribed can address impairments and functional deficits.[15–17]

Various classifications have been useful in guiding exercise prescription and in teaching patients to monitor and appropriately modify their home programs and activities of daily living (ADLs). In the classification of functional status proposed by the American College of Rheumatology, patients are divided into four groups based on their ability to perform self-care, vocational activities, and avocational activities (Display 12-2). Most exercise program studies that looked at exercise effects considered patients in functional class I, II, and occasionally, III.

Another classification scheme that may guide the therapist in exercise program design examines the radiologic and clinical evidence of disease progression (see Display 12-1 and Building Block 12-3).

DISPLAY 12-2
Classification of Functional Status of Patients with Rheumatoid Arthritis*

Class I: Completely able to perform usual ADLs (self-care, vocational, and avocational)*

Class II: Able to perform usual self-care and vocational activities, but limited in avocational activities

Class III: Able to perform usual self-care activities, but limited in vocational and avocational activities

Class IV: Limited in ability to perform usual self-care, vocational, and avocational activities

*Usual self-care activities include dressing, feeding, bathing, grooming, and toileting. Avocational (recreation, leisure) and vocational (work, school, homemaking) activities are patient desired and age- and sex-specific.

From Hochberg MC, Chang RW, Dwosh I, et al. The American College of Rheumatology 1991 revised criteria for the classification of global functional status in rheumatoid arthritis. Arthritis Rheum 1992;35:498–502.

BUILDING BLOCK 12-3

RA-1
A 54-year-old woman with a 30-year history of RA is referred to you with complaints of pain, weakness, fatigue, and an increasingly difficult time doing her half time job as a computer programming instructor, her house work, and cooking due to these factors. She lives with her husband in a one story house with five stairs with railing to enter the house. Her children are grown and gone, her husband does most of the heavy work around the house and is not currently working due to a job layoff, so they depend on her job for health insurance.

Her RA was originally treated with nonsteroidal anti-inflammatories, followed by steroidal treatment then colloidal gold, and finally with methotrexate. She has joint deformities in feet, hands, knees, and elbows. She has had multiple tendon transplants and fusions in her feet, tendon transplants in her hand, and has both elbow and knee ligament laxity. She reports that with the onset of the gold treatment and then methotrexate, the progression of joint deformities stopped. She is now taking methotrexate.

Her main complaint at this visit is bilateral shoulder pain, difficulty driving due to shoulder pain when holding and turning the wheel, and neck and shoulder pain when she turns her head. She is having increasing shoulder pain at the end of a work day.

Review of systems is unremarkable except for slight hypotension, and increased breath and heart rate from resting rates of 12 and 72 respectively to 20 and 90 after walking 200 ft. Gait is inefficient with hip hiking and trunk rotation initiating swing phase and lumbar hyperextension with rollover to toe-off phase of gait.

RA-2
Your patient is a 32-year-old, right (R) hand dominant female competitive tennis player. She was diagnosed 3 years ago with rheumatoid arthritis following episodes of pain and swelling in bilateral (B) hands and feet. She was started initially on prednisone and methotrexate. Prednisone was then withdrawn as methotrexate took effect. She is here now with complaints of R elbow pain playing tennis and using her arm at home for cooking and gardening. No other joint pain is reported except occasional brief twinges of left (L) elbow pain. She has not played tennis in 6 months and has stopped all gym exercise due to fear of aggravating her symptoms.

She has been taking methotrexate since the rheumatoid arthritis was diagnosed and had a cortisone injection to the area of the common extensor tendon origin 3 weeks ago. This gave her about 50% relief of pain at rest, but with any use, symptoms flare again. She takes no other medication and has no other significant medical history.

R medial and lateral epicondylar provocation testing is positive. R elbow and wrist range of motion (ROM) is normal though she complains of tightness with both wrist flexion and extension and palpation is positive for pain in both flexor and extensor muscle groups. Mild joint laxity is present with varus and valgus testing R > L elbow. The R elbow joint is warmer than the L per palpation.

Her goal is to return to double tennis and to household tasks including cooking and gardening, pain free.

1. For the patients listed in cases RA-1 and RA-2, write out instructions you would give them to recognize when they may be entering a stage of acute inflammation (either autoimmune- or activity-triggered) and what their actions should be.
2. To which functional class does the patient in case RA-1 belong? The patient in case RA-2

EXERCISE RECOMMENDATIONS FOR PREVENTION AND WELLNESS

There is no direct way to prevent rheumatoid arthritis. On the other hand, the literature suggests that certain factors including obesity, trauma, hypermobility, and inflammation correlate with the development of osteoarthritis.[5,7] An exercise regimen aimed at maintaining appropriate body weight, sustaining good postural alignment, developing good muscular strength and length, and correctly using joints in ADLs may be logical and desirable for joint protection. It has been demonstrated, for example, that a 10 lb weight loss was correlated with a 50% decrease in the likelihood of knee OA developing in women.[18] But to the extent that osteoarthritis has a genetic basis in some persons and, in some cases, is correlated with trauma, infection, and inflammation, exercise is not a guarantee against developing osteoarthritis. A major goal of treatment is to limit the progression of arthritic damage in the affected joint and in the joints showing adaptive changes to pathology at the primary joint. Intervention includes assessing and treating impairments and resulting functional losses in an attempt to avoid disablement.

THERAPEUTIC EXERCISE INTERVENTION FOR COMMON IMPAIRMENTS

Exercise programs to address common impairments and activity limitations affecting a person's ability to function in society are necessary. A recent review of randomized controlled studies on the effect of water exercise on hip and knee osteoarthritis showed short term effects on function, quality of life, and pain.[15] A large study of 220 participants looked at the effect of aerobic exercise on symptoms, function, aerobic fitness, and disease outcomes in patients with rheumatoid arthritis at 1, 6, and 12 weeks. Positive effects were found on walk time and grip strength, and overall fatigue, pain, and depression symptoms were positively influenced. There was no finding of increased disease activity with exercise.[16] Another recent study[17] of the effect of short term intensive training in post hospitalization patients with rheumatoid arthritis or following joint replacement in patients with osteoarthritis showed long term (52 week) gains in ROM and self-reported function.

In osteoarthritis, the goal of treatment is to decrease pain and any inflammation which is present, to restore normal joint flexibility, and to reestablish balance between muscle length and strength around the joint. Any adaptive changes in joints proximal, distal, or contralateral to the affected joint and its surrounding structures must also be addressed. Performance of basic functional tasks (e.g., sit to stand to sit, balance, timed walking, performance of household, vocational, and recreational activities) and optimization of cardiovascular fitness are the tasks of an exercise program designed for a patient with osteoarthritis.

For patients with rheumatoid arthritis, exercise program considerations are largely those outlined for osteoarthritis, but because of the variability of its course and because of the possible systemic involvement of the disease, careful monitoring by the physical therapist and the patient is necessary. Patients must be taught to recognize symptom development and the stage of the illness and to modify activity appropriately.

The patient with arthritis typically presents with pain, mobility impairment, imbalances in muscle length, and movement patterns contributing to impaired muscle performance, and cardiovascular endurance impairment. These factors should be evaluated bilaterally throughout the entire extremity joint chain and the trunk. It is equally important to look at functional movement patterns, including gait, stairs, sit to stand to sit, and manipulation of tools and the environment when hands are involved.

The exercise program must carry the effects of therapy beyond treatment of a localized joint problem to issues of function in an attempt to reverse the disablement process. In planning an exercise regimen, the impairment at the affected joint and secondary impairments and activity limitations must be addressed. Limitations may occur along a continuum of function, ranging from deficits in high-level athletic performance to an inability to perform self-care activities.

The aims of treatment are to decrease impairment while improving function. Functional improvement includes performance of ADLs and improved muscle and cardiovascular conditioning. Functional activities should be incorporated into the exercise routine to ensure that functional skills are mastered and carried into daily life in an attempt to reverse the disablement process. Joints should be protected during exercise and during functional activities. See Building Block 12-4.

Pain

It is important to address and minimize pain during therapeutic intervention, because pain may lead to other impairments. Joint pain and swelling together with splinting or guarding can inhibit periarticular muscle function and lead to disuse atrophy, suppress the normal protective reflex response, and cause further cartilage breakdown.[3,7,8,19,20] These changes can lead to inefficient movement patterns, thereby decreasing cardiovascular endurance and further limiting activity. The changes may also disrupt the soft tissue balance around the joint, affecting its stability, alignment, and active motion. When a joint is abnormally aligned, muscles can no longer generate peak force, contributing to strength deficits.

The use of exercise to restore muscle balance and joint range for cardiovascular conditioning and to improve functional status was associated with no increase in pain in some studies on the effect of exercise on arthritis[21,22] and with a decrease in pain in others.[13,23] Patients often present with some degree of pain in the affected joints, which may prevent exercise to the full extent possible or signal the presence of an inflammatory process. In either case, helping to control the pain during and after exercise can maximize possible exertion and help to control inflammatory processes. It is important to recognize that any exercise-induced pain necessitates modification of the exercise.

 BUILDING BLOCK 12-4

1. Write a problem list including at least two impairments to body function or structure; two activity, and two participation limitations for cases RA-1 and RA-2.
2. Write one goal for the patient in each case addressing activity and participation deficits.

Thermal modalities and electrical stimulation to control pain can be applied in conjunction with exercise in the clinic. When possible, the patient should be taught to apply them at home and be instructed about sources for these modalities. The patient should learn how to apply these treatments, because the chronic condition mandates a continued need for them, at least episodically. Heat application to muscles may be appropriate for the patient with rheumatoid arthritis before exercise. Ice applied to joints after exercise may also be appropriate for the patient with osteoarthritis and for the patient with rheumatoid arthritis, if tolerated. Transcutaneous nerve stimulation (TNS) may be useful in conjunction with other modalities in managing pain. TNS should be used with caution with exercise, because it could mask symptoms of overexertion. It has been suggested that regular exercise be scheduled for late morning or early afternoon, especially for patients with rheumatoid arthritis with stiffness early in the day and fatigue later in the day.[24]

Exercise Modification in Response to Pain and Fatigue

Systemic deconditioning, muscle and joint irritability, and possibly anemia characterize patients with inflammatory arthritis. Evaluation of the patient's response to treatment allows appropriate and timely modification of the exercise prescription. Irreversible changes such as cartilage loss, bony deformity, or ligament laxity, together with systemic symptoms such as fatigue or reduced cardiovascular capacity, require modification of exercise to avoid aggravation of joint irritation or undue fatigue. In the past, exercises that increased pain for longer than 2 hours after exercise were modified. It is now accepted that any exercise that increases joint pain should be modified or avoided.[25] The patient should be taught to differentiate between muscle reaction to exercise and joint pain. Undue fatigue after exercise in deconditioned patients with osteoarthritis and rheumatoid arthritis, and in patients with rheumatoid arthritis who may be functioning at a lower aerobic capacity indicates a need to further modify the exercise prescription.

It is necessary to keep in mind that fatigue can be either systemic or exercise-induced, or both. Instructions to the patient with a rheumatic disease might include sleep and rest guidelines.[26]

Compliance with exercise programs increases when exertion and pain are within acceptable limits for the patient.[7,14,21] The patient's reaction to exercise should be carefully monitored, and self-monitoring skills should be taught as part of the therapy program. See Building Block 12-5.

Impaired Mobility and Range of Motion

Osteoarthritis and rheumatoid arthritis often contribute to mobility impairment. ROM can be diminished by several factors:

- Stiffness and shortening of muscles or tendons from spasm, guarding, or habitual postures
- Capsular stiffness or contracture
- Loss of joint congruity because of bony deformity

These conditions lead to muscle imbalances that can initially limit joint range and lead to joint contractures and muscle weakness affecting the entire limb and eventually affecting the whole body. The therapist must be aware of the muscle groups most typically affected by osteoarthritis and rheumatoid

BUILDING BLOCK 12-5

1. Each of your patients in cases OA, RA-1, and RA-2 have been prescribed an exercise routine at their first visit. List at least two questions you would ask all of them at the beginning of their second visit regarding the routines.
2. The following scenarios exist during the second visit. List your response to them:

   A. In case OA, your patient noted increased pain with the exercise routine you prescribed at the last visit.
   B. In case RA-1 your patient reported no increase in shoulder pain, but an overall increase in fatigue in general and especially when she had a few late nights staying up to do her physical therapy exercises when the rest of her work at home was done.
   C. In case RA-2 your patient admits she didn't do her exercises.

arthritis in specific joints. Muscle shortening leads to weakness and joint malalignment. For example, in hip osteoarthritis, hip flexor shortening and hip flexor and extensor weakness are common (Table 12-2). A thorough musculoskeletal evaluation should indicate which of these factors are present.

Cartilage maintenance depends in part on joint movement.[19,20] Passive, active, and active-assisted ROM exercises are designed to ensure that affected joints move through the full range available to them and can be used with patients with osteoarthritis, chronic rheumatoid, and to some extent, subacute rheumatoid arthritis.

Passive ROM is rarely necessary, except in cases of acute joint exacerbation and of severe muscle weakness and inflammation in rheumatoid arthritis. These patients probably are in functional status classes III and IV and often need to be at rest. To avoid contracture and to ensure maintenance of full ROM, one or two repetitions of gentle passive movement through full available range each day is required. Repetitive passive ROM movements may increase joint inflammation.[24] For patients with rheumatoid arthritis who are in functional status classes I and II or who have osteoarthritis, active ROM exercises should be performed daily for affected joints.

When weakness prevents the patient from attaining full ROM, assistance from another person or another limb may be required to achieve full available range. Typically, patients start with 1 to 5 repetitions and progress to 10 each day.

When muscle shortening is the cause of range limitations, passive stretch controlled by the patient or clinician may be provided as long as the joint is stable. Considerations outlined in Chapter 6 regarding stabilization of proximal and distal attachment sites to avoid stressing joints above and below the target muscle are especially important in this population. In patients with rheumatoid arthritis for whom the integrity of muscle, tendon, or ligament is in question (especially in smaller joints), *gentle* active ROM exercises are preferable. As a safety measure, it is important that the patient be safely positioned while performing active ROM exercises to ensure they do not fall, lose control of a limb, or apply more force than is intended (Fig. 12-3).

TABLE 12-2	Common Patterns of Joint Restriction in Osteoarthritis and Rheumatoid Arthritis		
JOINT	**RESTRICTION**	**STRETCH**	**STRENGTHEN**
Hip (OA/RA)	• All planes, especially internal rotation and extension	• Flexors • Extensors • Internal and external rotators • Tensor fascia lata	• Abductors • Extensors
Knee (OA/RA)	• Extension	• Hamstrings (quadriceps)	• Quadriceps
Ankle and foot (RA)	• Ankle dorsiflexion • MTP flexion • PIP extension	• Ankle dorsiflexors and plantarflexors • Tarsal invertors and evertors • Toe flexors and extensors	• Toe extensors and flexors • Tibialis posterior • Abductors
Shoulder (RA)	• Abduction • Flexion • External and internal rotators	• Careful in deranged joints • PROM, AAROM, AROM	• External rotation • Biceps • Triceps
Elbow (RA)	• Extension lost early	• Careful in deranged joints • PROM, AAROM, AROM	• Biceps • Triceps
Hand and wrist (RA)	• MCP extension • Wrist extension • First web space	• Careful in deranged joints • ROM wrist daily • Stretch wrist flexors and extensors, forearm pronators and supinators, hand intrinsics	• Finger extensors • Wrist extensors

AAROM, active assisted range of motion; AROM, active range of motion; MCP, metacarpophalangeal joint; MTP, metatarsophalangeal joint; OA, osteoarthritis; PIP, proximal interphalangeal joint; PROM, passive range of motion; RA, rheumatoid arthritis; ROM, range of motion.

Data from Hicks JE. Exercise in patients with inflammatory arthritis and connective tissue disease. Rheum Dis Clin North Am 1990;16:845–870 and from Moskowitz RW, Goldberg VM. Osteoarthritis: clinical features and treatment. In: Schumaker HR Jr, ed. Primer on the Rheumatic Diseases. 10th Ed. Atlanta: Arthritis Foundation, 1993:188–190.

Ligament laxity can occur in the cervical spine of patients with rheumatoid arthritis, and special considerations, especially for stretching exercise, apply. A more detailed description of these precautions is given in the section "Precautions During Strengthening Exercises When Ligament or Capsular Laxity Exists."

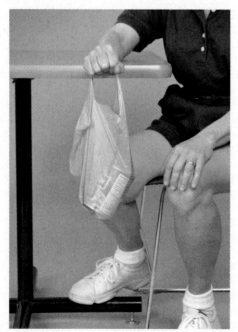

FIGURE 12-3. The patient performs an active range of motion exercise (wrist extension) with her arm and wrist firmly stabilized on the table for safety.

Patients who have rheumatoid arthritis with prolonged morning stiffness or osteoarthritis with the brief stiffness (<0.5 hour) common in the morning may benefit from instruction in a ROM and stretching routine targeting the stiff areas. This exercise can be done before retiring at night, in the morning after a warm shower, or during both periods.

Instruction of the patient in self-mobilization techniques as part of a home exercise program may be useful in cases of osteoarthritis in which capsular restriction limits movement but no acute joint irritation or bony block exists[27] (see Self-Management 12-1: Self-Mobilization of the Shoulder Joint). Capsular stiffness in patients with rheumatoid arthritis often results from joint distention, and further distractive forces on this inflamed and often weakened tissue should be avoided. When stability is good, passive application of grade 1 oscillations by a skilled therapist to relax periarticular spasm before passive or active ROM activities may be beneficial (see Chapter 7).

Impaired Muscle Performance

The same forces which lead to ROM losses affect, and can in turn themselves be affected, by muscle imbalances which occur around the involved joints.

Strengthening of weakened muscles is an important part of regaining muscle balance around the joint. It can be done isometrically, isotonically, or isokinetically (see Chapter 5). Each form of exercise has its place in rehabilitation of the arthritic joint, depending on the state of the joint. Isokinetic equipment is most readily available in a clinical setting and is not likely to be practical for independent exercise programs; it is not discussed here. See Building Block 12-6.

SELF-MANAGEMENT 12-1 *Self-Mobilization of the Shoulder Joint*

Purpose: To stretch the tight capsule and muscles around the shoulder, which are limiting movement

Position: Sit on a straight-back chair as shown, with a folded towel padding your arm.

Movement technique: Let your arm hang down.

Grasp it just above the elbow.

Repeat a gentle, rhythmic series of downward tugs, trying to keep your shoulder muscles relaxed.

Dosage

Repetitions _____

Frequency _____

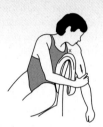

Isometric Exercise

Isometric exercise is most appropriate for acute flares in osteoarthritis and rheumatoid arthritis, but precautions to avoid increased intra-articular inflammation should be observed.

Isometric Exercise in Rheumatoid Arthritis Patients suffering acute exacerbations of rheumatoid arthritis are primarily at rest, are positioned to prevent deformity, and may have one or two daily applications of passive ROM applied to large joints and active ROM applied to small joints. In this stage, the preven-

---

BUILDING BLOCK 12-6

1. Your patient in case OA has demonstrated loss of both active and passive ROM of L knee extension with end of range pain. What objective tests would you use to determine the source of this restriction?
2. You prescribe an exercise routine to address soft tissue restrictions around the knee. What protective guidelines would you give your patient?
3. Your patient in case RA-1 complains of morning pain and stiffness "all over." What advice would you give them?
4. Your patient in case RA-1 is bed bound with an acute flare of symptoms. You are concerned about maintaining her shoulder ROM. What instruction would you give a family member caring for her? How would your advice differ if her finger joints were involved?
5. Both your patients in cases OA and RA-1 are found to have capsular tightness affecting joint ROM. How would your advice to them differ?

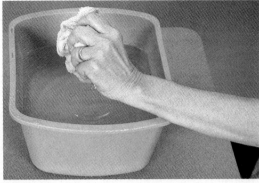

FIGURE 12-4. Squeezing a wet towel is an example of an isometric exercise that can strengthen an arthritic hand. The patient avoids movement into painful ranges or applying pain-causing pressure. Using warm water soothes joints.

tion of muscle atrophy is important. Muscle strength declines 3% each week in a patient at rest.[28] Because it appears that isometric contractions are associated with the least joint shear and intra-articular pressure increases,[29] this form of exercise is often prescribed in the acute and subacute phases of disease (Fig. 12-4). A single isometric contraction at two thirds of maximal effort, which is held for 6 seconds, increases strength in a normal person; three maximal contractions, with 20-second rest periods, performed three times each week increase strength in patients with rheumatoid arthritis.[24,30] However, one drawback is that maximal isometric contraction raises blood pressure.

As a means of increasing muscle strength without raising blood pressure significantly, Gerber and Hicks[31] described a program of brief isometric exercise (BRIME) of one to six isometric contractions, held for 3 to 6 seconds, with 20-second rests between contractions (see Self-Management 12-2: Brief Isometric Exercise—Isometric Quadriceps Contraction).

Isometric contractions performed at one joint angle only strengthen the muscle at that angle selectively.[32] For this reason, repetitions at various angles may be desirable. During an acute exacerbation of arthritis, it may be necessary to limit contraction to one joint angle to avoid stressing the joint.

Isometric Exercise in Osteoarthritis In the acutely painful osteoarthritic joint, especially if there is significant inflammation and swelling, intra-articular pressure and shear should be limited while preventing muscle atrophy. Isometric contractions are often the exercise of choice in this stage. The same considerations apply as for the patient with rheumatoid arthritis. Brief intense isometric exercises are appropriate when controlling blood pressure is an issue (see Selected Intervention12-1: Hand-to-Knee Pushes).

For the patient with an acute arthritic joint, the home program should start with five repetitions of 6-second contractions and assessment of the response. The patient can gradually increase repetitions to two sets of 15 if symptoms are not exacerbated. As acute pain, swelling, and inflammation resolve, movement into an isotonic routine is appropriate.

Dynamic Training

Dynamic muscle strengthening occurs when muscles contract as they shorten (i.e., concentric contractions) or lengthen (i.e., eccentric contractions), resulting in movement of the joint they cross. The advantages of dynamic exercise include increased movement of the joint, resulting in maintenance

SELF-MANAGEMENT 12-2 *Brief Isometric Exercise—Isometric Quadriceps Contraction*

Purpose: To maintain or slightly increase strength of quadriceps muscles during acute knee joint inflammation when the joint is otherwise held at rest and to avoid increasing blood pressure when this is a consideration

Position: Sit with the back supported or in a supine position; bend one knee and straighten the other.

Movement technique: Tighten the quadriceps of the straight leg.
Hold 3 to 6 seconds.
Rest 20 seconds.

Dosage

Repetitions _____

Frequency _____

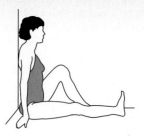

of capsular, ligament, and muscular flexibility and increased cartilage nutrition. Muscle strengthening occurs in all the joint ranges achieved during the exercise and results in a functionally more efficient muscle-joint complex. Joint stress and intra-articular pressure are higher than with isometric exercise.[29] Dynamic training is therefore appropriate for patients with chronic, subacute rheumatoid arthritis of classes I and II and for most patients with osteoarthritis.

In prescribing an exercise regimen, the use of low resistance and high repetition (to fatigue) in a motion arc that does not irritate the joint is preferred to high-load, low-repetition routines in which increased joint loading may cause joint inflammation.[24]

The use of free weights, machines, resistance tubing, and body weight in closed chain activities can be appropriate ways to apply resistance, but their limitations and advantages must be considered in relation to the individual needs of the patient. For example, resistance tubing is less likely to get out of control and torque a joint out of alignment than a free weight, but tubing resistance increases when it is stretched, just as end range movement is achieved and the exercising muscle is out of range of its mechanical advantage. Used correctly, machines offer the advantage of stabilizing the body and exercised joint but rarely offer a low enough resistance to allow a very deconditioned patient to use them. Closed chain exercises, which can range from minisquats to single-leg squat reaches, offer movement patterns which are the basis of function. Closed chain exercise may also be introduced through functional activities such as walking, stair climbing, sit to stand, bending, and squatting. Inclusion of these activities in the strengthening routine provides the clinician with an opportunity to confront safety issues involving balance and body mechanics while addressing daily activities. Bracing, assistive devices, and exercise intensity can then be considered in this context as well. The choice of resistance modality depends on the patient's presentation and the goal of treatment.

In general, start with low enough weight to allow three sets of 10 repetitions, with rest between sets and no resulting joint pain or swelling. The patient should gradually progress to 30 repetitions without rest and without symptom exacerbation and then increase the resistance and start the protocol again. See Building Block 12-7.

Impaired Aerobic Capacity

The effects of osteoarthritis and rheumatoid arthritis on joint structure can lead to a loss of functional movement patterns and affect cardiovascular fitness. Patients affected with either disease have decreased cardiovascular endurance, strength, walking time, and total work capacity compared with controls.[13,14,22,33]

SELECTED INTERVENTION 12-1
Hand-to-Knee Pushes

See Case Study No. 11

Although this patient requires comprehensive intervention as described in other chapters, only one exercise will be described. This exercise would be used in the early to intermediate phases of this patient's rehabilitation.

ACTIVITY: Standing hand-to-knee pushes

PURPOSE: To increase the muscle performance of the hip abductor (stance limb) and abdominal muscles

STAGE OF MOTOR CONTROL: Stability

MODE: Aquatic environment

POSTURE: Standing on one leg with your back against a wall, maintaining a proper lumbar alignment by pelvic tilting. Bend the opposite knee and flex the hip to approximately 90 degrees.

MOVEMENT: With the hand opposite your flexed hip, press isometrically against your knee. Maintain good spinal posture throughout the exercise. Hold for a count of three. Return to the start position.

DOSAGE: Perform five to seven repetitions with each knee, two to three sets to form fatigue.

EXPLANATION OF PURPOSE OF EXERCISE: Hip abductors on the stance limb are trained to maintain transverse plane pelvic position, while the abdominals work to maintain pelvic tilt against the isometric exercise. This exercise is performed in the upright position to enhance carryover to daily activities, but is performed in a gravity-lessened environment to reduce weight bearing on the single-stance limb.

BUILDING BLOCK 12-7

In the following scenarios describe the most appropriate exercise choice to address the listed problem. Include type of muscle contraction, number of repetitions, forms of resistance appropriate (if any), stretches and any precautions your patient should take.

1. Your patient in case RA-1 is now bed-bound with an acute flare of joint pain and swelling and systemic effects including fatigue and apparent myositis. Prescribe an exercise routine which is safe for her to do to preserve current quadriceps strength (remember her knees are hypermobile into extension due to ligament laxity).
2. Your patient in case OA is having problems walking up and down stairs with a step over step gait due to pain and perceived weakness.
3. Your patient in case RA-2 is having difficulty pulling open heavy doors, putting on her emergency brake, and using a pen to write for more than 8 to 10 minutes due to hand weakness and elbow pain.
4. List considerations which would guide your choice of exercises.

Addressing the cardiovascular endurance impairment of patients with arthritis has several benefits, including improved cardiorespiratory status and endurance,[32] improved sense of well-being,[21,34] and improved walk distance.[23] Cardiovascular training should be a major part of therapy programs for patients with osteoarthritis and chronic functional class I and II (possibly class III) rheumatoid arthritis.

Cardiovascular programs for patients with osteoarthritis or rheumatoid arthritis of the lower extremity weight-bearing joints need to be designed to minimize joints stress and shock, to encourage calcium uptake into bone, and to account for any balance difficulties. Several options are available, but adherence to a program is likely to be better when patients are able to pursue activities they find pleasurable.[35] Accessibility and cost factors may also be important for some people. Patient input into this aspect of the program design is important.

Water is a good medium for exercise and has demonstrated positive effects on pain, muscle strength, flexibility, depression, and anxiety.[21,36,37] Water provides a means of unloading joints; in waist-level water, the body weight is 50% of that on land, and in neck-level water, the body weight is 10%.[38] Water provides a medium that can resist or facilitate movement:

- It allows performance of movement patterns that may not be possible on land because of balance or strength deficits.
- It can relax muscles.
- It can modify pain perception through sensory stimulation.

Aquatic therapy can facilitate social interaction in class settings or during family recreation. This aspect may be an added benefit for a population that may be socially limited due to decreased participation in physical activities.

Cardiovascular work can come from walking in the shallow end of a pool, from the use of a foam noodle or float belt, which allows walking or running in deeper water, water

exercise classes, or swimming (Fig. 12-5). Swimming is best done by skilled persons with good form so that abnormal movement patterns of the back, neck, and shoulders are prevented. Use of a snorkel and swim mask can be beneficial for patients with cervical spine disorders.

Pool temperatures should be 82°F to 86°F for active exercise or 92°F to 98°F for pain relief and gentle ROM activities.[38] Local Arthritis Foundation offices provide a list of regional pools that meet requirements regarding such factors as temperature and accessibility. The Arthritis Foundation also sponsors water exercise classes taught by certified instructors. These classes are available to arthritis patients for a nominal fee. Information about these programs is available on The Arthritis Foundation web page, www.arthritis.org. See Chapter 16 for more information on aquatic rehabilitation.

Stationary or recreational bicycling is another form of low-impact exercise that can improve strength and cardiovascular conditioning. Bicycling is more effective than brisk walking or swimming for weight loss by obese patients needing to decrease the load on weight-bearing joints.[39] In an article on the use of biking in arthritis programs, Namey[40] discusses frame types, fit, and progression of exercise programs. He suggests an upright position on the bike with handle bars that are flat or that curve upward. He suggests that the seat should be high enough to allow the rider to have only a very mild bend in the knee at the bottom of the pedal stroke. It is worthwhile to have the rider take the bike to a bike store so that frame adjustments can be made for correct length from trunk to handlebars and for correct seat horizontal alignment (i.e., angled to allow neutral lumbar alignment unless the patient has a lumbar posterior element problem requiring flexion). Initial outings should be on level, low-traffic streets or trails, and they should be well within the ability of the rider in terms of strength and endurance. A helmet is a must.

A walking program can improve cardiovascular endurance. Several studies have shown additional benefits of a walking program for patients with arthritis including reduction of

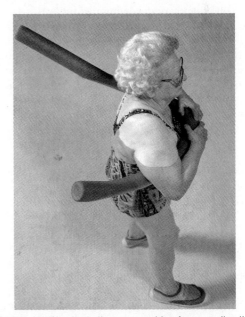

FIGURE 12-5. Walking in shallow water with a foam noodle allows the patient to improve cardiovascular endurance while unweighting arthritic joints. The deeper the water, the more unweighting.

pain, increase in flexibility and strength, and improvement of function.[21,23] Assessment for balance, safety, and current levels of function combined with advice regarding supportive footwear, acceptable walking surfaces, and progression of activities are necessary. Most neighborhoods have high school tracks that make an ideal exercise arena because of shock-absorbing level surfaces, easily calibrated distances, freedom from traffic hazards, and easy accessibility to a car to return home when the person becomes fatigued. Many shopping malls make their hallways available before hours for mall walking. This is ideal in bad weather or as a social opportunity, and it provides frequent opportunities for resting if necessary. In both settings, it is safer to use headphones for music or inspirational tapes than in public traffic areas, where the patient must attend to vehicular traffic. This form of exercise, however, is not without risk, because falls are always possible,[41] and an assistive device might be considered where balance is a problem.

The use of treadmills, cross-country ski machines, or rebounders (i.e., minitrampolines) offers options for low-impact, weight-bearing activity. This equipment requires more agility, balance, and coordination than outdoor or mall walking. Whichever form of exercise is chosen, cross-training can prevent boredom, stimulate different muscle groups, and alternate joint stress from session to session.

To modify exertion during training sessions, patients should be taught to monitor their heart rates or reliably apply the Borg perceived exertion rating technique[29] (see Chapter 6). They must also know their training parameters. Based on results of a study on aerobic exercise by patients with rheumatoid arthritis and osteoarthritis, Minor et al.[33] suggested that disease-related cellular changes in the muscle tissue of rheumatoid arthritis patients might contribute to low aerobic capacity. At similar prescribed heart rates, a patient with rheumatoid arthritis might be working at a higher percentage of aerobic capacity than a patient with osteoarthritis. Both patients, however, might be working at a higher capacity than a younger or more fit individual. Minor et al. in the same article, pointed out that high-intensity exercise is neither required nor appropriate for effective conditioning of deconditioned subjects.

Another useful form of monitoring for patients with rheumatic disease is the training index. Originally developed by Hagberg[42] for determining minimal beneficial cardiovascular fitness levels in cardiac patients, this tool was adapted by Burkhardt and Clark for use in patients with rheumatic disease. In this technique, the pulse during exercise is divided by the maximum heart rate (i.e., 220 minus the person's age) and multiplied by the number of minutes of exercise to yield the training index for that session of exercise. At the end of a week of exercise, daily training index values are added to give the total for the week. The recommended number of units is 42 to 90 per week to maintain cardiovascular fitness. This is a useful monitoring tool for tracking the level of activity and to coach patients in pacing exercise when needed (see Patient-Related Instruction 12-1: Determining the Training Index to Track the Level of Exertion).

The training index can have motivational value because it can serve as a tangible sign of progress. Tracking the training index may be especially motivating for patients who view aerobic exercise primarily as a means to weight loss, which is generally slower than most persons need for positive reinforcement and who then become discouraged and stop. The training index may also be useful for motivating patients who are at a very low level of activity, because they can see

Patient-Related Instruction 12-1

Determining the Training Index to Track the Level of Exertion

This is a simple way for you to keep track of how much exercise you are doing and whether you are (a) progressing in the amount you are doing and (b) whether you are gradually reaching a level of exertion that helps your heart and lungs stay healthy. Always pay attention to your symptoms, and modify exercise appropriately. Remember, every little bit you do adds up!

Your training index (TI) goal is 42 to 90 each week. As time goes on, this number may rise. You and your therapist will discuss this.

Max heart rate (MHR) = 220 minus your age.
Intensity = pulse with exercise divided by MHR.

Example: A 40-year-old woman who exercises three times each week:

- Session 1: pulse = 100 for 10 minutes of exercise
- Session 2: pulse = 110 for 15 minutes of exercise
- Session 3: pulse = 110 for 20 minutes of exercise

Her MHR = 220 − 40 = 180.

- Session 1: 100/180 = 0.55; 0.55 × 10 minutes = 5.5
- Session 2: 110/180 = 0.61; 0.61 × 15 minutes = 9.2
- Session 3: 110/180 = 0.61; 0.61 × 20 minutes = 12.2

Her total TI = 26.9

evidence of accumulated effort over time in a quantified manner. Introducing the training index in conjunction with a discussion of the benefits of aerobic exercise may be one more way to help the patient remain motivated.

Whatever form of cardiovascular exercise is chosen, it should be fun and satisfying for the patient. This is an important link in maintaining or regaining function, because the more closely training fits with patient goals, the more effective it is.

Special Considerations in Exercise Prescription and Modification

The impairments common to the patient with arthritis can pose specific challenges in designing a safe, effective exercise routine. The possibility of joint inflammation, laxity, and deformity in rheumatoid and osteoarthritis and of systemic effects in rheumatoid arthritis necessitate precautions during exercise. Pain in both conditions can interfere with function and therapeutic exercise, and it must be dealt with.

All positive findings from the initial evaluation should be considered when identifying the specific impairments to be addressed with exercise. These findings guide decisions about the prescription variables and necessary precautions which might include

- Protect joints during strengthening when ligament or capsular laxity exists (see below).
- Restore muscle balance when splinting, postural habit, or pain inhibition has selectively weakened muscle groups around one or more joints
- Normalize specific joint movement patterns
- Restore functional activities
- Treat pain and inflammation during and after exercise

- Take into account systemic variables such as fatigue levels, irritability of joints, and cardiovascular fitness, especially in the patient with rheumatoid arthritis

Precautions During Strengthening Exercises when Ligament or Capsular Laxity Exists

Joint instability caused by ligament laxity, muscle atrophy, or bony joint deformity can affect arthritic joints (see Figs. 12-1 and 12-2) and must be assessed during evaluation. Muscle strengthening around these joints can increase stability without external support, but it is undesirable to load these joints in a way that aggravates the instability. For example, in medial or lateral collateral ligament laxity of the knee, dynamic abductor or adductor strengthening without increased joint stress may be performed by placing the weight proximal to the knee joint rather than at the ankle. Other protective approaches may include bracing of the knee during exercise or the use of a closed chain pattern if proximal muscles are adequate to stabilize the knee in good alignment and the loading forces are tolerated by the joint.

In the small joints of the hand and foot, ligament laxity caused by the erosive effects of rheumatoid arthritis or asymmetric joint deformity from cartilage destruction and marginal spurring resulting from osteoarthritis need to be considered as carefully in exercise prescription as they are in instructions for joint protection during ADLs.

Restoration of function in hand, foot, and knee joints can be difficult in this context due to the relatively long lever forces of muscles crossing these joints where ligament laxity often is present. Intervention with exercise aimed at function in these joints will often have to be done in conjunction with ring splints, bracing, foot orthotics and special shoes, medication, therapeutic modalities, and the use of adaptive equipment. Functional use of pens, kitchen utensils, levers, and buttons (including keyboards) in hand rehab, for example, provide opportunities for a combination of strengthening and safe functional training (Figs. 12-6 and 12-7).

Ligament integrity during ROM activities is a crucial safety issue for the upper cervical spine. Rheumatoid arthritis can affect the ligaments of the upper cervical spine and middle

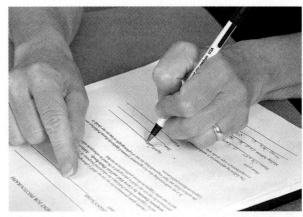

FIGURE 12-7. It is important to incorporate functional activities into the treatment plan. Here, the patient with arthritic fingers practices writing skills.

spine segments (i.e., C5 and C6 areas) and can cause erosion of the dens.[5] Any patient presenting with upper cervical spine instability or long tract signs should be referred to the physician for consideration of immobilization. Patients with a history of rheumatoid arthritis who do not have objective signs of cervical instability should be warned that any cervical spine ROM exercise that results in upper extremity pain or paresthesia or dizziness should be discontinued and they should consult their physicians.[25]

Joint protection can be approached through mechanisms that unload the joint, attenuate shock, and maximize neutral joint alignment. In addition to use of splints and braces, the following approaches may be implemented to decrease joint forces:

- Unweighting joints through the use of assistive devices (e.g., in hip osteoarthritis, use of a cane on the contralateral side to reduce joint reaction forces as much as 50%)[43]
- Attenuating shock forces in weight-bearing joints (e.g., viscoelastic insoles decreased impact vibration by 42% in tibias of experimental subjects)[44]
- Using a water medium[38] or unloading equipment in a clinic setting[45]

Weight reduction is an important goal of exercise for patients with pathologic joints and often a major goal of exercise programs. The Framingham studies indicated that obesity was a major predictor of the development of osteoarthritis[46] and that loss of as little as 10 lb decreased the risk of developing knee osteoarthritis by 50% in women.[18] Reduction of joint loading forces by weight loss decreases one of the stresses acting on the joint. Strengthening and recovery of joint reflex mechanisms offers increased joint protection, and normalizing joint alignment to as nearly neutral as possible distributes forces more symmetrically through the joints.[2]

Choosing exercise equipment that does not stress joints (e.g., cuff weights for upper extremity strengthening rather than free weights when there is wrist or finger joint instability), that can be of low enough resistance to ensure control of the joint by the patient (i.e., some machines do not start at a low enough weight setting for deconditioned individuals), and that encourages movement in physiologic patterns (e.g., shoulder abductor strengthening should be done in shoulder external rotation) contributes to patient safety during exercise. By understanding the factors necessary for good joint health, the therapist is able to design an exercise program that protects the

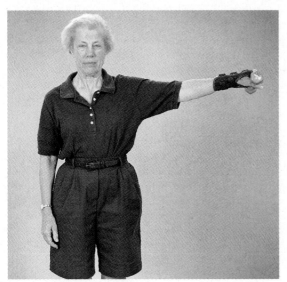

FIGURE 12-6. The patient uses a wrist brace to stabilize joints during exercise.

BUILDING BLOCK 12-8

1. Your patient in case OA was referred to you in part to establish a cardiovascular routine for help with weight control and hypertension. Design one possible routine which will also help him reach his goal of returning to play golf with friends. Set target heart rate and explain how you would teach him to monitor this. List precautions you would teach him.
2. Your patient in case RA-1 shows signs of cardiovascular deconditioning (increased heart and breathe rate with a 200-ft walk). Design a possible aerobic conditioning routine for her, including a way for her to judge her level of exertion and list precautions and protective devices you might suggest for her.

PATIENT EDUCATION

Chronically affected patients should be educated about their conditions during treatment and given self-help literature and information about community resources such as the Arthritis Foundation. Some treatments may be appropriately applied by family members or caregivers, and their involvement in treatment sessions to learn these techniques and to ask questions can be an efficient use of treatment time.

Working with patients with arthritis can be an exciting challenge to the physical therapist. This is a chance to apply the principles of exercise prescription in a situation demanding knowledge of joint and muscle pathology, the ability to do careful and complete assessment, the ingenuity to modify treatments to fit the determined requirements, and the ability to motivate patient cooperation. The benefit to the patient of this successful process can be an improvement in the quality of her life.

unhealthy joint from forces it is unable to resist while helping the patient achieve muscle balance around the affected joint in an effort to improve joint physiology. See Building Block 12-8.

Synthesis of Exercise Approach for the Patient with Rheumatic Disease in the Context of Adjunctive Therapies

Assessment of the functional use of affected joints (i.e., primary sites of disease and those with adaptive responses) indicates where abnormal movement patterns exist. Abnormal movement patterns can result from irreversible joint surface deformity or erosion of the capsule or ligaments. Abnormal movements also can be caused by muscle imbalance around joints earlier in the course of disease or in joints undergoing adaptive response to disease in a distant joint. Assessment of muscle balance between synergist and agonist or antagonist muscles (e.g., in the hip between iliotibial band and iliopsoas, in the shoulder between the deltoid and rotator cuff muscles) may be useful for designing a program aimed at restoring a muscle balance that allows the joint to function as close to the kinesiologic standard as possible. This approach decreases the energy required to function and contributes to healthier joint alignment.

To modify the processes leading to muscle atrophy and subsequent functional loss, a combination of medications (for pain and reduction of inflammation), therapeutic modalities, posture and body mechanics instruction, external bracing, and other support devices are often necessary. For example, a patient with osteoarthritis of the hip may be requested to temporarily use a cane to unload the painful joint; instructed in stretching of hip flexors and strengthening of weak hip abductors and extensors; educated in correct rest postures and lower extremity alignment with walking; and undergo joint mobilization to restore capsular mobility.

Coordination of Multiple Medical Interventions for Energy Conservation

A patient with more advanced or complicated arthritis may have a team consisting of a rheumatologist, orthopedic surgeon, psychologist, vocational counselor, orthotist, nurse, podiatrist, nutritionist, occupational therapist, and physical therapist. Demands made on the patient's time, energy, and financial resources by individual team members must be considered. Duplication of services should be avoided, whereas teamwork to provide positive functional outcomes should be practiced.

KEY POINTS

- Exercise can mitigate impairments that lead to functional deficits in patients with rheumatoid arthritis and osteoarthritis and has a positive effect on quality of life.
- The stability and mobility of a normal diarthrodial joint depend on the integrity of its anatomic parts. The disease processes of osteoarthritis and rheumatoid arthritis attack these anatomic parts and affect joint integrity and function.
- The pathology of one diarthrodial joint in a kinetic chain can adversely affect joints proximal and distal in that same chain and the contralateral joints. Exercise prescription should consider these joints when assessment indicates the need.
- Pain is a common impairment in patients with osteoarthritis or rheumatoid arthritis. Management of pain with therapeutic modalities, safe alignment, bracing, and pacing is a necessary component of exercise prescription.
- Joint movement is necessary for maintaining joint health. Passive, active assisted, and active ROM exercises are appropriate, and the choice depends on the severity of involvement of the joint.
- Isometric exercise is useful in maintaining strength of the muscles around an affected joint. It can be done without aggravating an inflamed joint and without raising blood pressure in patients when this is a consideration by using BRIMEs.
- Dynamic training offers the advantage of strengthening periarticular musculature through full joint range and increasing cartilage nutrition. Certain precautions must be followed, especially in strengthening muscles around unstable joints.
- Cardiovascular conditioning is frequently necessary for patients with osteoarthritis or rheumatoid arthritis. It has a positive effect on the quality of life. Following specified guidelines, it is possible to prescribe exercise that does not aggravate existing joint pathology.
- Because of inflammation and joint instability, exercise prescription must include special precautions such as joint bracing, nonjarring movements, conjunctive therapeutic modality use, and pacing.
- Patients' adherence to an exercise program often depends on their belief in the program and on sharing common goals with the therapist. For this reason, the therapist must be aware of patients' beliefs and goals during the treatment program.

REFERENCES

1. Berenbaum F. Osteoarthritis epidemiology, pathology and pathogenesis. In: Klippel John H, ed. Primer on Rheumatic Diseases. 12th Ed. New York, NY, Springer Publishing, 2001.
2. Brandt KD, Slemenda CW. Osteoarthritis epidemiology, pathology and pathogenesis. In: Schumacher HR Jr, ed. Primer on the Rheumatic Diseases. 10th Ed. Atlanta: Arthritis Foundation, 1993:184–187.
3. Allen ME. Arthritis and adaptive walking and running. Rheum Dis Clin North Am 1990;16:887–914.
4. Minor MA. Exercise in the management of osteoarthritis of the knee and hip. Arthritis Care Res 1994;7:198–204.
5. Anderson RJ. Rheumatoid arthritis clinical features and laboratory. In: Schumacher HR Jr, ed. Primer on the Rheumatic Diseases. 10th Ed. Atlanta: Arthritis Foundation, 1993:90–95.
6. Gerber L. Rehabilitation of patients with rheumatic diseases. In: Schumacher HR Jr, ed. Primer on the Rheumatic Diseases. 10th Ed. Atlanta: Arthritis Foundation, 1993:90–95.
7. Jokl P. Prevention of disuse muscle atrophy in chronic arthritides. Rheum Dis Clin North Am 1990;16:837–844.
8. Fahrer H, Rentsch HU, Gerber NJ, et al. Knee effusion and reflex inhibition of the quadriceps. J Bone Joint Surg Br 1988;70:635–638.
9. Sirca A, Susec-Michiel M. Selective type II fiber muscular atrophy in patients with osteoarthritis of the hip. J Neurol Sci 1980;44:149–159.
10. Lankhorst GJ, van de Stadt RJ, Van der Korst JK. The relationship of functional capacity, pain and isometric and isokinetic torque in osteoarthrosis of the knee. Scand J Rehabil Med 1985;17:167–172.
11. Felson DT, Zhang Y, Anthony JM, et al. Weight loss reduces the risk for symptomatic knee osteoarthritis in women. Ann Intern Med 1992;117:535–539.
12. Nordesjo LO, Nordgren B, Wigren A, et al. Isometric strength and endurance in patients with severe rheumatoid arthritis or osteoarthritis in the knee joints. Scand J Rheumatol 1983;12:152–156.
13. Fisher NM, Pendergast DR, Gresham GE, et al. Muscle rehabilitation: its effect on muscular and functional performance of patients with knee osteoarthritis. Arch Phys Med Rehabil 1991;72:367–374.
14. Bland JH, Cooper SM. Osteoarthritis: a review of the cell biology involved and evidence for reversibility. Management rationally related to known genesis and pathophysiology. Semin Arthritis Rheum 1984;14:106–132.
15. Bartels EM, Lund H, Hagen KB, et al. Aquatic exercise for the treatment of knee and hip osteoarthritis. Cochrane Database Syst Rev 2007;(4). Art. No: CD005523. DOI:10.1002/14651858.CD005523.pub2.
16. Neuberger GH, Aaronson LS, Gajewski B, et al. Predictors of exercise and effect of exercise on symptoms, function, aerobic fitness, and disease outcomes of rheumatoid arthritis. Arthritis Rheum 2007;57:943–952.
17. Bulthuis Y, Drossaers-Bakker W, Taal E, et al. Arthritis patients show long-term benefits from 3 233ks intensive exercise training directly following hospital discharge. Rheumatology 2007;46:1712–1717.
18. Roy S. Ultrastructure of articular cartilage in experimental immobilization. Ann Rheum Dis 1970;29:634–642.
19. Danneskiold-Samsoe B, Grimby G. The relationship between the leg muscle strength and physical capacity in patients with rheumatoid arthritis with reference to the influence of corticosteroids. Clin Rheumatol 1986;5:468–474.
20. Edstrom L, Nordemar R. Differential changes in type I and type II muscle fibers in rheumatoid arthritis. Scand J Rheumatol 1974;3:155–160.
21. Minor MA, Hewett JE, Webel RR, et al. Efficacy of physical conditioning exercises in patients with rheumatoid arthritis and osteoarthritis. Arthritis Rheum 1989;32:1396–1405.
22. Stenstrom C. Therapeutic exercise in rheumatoid arthritis. Arthritis Care Res 1994;7:190–197.
23. Kovar PA, Allegrante JP, MacKenzie CR, et al. Supervised fitness walking in patients with osteoarthritis of the knee. Ann Intern Med 1992;116:529–534.
24. Hicks JE. Exercise in patients with inflammatory arthritis and connective tissue disease. Rheum Dis Clin North Am 1990;16:845–870.
25. Lorig K, Fries JF. The Arthritis Help Book. 4th Ed. Reading, MA: Addison-Wesley, 1995:124.
26. Minor MA, Westby MD. Rest and Exercise in Clinical Care in the Rheumatic Diseases. 2nd Ed. Atlanta: American College of Rheumatology, 2001:179–184.
27. Kessler RM, Hertling D. Management of Common Musculoskeletal Disorders. Philadelphia, PA: Harper & Row, 1983:10–50.
28. Muller EA. Influence of training and of inactivity on muscle strength. Arch Phys Med Rehabil 1970;51:449–462.
29. Jayson MIV, Dixon SJ. Intra-articular pressure in rheumatoid arthritis of the knee. Part III: pressure changes during joint use. Ann Rheum Dis 1970;29:401–408.
30. Machover S, Sapecky AJ. Effect of isometric exercise on the quadriceps muscle in patients with rheumatoid arthritis. Arch Phys Med Rehabil 1966;47:737–741.
31. Gerber L, Hicks J. Exercise in the rheumatic diseases. In: Basmajian JV, ed. Therapeutic Exercise. Baltimore, MD: Williams & Wilkins, 1990:333.
32. McCubbin JA. Resistance exercise training for persons with arthritis. Rheum Dis Clin North Am 1990;16:931–943.
33. Minor MA, Hewett JE, Webel RR, et al. Exercise tolerance and disease related measures in patients with rheumatoid arthritis and osteoarthritis. J Rheumatol 1988;15:905–911.
34. Danneskiold-Samsoe K, Lyngberg K, Risum T, et al. The effect of water exercise therapy given to patients with rheumatoid arthritis. Scand J Rehabil Med 1987;19:31–35.
35. Jensen GM, Lorish CD. Promoting patient cooperation with exercise programs. Arthritis Care Res 1994;7:181–189.
36. Basia B, Topolski T, Kinne S, et al. Does adherence make a difference? Results from a community-based aquatic exercise program. Nurs Res 2002;51:285–291.
37. Patrick DL, Ramsey SD, Spencer AC, et al. Economic evaluation of aquatic exercise for persons with osteoarthritis. Med Care 2001;39:413–424.
38. McNeal RL. Aquatic therapy for patients with rheumatic disease. Rheum Dis Clin North Am 1990;16:915–929.
39. Gwinup G. Weight loss without dietary restriction: efficacy of different forms of aerobic exercise. Am J Sports Med 1987;15:275–279.
40. Namey TC. Adaptive bicycling. Rheum Dis Clin North Am 1990;16:871–886.
41. Gianini MJ, Protas EJ. Comparison of peak isometric knee extensor torque in children with and without juvenile rheumatoid arthritis. Arthritis Care Res 1993;6:82–88.
42. Hagberg JM. Central and peripheral adaptations to training in patients with coronary artery disease. Biochem Exerc 1986;16:267–277.
43. Neumann DA. Biomechanical analysis of selected principles of hip joint protection. Arthritis Care Res 1989;2:146–155.
44. Voloshin A, Wosk J. Influence of artificial shock absorbers on human gait. Clin Orthop Rel Res 1981;160:52–56.
45. Essenberg VJ Jr, Tollan M. Etiology and treatment of fibromyalgia syndrome. Orthop Phys Ther Clin North Am 1995;4:443–457.
46. Felson DT, Anderson JJ, Naimark A, et al. Obesity and knee osteoarthritis the Framingham study. Ann Intern Med 1988;109:18–24.

chapter 13
Therapeutic Exercise in Obstetrics

M.J. STRAUHAL

From the moment of conception, pregnancy profoundly alters a woman's physiology. Every system in her body changes during the childbearing year to provide for the diverse needs of fetal growth and development, meet the metabolic demands of pregnancy, and protect her normal physiologic functioning.[1-4] By considering these changes, the physical therapist can carefully implement a therapeutic exercise program that is safe for the mother and fetus. Therapeutic exercise may be prescribed to pregnant women for several reasons:

- Primary conditions unrelated to pregnancy
- Disorders related to the physiologic changes of pregnancy, such as back pain, faulty posture, or leg cramps
- Physical and psychologic benefits
- Preventive measures (Display 13-1)

Women are usually healthy and highly motivated at this time of their lives, and the physical therapist has the opportunity to introduce important lifestyle changes. Therapeutic exercise during this phase in life can play an important role in immediate intervention and in prevention of dysfunction and disease in the future.

DISPLAY 13-1
Possible Benefits of Prenatal Exercise

- Preservation or increase of maternal metabolic and cardiopulmonary capacities (fitness)
- Facilitation of labor, endurance for labor and delivery, possible decreased perception of pain, and improved relaxation
- Promotion of faster recovery from labor
- Promotion of good posture and body mechanics
- Prevention of injury and protection of connective tissue at risk because of laxity
- Prevention of low back pain, diastasis recti, and urinary incontinence
- Psychologic benefits—improved mood, body image, and self-esteem and reduction of postpartum depression
- Assistance in the management of gestational diabetes
- Prevention of excessive weight gain
- Improvement of muscle tone
- Decreased risk of venous stasis, DVT, varicose veins, edema, and leg cramps
- Decreased risk of bone loss because of high circulating estrogen levels
- Reduction of postdate deliveries

Data from references 5, 6, 40, 50, 60, 151, 190, and 191.

PHYSIOLOGIC CHANGES RELATED TO PREGNANCY—SUPPORT ELEMENT

Physiologic changes related to pregnancy include significant alterations in the maternal endocrine, cardiovascular, respiratory, and musculoskeletal systems.

Endocrine System

The endocrine system orchestrates the hormones that mediate changes in the soft tissue and smooth muscle. Various levels of relaxin, estrogen, and progesterone cause fluid retention, growth of uterine and breast tissue, greater extensibility and pliability of ligaments and joints, and a reduction in smooth muscle tone. Hormonal changes and structural adaptations alter gastrointestinal function.[3] Nausea, vomiting, changes in appetite, constipation, heartburn, and abdominal pain may interfere with a pregnant woman's ability and motivation to perform an exercise program.

The thyroid gland enlarges moderately during pregnancy because of hyperplasia of the glandular tissue and increased vascularity.[3] Basal metabolic rate increases during a normal pregnancy by as much as 15% to 30% by term (i.e., birth occurring between 38 and 42 weeks of gestation).[1-5] The pregnant woman requires approximately 300 kilocalories (kcal) more per day to meet this increased metabolic need.[1,2,4] Metabolic need is increased further (up to 500 kcal per day) in pregnant women who regularly exercise and with lactation (i.e., secretion of milk by the breasts).[1,2,6,7]

The thermoregulatory abilities of the body are affected by endocrine changes. Increased metabolism results in excess heat that is dissipated by peripheral vasodilation and acceleration of sweat gland activity. Thermoregulatory adaptations appear early in pregnancy and may protect fetal development and limit thermal stress in women who exercise during pregnancy.[8]

Gestational Diabetes Mellitus

The pancreas adapts to the increased nutrient demands of the mother and fetus. There is a progressive rise in insulin levels during pregnancy into the third trimester. The rise in the serum insulin level, which peaks at about 32 weeks' gestation, is a result of pancreatic islet hypertrophy.[6] Specific hormones promote maternal glucose production or decreased peripheral use of glucose to provide more fuel for the fetus.[6] Approximately 1% to 14% of pregnant women experience a failure of the pancreas to secrete insulin in sufficient quantity to take care of this glucose or they experience a failure of the body to properly use insulin, resulting in hyperglycemia (i.e., high blood sugar).[9-11] This is called gestational diabetes mellitus (GDM) and is considered the most common medical complication of pregnancy.[6,11]

The highest prevalence of GDM occurs at 24 to 40 weeks' gestation.[2] Risk factors for GDM include unmodifiable factors such as advanced maternal age, genetic background and family history of Type 2 diabetes mellitus, nonwhite ethnicity, and the number of previous pregnancies. Modifiable risk factors include obesity, physical inactivity, dietary fat, smoking, and certain drugs.[11] All pregnant women should be screened for diabetes, because it can occur even when no risk factors or symptoms are present. Management consists of diet, careful monitoring of glucose levels, and possibly insulin therapy.[6,11]

Cardiovascular conditioning exercise facilitates glucose use and reduces the amount of insulin needed to keep blood glucose levels normal, and it may play an important role in the management of GDM.[6,11–21] One study documented that women with GDM who trained with arm ergometry lowered their levels of glycemia better than with dietary changes alone.[17,18] Physical training may help avoid or delay insulin therapy.[22]

In 2004, the American Diabetes Association recommended that pregnant women without medical or obstetrical contraindications should be encouraged to exercise moderately as a part of preventing GDM.[23] Although a Cochrane review concluded that evidence was insufficient to recommend or advise against pregnant women with GDM exercising, Gavard and Artal's critical appraisal of the scientific literature suggests that exercise is protective against GDM and preeclampsia.[24–26] Further research is needed, because some studies show that prolonged strenuous exercise may induce hypoglycemia (i.e., low blood sugar) faster in the pregnant than in the nonpregnant woman.[27] Hypoglycemia means that levels of glucose in the bloodstream are too low to meet the body's energy needs. In pregnancy, hypoglycemia may develop in women whose bodies cannot adjust to the increased glucose requirements of the fetus, with or without exercise.[28] Some pregnant women feel better when they eat frequent, small, high-protein meals with an emphasis on complex carbohydrates (i.e., whole grains, fruits, and vegetables) rather than simple sugars (i.e., sweets).[29]

Even if there is no improvement of maternal glucose control, exercising three to four times each week for 30 minutes does improve cardiorespiratory fitness in pregnant women with GDM.[13] Since overt diabetes mellitus develops in 50% or more of women with GDM, they are at greater risk for cardiovascular complications.[6] Pregnancy provides an excellent opportunity to educate these patients, instruct them in an exercise program, and stress the importance of continuing exercise after delivery.[30,31] See Building Block 13-1.

Cardiovascular System

Maternal hemodynamic changes include a blood volume increase of 30% to 50% that peaks in the middle of the third trimester.[3,6,32] The increase in maternal blood volume varies with the size of the fetus and with multiple fetuses (e.g., twins, triplets).[6] In normal pregnancy, one sixth of the total maternal blood volume is within the uterine vascular system.[3] An increase in kidney blood flow improves removal of metabolic waste associated with fetal growth resulting in increased urine production and frequency. Increased skin blood flow helps with heat dissipation but makes the pregnant woman appear flushed.

Anemia

Hemoglobin levels fall progressively because of a greater increase in plasma than of red blood cells.[1,2,4–6] A deficiency in red blood cells, hemoglobin, or both is called anemia, and during pregnancy, this deficit is called physiologic dilutional anemia (i.e., 15% below nonpregnant levels).[6] Many cases of anemia are caused by iron deficiency, because the body uses iron to produce hemoglobin. In pregnancy, iron stores are heavily called on to increase blood volume and to provide hemoglobin for the placenta and fetus.[33–35] Women are usually prescribed supplemental iron to prevent anemia during pregnancy and during breast-feeding. Symptoms of mild iron deficiency may be experienced early in pregnancy and include fatigue, light-headedness, and decreased exercise tolerance.

Hemoglobin concentration determines the oxygen-carrying capacity of the blood. The amount of oxygen transferred across the placenta is influenced by maternal and fetal hemoglobin concentrations.[6] The relative difference between the red blood cell volume and the plasma volume does not interfere with oxygen distribution to various organs during pregnancy as might be expected. Changes in cardiac output, stroke volume, and heart rate contribute to an increase in oxygen distribution.[6] When a pregnant woman exercises, many of the variables that determine the transfer of oxygen across the placenta are affected. Physiologic adaptations to pregnancy and to exercise appear to be complementary and fetoprotective.[8,26,36–39]

Factors contributing to oxygen distribution include an increase in cardiac output by 30% to 50% and an increase in resting pulse by 8 beats per minute (bpm) in the early weeks of pregnancy to a plateau of about 20 bpm at 32 weeks.[1–3,6] During normal pregnancy, cardiac output is influenced by increased maternal weight, basal metabolic rate, and blood volume and by decreased arterial blood pressure and vascular resistance.

Hormonal changes influence the decrease in total systemic vascular resistance by 25% and in total peripheral vascular resistance by 30%. This helps to balance the change in cardiac output and produces an arterial blood pressure decrease of 5 to 10 mm Hg for the duration of the pregnancy.[1,2,4,5] Peripheral vasodilation keeps the blood pressure within normal limits despite the increase in blood volume during pregnancy.[3] See Building Block 13-2.

BUILDING BLOCK 13-1

Consider a 29-year-old pregnant woman at 32 weeks' gestation. She has just been diagnosed with GDM. What exercise advice might you give this patient to help her control her high blood sugar? What might you tell this patient about the effects of exercise during her pregnancy on her future health?

BUILDING BLOCK 13-2

Describe changes in the cardiovascular system that appear to be fetoprotective in the exercising woman.

Hypertension

Gestational hypertension affects 10% of pregnancies and can lead to preeclampsia or eclampsia (see Display 13-2). Women who are hypertensive during pregnancy are at greater risk of future cardiovascular or cerebrovascular events.[25] Pregnancy may lead to sedentary behavior and excessive weight gain, placing these women at increased risk for chronic diseases. It has been suggested that exercise may help prevent preeclampsia.[26,40] A Cochrane review, however, concluded that there was insufficient evidence on the effects of exercise for the prevention of preeclampsia and its complications.[41]

Supine Hypotensive Syndrome

Body position also influences hemodynamic changes. As pregnancy progresses, supine hypotension or inferior vena cava syndrome may develop when the backlying position is assumed.[42] The aorta and inferior vena cava may be occluded by the increased weight and size of the uterus (usually after the fourth month of pregnancy). The obstruction of venous return and subsequent hemodynamic adjustments from aortic compression decrease cardiac output.[1-4] Research suggests that a variety of factors are involved in determining the possible severity and significance of supine hypotensive syndrome (SHS).[42] Signs and symptoms of SHS are presented in Table 13-1. The American College of Obstetricians and Gynecologists (ACOG) recommends that pregnant women avoid the supine position after the first trimester.[43] A physical therapist with a thorough understanding of SHS and the rationale behind position changes can take a flexible approach to treatment and exercise in the supine position and reduce the alarm and paranoia occasionally associated with SHS.

Some women are asymptomatic during documented severe supine hypotension (arterial pressure of 80/40 mm Hg) or report symptoms before or after the hypotensive episode. The variability in signs and symptoms may reflect different degrees of reflex autonomic activation.[42] As many as 60% of women may experience symptoms at some time during pregnancy, but the incidence of true SHS is about 8%, with risk peaking at 38 weeks' gestation.[42] Kotila and Lee[44] estimated the incidence of severe cases of SHS to be <1% of the 2,000 women they studied. Other studies report that there is sufficient uteroplacental perfusion even if aortocaval circulation is diminished over time.[44] Uterine blood flow changes have been found to be significantly less during supine exercise compared to supine rest.[45]

The earliest sign of impending SHS is an increase in maternal heart rate and a decrease in pulse pressure. Spontaneous

TABLE 13-1 Supine Hypotensive Syndrome

SIGNS	SYMPTOMS	SIGNS IN SEVERE CASES
Pallor or cyanosis	Faintness	Unconsciousness
Muscle twitching	Dizziness	Incontinence
Shortness of breath	Restlessness	Impalpable pulses
Hyperpnea	Nausea and vomiting	A lifeless appearance
Yawning	Chest and abdominal discomfort or pain	Convulsions
Diaphoresis	Visual disturbances	Cheyne-Stokes respiration
Cold, clammy skin	Numbness or paresthesias in the limbs	
A wild expression	Headache	
Syncope	Cold legs	
	Weakness	
	Tinnitus	
	Fatigue	
	Desire to flex hips and knees	
	Anguish	

Data from references 34 and 36.

recovery usually occurs with a change in maternal position, even if very slight.[3,4,42] Maximum venous return and cardiac output are obtained in the left lateral recumbent position, but the right lateral recumbent position also reduces symptoms.[1,2,4,42]

SHS is confined almost exclusively to the supine position, although anatomic anomalies (e.g., bicornuate uterus, which has two horns or horn-shaped branches) may predispose a small number of women to symptoms in sidelying positions. Prolonged and motionless standing also can occlude the inferior vena cava and the pelvic veins during pregnancy, decreasing cardiac output, increasing venous pressure, and contributing to edema and varicosities in the lower extremities.[3]

Awareness of hemodynamic changes and SHS becomes important to the physical therapist when performing manual therapy techniques or prescribing exercises that require supine positioning or prolonged standing. Accommodating to a more upright or sidelying position (especially in the third trimester) or frequent position changes may be appropriate when working with patients at risk for SHS. Suggestions for position changes include placing a small wedge or pillow under the right hip in supine, raising the head and shoulders 20 to 30 degrees, semisitting, prone (on a special support or with use of pillows or wedge to decrease abdominal compression and ensure patient comfort), or quadruped (i.e., all-fours position). Changing positions from lying to upright should be done cautiously to decrease symptoms of orthostatic hypotension. Symptoms of SHS have disappeared with manual displacement of the uterus to the left or with lifting of the uterus in supine.[42] Conversely, SHS has been induced by abdominal pressure, which should be considered when positioning a patient in prone or when prescribing a maternal external support that may put pressure on the abdomen.[42] The physical therapist should encourage the pregnant woman to shift positions frequently during exercise, work, and treatment to avoid stasis and hypotension. Because supine positioning during labor has been associated with a lower fetal oxygen saturation, position changes apply to the laboring woman as well.[46] See Building Block 13-3.

Respiratory System

The respiratory system also adapts to the many changes of pregnancy. By 15 weeks' gestation, significant changes in lung volumes and capacities are present.[47] Hormonal changes produce increased mucus in the respiratory tract with associated increases in sinus and coldlike symptoms.[1,4] The upper respiratory tract may become predisposed to coughing and sneezing, increasing the likelihood of stress urinary incontinence in the pregnant woman with weak pelvic floor and abdominal muscles.

The diaphragm is displaced upward by about 4 cm, but diaphragmatic excursion is increased.[1,2,4,6] An increased pulmonary ventilation rate (i.e., the total exchange of air in the lungs measured in liters per minute) during pregnancy

is achieved by the woman breathing more deeply, increasing tidal volume (i.e., the amount of gases exchanged with each breath).[1–3,6] The respiratory rate increases only slightly (approximately 2 bpm), but there is an associated increase in respiratory minute volume, which is the amount of air inspired in 1 minute.[1–4,6] Lung compliance increases and airway resistance decreases from the relaxing effect of progesterone on smooth muscles.[6] This has been referred to as hyperventilation of pregnancy. Although arterial blood gases reflect an increase in oxygen and a decrease in carbon monoxide, causing mild respiratory alkalosis, this is not true hyperventilation. This mild maternal alkalosis promotes placental gas exchange and prevents fetal acidosis.[6] It may be perceived as dyspnea at rest and during exercise or as a decrease in the tolerance for exercise and exertion. In early pregnancy, it is unrelated to the encroachment of the uterus on the diaphragm. Later, as the lower costal girth is increased, greater breathing movement takes place at the middle costal and apical regions compared with the abdomen.[48]

Pregnancy is characterized by a 10% to 20% increase in oxygen consumption, which, combined with a reduction in functional residual capacity, results in a lower oxygen reserve.[6,49] Exercise produces an increased demand for oxygen and risks the possibility of blood flow being shunted from the uterus to the active skeletal muscles, although research has not proven this to be true.[6] Some studies show this increase in oxygen demand to be more dramatic during weight-bearing exercises, which are more energy costly in pregnancy because of the extra body weight.[6,50] With increasing body weight, more oxygen is required to exercise, and a woman reaches her maximal exercise capacity at a lower level of work.[50] Maximal exercise capacity of pregnant women may decline by approximately 20% to 25% in the second and third trimesters of pregnancy. Some evidence suggests, however, that pregnancy and advanced gestation are not associated with reduced aerobic work capacity or increased respiratory distress at any given work rate or ventilation during non–weight-bearing or weight-supported exercise.[6,47,51] Pregnant women may need to be advised to decrease workloads later in pregnancy, however, when fetal demand is at its greatest.[48]

PHYSIOLOGIC CHANGES RELATED TO PREGNANCY—BASE ELEMENT

Musculoskeletal System

The physical therapist is perhaps best suited to deal with the multiple musculoskeletal changes that occur in response to pregnancy. Many of these changes may make the childbearing woman more vulnerable to injury and pain.[52] Most women will experience some degree of musculoskeletal discomfort during pregnancy. Approximately 25% will have disabling symptoms.[53] Although the physiologic and morphologic changes in pregnancy are normal, musculoskeletal symptoms should not be considered normal despite the fact that they are common.

Optimal weight gain by the mother during pregnancy is important to pregnancy outcome, but a wide range in weight gain is compatible with good clinical outcomes.[1–4] The pattern of weight gain may also have important implications. Birth weight of the infant parallels maternal weight gain, and overweight and underweight women face increased risks during pregnancy. There are potential hazards for the mother

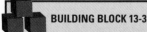

BUILDING BLOCK 13-3

SHS is a concern as pregnancy progresses. Describe the signs and symptoms of SHS and possible exercise adaptations for your pregnant patients.

and the infant when weight gain is restricted, and exercise should not be used to decrease weight. Both low birth weight (<2,500 g; <5 lbs. 5 oz.) and high birth weight (>4,000 to 4,500 g; 8 lb 13 oz to 9 lb 15 oz) are associated with poor fetal outcomes.[54] An average maternal weight gain of 12.5 kg (27.5 lb) is usually recommended during pregnancy, but the desirable range is related to prepregnancy weight status. ACOG supports the guidelines established by the National Academy of Sciences Institute of Medicine (IOM) that recommend a weight gain of 12.5 to 18 kg (27.5 to 40 lb) for underweight women, 11.5 to 16 kg (25 to 35 lb) for normal-weight women, and 7 to 11.5 kg (15 to 25 lb) for overweight women.[1] These figures are based on prepregnancy body mass index (i.e., weight in kilograms divided by the square of the height in meters). Recent studies have shown that lower gestational weight gain limits, especially among obese women, are associated with a decreased risk of adverse maternal and fetal outcomes.[55] Excessive weight gain during pregnancy and GDM are not only associated with obesity and diabetes later in life for the mothers but also with higher birth weight and obesity in their children.[6,56] Revisions to the IOM guidelines have been recommended.

The enlargement of the uterus and its contents, increases in blood volume and extracellular fluid, and an increase in breast tissue contribute to weight gain during pregnancy.[1,2] The nonpregnant uterus is approximately 6.5 cm long, 4 cm wide, and 2.5 cm deep and weighs 50 to 70 g.[1-3,50] By term, the uterus has dramatically increased to 32 cm long, 24 cm wide, and 22 cm deep and weighs about 1,100 g.[1-4] By the end of 12 weeks, the uterus becomes too large to remain wholly within the pelvis and becomes an abdominal organ.[1-3] It enlarges more rapidly in length than in width. This gradual increase in size and weight causes an upward and forward shift in the woman's center of gravity, which may result in an increased lumbar lordosis and compensatory thoracic kyphosis. Enlarging breasts gaining up to 500 mg each add to this tendency, and scapular adductors and upward rotators may become overstretched. As the shoulders become rounded, the head shifts forward, and posterior neck muscle activity increases to support the head. Posterior suboccipital muscles may also increase activity, extending the head on the neck to maintain eyes horizontal (i.e., optical righting reflex). The subcostal angle of the thorax increases from approximately 68 degrees in early pregnancy to approximately 103 degrees in late pregnancy to accommodate the fetus.[1-4,6] Expansion of the rib cage and the upward pressure of the enlarging uterus produces up to 4 cm of elevation of the diaphragm.[1-4] Chest circumference increases by 5 to 7 cm. In the last trimester, the trunk may rotate to the right (dextrorotation) as the growing uterus rotates to the right on its long axis. This most likely occurs because of the position of the rectosigmoid (lower portion of the sigmoid colon and upper portion of the rectum) on the left side of the pelvis.[1,2,6]

Changes in hormones contribute to joint laxity and subsequent hypermobility. This joint laxity contributes to increased foot pronation during pregnancy. Poor foot alignment affects the mechanics of the lower kinetic chain. Unlike other joints in the body that return to their normal prepregnancy position, the foot may not.[3] The postpartum woman may notice a permanent increase in shoe size. Since laxity and weight gain change foot biomechanics, pregnant women should be advised regarding proper footwear and possibly orthotics for support (see Chapter 21).

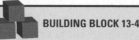

BUILDING BLOCK 13-4

Consider the physiologic and morphologic changes that result from pregnancy. Describe some of the changes that affect the musculoskeletal system and lead to postural changes and possible impairment.

Hormonal changes facilitating ligamentous laxity, softening of cartilage, and proliferation of synovium also influence postural changes. Postural changes in response to pregnancy can be further exaggerated by work, activities of daily living (ADLs), recreation, and exercise and can possibly contribute to injuries during more strenuous movement. Mechanical changes may aggravate preexisting conditions, so the therapist should not assume that a pregnant woman's complaints of aches and pains are always a result of the pregnancy. Musculoskeletal complaints associated with pregnancy and postpartum may not get serious consideration and the consequence may be underreferring to physical therapy in this population (see Building Block 13-4).

THERAPEUTIC EXERCISE INTERVENTION FOR WELLNESS

Every pregnant woman adapts differently to the physiologic changes of pregnancy. The physical therapist must consider age, level of fitness, previous and current exercise history, and concurrent adaptations to the changes of pregnancy when designing a therapeutic exercise program for the childbearing client.

Research focused on physical activity in the workplace has identified four physical stressors associated with an increased incidence of prematurity and low birth weight, both of which are factors of poor pregnancy outcome: quiet standing, long work hours, protracted ambulation, and heavy lifting.[52] The belief is that these activities cause intermittent but protracted reductions in uterine blood flow, thereby decreasing fetal nutrition. Research focused on recreational exercise during pregnancy has indicated an overall positive impact on pregnancy outcome.[8,57,58] The interaction between the physiologic adaptations to exercise and pregnancy appears to improve maternal cardiovascular reserve, maternal heat dissipation, placental growth, and functional capacity.[8,57] Women who engage in active exercise during pregnancy have fewer of the common discomforts associated with pregnancy, such as swelling, leg cramps, fatigue, shortness of breath, somatic complaints, insomnia, and anxiety.[8,59,60] In low-risk pregnancies, there are no apparent adverse pregnancy outcomes such as increased miscarriage, preterm labor, preterm birth, or intrauterine growth restriction associated with exercise.[8] Preterm birth, a major determinant of neonatal mortality and morbidity, has been shown to significantly reduce in women who exercised compared to sedentary women.[61] Other studies have shown a reduction in the duration of labor and incidence of obstetric complications during delivery associated with maternal exercise.[62-64] See Building Block 13-5.

BUILDING BLOCK 13-5

Describe workplace activities that may negatively affect pregnancy outcome.
Has research on exercise identified similar associations?

DISPLAY 13-3
Relative Contraindications or Limitations to Exercise During Pregnancy

1. Diabetes
2. Anemia or other blood disorder
3. Thyroid disease
4. Dilated cervix
5. History of preterm labor during previous pregnancy
6. Uterine contractions that last several hours after exercise
7. Sedentary lifestyle
8. Extreme obesity or underweight (including eating disorders, poor nutrition, and inadequate weight gain)
9. Overheating—high maternal core temperature may be associated with abnormal fetal development (teratogenesis) in the first trimester
   - Swimming pool temperatures should not exceed 85°F to 90°F (29.4°C to 32.2°C)
   - Avoid Jacuzzi temperatures above 101°F (38.5°C)
   - Avoid exercising in hot, humid weather or with fever
10. Breech presentation during the third trimester
11. Multiple gestations
12. Pulmonary disease (e.g., exercise-induced asthma, chronic obstructive pulmonary disease)
13. Peripheral vascular disease
14. Hypoglycemia
15. Cardiac arrhythmias or palpitations
16. Pain of any kind with exercise
17. Musculoskeletal conditions (e.g., diastasis recti, pubic symphysis separation, sacroiliac dysfunction)
18. Medication that alters maternal metabolism or cardiopulmonary capacity
19. Smoking, alcohol, recreational drug, and caffeine consumption

Data from references 6, 7, 50, and 60.

Studies on exercise during pregnancy vary regarding type, intensity, duration, and frequency of exercise and are therefore difficult to compare.[8,65] Current research, however, suggests that moderate aerobic exercise, carefully prescribed and monitored during pregnancy, is safe and beneficial for the mother (even if previously sedentary[66]) and the fetus.[5,6,8,32,36–39,57–60,62–64,66–75] Healthy, well-conditioned women can participate in a moderate- or high-intensity exercise program during pregnancy without adverse fetal or maternal outcomes.[76] A Cochrane review reported that regular aerobic exercise during pregnancy appeared to improve or maintain physical fitness.[77]

Concerns about exercise during pregnancy exist nonetheless (Table 13-2). Although many of these concerns are not substantiated by research, the guidelines for exercise err on the side of conservative management. Precautions and contraindications should be considered, and prudent guidelines should be followed when developing an exercise program for a pregnant woman.

Precautions and Contraindications

Pregnant and postpartum women should be advised to seek the approval of their health care providers (e.g., physician, midwife) before engaging in an exercise program. They should be screened for contraindications or risk factors for adverse maternal or perinatal outcome. Dietary intake, prepregnant BMI, and exercise history should be addressed.[78] Displays 13-2 and 13-3 detail the absolute and relative contraindications to exercise during pregnancy. Limitations or modifications of the exercise program may be recommended at any time during the pregnancy.[5,6,50,67] For example, a pregnant woman with preexisting pulmonary disease may be able to exercise, but her intensity level may vary over time as pregnancy-induced changes affect the respiratory system. In the presence of a specific relative contraindication, decisions regarding exercise should be made in conjunction with the patient's physician and guidelines referenced in Displays 13-4 and 13-5.

Exercise Guidelines

ACOG and the Melpomene Institute for Women's Health Research have published guidelines for exercise both during pregnancy and after delivery (Displays 13-4 and 13-5).[7,43,79]

TABLE 13-2 Exercise Risks During Pregnancy

MATERNAL	FETAL
Hypoglycemia	Hypoxia—possibility that blood flow will be shunted from the uterus in favor of exercising muscles
Chronic fatigue	Distress
Musculoskeletal injury from repetitive mechanical stress, changes in balance, and soft tissue laxity	Intrauterine growth retardation from alterations in energy and fat metabolism
Cardiovascular complications	Malformations
Spontaneous abortion	Hyperthermia secondary to maternal hyperthermia, increasing risk of neural tube defects and preterm labor
Preterm labor	Prematurity and reduced birth weight

Data from references 5–7, 40, 50, and 60.

DISPLAY 13-4
General Exercise Guidelines

- Exercise regularly, at least three times per week.
- Avoid ballistic movement, rapid changes in direction, and exercises that require extremes of joint motion.
- Include warm-ups and cooldowns.
- Avoid an anaerobic (breathless) pace.
- Strenuous activity should not exceed 30 minutes; 15- to 20-minute intervals are recommended to decrease the risk of hyperthermia. Ketosis and hypoglycemia are more likely to occur with prolonged strenuous exercise.
- Discourage vigorous exercise or exertion in high heat and humidity, with high pollution levels, and during febrile illness.
- Frequent change of positions may be required to avoid SHS but be careful of sudden changes in posture to reduce possible orthostatic hypotension.
- Avoid prolonged periods of standing, especially in the third trimester.
- Modify the intensity of exercise according to symptoms and stage of pregnancy.
- Do not exercise to exhaustion or undue fatigue. Adequate rest is important. Rest after exercise in the left lateral recumbent position for maximum cardiac output. Exercising to the point of fatigue or exhaustion may compromise the function of the uterus, with a detrimental effect on the fetus.
- Maintain metabolic homeostasis by adequate caloric intake. Increase it to 300 kcal per day for pregnancy alone, 500 kcal per day more for exercising during pregnancy, and 500 kcal per day more for lactation (may vary based on prepregnancy weight).
- Fluids should be taken before, after, and possibly during exercise to avoid dehydration.
- Avoid gastrointestinal discomfort by eating at least 1½ hours before an exercise workout.
- "No pain, no gain" does not apply to exercise during pregnancy.
- Low-resistance and high-repetition exercise is recommended. Avoid Valsalva maneuvers and encourage proper breathing during exercise.
- Maternal adaptations favor non–weight-bearing exercise instead of weight-bearing exercise.
- Postpartum progression into prepregnancy exercise routines should be gradual.
- Stop exercise or activity if unusual symptoms occur (see Display 13-5).

Data from references 1–7 and 60.

DISPLAY 13-5
Signs and Symptoms that Signal the Patient to Stop Exercise and Contact Her Physician

1. Pain of any kind
2. Vaginal bleeding
3. Uterine contractions that persist at 15-minute intervals or more frequently and are not affected by rest or change of position
4. Persistent dizziness, numbness, tingling
5. Visual disturbance
6. Faintness
7. Shortness of breath
8. Heart palpitations or tachycardia
9. Persistent nausea and vomiting
10. Leaking amniotic fluid
11. Decreased fetal activity
12. Generalized edema (rule out preeclampsia)
13. Headache (rule out hypertension)
14. Calf pain or swelling (rule out thrombophlebitis)

Data from references 1–7 and 60.

keep the maternal heart rate and blood pressure lower than with land exercise. Additionally, the buoyancy of water is supportive, and water is thermoregulating.[80–84]

The above guidelines are for the general population.[3,6,7,50,67,79,85–87] They differ from those given to the elite or professional athlete, whose risks and precautions are similar but whose training level may be more intense if closely supervised.[6,58,88,89] Healthy, well-trained pregnant athletes may benefit from training at vigorous levels while facilitating a more rapid return to competition postpartum.[90] Several activities should be discouraged or avoided during pregnancy.[5,6,50,67] For instance, the pregnant woman should be dissuaded from participating in competitive or contact sports. The following activities have the potential for high-velocity impact that may cause abdominal trauma and should be discouraged:

- Horseback riding
- Snow and water skiing
- Snow boarding
- Ice skating
- Diving
- Bungee jumping
- Heavy weight lifting
- High-resistance activities

Hyperbaric conditions, as in scuba diving, and activities that may promote extreme Valsalva maneuvers, such as weight lifting, should be avoided. The pregnant woman should not partake in activities that pose an increased risk of damaging joints, ligaments, and discs secondary to hormonal changes that already increase joint laxity (e.g., positions in which free weights may put joints into traction or stress the ligaments). The shift in the center of gravity along with increasing weight gain puts the pregnant woman at a higher risk for injury in sports that require balance and agility.[79] The pregnant woman should avoid activities and exercises in which loss of balance is increased (e.g., mountain climbing, gymnastics, downhill skiing, sliding into base), especially in the third trimester. Caution should also be used when exercising at high altitudes during pregnancy.[43,91,92]

Changing attitudes regarding exercise during pregnancy are reflected in ACOG's 2002 revision of its recommendations. In this update, ACOG recommended moderate exercise, 30 minutes or more per day, on most days of the week. The guidelines recommend that previously sedentary women could start a new exercise program during pregnancy. A gentle-paced water aerobics class may be an appropriate starting point for the beginner. Exercise in water offers several physiologic advantages for the pregnant woman.[80–82] The hydrostatic force of water, proportional to the depth of immersion, produces an increase in central blood volume by pushing extravascular fluid (edema) into the vascular spaces.[83] This may lead to increased uterine blood flow and serves to

Exercise Intensity

Exercise prescription regarding target heart rate or workout intensity, duration, and frequency during pregnancy remains controversial. There are drawbacks with using the target heart rate formula for the aerobic portion of an exercise session during pregnancy.[6,32,67,93] It usually is expressed as 60% to 90% of an individual's age-predicted maximum heart rate. Wisewell et al.[6] reported that the maximum heart rate in pregnant women is lower than this estimated value. In pregnancy, the maternal resting heart rate is elevated over nonpregnant values by 15 to 20 bpm.[4,6] Mitral valve prolapse occurs more frequently during pregnancy and may be aggravated by heart rates above 140 bpm.[6,50] With this in mind, recommendations for the general population include the reduction of exercise intensity during pregnancy by approximately 25%. A maximal heart rate of 60% to 75% of the age-predicted maximum is considered safe with a maximum maternal heart rate of 140 bpm for those just starting an exercise program and 160 bpm for those exercising prior to becoming pregnant.[6,67,93]

Exercise intensity may also be determined by the degree of respiratory distress or the rate of perceived exertion.[6] These levels correlate with maximal heart rate percentages:

Light: 40% to 50% of heart rate maximum
Moderate: 51% to 65% of heart rate maximum
Heavy: 66% to 80% of heart rate maximum

Conversing with ease during exercise indicates that a woman is exercising at the light to moderate intensity that is optimal for pregnancy.[6]

Endurance exercise has the additional benefit for pregnant women of preparing them for the increased exertion of labor and delivery. With fluctuation in the hormonal milieu, aerobic exercise is an excellent mood elevator. If key postural muscles, especially those of the pelvic floor, are weak, however, aerobic exercise can be detrimental because of the added stress to those structures. Water aerobics or bicycling is an appropriate form of cardiovascular fitness that may decrease stress on weak muscles and vulnerable joints.[80–82]

Exercise Classes

Prenatal wellness can be greatly enhanced by prenatal exercise classes. Physical therapists' understanding of the musculoskeletal system makes them ideal instructors. An individual approach with a focus on essential muscles affected by pregnancy makes these classes different from other community-based classes. Special certification is not required to teach classes, but continuing education in this area is recommended.

Prenatal exercise classes should address the physiologic changes that occur during pregnancy and the therapeutic exercises that prepare the body for these changes. Compliance with exercise is enhanced when clients understand that musculoskeletal dysfunction and associated discomfort may be prevented. Since women who have had one or more vaginal deliveries are at increased risk for chronic back pain, classes that target back pain prevention might be a cost-effective way to reduce disability and health care costs in the future.[94,95] Many women return to these exercise classes after delivery for continued socialization and support (see Chapter 4).

THERAPEUTIC EXERCISE INTERVENTION FOR COMMON IMPAIRMENTS

Focusing on the balance of muscle length and strength in key postural muscles in pregnant and postpartum women is extremely important. These muscles are most affected by the biomechanical changes of pregnancy. Length-associated changes arising from the typical kyphosis-lordosis posture can be prevented by addressing the posterior neck muscles, the middle and lower trapezius muscles, the transversus abdominis (TA), external and internal obliques (EO and IO, respectively), hip extensors, and the pelvic floor. Adaptive shortening is common in the anterior shoulder muscles, lumbar paraspinals, and hip flexors. Appropriate active and passive stretches should be prescribed for these areas. Lumbar, sacroiliac, and pubic symphysis problems may be greatly relieved by lumbopelvic stabilization exercises and by the use of external supports during pregnancy.[96–98]

Adjunctive Interventions

Pregnancy restricts the use of many modalities, especially ones that increase body heat. This is especially important over the abdomen or uterus.

Hot packs are generally safe to use on the back, neck, and extremities. Ultrasound may be considered at sites away from the uterus, especially when treating nonpregnancy related concerns (e.g., whiplash, peripheral joint, or muscular injury).[99] Continuous shortwave or microwave diathermy should not be applied to the low back, abdominal, or pelvic regions of the pregnant woman because of the possible thermal effect on the fetus.[99–101] This finding has only been documented in pregnant laboratory animals, and, for obvious reasons, the approach has not been tested on pregnant women.

Ice, when properly applied, should be encouraged for muscular and joint pain and inflammation during pregnancy. Electrical stimulation is typically contraindicated during pregnancy because some studies have shown that electrical stimulation applied to various parts of the body may induce labor. Transcutaneous electrical nerve stimulation (TENS) has been used for pain during labor and delivery. A recent position paper published by the Association of Chartered Physiotherapists in Women's Health (ACPWH) suggested that TENS could be used safely for musculoskeletal pain during pregnancy when other interventions have failed and when the alternative is a medication that would cross the placental barrier.[102] Manual therapy and muscle energy techniques may be used with caution considering the potential of ligamentous laxity. Heavy traction techniques and vigorous manipulations with pregnant patients should be avoided.[50]

Normal Antepartum Women

For the pregnant woman, postural awareness is vital when considering accommodations resulting from the shift in the center of gravity, weight gain, and possible joint hypermobility. Frequent attention to spine and pelvis alignment (see Chapters 9 and 17), scapular position (see Chapter 25), inner core facilitation (see Chapter 17), and patellofemoral function (see Chapter 20) can be effective in preventing length-associated changes in key muscles (Fig. 13-1). Postural faults may be perpetuated into the postpartum period,

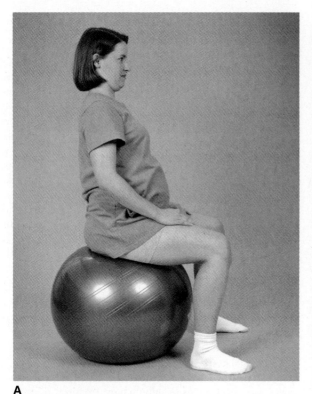
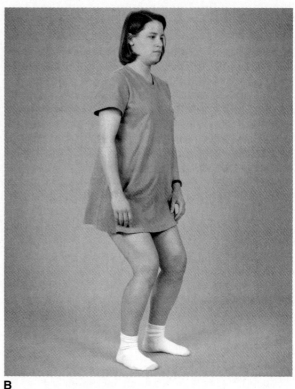

A   **B**

FIGURE 13-1. The pregnant woman is performing (A) chin tucks and (B) small knee bends to minimize length-associated changes.

especially when caring for the new infant. Proper body mechanics and joint protection should be stressed to decrease abnormal forces on joints that are at increased risk of injury because of hormonally induced laxity.

Sample musculoskeletal evaluations that incorporate adaptations for manual muscle testing and limit the number of body position changes for the pregnant client can be found in *Obstetric and Gynecologic Care in Physical Therapy*[49,103] and *Clinics in Physical Therapy: Obstetric and Gynecologic Physical Therapy*.[50]

Impaired Muscle Performance

Abdominal Strength   Goals for performing abdominal exercises during pregnancy include improvement of muscle balance and posture, support of the growing uterus, stabilization of the trunk and pelvis, and maintenance of function for more rapid recovery after delivery. It has been suggested that abdominal muscle strengthening exercises during pregnancy may reduce the development of a diastasis recti abdominis (DRA).[104] Most pregnant women can perform abdominal exercises in supine with frequent position changes. Exercises such as supine hip and knee flexion with hip abduction and lateral rotation (see Self-Management 17-3: Bent Knee Fall-Out) and progressive leg slides (see Self-Management 17-1: Supine Intrinsic Spinal Muscles Progression) are appropriate as long as the neutral spine position is maintained. In the case of an anterior pelvic tilt and lumbar lordosis, the client can be taught to use the abdominal muscles (particularly the EO) to tilt the pelvis in a posterior direction. This activity can be performed in a variety of positions (e.g., sitting, standing) and can be used to actively stretch the low back extensors while strengthening the abdominal muscles. Bilateral straight-leg

raising and leg-lowering exercises should be avoided during pregnancy because of the vulnerability of the vertebral joints and excessive pull on an overstretched abdomen. When a woman has SHS, the supine position should be avoided, and the use of sidelying, sitting, standing, and quadruped positions can be creatively used to train the patient in abdominal facilitation and neutral spine. The quadruped position is excellent for performing concentric and eccentric contractions of the abdominal muscles (see Self-Management 13-1: Quadruped Abdominal Exercise).

Pelvic Floor Strength   The pelvic floor muscles may undergo length-associated changes from the long-standing pressure of the growing uterus. Hormonally softened tissue further complicates the increased load on the pelvic floor. A vaginal birth or a lengthy and unproductive second stage of labor (i.e., pushing phase) before cesarean section poses problems for a vulnerable pelvic floor. There is the potential for direct trauma to the muscles with an episiotomy (an incision in the pelvic floor made during childbirth to enlarge the vaginal opening and allow faster delivery), tears, or lacerations. In addition, pudendal or obturator nerve stretch injuries may occur during delivery.

The importance of pelvic floor muscle strength cannot be overemphasized (see Chapter 18). It plays a vital role in supporting the internal organs (such as the rectum, vagina, and uterus) by preventing downward displacement (i.e., prolapse or pelvic relaxation). Pregnancy and postpartum pelvic floor dysfunction may manifest as pelvic organ prolapse, urinary or fecal incontinence, pelvic pain from muscle spasm, painful episiotomy, tears, or joint malalignment (sacrococcygeal involvement). A strong, coordinated pelvic floor may result in improved control and relaxation during the second stage of

SELF-MANAGEMENT 13-1 *Quadruped Abdominal Exercise*

Purpose: To train the patient in abdominal facilitation when backlying is uncomfortable or not possible (e.g., SHS)

Position: On hands and knees

Movement Technique:

1. Concentric contraction
   a. Inhale, allowing the abdomen to expand.
   b. While exhaling slowly, pull the tummy in while maintaining neutral spine. (To stretch back extensors, push the lower back up and tuck the chin down.)
2. Eccentric contraction.
   a. Slowly relax your tummy, and return to the starting position.

Dosage

Repetitions: _____

Frequency: _____

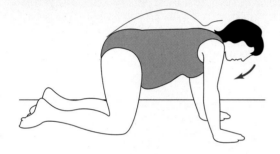

delivery[105] and in postpartum recovery. Attention to the pelvic floor muscles should occur early in the pregnancy and should continue throughout the duration of the pregnancy and postpartum phase[50,106] (see Chapter 18).

Impaired Joint Integrity and Muscle Length

Joint Hypermobility During pregnancy, there is a greater degree of joint laxity throughout the body. Studies looking at this in relation to serum relaxin levels are conflicting.[107] There are no studies reporting a higher incidence of exercise-induced injuries during pregnancy.[37,107]

Abdominal Muscle Length

Diastasis Recti Modifications to exercise for abdominal muscles are necessary for a woman with DRA.[106,108,109] In standing, the abdominal wall supports the uterus and maintains its longitudinal axis in relation to the axis of the pelvis.[2] The muscles of the abdomen that must lengthen to accommodate the enlarging uterus and growing fetus in pregnancy are the EO and IO, TA, and rectus abdominis. The linea alba is formed by the crossing fibers of the aponeuroses of these muscles, making a tendinous seam from the sternum to the symphysis pubis (SP). Hormonal changes and the increasing mechanical stress placed on these structures during pregnancy may result in a painless separation of the linea alba.[50] The rectus muscles separate in the midline, creating a DRA. The

prevalence of DRA has been estimated to be as high as 66% during pregnancy.[108]

The rectus muscles are normally about 2 cm apart above the umbilicus and are in contact with each other below the umbilicus. A separation greater than this is considered to be a DRA.[50,106,108,109] If severe, the anterior uterine wall may be covered by only skin, fascia, and peritoneum. If extreme, the gravid uterus drops below the level of the pelvic inlet when the woman stands. The pelvic inlet is bound posteriorly by the body of the first sacral vertebra (promontory), laterally by the linea terminalis, and anteriorly by the horizontal rami of the pubic bones and SP.[2] Descent of the fetal head below this point is called engagement and occurs normally during the last few weeks of pregnancy or during labor. Upright exercise should be restricted if engagement occurs at any other time during the pregnancy.[2]

The presence of a DRA potentially reduces the ability of the abdominal wall muscles to contribute to their role in trunk and pelvic girdle alignment, motion, and stability; support of pelvic viscera; and by way of increasing intra-abdominal pressure, forced expiration, defecation, urination, vomiting, and the second stage of labor (i.e., pushing).[50] Checking for a DRA should be done beginning in the second trimester and continue throughout the rest of the pregnancy and into the postpartum phase. To evaluate the abdominal wall for a DRA, the pregnant woman should lie in the supine hooklying position. With the chin tucked and arms extended to the knees, she should raise her head and shoulders until the scapulae clear the surface. The therapist checks for a central bulge in the abdomen and, with fingers placed cephalocaudally, measures the amount of separation between the rectus muscles 2 in above, 2 in below, and at the level of the umbilicus.[50,109] Each finger represents approximately 1 cm (Fig. 13-2).

A diastasis correction exercise can be performed to maintain alignment and discourage further separation. This is performed with the woman in supine hooklying position if she tolerates backlying (i.e., exclude SHS). With arms crisscrossed over the abdomen, the patient manually approximates the recti muscles toward midline, performs a posterior pelvic tilt, and slowly exhales while lifting her head. The scapulae should clear the surface[106] (see Self-Management 13-2: Correction of DRA). Exhalation prevents an increase in intra-abdominal pressure, engaging the TA first with a neutral spine.[50] The additional support of a large sheet folded lengthwise under the patient's back may be helpful as pregnancy progresses. The two ends of the sheet are brought up and crisscrossed over the abdomen to simulate support of the abdominal wall. The patient can grip each end of the sheet and pull outward to support the recti muscles toward the midline (see modification in Self-Management 13-2: Correction of DRA). If DRA is detected, patients are usually encouraged to avoid unsupported curl ups, trunk rotation exercises, and sitting straight up from a supine position, or jackknifing, because these activities may encourage further separation.

As an adjunct to therapeutic exercise, an external support in the form of an abdominal binder, lumbopelvic support, or sacroiliac belt can assist the patient in achieving improved body mechanics and postural alignment. When a diastasis is present, the external support helps to reestablish and maintain normal alignment of the abdominal wall and support

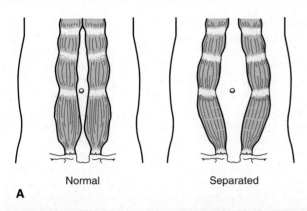

Normal   Separated

A

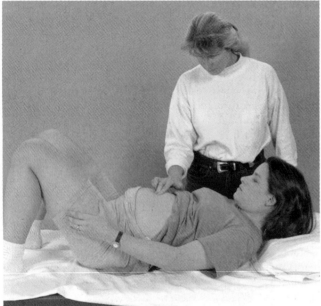

B

FIGURE 13-2. (A) Comparison of a normal abdomen with a DRA. (B) The therapist checks for a central bulge in the abdomen and measures the amount of separation between the rectus muscles.

the gravid uterus to prevent further stretch weakness. These supports are worn during upright exercises and ADLs. See Building Block 13-6.

Pelvic Floor Muscle Length

If coccyx pain is associated with pelvic floor tension myalgia, pelvic floor relaxation or "inversed command" must be emphasized.[110] After ruling out the possibility of referred pain from L5–S1, the patient can be taught a self-management

BUILDING BLOCK 13-6

Consider the pregnant patient who has a DRA at 28 weeks gestation. She has tried the supine DRA correction (Self-Management 14-2: Correction of DRA) but gets diaphoretic and dizzy when she lies supine. How might you address the DRA in this case?

SELF-MANAGEMENT 13-2 *Correction of DRA*

Purpose: To correct a DRA and improve the length-tension relationship of abdominals (rectus abdominis)

Position: Backlying with knees bent and feet flat. Cross hands over the midline.

Movement Technique:

1. Inhale.
2. As you exhale (engaging TA), rock your pelvis back (engaging RA), flattening your lower back.
3. Tuck your chin, and slowly raise your head off the surface while pulling the belly muscle toward the midline.
4. Slowly lower the head and relax.

Dosage
Repetitions: _____
Frequency: _____

Modification:

Fold a sheet lengthwise under your low back. Cross the sheet over the midline, holding the opposite ends in each hand. As you tuck your chin and slowly raise your head, pull outward on the ends of the sheet. As you lower your head and relax, release your grip on the sheet.

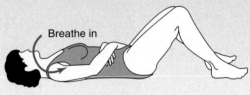

Breathe in

Starting position

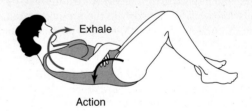

Exhale

Action

technique to relax the pelvic floor muscles. The patient is instructed to place her hand over the anal cleft, placing the middle finger in the cleft and the other fingers on the buttocks. As she pretends to "pass gas" gently without straining or bearing down, she should feel the anal cleft bulge out against the middle finger.[111] This lengthens the pelvic floor and should be practiced several times each day to recall the sensation. The use of a donut cushion or sitting with layers of towels under the thighs may be useful in keeping pressure off the coccyx.[50,111]

If pelvic floor muscle tension has caused sacrococcygeal malalignment, direct mobilization of this articulation may be performed to reduce pain.[112] This technique also is appropriate for a subluxed coccyx after childbirth.[49]

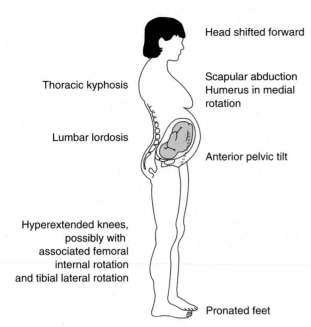

Head shifted forward

Thoracic kyphosis

Scapular abduction
Humerus in medial
rotation

Lumbar lordosis

Anterior pelvic tilt

Hyperextended knees,
possibly with
associated femoral
internal rotation
and tibial lateral rotation

Pronated feet

FIGURE 13-3. Incorrect posture during pregnancy.

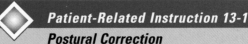

Patient-Related Instruction 13-1

Postural Correction

To correct posture during pregnancy, follow the steps below. Perform these steps simultaneously as often as you can—at least six times per day. Try them during different daily activities such as brushing your teeth, washing the dishes, or standing in line. Maintain them while performing exercises in the standing position.

1. Elongate the neck by drawing the chin back and keeping eyes level.
2. Lift your breastbone, ribs, and head without arching your lower back, as though you are trying to be taller. Breathe normally; do not hold your breath.
3. Pull your lower abdominal muscles in by pulling your belly button toward your spine. The pelvis should be in neutral position.
4. Unlock your knees, squeeze your buttock muscles to separate your knees, and turn your thighs slightly outward so that the kneecaps face the middle of your feet.
5. Pull "up and in" with the pelvic floor muscles.
6. Shift your weight slightly so half of your weight is on your heels and half is on the balls of your feet. Slightly lift the arches of your feet without rolling out on the sides of your feet.

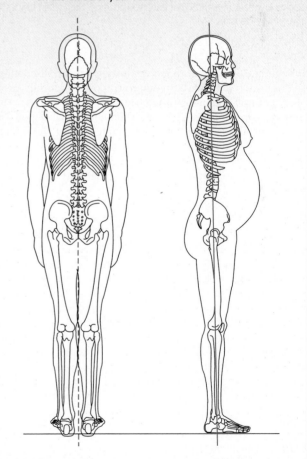

Impaired Posture—Biomechanical Element

Lumbar lordosis may result from pregnancy, or pregnancy may exaggerate a preexisting lordosis. Ideal postural alignment, as defined by Kendall et al.,[113] involves a minimal amount of stress and strain and is conducive to maximal efficiency of the body (refer to Chapter 9 for the definition of ideal alignment of the spine and pelvis). During pregnancy, the center of gravity shifts anteriorly, which may result in anterior rotation of the ilium. This accentuates and increases the normal anterior curve of the lumbar region, creating a lordosis (Fig. 13-3) (see Patient-Related Instruction 13-1: Postural Correction). Muscle weakness resulting from length-associated changes in the abdominal muscles and the hip extensor muscles results in poor control of the pelvis (in this case, an anteriorly tilted pelvis). However, adaptations to biomechanical changes during pregnancy vary from woman to woman. Anterior pelvic tilt and lumbar lordosis have not been consistently observed and are not necessarily associated with reports of pain.[95,114] Frequent inner core activation (see Patient-Related Instruction 17-1: How to activate your intrinsic spinal muscles) in various positions enhances muscular control and strength and the postural awareness required throughout the day to relieve pain and fatigue in the low back.

A lordosis at the thoracolumbar junction may cause mechanical stress on the muscles and ligaments, producing foraminal narrowing. The result may be radicular irritation manifesting as pain along the course of the iliohypogastric and ilioinguinal nerves anteriorly and posteriorly—a common referral source of pain for prepartum and postpartum women.[50] Radicular symptoms may also be experienced in the upper extremities, chest, and neck because of a compensatory thoracic kyphosis and increased cervical lordosis. Changes in the transverse diameter of the chest may mechanically aggravate preexisting costovertebral or thoracic joint dysfunction.

Thoracic kyphosis may develop during pregnancy and persist postpartum. Performing wall slides with the back to the wall (see Display 25-14, Fig.1) facilitates strengthening of the scapular upward rotators and the thoracic erector spinae and stretches the pectoral muscles. This exercise can reduce thoracic kyphosis and lift the rib cage off the uterus by promoting balance in length and strength of the anterior and posterior upper quarter muscles. Performing this exercise frequently

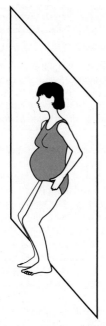

FIGURE 13-4. Wall abdominal isometrics. Standing with feet about 3 in from the wall, bend hips and knees to put hip flexors on slack. Pull belly button in toward the spine. Slowly straighten hips and knees while keeping low back in neutral (not flat back) position. Stop when low back moves into extension.

throughout the day can reduce postural pain and discomfort. Another useful exercise to improve posture during pregnancy is a wall abdominal isometric exercise (Fig. 13-4). This exercise helps to maintain tone in the abdominal region and normal hip flexor length, both of which support the lumbar curve and pelvic position. Frequent changes of position and proper posture and body mechanics during daily activities at home and at work apply to both pregnant and nonpregnant women.

Gait

Gait should be assessed for adaptations or muscle imbalances resulting from pregnancy. Three-dimensional motion analysis techniques investigating alterations in gait during pregnancy suggest that alterations in kinetic parameters may lead to overuse of various lower extremity muscle groups.[115] Increases in hip moment and power in the coronal and sagittal planes and increases in ankle moment and power in the sagittal plane may be due to increased use of hip abductors, hip extensors, and ankle plantar flexors. Although this appears to reflect compensations used to maintain a normal gait, they may contribute to lumbar, pelvic, and hip pain, as well as muscle cramps in the lower extremities and overuse impairments, especially in the underconditioned woman.

Pain

Approximately 50% to 90% of women experience back pain during pregnancy.[4,6,48,95,114,116] Many women with chronic back pain link the onset to pregnancy.[95,117,118] Back pain may occur at any time throughout the pregnancy but most commonly occurs between the fourth and the seventh months.[35] Back pain causes include:

- Biomechanical strain from increases and imbalances in joint loading resulting from increased body mass and dimension
- Postural changes, such as lumbar lordosis creating increased stress on the facet joints, posterior ligaments, and intervertebral disks
- Postural changes that aggravate preexisting spondylolisthesis, degenerative facet joint disease, lateral stenosis, and muscle imbalances
- Ligamentous laxity affecting the sacroiliac joints (SIJs), pubic symphysis, and sacrococcygeal joint
- Muscle fatigue from overload on key muscles including back extensors, abdominals, and pelvic floor

The relationship between postural changes during pregnancy and back pain is unclear.[114] Back pain is not entirely explained by biomechanical changes that can be measured by postural assessment. The source of pain is likely to be multifactorial, but there are common patterns of presentation. These are lumbar pain (LP), pelvic girdle pain (PGP), and nocturnal pain.[95,117,119–121] Inconsistencies in terminology and diagnostic criteria have made comparisons of prevalence, interventions, and outcomes difficult.[120]

Evaluation and exercise prescription for pregnancy back pain must be individualized. Higher levels of prepregnancy fitness and physical activity appear to decrease the risk for pregnancy-related LP and PGP.[95,117,119,122] Patients may need to be advised to adjust their exercise habits as the pregnancy progresses. Back pain and other pregnancy-related discomforts may be minimized by reducing the duration and intensity levels of exercises.[6,79]

Lumbar Pain LP is described as pain in the lumbar spine with or without radiation into the leg. It is aggravated by prolonged standing or sitting or repetitive lifting. LP responds to treatment focused on posture, body mechanics for ADLs, and exercise similar to the nonpregnant population (see Chapter 18). Several tests have been described to distinguish between LP and PGP.[95,117,123–125] Ronchetti et al. reported on diagnostic tests with acceptable intra- and interrater reliability, sensitivity, and specificity for the PGP population.[126] These include the posterior pelvic pain provocation test (or thigh thrust test), active straight leg raise test, hip abduction and adduction resistance test, the Patrick (Fabere) test, and palpation of the long dorsal sacroiliac ligament test. They concluded that each test provoked a particular aspect of PGP dysfunction. For diagnostic confirmation and assessment of PGP severity, a combination of tests is necessary.[126] See Building Block 13-7.

Pelvic Girdle Pain Recently published European guidelines on PGP propose that the diagnosis of PGP be reached after exclusion of lumbar, gynecologic, and urologic causes.[120]

BUILDING BLOCK 13-7

You have a 31-year-old pregnant patient who presents with complaints of low back pain. What tests might you use to assess this patient's impairment and distinguish her complaints from PGP?

They define PGP as pain that is experienced between the posterior iliac crest and the gluteal fold, particularly in the vicinity of the SIJs. The pain may radiate into the posterior thigh. Pain can occur in conjunction with the SP or exclusively in the SP.

Prevalence of PGP during pregnancy using this definition is about 20% and risks for its development are increased by a history of low back pain and previous pelvic trauma.[120] Other risk factors include PGP in a previous pregnancy, multiparity, a physically demanding job, and poor ergonomics.

The SIJ area has been described as the most common location of pregnancy back pain and is aggravated by extremes of hip and spinal movement and asymmetrical loading of the pelvis.[95,114,117,127] Patients with PGP commonly report difficulties with walking (waddle gait), standing, particularly single leg stance activities (dressing, stair climbing), activities that require a straddle (in/out of bath or car), rolling in bed, and sexual activities.

Pain in the pelvic joints may occur very early in pregnancy, possibly because of circulating hormones. Although the lumbar spine and the hip may refer pain into the pelvic region, a variety of alterations in SIJ and SP configuration and movement may produce impairment and functional limitations. There is evidence that the degree of joint and ligamentous laxity is not related to the amount of pain experienced in PGP.[120] Some women may be able to handle changes in the pelvic joints better than others, and decreased joint stability may be compensated for by muscle function.[120]

Gutke and colleagues reported an association between PGP and muscle dysfunction suggesting altered force closure of the pelvis and impaired joint stability.[121] Manual therapy techniques may be used to reduce asymmetry and abnormal motion. Muscle imbalances in the major muscles influencing lumbopelvic joint stability must be addressed (see Chapter 18). Randomized controlled trials have shown stabilizing exercises (those that incorporate specifically the transverse abdominis, multifidi, pelvic floor muscles, and hip muscles) to be effective interventions for PGP during pregnancy[128] and postpartum.[129,130]

Stretching techniques must be performed gently and cautiously because of possible joint hypermobility or true articular instability. An external support or belt may be appropriately applied to enhance stability of this region and the SP.[96–98]

The SP is the only bony junction in what Noble calls the "vulnerable midline."[106] This area includes the abdominal and pelvic floor muscles that are connected in midline by a tendinous seam. There is marked widening of the pubic symphysis by 28 to 32 weeks of gestation, from approximately 4 to 7 mm.[1] Widening begins early in pregnancy and facilitates vaginal delivery but can lead to pelvic discomfort and gait unsteadiness in late pregnancy. Wide leg motions or reciprocal movement of the lower extremities such as stair climbing or turning in bed may cause pain in a lax SP. If such pain occurs, leg exercises may need to be eliminated until the joint is stabilized. Symphysis pubis dysfunction (SPD) is best identified by palpation of the SP and by the modified Trendelenburg test of the pelvic girdle according to the European PGP guidelines.[120] The ACPWH recently released a collaborative document titled Pregnancy-Related Pelvic Girdle Pain that replaces their previous SPD recommendations.[131] This guide for pregnant and postpartum women includes general advice and information on physical therapy and exercise. Recommendations include avoidance of wide

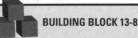

> **BUILDING BLOCK 13-8**
>
> Your patient has difficulty with walking, turning in bed, and getting in and out of her car. What exercises might you instruct this patient in to minimize her discomfort?

or reciprocal movements of the lower extremities, elimination of exercises or ADLs that provoke pain, and reduction of prolonged postures (sitting or standing). Vigorous stretching of the hip adductor muscles should also be avoided because this exercise may result in pubic symphysis separation.[132] See Building Block 13-8.

Nocturnal Back Pain   Nocturnal back pain is described as "cramplike" and is thought to be linked to increased blood volume and pressure on the inferior vena cava.[133] Decreasing venous flow could result in hypoxia of neural tissues. Position changes during sleep are recommended.

Other Sources of Pain   The round ligaments are two rounded cords that run from the superior angle of the uterus on either side to the labia majora. During pregnancy, these ligaments must stretch with the growing uterus and may intermittently spasm, causing sharp pain in the groin. This is especially true with sudden position changes. Gentle side stretching in tailor or regular sitting positions with arms overhead may relieve this discomfort (Fig. 13-5). This stretch may also help relieve heartburn and the feeling of shortness of breath as it lifts the rib cage upward and away from the pelvis.

Transient osteoporosis (TO) during pregnancy is self-limiting and spontaneously resolves postpartum.[134,135] Despite the rarity of fractures, pregnant women with TO may develop pain in the back, groin, hip, or lower extremities.[136] Careful attention should be paid to medical and family history because preexisting osteopenia and genetics play a role in the degree of bone loss.[137–139] Exercise history is vital in the differential diagnosis because a woman with compromised skeletal integrity, such as an amenorrheic athlete, may be at a higher risk for osteoporosis and fracture during pregnancy and lactation.[140,141]

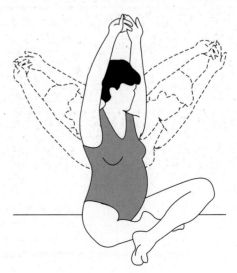

FIGURE 13-5. Gentle side stretching in tailor sitting.

Immobilization and inactivity are risk factors for TO and should be considered when treating a woman on bed rest for a high-risk pregnancy. Early recognition of TO and intervention with protective weight bearing are important in keeping the condition self-limiting and without long-term sequelae.[53]

Recovery time is stated in the literature to vary between 2 and 12 months postpartum and is compromised by lactation.[142,143] Profound detrimental effects on maternal bone mineral density during lactation are due to the cumulative effects of prolonged estrogen deficiency and calcium loss. Studies have not been able to show that lactation-induced bone loss is less in exercising women. More research is needed to address types of exercises (high impact and site specific) and exercise duration postpartum.[140] Lactation-induced osteopenia is reversible with cessation of breast-feeding.

High-risk Antepartum

When the outcome of pregnancy is adversely affected by maternal or fetal factors, the pregnancy is identified as high risk.[144,145] Bed rest is used in nearly 20% of all pregnancies to treat a wide variety of conditions. Bed rest may be prescribed when a pregnancy becomes complicated at conception, when preexisting maternal disease such as heart disease is present, or as the pregnancy advances. It is estimated that approximately one of four complicated pregnancies leads to the birth of a premature baby.[146]

Life Span Considerations

More women are choosing to delay childbearing until their fourth or fifth decade. Their decision may be influenced by a career, new marriage, financial security, and infertility problems.[147] Women who delay childbearing may expect good pregnancy outcome but higher incidence of obstetric complications.[148-154] These include preeclampsia, placenta previa, placental abruption, breech presentation, preterm delivery (before 32 weeks), and low birth weight. There is increased risk of operative delivery, including use of forceps, vacuum extraction, and cesarean section. Although pregnant women with diabetes and hypertension are at increased risk for adverse perinatal outcome irrespective of age, these complications increase almost linearly with age.[155]

The detrimental effects of inactivity in the form of bed rest vary according to the duration of bed rest, the patient's prior state of health and conditioning, and activity performed during bed rest. Much has been written about the effects of bed rest, many of which occur within the first 3 days. These effects include decreased work capacity, orthostatic hypotension, increased urine calcium (possibly leading to bone loss), decreased gastrointestinal motility (leading to constipation), and increased risk of deep venous thrombosis (DVT). Because maternal activity appears to modulate bone mineral acquisition during intrauterine life, bed rest may be detrimental to fetal as well as maternal bone health.[156] The theoretical basis for bed rest during a high-risk pregnancy is to promote uterine and placental blood flow and to reduce gravitational forces that may stimulate cervical effacement (i.e., obliteration of the cervix in labor, when only the thin external os remains) and dilation.[157-160] The left lateral recumbent (which maximizes blood flow to the mother and the fetus) or Trendelenburg position may be recommended. Bathroom privileges may be restricted. Typically, these patients report musculoskeletal, cardiovascular, and psychosocial complaints.

Even modest activity can reduce detrimental effects of bed rest.[144,145] Therapeutic exercises for this patient population focus on several features:

- Improvement of circulation
- Promotion of relaxation
- Avoidance of increased intra-abdominal pressure by minimizing abdominal contractions during exercise, basic ADLs, bed mobility, transfers, and self-care
- Avoidance of Valsalva maneuvers
- Prevention of decreased muscle tone and deconditioning effects
- Prevention of musculoskeletal discomfort

Activity guidelines for the high-risk antepartum patient are outlined in Display 13-6. Contraindications include increased

---

DISPLAY 13-6
Activity Guidelines for the High-Risk Antepartum Patient

1. Obtain approval from the health care provider before any exercise.
2. Tell the patient not to lift legs against gravity (including kicking off covers). Lower extremity movement may increase symptoms (e.g., increased bleeding, contractions, blood pressure, leakage of amniotic fluid). If symptoms increase, lower extremity exercises should be deferred first. Active assisted or passive range of motion exercises for the lower extremities may be appropriate.
3. Do not perform resisted lower extremity exercise.
4. Do unilateral exercises, except for ankles and wrists, to avoid stabilization by abdominal muscles.
5. Progress the number of exercises and repetitions gradually.
6. Do not overdo. Exercises may become more difficult as pregnancy progresses and fatigue increases or when medicated with tocolytics (medications used to stop or control preterm labor). You may need to modify exercises if tocolytics increase fatigue or give the patient the "jitters." Timing exercise further from dosage time is helpful.

7. Avoidance of abdominal contractions during exercise is necessary to help eliminate expulsion forces and uterine irritability, especially with preterm labor.
8. Avoid Valsalva maneuvers. Valsalva maneuvers are bearing-down efforts accompanied by holding the breath without exhalation (closed glottis). This increases the intra-abdominal pressure and pressure on the uterus. Valsalva maneuvers may be performed by a patient with abnormal respiratory rate and rhythm and may or may not include an abdominal contraction. A Valsalva maneuver must be avoided during bed mobility, transfers, exercises, or bowel movements to avoid irritating the uterus. The therapist instructs the patient to exhale on any effort.
9. Comfort measures include body mechanics and positioning in bed to support the spine and abdomen in proper alignment. In sidelying, pillows between the legs, under the abdomen, and behind the back and shoulders may be helpful. Frequent changes of position should be encouraged.
10. If symptoms increase with bed rest exercises, stop and report to the physician.

bleeding, contractions, blood pressure, or leakage of amniotic fluid; exacerbation of the condition (depends on the diagnosis); unstable conditions; and extreme cases when the patient should not move more than needed for basic care.

Impaired Muscle Performance

General strengthening and toning exercises help prevent or reduce decreased muscle tone and the deconditioning effects of bed rest. Frequent position changes in bed should be encouraged to avoid SHS and prevent musculoskeletal discomfort. Discomfort may be experienced because of static positioning, joint stiffness, and decreased circulation. Fluid retention and direct compression from immobility may lead to peripheral nerve impairments (these are discussed later in this chapter).

These strengthening and toning exercises can be done in the supine position:

- Neck rotation and side bending
- Gentle isometric neck extension into a pillow
- Shoulder presses down and back into a pillow
- Unilateral heel slides, hip internal rotation and external rotation, hip abduction and adduction, and terminal knee extension off a pillow
- Graded pelvic floor contractions if performed correctly (with minimal abdominal muscle activation or breath holding)

These strengthening and toning exercises can be done in the sidelying position:

- Unilateral shoulder circles (downward and backward), arm circles, hand and wrist active ROM, knee extension with hip flexed, partial knee to chest, and hip external rotation
- Unilateral resistive band (or light weights) for upper extremities only: biceps curl, triceps press, shoulder press, diagonal lift, shoulder extension, and horizontal abduction and adduction (avoid proprioceptive neuromuscular facilitation pattern D2 upper extremity extension with or without resistive band because it facilitates the abdominal muscles)
- Graded pelvic floor contractions

The support of a spouse, family, and friends can greatly reduce the anxiety and stress the high-risk antepartum patient may experience. Bed rest places the patient in the difficult position of limiting simple ADLs and limiting her roles as mother (if she has other children), spouse, and provider (unless she can work from her bed). The physiologic effects of stress can take its toll, and the patient and caregivers must understand the rationale for bed rest and importance of therapeutic exercise to enhance fetal and maternal outcomes. Most patients are home for this bed rest, although some women are hospitalized. A home visit to teach the patient and family proper exercise performance may be appropriate (see Self-Management 13-3: Sidelying Exercises for the Patient on Bed Rest and Patient-Related Instruction 13-2: Bed Mobility).

One study reported noncompliance of 33.8% for bed rest in the high-risk antepartum women they studied.[161] Reasons for noncompliance included not feeling ill, child care responsibilities, household demands, lack of support, having to work, and discomfort while on bed rest. Pregnancy outcomes were similar for women who did and did not adhere to bed rest

SELF-MANAGEMENT 13-3 *Sidelying Exercises for the Patient on Bed Rest*

Purpose:	To maintain strength of the lower extremities while on bed rest restrictions
Position:	Sidelying. Place a pillow under your head and between your knees.

Movement Technique:

1. Knee extension with the hip flexed. Begin with the hip partially flexed. Bend and straighten the knee as shown in Fig. A.
2. Knee extension with the hip extended. Begin with the hip in a straight position. Bend and straighten the knee as shown in Fig. B.
3. Knee-to-chest exercise. Slowly draw the knee up to the chest and then slide it back as shown in Fig. C.

Precaution:	Stop exercising if contractions or pain is experienced

Dosage

Repetitions: _____
Frequency: _____

(A) Knee extension with the hip flexed. (B) Knee extension with the hip extended. (C) Knee to chest.

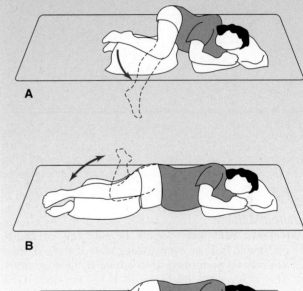

A

B

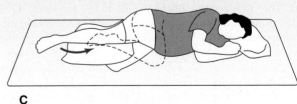

C

recommendations. Further research is needed to address the validity of the practice of bed rest as treatment for high-risk pregnancies.[161–165]

Because many high-risk pregnancies end in cesarean section deliveries, it may be an appropriate time to prepare the patient for cesarean recovery and rehabilitation. Discussion of cesarean section is provided later in this chapter.

Those women who have endured bed rest during their pregnancy may find that postpartum recovery is delayed. They

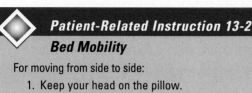

Bed Mobility

For moving from side to side:

1. Keep your head on the pillow.
2. Roll like a log.

For moving from lying to sitting using the "bed rest push-up":

1. Roll to one side.
2. Keeping your back straight, use your arms to push up to sitting while you swing your legs over the edge of the bed.
3. Reverse to lie back down.

Be sure to breathe and keep your stomach muscles relaxed. This helps to avoid Valsalva maneuvers. Never jackknife to sit.
    Bed-rest push-up

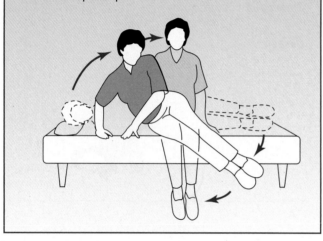

may experience greater muscle soreness and decreased muscle recovery time and may be more prone to musculoskeletal dysfunction.

Impaired Mobility

Circulation Exercises Supine or sidelying circulation exercises should be done every waking hour. If allowed, these exercises may be performed while sitting at the edge of the bed. This reduces the likelihood of lower extremity DVT. Ankle pumps and circles improve circulation by facilitating a pumping action in the muscles of the lower extremities. Gentle lower extremity isometrics may also help. However, the therapist must be extremely careful that the patient avoids increasing intra-abdominal pressure or blood pressure. Examples of lower extremity isometrics include quadriceps, gluteal, and adductor muscle exercises.

Pain (Stress)

Relaxation Exercises There are several ways of instructing relaxation exercises.[48,49,106] Two methods of relaxation require conscious recognition and release of muscle tension. The Mitchell method involves contraction of the opposing muscle groups to release stress-induced tension in muscles.[166] The Jacobson method, also known as progressive relaxation, involves alternately contracting and relaxing muscle groups progressively throughout the body.[167]

Visualization techniques or meditation may be helpful as a way to withdraw from the stress-producing situation temporarily. Diaphragmatic breathing and body awareness during exercises or ADLs also improve relaxation.[106]

Biofeedback and stretching are more active forms of relaxation. The patient is required to be mentally attentive to purposefully reduce a state of tension and recognize a state of relaxation. See Building Block 13-9.

Postpartum

Impaired Muscle Performance

Postpartum exercise is vital for the restoration of normal muscle function. Pelvic floor and abdominal contractions may be started within the first 24 hours after delivery to restore tone.

Even if a DRA was not present during pregnancy, a separation could have developed during the second stage of labor. A DRA does not always resolve spontaneously after delivery and may persist well into the postpartum phase. Immediate postpartum prevalence of DRA is about 35%.[168] Studies suggest that women who exercised during pregnancy are less likely to develop DRA.[168] DRA should be evaluated and reduced before aggressive abdominal strengthening begins. However, isometric activation and facilitation of these muscles in various positions are appropriate. It is important to remind the patient that these muscles may not provide adequate support initially for the trunk and low back, which are more vulnerable to injury.[169] Because of their synergistic relationship, persistent DRA beyond the childbearing years may play a role in the development of pelvic floor dysfunction.[170] In some cases, the temporary use of an abdominal binder is advisable.

Pelvic floor contractions immediately after delivery are essential in restoring muscle tone, reducing edema, facilitating circulation, and relieving pain, especially if an episiotomy has been performed or if the perineum was torn. The perineum comprises the pelvic floor and associated structures occupying the pelvic outlet; the area is bound anteriorly by the pubic symphysis, laterally by the ischial tuberosities, and posteriorly by the coccyx. The patient should be instructed to contract or "brace" the pelvic floor muscles with coughing, sneezing, or laughing; avoid Valsalva maneuvers when lifting the infant; and initially support the sutured perineum manually during defecation.

Pelvic floor strengthening should continue in the postpartum phase and beyond to restore muscle tone and to enhance normal bowel, bladder, and sexual functions. A systematic review reported that pelvic floor muscle exercises were effective in reducing or resolving urinary incontinence postpartum.[171] The supportive function of the pelvic floor is additionally challenged by lifting and carrying the infant and various pieces of child care equipment (e.g., stroller, infant seat, and diaper bag) (see Chapter 18).

Women with back pain during pregnancy are at high risk for back pain postpartum.[172–176] Studies suggest that attention be paid to muscles that influence spinal and pelvic stability including TA, pelvic floor, lumbar multifidus, hip rotators, and gluteus maximus[177–179] (see Chapters 17, 18, and 19).

Cesarean Recovery

A cesarean section (i.e., C-section) is the surgical delivery of the baby through the wall of the abdomen and the uterus after a horizontal (most preferred in the United States) or vertical incision has been made. The horizontal, or transverse, incision extends from side to side, just above the pubic hairline. This incision is preferred because there is less blood loss, it heals with a stronger scar, and it is less likely to result in complications in a subsequent vaginal delivery.[1–4,180] Vertical incisions are sometimes needed because of certain positions of the baby or placenta.

The rate for cesarean births in the United States is approximately 10% to 25%.[180] About 25% to 30% of these are performed because the pregnant woman has had a previous cesarean section.[181] Women may be encouraged to try a vaginal birth after cesarean (VBAC) delivery. Reasons to consider VBAC are less risk (this is controversial), shorter recovery time, and more involvement in the birth process.[181,182]

The cesarean procedure may be planned for reasons such as placenta previa (placement of the placenta below the fetus and over part or all of the cervix), breech presentation (presentation of the buttocks or feet of the fetus in the birth canal), and maternal illness or emergently for reasons such as fetal distress (a condition of fetal difficulty in utero detected by electronic fetal monitoring and fetal scalp sampling), prolapse of the umbilical cord, or failure to progress in labor. In childbirth classes, all women should be prepared for the possibility of a cesarean section birth. Some health care facilities have group classes before delivery for planned cesarean section patients. This class provides an excellent opportunity to educate and instruct patients in recovery after the procedure. They experience many of the same physical discomforts associated with major abdominal surgery but have the additional responsibility of caring for the newborn.

Exercises may begin within 24 hours after delivery but should be graded and based on the patient's comfort level.[106,183] Breathing exercises are important to keep lungs clear of mucus. Coughing may be painful, and "huffing" (by pulling the abdominals up and in) is recommended while splinting the incision. Pelvic rocking or bridging with a gentle twist from side to side may assist in alleviating discomfort from decreased intestinal motility. Lower extremity exercises help prevent DVT and orthostatic hypotension before early ambulation. Despite the absence of a vaginal delivery, the pelvic floor has undergone dramatic changes during the pregnancy, or there may have been a lengthy and unproductive trial of pushing. Pelvic floor exercises should be continued or initiated immediately. Gentle activity of the abdominal muscles stimulates healing of the incision and facilitates the return of muscle tone.

The patient can progress with abdominal exercises as tone increases and tissues tolerate added stress. Chronic pain and nerve entrapment may occur after a Pfannenstiel (transverse) incision.[184] Scar mobilization after sutures are removed (usually 3 to 6 days), or as comfort allows, assists proper healing and reduces adhesion formation. Postpartum precautions and exercises apply, but exercise is progressed more slowly. Attention to balanced upright posture is important, because pain and discomfort at the incision may prompt a protective flexed posture. TENS may be helpful in alleviating incisional pain.

Impaired Mobility and Muscle Length

The patient must accommodate to multiple body changes that occur rapidly. Weight loss and a change in the center of gravity produce postural readjustments. Ligaments and connective tissue may remain under hormonal influence for up to 12 weeks.[6]

If the mother is breast-feeding, the neck and upper back muscles are affected by the increased weight of the lactating breasts and by the positions assumed by the mother during nursing. Exercises that improve postural awareness and the length-tension properties of the anterior and posterior neck muscles (see Chapter 23) and scapular muscles, such as the lower and middle trapezius, are appropriate (see Chapter 25). Certain exercises may be uncomfortable for a nursing mother to perform because of breast tenderness (e.g., prone positioning). Attention should be paid to sitting posture and positioning of the baby during breast-feeding. The breast-feeding mother requires adequate caloric intake, fluids, and plenty of rest to produce milk for lactation. Exercise is an efficient way for the postpartum woman to return to prepregnancy weight.[185] Exercise does not adversely affect breast milk as long as she has adequate energy reserves (metabolic need increases by 500 kcal per day with lactation).[185]

Caring for an infant is physically demanding and involves repetitive lifting, feeding, and carrying. Proper body mechanics and attention to key postural muscles will prevent repetitive strain injuries.

Impaired Aerobic Capacity

When a woman has maintained good physical condition during pregnancy, her postpartum fitness is improved. If labor and delivery are uncomplicated, exercise can usually be resumed before the 6-week checkup.[50] Return to exercise should be gradual and based on her comfort level. Postpartum exercise guidelines are listed in Display 13-7.

Pain

If muscle tension in the pelvic floor is increased as a result of pain from an infected or poorly healed episiotomy or tear, the inversed command may be initiated. Modalities in the form of superficial heat, ultrasound, ice, TENS, and perineal massage may help to reduce discomfort.[48] Although pregnancy itself may be a factor in the development of lumbar disc disease, second-stage labor may markedly increase intradiscal pressure.[50] A disc protrusion may develop, or a preexisting protrusion may be exacerbated. This is treated with postural education, body mechanics, exercise, manual therapies, and modalities as in the general population, keeping in mind that hormonal changes persist for several weeks after delivery. The prevalence for low back pain or PGP after delivery is 5% to 37%.[126] Women with persistent PGP postpartum often had serious pain during pregnancy.[120]

Stress—Cognitive Element

Postpartum depression (postpartum blues) is one of the most common complications of childbearing.[186] The prevalence rate is 13% and may occur because of physiologic readjustments and endocrine upheaval. This transient depression may initially interfere with exercise performance, but physical exercise is also emerging as an effective intervention strategy.[186] Support and involvement of the spouse and family members can make a difference in the new mother's desire to exercise after delivery.[187] Group classes for postpartum exercise encourage mothers to exchange experiences and work through problems together. Many classes incorporate exercises that include the infant and the mother.

THERAPEUTIC EXERCISE INTERVENTION FOR COMMON IMPAIRMENTS
Nerve Compression Syndromes

Soft tissue edema is reported by 80% of pregnant women, usually in the last few weeks of pregnancy.[53] Nerve compression syndromes may arise during pregnancy because of fluid retention, edema, soft tissue laxity, and exaggerated postural changes. Special attention should be paid to blood pressure in these patients because these syndromes may be the first sign of increasing fluid resulting from preeclampsia (a condition of hypertension, edema, and proteinuria).

Intercostal Neuralgia

Intercostal neuralgia is the term used to describe unilateral, intermittent pain in the rib cage or chest from flaring of the rib cage. Exercises to relieve this discomfort include spinal elongation with arms overhead in supine, sitting, or standing positions and trunk side bending away from the pain.

Thoracic Outlet Syndrome

If muscle support is inadequate, spinal curves may become more pronounced as the center of gravity changes and the woman gains weight, especially in the breasts. The forward head and shoulder posture may lead to thoracic outlet syndrome (TOS), with compromise of the brachial plexus and subclavian vessels. A variant of TOS, called acroparesthesia, occurs when the neurovascular bundle becomes stretched over the first rib, which may be elevated in pregnancy. The woman may complain of pain, numbness, and tingling in the hand and forearm.[50]

Strengthening of the upper back and scapular muscles and lengthening of the pectoral muscles may assist in relieving symptoms (see Chapters 24 and 25). Support for the upper back and breasts in the form of a good brassiere and manufactured supports may be appropriate to decrease the load.[113] This is especially important after delivery for the nursing mother.

Carpal Tunnel Syndrome

Carpal tunnel syndrome of pregnancy usually disappears after delivery but may persist or develop in the postpartum phase if the woman is breast-feeding. It is addressed much the same as in the nonpregnant client (see Chapter 26), with a decrease in hand and wrist flexion activities, night use of resting splints, and exercises to keep fingers mobile and improve movement of fluids. Unlike patients with cumulative traumatype carpal tunnel syndrome, pregnant and breast-feeding clients typically have bilateral symptoms.

Lateral Femoral Cutaneous Nerve Entrapment

Lateral femoral cutaneous nerve entrapment (meralgia paresthetica) occurs in pregnancy when the nerve is compressed as it emerges from the pelvis at the inguinal ligament adjacent to the anterior superior iliac spine or where branches enter the tensor fascia lata. Adequate length in the tensor fascia lata, iliopsoas, and rectus femoris muscles is necessary to help prevent this condition. Exercises to balance the hip muscles may be appropriate (see Chapter 19). Lying on the unaffected side draws the uterus away from the compressed area and may further ease symptoms. Soft tissue techniques to reduce stiffness of the iliotibial band may also be helpful.

Tarsal Tunnel Syndrome

Tarsal tunnel syndrome, or posterior tibial nerve compression, occurs as a result of edema in the tarsal tunnel just posterior to the medial malleolus. Compression of the posterior tibial nerve produces numbness and tingling in the medial aspect of the foot and may also result in weakness of the flexor muscles of the toes.[6] Elevation and active foot and ankle exercises help to decrease edema and relieve compression. A posterior splint may be used to immobilize the ankle at night.

Peroneal Nerve Compression

The peroneal nerves wrap around the neck of the fibula and supply the muscles that dorsiflex the ankle. Prolonged squatting may compress these nerves and cause foot drop.[6] Pregnant women should be discouraged from prolonged squatting during exercise and during delivery. See Building Block 13-10.

BUILDING BLOCK 13-10

Your pregnant patient complains of numbness, tingling, pain, and burning at the anterolateral thigh. What is your potential physical therapy diagnosis? How would you incorporate therapeutic exercises as an intervention for this condition?.

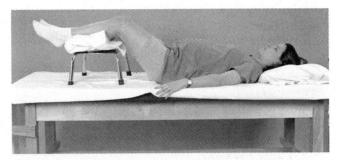

FIGURE 13-6. Elevation of feet to reduce varicosis. Note: The feet are higher than the heart to assist venous circulation. Place a wedge under the right hip to prevent SHS.

Other Impairments

Other impairments that may result from pregnancy include temporomandibular joint (TMJ) dysfunction, patellofemoral dysfunction, weight-bearing joint discomfort or dysfunction, and varicosis. Exercise interventions are presented in other chapters for some of these impairments, but guidelines for pregnancy should be carefully followed.

Temporomandibular Joint Dysfunction

TMJ dysfunction may be related to pregnancy. TMJ dysfunction can be caused during pregnancy by hypermobility resulting from increased laxity or may appear after delivery because of excessive tension in the face during the "pushing" phase of delivery[49] (see Chapter 22). Differential diagnosis for TOS and TMJ dysfunction would include appropriate tests for cervical dysfunction.

Patellofemoral Dysfunction

Patellofemoral dysfunction and pain may occur from the added stress of weight gain and fluid retention, especially with preexisting muscle weakness. Knee hyperextension and foot pronation are common in pregnancy, possibly because of the change in the center of gravity, which results in additional stress on the knees. Kinematic studies show that patellofemoral force increases by 83% in a pregnant woman rising from a chair without the use of her upper extremities.[6] Enlargement of the uterus causes a reduction in hip flexion and repositions the center of mass farther from the axis of rotation. Greater muscular effort is therefore required to move from sit to stand, which translates into increased force across the joint. This muscular effort is reduced if the pregnant woman uses her arms to rise from a chair or avoids low seating (see Chapter 20).

Weight-Bearing Joint Discomfort or Dysfunction

Weight gain in pregnancy increases the stress on weight-bearing joints, causing discomfort in normal joints or potentially increasing dysfunction in joints with preexisting arthritis or instability. Stair climbing produces forces of three to five times the body weight in the hip and knee joints. In a woman who increases her weight by 20% in pregnancy, forces on her weight-bearing joints may increase by 100%[50] (see Chapters 19 and 20).

Varicosis

Venous pressure in the lower body increases with advancing pregnancy. Venous distention and stasis contribute to varicosities of the lower extremities and vulvar region.[4] Frequent foot and ankle exercises help to alleviate edema and muscle cramps, especially if the patient is sedentary or sits on the job. They also help reduce the likelihood of lower extremity DVT. Patients should be advised to elevate the lower extremities higher than the heart to assist venous circulation (Fig. 13-6). The quadruped position reduces stress on the lower extremity vascular structures, and sidelying positions decrease compression of the inferior vena cava. Because long periods of static standing increase compressive forces of the weight of the fetus on the vascular system, the patient should sit instead of stand when she has the option. Immersion in water has also been shown to mobilize extravascular fluid and reduce edema.[83,188] Compression stockings should be considered.

LAB ACTIVITIES

1. Your patient is 20 weeks' pregnant and complains of sharp pain in the right SIJ with transitional movement. With your partner, perform tests and measures to assess her dysfunction.
   - Discuss adjunctive interventions that may be appropriate and safe to use on this patient.
   - Demonstrate positioning for treatment and exercise. Make appropriate modifications if SHS is present.
2. With your partner, demonstrate evaluation of the abdominal muscles for a DRA and the appropriate corrective exercise. Discuss other treatment options for a DRA and the advice you would give to the postpartum patient with a DRA regarding basic ADLs.
3. Discuss possible reasons for a pregnancy becoming high risk. Demonstrate exercises that could be taught to a pregnant woman on bed rest.
4. Design an exercise class for healthy pregnant women. Use the general exercise guidelines in Display 13-4.
   - Consider the safety of your class participants. How will you screen participants for possible contraindications or restrictions to exercise?

(continued)

LAB ACTIVITIES *(Continued)*

i. Develop a screening tool utilizing the information in Displays 13-2 and 13-3

ii. Would you require participants to get a physician referral/approval before being allowed to participate in the class?

- Identify barriers to exercise your class participants might encounter.
- Possible answers: fatigue, limited time, limited resources for child care, lack of exercise knowledge, fear of harming the baby.
- Describe the possible physical and psychological benefits of exercise to your class participants. Use the information in Display 13-1 to guide you.
- Describe the possible benefits of exercise during pregnancy on the future health.
- Possible answers: possible decrease in onset of diabetes mellitus, cardiovascular disease, and postpartum depression; rapid return to prepregnancy weight; decrease in obesity.
- How will you motivate your class to participate in exercise?
  Possible answers:
  i. Emphasize the benefits of exercise on both maternal and fetal health
  ii. Help participants to identify supportive family members and friends
  iii. Encourage social interaction within the class
  iv. Help them to set realistic goals
  v. Suggest that they may be setting a positive example for other family members (spouse, other children at home)
- Simply describe the physiologic changes that occur in various systems of the body during pregnancy.

Possible answers:

Endocrine System

i. Hormonal changes affecting growth of tissue, ligamentous laxity, gastrointestinal function, and pancreatic function possibly resulting in GDM

ii. Thyroid changes affecting metabolism and thermoregulatory function

iii. Cardiovascular system

iv. Increase in blood volume

v. Change in hemoglobin levels possibly resulting in anemia

vi. Increase in cardiac output

vii. Decrease in vascular resistance

Respiratory System

i. increase in mucus production

ii. change in diaphragm position

iii. increase in pulmonary ventilation rate

iv. increase in oxygen consumption

Musculoskeletal System

i. postural changes associated with increased weight in uterine and breast tissue possibly resulting in muscular and joint discomfort

ii. a change in weight distribution affecting weight-bearing joints

iii. joint laxity possibly resulting in less protection for the joints

iv. swelling and fluid accumulation possibly resulting in nerve compression syndromes

- Consider the musculoskeletal changes associated with pregnancy. What strengthening exercises might you want to include in your class to target key muscles?
  Possible answers: abdominal muscles [especially transversus abdominis], pelvic floor muscles, posterior cervical muscles, mid and lower trapezius, hip extensors, consider strengthening the upper extremity musculature to prepare your clients for the future demands of caring for their infant.
- What flexibility exercises would you include?
  Possible answers: anterior shoulder muscles, lumbar paraspinals, hip flexors.
- What precautions might you provide to your class regarding flexibility exercise/stretching?
  Possible answers: ligamentous laxity may lead to excessive stress on the joints, avoid extreme ranges of motion, move slowly into end ranges of stretch, avoid ballistic movements.
- Include modifications in your class for a variety of complications that might occur.

SHS
Answer: see Table 13-1.

DRA
Answer: teach your class a self-check for DRA by having them lie supine hooklying, place fingers between the rectus muscle bellies at the umbilicus and lift their head; teach those with DRA the correction technique in Self-Management 13-2: Correction of DRA.

Pelvic floor muscle weakness and associated urinary incontinence
Answer: teach Kegals, see Chapter 18.

Pelvic floor muscle tension.
Answer: teach "inversed command" by having the client place her middle finger at the anal cleft and "pretend to pass gas" to allow the pelvic floor muscles to lengthen.

PGP
Answer: avoid single leg standing or stepping exercises, teach getting in and out of exercise positions with legs together, consider recommending a support belt.

Lower extremity edema
Answer: elevation of legs for exercises such as ankle pumps and ankle circles to enhance fluid distribution, consider recommending compression stockings for upright exercise and activities.

(continued)

LAB ACTIVITIES *(Continued)*

Stages of pregnancy
Answer: advise clients to adjust exercises as pregnancy progresses, reduce exercise duration and intensity levels to minimize pain and discomfort.
- How will you incorporate promotion of cardiovascular fitness into your class?
Possible answer: low impact exercise such as walking, encourage aquatic exercise.
- Instruct your class in methods to monitor exercise intensity and give them target heart rate limits.
Answer: Rate of Perceived Exertion, "talk test"—the client must be able to hold a conversation while exercising, maximum target HR for beginners 140 bpm and for previous exercisers 160 bpm.

- What signs and symptoms should your class be aware of as a signal to stop exercising and contact their health care provider?
Answer: see Display 13-5.
- How will you prepare your class for the postpartum phase of childbearing?
Possible answers: address posture and body mechanics as it relates to breast-feeding, child care, and baby equipment; provide information and resources on postpartum depression; advise them to seek intervention for musculoskeletal dysfunction; encourage them to return to exercise with approval of their health care provider and with special consideration to the pelvic floor and abdominal muscles; use Display 13-7.

CASE STUDY 13-1

The patient is a 34-year-old married woman in her second trimester of pregnancy. She has a 3-year-old and 6-year-old at home and she works part-time as an administrative assistant. During the past few weeks, she has noticed the progressive onset of pelvic pain and subsequent limitation in ADLs.

PMH: coccyx injury from slipping on the ice during her teen years, mild LBP during her previous pregnancy

Obs: waddle gait, + modified Trendelenburg

IMPAIRMENTS

Pain in the right SIJ with radiation into the right posterior thigh, pain at the SP, instability of pelvic girdle joints, antalgic gait

LIMITATIONS

Walking long distances, stair climbing, getting dressed, getting in and out of the car, bed mobility, sexual activity

RESTRICTIONS

Unable to participate in her pregnancy exercise class, unable to perform household chores and care for her two children at home in their two-story house, unable to drive children to sports activities, unable to drive to work

1. What is the most probable physical therapy diagnosis for this patient?
2. What immediate advice might you give to this patient regarding her ADLs?
3. The patient and her family live in a two-story house. What suggestions might you give to the patient regarding her functional independence in the home?
4. Describe the important muscle groups you would emphasize during exercise instruction with this patient.
5. What adjunctive interventions might you consider for this patient?
6. Using the list of limitations and restrictions, create some functional goals for this patient.

KEY POINTS

- The many physiologic changes that occur during pregnancy affect a woman's ability and motivation to exercise.
- By following precautions, contraindications, and guidelines, a safe therapeutic exercise program may be established for pregnant women.
- Exercise during pregnancy has many benefits and may prevent or assist in the treatment of common impairments.
- Therapeutic exercise during pregnancy focuses on key postural muscles most affected by the biomechanical changes of pregnancy.
- A high-risk pregnancy may require bed rest; however, specific exercises may be performed and are beneficial.
- Therapeutic exercise is beneficial for postpartum recovery, even if a cesarean section has been performed.

CRITICAL THINKING QUESTIONS

1. The pregnant woman is positioned in supine for a manual therapy technique. Her face begins to lose color, and she complains of faintness.
   a. Should you continue with the technique but move very gently?
   b. Should you offer the patient a glass of water?
   c. Should you have her lie on her side until the symptoms resolve?
   d. Would you proceed with the technique after the symptoms resolved?
   e. What are some possible position changes you could make other than sidelying that could alleviate symptoms?
   f. Can you treat the patient in positions other than supine?

2. A 32-year-old woman, 6 weeks after delivery of her second child, experienced severe lower quadrant pain while lifting a stroller into the trunk of her car.

a. List possible causes for her pain.

b. What specific muscle groups would you assess, and what treatment options would you consider?

3. The pregnant patient is being instructed in an exercise program to improve her posture. She begins to experience contractions.

a. Should you stop the exercise and send the patient home?

b. Should you have the patient lie in left lateral recumbent position until the contractions stop? Would you then proceed?

c. Should you call the patient's doctor immediately?

d. What is your advice to the patient regarding performance of her exercise program?

REFERENCES

1. Cunningham FG, MacDonald PC, Gant NF, et al. Williams Obstetrics. 20th Ed. Stanford, CT: Appleton & Lange, 1997.

2. Cunningham FG, MacDonald PC, Gant NF. Williams Obstetrics. 18th Ed. Norwalk, CT: Appleton & Lange, 1989.

3. Bobak IM, Jensen MD, Zalar MK. Maternity and Gynecologic Care. 4th Ed. St. Louis: CV Mosby, 1989.

4. Scott JR, DiSaia PJ, Hammond CB, et al., eds. Danforth's Obstetrics and Gynecology. 7th Ed. Philadelphia, PA: J.B. Lippincott, 1994.

5. Wolfe LA, Amey MC, McGrath MJ. Exercise and pregnancy. In: Torg JS, Separd RJ, eds. Current Therapy in Sports Medicine. 3rd Ed. St. Louis, MO: Mosby, 1995.

6. Artal Mittelmark R, Wisewell RA, Drinkwater BL, eds. Exercise in Pregnancy. 2nd Ed. Baltimore, MD: Williams & Wilkins, 1991.

7. American College of Obstetricians and Gynecologists. Exercise during pregnancy and the postpartum period. ACOG Technical Bull 1994;189.

8. Morris SN, Johnson NR, Exercise during pregnancy. J Reprod Med 2005;50:181–188.

9. Avery MD, Rossi MA. Gestational diabetes. J Nurse Midwife 1994;39:9S–19S.

10. Weller KA. Diagnosis and management of gestational diabetes. Am Fam Physician 1996;53:2053–2062.

11. Menato G, Simona B, Signorile A, et al. Current management of gestational diabetes mellitus. Expert Rev Obstet Gynecol 2008;3:73–91.

12. Bung P, Artal R. Gestational diabetes and exercise: a survey. Semin Perinatol 1996;20:628–633.

13. Avery MD, Leon AS, Kopher RA. Effects of a partially home-based exercise program for women with gestational diabetes. Obstet Gynecol 1997;89:10–15.

14. Jovanovic-Peterson L, Peterson CM. Exercise and the nutritional management of diabetes during pregnancy. Obstet Gynecol Clin North Am 1996;23:75–86.

15. Jackson P, Bash DM. Management of the uncomplicated pregnant diabetic client in the ambulatory setting. Nurse Pract 1994;19:64–73.

16. Bung P, Artal R, Khodiguian N, et al. Exercise in gestational diabetes: an optional therapeutic approach? Diabetes 1991;40(Suppl 2):182–185.

17. Jovanovic-Peterson L, Peterson CM. Is exercise safe or useful for gestational diabetic women? Diabetes 1991;40(Suppl 2):179–181.

18. Jovanovic-Peterson L, Durak E, Peterson CM. Randomized trial of diet versus diet plus cardiovascular conditioning on glucose levels in gestational diabetes. Am J Obstet Gynecol 1990;162:754–756.

19. Horton ES. Exercise in the treatment of NIDDM: applications for GDM? Diabetes 1991;40(Suppl 2):175–178.

20. Bung P, Bung C, Artal R, et al. Therapeutic exercise for insulin requiring gestational diabetics: effects on the fetus—results of a randomized prospective longitudinal study. J Perinat Med 1993;21:125–137.

21. Winn HN, Reece EA. Interrelationship between insulin, dietary fiber, and exercise in the management of pregnant diabetics. Obstet Gynecol Surv 1989;44:703–710.

22. Garcia-Patterson A, Martin E, Ubeda J, et al. Evaluation of light exercise in the treatment of gestational diabetes. Diabetes Care 2001;24:2006–2007.

23. American Diabetes Association. Position statement on gestational diabetes mellitus. Diabetes Care. 2004;27(Suppl 1):S88–S90.

24. Ceysens G, Rouiller D, Boulvain M. Exercise for diabetic pregnant women. Cochrane Database Syst Rev 2006;3:CD004225.

25. Garovic VD, Hayman SR. Hypertension in pregnancy: an emerging risk factor for cardiovascular disease. Nat Clin Pract Nephrol 2007;3:613–622.

26. Gavard JA, Artal R. Effect of exercise on pregnancy outcome. Clin Obstet Gynecol 2008;51:467–480.

27. Bessinger RC, McMurray RG, Hackney AC. Substrate utilization and hormonal response to moderate intensity exercise during pregnancy and after delivery. Am J Obstet Gynecol 2002;186:757–764.

28. Field JB. Exercise and deficient carbohydrate storage and intake as causes of hypoglycemia. Endocrinol Metab Clin North Am 1989;18:155–161.

29. Carlson KJ, Eisenstat ST, Zipporyn T, eds. The Harvard Guide to Women's Health. Cambridge, MA: Harvard University Press, 1996.

30. Clapp J. Effect of dietary carbohydrate on the glucose and insulin response to mixed caloric intake and exercise in both nonpregnant and pregnant women. Diabetes Care 1998;21(Suppl 2):B107–B112.

31. Carpenter MW. The role of exercise in pregnant women with diabetes mellitus. Diabetes Care 2000;43:56–64.

32. Shangold M, Mirkin G, eds. Women and Exercise: Physiology and Sports Medicine. Philadelphia: FA Davis, 1994.

33. Lops VR, Hunter LP, Dixon LR. Anemia in pregnancy. Am Fam Physician 1995;51:1189–1197.

34. Engstrom JL, Sittler CP. Nurse-midwifery management of iron-deficiency anemia during pregnancy. J Nurse Midwife 1994;39:205–345.

35. Scholl TO, Hediger ML. Anemia and iron-deficiency anemia: complication of data on pregnancy outcome. Am J Clin Nutr 1994;59:492S–500S.

36. Wang TW, Apgar BS. Exercise during pregnancy. Am Fam Physician 1998;57:1846–1852.

37. Clapp JF. Exercise during pregnancy: a clinical update. Clin Sports Med 2000;19:273–286.

38. Heffernan AE. Exercise and pregnancy in primary care. Nurse Pract 2000;25:42–60.*

39. Clapp JF, Stepanchak W, Tomaselli J, et al. Portal vein blood flow—effects of pregnancy, gravity and exercise. Am J Obstet Gynecol 2000;183:167–172.

40. Dempsey JC, Butler CL, Williams MA. No need for a pregnant pause: physical activity may reduce the occurrence of gestational diabetes mellitus and preeclampsia. Exerc Sport Sci Rev 2005;33:141–149.

41. Meher S, Duley L. Exercise or other physical activity for preventing pre-eclampsia and its complications. Cochrane Database Syst Rev 2006;(2):CD005942.

42. Kinsella SM, Lohmann G. Supine hypotensive syndrome. Am J Obstet Gynecol 1994;83:774–787.

43. The American College of Obstetricians and Gynecologists. Exercise during pregnancy and the postpartum period. ACOG Committee Opinion No. 267. 2002;99:171–173.

44. Kotila PM, Lee SN. Effects of Supine Position During Pregnancy on the Fetal Heart Rate [thesis]. Forest Grove, OR: Pacific University, 1994.

45. Jeffreys RM, Stepanchak W, Lopez B, et al. Uterine blood flow during supine rest and exercise after 28 weeks of gestation. Internat J Obstet Gynaec 2006;113:1239–1247.

46. Carbonne B, Benachi A, Leeque ML, et al. Maternal positions during labor: effects on fetal oxygen saturation measured by pulse oximetry. Obstet Gynecol 1996;88:797–800.

47. Jensen D, Webb KA, Wolfe LA, et al. Effects of human pregnancy and advancing gestation on respiratory discomfort during exercise. Respir Physiol Neurobiol 2007;156:85–93.

48. Polden M, Mantle J. Physiotherapy in Obstetrics and Gynecology. Oxford: Butterworth-Heinemann, 1990.

49. O'Connor LJ, Gourley RJ. Obstetric and Gynecologic Care in Physical Therapy. Thorofare, NJ: Slack, 1990.

50. Wilder E, ed. Clinics in Physical Therapy. Vol 20. Obstetric and Gynecologic Physical Therapy. New York: Churchill Livingstone, 1988.

51. Jensen D, Webb KA, O'Donnell DE. Chemical and mechanical adaptations of the respiratory system at rest and during exercise in human pregnancy. Appl Physiol Nutr Metab 2007;32:1239–1250.

52. Heckman JD, Sassard R. Musculoskeletal considerations in pregnancy. J Bone Joint Surg Am 1994;76:1720–1730.

53. Borg-Stein J, Dugan S. Musculoskeletal disorders of pregnancy, delivery and postpartum. Phys Med Rehabil Clin N Am 2007;459–476.

54. Kaiser L, Allen LH. Position of the American Dietetic Association: nutrition and lifestyle for a healthy pregnancy outcome. J Am Diet Assoc 2008;108:553–561.

55. Cedergren MI. Optimal gestational weight gain for body mass index categories. Obstet Gynecol 2007;110:759–764.

56. Hui AL, Ludwig SM, Gardiner P, et al. Community-based exercise and dietary intervention during pregnancy: a pilot study. Can J Diabetes 2006;30:169–175.

57. Clapp JF. Pregnancy outcome: physical activities inside versus outside the workplace. Semin Perionatol 1996;20:70–76.

58. Clapp JF. A clinical approach to exercise during pregnancy. Clin Sports Med 1994;13:443–458.

59. Horns PN, Ratcliffe LP, Leggett JC, et al. Pregnancy outcomes among active and sedentary primiparous women. J Obstet Gynecol Neonat Nurs 1996;25:49–54.

60. Sternfeld B, Quesenberry CP Jr, Eskenazi B, et al. Exercise during pregnancy and pregnancy outcome. Med Sci Sports Exerc 1995;27: 634–640.

61. Hegaard HK, Hedegaard M, Danum P, et al. Leisure time physical activity is associated with a reduced risk of preterm delivery. Am J Obstet Gynecol 2008;198:180.e1–180.e5.

62. Botkins C, Driscoll CE. Maternal aerobic exercise: newborn effects. Fam Pract Res J 1991;11:387–393.

63. Clapp JF III. The course of labor after endurance exercise during pregnancy. Am J Obstet Gynecol 1990;163:1799–1805.

64. Beckmann CR, Beckmann CA. Effects of a structured antepartum exercise program on pregnancy and labor outcome in primiparas. J Reprod Med 1990;35:704–709.

65. Chasen-Taber L, Evenson KR, Sternfeld B, et al. Assessment of recreational physical activity during pregnancy in epidemiologic studies of birthweight and length of gestation: methodologic aspects. Women Health 2007;45:85–107.

66. Marquez-Sterling S, Perry AC, Kaplan TA, et al. Physical and psychological changes with vigorous exercise in sedentary primigravidae. Med Sci Sports Exerc 2000;32:58–62.

67. Kulpa P. Exercise during pregnancy and postpartum. In: Agostini R, ed. Medical and Orthopedic Issues of Active Athletic Women. Philadelphia, PA: Hanley & Belfus, 1994.

68. Wolfe LA, Walker RM, Bonen A, et al. Effects of pregnancy and chronic exercise on respiratory responses to graded exercise. J Appl Physiol 1994;76:1928–1936.

69. Zeanah M, Schlosser SP. Adherence to ACOG guidelines on exercise during pregnancy: effect on pregnancy outcome. J Obstet Gynecol Neonat Nurs 1993;22:329–335.

70. McMurray RG, Mottola MF, Wolfe LA, et al. Recent advances in understanding maternal and fetal responses to exercise. Med Sci Sports Exerc 1993;25:1305–1321.

71. Wolfe LA, Mottola MF. Aerobic exercise in pregnancy: an update. Can J Appl Physiol 1993;18:119–147.

72. Clapp JF III. Exercise and fetal health. J Dev Physiol 1991;15:9–14.

73. Sady SP, Carpenter MW. Aerobic exercise during pregnancy: special considerations. Sports Med 1989;7:357–375.

74. Clapp JF III. The effects of maternal exercise on early pregnancy outcome. Am J Obstet Gynecol 1989;161:1453–1457.

75. Hall DC, Kaufmann DA. Effects of aerobic and strength conditioning on pregnancy outcomes. Am J Obstet Gynecol 1987;157:1199–1203.

76. Kardel KR, Kase T. Training in pregnant women: effects on fetal development and birth. Am J Obstet Gynecol 1998;178:280–286.

77. Kramer MS, McDonald SW. Aerobic exercise for women during pregnancy. Cochrane Database of Syst Rev 2002;(2):CD000180.

78. Penney DS. The effect of vigorous exercise during pregnancy. J Midwifery Womens Health 2008;53:155–159.

79. The Melpomene Institute for Women's Health Research. The Bodywise Woman. New York: Prentice Hall Press, 1990.

80. Ruoti RG, Morris DM, Cole AJ. Aquatics Rehabilitation. Philadelphia, PA: Lippincott-Raven Publishers, 1997.

81. Katz VL. Water exercise in pregnancy. Semin Perinatol 1996;20:285–291.

82. Smith SA, Michel Y. A pilot study on the effects of aquatic exercises on discomforts of pregnancy. JOGNN 2006;35:315–323.

83. Kent T, Gregor J, Deardoff L, et al. Edema of pregnancy: a comparison of water aerobics and static immersion. Obstet Gynecol 1999;94:726–729.

84. McMurray RG, Katz VL. Thermoregulation in pregnancy. Sports Med 1990; 10:146–158.

85. Bell R, O'Neill M. Exercise and pregnancy: a review. Birth 1994;21:85–95.

86. Yeo S. Exercise guidelines for pregnant women. Image J Nurs Sch 1994;26: 265–270.

87. Treyder SC. Exercising while pregnant. J Orthop Sports Phys Ther 1989; 10:358–365.

88. Hale RW, Milne L. The elite athlete and exercise in pregnancy. Semin Perinatol 1996;20:277–284.

89. Wiswell RA. Applications of methods and techniques in the study of aerobic fitness during pregnancy. Semin Perinatol 1996;20:213–221.

90. Kardel KR. Effects of intense training during and after pregnancy in top-level athletes. Scand J Med Sci Sports 2005;15:79–86.

91. Huch R. Physical activity at altitude in pregnancy. Semin Perinatol 1996; 20:304–314.

92. Entin PL, Coffin L. Physiological basis for recommendations regarding exercise during pregnancy at high altitude. High Alt Med Biol 2004;5:321–334.

93. Mottola MF, Davenport MH, Brun CR, et al. VO_2 peak prediction and exercise prescription for pregnant women. Med Sci Sports Exerc 2006;1389–1395.

94. Levangie PK. Association of low back pain with self-reported risk factors among patients seeking physical therapy services. Phys Ther 1999;79:757–766.

95. Perkins J, Hammer RL, Loubert PV. Identification and management of pregnancy-related low back pain. J Nurse Midwifery 1998;43:331–340.

96. Depledge J, McNair PJ, Keal-Smith C, et al. Management of symphysis pubis dysfunction during pregnancy using exercise and pelvic support belts. Phys Ther 2005;85:1290–1300.

97. Nilsson-Wikmar L, Holm K, Oijerstedt R, et al. Effect of three different physical therapy treatments on pain and activity in pregnant women with pelvic girdle pain: a randomized clinical trial with 3, 6, and 12 months follow-up postpartum. Spine 2005;30:850–856.

98. Kalus SM, Kornman LH, Wuinlivan JA. Managing back pain in pregnancy using a support garment: a randomised trial. BJOG 2008;115:68–75.

99. Michlovitz SL, ed. Thermal Agents in Rehabilitation. 2nd Ed. Philadelphia, PA: FA Davis, 1990.

100. Edwards MJ. Congenital defects in guinea pigs: prenatal retardation of brain growth of guinea pigs following hyperthermia during gestation. Teratology 1969;2:329.

101. Smith DW, Clarren SK, Harvey MAS. Hyperthermia as a possible teratogenic agent. J Pediatr 1978;92:878.

102. ACPWH guidance on the safe use of Transcutaneous Electrical Nerve Stimulation (TENS) for musculoskeletal pain during pregnancy. 2007; www.acpwh.org.uk

103. Stephenson RG, O'Connor LJ. Obstetric and Gynecologic Care in Physical Therapy. 2nd Ed. Thorofare, NJ: Slack, 2000.

104. Chiarello CM, Falzone LA, McCaslin KE, et al. The effects of an exercise program on diastasis recti abdominis in pregnant women. J Womens Health Phy Ther 2005;29:11–16.

105. Salvesen KA, Morkved S. Randomised controlled trial of pelvic floor muscle training during pregnancy. BMJ 2004;329:378–380.

106. Noble E. Essential Exercises for the Childbearing Years. Harwich, MA: New Life Images, 1995.

107. Schauberger CW, Rooney BL, Goldsmith L, et al. Peripheral joint laxity increases in pregnancy but does not correlate with serum relaxin levels. Am J Obstet Gynecol 1996;174:667–671.

108. Boissannault J, Blaschak M. Incidence of diastasis recti abdominis during the childbearing years. Phys Ther 1988;68:1082.

109. Bursch S. Interrater reliability of diastasis recti abdominis measurement. Phys Ther 1987;67:1077.

110. Sinaki M, Merrit JL, Stillwell GK. Tension myalgia of the pelvic floor. Mayo Clin Proc 1977;52:717–722.

111. Mayo Clinic. Home Instructions for Relief of Pelvic Floor Pain. Rochester, MN: Mayo Foundation for Medical Education and Research, 1989.

112. Hansen K. Sacrococcygeal instability in pregnancy. Obstet Gynecol Phys Ther 1993;17:5–7.

113. Kendall FP, McCreary EK, Provance PG. Muscles Testing and Function. Baltimore, MD: Williams & Wilkins, 1993.

114. Franklin ME, Conner-Kerr T. An analysis of posture and back pain in the first and third trimesters of pregnancy. J Orthop Sports Phys Ther 1998;28:133–138.

115. Foti T, Davids JR, Bagley A. A biomechanical analysis of gait during pregnancy. J Bone Joint Surg 2000;82-A:625–632.

116. Kelly-Jones A, McDonald G. Assessing musculoskeletal back pain during pregnancy. Prim Care Update Obstet Gynecol 1997;4:205–210.

117. Ostgaard HC, Zetherstrom G, Roos-Hansson E, et al. Reduction of back and posterior pelvic pain in pregnancy. Spine 1994;19:894–900.

118. Sihvonen T, Huttunen M, Makkonen M, et al. Functional changes in back muscle activity correlated with pain intensity and prediction of low back pain during pregnancy. Arch Phys Med Rehabil 1998;79:1210–1212.

119. Colliton J. Back pain and pregnancy. Physician Sports Med 1996;24:89–93.

120. Vleeming A, Albert HB, Ostgaard HC, et al. European guidelines for the diagnosis and treatment of pelvic girdle pain. Eur Spine J 2008;6: 794–819.

121. Gutke A, Ostgaard HC, Oberg B. Association between muscle function and low back pain in relation to pregnancy. J Rehabil Med 2008;40:304–311.

122. Mogren IM. Previous physical activity decreases the risk of low back pain and pelvic pain during pregnancy. Scand J Public Health 2005;33:300–306.

123. Ostgaard HC, Zetherstrom G, Roos-Hansson E. The posterior pelvic pain test in pregnant women. Eur Spine J 1994;3:258–260.

124. Mens JMA, Vleeming A, Snijders CJ, et al. Reliability and validity of the active straight leg raise test in posterior pelvic pain since pregnancy. Spine 2001;26:1167–1171.

125. Vleeming A, DeVries HJ, Mens JMA, et al. Possible role of the long dorsal sacroiliac ligament in women with peripartum pelvic pain. Acta Obstet Gynecol Scand 2001;81:430–436.

126. Ronchetti I, Vleeming A, van Wingerden JP. Physical characteristics of women with severe pelvic girdle pain after pregnancy. Spine 2008;33:E145–E151.

127. Berg G, Hammar M, Moller-Nielson J, et al. Low back pain during pregnancy. Obstet Gynecol 1988;71:71–75.

128. Elden H, Ladfors L, Olsen MF, et al. Effects of acupuncture and stabilizing exercises among women with pregnancy – related pelvic pain: a randomised single blind controlled trial. BMJ 2005;330:761–764.

129. Stuge B, Laerum E, Kirkesola G, et al. The efficacy of a treatment program focusing on specific stabilizing exercises for pelvic girdle pain after pregnancy: a randomized controlled trial. Spine 2004;29:351–359.

130. Stuge B, Veierod MB, Laerum E, et al. The efficacy of a treatment program focusing on specific stabilizing exercises for pelvic girdle pain after pregnancy: a two-year follow-up of a randomized clinical trial. Spine 2004;29:E197–E203.

131. Pregnancy-Related Pelvic Girdle Pain. The Association of Chartered Physiotherapists in Women's Health 2007. acpwh.org.uk

132. Callahan J. Separation of the symphysis pubis. Am J Obstet Gynecol 1953; 66:281–293.

133. Fast A, Weiss L, Parich S, et al. Night backache in pregnancy—hypothetical pathophysiological mechanisms. Am J Phys Med Rehabil 1989;68: 227–229.

134. Fingeroth RJ. Successful operative treatment of a displaced subcapital fracture of the hip in transient osteoporosis of pregnancy. A case report and review of the literature. J Bone Joint Surg 1995;77:127–131.

135. Samdani A, Lachmann E, Nagler W. Transient osteoporosis of the hip during pregnancy: a case report. Am J Phys Med Rehabil 1998;77:153–156.

136. Smith R, Athanasou NA, Ostlere SJ, et al. Pregnancy-associated osteoporosis. Q J Med 1995;88:865–878.

137. Dunne F, Walters B, Marshall T, et al. Pregnancy associated osteoporosis. Clin Endocrinol 1993;39:487–490.

138. Carbone LD, Palmiere GM, Graves SC, et al. Osteoporosis of pregnancy: long-term follow-up of patients and their offspring. Obstet Gynecol 1995;86:664–666.

139. Khastgir G, Studd JW, King H, et al. Changes in bone density and biochemical markers of bone turnover in pregnancy-associated osteoporosis. Br J Obstet Gynecol 1996;103:716–718.
140. Little KD, Clapp JF. Self-selected recreational exercise has no impact on early postpartum lactation-induced bone loss. Med Sci Sports Exerc 1998;30:831–836.
141. Keen AD, Drinkwater BL. Irreversible bone loss in former amenorrheic athletes. Osteoporosis Int 1997;7:311–315.
142. Funk JL, Shoback DM, Genant HK. Transient osteoporosis of the hip in pregnancy: natural history of changes in bone mineral density. Clin Endocrinol 1995;43:373–382.
143. Sowers M. Pregnancy and lactation as risk factors for subsequent bone loss and osteoporosis. J Bone Mineral Res 1996;11:1052–1060.
144. Pipp LM. The exercise dilemma: considerations and guidelines for treatment of the high risk obstetric patient. J Obstet Gynecol Phys Ther 1989;13:10–12.
145. Frahm J, Davis Y, Welch RA. Physical therapy management of the high risk antepartum patient: physical and occupational therapy treatment objectives and program, part III. Clin Manage Phys Ther 1989;9:28–33.
146. Gilbert ES, Harmann JS. Manual of High Risk Pregnancy and Delivery. St. Louis: Mosby, 1993.
147. Barnes LP. Pregnancy over 35: special needs. MCN Am J Matern Child Nurs 1991;16:272.
148. Kozinszky Z, Orvos H, Zoboki T, et al. Risk factors for cesarean section of primiparous women aged over 35 years. Acta Obstet Gynecol Scand 2002;81:313–316.
149. Astolfi P, Zonta LA. Delayed maternity and risk at delivery. Paediatr Perinat Epidemiol 2002;16:67–72.
150. Seoud MA, Nassar AN, Usta IM, et al. Impact of advanced maternal age on pregnancy outcome. Am J Perinatol 2002;19:1–8.
151. Ziadeh S, Yahaya A. Pregnancy outcome at age 40 and older. Arch Gynecol Obstet 2001;265:30–33.
152. Jolly M, Sebire N, Harris J, et al. The risks associated with pregnancy in women aged 35 years or older. Human Reprod 2000;15: 2433–2437.
153. Abu-Heija AT, Jallad MF, Abukteish F. Maternal and perinatal outcome of pregnancies after the age of 45. J Obstet Gynaecol Res 2000;26:27–30.
154. Gilbert WM, Nesbitt TS, Danielsen B. Childbearing beyond age 40: pregnancy outcome in 24,032 cases. Obstet Gynecol 1999;93:9–14.
155. Vankatwijk C, Peeters LL. Clinical aspects of pregnancy after the age of 35 years: a review of the literature. Hum Reprod Update 1998;4:185–194.
156. Growth and bone development. Nestle Nutrition Workshop Series: paediatric programme. 2008;61:53–68.
157. Goldenberg RL, Cliver SP, Bronstein J, et al. Bed rest in pregnancy. Obstet Gynecol 1994;84:131.
158. Maloni JA, Kasper CE. Physical and psychosocial effects of antepartum hospital bed rest: a review of the literature. Image J Nurs Sch 1991;23:187–192.
159. Maloni JA, Chance B, Zhang C, et al. Physical and psychosocial side effects of antepartum hospital bed rest. Nurs Res 1993;42:197–203.
160. Maloni JA. Home care of the high-risk pregnant woman requiring bed rest. J Obstet Gynecol Neonat Nurs 1994;23:696–706.
161. Josten LE, Savik K, Mullett SE, et al. Bed rest compliance for women with pregnancy problems. Birth 1995;22:1–12.
162. Schroeder CA. Women's experience of bed rest in high-risk pregnancy. Image J Nurs Sch 1996;28:253–258.
163. Maloni JA. Bed rest and high-risk pregnancy: differentiating the effects of diagnosis, setting, and treatment. Nurs Clin N Am 1996;31:313–325.
164. Smithing RT, Wiley MD. Bedrest not necessarily an effective intervention in pregnancy. Nurse Pract Am J Primary Health Care 1994;19:15.
165. Bogen JT, Gitlin LN, Cornman-Levy D. Bedrest treatment in high-risk pregnancy: implications for physical therapy. Platform Presentation at the American Physical Therapy Association Combined Sections Meeting, February 1997; Dallas, TX.
166. Mitchell L. Simple Relaxation. 2nd Ed. London: John Murray, 1987.
167. Jacobson E. Progressive Relaxation. Chicago: University of Chicago Press, 1938.
168. Candido G, Lo T, Janssen PA. Risk factors for diastasis of the recti abdominis. J Assoc Chartered Physiotherapists in Women's Health 2005;97:49–54.
169. Coldron Y, Stokes MJ, Newham DJ, et al. Postpartum characteristics of rectus abdominis on ultrasound imaging. Man Ther 2008;13:112–121.
170. Spitznagle TM, Leong FC, Van Dillen LR. Prevalence of diastasis recti abdominis in a urogynecological patient population. Int Urogynecol J 2007;18:321–328.
171. Haddow G, Watts R, Robertson J. The effectiveness of a pelvic floor muscle exercise program on urinary incontinence following childbirth: a systematic review. International J Evid Based Healthc 2005;3:103–146.
172. Mens JMA, Vleeming A, Snijders CJ, et al. Responsiveness of outcome measurements in rehabilitation of patients with posterior pelvic pain since pregnancy. Spine 2002;27:1110–1115.

173. Brynhildsen J, Hansson A, Persson A, et al. Follow- up of patients with low back pain during pregnancy. Obstet Gynecol 1998;91:182–186.
174. Richardson C, Jull G, Hodges P, et al. Therapeutic \Exercise For Spinal Segmental Stabilization In Low Back Pain. Edinburgh, Scotland: Churchill Livingstone, 1999.
175. Mens JMA, Vleeming A, Stoeckart R, et al. Understanding peripartum pelvic pain. Spine 1996;21:1363–1369.
176. Mens JMA, Snijders CJ, Stam HJ. Diagonal trunk muscle exercises in peripartum pelvic pain: a randomized clinical trial. Phys Ther 2000;80:1164–1173.
177. Hides JA, Richardson CA, Jull GA. Multifidus muscle recovery is not automatic after resolution of acute, first-episode low back pain. Spine 1996; 21:2763–2769.
178. Sapsford RR, Hodges PW. Contraction of the pelvic floor muscles during abdominal maneuvers. Arch Phys Med Rehabil 2001;82:1081–1088.
179. Sapsford RR, Hodges PW, Richardson CA, et al. Co-activation of the abdominal and pelvic floor muscles during voluntary exercises. Neurourol Urodyn 2001;20:31–42.
180. American College of Obstetricians and Gynecologists. Cesarean Birth. ACOG patient education pamphlet AP06. Washington, DC: American College of Obstetricians and Gynecologists, 1983.
181. American College of Obstetricians and Gynecologists. Vaginal Birth After Cesarean Delivery. ACOG patient education pamphlet AP070. Washington, DC: American College of Obstetricians and Gynecologists, 1990.
182. Rangelli D, Hayes SH. Vaginal birth after cesarean: the role of the physical therapist. J Obstet Gynecol Phys Ther 1995;19:10–13.
183. Gent D, Gottlieb K. Cesarean rehabilitation. Clin Manage Phys Ther 1985; 5:14–19.
184. Loos MJ, Scheltinga MR, Mulders LG, et al. The Pfannenstiel incision as a source of chronic pain. Obstet Gynecol 2008;111:839–846.
185. Scott S. Exercise in the postpartum period. Health Fitness 2006;10:40–41.
186. Shaw E, Kaczorowski J. Postpartum care – what's new? Curr Opin Obstet Gynecol 2007;19:561–567.
187. Hinton PS, Olson CM. Postpartum exercise and food intake: the importance of behavior-specific self efficacy. J Am Diet Assoc 2001;101:1430–1437.
188. Katz VL, Ryder RM, Cefalo RC, et al. A comparison of bed rest and immersion for treating the edema of pregnancy. Obstet Gynecol 1990;75:147–151.
189. Knee-chest exercises and maternal death [No authors listed]. Med J Aust 1973;1:1127.
190. Nelson P. Pulmonary gas embolism in pregnancy and the puerperium. Obstet Gynecol Surv 1960;15:449–481.
191. Weiss Kelly AK. Practical exercise advise during pregnancy: guidelines for active and inactive women. Phys Sports Med 2005;33(6).

SUGGESTED READINGS

Clapp JF. Exercising Through Your Pregnancy. Champaign, IL: Human Kinetics, 1998.
Myers RS, ed. Saunders Manual of Physical Therapy Practice. Chapters 22 and 23. Philadelphia: WB Saunders, 1995.
Nobel E. Essential Exercises for the Childbearing Year. 4th Ed. Harwich, MA: New Life Images, 1995.
Nobel E. Marie Osmond's Exercises for Mothers-To-Be. New York: New American Library, 1985.
Nobel E. Marie Osmond's Exercises for Mothers and Babies. New York: New American Library, 1985.
Pauls JA. Therapeutic Approaches to Women's Health. Gaithersburg, MD: Aspen Publishers, 1995.
Simkin P, Whalley J, Kepler A. Pregnancy, Child Birth and the Newborn: The Complete Guide. Deephaven, MN: Meadowbrook Press, 1991.

RESOURCES

American College of Obstetricians and Gynecologists (ACOG), 409 12th Street, SW, Washington, DC 20024-2188; (202) 638-5577.
American College of Sports Medicine, P.O. Box 1440, Indianapolis, IN 46206; (317) 637-9200.
American Physical Therapy Association, Section on Women's Health, P.O. Box 327, Alexandria, VA 22313; (800) 999-2782 ext. 3237.
Melpomene Institute for Women's Health Research, 1010 University Avenue, St. Paul, MN 55104; (612) 642-1951.

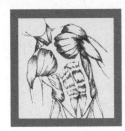

chapter 14

Closed Kinetic Training

SUSAN LYNN LEFEVER

Historically, the concepts and principles involving the disciplines of human kinesiology and the biomechanics of movement have been inextricably woven into the study of mechanical engineering. The kinetic chain concept originated in 1955, when Steindler[1] used mechanical engineering theories of closed kinematic and link concepts to describe human kinesiology. In the link concept, rigid overlapping segments are connected in a series by movable joints. This system allows for predictable movement of one joint based on the movement of the other joints and is considered a closed kinematic chain.[2,3] In the lower extremity of the human body, each bony segment can be viewed as a rigid link; bones of the foot, lower leg, thigh, and pelvis are seen as rigid links. Similarly, the subtalar, talocrural, tibiofemoral, and hip synovial joints act as the connecting joints.

Applying these concepts to human movement, Steindler[1] observed that two types of kinetic chains exist, depending on the loading of the "terminal joint." Steindler classified these as an open kinetic chain (OKC) and a closed kinetic chain (CKC). He observed that muscle recruitment and joint motions were different when the foot or hand was free to move or met considerable resistance. An OKC was described when the end segment is free to move (e.g., swing limb during gait, waving the hand).[1] In the CKC, "the terminal joints meet considerable external resistance which prohibits or restrains its free motion" (e.g., descending stairs, upper extremity during crutch walking).[1] Display 14-1 summarizes characteristics common to OKC and CKC.

The use of CKC exercises in rehabilitation began in the 1980s, when physicians began looking for safe ways to rehabilitate the quadriceps mechanism in patients after anterior cruciate ligament (ACL) reconstruction. During the 1960s and 1970s,[4,5] documentation in the biomechanics literature demonstrated an increase in the anterior shear forces during the last 30 degrees of OKC knee extension. Numerous researchers[6–10] thought that this increase in anterior shear placed a detrimental strain on the healing graft that could compromise the surgical result.

Using cadaveric experiments, Grood et al.[8] documented increased anterior tibial translation with OKC knee extension and subsequently suggested exercising in an upright posture to use the "forces of weight bearing" to minimize anterior tibial translation. Stability is enhanced in the weight-bearing position because of increased joint compressive forces, improved joint congruency, and muscular co-contraction.

Henning et al.[9] supported this hypothesis by the findings of an in vivo ACL strain study. By placing a strain gauge in the ACL of two volunteers, the amount of strain across the ACL was measured during various exercises, including isometric knee extension at 0 and 22 degrees and such daily activities

---

 DISPLAY 14-1
Characteristics Common to CKC and OKC Activities

The following characteristics are common to CKC activities:

- Interdependence of joint motion (i.e., knee flexion depends on ankle joint dorsiflexion)
- Motion occurring proximal and distal to the axis of the joint in a predictable fashion (e.g., knee flexion is accompanied by hip flexion, internal rotation, and adduction and by ankle joint dorsiflexion and internal tibial rotation)
- Recruitment of muscle contractions that are predominantly eccentric, with dynamic muscular stabilization in the form of co-contraction
- Greater joint compressive forces resulting in decreased shearing
- Stabilization afforded by joint congruency
- Normal posture (weight bearing) and muscle contractions
- Enhanced proprioception because of the increased number of stimulated mechanoreceptors

The following are characteristics common to OKC activities:

- Independence of joint motion (e.g., knee flexion is independent of ankle joint position)
- Motion occurring distal to the axis of the joint (e.g., knee flexion results with motion of only the lower leg)
- Muscle contractions that are predominantly concentric
- Greater distraction and rotary forces
- Stabilization afforded by outside means
- Activation of mechanoreceptors limited to the moving joint and surrounding structures

as walking and stationary biking. It was found that isometric knee extension at 0 and 22 degrees placed more strain on the ACL than walking or stationary biking.

Although most of the scientific literature concerning CKC activities is focused on quadriceps rehabilitation after ACL reconstruction, contrasting research by Hungerford and Barry[11] evaluated patellofemoral contact pressure areas during OKC and CKC exercises. The investigators believed an OKC extension exercise, performed in the 0- to 30-degree range of knee flexion, resulted in high patellofemoral contact pressures because of the decreasing patellofemoral contact area with an increasing length of the moment arm as the limb assumed a more horizontal position. They concluded that OKC extension exercises against resistance produce nonphysiologic loading of patellar articular cartilage. Even relatively small loads, which are commonly used in physical therapy departments, produce pressures far in excess of normal activities, such as stair climbing or squatting.[11]

PHYSIOLOGIC PRINCIPLES OF CLOSED KINETIC TRAINING

Three major physiologic principles supporting the use of CKC training include muscular factors, biomechanical factors, and neurophysiologic factors.

Muscular Factors

CKC exercises stimulate muscular co-contractions, thereby enhancing stability in the weight-bearing position.[3–7,12,13] For example, weight-bearing activities decrease the amount of anterior shear across the ACL[5–9,14] as a result of co-contraction of the hamstring musculature. This provides dynamic stabilization that results in improved postural holding and additional support for the joint.[15–17] The type of muscular contractions in the closed chain setting is predominately eccentric in nature, followed by co-contractions and finally concentric muscle function.

Stretch Shortening Cycle

One method of training the neuromuscular system to perform this sequence of muscle contractions is referred to as plyometric training. Plyometric training is a method of training the neuromuscular system to increase power (i.e., work per time). This is accomplished by combining speed and strength of muscular contractions.[18–21] The increased power occurs from storing energy during the eccentric phase and immediately using this stored energy during the concentric phase. Plyometric exercises involve rapid closing and opening of the kinetic chain[3] and are routinely prescribed as part of the rehabilitation of athletes after orthopedic injuries.

A frequent goal of rehabilitation of athletes is to return their ability to change forward energy into vertical height, as in blocking a volleyball or dunking a basketball. The basic premise is that a muscle can perform more positive (concentric) work if it is stretched (eccentrically loaded) immediately before shortening. This is referred to as the stretch-shortening cycle (SSC).[18,21,22] Mechanically, the elastic components of the muscle and tendon (i.e., myosin, actin, and other proteins) that are arranged in series are stretched during the eccentric portion, thereby storing energy. During the concentric portion, this energy is released as the elastic components return

to their resting length.[2,18,21,22] This is similar to the way a spring stores energy as it is stretched and releases the energy as it returns to its resting length. It is believed that activation of the muscle spindle, inhibition of the Golgi tendon organs through the stretch reflex, and a marked increase in the chemical energy enhance muscular contraction.[17,21–23] The result is improved neural efficiency and neuromuscular control with increased tolerance to stretched loads (i.e., decreased injury) and an increase in the explosive ability of muscular contractions.[2,18,21] CKC activities that stimulate the use of the SSC include running, jumping activities, box drills, and skipping. (See Building Block 14-1.)[3]

Biomechanical Factors

Biomechanical factors contributing to joint stability include the geometry of the joint surfaces, joint approximation, and stimulation of joint receptors. For example, the geometry of the joint surfaces appears to aid in the decrease of anterior tibial displacement in the loaded knee joint.[17,24] Additionally, CKC activities at the talocrural joint increase ankle joint approximation, enhancing joint congruency and contributing to joint stability.[25]

Joint Surface Geometry

Understanding the geometry of the joint surfaces also allows the clinician to more fully understand the osteokinematics associated with CKC function. Osteokinematically, the distal segment moves through a greater range of motion (ROM) more rapidly than the proximal segment.[26] For example, knee flexion is associated with obligatory internal tibial rotation.

Understanding the influence of foot and ankle biomechanics on the entire kinetic chain is essential to ensure accurate prescription of CKC exercises. A brief description of how motion of the subtalar joint can influence the kinetic chain is provided to illustrate proper CKC training. Closed-chain pronation of the subtalar joint results in calcaneal eversion and talar plantar flexion and adduction[27] (Fig. 14-1). The alignment of the talus in the ankle mortise dictates that in a CKC setting motion of the lower leg must follow the motion of the talus. That is, as the talus plantar flexes and adducts, the lower leg internally rotates as the fibular head translates superiorly and anteriorly. This results in talocrural joint dorsiflexion and

> ### BUILDING BLOCK 14-1
>
> Consider a 16-year-old high school basketball player recovering from a lateral ankle sprain. He is 8 weeks post injury and is preparing to return to his sport.
>
> 1. Describe one easy plyometric exercise in the sagittal plane to help him begin plyometric training. Include dosage.
> 2. Utilizing the quick stretch component of plyometric exercises, modify this exercise to enhance the amount of stored energy.
> 3. Describe one advanced frontal plane plyometric exercise to help him safely reach his long-term goal of returning to playing basketball.

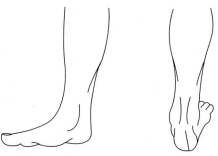

FIGURE 14-1. Closed-chain pronation: calcaneal eversion, talar plantar flexion, and adduction.

knee flexion with a valgus stress (Fig. 14-2). Motion occurring up the chain continues with femoral adduction and internal rotation as the hip moves into flexion.[28–30] The pelvis tilts anteriorly and internally rotates in phase with the limb (the tibia, femur, and pelvis all internally rotate, with the distal segment moving faster and through a greater ROM) as the lumbar spine extends and counterrotates.[29] A very important concept to understand with closed chain function is that frontal plane movements of calcaneus (inversion/eversion) result in transverse plane movement of the entire limb (external/internal rotation). (The subtalar joint acts like a torque converter.)[27] (See Building Block 14-2A.)

Jackson[29] describes the pelvis as the next triplane joint that has an intimate relationship with the subtalar joint. He feels that the pitch of the subtalar joint axis dictates the amount of transverse and frontal plane rotation occurring at the pelvis and throughout the lower limb. The average axis of the subtalar joint is 42 degrees midway between the sagittal and transverse planes (see Chapter 21), thus promoting fairly equal amounts of transverse plane motion of the limb (hip external/internal rotation) and frontal plane motion of the subtalar joint (inversion/eversion). A high subtalar joint axis results in increased transverse plane motion of the pelvis and entire lower extremity. This configuration results in subtalar joint supination and the predictable movements of the entire lower extremity. As the subtalar joint supinates, motions up the chain include tibial external rotation, knee extension, femoral external rotation, and abduction and external rotation of the

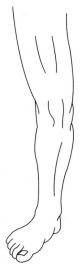

FIGURE 14-2. Closed-chain pronation: internal rotation of the lower leg and flexion with valgus stress at the knee.

BUILDING BLOCK 14-2A

The subtalar joint acts as a torque converter changing frontal plane motion of the foot (subtalar joint inversion/eversion) into transverse plane motion of the limb (external/internal rotation of the hip). Describe two transverse plane exercises at the hip to help decrease frontal plane motion of the foot.

BUILDING BLOCK 14-2B

Observation of a patient with the diagnosis of low back pain during the gait cycle reveals an increase in the amount of pelvic rotation and a decrease in the amount of subtalar joint pronation.

You suspect this patient may have a ___ subtalar joint axis.

1. Describe the relationship between the patient's diagnosis and limb mechanics
2. What posture should you exercise the hip and knee in to help decrease stress on the lower back?

ilium.[27,29] The clinical significance of a high subtalar joint axis is that the limb has difficulty with shock attenuation.[28] This lack of shock attenuation should alter the type and dosage of CKC exercises the clinician prescribes during lower extremity rehabilitation. (See building block 14-2B.)

A low subtalar joint axis results in more frontal plane motion of the pelvis and lower extremity.[29] Excessive subtalar pronation results in an increase in the frontal plane motions of femoral adduction and an increased valgus stress on the knee. The clinical result is a limb that is inefficient during propulsion.[28] When prescribing CKC exercises for the patient with a low subtalar joint axis, the clinician should position the foot in subtalar joint neutral (see Chapter 21) before beginning the exercise and have the patient maintain that foot position during the exercise. (See Building Block 14-2C.) Foot and ankle motion influences hip, knee, and pelvic motion; therefore, initiation of exercises in one segment of the lower extremity

BUILDING BLOCK 14-2C

Observation of a patient with the diagnosis of patellofemoral pain syndrome during the gait cycle reveals an increase in the amount of frontal plane foot and limb motion.

You suspect this patient may have a ___ subtalar joint axis?

1. Describe the relationship between the patient's diagnosis and limb mechanics
2. What posture should you exercise the hip and foot in to help decrease stress on the knee?

CASE STUDY 14-1

The patient is a 28-year-old male roofing contractor with c/o L medial shin pain and the diagnosis of posterior tibialis tendinitis. States pain is worse at work with climbing ladders and working on a steep pitched roof. Pain has been getting worse over the past month. Recreational activities include jogging × 3 weekly 30 to 40 minutes which he has been unable to do secondary to the pain. Pain is a 5 on a 0 to 10 scale. Rest and Nonsteroidal Anti-inflammatories (NSAIDs) have not been helpful.

PMH: Hernia operation × 4 years ago, intermittent low back pain

Obs: The patient ambulates with a toe-out position on the left, with a normal base of support. Additionally, his gait reveals an inverted position of the heel at initial contact with subtalar joint eversion to vertical and prolonged subtalar joint pronation through early to mid stance without midfoot collapse and with minimal lowering of medial longitudinal arch height. During the later part of the propulsive phase of gait the patient demonstrates a medial heel whip.

EXAMINATION

MMT: Normal throughout except: L hip abduction 4/5, hip external rotation 4–/5, posterior tibialis 4–/5 +pain

ROM: Normal throughout except: Bilateral decreased talocrural joint dorsiflexion by 50%

Plantar Callus Pattern: Lateral border of the heel, pinch on great toe

Weight-Bearing Alignment: External tibial rotation, vertical calcaneal position.

Weight-Bearing Examination: Neutral (subtalar neutral) calcaneal position 10 degrees varus, relaxed calcaneal position vertical. Navicular drop (sit to stand) 7 mm.

ACTIVITY LIMITATIONS

1. Patient unable to work safely on pitched roofs.
2. Patient unable to climb frequently up and down ladders.
3. Patient unable to run/walk more than 10 minutes.
4. Patient unable to stand for more than 40 minutes

PARTICIPATION RESTRICTIONS

1. Has been decreasing hours at work over the past month
2. Unable to participate in recreational activities

---

kinetic chain results in predictable movement of the other segments. The distal segment moves through a greater ROM and more rapidly than the proximal segment.[29]

Case Study 14-1 and Building Blocks 14-2D and 14-2E will be used to illustrate the influence of motion on the kinetic chain.

Electromyographic (EMG) studies by Perry[31] show that the gluteus medius and, to a lesser extent, the gluteus maximus and posterior tibialis are active in the stance leg during midstance of the gait cycle. Because hip external rotation effects foot supination, these findings suggest that clinicians should encourage the patient to contract the hip musculature during stance phase of gait to enhance supination of the subtalar joint.

Wolff's Law

Additional support for using CKC exercises in rehabilitation is provided by the constant remodeling of tissues.[2] Wolff's Law states that bone remodels according to the stresses placed on it. Areas of increased stress result in bone deposition. Related research in the field of osteoporosis has shown that early pubertal girls placed on a jumping program for 7 months had an increase in bone cross-sectional area in the femoral neck and intertrochanter regions.[32]

This theory has been extended to the remodeling of soft tissues. Collagen fibers organize themselves along lines of mechanical stress.[2] This is of particular importance when rehabilitating patients after ligamentous injuries. A gradual change in the mechanical stress through the injured tissue along biomechanically consistent lines can help strengthen the injured tissue and help it to resist reinjury.[2] It is important to place gradual mechanical stress on healing soft tissues by

---

BUILDING BLOCK 14-2D

1. Using the information in the Display box 14-1, Case study 14-1, and the short-term goal of teaching the patient how to supinate the subtalar joint, describe two joining segments in the kinetic chain which can be used to accomplish this goal.
2. Describe two or three CKC exercises to help this patient reach his goal.
3. How would you progress these exercises as his symptoms subsided?
4. How would you change these exercises to encourage eccentric muscle function of posterior tibialis?

BUILDING BLOCK 14-2E

Consider the patient in Case Study 14-1 to answer the following questions.

1. Given the history and examination findings, what are some signs and symptoms that are compatible with abnormal closed chain function?
2. Does the pathology match his abnormal closed chain mechanics? Why or why not?
3. Write some possible short term and long term goals for this patient.

BUILDING BLOCK 14-3

Using Wolff's Law of constantly remodeling tissues, progress a patient using CKC training techniques with an Achilles tendinitis through the stages of healing to accomplish the goal of pain-free with jumping.

BUILDING BLOCK 14-4

Name a pathology requiring neural adaptation of the nervous system and describe two different CKC exercises to assist this patient with Lower Extremity (LE) strengthening.

placing them in functional positions throughout the rehabilitation process. For example, when rehabilitating a patient with a medial deltoid ligament sprain to the ankle, the position of the foot during CKC exercises is important for controlling the amount of stress placed on the healing tissue. Allowing the subtalar joint to excessively pronate during the exercise places an undesirable stress on the healing medial deltoid ligament. (See building block 14-3.)

Neurophysiologic Factors

Neurophysiologic support for using CKC activities in rehabilitation is provided by stimulation of the proprioceptive system. Proprioception is a specialized form of touch and is composed of the sensation of joint movement (i.e., kinesthesia) and of joint position (i.e., joint position sense).[33] The sensory receptors consist of mechanoreceptors and nociceptors found in muscles, joints, periarticular structures, and skin. Four major types of joint receptors, the muscle spindle, the Golgi tendon organs, and cutaneous receptors have been identified as structures providing sensory input to the central nervous system (CNS).[34] Deformation and loading of the soft tissues surrounding a joint trigger the mechanoreceptors to convert this mechanical energy to electrical impulses.[33,35] The electrical impulses are transmitted to and integrated by the CNS to produce a motor response.[34–36]

CKC activities use the force of gravity to stimulate these receptors. Borsa hypothesized that a loss of mechanoreceptor feedback after joint injury results in the loss of protective muscular co-contraction, contributing to a cycle of repeated ligamentous injury and further joint instability.[37] The use of CKC activities during rehabilitation can stimulate these mechanoreceptors.[34,38] By encouraging muscular co-contractions through CKC exercises, the cycle of repeated ligamentous injury may be disrupted.[38]

Balance

The goal of restoring balance mechanisms after a joint injury provides additional neurologic support for the use of CKC activities. Balance (i.e., postural control) is the ability of the body to maintain the center of mass over the base of support without falling.[39] This is an important motor skill. An individual senses body position relative to gravity by combining visual, vestibular, and somatosensory (i.e., proprioceptive) inputs.[39] Small adjustments in the ankle, hip, and knee are used to maintain the line of gravity over the base of support.[38,40,41] In a CKC movement, indirect forces from muscles of adjacent segments are transferred to and received from adjoining segments. The position of an adjoining segment of the kinetic chain can assist with proprioceptive input, helping to maintain equilibrium.[39] CKC activities focusing on balance and postural control should be an important part of any upper or lower extremity program, particularly one with the goal of restoring normal kinesthesia (see Chapter 8).

Neural Adaptation

Neural adaptation involves changes in the ability of the nervous system to recruit the appropriate muscles to obtain a desired result.[42] When beginning a new exercise program, the strength gains that occur in the first few weeks can be attributed to improved coordination from neural adaptation as the person becomes more efficient in performing the activity.[42]

Continued practice of patterned motion requires less and less cognitive awareness, until it eventually becomes automatic or habitual and can be performed with ease.[12,22] Using functional CKC activities enhances the nervous system's ability to recruit groups of muscles to work together. Neural pathways that closely replicate functional demands are created. Proponents of motor learning describe the process of learning a new movement as beginning on a conscious cognitive level and, with repetition, moving to a more subconscious level. Rehabilitative programs should enhance functional outcomes by including functional CKC activities. For example, a quadriplegic patient must learn to use his or her upper body to perform transfers from the wheelchair to the bed. Therefore, a new neural pathway of using the upper extremity in a closed fashion becomes necessary. Seated CKC triceps dips would be an appropriate activity to include in this patient's rehabilitation program to enhance development of this pathway. (See Building Block 14-4.)

Specificity of Training

CKC training relies on the principle of the specificity of training.[15,40,42] Studies involving strength training have shown that a greater increase in strength was measured when the test activity was similar to the actual training exercise.[42,43] This approach involves the use of the specific adaptations to imposed demands (SAID) principle.[44,45] Changes in the neuromuscular system can be accomplished by applying a specific type of mechanical stress (i.e., imposed demands) to that system. In response to the stress, the body makes specific adaptations in muscle recruitment patterns. Using CKC training helps to replicate the imposed demands of activities of daily living and uses a more natural recruitment pattern of an eccentric muscle contraction to decelerate or control a movement, followed by a concentric muscle contraction. Using a 4-in step to perform step-up exercises to gain the lower extremity hip and thigh strength needed to improve the functional performance of ascending stairs is an example of using the SAID principle with a CKC activity. (See Building Block 14-5.)

EXAMINATION AND EVALUATION

The evaluation of functional activities and documentation of improvements in function are critical issues facing the physical therapy profession. Many insurance companies base

BUILDING BLOCK 14-5

Discuss three characteristics unique to CKC training that most aptly apply to the patient with:

1. That presents with an unstable knee
2. Returning to a collegiate sport
3. s/p Cerebral Vascular Accident (CVA) with R hemiplegia

reimbursement of physical therapy services on documented improvements in function. Testing of CKC activities can be both static and dynamic.

Standardization Tools

In the Lower Extremity Functional Profile, Gray and Team Reaction[46] attempted to set standards for the measurement and documentation of functional testing in a CKC setting. The tests are designed with a set of rules using clear and consistent terminology and standards that can be easily documented. The tests evaluate the functional movements of static and dynamic balance, amount of motion (i.e., excursion), and distance moved in a CKC environment.[46] Tests for the sport activities of step, hop, and jump also are presented.[46] Other researchers have devised functional tests for both the upper and the lower extremity to determine the readiness of an athlete to return to recreational activities.[47–50] A few CKC submaximal tests can indicate the safety of performing plyometric exercises.[18,23] For example, before initiation of plyometric activities, Albert[18] and the National Strength and Conditioning Coaches Association[23] recommend that a person should be able to long jump his or her height in distance. Evaluation of patients from a CKC approach is useful when dealing with adolescents to ensure that their immature muscular and skeletal systems can handle the stress of increased loads. Comparative results of functional testing can be obtained from pretest and posttest values or by comparing right and left values.[46]

CKC training has the unique advantage of "becoming the test"; the test becomes the exercise, and consequently, the exercise becomes the test. An example is testing of static balance. The patient presents with difficulty in single-limb stance during gait. The patient is asked to balance with shoes off, eyes open, on one limb. Measurement is taken of the amount of time balance is achieved. The test ends when an alteration in position of the stance limb, the non–weight-bearing limb touches, or after 30 seconds. If less than optimal performance occurs, this activity becomes part of the patient's home exercise program. After the 30-second limit is reached, the difficulty of the test can be enhanced.[46]

Another example of an exercise is an excursion test in single-limb stance. Excursion tests are designed to measure the amount of motion that can be controlled at a joint.[46] For example, consider a patient who presents with decreased stride length on the left during gait. Beginning on the left leg, the patient is asked to extend the left hip with a successful return to the standing position while maintaining the single-limb stance. The degree of hip extension in the sagittal plane is measured. If limited hip extension is measured, this activity becomes part of the patient's home exercise program.[46]

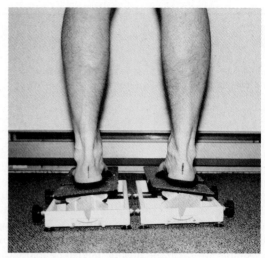

FIGURE 14-3. Posterior view using ProWedgeIt.

Another potential examination tool, the ProWedgeIt (Biomechanical Services Corporation) (see Fig. 14-3), has become available permitting the evaluation of CKC activities by altering the position of the foot in the frontal plane. This type of examination tool can be used to assess improvement in the patient's function with his or her foot held in a certain posture. For example, a patient that demonstrates excessive subtalar joint pronation during stance may have a reduced medial reach. When retested using the ProWedgeIt with the subtalar less pronated, an improvement in the medial reach should be evident. This may be helpful when deciding if any frontal plane assistance in the form of a function foot orthosis would be helpful (Fig. 14-4).

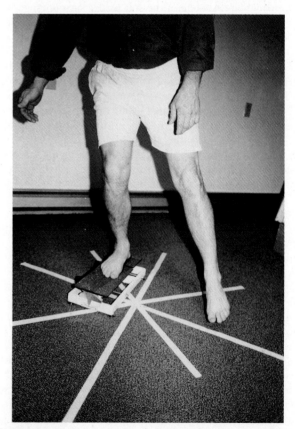

FIGURE 14-4. Medial reach using ProWedgeIt (Biomechanical Services, Inc.; Brea, CA 92821).

CASE STUDY 14-2

Patient is a 60-year-old female who c/o bilateral medial plantar heel pain L > R. Patient complains of significant heel pain the first thing in the morning or when she arises in the middle of the night requiring her to "shuffle to the bathroom." Once she is up and moving her heel, pain subsides unless she is on her feet for sustained activities or for a prolonged amount of time. Pain is rated at a 6 on 0 to 10 scale. Footwear includes 3-year-old casual shoes, open-toe slingback sandals with a 1-in heel, "unbranded" 2-year-old walking shoes.

PMH: Type II diabetic × 5 years controlled by diet and exercise. Left bunionectomy × 2 years ago; high blood pressure which is controlled with medication.

Obs: Mild truncal obesity. The patient demonstrates a bilateral Trendelenberg gait pattern, with a wide base of support and an increase in the toe-out angle of her gait. Additionally, her gait reveals excessive and prolonged subtalar joint pronation with midfoot collapse throughout stance resulting in abduction of the forefoot on the rearfoot and loss of medial longitudinal arch height. During the later part of the propulsive phase of the gait cycle, the patient demonstrates a medial heel whip, thus shifting her weight to the lateral aspect of her foot.

MMT: Normal throughout except: Bilateral hip abduction 4–/5, hip external rotation 3+/5, hip extension 4–/5

ROM: Normal throughout except: B decreased talocrural joint dorsiflexion by 50% and decreased hip internal rotation and extension by 50%.

Non–weight-bearing FF to RF Foot Alignment: Perpendicular

Weight-Bearing Alignment: Bilateral anterior pelvic tilt, with slight hip flexion, internal medial femoral rotation, knee valgus, external tibial rotation, calcaneal eversion, and lowered medial longitudinal arch.

Weight-Bearing Examination: Neutral (subtalar neutral) calcaneal position 2 degrees varus, relaxed calcaneal position 10 degrees everted. Navicular drop (sit to stand) > 10 mm.

ACTIVITY LIMITATIONS

1. Very painful first few steps in the morning
2. Patient unable to walk more than ¼ mile without stopping to rest.
3. Patient unable to bear weight for longer than 20 minutes.

PARTICIPATION RESTRICTIONS

1. Patient unable to maintain household and perform gardening activities and volunteer activities.
2. Patient unable to participate in her regular exercise program, both a primary social outlet and necessary to control her type II diabetes.

THERAPEUTIC EXERCISE INTERVENTION

CKC training is a valuable form of exercise for enhancing patient's ability to function in their work, home, or recreational environments. Rehabilitation of muscular strength and neuromuscular coordination must take into account the position and function of the entire kinetic chain. The position of an adjacent segment directly affects the muscular contraction and applied force throughout the involved region. No longer is there rehabilitation of a "knee patient." A study by Bullock-Saxton[51] supports this concept. The researcher compared two groups: an injured group who had sustained severe unilateral ankle sprains and a matched uninjured, control group. Changes in sensory perception (i.e., vibration) and motor response (i.e., hip extensor firing pattern) were found. The results showed significant delays in gluteus maximus recruitment on the ipsilateral and contralateral sides in the injured group.[51] (See Case Studies 14-2 and 14-3, and Building Block 14-6.)

Rehabilitation of a patient with a knee injury focuses on functional limitations and rehabilitation of the entire limb. Resolving these functional limitations includes weight-bearing activities under task-specific conditions. The flexibility, simplicity, and creativity associated with CKC training afford countless possibilities for exercises to be included in a home exercise program. (See Building Block 14-7.)

To assist the clinician in prescribing appropriate CKC exercises, this section is divided into elements of the movement system, activity or technique, and dosage guidelines.

Elements of the Movement System

Base Element

Impairments in the base element of the movement system (e.g., muscle performance, ROM, muscle flexibility, joint mobility and integrity) can be dealt quite well with CKC exercise.

Muscle performance must be at least at a functional level in the target muscles to participate in upright closed chain activities. The higher the demand for muscle performance, the higher the muscle grade must be to perform the activity with precision. Clinicians should be cautious in prescribing CKC activities when the muscle performance cannot support optimal performance of the activity. OKC activities, in gravity-assisted, gravity-reduced, or gravity-eliminated positions, may be necessary until the muscle performance improves to a functional level. For example, if gluteus medius strength is <3/5, a step-up or step-down activity may be performed with a faulty Trendelenburg pattern. In this case, a better choice may be to perform prone hip abduction (see Chapter 19) until 3 to 3+/5 muscle grade is achieved before prescribing a step-up or step-down activity. Eventually, performing the step-up or step-down with a level pelvis is more important than compromising the quality of the exercise for the sake of performing a CKC exercise.

ROM, muscle length, and joint mobility and integrity impairments can also be treated quite well with CKC activities. When choosing a specific type of CKC exercise the clinician must take into consideration the relationship

CASE STUDY 14-3

The patient is a 17-year-old female high school soccer player who c/o right posterior lateral hip pain × 2 weeks she has a diagnosis of greater trochanteric bursitis. The patient complains of hip pain while running which is worse when she begins running. Once she is warmed up and moving, her hip pain subsides unless she is on her feet for sustained activities or for a prolonged amount of time. Pain is rated at a 6 on 0 to 10 scale. She is pain free with non–weight-bearing activities. She is trying to win a college scholarship in soccer.

PMH: Unremarkable, tonsillectomy age 5 years old

Obs: The patient demonstrates a bilateral Trendelenberg gait pattern, with a wide base of support and an increase in the toe-out angle of her gait. Additionally, her gait reveals excessive and prolonged subtalar joint pronation with midfoot collapse throughout stance resulting in abduction of the forefoot on the rearfoot and loss of medial longitudinal arch height. During the later part of the propulsive phase of gait the patient demonstrates a medial heel whip, thus shifting her weight to the lateral aspect of her feet.

MMT: Normal throughout except: Bilateral hip abduction 4–/5, hip external rotation 3+/5, hip extension 4–/5

ROM: Normal throughout except: Bilateral decreased talocrural joint dorsiflexion by 50% and decreased hip internal rotation and extension by 30%.

Non–weight-bearing FF to RF Alignment: FF varus 10 degrees

Weight-Bearing Alignment: Bilateral anterior pelvic tilt, with slight hip flexion, internal medial femoral rotation, knee valgus, external tibial rotation, calcaneal eversion, and lowered medial longitudinal arch.

Weight-Bearing Examination: Neutral (subtalar neutral) calcaneal position vertical, relaxed calcaneal position 10 degrees everted. Navicular drop (sit to stand) > 10 mm.

ACTIVITY LIMITATIONS

1. Patient unable to walk/run more than 10 minutes without stopping to rest.
2. Patient unable to bear weight for longer than 20 minutes.

PARTICIPATION RESTRICTIONS

1. Patient unable to participate in her regular exercise program, both a primary social outlet and possible scholarship for college soccer.

between the movement of the proximal and distal segments. The relationship of the proximal and distal segments affects the movement of the limb as a whole. In a CKC functional activity, the proximal segment is moving on a more stationary distal segment. For example, closed-chain knee extension is performed by the medial aspect of the femur moving posteriorly, with an internal rotation component, over a fixed tibia. Similarly, in a closed-chain setting ankle joint dorsiflexion is accomplished by the tibia and fibula moving over the talus. Because motion occurs both proximally and distally to the axis

of rotation, ankle joint dorsiflexion is often accompanied by subtalar joint pronation.

Osteokinematically, the distal segment moves through a greater ROM more rapidly than the proximal segment.[29] For example, knee flexion is coupled with obligatory internal tibial rotation. To perform CKC knee flexion, the tibia must internally rotate more than the femur. If this rotation does not occur, the knee is unable to flex. The concept of the proximal segment moving over the distal segment becomes important when mobilizing joints after periods of immobilization. Standard mobilization techniques describe mobilization of the distal segment.[52] During function, the proximal segment is moving over the distal segment. Mobilizing joints, particularly those of the foot and ankle, in accordance with this principle can enhance function.[53,54] Incorporating CKC activity after

BUILDING BLOCK 14-6

Consider the patients in Cases 14-2 and 14-3 to answer the following questions.

1. What are the common examination findings between both case studies?
2. What examination findings are different and significant to abnormal gait?
3. Using the principles of CKC function, how does the influence of the weak hip musculature in case #2 contribute to her pathology? Does the pathology match her abnormal closed chain mechanics?
4. Using the principles of CKC function, how does the influence of the forefoot varus alignment in case #3 contribute to her pathology? Does the pathology match her abnormal closed chain mechanics?
5. Describe two hip CKC exercises in the frontal plane to improve the valgus position at the knee.

BUILDING BLOCK 14-7

Consider the patient in the Building Block 20-4 with the MCL injury

1. Design two or three foot exercises to help her Medial Collateral Ligament (MCL) injury recover in a biomechanically consistent fashion using the principles of CKC function.
2. What additional aids can be used during the rehabilitation process to assist her with improved limb biomechanics to help assist in the healing of the injured tissue?

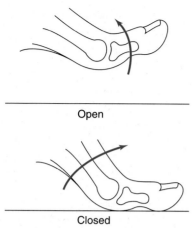

FIGURE 14-5. Incorporating closed kinetic chain activity to improve ROM for the first metatarsal phalangeal joint.

joint mobilization should be considered to ensure proper CKC kinematics and recruitment patterns in newly gained ROM (Fig. 14-5). (See building block 14-8.)

Modulator Element

Impairments in the modulator element (e.g., neuromuscular control) can be effectively managed with CKC activities. For example, controlling knee flexion in a CKC position requires muscular control of rotation of the tibia from below and of the femur from above. The tibia internally rotates through a larger excursion while the femur remains relatively laterally rotated as the knee flexes. If the femur and tibia rotated the same amount with the same speed, no relative motion would have occurred (Fig. 14-6). Coordinated knee flexion is accomplished by controlling the rate and amount of subtalar joint pronation by eccentric contraction of the deep posterior calf muscle group and excessive hip internal rotation by eccentric contraction of the hip lateral rotators.

Biomechanical Element

The biomechanical element of the movement system is probably the element most affected by CKC training. To take full advantage of the benefits of CKC activities, some biomechanical elements to consider include

- Placement of the center of mass
- Placement of the foot

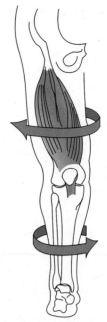

FIGURE 14-6. Relative rotation of the distal and proximal segments.

Performing a knee flexion-extension exercise in a closed chain position can strengthen different muscle groups, depending on where the center of mass is placed relative to the knee. Figure 14-7 shows an example of a minisquat with the center of mass placed directly above the knee. The knee extensors must work to control the movement. In Figure 14-8, the center of mass is located behind the knee, resulting in more stress placed on the hip extensors to control the movement. Figure 14-9 shows a knee flexion-extension exercise in which the pelvis is forward relative to the knee. In this example, the gastrocnemius must work to control the knee movement. This is true in the daily activities of stair climbing, sit to stand movement, and forward progression of the body over the stance limb during the gait cycle. When prescribing these CKC activities, placement of the center of mass can directly influence muscle recruitment. (See Building Block 14-9.)

Placement of the foot can also influence the efficiency of performing CKC exercises. When the subtalar joint is permitted to pronate excessively, internal rotation of the entire lower limb

---

BUILDING BLOCK 14-8

Consider a 29-year-old female who sustained a right tri-malleolar ankle fracture and underwent Open Reduction Internal Fixation (ORIF) 6 weeks ago. One of your short-term goals is to improve ankle joint Active Range of Motion (AROM) into Dorsiflexion (DF) by 5 and plantarflexion by 10

1. Using the CKC characteristic of the proximal segment moving over a more fixed distal segment, describe how you would perform joint mobilization techniques to obtain your short-term goals.
2. Describe a CKC exercise to isolate ankle joint dorsiflexion while limiting subtalar joint pronation.

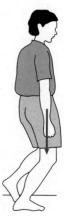

FIGURE 14-7. The center of mass is located directly over the knee.

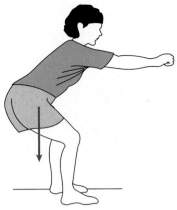

FIGURE 14-8. The center of mass is located behind the knees.

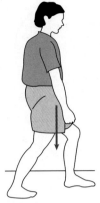

FIGURE 14-9. The center of the mass is located in front of the knee of the back leg.

occurs with a resultant increased valgus stress at the knee.[28,55] This may contribute to patellofemoral pain or interrupt the healing of a medial collateral ligament strain. External devices can be used to position the foot and consequently the entire lower extremity in a better position. An external device to support the subtalar joint in a neutral or slightly supinated position when stretching the gastrocnemius in a CKC position can be used to limit subtalar pronation and enhance dorsiflexion of the talocrural joint (see Figs. 14-10 and 14-3).

Activity or Technique

When choosing rehabilitative activities, it is important to consider the mode or method, postures, and the specific movement pattern necessary for the patient to achieve his or her optimum function. Different modes can be used while performing different types of kinetic chain exercises. Conversely, one could look at CKC training as a mode in and of itself. For example, CKC training could be the mode used to rehabilitate ROM, balance, or muscle performance impairments. If proprioceptive training is chosen, the mode can be a balance board, foam pad, or dynamic single-limb stance; however, the mode will be applied in a CKC posture. The initial and ending postures might include ambulating with a wide base of support ending with a narrow base of support. The movement should be specifically defined through a given range.

Dosage

There are a number of dosage parameters that can be changed to evoke an appropriate outcome using CKC activities. These include type of contraction, intensity, speed, duration, frequency, sequence, environment, and feedback.

BUILDING BLOCK 14-9

1. Using the biomechanical element of placement of the center of mass, describe two different variations of the forward lunge exercise.
2. How might the Center of Mass (COM) and the muscle firing pattern be altered in each condition?

Different types of muscle contractions can be used during different types of kinetic chain exercises. For example, if concentric muscle strength of the quadriceps muscle was the goal of rehabilitation and CKC training was the mode of activity, stationary cycling would be an appropriate activity. Stationary cycling employs the use of a CKC movement; the foot is fixed to a pedal, and the foot meets resistance, but the foot is free to move, resulting in a predominance of concentric muscle contraction.[14,56] Additional examples of similar types of CKC exercises using concentric muscle contraction of the hip and knee extensors include the use of a stair-climbing machine and knee extension using the seated leg press.

If, on the other hand, eccentric quadriceps muscle strength was a goal of rehabilitation and stepping exercises were the mode of the activity, a step-down would be a good choice. When analyzing functional activities such as walking,

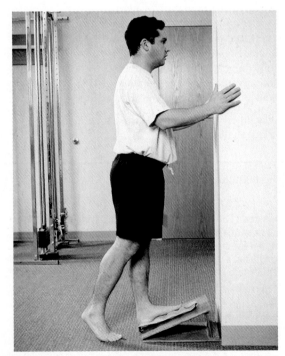

FIGURE 14-10. Supporting the subtalar joint in a neutral or slightly supinated position enhances ankle-talocrural joint dorsiflexion.

BUILDING BLOCK 14-10

Consider the previous female patient who sustained a right trimalleolar ankle fracture and underwent ORIF 3 weeks ago. One of your short-term goals is to progress the patient weight bearing (WB) status by 25% of body weight per week.

Using CKC exercises, how could you safely progress this patient to reach the short-term goal? What is your rational?

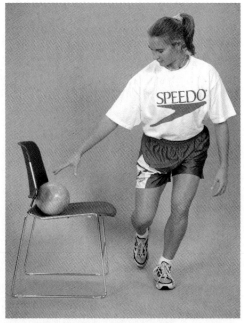

FIGURE 14-11. A lateral reach during a single-leg stance challenges the frontal plane.

descending stairs, or sitting from standing, determining the type of muscle contractions and joint motions necessary to complete the task should help guide the decision-making process about the type of kinetic chain exercise to prescribe.

The variables of force (intensity), speed, duration frequency, sequence, and environment must be considered, alone and in combination when using CKC exercises in a rehabilitation program.[39,46] Chapter 2 further details the gradation of exercise. (See Building Block 14-10.)

Earlier in the rehabilitative process, muscle performance, neuromuscular control, and the healing tissue's tolerance to stress are less developed. Both intensity and environment can be manipulated to place a gradual stress on the healing tissues. The intensity should begin low in a gravity-assisted, gravity-eliminated, or gravity-reduced posture. As the injured tissue heals and muscle performance and coordination develop, mechanical stress can be increased by increasing the weight-bearing forces.

CKC exercises should be performed slowly and in a controlled manner and then progressed as the healing tissue can tolerate stress and neuromuscular control improves. Frequently, the duration of CKC exercises is measured in time versus number of repetitions and the exercise is stopped when the patient can no longer demonstrate proper performance of the activity. Curwin and Stanish[57] support the theory that proper rehabilitation of patients with tendinitis injuries incorporates eccentric loading of the musculotendinous unit with high velocity movements. Researchers[57] believe that the inability of the musculotendinous unit to control the eccentric load contributes to tendinitis injuries.

When developing a plyometric training program general guidelines for implementation include an inverse relationship between the volume of exercises performed and the intensity of the activities. That is to say that as the intensity increases the duration and frequency decrease. Likewise, as the duration and frequency increase the intensity decreases.[18] Plyometric exercises are demanding and should be performed no more than twice weekly.

The ability to sequence complex movements in multiple directions is required in activities of daily living and athletic activities. Initiation of CKC exercises should begin in a single plane and then progress to include all three cardinal body planes. An example of challenging the frontal plane during single-leg stance is lateral reach (Fig. 14-11). An example of challenging the transverse plane during single-leg stance is reaching with trunk rotation to the right (Fig. 14-12). Additional activities using an external object (e.g., dribbling a basketball) should be incorporated to further challenge patients according

to their functional needs. Sequencing of plyometric exercises should begin with jumps in place and progress through bounding, skipping, and, finally, depth jumping.[18]

Acquiring good postural control is important for efficient function and safety. The use of full-length mirrors to help the patient maintain good biomechanical alignment is a good source of biofeedback to ensure proper performance. Additionally, the patient may initially need the use of an external support mechanism while performing balance and

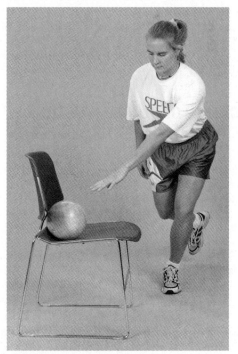

FIGURE 14-12. Reaching with trunk rotation to the right during a single-leg stance challenges the transverse plane.

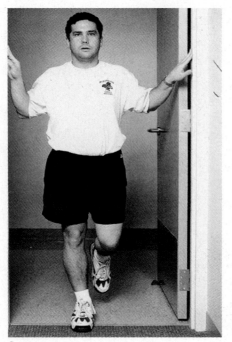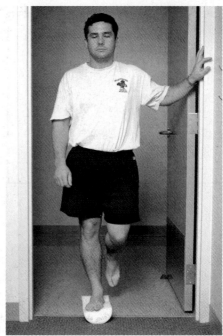

A   **B**

FIGURE 14-13. (A) Balance exercise using external support. (B) By altering the surface (use of a foam pad), the exercise becomes more challenging.

postural control. Gradation of the activity occurs by gradually removing the external support. For example, improving static single-limb balance can be performed in a doorway, with the shoe on and touching the doorway with both hands. As balance and the patient's confidence improve, the activity is progressed and the external support is removed. The shoe is removed, followed by touching the doorway with only one hand, progressing to not touching the doorway during the exercise. Closing the eyes continues to remove external support, as does altering the supporting surface by placing a foam pad beneath the foot. The foam pad alters the mechanoreceptor input and the ground reaction force to the limb (Fig. 14-13).

APPLICATION OF CLOSED KINETIC CHAIN EXERCISES

Selected techniques of both lower extremity and upper extremity CKC exercises are presented to demonstrate the treatment principles and stimulate creativity when using CKC activities as an integral part of a home exercise prescription. The most commonly prescribed CKC exercises for the lower extremity involve some type of step-down, squatting and lunging activities. During this type of exercise the hip and knee extensors work to decelerate the hip and knee flexion during the lowering phase while the ankle joint supinators assist with decelerating the foot in this phase. Controlling motion at the foot helps with controlling limb rotation. The deep hip lateral rotators work to decelerate the medial rotation of the femur. In the rising phase of the exercise the same muscles work concentrically. Stabilization (isometric contractions) is performed by the inner core from above.

Lower Extremity Examples and Progression

Research in the field of sports medicine has focused on factors leading to the increased incidence of ACL injuries in female athletes involved in jumping and cutting sports. Research by Hewett[58] evaluated landing techniques of female athletes and found a decrease in the knee flexor moment, increase in the abduction/adduction stress at the knee, and an increase in peak landing forces. A 6-week jump training program using plyometric exercises was designed to decrease landing forces

---

DISPLAY 14-2
Sample Jumping Program

EXERCISES	REPETITIONS/AMOUNT OF TIME	
Phase I: Basic Mechanics	Week 1	Week 2
1. Vertical jumps	20 seconds	25 seconds
2. Tuck jumps	20 seconds	25 seconds
3. Broad jumps	5 reps	10 reps
4. Squat jumps	10 seconds	15 seconds
5. Skipping in place	20 seconds	25 seconds
Phase II: Training	Week 3	Week 4
1. Vertical jumps	30 seconds	30 seconds
2. Tuck jumps	30 seconds	30 seconds
3. Jump, jump, jump	5 reps	8 reps
4. Squat jumps	20 seconds	20 seconds
5. Skipping for distance	1 run	2 runs

Adapted from Hewett T, Stroupe A, Nance T. Plyometric training in female athletes. Am J Sports Med 1996;24:765–773.

by teaching neuromuscular control of the lower limb during landing.[55,58,59] These training programs resulted in a decrease in ACL injuries of female athletes. A sample of the jump training program is shown in Display 14-2. The decision to increase the progression is based on the athlete's proficiency in landing the jumps.

All closed-chain exercises are not functional. Similarly, all open-chain exercises should not be dismissed because they are non–weight-bearing activities.[2] A more pragmatic approach to choosing rehabilitation activities should be investigated; it is sometimes appropriate during rehabilitation to prescribe nonfunctional CKC exercises.[60] For example, consider a patient who is unable to stand from a seated position. The patient presents with concentric quadriceps and hip extensor muscle weakness, mild anterior knee joint laxity, moderate tibiofemoral arthritis, and limited ankle dorsiflexion. Exercise could include stationary cycling because it requires concentric quadriceps, and hip extensor muscle contraction affords joint stability, decreases joint compressive forces, and allows the ankle to move freely.

Sample exercises for ROM, joint mobility, balance, and muscle performance impairments are shown in Figures 14-10 and 14-13 and in all of the Self-Management displays 14-1 to 14-24 in this chapter.

SELF-MANAGEMENT 14-1 *Improving Hip Mobility—Backward Lunge*

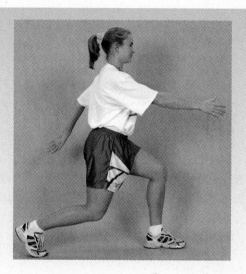

Purpose:	To improve backward movement of your hip
Precautions and Contraindications:	Pain on exertion, acute injury, lumbar spine anteroposterior instability
Position:	Standing with feet shoulder width apart, knees over second toes
Movement Technique:	Maintain arch height.
	Lunge backward, and maintain a neutral spine position.
	Extend the hip.
	Hold for ___ seconds.
	Slowly return to the start position.

Dosage
Repetitions: _____
Frequency: _____

SELF-MANAGEMENT 14-2 *Foot Intrinsic Muscle Strengthening*

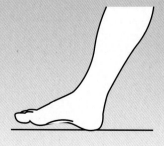

Purpose:	To improve foot strength through the arch of your foot
Precautions and Contraindications:	Pain on exertion, acute injury
Position:	Begin seated; progress to single-leg stance
Movement Technique:	Maintain arch height
	Tighten the muscles in your arch
	Do not push the ball of your foot into the floor
	Hold for ___ seconds

Dosage
Repetitions: _____
Frequency: _____

SELF-MANAGEMENT 14-3 *Hip Strengthening—Sagittal Plane*

Purpose:	To strengthen the muscles in the front part of your thigh
Precautions and Contraindications:	Pain on exertion, acute injury
Position:	Single-leg stance on ___ -in box
Movement Technique:	Maintain arch height
	Step forward with the non–weight-bearing limb
	Control hip and knee flexion of the stance limb
	Take ___ seconds to complete the exercise
	Slowly return to the start position

Dosage
   Repetitions: _____
   Frequency: _____

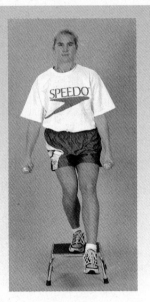

 SELF-MANAGEMENT 14-4 *Hip Strengthening—Transverse Plane*

Purpose:	To strengthen your hip rotator muscles.
Precautions and Contraindications:	Pain on exertion, acute injury, lumbar spine rotational instability
Position:	Single-leg stance on ___-in box
Movement Technique:	Maintain arch height
	Externally rotate the non–weight-bearing limb
	Control internal rotation of the stance limb
	Take ___ seconds to complete the exercise
	Slowly return to the start position

Dosage
   Repetitions: _____
   Frequency: _____

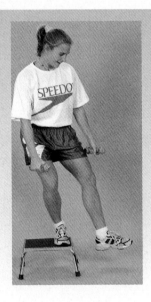

SELF-MANAGEMENT 14-5 *Hip Strengthening—Frontal Plane*

Purpose:	To strengthen your outside hip muscles
Precautions and Contraindications:	Pain on exertion, acute injury
Position:	Single-leg stance
Movement Technique:	Maintain arch height
	Place resistive band around waist and anchor securely
	Laterally lunge on the non–weight-bearing limb
	Control adduction of the stance limb
	Take ____ seconds to complete the exercise
	Slowly return to the start position

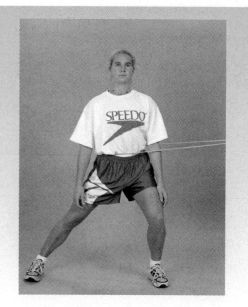

Dosage
    Repetitions: _____
    Frequency: _____

SELF-MANAGEMENT 14-6 *Quadriceps Strengthening >30 Degrees (Wall Squats)*

Purpose:	To strengthen the muscles around your knee and in the front part of your thigh
Precautions and Contraindications:	Pain on exertion and acute injury of posterior cruciate ligament (should consider supine leg press).
Position:	Standing approximately 2 ft from the wall, with feet shoulder width apart, knees over second toes
Movement Technique:	Maintain arch height.
	Stand with the back against the wall.
	Slowly slide down the wall, bending the knees, stopping at degrees.
	Maintain knees over second toes.
	Hold for 6 seconds.
	Take 4 seconds to complete the exercise.
	Slowly return to the start position.

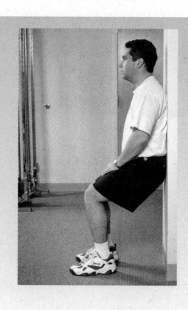

Dosage
    Repetitions: _____
    Frequency: _____

SELF-MANAGEMENT 14-7 **Quadriceps Strengthening 0 to 30 Degrees (Retro-walking)**

Purpose:	To strengthen the muscles around your knee and in the front of your thigh and to improve your balance
Precautions and Contraindications:	Pain on exertion, acute injury, and balance difficulties
Position:	Standing on the treadmill, with feet at the normal angle and base of gait, holding onto the side railing
Movement Technique:	Walk backward, extending the right hip and landing on the ball of the right foot.
	Extend the right knee, pressing the right heel into the bed of the treadmill.
	Repeat the sequence by extending the left hip.

Dosage
Repetitions: _____
Frequency: _____

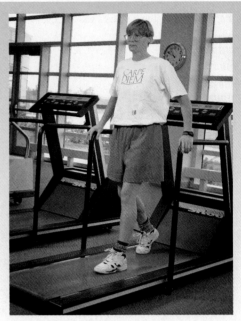

Positioning on treadmill

 SELF-MANAGEMENT 14-8 **Calf Strengthening—Single-Leg Heel Raise**

Purpose:	To strengthen your calf muscles and improve your balance
Precautions and Contraindications:	Pain on exertion, acute injury, and severe balance disorders
Position:	Single-limb stance
Movement Technique:	Maintain arch height
	Place a ball or rolled-up sock between the ankles
	Keeping your knee straight, squeeze the sock and raise the heel off the floor
	Try to keep the weight evenly distributed over the first and fifth toes
	Take ___ seconds to raise heel off the ground
	Take ___ to slowly return to the start position

Dosage
Repetitions: _____
Frequency: _____

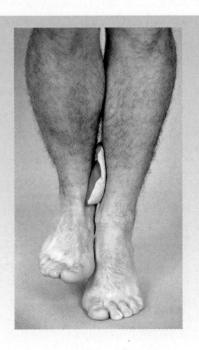

SELF-MANAGEMENT 14-9 *Quadriceps Strengthening >30 Degrees (Forward Lunge)*

Purpose:	To strengthen the muscles around your knee and in the front part of your thigh
Precautions and Contraindications:	Pain on exertion and acute injury
Position:	Standing with feet shoulder width apart, knees over second toes
Movement Technique:	Maintain arch height
	Lunge forward
	Keep the knee over the second toe and behind the ankle
	Bend the knee forward until the thigh becomes parallel to the ground
	Hold for 6 seconds
	Take 4 seconds to perform the exercise
	Slowly return to the start position

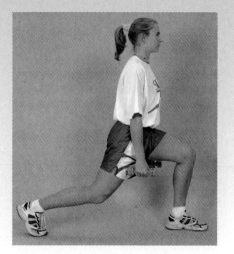

Dosage
  Repetitions: _____
  Frequency: _____

 SELF-MANAGEMENT 14-10 *Quadriceps Strengthening 0 to 30 Degrees (Closed Kinetic Chain Short-Arc Quads)*

Purpose:	To strengthen the muscles around your knee
Precautions and Contraindications:	Pain on exertion and acute injury
Position:	Standing with feet shoulder width apart and with the affected knee over the second toe, place the ball behind the knee and the heel against the wall

Movement Technique:	Maintain arch height
	Try to straighten your knee by pushing the back of your knee into the ball
	Hold this position for 6 seconds
	Slowly return to the start position

Dosage
  Repetitions: _____
  Frequency: _____

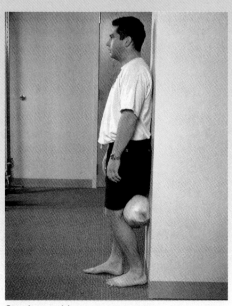

Starting position

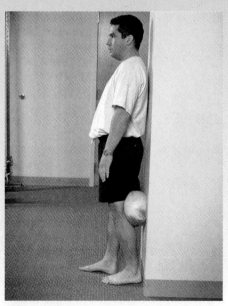

Ending position

SELF-MANAGEMENT 14-11 *Lumbar Spine Strengthening*

Purpose: To strengthen your lower back and buttock muscles

Precautions and Contraindications: Pain on exertion and acute injury

Position: Kneeling on hands and knees

Movement Technique:
Maintain neutral spine
Slowly extend your ___ arm and ___ leg

Stabilize the pelvis on the weight-bearing limb

Stabilize the shoulder girdle with the weight-bearing arm

Hold ___ seconds

Slowly return to the start position

Dosage
Repetitions: _____
Frequency: _____

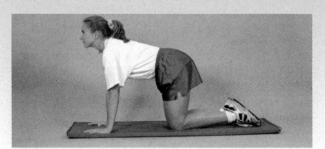

Starting position

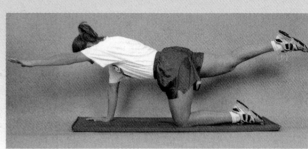

Ending position

SELF-MANAGEMENT 14-12 *Hip Strengthening—Backward Lunge with Tubing*

Purpose: To strengthen your hip and buttock muscles

Precautions and Contraindications: Pain on exertion, acute injury, and lumbar spine anteroposterior instability

Position: Standing with feet shoulder width apart, knees over second toes

Movement Technique:
Maintain arch height
Place Thera-Band around the waist

Lunge backward, and maintain a neutral spine position

Extend the hip

Hold for ___ seconds

Slowly return to the start position

Dosage
Repetitions: _____
Frequency: _____

Starting position

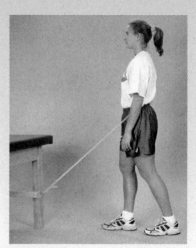

Ending position

SELF-MANAGEMENT 14-13 Hip Strengthening—Backward Squat

Purpose:	To strengthen your hip and buttock muscles eccentrically
Precautions and Contraindications:	Pain on exertion and acute injury
Position:	Standing with feet shoulder width apart, knees over second toes
Movement Technique:	Maintain arch height
	Place a tall chair directly behind you
	Sit backward onto the chair, pivoting around your knees
	As you sit back, move your arms forward to counterbalance the sitting motion
	Slowly return to the start position

Dosage

Repetitions: _____

Frequency: _____

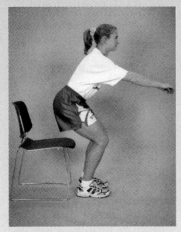

Starting position

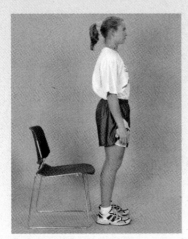

Ending position

SELF-MANAGEMENT 14-14 Calf Strengthening—Forward Lean

Purpose:	To strengthen your calf muscles and to improve your balance
Precautions and Contraindications:	Pain on exertion and acute injury
Position:	8 to 10 in from a wall, single-limb stance
Movement Technique:	Maintain arch height.
	Place hands in front of your chest to catch yourself.
	Keeping your knee straight, lean forward, leading with your waist.
	Use your gastrocnemius muscle to control the forward motion.
	Slowly return to the start position.

Dosage

Repetitions: _____

Frequency: _____

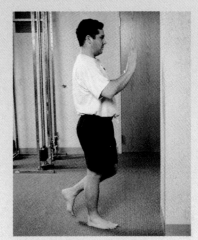

Starting position

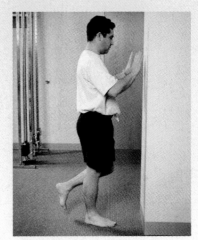

Ending position

SELF-MANAGEMENT 14-15 *First Ray Stability—Windlass Mechanism*

Purpose:	To strengthen the muscles supporting the arch of your foot
Precautions and Contraindications:	Pain on exertion and acute injury
Position:	Begin seated, progress to normal walking stride
Movement Technique:	Maintain arch height.
	Extend *only* the hallux.
	Gently push the knuckle of your big toe onto the floor.
	Hold ___ seconds.

Dosage
Repetitions: _____
Frequency: _____

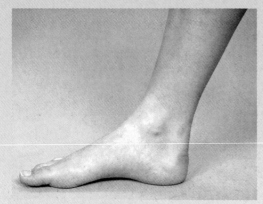

Starting position

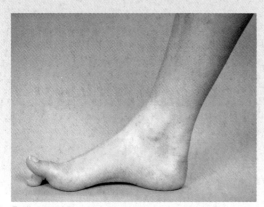

Ending position

 SELF-MANAGEMENT 14-16 *Subtalar Joint and Midtarsal Joint Pronation*

Purpose:	To improve controlled movement of your heel and the arch of your foot
Precautions and Contraindications:	Pain on exertion and acute injury
Position:	Begin seated, progress to normal walking stride
Movement Technique:	Extend *only* the lateral four toes in a smooth and controlled manner.
	Gently try to lift the lateral border of your foot off the floor.
	Take ___ seconds to **complete this exercise.**

Dosage
Repetitions: _____
Frequency: _____

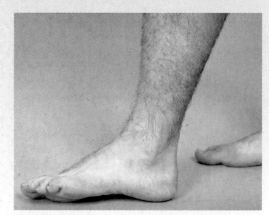

Starting position

Ending position

SELF-MANAGEMENT 14-17 *Subtalar Joint Pronation*

Purpose: To promote controlled movement of your heel and improve your balance

Precautions and Contraindications: Pain on exertion, acute injury, and severe balance disorder

Position: Single-leg stance

Movement Technique:

Place Thera-Band around the outside of the foot and attach it to an immovable object.

Raise the heel off the floor.

As you return, equalize the heel to the floor and control the motion of the Thera-Band, pulling the subtalar joint into a pronated position.

Take ___ seconds to complete this exercise.

Dosage
Repetitions: _____
Frequency: _____

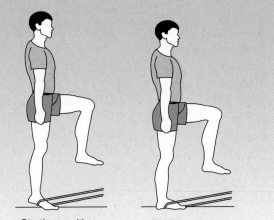

Starting position   *Ending position*

 SELF-MANAGEMENT 14-18 *Hip Strengthening—Transverse Plane*

Purpose: To strengthen your hip rotator muscles

Precautions and Contraindications: Pain on exertion, acute injury, lumbar spine rotational instability

Position: Single-leg stance; place non–weight-bearing limb on a wheeled stool

Movement Technique:

Maintain arch height.

Externally rotate the non–weight-bearing limb.

Control internal rotation of the stance limb.

Take ___ seconds to complete this exercise.

Slowly return to the start position.

Dosage
Repetitions: _____
Frequency: _____

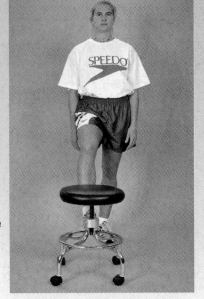 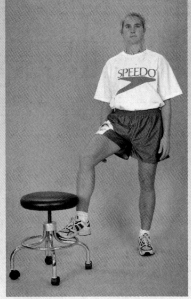

Starting position   *Ending position*

SELF-MANAGEMENT 14-19 *Quadriceps Strengthening 0 to 30 Degrees (Standing Stationary Cycling)*

Purpose:	To strengthen the muscles around your knee and in the front part of your thigh
Precautions and Contraindications:	Pain on exertion, acute injury, balance difficulties
Position:	Standing on the pedals of the bike
Movement Technique:	Begin pedaling in an upright position.
	Use the quadriceps muscle to control the knee as it moves into extension.

Dosage
  Repetitions: _____
  Frequency: _____

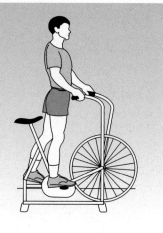

SELF-MANAGEMENT 14-20 *Glenohumeral Co-Contraction*

Purpose:	To stabilize the muscles around your shoulder when it is newly injured and painful
Precautions and Contraindications:	Pain on exertion, balance difficulties
Position:	Standing hands supported on a table

Movement Technique:	Weight shift sagittal, frontal, and transverse planes.
	Use co-contraction of the muscles surrounding the glenohumeral joint.

Dosage
  Repeat: _____ sec/min
  Frequency: _____

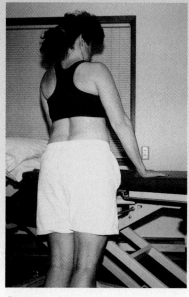

Starting position

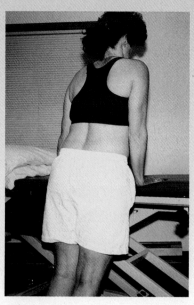

Ending position

SELF-MANAGEMENT 14-21 *Glenohumeral Dynamic Stability*

Purpose: To stabilize the muscles around your shoulder, as your shoulder pain lessens

Precautions and Contraindications: Pain on exertion, acute injury

Position: Quadruped injured hand weight bearing on soft 6-in ball

Movement Technique: Weight shift on to injured arm and move the ball in sagittal, frontal, and transverse planes

Enhance dynamic stability with controlled mobility by using axial compression and a moveable boundary.

Dosage

Repeat _____ sec/min
Frequency: _____

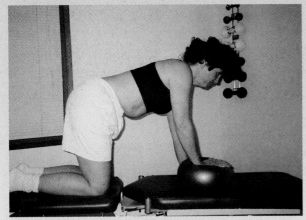

Starting position

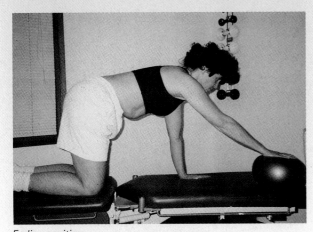

Ending position

SELF-MANAGEMENT 14-22 *Scapulothoracic Stability*

Purpose: To improve the function of your scapular muscles

Precautions and Contraindications: Pain on exertion

Position: Standing with injured arm in scapular plane at shoulder height, elbow extended, push into the wall encouraging scapular protraction

Movement Technique: Straight arm push up against the wall with a "plus"

Recruitment of serratus anterior to promote scapulothoracic stability while using axial compression.

Dosage

Repeat _____ sec/min
Frequency: _____

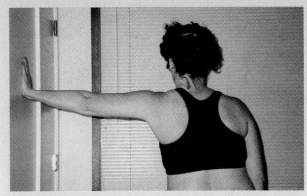

Starting position

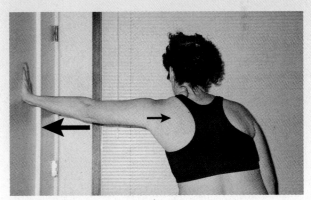

Ending position

SELF-MANAGEMENT 14-23 *Glenohumeral Internal Rotation*

Purpose: To improve the stability of your shoulder and gain internal rotation mobility

Precautions and Contraindications: Pain on exertion

Position: Standing with injured side toward the wall, injured arm in scapular plane at shoulder height elbow extended

Movement Technique:
Push into the wall with ____ hand

Tighten abdominal muscles

Reach beneath injured arm with opposite hand

Hold for 15 seconds to 30 seconds

Dosage
Repetitions: _____
Frequency: _____

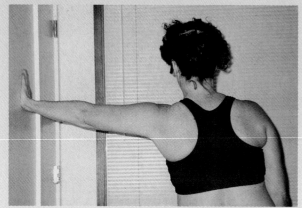

Starting position

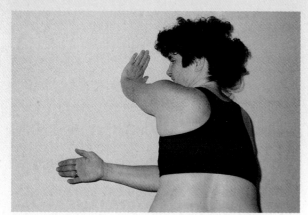

Ending position

SELF-MANAGEMENT 14-24 *Thoracic Spine Extension/Glenohumeral Joint Stability*

Purpose: To improve the mobility of your thoracic spine and stability of your shoulder to improve your posture

Precautions and Contraindications: Pain on exertion

Position: Quadruped

Movement Technique:
Tighten abdominal muscles

Push into the floor spreading the area between your shoulder blades

Bring the top of your head and tailbone toward each other

Hold for 15 to 30 seconds

Reverse the movement squeezing the shoulder blades together sinking in the area between your shoulder blades

Lengthen through the top of your head and tailbone

Hold for 15 seconds to 30 seconds

Repeat the exercise trying to move one vertebra at a time

Dosage
Repetitions: _____
Frequency: _____

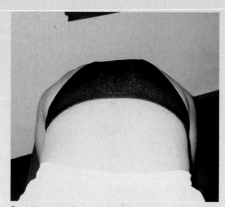

Starting position

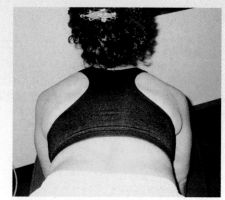

Ending position

Upper Extremity Examples and Progression

Research has been done to evaluate the necessity to perform CKC exercises for the upper extremity. Intramuscular EMG data have shown that a number of closed or partially closed activities should be incorporated into a shoulder rehabilitation program.[61,62] CKC activities have been shown to improve neuromuscular control of the upper extremities.[63] Additional studies have evaluated the importance of having a "stable base" for performing skill activities.[63,64] The results of these studies confirm the findings of Sullivan et al.[12] concerning the concepts of the stages of motor control. First, stability is necessary in the form of co-contraction around the glenohumeral and scapulothoracic joints, progressing to controlled mobility with proper scapulothoracic rhythm. Consider the patient who presents with left arm hemiplegia and with a subluxated humeral head with anterior ligamentous laxity, poor stability of the humeral head in the glenoid fossa, poor scapulothoracic rhythm, and altered kinesthesia. Exercise should include upper extremity weight bearing with weight shifting to improve stability and enhance kinesthesia. The progression of this exercise could go as follows. Begin with a standing weight shift exercise in the sagittal, frontal, and transverse planes, with both hands on the table and eyes open. Duration could be for 10 seconds increasing to 1 minute. Progression of this exercise from eyes open to eyes closed and adding proprioceptive neuromuscular facilitation manual techniques to stimulate co-contraction and rhythmic stabilization of the muscles around the glenohumeral joint after the patient could master an effective cocontraction changing the surface to a less stable base (standing on a wobble board in both the frontal and sagittal planes) would make this a more challenging activity. The addition of making the weight-bearing arm resist a more challenging environment would follow in sequence with the addition of moveable boundary (weight bearing onto a ball) external axial load.

Additional studies have demonstrated the necessity of an efficient kinetic chain to accomplish these complex skill movements by generating, transferring, and regulating forces created in the legs and trunk to the hand.

PRECAUTIONS AND CONTRAINDICATIONS

When choosing CKC training as a method of rehabilitation, the patient's safety is a primary concern. A rehabilitation program should begin submaximally and progress to functional goals the patient can tolerate. To safely progress a patient through the rehabilitative process, it is necessary to incorporate criteria for gradation of the exercise. When substitution of another component in the chain occurs and the intended link is unable to perform the activity, the exercise should be altered to an easier level.[33] For example, a patient could perform a lateral step-down from a 6-in step with the instruction to keep his or her knee over the second toe and could continue until a substitution occurred. Inability to keep the knee over the second toe or an increase in symptoms would result in modifying the step-down. The exercise should be stopped on a 6-in step and continued on a 4- or 2-in step. Proper performance of the exercise should be stressed over the number of repetitions.

Additional precautions when using CKC exercises include pain, joint effusion, and the inability of joints to handle the compressive forces. Environmental conditions must be evaluated so that the activities are performed on a flat, hard surface with appropriate footwear.

KEY POINTS

- CKC exercises use the forces of weight bearing and the effect of gravity to simulate functional activities.
- Common characteristics of CKC activities include interdependence of joint motion, motion occurring proximal and distal to the axis of rotation, greater joint compressive forces, stabilization afforded by joint congruency, recruitment of muscle contractions, and eccentric followed by concentric muscle contractions to provide a more normal functional pattern.
- Proximal segments move over more fixed distal segments.
- CKC training of the lower extremity involves movement of the foot, ankle, knee, hip, and pelvis in a predictable sequence.
- The success of using CKC activities in the rehabilitation of patients begins with understanding the kinetics and kinematics of the joints and subsequent kinesiology when the distal segment is attached to a supporting surface.

CRITICAL THINKING QUESTIONS

1. Consider Case Study No. 6 in Unit 7.
   a. Describe the relationship between this patient's knee mobility impairment and its effect on the ipsilateral hip, ankle, and subtalar joints.
   b. Choose a specific goal and design a treatment program using three different CKC exercises. Include modulator and biomechanical factors.
   c. If this patient was returning to play basketball, design a plyometric exercise program to return this patient safely to his sport.
2. Consider Case Study No. 4 in Unit 7.
   a. Describe three CKC exercises to improve his impairments

LAB ACTIVITIES

1. Choose three closed- or partially closed-chain exercises (one for each segment of the lower extremity) and adapt each exercise to patients with the following injuries. Be prepared to demonstrate the exercises, give written home instructions (including dosage and precautions), and explain the scientific basis of your selection.
   a. Subacute extensor mechanism dysfunction in a college athlete
   b. Extensor mechanism dysfunction in a 70-year-old sedentary woman
   c. Acute, excessive pronation of the subtalar joint in a 15-year-old recreational athlete
   d. Chronic, excessive pronation of the subtalar joint and excessive pronation in a diabetic, hypertensive, slightly obese 60-year-old man who is moderately active
   e. ACL-deficient knee in a 45-year-old firefighter who is preparing for return to work in 2 weeks
   f. ACL-reconstructed knee with medial collateral ligament strain 6 weeks after surgery
2. Choose three CKC exercises for the upper extremity. Incorporate at least two proprioceptive neuromuscular facilitation elements in your treatment for the following patients:
   a. A 17-year-old high school senior softball player with an anterior instability of the glenohumeral joint, who has a good chance for a college scholarship if she performs well this season
   b. Chronic faulty movement pattern of the glenohumeral joint with dominance of the axiohumeral rotators (pectoralis major and latissimus dorsi) over the scapulohumeral rotators in a 48-year-old carpenter
3. Using the principle of the proximal segment moving over a fixed distal segment, mobilize the tibiofemoral joint to gain knee extension and talocrural joint to obtain dorsiflexion. Develop one CKC activity to be used as a home exercise to maintain mobility of each joint.
4. Develop an activity changing the center of mass over the base of support to alter muscle recruitment of the hamstrings, quadriceps and gluteals, and gastrocnemius and soleus in squat, sit-to-stand, and step-up activities.
5. Analyze the influence of forcing an excessively toed-in position of a patient with a naturally toed-out stance position on the ACL at the knee.
6. Develop five activities for each plane to enhance movement in the frontal, transverse, and sagittal planes during single-limb stance.
7. Describe the effect of subtalar joint supination on the osteokinematics of the ankle and hip.

REFERENCES

1. Steindler A. Kinesiology of the Human Body Under Normal and Pathological Conditions. Springfield, IL: Charles C Thomas, 1973.
2. Snyder-Mackler L. Scientific rationale and physiological basis for the use of closed kinetic chain exercise in the lower extremity. J Sport Rehabil 1996;5:2–12.
3. Wilk KE, Naiquan Z, Glenn SF, et al. Kinetic chain exercise: implications for the anterior cruciate ligament patient. J Sport Rehabil 1997;6:125–140.
4. Lindal O, Movin A. The mechanics of the knee joint. Acta Orthop Scand 1967;38:226–234.
5. Smidt GL. Biomechanical analysis of knee flexion and extension. J Biomech 1973;6:79–92.
6. Paulos L, Noyes FR, Grood ES, et al. Knee rehabilitation after anterior cruciate ligament reconstruction and repair. Am J Sports Med 1981;9:140–143.
7. Arms SW, Pope MH, Johnson RJ, et al. The biomechanics of the anterior cruciate ligament rehabilitation and reconstruction. Am J Sports Med 1984;12:8–18.
8. Grood ES, Suntay WT, Noyes FR, et al. Biomechanics of the knee-extension exercise. Effect of cutting the anterior cruciate ligament. J Bone Joint Surg 1984;66A:725–734.
9. Henning CE, Lynch MA, Glick KR. An in vivo strain gauge study of elongation of the anterior cruciate ligament. Am J Sports Med 1985;13:22–26.
10. Renstrom P, Arms SW, Stanwyck TS, et al. Strain within the anterior cruciate ligament during hamstring and quadriceps activity. Am J Sports Med 1986;14:83–87.
11. Hungerford DS, Barry M. Biomechanics of the patellofemoral joint. Clin Orthop 1979;144:9–15.
12. Sullivan PE, Markos PD, Minor MAD. An Integrated Approach to Therapeutic Exercise Theory and Clinical Application. Reston, VA: Reston Publishing Company, 1982.
13. Knott M, Voss DE. Proprioceptive Neuromuscular Facilitation. 2nd Ed. New York, NY: Harper & Row, 1968.
14. Wozniak-Timmer CA. Cycling biomechanics: a literature review. J Orthop Sports Phys Ther 1991;14:106–113.
15. Palmitier RA, An KN, Scott SG, et al. Kinetic chain exercises in knee rehabilitation. Sports Med 1991;11:402–413.
16. Lutz GE, Palmitier RA, An KN, et al. Comparison of tibiofemoral joint forces during open-kinetic-chain and closed-kinetic-chain exercises. J Bone Joint Surg Am 1993;75:732–739.
17. Yack HJ, Collins CE, Whieldon TJ. Comparison of closed and open kinetic chain exercise in the anterior cruciate ligament-deficient knee. Am J Sports Med 1993;21:49–53.
18. Albert M. Eccentric Muscle Training in Sports and Orthopaedics. New York, NY: Churchill Livingstone, 1991.
19. Voight ML, Cook G. Clinical application of closed kinetic chain exercise. J Sport Rehabil 1996;5:25–44.
20. Komi PV, Bosco C. Utilization of stored elastic energy in leg extensor muscles by men and women. Med Sci Sports Exerc 1978;10:261–268.
21. Enoka R. Neuromechanical Basis of Kinesiology. Champaign, IL: Human Kinetic Books, 1988.
22. Bosco C, Komi P. Potentiation of the mechanical behavior of the human skeletal muscle through prestretching. Acta Physiol Scand 1979;106:467–472.
23. National Strength and Conditioning Coaches Association (NSCCA). Plyometric Training: Understanding and Coaching Power Development for Sports [video tape]. Lincoln, NE: National Strength and Conditioning Association, 1989.
24. Markolf KL, Bargar WL, Shoemaker SC, et al. The role of joint load in knee stability. J Bone Joint Surg Am 1981;63:570–585.
25. Stormont DM, Morrey BF, An K, et al. Stability of the loaded ankle. Am J Sports Med 1985;13:295–300.
26. Roy S, Irvin R. Sports Medicine: Prevention, Evaluation, Management and Rehabilitation. New York, NY: Prentice-Hall, 1983.

27. Root ML, Orien WP, Weed JH. Normal and Abnormal Function of the Foot, Vol II. Los Angeles, CA: Clinical Biomechanics Corporation, 1971.
28. Inman VT, Ralston HJ, Todd F. Human Walking. Baltimore, MD: Williams & Wilkins, 1981.
29. Jackson RJ. Functional Relationships of the Lower Half. Middleburg, VA: Richard Jackson Seminars, 1995.
30. Mann RA, Hagy J. Biomechanics of walking, running and sprinting. Am J Sports Med 1980;8:345–350.
31. Perry J. Gait Analysis: Normal and Pathological Function. Thorofare, NJ: Slack, 1992.
32. Petit MA, McKay HA, MacKelvie KJ, et al. A randomized school-based jumping intervention confers site and maturity-specific benefits on bone structural properties in girls: a hip structural analysis study. J Bone Mineral Res 2002;17:363–372.
33. Lephart SM, Pinccivero DM, Jorge LG, et al. The role of proprioception in the management and rehabilitation of athletic injuries. Am J Sports Med 1997;25:130–137.
34. Grigg P. Peripheral neural mechanisms in proprioception. J Sport Rehabil 1994;3:2–17.
35. Barrack RL, Lund PJ, Skinner HB. Knee joint proprioception revisited. J Sport Rehabil 1994;3:18–42.
36. Umphred DA, McCormack GL. Classification of common facilitatory and inhibitory treatment techniques. In: Umphred DA, ed. Neurological Rehabilitation. 2nd Ed. St. Louis, MO: CV Mosby, 1990.
37. Borsa PA, Lephart SM, Mininder SK, et al. Functional assessment and rehabilitation of shoulder proprioception for glenohumeral instability. J Sport Rehabil 1994;3:84–104.
38. Harter RA. Clinical rationale for closed kinetic chain activities in functional testing and rehabilitation of ankle pathologies. J Sport Rehabil 1996;5:13–24.
39. Nashner L. Practical biomechanics and physiology of balance. In: Jacobson G, Newman C, Kartush J, eds. Handbook of Balance Function and Testing. St. Louis, MO: Mosby-Year Book, 1993.
40. Irrgang JJ. Closed Kinetic Chain Exercises for the Lower Extremity: Theory and Application. LaCrosse, WI: Sports Physical Therapy Home Study Course, Sports Physical Therapy Section of the American Physical Therapy Association, 1994.
41. Guskiewicz KM, Perrin DH. Research and clinical applications of assessing balance. J Sport Rehabil 1996;5:45–63.
42. Sale DG. Neurological adaptation to strength training. In: Komi PV, ed. Strength and Power in Sport. Oxford: Blackwell Scientific Publications, 1992.
43. Sale DG, MacDougall D. Specificity in strength training: a review for the coach and athlete. Can J Appl Sports Sci 1981;6:87–92.
44. Kegerreis S. The construction and implementation of functional progressions as a component of athletic rehabilitation. J Orthop Sports Phys Ther 1983;5:14–19.
45. Roy S, Irvin R. Sports Medicine: Prevention, Evaluation, Management and Rehabilitation. New York, NY: Prentice-Hall, 1983.
46. Gray GW. Team Reaction: Lower Extremity Functional Profile. Adrian, MI: Wynn Marketing, 1995.
47. Mangine RE, Kremchek TE. Evaluation-based protocol of the anterior cruciate ligament. J Sport Rehabil 1997;6:157–181.
48. Lephart SM, Perrin DH, Fu FH, et al. Functional performance tests for the anterior cruciate insufficient athlete. J Athletic Training 1991;26:44–49.
49. Risberg MA, Ekeland A. Assessment of functional tests after anterior cruciate ligament surgery. J Orthop Sports Phys Ther 1994;19:212–217.
50. Goldbeck TG, Davies GJ. Test-retest reliability of the closed kinetic chain upper extremity stability test: a clinical field test. J Sport Rehabil 2000;9:35–45.
51. Bullock-Saxton JE. Local sensation changes and altered hip muscle function following severe ankle sprain. Phys Ther 1994;74:17–31.
52. Kaltenborn FM. Mobilization of the Extremity Joints, Examination and Basic Treatment Techniques. Oslo: Olaf Norlis Bokhandel, Universitetsgaten Oslo, 1980.
53. Mulligan BR. Manual Therapy "NAGS", SNAGS", "MWMS", etc. Wellington, New Zealand: Plane View Services Ltd, 1999.
54. Hoke BR, Lefever-Button S. When the Feet Hit the Ground … Take the Next Step. Toledo, OH: American Physical Rehabilitation Network, 1994.
55. Silvers HJ, Mandelbaum BR. Are ACL tears preventable in the female athlete? Medscape Orthopaed Sports Med 2002;6(2); www.medscape.com/viewarticle/439586.
56. Jorge M, Hall ML. Analysis of EMG measurements during bicycle pedalling. J Biomech 1986;19:683–694.
57. Curwin S, Stanish W. Tendinitis: Its Etiology and Treatment. Lexington, MA: Collamore Press, 1984.
58. Hewett T, Stroupe A, Nance T. Plyometric training in female athletes. Am J Sports Med 1996;24:765–773.
59. Hewett TE, Lindenfeld TN, Riccobene JV, et al. The effect of neuromuscular training on the incidence of knee injury in female athletes. Am J Sports Med 1999;27:699–706.
60. Snyder-Mackler L, Delitto A, Bailey SL, et al. Strength of the quadriceps femoris muscle and functional recovery after reconstruction of the anterior cruciate ligament. J Bone Joint Surg Am 1995;77:1166–1173.
61. Townsend H, Jobe FW, Pink M, et al. Electromyographic analysis of the glenohumeral muscles during a baseball rehabilitation program. Am J Sports Med 1991;19:264–272.
62. Moseley JB, Jobe FW, Pink M, et al. EMG analysis of the scapular muscles. Am J Sports Med 1992;20:128–134.
63. Ubinger ME, Prentice WE, Guskiewicz KM. The effect of closed kinetic chain training on neuromuscular control in the upper extremity. J Sport Rehabil 1999;8:184–194.
64. Glousman R, Jobe FW, Tibone JE, et al. Dynamic electromyographic analysis of the throwing shoulder with glenohumeral instability. J Bone Joint Surg Am 1988;70:220–226.

RECOMMENDED READINGS

Beckett ME, Massie DL, Bowers KD, et al. Incidence of hyperpronation in the ACL injured knee: a clinical perspective. J Athl Training 1992;27:58–60.
DeCarlo M, Shelbourne KD, McCarroll JR. Traditional versus accelerated rehabilitation following ACL reconstruction: a one year follow-up. J Orthop Sports Phys Ther 1992;15:309–316.
Irrgang JL, Whitney SL, Cox ED. Balance and proprioceptive training for rehabilitation of the lower extremity. J Sport Rehabil 1994;3:68–83.

chapter 15

Proprioceptive Neuromuscular Facilitation

KYLE M. YAMASHIRO AND RAFAEL F. ESCAMILLA

HISTORY AND BACKGROUND

Proprioceptive Neuromuscular Facilitation (PNF) uses proprioceptive (sensory receptors found in muscles, tendons, joints, and the inner ear that detect body and limb motion or position) input to improve (facilitate) neuromuscular function during human movement. Neuromuscular function is enhanced by providing resistance during concentric, eccentric, and isometric muscle actions, thereby enhancing muscle strength and endurance, balance and posture, and stability and mobility. Neuromuscular function is also enhanced during stretching techniques, thus improving joint range of motion and muscle flexibility.

PNF was developed by Neurophysiologist Dr. Herman Kabat near the mid-1940s. Prior to PNF, rehabilitation was typically done one joint and muscle at a time. Based on neurophysiologic principles previously established in the early 20th century by Physiologist Charles Sherrington, in 1946 Dr. Kabat began to look for natural movement patterns for rehabilitating the muscles of polio patients and soon thereafter discovered that typical human movement patterns involved diagonal patterns employing multiple muscles and joints. Basic neurophysiologic principles for PNF involved autogenic inhibition, reciprocal inhibition, successive induction, and irradiation. Autogenic inhibition results in inhibition of the agonist with agonist contraction due to stimulation of the golgi tendon organ. Reciprocal inhibition results in the inhibition of the agonist muscle when the antagonist muscle is stimulated. Successive induction results in increased activity in the agonist immediately after activity in the antagonist. Irradiation results in the overflow or spread of energy from stronger segments to weaker segments.

Around 1950, physical therapists, Maggie Knott and Dorothy Voss, began working with Dr. Kabat in developing PNF principles and techniques, and they began presenting these principles and techniques at PNF workshops in the early 1950s. Moreover, in the mid- to late 1950s, Mrs. Voss, Mrs. Knott, and Dr. Kabat began publishing their work on PNF in physical therapy, occupational therapy, and physical medicine scientific journals.[1,2] In the 1960s, Physical Therapy programs at Universities began teaching PNF principles and techniques. In the late 1970s, PNF principles and techniques began to be employed by athletes to increase joint range of motion and muscle flexibility and strength, and in the 1980s PNF research studies relative to athletes and athletic performance were published in sports physical therapy and sports medicine journals.[3–7] PNF continues to be used currently in a variety of physical therapy settings, such as orthopaedic, neuro, and pediatric settings.

PNF EVIDENCE

The preponderance of PNF research in the peer review scientific literature examined the effectiveness of PNF stretching techniques, such as contract-relax, hold-relax, and hold-relax with agonist contraction, on neuromuscular function, joint range of motion, and muscle flexibility. While PNF, static, and ballistic stretching have all been shown to improve joint range of motion, PNF stretching appears to produce the greatest range of motion gains.[8–12] Moreover, PNF stretching has been shown to be effective in increasing both passive and active joint range of motion.[12]

A summary of the PNF stretching literature[12] suggests that contract-relax, hold-relax, and hold-relax with agonist contraction are all effective in improving joint range of motion. However, there are limited data that suggest that hold-relax with agonist contraction may be slightly more effective compared to contract-relax and hold-relax.[12] A minimum of 1 repetition performed twice per week for 4 to 12 weeks is suggested to improve joint range of motion.[11] Only 20% of a maximum static contraction of the target muscle being stretched is required for joint range of motion improvement, and this contraction should be maintained for a minimum of 3 seconds.[12] While employing a higher intensity static contraction (e.g., 80% to 100% of maximum contraction) for a longer period of time (e.g., 5 to 10 seconds) may not significantly improve joint range of motion compared to lower intensity and duration stretching, higher intensity and duration isometric or dynamic contraction has been shown to result in greater muscular strength and power and improved stiffness in the musculotendinous unit.[12] Joint range of motion has been shown to improve with contraction durations between 3 and 15 seconds, although longer contraction durations (e.g., 10 to 20 seconds) have been shown to result in greater joint range of motion gains.[12,13] Stretch duration is typically between 10 and 30 seconds.[20]

Mahieu et al.[14] reported that the increased joint range of motion observed after PNF stretching could not be explained by changes in the musculotendinous tissue that was stretched but rather was explained by an increase in stretch tolerance. This is supported by data provided by Mitchell et al.,[15] which demonstrated that an increase in stretch tolerance occurred after employing the contract-relax PNF stretching technique. Moreover, these authors suggested that at least four repetitions of contract-relax stretching are needed to get the greatest improvement in range of motion.

Rowlands et al.[16] reported that 4 weeks of PNF hold-relax stretching resulted in significantly increased ankle range of motion, maximal isometric strength, rate of force development, and stiffness of the musculotendinous unit. These authors suggested that the increased stiffness in the musculotendinous unit after PNF training is explained by adaptations to the maximal isometric muscle contractions that occurred during the hold-relax stretching technique. Moreover, they suggested that because a stiffer musculotendinous unit system is related to an improved the ability to store and release elastic energy, PNF stretching would benefit certain athletic performance due to a reduced contraction time or greater mechanical efficiency. Data from the above studies suggest that the changes in the ability to tolerate stretch and the viscoelastic properties of the stretched muscle, both induced by PNF procedures, are possible mechanisms which result in enhanced joint range of motion and muscle flexibility from PNF stretching techniques.

Data from the PNF stretching literature do not support the common belief that contraction of a muscle immediately prior to stretching that muscle (autogenic inhibition), or contraction of the antagonist muscle groups at the same time the agonist muscles are being stretched (reciprocal inhibition), produces relaxation (inhibition) of the stretched muscle by stimulating sensory receptors (e.g., golgi tendon organ) within the musculotendinous unit.[17] It has been reported from the literature that following contraction of a stretched muscle, inhibition of the stretch muscle only lasts approximately 1 second.[17] Moreover, decreases in the response amplitude of the Hoffmann and muscle stretch reflexes following a contraction of a stretched muscle may not be due to the activation of golgi tendon organs, as commonly believed, but instead may be due to presynaptic inhibition of the muscle spindle sensory signal.[17]

Manoel et al.[18] reported that dynamic stretching may increase acute muscular power to a greater degree than static and PNF stretching. Moreover, Bradley et al.[19] reported that vertical jump performance was decreased for 15 minutes after static or PNF stretching, whereas ballistic stretching has little effect on jumping performance. Church et al.[20] also reported a decrease in vertical jump performance subsequent to employing PNF stretching as part of a warm-up. It can be concluded from these data[19,20] that both PNF and static stretching should not be performed immediately prior to performing explosive athletic movements similar to the vertical jump. Marek et al.[21] examined the acute effects of static and PNF stretching on muscle strength and power output, and reported that the short term effects of both static and PNF stretching resulted in diminished muscle strength and power during maximum effort isokinetic knee extension at angular velocities of 60 degrees per second and 300 degrees per second.

Employing PNF resistance techniques have also been shown to be effective in enhancing the neuromuscular system.[22] For example, it has been suggested that employing reversal of patterns PNF techniques may increase the rate of force development in older individuals, which may help functional activities, such as going up and down stairs, as well as reduce the risk of falls.[22] Nelson et al.[23] reported that compared to weight training, PNF resistance training resulted in greater gains in knee and elbow extensor strength, throwing distance, and vertical jump.

PHILOSOPHY AND PRINCIPLES OF PNF

The basis of the PNF philosophy is the idea that all human beings, including those with disabilities have untapped existing potential.[1] The treatment approach is always positive and focuses on what the patient can do, on a physical and psychological level. The PNF approach is holistic, integrating sensory, motor, and psychological inputs to ensure every treatment is directed toward the human being, not a specific problem. PNF attempts to provide a maximal response for increasing strength, flexibility, coordination, and functional mobility. PNF patterns are more concerned with mass body movements as opposed to specific muscle actions. These patterns are composed of both diagonal and rotational exercise patterns that are similar to the motions required for activities of daily living, functional mobility, and even athletic performance.

Many believe that the patterns of PNF must be known to treat within the concept of PNF. Meaning there are over 100 different patterns, hand holds, variations, and modifications as well as terminology (e.g., D1, D2, bilateral asymmetrical upper extremity). More importantly, is understanding the use of the appropriate procedures and basic techniques. It is the goal of this chapter to share with the student and the clinician how to utilize PNF procedures and techniques when applying manual therapeutic exercise. Only a few basic PNF patterns are shown in a simplified form to allow the learner to practice applying manual therapeutic exercises. For further refinement of PNF skills the learner should consult the text by Voss and Knott[2] and should seek out the opportunity to practice with a skilled practitioner.

PNF PROCEDURES

The premise underlying PNF basic procedures is enhancing the patient's postural responses or movement patterns. The goal of each treatment is to facilitate or ease achievement of a movement or posture. These procedures can be utilized with most patients regardless of medical diagnosis. The examination and evaluation will determine the specific procedures utilized as well as any necessary modifications.

Manual Therapeutic Exercise Using PNF Procedures

The therapist must utilize correct manual contacts, body positioning, verbal cues, and visual cues during PNF applications. One advantage of manual therapeutic exercise is the ability to continuously assess the patient's movement or posture. This ongoing assessment allows for immediate modification of the activity. During a treatment session, the clinician can influence all or some of the following:

- the magnitude of resistance
- type of contraction
- traction or compression to a joint, promoting movement or stability
- the direction of the movement or pattern
- whether the treatment is direct or indirect

Manual Contacts

Motor responses are often influenced by the stimulation of skin and other receptors. The therapist can therefore enhance the appropriate motor response through the proper use of manual contact. The patient's position must also be considered in an effort to avoid postural positions that may conflict

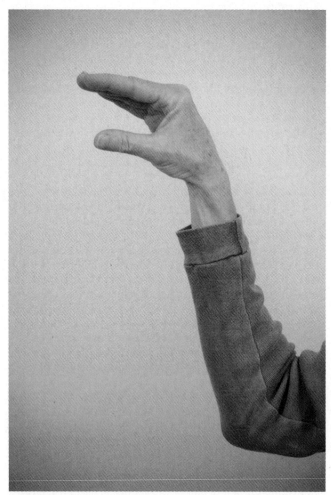

FIGURE 15-1. Lumbrical grip.

with the desired movement (e.g., a patient with extensor tone may be placed in sidelying instead of supine when facilitating hip flexion).

- *Strength or power*: When the therapist applies proper contact to the segment being facilitated, the patient often demonstrates increased strength of contraction.
- A common grip to use is the *"lumbrical grip"*; this allows a broad surface of contact which controls motion, and avoids squeezing the patient. See Figure 15-1.

Body Position and Mechanics

The clinician's body position and the use of good body mechanics are essential when using PNF. The clinician's body should be positioned at either end of the desired movement, with the shoulders and hips facing in the direction of the movement. Their forearms should always be pointed in the direction of the desired movement. Several key points on the use of proper body mechanics are important to provide an effective treatment and to prevent injuries to the clinician. First, the movement of the therapist must be a mirror image of the patient's movement. Second, maintain a neutral spine with movement occurring from the hips and legs. Third, weight shift in the direction of movement. Fourth, and most importantly, the resistance comes from the trunk and pelvis, not the extremities.

Verbal Cues

Verbal cues should be brief, clear, concise, and appropriate for the needs and comprehension of the patient. The volume of the command is dependent on the effort of the movement; the therapist should use louder commands for stronger contractions and softer commands for stability or relaxation. The timing is very important with the command usually given just before the movement takes place or repeated as needed to facilitate a weak component or for emphasis.

Visual Stimulus

Visual input increases motorneuron excitability in the muscles which are responsible for the movement. Vision facilitates coordination of the head and in turn will facilitate a stronger contraction from the trunk (e.g., resisted shoulder abduction at 90 degrees will be stronger with more trunk activity when the subject is looking at the tested arm compared to when he or she looks away from the arm).

Appropriate Resistance

The most important fundamental basis when applying manual therapeutic exercises is using *appropriate resistance*. Resistance is used to facilitate the muscle to contract to improve motor control and improve strength. The magnitude of the facilitation is directly related to the amount of resistance applied. Facilitation of the agonist will increase the response of the specific muscle and synergistic muscles at the same joint and neighboring joints. When using none to light resistance the antagonists are usually inhibited. Increasing the resistance in the agonist will cause muscle activity in the antagonist groups as well (cocontraction).[24]

Manual therapeutic exercise allows the therapist to determine the amount of resistance that demands maximal effort from the patient without breaching the intention of the effort. The levels of resistance include: passive range of motion (PROM), active assisted range of motion (AAROM), and resistive range of motion which can be applied with light, medium, or maximal resistance and/or resistance can be applied to inhibit the antagonist (reciprocal inhibition). The advantage of manual resistance is that the clinician can assess and then vary the resistance throughout the range depending on the patient's ability. In other words, the patient may require assistance or light resistance at the initiation of movement while resistance can increase in the mid range followed by less resistance again at the end range. The clinician can also select a specific range to emphasize volitional control of the patient. For example, in a patient with incomplete paraplegia, the therapist may choose to treat volitional control of hip extension from 70- to 30-degree flexion, knowing that at 15 degrees spasticity of the hip extensor muscles occurs.

PNF Utilizes Two Types of Contractions

Isotonic—implies movement: This is active voluntary movement with the "intention" of contraction to produce motion (dynamic). This can be either concentric or eccentric. The resistance must be applied so that the motion can occur in a smooth and coordinated manner. *Isometric*—implies posture: the "intention" of co-contraction, holding, or stabilizing amount of resistance which can be equaled so that no joint motion occurs. In motor learning, isotonic and the ability to move precede isometric and the ability to maintain posture. However, in normal neuromuscular activity there must be

BUILDING BLOCK 15-1
Approximation and Co-contraction

Wendy is a 14-year-old volleyball player with pain in the right shoulder and scapular winging. Assess her movement in shoulder elevation. You note throughout the range of motion her scapula is unstable. Design an exercise to improve this problem using approximation and co-contraction.

a balance of both: movement is necessary for posture and posture is necessary for movement.

Irradiation

Irradiation refers to the overflow of response to a stimulus. This response can facilitate or inhibit a contraction in the synergistic muscles and patterns of movement.[25] The muscular response and the spread of stimulation will increase as the intensity and the duration increases.[26] Therefore, weaker muscle groups will gain from stronger muscle while working synergistically in muscle groups or patterns.[27]

Traction and Approximation

Traction and approximation stimulate joint receptors and should be used with directional resistance. *Traction* is a manual distraction of the joint surface which promotes movement and is useful with pulling and reaching motions. *Approximation is* a manual compression of joint surfaces, facilitates co-contraction which promotes stability and is used with pushing activities. Traction should be applied throughout the entire range of the agonist. Compression should be applied light then progressively heavier (see Building Block 15-1).

Patterns of Facilitation

The brain generates and organizes mass movement patterns rather than individual muscle contractions. PNF utilizes mass movement patterns. Human motion is patterned and rarely involves straight plane movements because all muscles are oriented in a diagonal and spiral direction. Therefore, most human movement involves three pivots of motion occurring at all joints:

Flexion or extension: Major excursion of range
Abduction or adduction: Medium excursion of range
Rotation: Smallest excursion of range but the most
    important.

With all extremity movement whether unilateral or bilateral, there is rotation of the trunk and pelvis. Rotation of the trunk in the spiral and diagonal pattern will produce greater strength and a longer lever arm than in the straight plane pattern. The longer the lever arm the more efficient the movement pattern.

Quick Stretch

A quick stretch facilitates the muscle's ability to contract with greater force. The stretch reflex is evoked by a gentle but quick stretch to a muscle under tension (stimulating muscle spindles). It can be applied two ways: First, a quick stretch is

applied to all components simultaneously of the entire pattern in its lengthened position to initiate the movement (e.g., Wind-up of a pattern: hip: extension, abduction, internal rotation, knee: extension, ankle: plantarflexion, eversion, and toe plantarflexion). Alternatively, a quick stretch can be applied to a muscle that is already contracting in an effort to strengthen a response. It is important to maintain resistance immediately following the quick stretch; otherwise, it will result in inhibition of the agonist muscle. Quick stretch is a key component to PNF; however, it is a very difficult skill to perform and is not emphasized in this chapter. If the practitioner performs quick stretch incorrectly, it may cause damage to other structures that are also on tension (e.g., joint capsule, ligament, and nerves). The timing and amount of applied quick stretch requires many hours of practice and a skilled practitioner to supervise.

EVALUATION AND TREATMENT IMPLEMENTATION

Working within the PNF philosophy the first emphasis is on what the patient *can do* in order to facilitate the functional goals. In other words, for a patient with a right hemiparesis, the clinician can utilize the strength and movement available in the left upper and lower extremity to facilitate rolling to the right.

The clinician must also note whether the patient's functional problem is *static* inability to maintain position) or *dynamic* (loss of ability to move or control motion). Finally, the clinician must identify the specific reason for the functional loss, that is, pain, weakness, loss of sensation, or lack of motor control.

After determining the patient's goals, the clinician can now determine whether treatment sessions should emphasize Direct Treatment or Indirect Treatment.

Direct Treatment

The use of techniques on the affected limb, muscle, or motion (e.g., to increase right hip flexion strength the therapist may apply resistance directly on the right thigh resisting hip flexion).

Indirect Treatment

The use of techniques on the unaffected limb, muscle, or motion. Literature has confirmed the effectiveness of indirect treatment initiated on the strong and pain-free part of the body to increase muscle tension and EMG activity on the affected parts of the body. Therefore, the clinician can use techniques on the unaffected parts of the body to direct irradiation to the affected parts of the body (e.g., the patient with right hip flexor weakness, the therapist may involve the left lower extremity and resist bilateral hip flexion thereby facilitating right hip flexor activity).

MANUAL THERAPEUTIC EXERCISE USING PNF TECHNIQUES

The goals of the PNF techniques are to promote movement, facilitate stability, or to gain ROM/flexibility. These techniques are grouped into Movement, Stability, and Flexibility.

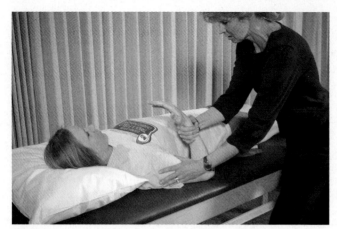

FIGURE 15-2. End range: elbow flexion. Command: "Hold."

Movement

Replication Rrepeated Contractions

Purpose   To teach the patient the expected outcome of the activity or movement. It is also utilized as an excellent assessment tool for the physical therapist to "feel" the patient's ability to hold at the end range of motion. The patient is placed in the end position (agonist muscle in its shortened length) and asked to hold while the therapist applies "demand" to all the components of desired direction resulting in simultaneous joint stimulation (Fig. 15-2). The patient is then moved (either passively or actively) slightly back into the diagonal from which he moved through and asked to actively return to the end position. Each replication of the movement starts progressively closer toward the beginning of the pattern of movement to challenge the patient through more range for a repeat finish (see Building Block 15-2).

Rhythmic Initiation

Purpose   To teach the patient movement sensation through passive, active-assistive, and resisted movement in the same direction or pattern. This is primarily used to enhance the patient's ability to initiate movement. It is also a useful tool when motor learning or communication problems exist by allowing the patient to look and "feel" the desired movement, thereby decreasing frustration. This technique is also beneficial for patients who have a fear of moving due to pain. Rhythmic Initiation allows the physical therapist to evaluate the patient's ability and willingness to be moved, and is a good assessment tool. This technique was developed to focus on the agonist muscle group only during unidirectional movement (see Building Block 15-3). Commands should progress as follows; "Let me move you," "Help me to move you," "Now, you do it." See Figure 15-3.

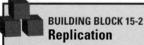

BUILDING BLOCK 15-3
Rhythmic Initiation

Mr. Jones has right upper quadrant hemiparesis and is having difficulty rolling to his left. Assess his rolling movement. The therapist noted that he is able to use his pelvis and lower body efficiently. However, his right upper extremity and his upper quadrant are lagging behind and his trunk is unable to engage in flexion. Describe how you might use rhythmic initiation to facilitate rolling.

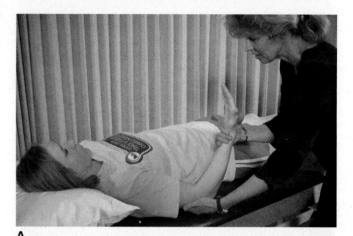

A

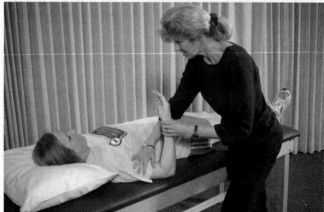

B

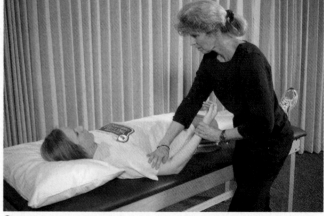

C

FIGURE 15-3. (A) "Let Me Move You." (B) "Help Me Move You." (C) "Pull-up."

BUILDING BLOCK 15-2
Replication

Mr. Jones suffered a CVA and is having difficulty with eating using his right hand secondary to weakness in the right UE especially the hand. He often drops the fork from his hand. Come up with a strategy to improve this functional activity using replication.

DISPLAY 15-1
Combination of Isotonics

John is an 18-year-old baseball player who is at the end stages of his labral repair rehab and is now ready to begin a throwing program. Prior to surgery his pain occurred during the follow through while his arm was decelerating.

- Assess his throwing motion: You note that his wind up phase and acceleration phases are good, however you note that in the follow through, the deceleration phase, he has a slightly flexed elbow (short arming) instead of full shoulder and elbow extension. This is resulting in decreased velocity and inefficiency.
- Position the player supine to the start of the D2 flexion pattern: (see Table 15-1 for D2 flexion pattern) shoulder extended, adducted, and internally rotated, elbow extended.
- Move the patient through the pattern to the end position (D2 shoulder flexion, abducted, and externally rotated and elbow still in extension.
- Return the patient to the start of the pattern.
- Command "Pull up!" (loud voice). This is the concentric phase while the muscles are shortening during contraction to the end position.
- "Now Hold!"(normal voice) Isometric phase: muscles are contracting but no change in muscle length. This transition from a concentric contraction and preparing for the eccentric phase.
- "Let me bring you down slowly!" (a little softer tone) and return the patient to the start of the position. Eccentric phase the muscles are contracting while lengthening. Emphasis on the decelerating muscles.
- Repeat six to eight repetitions.
- Now reassess his throwing.

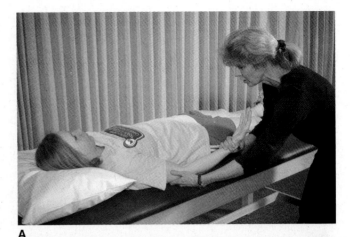

A

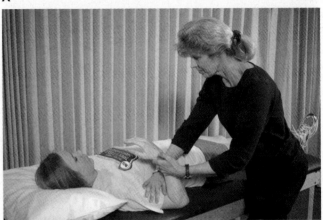

B

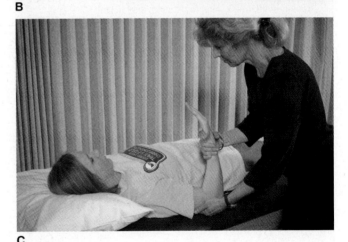

C

FIGURE 15-4. (A) Concentric biceps—"Pull up!" (B) Isometric biceps—"Hold." (C) Eccentric biceps—"Let me pull you down... Slowly."

Combination of Isotonics

Purpose To emphasize control and quality of movement of the agonists by changing the muscle dynamic contraction intent (see Display 15-1). The intention of the isotonic contractions employ combinations of concentric and eccentric muscle actions, without any relaxation, to promote smooth, coordinated functional movement. See Figure 15-4.

Reversals of Patterns (Slow Reversals and Agonists Reversals)

Purpose To facilitate dynamic movement reversals of antagonistic patterns through a full range of motion, teach reversals of movement, and improve endurance. These reversals may or may not involve an initial "quick stretch" from elongated muscle tissue at beginning range. The patient is asked to dynamically move through the pattern to end range and then reverse and move through the range of the antagonistic pattern. The end of one pattern is the beginning of the other pattern (Fig. 15-5). When performing this technique in this manner the patient's energy level accelerates during the pattern but drops to negligible at the completion of the diagonal while the therapist is repositioning grips and elongating tissue for the "stretch" of the return pattern. Each directional movement is initiated by the physical therapist's command or "quick stretch" (see Display 15-2).

Stability

Rhythmic Stabilization

Purpose To promote stability of a body part in a specific range. This technique uses continuous alternating demands to isometric contractions and co-contractions. Little to no motion occurs while patient tries to maintain body position. Muscle demands must be very slow and specific. For example, a physical therapist may apply simultaneous resistance to the anterior left shoulder and posterior right shoulder for a few seconds before switching the resistance to the posterior left shoulder

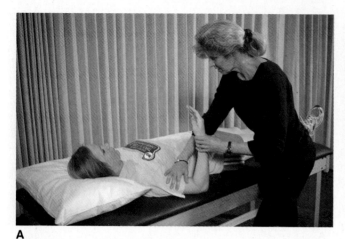
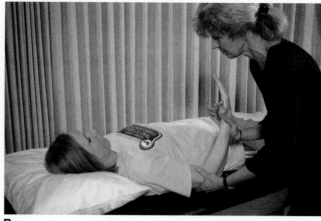

A   **B**

FIGURE 15-5. (A) Concentric biceps—"Pull up." (B) Concentric triceps—"Push Down."

 DISPLAY 15-2
Reversal of Antagonist

Larry had a total knee replacement 3 months ago and you note that he is still walking with a slow cadence and a stiff legged gait. He has full knee ROM, good strength in both quadriceps and hamstrings, and has no pain.

- Assess his knee movement in sitting and noted that he slowly moves his knee into extension and returns into knee flexion slowly.
- Position him sitting on the table facing you.
- Place your left hand just above the anterior ankle joint; this will facilitate extension. Place your right hand on the posterior region of the ankle joint, facilitating knee flexion.
- Ask Larry to "Kick up" and "Pull back." Starting slow then progressively increase the speed of contraction to fast.
- Reassess his walking.

and the anterior right shoulder. The physical therapist's movements should be smooth, fluid, and continuous. The physical therapist may also provide traction or approximation, particularly when making rotational demand switches (Fig. 15-6). At no time between the changing muscle contractions is there relaxation of the body part being worked (see Self-Management 15-1: Improve Scapular Stabilization Progression).

 SELF-MANAGEMENT 15-1 *Improve Scapular Stabilization Progression*

Purpose: To enhance the stability of the scapula by applying rhythmic stabilization for a home program to strengthen the upper and lower fibers of the serratus anterior to improve scapular stability for upper extremity functional activities.

Position: Place the hands on the floor and get into a push up plus (scapular protraction), neutral spine position with your feet in a wide base position

Movement Technique:

Level 1: Maintain scapular protraction, neutral spine, and both hands on the floor, weight shift from right to left upper extremity. Perform the weight shifts 10× to each arm without rest.

Level 2: Using the same position as above, now use a narrow base with both ankles touching. Perform the weight shifts 10× to each side.

Level 3: Maintain the push up plus position and use the above narrow base position.

Lift one leg at a time in the straight position approximately 3 in off the floor. Perform alternate leg lifts 10× each leg.

Level 4: Now place hands on a basketball, maintain the push up plus position, and close your eyes. Perform alternate leg lifts 10× each leg.

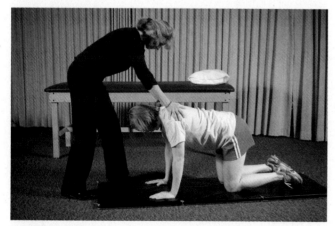

FIGURE 15-6. Stability in quadruped. Approximation and co-contraction through the UEs. "Hold."

Fred is a football player who suffered a moderate hamstring strain on his right about 6 weeks ago. He is ready to return to practice but you notice as he is running he has a short stride length on the right side.

- Position him supine on the table
- Therapist position: Standing at the foot of the table and raising his right leg in the straight leg position
- Take to end range and then back off
- "Push into my hands for 15 seconds." The patients contracts the agonist hamstrings
- "Relax and let me move you." Return to the end position
- Reevaluate his running

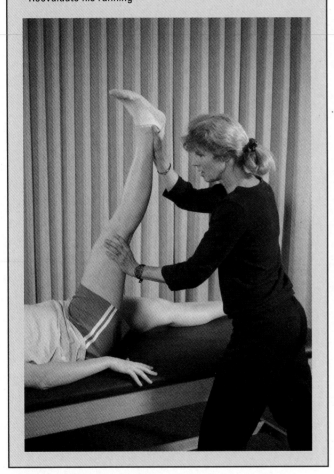

Flexibility

Contract-Relax

Purpose   To release tight musculature, that is inhibiting range of motion. The technique is a resisted contraction of an agonist group of muscles through a variable range of motion (concentric muscle action), followed by an immediate passive movement and stretch of the same muscle in the opposite direction of the contraction (see Display 15-3).

Ms. Smith is a 50-year-old female who has a right shoulder adhesive capsulitis. She is improving with shoulder elevation and is now able to elevate her arm actively to 100 degrees and her end range of motion is 105 degrees passively. Describe exercises for her using activities to increase flexibility.

Hold-Relax with Antagonist Contraction

Purpose   To release tight musculature, that is inhibiting range of motion. The technique is the same as the Contract-Relax technique, except the antagonist muscle contracts to aid in the stretch of the agonist muscle (see Building Block 15-4).

Step 1: Take to end range and back off
Step 2: "Now pull up and hold for 15 seconds." Patient actively pulls the leg into further flexion.
Step 3: "Let me move you." Therapist moves further into the range.

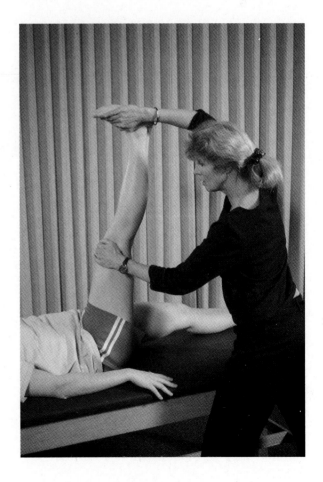

TABLE 15-1 **PNF Summary of Upper Extremity D1 and D2 Diagonal Patterns**

UPPER EXTREMITY PATTERN	D1 FLEXION	D1 EXTENSION
Scapula	Anterior Elevation	Posterior Depression
Shoulder	Flexion Adduction External Rotation	Extension Abduction Internal Rotation
Elbow	Varies	Varies
Forearm	Supination	Pronation
Wrist	Flexion	Extension
Fingers	Flexion	Extension

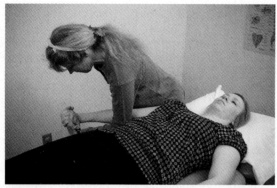

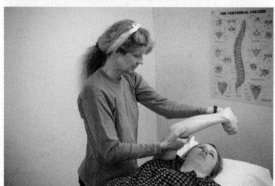

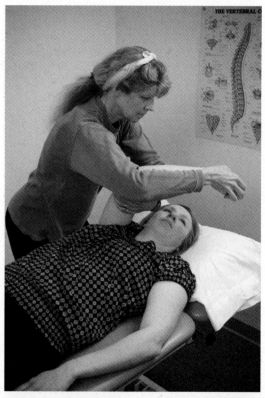

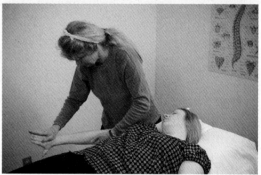

UPPER EXTREMITY PATTERN	D2 FLEXION	D2 EXTENSION
Scapula	Posterior Elevation	Anterior Depression
Shoulder	Flexion Abduction External Rotation	Extension Adduction Internal Rotation
Elbow	Varies	Varies
Forearm	Supination	Pronation
Wrist	Extension	Flexion
Fingers	Extension	Flexion

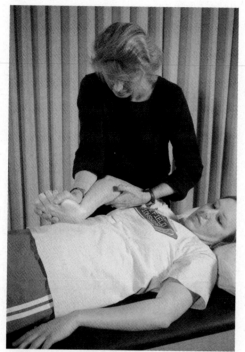
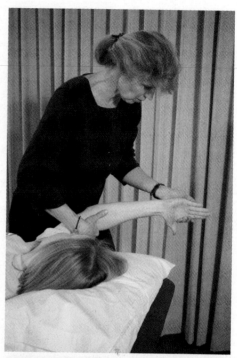
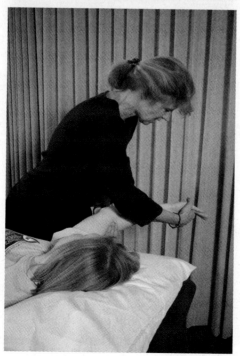
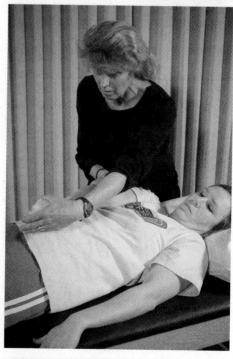

TABLE 15-2 PNF Summary of Lower Extremity D1 and D2 Diagonal Patterns

LOWER EXTREMITY PATTERN	D1 FLEXION	D1 EXTENSION
Pelvis	Anterior Elevation	Posterior Depression
Hip	Flexion Adduction External Rotation	Extension Abduction Internal Rotation
Knee	Varies	Varies
Ankle	Dorsiflexion	Plantar Flexion
Foot	Inversion	Eversion
Toes	Extension	Flexion

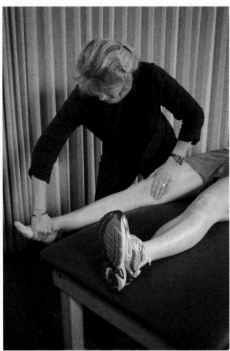

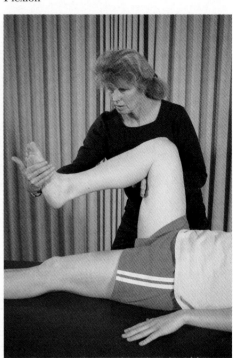

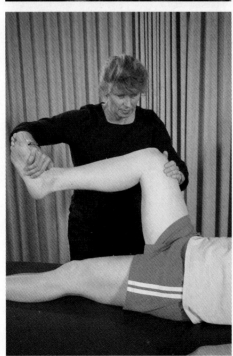

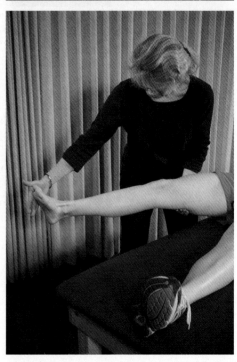

LOWER EXTREMITY PATTERN	D2 FLEXION	D2 EXTENSION
Pelvis	Posterior Elevation	Anterior Depression
Hip	Flexion Abduction Internal Rotation	Extension Adduction External Rotation
Knee	Varies	Varies
Ankle	Dorsiflexion	Plantar Flexion
Foot	Eversion	Inversion
Toes	Extension	Flexion

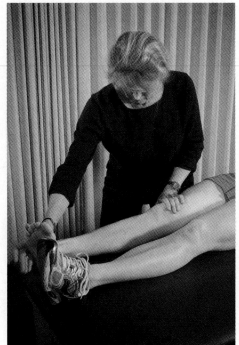

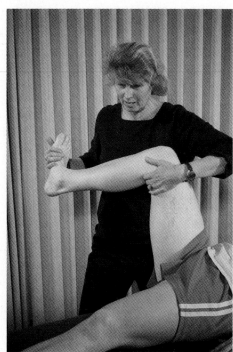

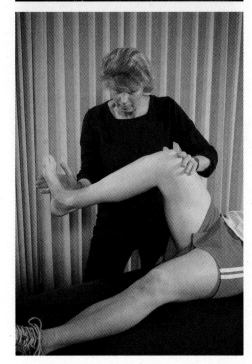

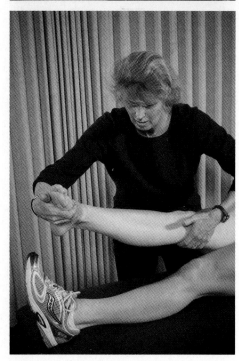

LAB ACTIVITIES

Manual Contacts

DIRECTION OF MOVEMENT

a. Have your partner in the supine position with eyes closed.
b. Raise the right forearm to 90 of elbow flexion and supination
c. Manual contact no. 1: Wrap entire hand around the forearm:
   Command: "Hold that position"
d. Manual contact no. 2 using a lumbrical grip on flexor surface only:
   Command: "Hold that position"... now pull up!
e. Manual contact no. 3 using a lumbrical grip on the extensor surface only:
   Command "Hold that position... now push down!"
   1. Which manual contacts facilitated specific muscle activity?
   2. Which manual contact was difficult to facilitate the direct line of movement?

STRENGTH OF CONTRACTION

a. Use manual contact no. 2: apply light pressure, and then slowly increase the pressure.
b. Repeat elbow flexion five times, start with a soft voice and raise your voice with each repeat
   1. Does the patient respond to the pressure of the manual contact?
   2. Does the voice of the therapist facilitate the patient's contraction?
c. Now have the patient hold at 90 degrees of elbow flexion.
   1. Begin with light resistance to the biceps. Note biceps and triceps muscle tension
   2. Now increase to maximal resistance. Note that although resisting elbow flexion irradiation occurs into the triceps muscle as well.

APPROPRIATE RESISTANCE AND SPEED OF CONTRACTION

a. *Try the following resistance guide to facilitate elbow flexion*: perform:
   1. PROM, AAROM, light resistance, medium resistance, and finally maximal resistance.
   2. Now control the speed of contraction from slow to medium speed to fast speed.
The result of each resistance should be a smooth and coordinated movement

Irradiation

a. The clinician stands in front of a patient who is sitting at the edge of a table. Have the patient raise their arms to 90 degrees of shoulder flexion, elbows extended and fingers interlocked.

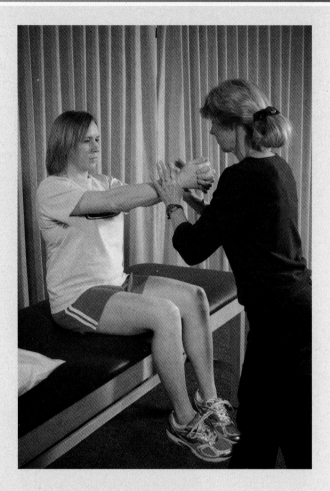

b. The clinician resists up into both arms of the patient and increases the static resistance and duration.
   1. Note the irradiation occurring in the hip flexors.
   2. Note the irradiation into the trunk
c. Try resisting just one arm in the same position.
   1. Is there more or less trunk activity with one arm compared to both arms?
   2. Irradiation through the trunk will increase when involving two extremities

Mass Movement Pattern

a. Stand facing your partner, throw a ball and follow through to the same side hip.
b. Throw the ball and follow through to the contralateral hip.
   1. Compare: Ball velocity of the throw
   2. Compare the mass movement pattern from the feet, knees, hip, trunk, shoulders, and neck

Manual Therapy:

List the advantages of manual therapeutic exercises.
List the disadvantages of manual therapeutic exercises

(continued)

LAB ACTIVITIES (Continued)

Patient Problem

Ms. Spock is a 54-year-old lady that suffered a CVA with mild to moderate right sided hemiparesis. She is having difficulty with sit to stand.

Evaluation

- She has good ROM in all extremities.
- Upper body strength is 5/5 on the left, 4/5 on the right, weak grip
- Lower body strength is 5/5 on the left, 3+/5 on the right
- Balance: sitting: good slight lean to the right
- Balance: Standing: fair +: leans to the right, and center of gravity is behind base of support. Requires a walker for independent standing and gait. Requires Stand by assist without walker

Functional Assessment: Sit to stand and return

- It takes approximately 10 seconds to sit to stand from a chair.
- She has a tendency to lean to the weak side as she is standing but is able to maintain balance
- Weight is through the heels not the forefoot.
- Inadequate forward trunk lean
- She uses a walker for gait
- Return to sitting you note she "plops" back into the chair

Goal: Safe and efficient sit to stand and return.
Design a treatment plan and progression

- What techniques would you apply in the treatment
- How would you facilitate the progression: sitting forward trunk lean, sit to stand, weight shift to the forefoot, return to sitting with a controlled movement to the chair.
- Design a safe home program she can do independently.

KEY POINTS

- The advantage to manual therapeutic exercise is the ability to constantly assess the patient's movement or posture which allows for immediate modification of the treatment or resistance.
- The clinician can influence variables such as the magnitude of resistance, type of contraction, joint compression or distraction, movement or stability emphasis and the direction of the movement or pattern.
- PNF is a manual therapy approach that attempts to provide a maximal response for increasing strength, flexibility, coordination, and functional mobility. PNF patterns are more concerned with mass body movements as opposed to specific muscle actions.
- These patterns are composed of both diagonal and rotational exercise patterns that are similar to the motions required for activities of daily living, functional mobility, and even athletic performance.

CRITICAL THINKING QUESTIONS

1. How does the clinician know they are applying too much resistance?
2. Which technique should always be utilized when facilitating movement?
3. Which technique should be applied when attempting to gain ROM?
4. Which technique should be applied to improve sitting balance?
5. Give an example of how to apply a direct treatment and an indirect treatment to facilitate trunk flexion.
6. What are two advantages to using manual therapeutic exercise?
7. What are two disadvantages of manual therapy exercise?

REFERENCES

1. Kabat H, Mc Leod M, Holt C. The practical application of proprioceptive neuromuscular facilitation. Physiotherapy 1959;45:87–92.
2. Voss DE, Knott M. Patterns of motion for proprioceptive neuromuscular facilitation. Br J Phys Med 1954;17:191–198.
3. Engle RP, Canner GC. Proprioceptive neuromuscular facilitation (PNF) and modified procedures for anterior cruciate ligament (ACL) instability. J Orthop Sports Phys Ther 1989;11:230–236.
4. Godges JJ, Macrae H, Longdon C, et al. The effects of two stretching procedures on hip range of motion and gait economy. J Orthop Sports Phys Ther 1989;10:350–357.
5. Prentice WE. An electromyographic analysis of the effectiveness of heat or cold and stretching for inducing relaxation in injured muscle. J Orthop Sports Phys Ther 1982;3:133–140.
6. Rees SS, Murphy AJ, Watsford ML, et al. Effects of proprioceptive neuromuscular facilitation stretching on stiffness and force-producing characteristics of the ankle in active women. J Strength Cond Res 2007;21:572–577.
7. Voss DE. Proprioceptive neuromuscular facilitation application of patterns and techniques in occupational therapy. Am J Occup Ther 1959;13:191–194.
8. Etnyre BR, Abraham LD. Gains in range of ankle dorsiflexion using three popular stretching techniques. Am J Phys Med 1986;65:189–196.
9. Ferber R, Osternig L, Gravelle D. Effect of PNF stretch techniques on knee flexor muscle EMG activity in older adults. J Electromyogr Kinesiol 2002;12:391–397.
10. Funk DC, Swank AM, Mikla BM, et al. Impact of prior exercise on hamstring flexibility: a comparison of proprioceptive neuromuscular facilitation and static stretching. J Strength Cond Res 2003;17:489–492.
11. Sharman MJ, Cresswell AG, Riek S. Proprioceptive neuromuscular facilitation stretching: mechanisms and clinical implications. Sports Med 2006;36:929–939.
12. Shellock FG, Prentice WE. Warming-up and stretching for improved physical performance and prevention of sports-related injuries. Sports Med 1985;2:267–278.
13. Sady SP, Wortman M, Blanke D. Flexibility training: ballistic, static or proprioceptive neuromuscular facilitation? Arch Phys Med Rehabil 1982;63:261–263.
14. Mahieu NN, Cools A, De Wilde B, et al. Effect of proprioceptive neuromuscular facilitation stretching on the plantar flexor muscle-tendon tissue properties. Scand J Med Sci Sports 2009 Aug;19(4):553–556.
15. Mitchell UH, Myrer JW, Hopkins JT, et al. Acute stretch perception alteration contributes to the success of the PNF "contract-relax" stretch. J Sport Rehabil 2007;16:85–92.
16. Rowlands AV, Marginson VF, Lee J. Chronic flexibility gains: effect of isometric contraction duration during proprioceptive neuromuscular facilitation stretching techniques. Res Q Exerc Sport 2003;74:47–51.
17. Chalmers G. Re-examination of the possible role of Golgi tendon organ and muscle spindle reflexes in proprioceptive neuromuscular facilitation muscle stretching. Sports Biomech 2004;3:159–183.

18. Manoel ME, Harris-Love MO, Danoff JV, et al. Acute effects of static, dynamic, and proprioceptive neuromuscular facilitation stretching on muscle power in women. J Strength Cond Res 2008;22:1528–1534.

19. Bradley PS, Olsen PD, Portas MD. The effect of static, ballistic, and proprioceptive neuromuscular facilitation stretching on vertical jump performance. J Strength Cond Res 2007;21:223–226.

20. Church JB, Wiggins MS, Moode FM, Crist R. Effect of warm-up and flexibility treatments on vertical jump performance. J Strength Cond Res 2001;15: 332–336.

21. Marek SM, Cramer JT, Fincher AL, et al. Acute effects of static and proprioceptive neuromuscular facilitation stretching on muscle strength and power output. J Athletic Training 2005;40(2):94–103.

22. Gabriel DA, Kamen G, Frost G. Neural adaptations to resistive exercise: mechanisms and recommendations for training practices. Sports Med 2006;36: 133–149.

23. Nelson AG, Chambers RS, McGown CM, et al. Proprioceptive neuromuscular facilitation versus weight training for enhancement of muscular strength and athletic performance. J Orthop Sports Phys Ther 1986;7:250–253.

24. Gelhorn E, Loofbourrow GN. Proprioceptively induced reflex patterns. AM J Physiology 1948;154:433–438.

25. Kabat H. Prorioceptive facilitation in therapeutic exercise. In: Licht S. Johnson EW, eds. Therapeutic Exercise. 2nd Ed. Baltimore, MD: Waverly, 1961.

26. Sherrington C. The integrative action of the nervous system. 2nd Ed. New Haven, CT: Yale University Press, 1947.

27. Hildebrandt FA. Application of the overload principle to muscle training in man. Arch Phys Med Rehab 1958;37:278–283.

chapter 16
Aquatic Physical Therapy

LORI THEIN BRODY

Although water has been used therapeutically for centuries, only recently has its use become widespread in the rehabilitation community. Traditionally, water therapy has been limited to whirlpools used to debride wounds or to apply heat or cold treatments. However, the unique buoyant and resistive properties of water make it a useful tool for therapeutic exercise. The advantages of unloading and of immersion in a resistive medium are well recognized, and the use of water as a rehabilitative medium continues to grow. As a result, the body of knowledge surrounding aquatic rehabilitation has expanded tremendously. As with land-based exercises, different techniques, schools of thought, and approaches have been developed. The Halliwick method, the Bad Ragaz Ring method, Watsu, and Ai Chi are all examples of approaches to rehabilitation in the water. Further information on resources for these techniques can be found in the "Additional Resources" section at the end of the chapter.

As with other approaches to therapeutic exercise, it is important to realize that water is a tool, with advantages and disadvantages. Not all patients are appropriate candidates for aquatic rehabilitation. The strengths and weaknesses of each treatment modality must be matched to the needs of the patient. Because water is such a unique environment, the clinician should get in the pool and experience the effects of different exercises before prescribing them for patients. Often, aquatic exercises that appear to be simple can be quite difficult, and exercises that are difficult on land are easy to perform in the pool. The trunk stabilizing muscles are challenged with most arm and leg exercises and represent a very different task from the same activity performed on land.

Aquatic physical therapy can be defined as the use of an aquatic medium to achieve physical therapy goals. The purpose of this chapter is to acquaint the reader with the fundamental principles of therapeutic exercise in the water. It is intended to provide the framework for integration of water-based and land-based exercises to treat impairments, activity limitations, and participation restrictions.

PHYSICAL PROPERTIES OF WATER

The physical properties of water provide countless options for rehabilitation program design. Be familiar with these properties and the intended or unintended effects that may result from their interaction. For example, the effect of buoyancy on gait is that of unweighting, thereby reducing the amount of physical work of walking. However, this reduction may be offset by the frontal resistance encountered because of the water's viscosity. As such, the clinician and patient should clearly define the goals of any given exercise in the pool to ensure progress toward overall functional goals.

Buoyancy

Archimedes' principle states that an immersed body at rest experiences an upward thrust equal to the weight of the same fluid volume it displaces.[1] As such, rather than a downward force resulting from gravity and body weight, individuals in the pool experience an upward force (i.e., buoyancy) related to water depth and specific gravity. The specific gravity of an object (or an individual) is its density relative to that of water.[1] The specific gravity of water is almost exactly 1 g/cm³; therefore, anything with a specific gravity >1 g/cm³ sinks, and anything less floats. This property forms the scientific basis for underwater weighing to determine body composition. The specific gravity of a person is determined by the relationship between lean body mass and body fat. Individuals with a higher relative lean body mass are more likely to sink, and those with a higher relative body fat have a tendency to float. These differences can be balanced by the appropriate use of water depth, flotation equipment, and waterproof weight equipment.

Buoyancy acts through the center of buoyancy, which is the center of gravity of the displaced liquid. If the body weight and the displaced fluid weights are unequal, a rotation about the center of buoyancy occurs until equilibrium is reached. The moment of buoyancy is the product of the force of buoyancy and the perpendicular distance from the center of buoyancy to the axis of rotation. As on land, the greater the distance, the greater is the force needed to move the limb.

Buoyancy is one property of water that can be used to progress therapeutic exercise. The four main variables that can be manipulated to alter resistance or assistance are

1. Position or direction of movement in the water
2. Water depth
3. Lever arm length
4. Flotation or weighted equipment use

Position and Direction of Movement
As with gravity, patient position and direction of movement can greatly alter the amount of assistance or resistance. Activities in the water can be buoyancy-assisted, buoyancy-supported, or buoyancy-resisted (Fig. 16-1). Movements toward the surface of the water are considered to be buoyancy-assisted exercises and are similar to gravity-assisted exercises on land. In this case, the movement is assisted by the water's buoyancy. In the standing position, shoulder abduction and flexion, as well as the ascent phase of a squat, are considered buoyancy-assisted exercises. In a prone position, hip extension can be buoyancy-assisted.

355

CASE STUDY 16-1

HISTORY: The patient is a 57-year-old female who fell 8 weeks ago and sustained a right bimalleolar fracture. She was treated with open reduction internal fixation and placed in a boot. Over the following 6 weeks, her weight-bearing status was gradually increased. She is now full weight bearing (FWB) and is instructed to wean herself from the walking boot. She is apprehensive about walking without the boot. She feels like her ankle is stiff, weak and that she has poor balance. She is otherwise healthy although she has mild degenerative joint disease in both knees. She reports that her knees are bothering her more since walking in the boot and because she has been unable to exercise regularly. She hopes to return to walking 3 mi per day for routine exercise.

EXAMINATION: Patient 65 in tall, weighing 150 lb. Ambulates with a slight limp in walking boot. Unable to walk FWB without boot. AROM from 0- to 30-degree dorsi/plantar flexion and 10-degree eversion to 15-degree inversion. Decreased AP glide of talus in mortise. Joint stable. Significant atrophy and strength of 4/5 throughout with discomfort but no frank pain. No neurologic signs. Unable to single-leg balance on involved limb.

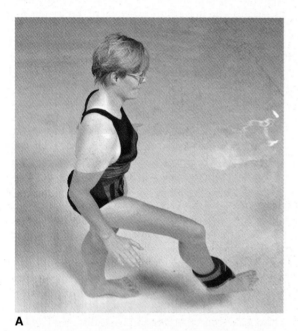

A

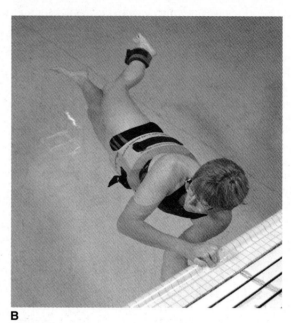

B

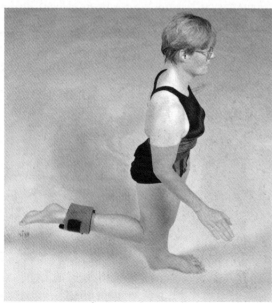

C

FIGURE 16-1. (A) Buoyancy-assisted knee extension. In a standing position with the hip flexed, knee extension is assisted by buoyancy. (B) Buoyancy-supported knee extension. In a sidelying position, knee extension is neither assisted nor resisted by buoyancy, but moves through a range perpendicular to buoyancy. (C) Buoyancy-resisted knee extension. In a standing position with the knee flexed, the motion from flexion to extension becomes resisted by the water's buoyancy.

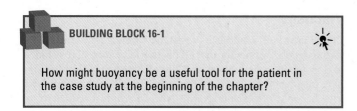

BUILDING BLOCK 16-1

How might buoyancy be a useful tool for the patient in the case study at the beginning of the chapter?

Movements parallel to the bottom of the pool are considered buoyancy supported and are similar to gravity-minimized positions on land. These movements are neither resisted nor assisted by buoyancy. In a standing position, horizontal shoulder abduction is an example of such an activity. Hip and shoulder abduction in a supine position are also examples of buoyancy-supported activities.

Movements toward the bottom of the pool are buoyancy-resisted exercises. In a supine position, shoulder and hip extension are buoyancy-resisted activities, and the descent phase of a squat is resisted in a standing position. The ability of the clinician to position the patient a number of ways allows for a multitude of assisted, supported, and resisted activities (see Building Block 16-1).

Water Depth

The water's depth is another variable that can alter the amount of assistance or resistance offered. For example, performing a squat in waist-deep water is easier than hip-deep water. Less support is provided by buoyancy in the shallower water. Walking can be easier or harder in deeper water, depending on the individual's impairment or disability. Someone with pain because of degenerative joint disease may find walking in deeper water easier because of the additional unloading of buoyancy, and someone with muscular or cardiovascular weakness may find the additional frontal resistance of deeper water more difficult. Estimates of percentage weight bearing at various depths have been obtained by Harrison et al.[2] The amount of weight bearing depends on the body composition of the patient, the water's depth, and the walking speed. Fast walking can increase the loading over the static condition by as much as 76%.[2] Occasionally, water depth options are limited by the available facilities. Modifications can be made by adding buoyant equipment to unload or by adding resistive equipment to increase frontal resistance.

Lever Arm Length

Just as with exercise on land, the lever arm length can be adjusted to change the amount of assistance or resistance. Performing buoyancy-assisted shoulder abduction in a standing position is easier with the elbow straight (i.e., long lever) than with the elbow flexed (i.e., short lever). Conversely, buoyancy-resisted shoulder adduction is more difficult with the elbow extended because of the long lever arm (Fig. 16-2).

Buoyant Equipment

To further increase the amount of assistance or resistance, buoyant equipment can be added to the lever arm (Fig. 16-3). Additionally, as the buoyancy of the equipment increases, the resistance also increases. A buoyant "bell" in the hand during shoulder abduction increases the assistance from buoyancy

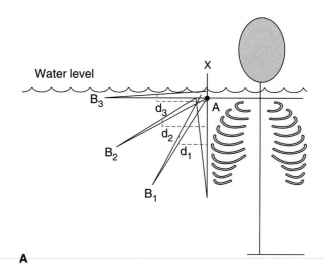

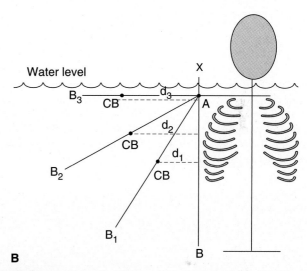

FIGURE 16-2. (A) The effect of buoyancy on shoulder abduction with a shortened lever arm (elbow bent). (B) The effect of buoyancy on shoulder abduction with a long lever arm (elbow extended). Increasing the lever arm increases the distance from the center of rotation, thereby increasing the resistance or assistance. (Adapted from Skinner AT, Thomson AM, eds. Duffield's Exercise in Water. 3rd Ed. London: Bailliere Tindall, 1983.)

while increasing resistance to the adduction return motion. Buoyant cuffs can be added anywhere along the lever arm to adjust the quantity and location of assistance or resistance (Fig. 16-4). Buoyant equipment is also used to support individuals in supine or prone positions as they perform exercises. Because buoyancy works in the direction opposite that of gravity, any land activity that would be resisted by gravity is assisted by buoyancy and vice versa.

Hydrostatic Pressure

The pressure exerted by the water at increasing depths (i.e., hydrostatic pressure) accounts for the cardiovascular shifts seen with immersion and for the purported benefit of edema control. Pascal law states that the pressure of a fluid is exerted on an object equally at a given depth.[1] The pressure increases with the density of the fluid and with its depth. Hydrostatic pressure is greatest at the bottom of the pool because of the

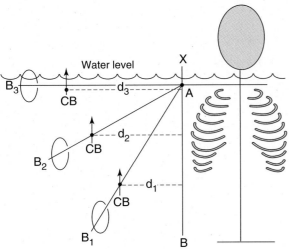

FIGURE 16-3. The effect of buoyancy with the addition of a float in the hand. The distance from the axis of rotation is further increased, thereby increasing the resistance or assistance. (Adapted from Skinner AT, Thomson AM, eds. Duffield's Exercise in Water. 3rd Ed. London: Bailliere Tindall, 1983.)

weight of the water overhead. As such, the pool may be a good exercise option for individuals with lower extremity edema or joint effusion. The hydrostatic pressure also produces centralization of peripheral blood flow, which alters cardiac dynamics. This is discussed later in this chapter under "Physiologic Responses to Immersion."

Viscosity

The viscosity of a fluid is its resistance to adjacent fluid layers sliding freely by one another.[1] This friction causes a resistance to flow when moving through a liquid. Viscosity is of little significance when stationary. The viscous quality of water allows it to be used effectively as a resistive medium because of its hydrodynamic properties. Turbulent flow is produced when the speed of movement reaches a critical velocity.[3] Eddies are formed in the wake behind the moving object, creating drag that is greater in the unstreamlined object than in streamlined objects (Fig. 16-5). In turbulent flow, resistance is proportional to the velocity squared, and increasing the speed of movement significantly increases the resistance. When moving through the water, the body experiences a frontal resistance proportional to the presenting surface area. Resistance can be increased by enlarging the surface area. The clinician has two variables to alter resistance produced by viscosity: the velocity of movement and the surface area or streamlined nature of the object. Both speed and surface area affect force production when using viscosity as resistance.

Velocity of Movement

Turbulence and resultant drag are created when movement reaches a critical velocity. Slow movement through the water produces little drag, and resistance is minimal. Buoyancy may be a more significant resistive or assistive property than viscosity during slow movement. However, when moving rapidly through the water, much resistance can be encountered that is proportional to the speed of movement. Individuals

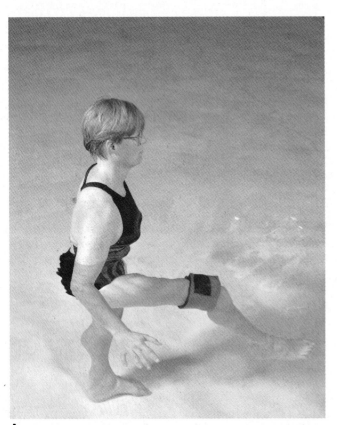
A

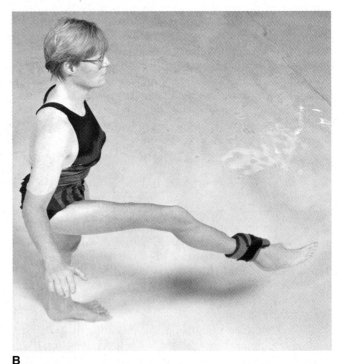
B

FIGURE 16-4. (A) Buoyant cuff added to the knee provides some assistance to hip flexion. (B) A buoyant cuff added at the ankle provides greater hip flexion assistance.

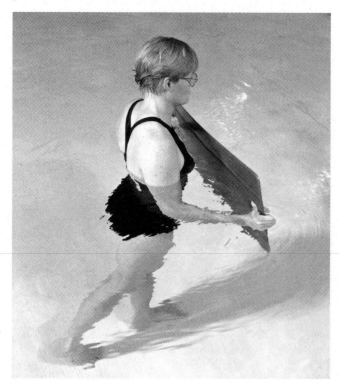

FIGURE 16-5. Using a plow while walking increases the surface area, creating eddies and drag.

can progress resistance incrementally by gradually increasing the speed of exercise. This allows multiple gradations of an exercise rather than finite increases in weight, as is frequently necessary in land programs.

A study comparing shoulder muscle activation at 30 degrees per second, 45 degrees per second, and 90 degrees per second in the water and on land highlights this property.[4] The percent of maximal voluntary contraction of the shoulder muscles was consistently higher on land at 30 degrees per second and 45 degrees per second, whereas those values were higher in water at 90 degrees per second (Table 16-1). This finding suggests that as the speed of movement through the water increases, so does the resistance. Slow movements produce muscle activation that is below those levels

achieved against gravity on land, whereas fast movements exceed the muscle activation of comparably paced land-based movements.

Surface Area

In addition to altering the speed of movement, resistance can be modified by changing the object shape to provide more or less turbulence. The body can be positioned to alter turbulence, or equipment can be added. For example, less resistance is encountered in sidestepping than in forward or backward walking because of the more streamlined shape in frontal plane movement. Performing shoulder internal and external rotation with the elbows bent to 90 degrees with the forearms pronated produces much less resistance than performing this exercise with the forearms in neutral (Fig. 16-6A and B). Adding resistive gloves further increases the resistance (Fig. 16-6C). Changing the pitch of the hand slightly between neutral and pronation alters the surface area and resultant resistance. This provides a multitude of resistive positions. A study of the Hydro-Tone (Hydro-Tone Fitness Systems, Inc., Huntington Beach, CA) resistive bells found that their orientation and water velocity both had a significant effect on force production.[5] Approximately 50% more force is produced when the bell is oriented at 45 degrees compared with 0 degrees at fast speeds. At slow speeds, the orientation made little difference in force production. Other equipment to increase the surface area and resultant turbulence are fins for the feet, a plow for resistive walking or other pushing and pulling activities, resistive bells and boots, and paddles or pinwheels (Fig. 16-7). A study using the Hydrotone (Hydro-Tone Fitness Systems, Inc., Huntington Beach, CA) boots showed increased drag compared with a barefoot condition[6–8] (see Building Block 16-2).

PHYSIOLOGIC RESPONSES TO IMMERSION

Significant physiologic changes occur with immersion at various depths. Be aware of the changes that occur despite changes known to occur with exercise. These responses may produce desirable effects (e.g., control of lower extremity edema) or undesirable effects (e.g., limitation of lung expansion). Choose the appropriate water depth based on

TABLE 16-1 Shoulder Muscle Activation (Electromyographic) During Arm Elevation in the Scapular Plane on Land and in Water. Data are Mean Percentage of Maximal Voluntary Contraction				
MUSCLE	**TEST CONDITION**	**30 DEGREES/SECOND**	**45 DEGREES/SECOND**	**90 DEGREES/SECOND**
Supraspinatus	Land	16.68	17.46	22.79
	Water	3.93	5.71	27.32
Infraspinatus	Land	11.10	10.76	15.03
	Water	2.28	2.89	21.06
Subscapularis	Land	5.96	6.83	7.45
	Water	1.49	2.26	10.73
Anterior deltoid	Land	15.88	18.82	22.09
	Water	3.61	43.49	32.83
Middle deltoid	Land	6.22	7.64	10.07
	Water	1.60	2.53	17.39
Posterior deltoid	Land	2.25	2.24	4.23
	Water	0.75	0.91	6.56

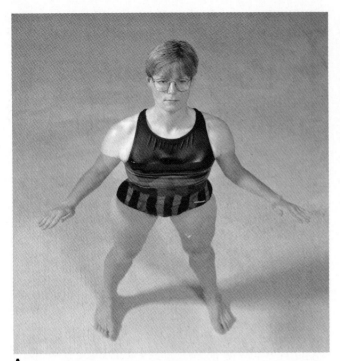

A

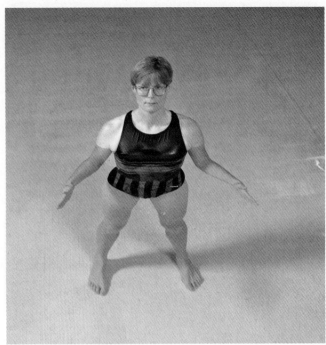

B

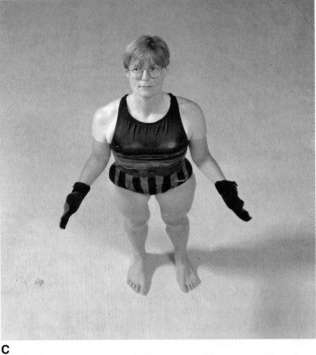

C

FIGURE 16-6. The amount of shoulder internal and external rotation resistance is less with (A) forearm pronation than with (B) forearm neutral. (C) Resistance can be further increased by the addition of gloves.

the specific health status of the patient and on the patient's physical therapy goals.

Effects of Hydrostatic Pressure

Immersion alone is not a benign action. The hydrostatic pressure encountered results in changes in cardiovascular dynamics even before exercise is initiated (Display 16-1). Immersion to the neck results in centralization of peripheral blood flow.[9–] [13] Risch et al.[12] found that immersion to the diaphragm raised heart volume by approximately 130 mL, and further immersion to the neck increased heart volume by another 120 mL. Intrapulmonary blood volume increases 33% to 60%, and vital capacity has been shown to decrease by 8%.[12] Immersion to the neck also increased central venous pressure at the height of the right atrium from 2.5 to 12.8 mm Hg.[12] The blood volume shift results in increased right atrial pressure of 12 to 18 mm Hg and increased left ventricular end-diastolic volume

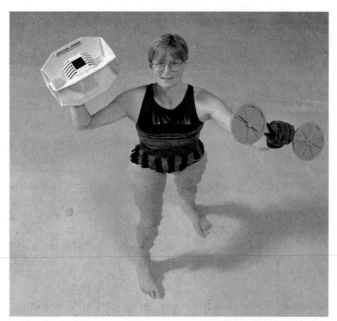

FIGURE 16-7. A variety of equipment is available to increase the surface area of moving limbs.

DISPLAY 16-1
Physiologic Changes with Immersion

1. Decreased:
   Peripheral blood flow
   Vital capacity
2. Increased:
   Heart volume
   Intrapulmonary blood volume
   Right atrial pressure
   Left ventricular end-diastolic volume
   SV
   CO
3. Decreased or unchanged HR

(i.e., cardiac preload).[10,11,13] The cardiac preload produces a stroke volume (SV) increase through the Frank-Starling reflex. Studies have shown an SV increase of 35% and a cardiac output (CO) increase of 32% while immersed to the neck.[9,13] The heart rate (HR) remains unchanged or decreases because of the relationship of HR, SV, and CO such that HR × SV = CO. Risch et al.[12] demonstrated that raising the water depth from the symphysis pubis to the xiphoid decreased the HR 15%. These HR changes depend on the depth of immersion, the individual's comfort level in the water, water temperature, and type and intensity of exercise.

The cardiovascular changes resulting from centralization of blood flow are graded, and they occur with simple immersion before the onset of exercise. This accounts for much of the variability in HR changes with water exercise reported in the literature. The hydrostatic indifference point is located approximately at the diaphragm and represents the point at which the increase in hydrostatic pressure in the lower extremities and abdomen is precisely countered by the hydrostatic pressure of the water.[12] The effect of hydrostatic pressure on cardiovascular changes depends on the depth of immersion and on body position. For example, when the water level drops below the symphysis pubis, the positive effects of prevention of lower extremity edema are negated. The clinician should match the needs of the patient (e.g., prevention of edema, cardiac history) with the risks and benefits

BUILDING BLOCK 16-2

The patient from the case study is starting a walking program in the pool. Which walking movements will facilitate ankle mobility? What factors should be considered when determining the speed and depth for the walking exercise?

of the various treatment modalities. For example, a patient with no significant cardiac history and ankle swelling would benefit from immersion in deeper water, whereas a patient with known cardiac disease and no lower extremity edema should be treated in more shallow water.

Effects of Water Temperature

Water temperature, as with hydrostatic pressure, alters the cardiovascular challenge to the immersed subject in a depth-related fashion. Water that is too warm or too cold can add a significant thermal load to the cardiovascular system. Choukroun and Varene[14] found CO to be unchanged from 25°C to 34°C (77°F to 93°F) but significantly increased at 40°C (104°F); oxygen consumption was significantly increased at 25°C (77°F). Several studies have found a decreased HR in subjects exercising in cold water, and exercising in very warm water can increase HR.[15–19] Thermoneutral temperature is suggested to be approximately 34°C.[17–19] Most pool temperatures range from 27° to 35°C (81°F to 95°F). Know the current pool temperature and potential effects on the patient.

PHYSIOLOGIC RESPONSES TO EXERCISE AND IMMERSION

In addition to the effects of immersion alone on cardiovascular dynamics, the clinician must consider the combination of changes resulting from immersion and changes resulting from exercise. Training in water produces physiologic adaptations similar to training on land, and aquatic training can be used to increase or maintain cardiovascular condition.[13,20–24] Deep-water running has been shown to maintain an individual's maximum oxygen consumption and 2-mi run time over a 6-week training period.[24] The pool can be used as a cardiovascular training tool alone or in combination with land-based training, providing the individual recovering from injury with alternative training mediums.

When training in the pool, the cardiac preload resulting from central volume increases persists despite the vascular shifts known to occur with exercise.[10] Despite the increase in blood flow to the working muscles (i.e., peripheralization of blood flow), the increased cardiac load resulting from hydrostatic pressure (i.e., centralization of blood flow) still occurs. Most studies have found the HR to be lower or unchanged compared with similar cardiovascular activity on land.[121,25–28] The depth of immersion affects the degree of cardiac changes, with increasing depth producing greater cardiovascular changes. Subjects studied while walking and jogging in ankle-, knee-, thigh-, and waist-deep water were found to work harder with increasing immersion up to the waist, at which point the increased resistance (resulting from increased surface area) was partially offset by buoyancy.[29] Running and jogging in waist-deep water produces the same HR and oxygen consumption changes as exercise on land.[30,31] However, exercise while immersed to the neck will produce a HR of 8 to 11 beats per minute lower than similar land-based exercise.[28,32]

Both shallow-water running and deep-water running can be used for cardiovascular training. As with on land, a linear relationship between HR and cadence exists for deep-water running.[33] Mechanically, shallow-water running more closely resembles land-based running because of the foot contact on the bottom, but contact may also cause impact or friction problems.

When performing resistive exercise in the pool, be sure to realize that most muscle contractions are concentric because of the negation of gravity. Eccentric contractions can be generated if the water is shallow enough to minimize the effects of buoyancy, by manually resisting the force of buoyancy in an eccentric fashion, or by using a lot of buoyant equipment. For example, performing a squat exercise in thigh-deep water requires eccentric contractions in the lowering phase, but performing the same exercise in waist-deep water negates most of gravity's effects. If enough flotation equipment is used, an exercise can require eccentric resistance against buoyancy. With large flotation devices in the hand, the motion of shoulder abduction becomes an eccentric contraction of the shoulder adductors, resisting the upward force of buoyancy.

EXAMINATION AND EVALUATION FOR AQUATIC REHABILITATION

The clinician must perform a full land-based examination. This is the same evaluation the clinician performs when designing a land-based program. As always, choose tests and measures based upon the patient history and systems review. Additionally, be sure to consider the physical properties of

---

DISPLAY 16-2
Patient Screen for Aquatic Rehabilitation

1. Basic safety
   Ability to enter/exit the pool safely
   Comfort in the water
   Ability to put face in the water
   Rhythmic breathing/bobbing
   Ability to supine and prone float and recovery
   Turning over
2. Precautions to aquatic environment
   Cardiac history
   Fear of the water
   Any precautions to land exercise (i.e., diabetes)
   Limited lung capacity
3. Contraindications to aquatic environment
   Fevers, infections, rashes
   Open wounds without Bioclusive dressing
   Incontinence without protection
   Unstable cardiac conditions

BUILDING BLOCK 16-3

What are the important aspects of the examination in terms of mobility and safety for the patient in the case study?

---

the water and the physiologic effects of immersion when determining the appropriateness of aquatic physical therapy for the patient (see Display 16-2). Will the patient benefit from the properties of buoyancy or hydrostatic pressure (i.e., relief of weight bearing or swelling control)? Will the centralization of blood flow place the patient at risk? Look for impairments that might alter the patient's relative density and ability to float. For example, a patient with paraparesis may need flotation to keep his or her legs from sinking when supine. Identify pathology or impairments that might affect the patient's ability to tolerate the hydrostatic pressure against the chest wall. Patients with decreased lung capacity may have difficulty breathing resulting from this pressure. Watch for sensory impairments that might alter the patient's ability to tolerate the touch of the pool floor, walls or water, or the visual or auditory sensory stimulation found in a pool.

Be sure to assess the patient's safety in the pool environment. Will the patient be able to traverse a wet shower room and pool deck? Will he or she be able to don and doff a swim suit? Are there safe mechanisms for transfer in and out of the pool, given the patient's physical capabilities? What is the patient's comfort level in the pool? Is he or she able to float and recover, blow bubbles, and immerse the face in the water? Is the patient able to regain balance comfortably if he or she loses it in the water? The patient's safety is paramount in the pool, just as on land (see Building Block 16-3).

THERAPEUTIC EXERCISE INTERVENTION

After determination of the appropriateness of aquatic physical therapy with the patient, specific physical therapy goals must be developed. These goals should be written to address the specific impairments and activity limitations identified. Aquatic exercise has been shown to improve impairments and activity limitations in individuals with various diseases and to improve the fitness of older women.[34,35] Patients with rheumatic disease showed significant improvement in premean and postmean scores of active joint motion and the Functional Status Index.[34] The decreased pain and difficulty with daily activities contributed significantly to the overall increased functional status and active joint motion. Elderly women participating in a 12-week water exercise class demonstrated significant improvements in oxygen consumption, muscular strength, agility, skinfold thickness, and cholesterol as compared with a control group.[35] A group of patients with coronary artery disease improved stress test time, oxygen consumption, and muscle strength after a 4-month aquatic exercise program.[36] However, improvements were lost after a 4-month detraining period, suggesting the need for continued exercise through the lifetime.

Research in individuals with arthritis has shown aquatic rehabilitation to be efficacious and cost-effective. Significant reductions in pain along with improvements in strength and function have been noted in patients with osteoarthritis of the hip or knee.[37–39] Additionally, compliance with the water therapy tends to be higher than with land therapy.[38,40,41] Other research has found significant improvements in measures of range of motion (ROM), thigh girth, pain scales, and 1-mi walk test in patients with knee osteoarthritis, with the aquatic group showing significantly lower pain levels than the land group.[42] The results reinforce the notion that patients can improve strength and function effectively in either a land or aquatic environment. The key is the ability to provide a comprehensive program, whether on land, in the water, or some combination of both.

Pools are expensive to build, staff, and maintain. A study of the cost-effectiveness of water-based therapy for lower limb osteoarthritis found a favorable cost-benefit ratio as measured by a reduction in Western Ontario and McMaster Osteoarthritis Index (WOMAC) pain as the measure of benefit.[37]

Although structured aquatic physical therapy for people with musculoskeletal impairments and activity limitations is relatively new, there is evidence supporting the clinical and cost-effectiveness of this intervention. A Cochrane Review examining the effectiveness of aquatic physical therapy for the treatment of hip and knee osteoarthritis is ongoing.[43] Improvements in impairments and activity limitations are reasonable rehabilitation goals. The following sections describe principles of aquatic physical therapy to treat common impairments.

Mobility Impairment

Exercises to improve joint mobility and ROM are easily performed in the water. The general muscular relaxation, support of buoyancy, and hydrodynamic forces occurring in water interact to provide an environment conducive to mobility activities. Be aware of the potential for overstretching while in the water. When designing a mobility program in the pool, the primary considerations are the following:

1. The force of buoyancy and its effect on the desired motion (assisting, supporting, or resisting)
2. The available ROM at the joint
3. The direction of the desired motion
4. The need for any flotation or weighted equipment

Progress simple ROM exercises addressing impairments to activities directed toward activity limitations and disabilities as quickly as possible. For example, progress exercises to increase hip and knee motion to normal ambulation as soon as possible.

Buoyancy is the physical property used most often to facilitate ROM. Use lever arm length and buoyant equipment to increase or decrease the amount of assistance from buoyancy. For example, hip flexion, shoulder flexion, and shoulder abduction are motions assisted by buoyancy in a vertical position. High marching steps can be performed with the knee flexed or extended, with or without flotation equipment to improve hip flexion ROM. As soon as motion and weight bearing allow, progress this activity to normal walking, running, or bicycling, depending on the patient's needs. Perform traditional stretching using static structures in the pool such as steps, pool sides, and bars (Fig. 16-8).

Be alert to the use of proper technique when performing any exercise in the pool. Because of the water's refraction, it may be difficult to see the patient's posture and mechanics during exercise. The maintenance of proper spine position and osteokinematics during ROM activity is essential for the progression to functional exercises. Observe the patient's exercise mechanics on land to ensure proper performance before pool exercise. Selected Interventions 16-1 and 16-2 present

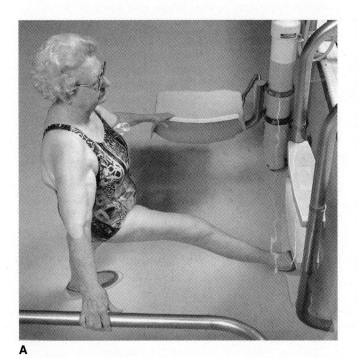
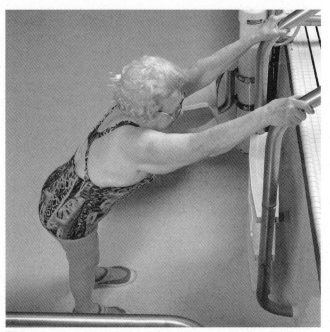

A   **B**

FIGURE 16-8. Stretching exercises for (A) hamstring muscles and (B) shoulder extensors can be performed using bars or the pool edge.

SELECTED INTERVENTION 16-1
Aquatic Therapy to Improve Upper Extremity Mobility

See Case Study No. 4

ACTIVITY: Shoulder internal rotation stretching

PURPOSE: To increase mobility in internal rotation and extension

ELEMENT OF THE MOVEMENT SYSTEM: Base

STAGE OF MOTOR CONTROL: Mobility

POSTURE: Standing in waist-deep water holding a buoyant barbell behind the back

MOVEMENT: Squat slightly and bring the hands closer together to increase the stretch

SPECIAL CONSIDERATIONS: Substitution such as forward trunk flexion or scapular protraction must be avoided. The patient should feel a medium to moderate stretching sensation.

DOSAGE: The patient should hold stretch for 30 seconds

EXPLANATION OF CHOICE OF EXERCISE: This exercise was chosen to increase shoulder mobility as one component of a comprehensive mobility, strength, and endurance program

performed in the pool. This program is balanced with a home exercise program.

FUNCTIONAL MOVEMENT PATTERNS TO REINFORCE GOAL OF SPECIFIC EXERCISES: Reaching behind the back for hygiene, tucking in shirt, and hooking brassiere

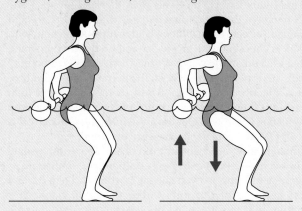

Starting position   Ending position

SELECTED INTERVENTION 16-2
Aquatic Therapy to Improve Lower Extremity Mobility

See Case Study No. 6

Although this patient requires comprehensive intervention as described in previous chapters, one specific exercise related to aquatic therapy will be described.

ACTIVITY: Lunge walking

PURPOSE: To increase mobility in the hip, knee, and ankle, and force or torque generation and endurance in the lower extremities

RISK FACTORS: No appreciable risk factors

ELEMENTS OF THE MOVEMENT SYSTEM: Base

STAGE OF MOTOR CONTROL: Controlled mobility

MODE: Mobility and resisted activity in a gravity lessened environment

POSTURE: Maintain an upright trunk throughout the exercise

MOVEMENT: Walking in a normal heel-toe gait pattern, exaggerating the knee flexion of the loading response to 60 to 80 degrees of flexion, followed by full extension at midstance.

SPECIAL CONSIDERATIONS: Ensure an upright trunk avoiding forward lean. Avoid knee flexion beyond 80 degrees of flexion, and maintain a vertical tibia during the knee flexion component.

DOSAGE: Repetitions to form fatigue; performed two to three times per week

EXPLANATION OF CHOICE OF EXERCISE: This exercise was chosen to improve mobility at the hip, knee, and ankle, as well as dynamic muscular control at these joints. This movement was chosen to emphasize the knee flexion component in the loading response phase of gait.

FUNCTIONAL MOVEMENT PATTERN TO REINFORCE GOAL OF EXERCISE: Normal gait, ascending and descending stairs, and getting in and out of chair

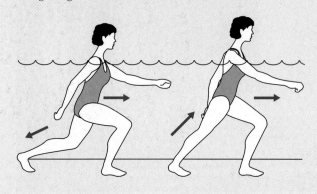

Starting position   Ending position

BUILDING BLOCK 16-4

> **BUILDING BLOCK 16-4**
>
> Describe an aquatic program to increase this patient's ankle mobility. Progress it from simple mobility exercises to more functional exercises.

examples of aquatic exercises that may be prescribed for clients with mobility impairment (see Building Block 16-4).

Muscle Strength/Power/Endurance Impairment

Although buoyancy is the primary tool used to increase mobility, viscosity and hydrodynamic properties provide the greatest challenge to strength and endurance. These forces have been proven to increase muscle strength following an aquatic resistive exercise program.[44–46] The turbulence created during motion produces the greatest resistance and is influenced by the surface area, object shape, and speed of movement. The strength training principles and progressions used in water-based activities are the same as those used on land. These include variables such as frequency, intensity, and duration. As with techniques to increase mobility, progress traditional strength and endurance training exercises to address activity limitations and disabilities as quickly as possible. For example, progress simple viscosity-resisted hip extension and knee extension exercises to normal gait or rising from a chair as quickly as possible. Calisthenics, open kinematic chain, closed kinematic chain, diagonal patterns, and motor control exercises can be performed effectively in the pool.

Because the patient is immersed in a resistive medium, exercise in any direction can be resistive if given a critical velocity. A resistive motion in any direction requires a counterforce to stabilize against the turning effects of the center of buoyancy. For example, an individual standing in shoulder-deep water performing bilateral shoulder flexion from neutral to 90-degree flexion is pushed backward by the force generated with the arms (see Self-Management 16-1: Bilateral Shoulder Flexion). The leg and trunk stabilizers must fire to counteract and keep the individual from falling over. This can be an effective technique to train trunk stabilization. It is easy to overlook the additional muscular work necessary to provide stabilization against resistive movements in the pool, and this demand probably contributes to the overwork experienced by many patients. Be aware of which muscle groups are providing stability, the quantity of stabilization necessary, and the position or posture of the joints being stabilized. In the absence of external support (e.g., hand hold, wall support), nearly any upper or lower extremity exercise places significant demands on the hip and trunk stabilizers.

As with exercises to increase mobility, equipment can be used to enhance resistive exercise. Buoyant cuffs or bells can be used to increase the resistance against buoyancy, and paddles, gloves, and other surface area–enhancing equipment can increase the resistance resulting from turbulence. It is important that the quality of the exercise not be sacrificed for an increase in resistance (see Self-Management 16-2:

SELF-MANAGEMENT 16-1 *Bilateral Shoulder Flexion*

Purpose:	Increased muscular strength and endurance in shoulder flexors and extensors. Increased trunk stability
Position:	Standing with the feet in stride, arms at the side, and palms facing forward
Movement Technique:	
	Level 1: Bring arms forward together; then turn palms facing backward and push arms backward. Turn palms forward and repeat.
	Level 2: As above, but with feet in stance
	Level 3: As above, with addition of resistive equipment
	Level 4: As above, but standing on one leg
	Level 5: As above, with eyes closed

Dosage
Repetitions: _____
Frequency: _____

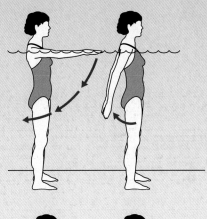

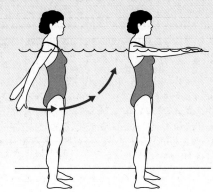

Bell Push-Downs). As resistance is increased, patients may alter their technique or posture to accommodate the resistance change. For example, adding gloves to bilateral shoulder horizontal abduction and adduction can increase the postural sway so much that the patient cannot maintain balance.

SELF-MANAGEMENT 16-2 *Bell Push-Downs*

Purpose: Increased abdominal strength
Increased trunk stability
Increased shoulder and arm strength

Position: Standing in chest-deep water, arms straight out in front with hands on a Styrofoam bell

Movement Technique:

Level 1: Tighten abdominal muscles and pull bell straight down toward legs. Control the bell on the way back up.

Level 2: Move to deeper water.

Level 3: Increase size of buoyant bell.

Dosage
Repetitions: _____
Frequency: _____

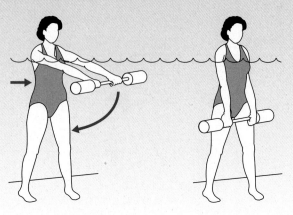

Starting position   *Ending position*

Cardiovascular endurance can be increased in several ways, relying on the same principles of overload and progression used in land-based programs. The activity must be of sufficient intensity and duration, use primarily large muscle groups, and should be performed three to five times per week. Deep-water activities are especially useful for individuals with weight-bearing limitations. Deep-water running, bicycling, cross-country skiing, and vertical kicking are only a few of the activities that can be performed continuously or as intervals. Traditional swimming strokes complement these lower extremity dominant exercises. Shallow-water running makes an excellent cardiovascular conditioning exercise if

BUILDING BLOCK 16-5

Design a beginning strengthening program for the case study patient, including activities that provide both direct resistance to the involved muscles as well as indirect challenges to the muscles.

SELF-MANAGEMENT 16-3 *Single-Leg Kicks*

Purpose: Increased hip mobility
Increased hip and knee muscle strength and endurance
Increased single-leg balance

Position: Standing on one leg in a neutral spine posture with abdominal muscles tightened. The non–weight-bearing leg should be straight at the knee and flexed at the ankle. If working primarily on balance, stand near the edge, but do not hold on to steady yourself. Otherwise, hold on to the side for support.

Movement Technique:

Level 1: Kick leg forward and back, ensuring proper spine position. Avoid arching your back as your leg comes back, and avoid letting your trunk sway.

Level 2: Add resistive equipment to foot or ankle.

Dosage
Repetitions: _____
Frequency: _____

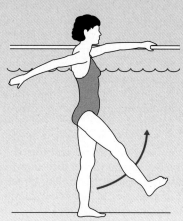

Starting position

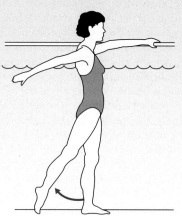

Ending position

impact is tolerated. Appropriate aquatic footwear must be worn when shallow-water running for any length of time. This can include an inexpensive surf shoe or a more expensive aquatic exercise shoe. This minimizes the likelihood of impact injuries and friction injuries to the bottom of the foot.

Balance Impairment

The supportive medium of the water and its destabilizing forces provide an ideal environment for balance training. Other individuals in the pool create turbulence and create destabilizing forces.[46] These forces can also be created by an individual's own movements. For example, kicking one leg forward produces a force pushing the individual backward

(see Self-Management 16-3: Single-Leg Kicks). The forward movement must be countered with balance responses. The increased reaction time makes these types of training movements especially useful for individuals with poor balance. Movements occur more slowly in the pool resulting from the water's viscosity. As such, when balance is lost, the fall is slowed dramatically, giving the individual time to react and respond.

A variety of balance activities performed on land can be adapted to the pool. Any single-leg stance exercise with concurrent movement of the arms, opposite leg, or both can provide a wealth of balance exercise. Single-toe raises, step-ups, and simple single-leg balance exercises can be performed with and without equipment (see Self- Management 16-4: Three-step Stop). Selected Intervention 16-3: Aquatic

 SELF-MANAGEMENT 16-4 *Three-Step Stop*

Purpose: Increased dynamic balance
Increased trunk stability
Increased lower extremity strength
Increased single-leg balance

Position: Standing on both legs in a neutral spine posture, with abdominal muscles tightened. Take three steps forward beginning with your right leg, then stop and balance on your right leg. Step back with the left leg for three steps, stopping to balance on the left leg. After several repetitions, switch to stepping with the left leg first.

Movement Technique:

Level 1: Use your arms as needed for balance.

Level 2: Place your arms across your chest.

Level 3: Close your eyes.

Dosage
Repetitions: _____
Frequency: _____

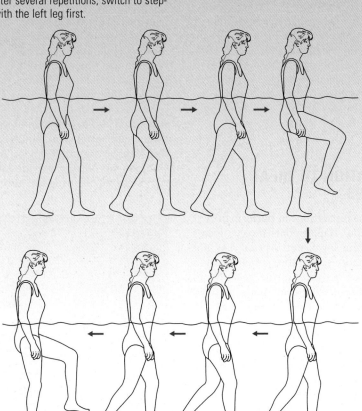

SELECTED INTERVENTION 16-3
Aquatic Therapy to Improve Balance

See Case Study No. 1

ACTIVITY: Single-leg balance in chest-deep water

PURPOSE: Train single-leg balance through entire lower extremity and trunk without full weight on the limb.

RISK FACTORS: No appreciable risk factors

ELEMENT OF THE MOVEMENT SYSTEM: Modulator

STAGE OF MOTOR CONTROL: Stability

POSTURE: Single-leg stance with arms in a comfortable position; lumbopelvic region in neutral and knee in slight flexion

MOVEMENT: None; simply maintain balance

DOSAGE: Repetitions to form fatigue or pain; attempt to hold as long as possible

FUNCTIONAL MOVEMENT PATTERN TO REINFORCE GOAL OF SPECIFIC EXERCISE: Single-leg stance of gait cycle

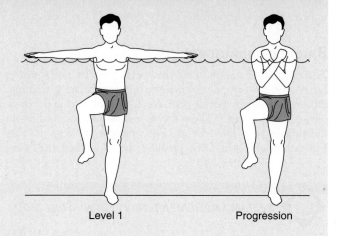

Level 1   Progression

Therapy to Improve Balance presents a sample of an aquatic exercise that may be prescribed for the client with balance impairment.

Research comparing the effects of balance training on land and in water found both mediums to result in improvements in the center of pressure variables, suggesting that balance training can be equally effective when performed in water.[47] The effects of a water-based program on balance, fear of falling, and quality of life was performed in community-dwelling older women with osteopenia or osteoporosis.[48] After a 10-week water-based and self-management program, the intervention group showed significant improvement over the control group in balance and quality of life, but not in fear of falling.

AQUATIC REHABILITATION TO TREAT ACTIVITY LIMITATIONS

Activity limitations represent restrictions in performance at the level of the whole person. Impairments involve losses at the tissue, organ, or system level, but may or may not contribute to activity limitations. As the patient makes improvements in impairments, activities in the pool should be modified to emphasize the activity limitations. Activity limitations related to posture or position can be addressed in the pool. If prolonged sitting is a functional limitation, a variety of sitting activities can be performed in the pool. Many pools contain steps where the patient can sit with various levels of depth (i.e., unloading). Chairs can be submerged in the pool, and buoyant equipment for sitting is available (Fig. 16-9). As sitting tolerance increases, the depth of water should be decreased, thereby more closely representing land situations. This same principle may be applied to deficiencies in prolonged standing or other positional limitations.

Activity limitations related to specific movement patterns (e.g., gait, forward reaching) respond well to aquatic rehabilitation. Unloading the lower extremity or spine alone is frequently adequate to normalize gait mechanics. Verbal or tactile cuing may be necessary if gait changes have existed for some time. Any impairments such as limitations in motion, endurance, or strength must be addressed concurrently. As normal pain-free gait mechanics are achieved, the water depth should begin decreasing to replicate the land-based environment. Similarly, other activity limitations in movement can be addressed in the same manner. For the individual with difficulty performing forward reaching, this activity can be assisted by buoyancy, which is progressed to buoyancy-supported and to buoyancy-resisted activity. Repetitive trunk flexion and extension, lifting, pushing, pulling, and squatting can be progressed in the same fashion (Fig. 16-10). Components of basic activities of daily living and instrumental activities of daily living can also be reproduced in the pool.

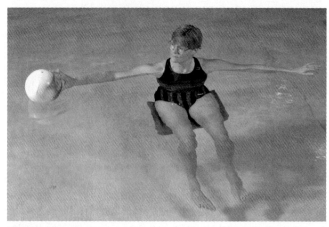

FIGURE 16-9. Posture exercises and reaching activities can be performed while sitting on flotation equipment.

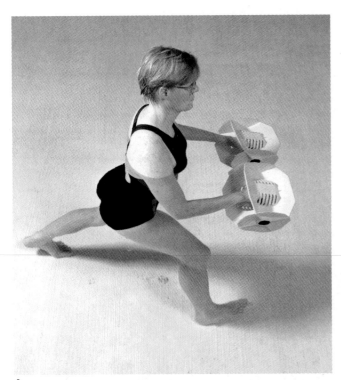
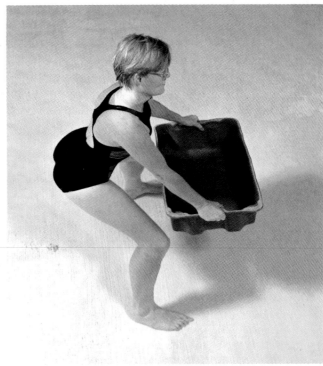

A   **B**

FIGURE 16-10. Work conditioning exercises such as (A) pushing and (B) lifting can be reproduced in the pool.

COORDINATING LAND AND WATER ACTIVITIES

One of the questions frequently asked by clinicians concerns the integration of water- and land-based activities. How much activity should be performed in the water, and when should land-based activity be incorporated? The advantages and disadvantages of aquatic rehabilitation and land rehabilitation should be matched to the needs of the individual patient, keeping in mind that humans function in a gravity environment. Because it is difficult to reproduce lower extremity eccentric muscle contractions in the pool, the patient should be progressed to land-based activities as quickly as tolerated. Early on, the patient may tolerate little land-based activity because of pain. Aquatic rehabilitation occupies most of the program at this time. As the patient is able to tolerate land-based activity, these exercises should be incorporated into the program. The quantity of water-based activity may remain unchanged, increase if tolerated, or decrease as the quantity of land-based exercise increases. The exact proportion and quantity of both land and water activity is determined by the needs and response of the patient. Occasionally, individuals respond better to alternate days in the pool, but others can progress to daily land-based exercises and discontinue pool exercise. The exercise program should be matched to the needs of the patient, with the goal of progressing to land-based exercise.

PATIENT-RELATED EDUCATION

As with land-based exercise, patient education is a key component of the aquatic physical therapy program. The education program begins before entry into the water with a discussion of the fundamental properties of the water and the patient's expectations. Ensure patient comfort in the water; this is enhanced by educating the patient about the anticipated experience in the water. Identify the areas of entry and exit from the pool, the water's depth, and any other important safety features (e.g., drop-offs, gutters, bars). Also familiarize the patient with the exercise program on land before entering the water to ensure proper exercise performance.

As the patient enters the water and the rehabilitation program proceeds, use this time as an opportunity to teach the patient about the expected benefits of the exercise. For example, when performing activities in single-leg stance, the patient frequently complains of an inability to maintain balance. Emphasize that developing balance is the purpose of the exercise and that any modification of the exercise to further destabilize the person is a progression of the exercise. When surface area–enhancing equipment is added, explain to the patient that it will increase the difficulty of the exercise. This also educates the patient on appropriate exercise program progression, and when the program is continued independently, the patient is able to self-manage and progress his or her own exercise program.

PRECAUTIONS/CONTRAINDICATIONS

Some absolute and relative contraindications to exercise in the water exist. Individuals with excessive fear of the water, open wounds, rashes, active infections, incontinence, or tracheostomy should not be admitted to the pool. However, some physicians allow patients with open wounds to participate in aquatic rehabilitation with use of a Bioclusive dressing. This is commonly seen in patients with postoperative incisions.

LAB ACTIVITIES

Pool Activities

1. Upper extremity
   a. Using a variety of positions (e.g., supine, prone, standing) and equipment (e.g., buoyant, resistive, wall, railings), develop an exercise program to increase a patient's shoulder, elbow, forearm, and wrist ROM in all available ranges. Do this for a variety of motion limitations (i.e., minimal loss to significant motion loss).
   b. Using a variety of positions and equipment, develop an exercise program to increase a patient's shoulder, elbow, forearm, and wrist strength and function. Progress from isometric exercise through a functional progression to activities of daily living, work, or sports. Perform open-and closed-chain exercises.
2. Lower extremity
   a. Using a variety of positions (e.g., supine, prone, standing) and equipment (e.g., buoyant, resistive, wall, railings) develop an exercise program to increase a patient's hip, knee, and ankle ROM in all available ranges. Do this for a variety of motion limitations (i.e., minimal loss to significant motion loss).
   b. Using a variety of positions and equipment, develop an exercise program to increase a patient's lower extremity strength and function. Progress from isometric exercise through a functional progression to activities of daily living, work, or sports. Perform open- and closed-chain exercises.
3. Trunk
   a. In an upright position, establish a neutral spine position and ambulate forward, backward, sidestepping, and braiding patterns. Vary step length, and observe resultant changes in ROM.
   b. In an upright position, perform a variety of upper extremity exercises, and observe the challenges to the trunk stabilizers. Perform exercises with a wide stance, narrow stance, and standing on one leg.
   c. In an upright position, perform a variety of lower extremity exercises, and observe the challenges to the trunk stabilizers. Notice the differences between sagittal plane and frontal plane motions.

Land Activities

Develop land-based and aquatic rehabilitation programs for the following patient problems. Progress the program from the acute phase through to a functional progression.

PATIENT No. 1

A 54-year-old man has L4–5 discogenic back pain. The patient has had recurrent episodes of pain over several years but has always been able to self-treat with a home exercise program designed by a physical therapist. Two weeks ago, the patient took a vacation requiring a long plane flight, followed by sleeping in a bed with a poor mattress. This patient has been unable to relieve the symptoms with self-treatment. His primary complaint is low back pain with occasional radicular pain to the left knee. Symptoms do not extend beyond the knee. The patient desires to return to walking as exercise and recreational golf. He works at a desk job.

Examination reveals an easily correctable lateral shift to the right, with decreased active and passive ROM in extension, left sidebending, and left rotation. Active motion is limited in flexion. Dural signs are positive for radicular symptoms, but deep tendon reflexes and sensation are intact throughout. The low back is diffusely tender, with a protective muscle spasm in the left erector spinae. Lower extremity strength is 5/5 to single repetition testing throughout.

PATIENT No. 2

A 60-year-old woman presents after a right proximal humeral fracture, which was cared for with sling immobilization for 6 weeks. She has a history of mild degenerative joint disease at the acromioclavicular joint. She is right-handed and complains primarily of an inability to perform her daily activities because of motion loss and shoulder pain. Her goals are to return to activities of daily living, golf, and gardening.

Examination reveals loss of motion in all shoulder motions in a capsular pattern. Elbow, wrist, and hand motions are normal. Strength tests are limited by shoulder pain. Accessory motion is slightly decreased compared with the left in anterior, posterior, and inferior directions. Strength and sensation are normal throughout the rest of the right upper extremity.

PATIENT No. 3

A 17-year-old girl is seen 6 weeks after abrasion chondroplasty for an acute osteochondral lesion on the weight-bearing surface of her right knee medial femoral condyle. Her goals are to return to basketball, softball, and volleyball. She is partial weight bearing (50%) and can be progressed by 25% every 2 to 3 weeks until full weight bearing is achieved.

Active motion of the knee is S:0-10-90 and passive motion is S:0-5-100 with an empty end-feel. She maintains a 1+ effusion and has 4+/5 strength to manual muscle test, with visible atrophy of the quadriceps. Hamstring muscle testing is 4+/5, gluteus maximus is 4+/5, and gluteus medius 4/5. She ambulates with an antalgic gait pattern with bilateral axillary crutches. Overall, she has a varus knee alignment.

Be aware of precautions to exercising in the water. The cardiovascular changes occurring with immersion should be of concern for the patient with a cardiac history. The hydrostatic pressure also limits chest expansion in those immersed in neck-deep water. This can create breathing difficulties for patients with pulmonary impairments or activity limitations. The hydrostatic pressure against the chest wall also can cause a sensation of an inability to breathe in persons who are uneasy in the water. The hydrostatic pressure produces diuresis, which can be avoided by emptying the bladder before entry to the pool.

Be alert to medical emergencies in the pool. It may be more difficult to respond to an emergency in the water, and an action plan must be in place. Be sure to know and practice safe removal of the patient from the water, and know the guidelines for implementing cardiopulmonary resuscitation in the pool.

Because of the sense of mobility experienced when exercising in the pool, many patients tend to overwork. Overexercise may occur because of the reduced gravity environment, the support of buoyancy, and the muscular relaxation associated with immersion, hydrostatic pressure, and water temperature. Frequently, the signs and symptoms of overwork do not manifest until later in the day or the next day. It therefore is better to err on the conservative side and underestimate the appropriate amount of exercise rather than overestimate.

KEY POINTS

- The pool provides a unique environment for the rehabilitation of individuals with a variety of impairments, activity limitations, and disabilities.
- The properties of buoyancy and viscosity can be used in a number of ways to achieve physical therapy goals.
- The effects of hydrostatic pressure and water temperature on the physiologic responses to activity must be considered to ensure patient safety.
- The water's viscosity provides much resistance and can be fatiguing for deconditioned individuals.
- Because a range of activities, from mobility and stretching to resistive and cardiovascular exercise, can be performed in the pool, aquatic therapy can progress from the early stages through functional progression.
- Balance is challenged with nearly every arm and leg movement in the pool, and the effects of exercises on the trunk and leg stabilizers must be considered when designing the exercise program.
- The pool program must be balanced by a well-designed land-based program to ensure proper transition back to the land environment.

CRITICAL THINKING QUESTIONS

1. How can the difficulty of the first selected intervention exercise (single-leg balance) be increased using the following?
   a. Arms
   b. Legs
   c. Equipment
   d. Other sensory systems
2. What factors might limit the patient's ability to perform this exercise?
3. How is this exercise changed in different water depths?
   a. Waist deep
   b. Neck deep
4. How is the exercise in Self-Management: Bell Push-Downs changed in different water depths?
   a. Chest deep
   b. Neck deep
5. How can mobility in internal rotation be improved while keeping the shoulders immersed?

REFERENCES

1. Beiser A. Physics. 2nd Ed. Menlo Park, CA: The Benjamin/Cummings Publishing Co., Inc., 1978.
2. Harrison RA, Hillman M, Bulstrode S. Loading the lower limb when walking partially immersed: implications for clinical practice. Physiotherapy 1992;78:164–166.
3. Skinner AT, Thomson AM, eds. Duffield's Exercise in Water. 3rd Ed. London: Bailliere Tindall, 1983.
4. Kelly BT, Roskin LA, Kirkendall DT, et al. Shoulder muscle activation during aquatic and dry land exercises in nonimpaired subjects. J Orthop Sports Phys Ther 2000;30:204–210.
5. Law LAF, Smidt GL. Underwater forces produced by the Hydro-Tone bell. J Orthop Sports Phys Ther 1996;23:267–271.
6. Poyhonen T, Keskinen K, Hautala A, et al. Determination of hydrodynamic drag forces and drag coefficients on human leg/foot model during knee exercise. Clin Biomech 2000;15(4):256–260.
7. Poyhonen T, Keskinen K, Kyrolainen, H, et al. Neuromuscular function during therapeutic knee exercise under water and on dry land. Arch Phys Med Rehabil 82(10) 2001;1446–1452.
8. Poyhonen T, Kyrolainen H, Keskinen K, et al. Electromyographic and kinematic analysis of therapeutic knee exercises under water. Clin Biomech 2001;16(6):496–504.
9. Arborelius M, Balldin UI, Lilja B, et al. Hemodynamic changes in man during immersion with the head above water. Aerospace Med 1972;43:592–598.
10. Christie JL, Sheldahl LM, Tristani FE, et al. Cardiovascular regulation during head-out water immersion exercise. J Appl Physiol 1990;69:657–664.
11. Green GH, Cable NT, Elms N. Heart rate and oxygen consumption during walking on land and in deep water. J Sports Med Phys Fitness 1990;30:49–52.
12. Risch WD, Koubenec HJ, Beckmann U, et al. The effect of graded immersion on heart volume, central venous pressure, pulmonary blood distribution, and heart rate in man. Pflugers Arch 1978;374:115–118.
13. Sheldahl LM, Tristani FE, Clifford PS, et al. Effect of head-out water immersion on response to exercise training. J Appl Physiol 1986;60:1878–1881.
14. Choukroun ML, Varene P. Adjustments in oxygen transport during head-out immersion in water at different temperatures. J Appl Physiol 1991;68:1475–1480.
15. Craig AB, Dvorak M. Thermal regulation of man exercising during water immersion. J Appl Physiol 1968;25:28–35.
16. Craig AB, Dvorak M. Comparison of exercise in air and in water at different temperatures. Med Sci Sports Exerc 1969;1:124–130.
17. Golden C, Tipton MJ. Human thermal responses during leg-only exercise in cold water. J Physiol 1987;391:399–405.
18. Golden C, Tipton MJ. Human adaptation to repeated cold immersions. J Physiol 1988;396:349–363.
19. Sagawa S, Shiraki K, Yousef MK, et al. Water temperature and intensity of exercise in maintenance of thermal equilibrium. J Appl Physiol 1988;2413–2419.
20. Avellini BA, Shapiro Y, Pandolf KB. Cardio-respiratory physical training in water and on land. Eur J Appl Physiol 1983;50:255–263.
21. Hamer PW, Morton AR. Water running: training effects and specificity of aerobic, anaerobic, and muscular parameters following an eight-week interval training programme. Aust J Sci Med Sport 1990;21:13–22.
22. Vickery SR, Cureton KG, Langstaff JL. Heart rate and energy expenditures during aqua dynamics. Physician Sports Med 1983;11:67–72.
23. Whitley JD, Schoene LL. Comparison of heart rate responses: water walking versus treadmill walking. Phys Ther 1987;67:1501–1504.
24. Eyestone ED, Fellingham G, George J, et al. Effect of water running and cycling on maximum oxygen consumption and 2-mile run performance. Am J Sports Med 1993;21:41–44.
25. Connelly TP, Sheldahl LM, Tristani FE, et al. Effect of increased central blood volume with water immersion on plasma catecholamines during exercise. J Appl Physiol 1990;69:651–656.
26. McMurray RG, Berry MJ, Katz VL, et al. Cardiovascular responses of pregnant women during aerobic exercise in the water: a longitudinal study. Int J Sports Med 1988;9:443–447.
27. Town GP, Bradley SS. Maximal metabolic responses of deep and shallow water running in trained runners. Med Sci Sports Exerc 1991;23:238–241.

28. Shono T, Fujishima K, Hotta N, et al. Physiological responses and RPE during underwater treadmill walking in women of middle and advanced age. J Physiol Anthropol Appl Human Sci 2000;19(4):195–200.

29. Gleim GW, Nicholas JA. Metabolic costs and heart rate responses to treadmill walking in water at different depths and temperatures. Am J Sports Med 1989;17:248–252.

30. Evans BW, Cureton KJ, Purvis JW. Metabolic and circulatory responses to walking and jogging in water. Res Q 1978;49:442–449.

31. Yamaji K, Greenley M, Northey DR, et al. Oxygen uptake and heart rate responses to treadmill and water running. Can J Sports Sci 1990;15:96–98.

32. Svedenhag J, Seger J. Running on land and in water: comparative exercise physiology. Med Sci Sports Exerc 1992;24:1155–1160.

33. Wilder RP, Brennan D, Schotte DE. A standard measure for exercise prescription for aqua running. Am J Sports Med 193;21:45–48.

34. Templeton MS, Booth DL, O'Kelly WD. Effects of aquatic therapy on joint flexibility and functional ability in subjects with rheumatic disease. J Orthop Sports Phys Ther 1996;23:376–381.

35. Takeshima N, Rogers ME, Watanabe E, et al. Water-based exercise improves health-related aspects of fitness in older women. Med Sci Sports Exerc 2002;33:544–551.

36. Tokmakidis SP, Spassis AT, Volaklis KA. Training, detraining and retraining effects after a water-based exercise program in patients with coronary artery disease. Cardiology 2008;111(4):257–264.

37. Cochrane T, Davey R, Matthes Edwards S. Randomised controlled trial of the cost-effectiveness of water-based therapy for lower limb osteoarthritis. Health Technol Assess 2005;9(31):1–114.

38. Foley A, Halbert J, Hewitt T, et al. Does hydrotherapy improve strength and physical function in patients with osteoarthritis: a randomised controlled trial comparing a gym based and a hydrotherapy based strengthening program. Ann Rheum Dis 2003;62:1162–1167.

39. Silva L, Valim V, Pessanha A, et al. Hydrotherapy versus conventional land-based exercise for the management of patients with osteoarthritis of the knee: a randomized clinical trial. Phys Ther 2008;88(1):12–21.

40. Hinman R, Heywood S, Day A. Aquatic physical therapy for hip and knee osteoarthritis: results of a single-blind randomized controlled trial. Phys Ther 2007;87(1):32–43.

41. Fransen M, Nairn L, Winstanley J, et al. Physical activity for osteoarthritis management: a randomized controlled clinical trial evaluating hydrotherapy or Tai Chi classes. Arthritis Rheum 2007;57(3):407–414.

42. Wyatt F, Milam S, Manske R, et al. The effects of aquatic and traditional exercise programs on persons with knee osteoarthritis. J Strength Cond Res 2001;15:337–340.

43. Bartels E, Lund H, Hagen K, et al. Aquatic exercise for the treatment of knee and hip osteoarthritis. (Protocol) Cochrane Database Syst Rev 2007 Oct 17;(4):CD005523.

44. Tsourlou T, Benik A, Dipla K, et al. The effects of a twenty-four-week aquatic training program on muscular strength performance in health elderly women. J Strength Cond Res 2006;20(4):811–818.

45. Ruoti RG, Troup JT, Berger RA. The effects of nonswimming water exercises on older adults. J Orthop Sports Phys Ther 1994;19:140–147.

46. D'Aquisto L, D'Aquisto D, Renne D. Metabolic and cardiovascular responses in older women during shallow water exercise. J Strength Cond Res 2001;15(12–19).

47. Roth A, Miller M, Ricard M, et al. Comparisons of static and dynamic balance following training in aquatic and land environments. J Sport Rehabil 2006;15(4):299–311.

48. Devereux K, Robertson D, Briffa N. Effects of a water-based program on women 65 years and over: a randomised controlled trial. Aust J Physiother 2005;51(2):102–108.

ADDITIONAL RESOURCES

Aquatic Physical Therapy Association: aquaticpt@assnoffice.com
Aquatic Resources Network: www.aquaticnet.com
Halliwick Method: www.halliwick.net
Ruoti R, Morris D, Cole AJ. Aquatic Rehabilitation. Philadelphia, PA: Lippincott Williams and Wilkins, 1997.

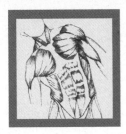

chapter 17

The Lumbopelvic Region

CARRIE M. HALL

Despite tremendous research on the topic of low back pain (LBP), the optimal treatment for patients with LBP remains largely enigmatic. Randomized clinical trials have failed to find consistent evidence for improved treatment outcomes with many treatment approaches commonly used by physical therapists and other practitioners including various forms of exercise, manual therapy, and traction.[1–3]

Underlying the difficulty in demonstrating the treatment effects of conservative management is the lack of consensus about classification of patients with lumbopelvic syndromes. Without a valid and reliable classification system, guidelines regarding conservative management for the patient with lumbopelvic syndrome–related signs and symptoms remain inexact.[4,5] As a result, the development of valid classification methods to assist the physical therapy management of patients with LBP has been recognized as a research priority.[6–15] There is growing evidence that the use of a classification approach to physical therapy management results in better clinical outcomes than the use of alternative management approaches. In 1995, Delitto et al.[7] proposed a classification system intended to inform and direct the physical therapy management of patients with LBP. The system described four classifications of patients with LBP (manipulation, stabilization, specific exercise, and traction). Each classification could be identified by a unique set of examination criteria and was associated with an intervention strategy believed to result in the best outcomes for the patient. The system was based on expert opinion and research evidence available at the time. A substantial amount of research has emerged in the years since Delitto's publication, including the development of clinical prediction rules, providing new evidence for the examination criteria used to place a patient into a classification and for the optimal intervention strategies for each classification. As research emerges, new evidence should continually be incorporated into existing classification systems. A case in point, in 2007, Fritz et al.[15] presented a clinical commentary reviewing Delitto's classification system, the evolution and status of the system, and discussed the implications for the classification of patients with low back pain. However, the classification scheme presented by Fritz is only one of many presented in the literature.[16–19]

It appears that outcomes of physical therapy care can be improved when patients are classified appropriately and treated accordingly, despite the method of classification that is used. At the time of this publication, the physical therapist is urged to remain aware of the current research regarding classification, and base intervention, and more specific to this text—therapeutic exercise intervention—on a thorough and systematic examination and evaluation process and focus the diagnosis on the underlying *cause(s)* of the presenting activity limitations and participation restrictions. Traditionally, the medical model has attempted to classify individuals based on a pathoanatomical source of symptoms; however, identifying relevant pathology in patients with LBP has proved elusive and is believed to be identified in <10% of cases.[20] Diagnostic imagery, such as radiography, magnetic resonance imaging, and computed tomography scans, produces substantial numbers of false positive findings, indicating pathology in asymptomatic individuals.[21] Effective intervention cannot be limited to treatment of pathology or disease; it must also address the disturbance in body functions and structures most closely associated with the underlying cause of the patient's reduced activity and participation levels. Exercise prescription should be based on individual and ongoing assessment of the activity and participation levels and associated body functions and structures. Despite the wide variety of exercises that are prescribed for the low back, evidence-based data to justify choices are not as complete as one may think or expect. The professional challenges regarding exercise prescription require the blend of knowledge, experience, and research.

REVIEW OF ANATOMY AND KINESIOLOGY

Prerequisite to sound clinical decision making in the patient management process (see Chapter 1) is an extensive knowledge of anatomy and kinesiology. The anatomy and kinesiology of the lumbopelvic region have received considerable attention in the literature,[22–26] which has enhanced clinical understanding of the function of the lumbopelvic region and emphasized the integrated nature of normal movement between the trunk and extremities. To properly examine, evaluate, diagnose, and treat the lumbopelvic region, in-depth knowledge of all aspects of the movement system involved in

LBP is essential. It is beyond the scope of this text to provide a complete review of the anatomy and kinesiology of the lumbopelvic region; thus, the review will be limited to myology. Further elaboration of anatomy and kinesiology can be found on the Web site.

Myology

Optimal function of the lumbopelvic region requires an integration of the musculature of the posterior and anterior aspects of the spine, pelvis, and hips. In addition, the latissimus dorsi influences lumbopelvic mechanics. Because of the integration of musculature spanning the lumbopelvic region, myology is addressed in an integrated format for the entire region.

Posterior Lumbopelvic Myology

The thoracolumbar fascia (TLF) and its powerful muscular attachments play an important role in stabilization of the lumbopelvic region.[27,28] Numerous muscular attachments into the TLF have been described, including attachments of transversus abdominis (TrA) and some fibers of the internal obliques (IO) into the lateral raphe portion of the TLF and attachments of gluteus maximus, latissimus dorsi, erector spinae, and biceps femoris into the posterior layer of TLF (Fig. 17-1). This pattern suggests that the hip, pelvic, and leg muscles interact with arm and spinal muscles through the TLF.[27] The gluteus maximus and latissimus dorsi may conduct forces contralaterally through the posterior layer of the TLF, and the action of these two muscles may be linked to provide support to the sacroiliac joint (SIJ) and lumbar spine during gait and rotation of the trunk. This integrated system has also been proposed as a method of load transference between the spine and hips, in which the TLF is a centrally placed structure for the interaction of muscles from each region.

The spinal extensors may be broadly categorized as superficial muscles (i.e., iliocostalis), which travel the length of the spine and attach to the sacrum and pelvis, and deep muscles (i.e., longissimus and lumbar multifidus [LM]), which span the lumbar segments. Even though the superficial spinal extensors do not attach directly to the lumbar spine, they have an optimal lever arm for lumbar extension by virtue of

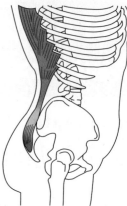

FIGURE 17-2. When viewed from the side, the superficial erector spinae can be seen to course superiorly and posteriorly from its point of origin at the pelvis to its attachment to the ribs. Elongation of the muscle occurs when the thorax (on the same side as the superficial erector spinae) is brought even further posterior, or the iliac crest on the same side is brought forward. Shortening of the superficial erector spinae occurs with thorax or pelvis movement opposite those just described. (Adapted from Porterfield JA, DeRosa C. Mechanical Low Back Pain: Perspectives in Functional Anatomy. 2nd Ed. Philadelphia, PA: WB Saunders, 1998.)

their attachments (Fig. 17-2). By pulling the thorax posteriorly, they can create an extension moment at the lumbar spine. They function eccentrically to control descent of the trunk during forward bending and isometrically to control the position of the lower thorax with respect to the pelvis during functional movements.[29,30] The attachment of the superficial spinal extensors also influences SIJ mechanics. Because of the attachment of the erector spinae aponeurosis to the sacrum, the pull of the erector spinae tendon on the dorsal aspect of the sacrum induces a flexion moment (i.e., nutation) of the sacrum on the ilium (Fig. 17-3).

The deep erector spinae have a poor lever arm for spine extension but are aligned to provide a dynamic counterforce to the anterior shear force imparted to the lumbar spine from gravitational force (Fig. 17-4). The attachment of the LM to the spinous process provides a good lever arm for spinal extension (Fig. 17-5). During forward-bending motions, this

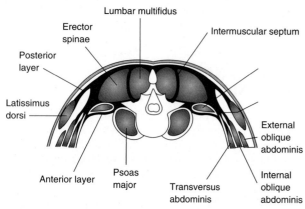

FIGURE 17-1. Cross-section of the lumbar spine showing layers of the trunk musculature. (Adapted from Porterfield JA, DeRosa C. Mechanical Low Back Pain: Perspectives in Functional Anatomy. 2nd Ed. Philadelphia, PA: WB Saunders, 1998.)

Lumbar multifidus
Erector spinae
Intermuscular septum
Posterior layer
Latissimus dorsi
Anterior layer
Psoas major
Transversus abdominis
Internal oblique abdominis
External oblique abdominis

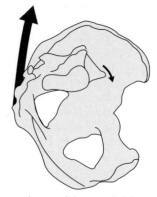

FIGURE 17-3. The attachment of the superficial erector spinae to the sacrum provides a potential force for sacral nutation (sacral flexion). Because nutation increases sacral stability, the superficial erector spinae may play a role in force closure of the sacroiliac joint. (Adapted from Porterfield JA, DeRosa C. Mechanical Low Back Pain: Perspectives in Functional Anatomy. 2nd Ed. Philadelphia, PA: WB Saunders, 1998.)

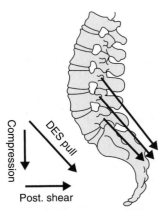

FIGURE 17-4. Because the deep erector spinae (DES) attach close to the axis of lumbar motion, the muscle group provides a dynamic posterior shear and compression force (*arrows*). This muscle can provide a force to prevent anterior translation. (Adapted from Porterfield JA, DeRosa C. Mechanical Low Back Pain: Perspectives in Functional Anatomy. 2nd Ed. Philadelphia, PA: WB Saunders, 1998.)

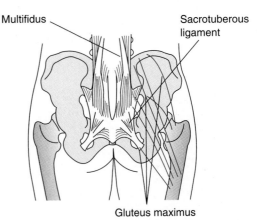

FIGURE 17-6. Anatomic relationship of lumbar multifidus (LM) to the sacroiliac joint, sacrotuberous ligament, and gluteus maximus. The LM attaches to the TLF primarily through a raphe separating the multifidus and gluteus maximus. The anterior border of the raphe is anchored to the SIJ capsule and the posterior border of the raphe becomes part of the TLF. Tendinous slips of the multifidus pass under the long dorsal SI ligament to join with the sacrotuberous ligament; these connections are thought to integrate the LM into the ligamentous support system of the SIJ. (Adapted from Porterfield JA, DeRosa C. Mechanical Low Back Pain: Perspectives in Functional Anatomy. 2nd Ed. Philadelphia, PA: WB Saunders, 1998.)

muscle contributes to controlling the rate and magnitude of flexion and anterior shear.[31] Because of its deep location, short fiber span, and oblique orientation, the LM is thought to stabilize against flexion and rotation forces on the lumbar spine.[32,33] Several studies have illuminated its relationship with the vertebral segment.[34–36] In a study of normal subjects without LBP, it seems that the deep fibers of the multifidi, along with the TrA, are the first muscles to become active when a limb is moved in response to a visual stimulus and fire independent of limb movement direction to control intervertebral movement.[37] The superficial fibers are also activated before the muscles that move the limb, but the timing of this seems to be dependent on the direction the limb is moved to assist with control of spinal orientation.[37] The LM also contributes to dynamic stability of the SIJ. Because it is attached to the sacrotuberous ligament, tension on the ligament imparted as a result of LM muscle contraction potentially increases the ligamentous stabilizing mechanisms of the SIJ (Fig. 17-6).

The effect of dysfunction of this muscle, discussed in detail in a later section, further emphasizes its important role in spine stabilization.

Anterior Lumbopelvic Myology

One of the most important muscle groups contributing to mobility and stability of the lumbopelvic region is the abdominal wall mechanism. The abdominal wall consists of, superficial to deep, the rectus abdominis (RA), external oblique (EO), IO, and TrA. The RA, EO, and IO appear to serve a relatively more dynamic role than the TrA.

The TrA is circumferential, situated deeply, and has attachments to the TLF, the sheath of RA, the diaphragm, iliac crest, and the lower six costal surfaces.[38] Because of its unique anatomic features, such as its deep location, its link to fascial support systems, its fiber type distribution, and its possible activity against gravitational load during standing and gait, the TrA is an important stabilizing muscle for the lumbar spine.[39–47] The TrA activates before the onset of limb movement in persons without LBP, but this function is lost in those with LBP.[39,48] Current theory suggests that this muscle is a key background stabilizing muscle for the lumbar spine and that the emphasis of specific exercises for the abdominal wall should involve specific recruitment of the TrA instead of general strengthening or endurance. Exercises of this nature are described in detail in a subsequent section of this chapter.

The oblique abdominal muscles working synergistically provide an anterior oblique sling and, together with the posterior oblique sling (i.e., TLF and associated structures), they assist in stabilization of the lumbar spine and pelvis in an integrated system of myofascial support.[49,50] The right EO works synergistically with the left IO to produce rotation to the left and to prevent excessive rotation when necessary. The LM must synergically contract to prevent flexion imposed by the obliques so that pure rotation or transverse-plane stabilization can occur. The inferior and medial directions of the

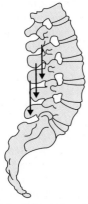

FIGURE 17-5. Because of the LM insertion, there is a large vertical vector for extension, with a small horizontal vector indicating it is a stabilizer of rotation rather than horizontal rotation being its primary function. The primary vector is to provide posterior sagittal rotation. The primary rotators of the trunk are the oblique abdominals that, by virtue of their vertical vector, cause a flexion moment as well as rotation, which is stabilized by the LM. (Adapted from Bogduk N, Twomey LT. Clinical Anatomy of the Lumbar Spine. Edinburgh: Churchill Livingstone, 1987.)

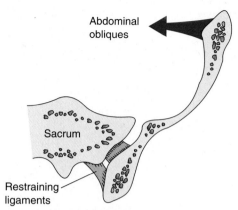

FIGURE 17-7. Contraction of the abdominal oblique muscles acting over the fulcrum of the interosseous ligament increases sacroiliac joint stability and pubic symphysis compression. (Adapted from Porterfield JA, DeRosa C. Mechanical Low Back Pain: Perspectives in Functional Anatomy. 2nd Ed. Philadelphia, PA: WB Saunders, 1998.)

fibers of the EO are positioned to prevent anterior pelvic tilt and anterior pelvic shear. With respect to the SIJ, the oblique abdominals provide compressive forces between the two pubic bones and at the SIJ posteriorly (Fig. 17-7).

Associated Pelvic, Hip, and Upper Extremity Myology

Twenty-nine muscles originate or insert into the pelvis. Twenty of these link the pelvis with the femur, and nine link the pelvis with the spine. This implies that significant forces can be generated through the pelvis and subsequently through the lumbar spine by various combinations of knee and hip muscle activity.

The iliacus and psoas major have significant attachments to the spine and pelvis. If not counterstabilized by the abdominal muscles, the iliacus can exert an anterior rotation force on the pelvis. If not counterstabilized by the deep erector spinae, LM, and abdominal muscles, the psoas major can exert an anterior translational force on lumbar segments.

The fibers of the gluteus maximus muscle run perpendicular to the plane of the SIJ and blend with the TLF and the contralateral latissimus dorsi.[23] Compression of the SIJ occurs when the gluteus maximus and the contralateral latissimus dorsi contract. This oblique system crosses the midline and is believed to be a significant contributor to load transference through the pelvic girdle during rotational activities and during gait.[23,49] The TLF is tensed by contraction of gluteus maximus, latissimus dorsi, and erector spinae muscles.

In addition to the attachment to the ischial tuberosity, the long head of the biceps femoris attaches to the sacrotuberous ligament. Contraction of the biceps femoris increases tension of the sacrotuberous ligament and pulls the sacrum against the ilium, effectively increasing the stability of the SIJ.[43]

In standing and walking, the pelvic girdle is stabilized on the femur by the coordinated action of the ipsilateral gluteus medius and minimus and by the contralateral adductor muscles. Indirectly, by maintaining a relationship between the hip, pelvis, and lumbar spine in the frontal plane, the gluteus medius, gluteus minimus, and adductors contribute to lumbar spine stability. Although these muscles are not directly involved in force closure of the SIJ, they play a significant role in pelvic girdle function.

The piriformis is considered to be part of the deep hip lateral rotator group and pelvic floor. It appears to play a vital role for stabilization of the SIJ. The piriformis attaches to the sacrum, the anterior surface of the sacrotuberous ligament, and the medial edge of the SIJ capsule. This muscle anchors the apex of the sacrum and controls sacral nutation.

The link of pelvic floor function and lumbopelvic function should not be underestimated. The pelvic floor forms the base of the abdominal cavity, so pelvic floor muscles must contract during tasks that elevate intraabdominal pressure to maintain continence and contribute to pressure increases. In subjects without LBP, strong voluntary abdominal muscle contraction caused pelvic floor muscle activity at the same intensity as maximal pelvic floor muscle effort. The pelvic floor does not simply respond to increases in intraabdominal pressure; instead, the pelvic floor muscles contract before the abdominal muscles.[51] One investigator found that some patients with chronic low back pain (CLBP) were unable to recruit the TrA without prior contraction of the pelvic floor.[44]

Gait

Gait is a vital functional activity. Table 17-1 displays the biomechanics and muscle function of the gait cycle of the lumbopelvic region.

EXAMINATION AND EVALUATION

The purpose of any examination/evaluation is to establish a diagnosis of the *source* (pathoanatomic diagnosis), if possible, and the underlying *cause* (pathomechanical diagnosis) of the presenting signs, symptoms, activity limitations and participation restrictions. However, the specific *source* of symptoms originating in the lumbopelvic region is difficult to diagnose. A pathoanatomic diagnosis is possible for approximately 70% of patients with CLBP if those patients with documented psychologic aggravation of their symptoms are excluded.[52] Even when a pathoanatomic diagnosis is provided, it cannot, in and of itself, guide decisions regarding intervention in the management of lumbopelvic conditions. Structural changes do not necessarily correlate with or predict levels of pain or disability.[53] Removal or correction of structural abnormalities of the lumbar spine may fail to cure or even worsen painful conditions.[54] Without a diagnosis that can guide patient management, use of a traditional pathoanatomic model (i.e., one that implies symptoms should be proportional to organ pathology) is limited.

The goal of the physical therapy examination is to determine the pathomechanical cause(s) of the patient's activity limitations and participation restrictions. However, that being said, examination can lead the examiner to a pathoanatomic diagnosis for the small percentage of patients in whom a precise structural fault can be ascribed. A pathoanatomic diagnosis can only be made by correlating the physical examination findings with the history and medical findings (i.e., radiographic, neurologic, and laboratory study results).

A pathomechanic approach to diagnosis of LBP is valuable for several reasons:

- It reveals to the examiner and the patient the type and direction of the mechanical stress that correlates with symptoms.
- It reveals physiologic impairments that correlate with the mechanical stress.

TABLE 17-1   Kinematics and Muscle Activity of the Gait Cycle in the Lumbopelvic Region

PHASES OF THE GAIT CYCLE	RANGE OF MOTION LUMBAR SPINE	RANGE OF MOTION PELVIC GIRDLE[a]	MUSCLE ACTIVITY LUMBAR SPINE[b]	MUSCLE ACTIVITY PELVIC GIRDLE[c]
Initial contact	Sidebending ipsilateral/ rotation contralateral	Small cranial/caudal shear; ipsilateral innominate rotates posteriorly/contralateral innominate rotates anteriorly	Bilateral erector spinae	HS, gluteus maximus[d]
Loading response	As at initial contact			
Midstance	As at initial contact	Ipsilateral innominate rotates anteriorly toward neutral; contralateral innominate rotates posteriorly toward neutral		
Terminal stance	Preparing for initial swing	Ipsilateral innominate rotates anteriorly past neutral; contralateral innominate rotates posteriorly	Bilateral erector spinae[e]	
Preswing	Preparing for initial swing			
Initial swing	Contralateral side-bend/ ipsilateral rotation			
Midswing	As initial swing			
Terminal swing	As initial swing			

[a]The motion of the sacrum between the two innominates and adjacent fifth lumbar vertebra has been described as a complex, polyaxial, torsional movement that occurs about the oblique axes. (Greenman PE. Principles of Manual Medicine. Baltimore, MD: Williams & Wilkins, 1989; Beal MC. The sacroiliac problem: review of anatomy, mechanics and diagnosis. J Am Osteopath Assoc 1982;81:667–679.)

[b]Discrepancy exists regarding activity of RA and obliqui externus and internus, perhaps because of speeds of walking during testing conditions. (Waters RL, Morris JM. Electrical activity of muscles of the trunk during walking. J Anat 1972;111:191–199; Sheffield FJ. Electromyographic study of the abdominal muscles in walking and other movements. Am J Phys Med 1962;41:142–147.) TrA and LM appear to be linked with the control of stability of the spine against the perturbation produced by the movement of the limbs and should be considered as active during the gait cycle. (Hodges PW, Richardson CA. Contraction of the abdominal muscles associated with movement of the lower limb. Phys Ther 1997;77:132–144.)

[c]Much of the muscle activity occurring across the pelvic girdle during gait is discussed in Chapter 20. Additional information regarding the link between the hip, the lumbopelvic region, and the upper extremity are provided in this table.

[d]HS activity increases the tension in the sacrotuberous ligament and contributes to the force closure mechanism of the pelvic girdle with loading of the limb. (Wingarden JP, Vleeming A, Snidjers CJ, et al. A functional-anatomical approach to the spine-pelvis mechanism: interaction between the biceps femoris muscle and the sacrotuberous ligament. Eur Spine J 1993;2:140; Snijders CJ, Vleeming A, Stoeckart R. Transfer of lumbosacral load to iliac bones and legs. Part 1: biomechanics of self-bracing of the sacroiliac joints and its significance for treatment and exercise. Clin Biomech 1993;8:285–300; Vleeming A, Stoeckart R, Snijders CJ. The sacrotuberous ligament: a conceptual approach to its dynamic role in stabilizing the sacroiliac joint. J Clin Biomech 1989;4:201–203.) Gluteus maximus becomes active with counter-rotation of the trunk and arm swing forward, resulting in lengthening of the contralateral latissimus dorsi muscle. Shortly thereafter, the arm swings backward, causing contraction of the contralateral latissimus dorsi. Lengthening and contraction of the latissimus dorsi contributes to increased tension in the TLF and thereby contributing to further force closure mechanism of the SIJ. (Lee D. Instability of the sacroiliac joint and the consequences to gait. J Manual Manipulative Ther 1996;4:22–29.) Gluteus maximus activity is key to force closure stabilizing mechanisms within the pelvis; loss of function of the gluteus maximus can hinder stability of the SIJ (Inman VT, Ralston HJ, Todd F. Human Walking. Baltimore, MD: Williams & Wilkins, 1981.)

[e]Battye CK, Joseph J. An investigation by telemetering of the activity of some muscles in walking. Med Biol 1966;4:125–135.

- It screens for pathology and anatomic and psychologic impairments that affect the prognosis.
- It becomes the basis for a therapeutic exercise program and for posture and movement retraining.
- It may improve research by denoting homogenous subgroups for treatment outcome studies.[55]

The key to pathomechanical testing of the lumbopelvic region is determining the postures and movements that correlate with the patient's signs or symptoms.[55] It can then be deduced what type and direction of forces exceed the tissue tolerance or adaptability and lead to mechanical or chemical stimulation of the nociceptive system. Physiological impairments that contribute to the pathomechanical cause can be determined and linked to the activity and participation restrictions because the diagnosis is based on the underlying mechanical cause of symptoms. For example, if it is determined that prolonged, excessive, or repeated extension of the lumbar spine is the underlying cause of symptoms, the patient will be guided to adjust postures (i.e., lordotic sitting posture) and movements (i.e., lumbar extension associated with overhead arm movements) and activities (i.e., swimming, running) associated with extension.

With all examination/evaluation processes, if the examiner is unable to correlate the history and physical examination findings with a mechanical cause, the source of the symptoms may be nonmechanical, and referral to a medical practitioner is indicated for further diagnostics (see Appendix 1).

The clinician examining a patient with a lumbopelvic syndrome has the responsibility of answering three critical questions by the end of the initial examination:

1. Is there a systemic or visceral disease underlying the pain (see Appendix 1)?
2. Is there evidence of neurologic compromise that represents a surgical emergency (e.g., cauda equina symptoms)?
3. Are there mechanical findings that guide conservative management?

DISPLAY 17-1
History Items in Patients with LBP or SIJ Syndrome

Disk Disease[190]

- Low back pain
- Burning, stabbing, "electrical" pain down the leg
- Numbness or paresthesia (sensitivity 30% to 74% for paresthesia)*
- Aggravated by increased intradiskal pressure or specific movements
- Substantial but not complete relief with rest
- Radicular distribution pain (sensitivity of 95% for sciatic distribution of pain)[21]
- Leg pain greater than back pain
- Pain superficial and sharp rather than less well-defined, dull, aching
- Sensitivity for sciatic distribution of pain of 79% to 95%*

ZJ Syndrome

- ZJs do not cause referred pain exclusively in the central lumbar spine**
- ZJs may refer pain into the leg below the knee possibly due to segmental facilitation as a result of nociceptive input from a painful structure elsewhere in the affected segment***

SIJ Syndrome

- Groin pain**
- Pain inferior to the posterior superior iliac spine (PSIS)****
- Radicular symptoms may occur as a result of extravasation of inflammatory mediators through a capsular recess or tear to adjacent neural structures[†]

Cauda Equina Syndrome[200]

- Sensitivity of 95% for urinary retention[21]

- Sensitivity higher than 80% for motor weakness and decreased sensation in the legs[21]
- LBP
- Bilateral or unilateral sciatica
- Sensitivity of 75% for saddle area hyperesthesia[21]
- Sexual dysfunction (decreased sensation during intercourse, decreased penile sensation, and impotence)
- L5–S1 central disk herniation may cause no motor or reflex changes in the legs

Stenotic Syndrome[21]

- 60% sensitivity for neurogenic claudication
- 85% sensitivity for leg pain
- 60% sensitivity for neurologic abnormalities

Van den Hoogen HMM, Koes BW, Van Eijk JTM, et al. On the accuracy of history, physical examination, and erythrocyte sedimentation rate in diagnosing low back pain in general practice. Spine 1995;19:1132–1137.

**Schwarzer AC, April CN, Derby R, et al. Clinical features of patients with pain stemming from the lumbar zygophyseal joints. Spine 1994;19:1132–1137.*

***Mooney V, Robertson J. The facet syndrome. Clin Orthop 1976;115:149–156.*

****Fortin JD, Dwyer AP, West S, et al. Sacroiliac joint: pain referral maps upon applying a new injection/arthrography technique, part I: asymptomatic volunteers. pine 1994;19:1483–1489; Fortin JD, Pier J, Falco F. Sacroiliac joint injection: pain referral mapping and arthrographic findings. In: Vleeming A, Mooney V, Dorman T, et al., eds. Movement, Stability & Low Back Pain. New York, NY: Churchill Livingstone, 1997.*

[†]Fortin JD, Pier J, Falco F. Sacroiliac joint injection: pain referral mapping and arthrographic findings. In: Vleeming A, Mooney V, Dorman T, et al., eds. Movement, Stability & Low Back Pain. New York, NY: Churchill Livingstone, 1997.

Data collected from the history and physical examination should provide an answer to all three questions. A hypothesis as to the diagnosis can be generated and a plan of care established. The underlying source and/or cause diagnosis will drive the total plan of care, particularly the therapeutic exercise portion. For that reason, we will review the conceptual framework behind each portion of the examination as it relates to therapeutic exercise intervention.

Patient History

Making an accurate diagnosis is, to a large extent, dependent on having a clear understanding of the patient's medical history and current symptoms. In addition to the general data collected from a patient/client history as defined in Chapter 2, special questions regarding symptoms related to the low back can begin the clinical reasoning process toward diagnosis. Research on validity of history findings with respect to LBP generally uses a pathoanatomic classification system. The research presented in Display 17-1 uses diagnostic labels of disk disease, ZJ syndrome, SIJ syndrome, cauda equina syndrome, and stenotic syndrome. For detailed list of questions, please refer to Magee's text.[56]

Screening Examination

Symptoms originating in the lumbopelvic region often are experienced elsewhere in the lower quadrant and symptoms mimicking lumbopelvic origin dysfunction can originate in

visceral tissues (see Appendix 1). It is for these reasons that a lumbopelvic screen is recommended before any lumbopelvic or lower quadrant examination. The purpose of the screening examination is to determine whether symptoms experienced in the lower quadrant are originating in the lumbopelvic region. If it is determined that symptoms are stemming from the lumbopelvic region, a more thorough lumbopelvic examination and evaluation is indicated. Display 17-2 lists the tests that should be included in any lumbopelvic screening examination.

DISPLAY 17-2
Lumbopelvic Scan Evaluation

Observation: Posture scan in standing and sitting, local signs of skin color, texture, scars, soft-tissue contours
Active range of motion (with overpressure if indicated): In standing, flexion, extension, lateral flexion; in sitting, rotation
Stress tests: Supine lumbar compression and distraction, supine sacroiliac joint compression and distraction, sidelying sacroiliac joint compression, prone lumbar torsion stress
Provocative test: Prone posteroanterior pressure to the lumbar spine
Palpation: Palpate-related lumbar-pelvic-hip musculature, assessing for tone changes, lesions, and pain provocation
Dural mobility tests: Slump test, straight-leg raise, prone knee flexion
Neurologic testing: Key muscles (see Table 18-3), reflexes, dermatomes

Tests and Measures

The following sections describe, in alphabetical order, the tests and measures highlighted in any lumbopelvic examination/evaluation. The tests and measures must be individualized based on the data collected from the history, systems review, and screening examination. Additional tests and measures may be included on a case-by-case basis. The reader is referred to the *Guide to Physical Therapist Practice* for a detailed list of physical therapy tests and measures.[57]

Anthropometric Characteristics

Anthropometric characteristics may be of interest, whereas an individual's unique anthropometric characteristics can be a risk factor in developing certain types of lumbopelvic syndromes. For example, the anthropometric characteristics of a male with broad shoulders, narrow pelvis, and high center of mass promote lumbar flexion versus hip flexion during forward bend movements. This may pose as a risk factor in developing LBP.[58] In addition, he may have difficulty returning to a job requiring bending and lifting without careful attention to body mechanics limiting lumbar flexion forces.

Ergonomics and Body Mechanics

An assessment of a patient's job-related duties and physical demands should include ergonomic and body mechanic assessment. This may include assessing material handling capabilities, such as lifting incrementally increasing weights at different heights. Assessment of non–material handling capabilities includes tasks such as sitting or standing tolerance, or work station ergonomics. These kinds of assessments are often termed functional capacity evaluations (FCEs). FCEs can be purchased or designed in the clinic and may use expensive mechanical devices interfaced with computers, or inexpensive handmade boxes, crates, and push/pull sleds. One important point to maintain concerning the validity of a FCE is that an FCE, conducted from 2 to 4 hours over 1 to 2 days of a person's life at a given point in time, cannot predict a person's capacity to work for 8 to 10 hours per day, 4 to 6 days per week, 52 weeks per year. At best, the FCE may simulate certain skills and capacities needed to perform the job. The FCE should be used as one aspect of the injured person's examination, not as a complete evaluation in and of itself.

Gait/Balance

Gait is a complex functional movement pattern that can indicate pathomechanical factors contributing to lumbopelvic signs or symptoms, particularly if the patient reports that walking increases or decreases symptoms. The relationship of other regions to the lumbopelvic region is important in ascertaining the mechanical stress imposed on the lumbar spine. For example, a hypomobile supinated foot that does not adequately pronate during the stance phase of gait may increase compressive stress on the lumbar spine, whereas a hypermobile pronated foot may induce a transverse-plane stress on the lumbar spine by creating a short limb during the stance phase of gait. Video analysis can be an efficient tool to evaluate the complex interaction of multiple regions on the lumbar spine during walking or running. Incorporating findings from a gait evaluation to other tests of measures can assist the practitioner in developing a specific exercise program to remediate the impairments related to gait deviation. Once

quality of gait improves, it can be used as more effective activity to improve endurance and serve as a graded exercise to reduce fear avoidance behaviors.[59]

Muscle Performance

The ability for the abdominal, spinal extensor, and pelvic girdle muscles to carry out functions of mobility and stability must be carefully assessed to ascertain the pathomechanics of the lumbopelvic region. Muscle performance testing includes tests of strength, power, and endurance adequate for each individual to carry out his or her desired controlled mobility (basic activities of daily living [BADLs]) and skill-level activities (instrumental activities of daily living [IADLs]).

Assessment of the force- or torque-generating capability of the spinal extensor and abdominal muscle groups can be performed with traditional manual muscle testing procedures as described by Kendall et al.[60] Because of the numerous details regarding accurate assessment of the abdominal muscles, Kendall's work should be reviewed to ensure optimal manual muscle testing results.

Although objective information about muscle force or torque production can be gathered from isokinetic testing, gross strength testing by this method may not be sensitive to the function of the deeper musculature surrounding the spine. Whereas many studies demonstrate an unequivocal relationship between impaired function of the deep abdominal and LM muscles and LBP, studies comparing gross trunk strength in normal or LBP patients have not consistently demonstrated such a relationship.[61–66] This difference may reflect the inherent limitations in conclusions that can be ascertained from studies examining maximal trunk strength in persons with LBP. For example, pain can hinder maximal effort, and a test of a patient with LBP may be more a test of the patient's tolerance to pain. This design problem may be responsible for the varied and seemingly contradictory results of trunk muscle strength reported in the literature.

Isokinetic testing of trunk muscle strength also focuses largely on the assessment of muscles primarily involved in and capable of producing large torques about the spine (e.g., RA, thoracolumbar erector spinae) rather than on muscles considered to provide stability and fine control (e.g., TrA and LM).[67,68] Most studies focus on maximal voluntary contractions, which are rarely carried out during the ADLs. In the CLBP population, sudden, unexpected, and insignificant movement at low load can exacerbate symptoms just as commonly as tasks involving maximal exertion.[69,70]

Isokinetic and traditional manual muscle testing may not be sensitive enough to assess the muscle performance of the deep trunk muscles (i.e., TrA and LM). Testing of trunk muscle strength should also consider the function of the deeper musculature. Tests that examine the ability of the deep trunk muscles to stabilize against various directional forces during active extremity movement can provide the clinician with an indication of their muscle performance.[8,71] High repetitions can provide an indication of the endurance of the trunk muscles. When the spine is unable to remain stable against a specific direction of force, it can indicate a lack of motor control, force or torque production, or fatigue (depending on the focus of the test) of the associated trunk muscle(s).

In theory, resisted testing of the trunk muscles can also provide information about the integrity of the trunk muscles relative to imposed strain. However, resisted testing of the trunk muscles can also provoke other pain-sensitive structures and result in a weak and painful test, making it difficult to use resisted testing as a differential diagnostic test for trunk muscle strain.

Muscle strength testing of pelvic girdle and pelvic floor muscles can provide pertinent information about factors that may contribute to lumbopelvic dysfunction. For example, weakness in the gluteus medius results in excessive hip adduction and pelvic drop in the single-limb support phase of gait, which can impose frontal or transverse plane stress on the lumbopelvic region and thereby contribute to lumbopelvic impairment or pathology. Chapters 18 and 19, respectively, provide recommendations for pelvic floor and pelvic girdle muscle performance testing.

Neurologic Testing: Tests for Motor Function and Sensory and Reflex Integrity

A thorough neurologic examination for the lumbopelvic region consists of three parts. An *upper motor neuron screening* is indicated when cord compression is suspected. An upper lumbar central herniation may result in spinal cord compression. A central herniation in the lower lumbar spine can cause compression to the cauda equina and therefore should not result in upper motor neuron signs.

Sufficient compression on the nerve root may result in decreased conductive function of the nervous system; *neuroconductive testing* may reveal segmentally related sensory changes, motor changes, and deep tendon reflex changes.[72] Testing motor function can indicate a pattern of muscle weakness from a specific disk level or peripheral nerve. Table 17-2 indicates the key muscles with the corresponding nerve root and peripheral nerve innervation.

The third part includes *neurodynamic tests* that examine the movement and tensile abilities of the nervous system. Examples of neurodynamic tests include the straight leg raise (SLR), prone knee bend (PKB), and slump maneuver. The clinician administering these tests should be skilled in the specialized features of handling and sequencing the components of the test and must understand what is considered to be a normal or acceptable response. Butler[73] describes the technique and rationale for neurodynamic tests in the lumbopelvic region. Deyo et al.[21] noted a sensitivity of 80% and specificity of 40% for the SLR in diagnosis of low lumbar disk

herniation. The SLR test is most appropriate for testing the L5 and S1 nerve roots. Irritation of the higher lumbar roots is tested by the PKB or femoral nerve stretch test; reliability and validity of the PKB are unknown.[21]

Pain

The clinician examines pain in the lumbopelvic region with respect to many variables:

- Measurement of pain with respect to the level of disability it imposes on an individual with LBP, and therefore can be used as an indicator of outcome
- Examination techniques used to diagnose whether the pain is originating in the lumbopelvic region and, if possible, determine the potential source(s) of the pain
- Examination techniques to determine the potential cause(s) of pain
- Examination techniques and clinical reasoning to determine the impact of pain on the physiologic function of the lumbopelvic region

Because the United States, in common with other Western nations, is trying to restrain the costs of health care, it is more important than ever for clinicians to demonstrate that the care they deliver is both efficient and effective. Pain scales are a common method for assessing patient outcome in back pain. At least 22 scales have been reported in the literature.[74] However, the presence of pain alone is a narrow definition of health outcome that correlates poorly with physical function.[75] Waddell and Main[76] stated that in evaluating the severity of LBP, three recordable, clinical components must be differentiated: pain, physical impairment, and disability. (See: "Work [Job/School/Play], Community, and Leisure Integration or Reintegration (Including IADLs)" for further discussion regarding measures of disability.)

Efficient allocation of health care resources can be augmented by an outcome measure that can predict those patients whose outcomes are likely to be poor. Those individuals can be redirected to more appropriate intervention. Waddell developed a list of nonorganic signs that can be used as a predictor of outcome for patients with lumbopelvic disabilities.[77,78] Waddell et al.[78] identified five nonorganic signs, and each can be detected by one or two tests. The tests assess a patient's pain behavior in response to certain maneuvers (Table 17-3). A patient presenting with a high Waddell score (i.e., 3–5 of 5 positive nonorganic signs) is believed to have a clinical pattern of nonmechanical, pain-focused behavior. The patient has significant enough psychologic impairments that intervention focused on physiologic and anatomic impairments alone probably cannot produce a successful outcome. A high Waddell score can be used as a predictor of functional outcome, as indicated by a low rate of return to work.[107] However, the practitioner must interpret this finding with caution.[78] A high Waddell score only indicates a high degree of nonorganic or psychologic impairments. It does not signify malingering, which is a judgment, not a medical or psychologic diagnosis.[77–80] Patients with a high Waddell score should be referred to the appropriate practitioner for treatment before or in conjunction with further physical therapy intervention.

In addition to measurement of pain in relation to outcome data, the clinician should also attempt to determine whether or not the lumbar spine or pelvis is indeed the source of the pain. After it has been determined that the lumbopelvic region is the

---

TABLE 17-2 Key Muscles and Corresponding Nerve Root and Peripheral Nerve in the Lumbopelvic Region

KEY MUSCLE	NERVE ROOT	PERIPHERAL NERVE
Psoas	L2 (3)	Femoral nerve
Quadriceps	L3 (4)	Femoral nerve
Tibialis anterior	L4 (5)	Deep peroneal
Extensor hallucis	L5 (S1)	Deep peroneal
Gluteus medius	L5 (S1)	Superior gluteal
Peroneii	L5 (S1)	Superficial peroneal
Medial hamstring	L5 (S1)	Sciatic
Gastrocnemius	S1 (S2)	Tibial
Peroneii	S1	Superficial peroneal
Lateral hamstring	S1	Sciatic
Gluteus maximus	S2	Inferior gluteal
Bladder and rectum	S4	

TABLE 17-3	Waddell Signs
TEST	**SIGNS**
Tenderness	Superficial—the patient's skin is tender to light pinch over a wide area of lumbar skin
	Nonanatomic—deep tenderness felt over a wide area, not localized to one structure
Simulation tests	Axial loading—light vertical loading over patient's skull in the standing position causes lumbar pain
	Acetabular rotation—back pain is reported when the pelvis and shoulders are passively rotated in the same plane as the patient stands; considered to be a positive test result if pain is reported within the first 30 degrees
Distraction tests	Straight-leg-raise discrepancy—marked improvement of straight-leg raising on distraction compared with formal testing
	Double-leg raise—when both legs are raised after straight-leg raising, the organic response is a greater degree of double-leg raising; patients with a nonorganic component demonstrate less double-leg raise compared with the single-leg raise
Regional disturbances	Weakness, cogwheeling, or giving way of many muscle groups that cannot be explained on a neurologic basis
	Sensory disturbance—diminished sensation fitting a "stocking" rather than a dermatomal pattern
Overreaction	Disproportionate verbalization, facial expression, muscle tension and tremor, collapsing, or sweating

From Karas R, McIntosh G, Hall H, et al. The relationship between nonorganic signs and centralization of symptoms in the prediction of the return to work for patients with low back pain. Phys Ther 1997;77:356. Reprinted with permission of the American Physical Therapy Association.

source of pain, even if the exact source of the pain cannot be diagnosed, attempts must be made to determine the mechanical cause of the pain. The complexity of understanding the causes or mechanisms of pain is beyond the scope of this text. Much controversy exists about whether chemical or mechanical mechanisms initiate and perpetuate pain and about exactly what neurophysiologic and biochemical processes are responsible for pain. The role of the therapist is to determine whether mechanical interventions can alter pain. During the examination process, the therapist can observe precise stabilization and movement patterns and correlate faulty patterns with the onset of or increase in pain. If altering the pattern of stabilization or movement reduces or eliminates the pain, the specific faulty movement patterns responsible for the pain can be diagnosed.[8]

Posture

The therapist should perform a cursory evaluation of the patient's standing or sitting postures during the history portion of the examination. Posture also is examined formally as part of the evaluation process. The patient is aware of the scrutiny during the formal examination and may assume what he or she considers to be proper posture or posture that depicts the painful or emotional state he or she wishes to portray. The posture portrayed during this examination may be unconscious or intentional, and the motivation is not always easily discerned. Observation of posture without the patient's knowledge can be more revealing of the true contribution of posture to his or her signs and symptoms.

More specific examination should include standing, sitting (supported and unsupported), and recumbent postures. Several things should be observed, including head position, shoulder girdle position, spine curves (i.e., cervical, thoracic, and lumbar), and lumbopelvic, hip, knee, ankle-foot alignment should be examined about all three planes. In standing, the examiner is looking for asymmetry and possible relationships between segmental regions (e.g., foot pronation and genu valgum on the side of a low iliac crest and apparent short limb). Bony landmarks are assessed to visualize the position of the pelvis, including the iliac crest, posterior superior iliac spines (PSISs), anterior superior iliac spines (ASISs), and pubic symphysis. Ideal pelvic alignment is best visualized through the ASIS and pubic symphysis in the frontal plane.[60]

A hypothesis can be developed regarding the contribution of faulty lumbopelvic alignment to the pathomechanical cause of symptoms and the relationship of other body regions in perpetuating the faulty lumbopelvic alignment. Correction of alignment can reduce pathomechanical stress in the lumbopelvic region and therefore reduce or eliminate symptoms. This is an early step toward the diagnosis of a pathomechanical cause of lumbopelvic activity limitations and participation restrictions. However, posture is not always a good indicator of the pathomechanical stress causing lumbopelvic symptoms. For example, a person with spinal stenosis may have a flat lumbar spine and yet incur symptoms with extension forces on the lumbar spine due to the narrowed spinal canal or lateral foramina.

Other hypotheses can be developed about muscle lengths. Assumptions can be made regarding muscle-fascial structures that are too long based on joint position, such as a long EO in an anterior pelvic tilt (Fig. 17-8). Muscle length testing is indicated to determine whether muscles are short because of joint position (e.g., specifically which hip flexors are short in anterior pelvic tilt). Additionally, the results of positional strength tests should correlate with muscle length hypotheses.

Range of Motion, Muscle Length, and Joint Mobility

ROM tests of the lumbopelvic region should not only assess the ROM of the lumbar spine, but also the pelvic-femoral complex and the relationship between the ROM of the hip and lumbar spine. The interrelationship of ROM with other regions of the body (e.g., thoracic spine and upper extremity) is also of interest. Muscle length testing of the spine, upper, and lower quarters should also be included. Mobility tests of the lumbopelvic region determine the intervertebral mobility/stability (passive intervertebral motion [PIVM] testing) of the spine and mobility/stability of the SIJ.

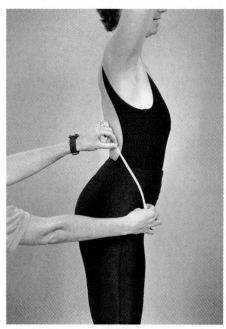

FIGURE 17-8. The lordotic posture and anterior pelvic tilt elongate the EO.

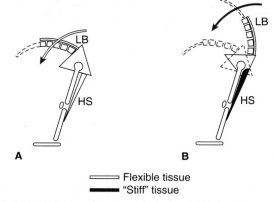

==== Flexible tissue
━━━ "Stiff" tissue

FIGURE 17-9. (A) Normal lumbopelvic rhythm. (B) Reduced extensibility of the HSs can alter lumbar-pelvic range of motion. Stiffness from the HSs slows the rate and can potentially restrict the range of pelvic motion, resulting in excessive flexion stress of the lumbar spine. (Adapted from Calliet R. Low Back Pain. 3rd Ed. Philadelphia, PA: FA Davis, 1981.)

ROM testing is performed in standing for flexion and extension, lateral flexion, and quadrant movements; it is performed in sitting for rotation. Overpressure can be used to reproduce symptoms. The intent of ROM testing is fourfold:

1. To determine the patient's willingness to move
2. To reproduce symptoms
3. To determine the quantity of motion in the lumbar-pelvic-hip complex
4. To determine the quality of movement by assessing the relationship between the various regions of the spine and the pelvic-hip complex

Chapter 19 describes hip ROM testing. The purpose of hip ROM testing is to determine reduced ROM in the hip that may contribute to compensatory spine motion, thereby imposing a pathomechanical stress on the lumbar spine. For example, a hip that has reduced ROM in extension may cause compensatory spine extension, particularly during the terminal stance phase of gait or in the final phase of return from a forward bend.

Active hip ROM testing can be used to assess movement patterns of the hip and stabilization patterns of the lumbopelvic region.[8] Faulty patterns can induce a pathomechanical stress on the lumbar spine and provoke symptoms. Correction of faulty patterns of lumbopelvic stabilization should reduce symptoms if the faulty pattern is contributing to pathomechanical stress on the affected structures. In this way, these tests can also be used to clear the hip joint of any possible involvement. If correction of lumbopelvic stabilization reduces symptoms, it is unlikely that the hip is the source of symptoms.

Thoracic ROM testing is described in Chapter 24. The purpose of thoracic ROM testing is to determine whether reduced ROM of the thoracic spine is contributing to compensatory motion in the lumbopelvic region (e.g., reduced or stiff thoracic spine rotation could induce increased stress to the lumbar spine during transverse plane movement patterns).

Tests of muscle extensibility across the pelvis and hip are described in Chapter 19. Data obtained from these tests provide the clinician with additional information about potential causes of pathomechanical stress on the lumbar spine. For example, during forward bending, stiff hamstrings (HSs) can restrict pelvic forward rotation, resulting in flexion stress (Fig. 17-9B) on the lumbar spine.

Although not direct measures of trunk muscle extensibility, lumbopelvic forward bending, backward bending, and lateral flexion can test for posterior, anterior, and lateral trunk extensibility, respectively. Assessment of postural alignment can lead to a hypothesis about excessive trunk muscle length (see the "Posture Examination" section).

One type of ROM testing unique to the lumbar region was developed by McKenzie.[81] This method is based on the assumption that sustained or repeated movements may affect nuclear position, resulting in centralization or peripheralization of symptoms. McKenzie defined the centralization phenomenon as "the situation in which pain arising from the spine and felt laterally to the midline or distally, is reduced and transferred to a more central or near midline position when certain movements are performed."[81] Peripheralization is the opposite phenomenon whereby pain arising from the spine and felt proximally and to the midline is increased and transferred laterally and distally when certain movements are performed. McKenzie's theory presumes that as long as the annulus and disk are intact, an offset load on the disk in a lesion-specific direction of spinal movement may apply a reductive force on a displaced nuclear fragment, directing it toward a more central location (i.e., "centralization"), thereby reducing symptom-generating stress on neural or other nociceptive structures.[81]

Joint mobility tests of the lumbar region or PIVM tests come in three categories: passive physiologic intervertebral motion (PPIVM), passive accessory intervertebral motion (PAIVM), and segmental stability tests. PIVM testing is used to determine relative mobility (e.g., hypermobility versus hypomobility) and to stress the related spine and pelvic joints in an attempt to determine end feel, assess irritability, assess stability, and provoke symptoms. Meadows provides descriptions of these tests and defines PAIVM as the passive assessment of an intervertebral joint through its glides, whereas stability tests attempt to examine segmental translatory mobility.[72] Research shows at best moderate intrarater reliability and poor interrater

TABLE 17-4 Descriptive Information for Selected Back-Specific Functional Instruments

INSTRUMENT	CONTENT	SCORING	COMPLETION TIME
Oswestry Low Back Disability Score	Pain intensity, interference with sleep, self-care, walking, sitting, standing, lifting, sex life, traveling, social life.	0–100	5 minutes
Million Visual Analogue Scale	Pain intensity, interference with physical activities, interference with work, overall handicap.	0–100	5–10 minutes
Roland Morris Disability Questionnaire	Physical activities, housework, mobility, dressing, getting help, appetite, irritability, pain severity.	0–24	5 minutes
Waddell Disability Index	Heavy lifting, sitting, walking, standing, social life, travel, sex life, sleep, footwear.	0–9	5 minutes
Low Back Outcome Score	Current pain, employment, domestic and sport activities, use of drugs and medical services, rest, sex life, five daily activities.	0–75	5 minutes

Adapted from Kopec KA. Measuring functional outcomes in persons with back pain. Spine 2000;25:3110–3114.

reliability.[82] Reliability improves when a positive response includes both perceived changes in ROM and provocation of symptoms rather than just decreased mobility.[83,84] A combination of PPIVM and PAIVM tests correctly identified dysfunctional levels diagnosed with intra-articular infiltration.[85]

Regarding the SIJ, a battery of tests has been suggested to rule out or confirm a suspected diagnosis of SIJ dysfunction.[86] A criteria of at least three of four tests with positive results is required to determine the presence of SIJ dysfunction: standing flexion, PKB, supine-to-long sitting, and palpation of the PSIS in sitting. Passive physiologic motion (PPM) tests of the pelvis include anterior and posterior innominate rotation.[100] Passive accessory motion (PAM) tests refer to the passive assessment of a joint by way of glides and in the SIJ can be used to test stability.[87]

All ROM, muscle length, and mobility/stability tests should assess the effect that altered motion or stabilization strategies of the examined region have symptoms. For example, an increased extension moment may be imposed on the L5 segmental level during prone hip extension because of relatively less extension mobility available at the hip. By determining which spinal segmental levels (e.g., L5), the associated anatomic regions (e.g., the hip), and the sources of structural limitation (e.g., muscle, capsule, bone), a specific intervention plan can be developed to address the related physiologic impairments. Addressing the impairments associated with lumbar extension can improve the patient tolerance to walking or running (activity and participation restriction).

Work (Job/School/Play), Community, and Leisure Integration or Reintegration (Including IADLs)

This category of tests and measures includes the measurement of participation restriction. Waddell and Main[76] proposed that in evaluating the severity of LBP, three recordable clinical illness components must be differentiated (see "Pain" category), one of those being disability. The following list is limited to validated functional questionnaires that were designed by selecting items relevant to back pain:

1. Oswestry Low Back Disability Score[88]
2. Million Visual Analogue Scale[89]
3. Roland Morris Disability Questionnaire[90]
4. Waddell Disability Index[76]
5. Clinical Back Pain Questionnaire (Aberdeen Low Back Scale)[74]
6. Lumbar Spine Outcomes Score (LSOQ)[75,91,92].

Descriptive information for the selected measures is given in Table 17-4. Problems in the assessment of outcome for patients with LBP have been subject to considerable recent investigation with little agreement in the literature concerning which outcome measure to use, with few reports using the same criteria for assessing patients.[93,94] The LSOQ (Display 17-3) appears to be acceptable to patients, easy to administer, highly reliable, valid, and responsive. It provides information on demographics, pain severity, functional disability, psychological distress, physical symptoms, health-care utilization, and satisfaction. It should be considered for use in both clinical and research applications as well as regulatory review involving patients with LBP complaints.[92]

THERAPEUTIC EXERCISE INTERVENTION FOR COMMON IMPAIRMENTS OF BODY FUNCTIONS

It is not usually possible or desirable to set up a particular exercise regimen for the lumbar spine and SIJ based solely on the pathology or medical diagnosis. We need to remain critical in our thinking and application of specific therapeutic exercise techniques to ensure that clinical efforts are being expended in the most efficacious manner for a given patient. It is prudent to avoid becoming overly dogmatic about the application of a single therapeutic exercise approach to the nonhomogenous group of patients with LBP. Therapeutic exercise intervention must be prescriptive and based upon each individual's unique combination of structural, physiological and psychological impairments and activity and participation restrictions.

Because this text is not presenting a treatment approach related to a specific classification system, the exercises are based on the impairments of body functions detailed in Unit 2 and are presented in alphabetical order. Impairments of body functions have been separated for clarity of presentation, though, in reality, patients most often present with a complex interaction of pathology and structural, physiological and psychological impairments. The exercise examples are not meant to demonstrate a comprehensive approach to the treatment

---

DISPLAY 17-3
The Low Back Outcome Score

Please mark on the line below how much pain you have had from your back on average over the past week.

0	1	2	3	4	5	6	7	8	9	10

No pain at all   Maximum pain possible

Please tick the answer which most closely describes you on each of the following six sections.

At present are you working
Full time at your usual Job	☐ 9
Full time at a lighter job	☐ 6
Part time	☐ 3
Not working/unemployed	☐ 0
Disability benefit	☐ 0
Housewife/student/retired	☐ score as for chores

At present can you undertake household chores or odd jobs
Normally	☐ 9
As much as usual but more slowly	☐ 6
A few, not as many as usual	☐ 3
Not at all	☐ 0

At present can you undertake sports or active pursuits (e.g., dancing)
As much as usual	☐ 9
Almost as much as usual	☐ 6
Some, much less than usual	☐ 3
Not at all	☐ 0

Do you have to rest during the day because of pain?
Not at all	☐ 6
A little	☐ 4
Half the day	☐ 2
Over half the day	☐ 0

How often do you have a consultation with a doctor or have any treatment (e.g., physiotherapy) for your pain?
Never	☐ 6
Rarely	☐ 4
About once a month	☐ 2
More than once a month	☐ 0

How often do you have to take pain killers for your pain?
Never	☐ 6
Occasionally	☐ 4
Almost every day	☐ 2
Several times each day	☐ 0

Please tick the box that best describes how much your back pain affects the following activities.

	NO EFFECT	MILDLY/ NOT MUCH	MODERATELY/ DIFFICULT	SEVERELY/ IMPOSSIBLE
Sex life	☐ 6	☐ 4	☐ 2	☐ 0
Sleeping	☐ 3	☐ 2	☐ 1	☐ 0
Walking	☐ 3	☐ 2	☐ 1	☐ 0
Traveling	☐ 3	☐ 2	☐ 1	☐ 0
Dressing	☐ 3	☐ 2	☐ 1	☐ 0

Pain scale readings are equivalent to the following scores: 0–2 = 9; 3–4 = 6; 5–6 = 3; 7–10 = 0. Patients are placed in one of four outcome categories based on overall scores: 65 or higher (excellent), 50 or higher (good), 30 or higher (fair), and lower than 30 (poor).

Adapted from Holt AE, Shaw NJ, Shetty A, et al. The reliability of the Low Back Outcome Score for Back Pain. Spine. 2002;27:206–210.

---

of physiologic impairments; they were chosen to illustrate principles and a reasonable approach to the use of exercise for the lumbopelvic region. Principles related to work-conditioning programs, although often used in addressing lumbopelvic dysfunction, are not covered in this text.

Aerobic Capacity Impairment

Aerobic capacity impairment can be considered a secondary condition resulting from the incapacitation associated with CLBP or a risk factor contributing to the development of CLBP. Research supports the fact that aerobic exercise alone is not enough to prevent recurrence of LBP, although aerobic exercise is beneficial for patients with lumbopelvic syndromes.[40] Aerobic exercise enhances healing, assists with weight loss, and has favorable psychologic effects, such as reduction of anxiety and depression.[98]

Typically, the patient is limited by musculoskeletal pain in working at the optimal target heart rate necessary for producing aerobic gains. Aerobic exercise is initially prescribed "to tolerance" and is progressively increased as the patient's signs and symptoms improve to 60% to 80% of age-predicted maximal heart rate (220 – age) for 30 to 50 minutes, three times per week. The mode of exercise (e.g., biking, swimming, walking, jogging) should be based on the patient's desires and the postures and movements that relieve symptoms. For example, if walking relieves pain, but sitting increases pain, walking should be encouraged and biking should be discouraged. If weight-bearing aerobic exercise is chosen, the physical therapist may need to counsel the patient in choosing proper footwear to ensure the best weight-bearing dynamics possible. Orthotic prescription may be necessary to optimize ground reaction forces (see Chapter 21). If weight-bearing exercise is unbearable, water is often a well-tolerated medium for aerobic exercise by a person with lumbopelvic dysfunction (see Chapter 16). Another option is to walk with some type of unloading mechanism either through harness apparatus or the use of crutches, walker, grocery cart, or stroller.

Balance and Coordination Impairment

The functional importance of proprioceptive training has been emphasized during rehabilitation of the spine.[96] Protection of the musculoskeletal system relies in part on adequate proprioception and reaction time of the neuromuscular system. This requires fine adjustments in neuromuscular activation patterns in response to a fluctuating load. True stability of the spine at the skill level requires precise and rapid responses to perturbations in the load imposed on the spine.

There is evidence that LBP patients may be prone to excessive postural sway, poor balance reactions, and altered strategies for balance.[97,98] Patients with LBP showed poor standing balance with altered postural adjustment strategy and increased visual dependence. The LBP group demonstrates reduced dependence on the hip strategy for postural control. The reduced utilization of the hip strategy may be due to reduced motion of the lumbar spine and hip as a result of increased activity of lumbopelvic muscles. Several EMG studies have reported increased activation of the erector spinae muscle in study participants with LBP during tasks such as trunk flexion,[99–103] and the absence of relaxation of the erector spinae at the end of range of trunk flexion (the "flexion-relaxation" phenomenon) has been shown to be associated with reduced intervertebral motion.[100] In contrast to the increased activation of the superficial trunk muscles, activity of the intrinsic spinal muscles has been found to be either decreased or delayed in patients with LBP. In people with LBP, impairment of the LM muscle has been reported as decreased activity[104] and reduction in size.[34,105] Similarly, activity of the deep abdominal muscle, transversus abdominus, has been found to be delayed in study participants with LBP.[106–108] The association of impairment of intrinsic spinal muscle activity with hyperactivity of the lumbosacral muscle in study participants with LBP is still unclear. However, it is possible that the hyperactivity of the lumbosacral muscle could be a cause or a compensation for the deficiency of the intrinsic spinal muscle function. Regardless, increased activity of the lumbosacral muscles is likely to restrict the range and pace of trunk-on-hip motion in response to postural perturbation. The reduced hip strategy (i.e., decreased anteroposterior shear force) identified when subjects stood on short base may be due to this mechanism. Other possible explanations for reduced hip strategy such as fear of movement cannot be excluded and require further investigation.

Authorities acknowledge the necessity of balance work in the rehabilitation of lumbopelvic patients, particularly when dealing with hypermobility and instability impairments.[109] Gym balls, wobble boards, slide boards, and foam rolls can be used to enhance proprioception and teach optimal balance strategies (e.g., use of intrinsic and superficial muscles as needed versus superficial only, improved use of hip strategy, decreased reliance on visual feedback). Aspects of proprioceptive training can be incorporated at any stage of rehabilitation, as illustrated by examples focusing on balance and coordination discussed in other sections of this chapter. After an activity is performed correctly on a stable surface, the patient can be positioned on a moving base of support, such as a gym ball (Fig. 17-10) or foam roll (Fig. 17-11). Any activity challenging balance and proprioception must be performed with precision, emphasizing correct body position and recruitment strategies. The rate of movement is progressed while accuracy is maintained.

One example of a high-level exercise challenging balance and coordination is standing on a half or full foam roller (the latter is the most difficult). The patient is instructed to shift

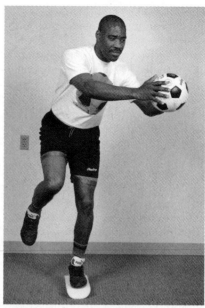

FIGURE 17-11. Standing on two foam rolls is easier than standing on one foam roll. For the stability phase, the goal is to reach to the side through rotation of the feet and hips with the spine in neutral. For controlled mobility, the goal is to move the feet, hips, thoracic, and lumbar spine in a combined rotational movement pattern. However, movement should be emphasized at the feet, hips, and thoracic spine, with very little rotation occurring in the lumbar spine.

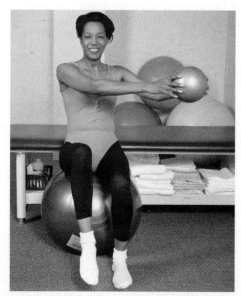

FIGURE 17-10. Sitting on a gym ball can add an element of difficulty to the stability phase of lumbo-pelvic exercise. Care must be taken to ensure quality of recruitment strategy as dominant strategies may emerge on the unstable surface.

his or her weight from side to side and forward to back from the ankles as trunk stability is maintained. Another variation is performance of squatting motions or upper extremity motions individually and then combined after proper trunk stabilization is accomplished. The ankles, knees, and hips are used as the fulcrum points for balance instead of the low back.

Muscle Performance Impairment

Treatment of general muscle performance impairments in the lumbopelvic region has limitations. Evidence suggests that muscular dysfunction in the presence of lumbopelvic syndromes does not so much affect the strength of the trunk musculature as it influences the patterns of trunk muscle recruitment.[110–113] Subtle shifts in the patterns of muscle recruitment result in some muscles being relatively underused in the force couple, whereas other muscles relatively dominate the force couple.[8] The cause and effect relationships of these subtle shifts in muscle recruitment patterns cannot be determined and should be thought of as part of a continuous cycle of altered recruitment strategies and movement patterns.

Lack of muscle endurance has been shown to also be a prime impairment in muscle performance. Many investigators have reported diminished trunk muscle endurance and increased rates of muscular fatigue in LBP patients compared with individuals without LBP, even when strength measures testing results are within normal limits.[65,66,111,114] Sophisticated electromyographic testing using a technique called power spectrum analysis has identified that the LM is the back extensor most susceptible to endurance changes.[112,115] These studies indicate the need to provide an endurance training component in the course of a total rehabilitation program. No special exercise recommendations are needed, because the dosage can be modified for exercises prescribed for force or torque production to satisfy endurance goals (i.e., higher repetitions with lower loads).

Mechanisms such as muscle strain, pain, inflammation, neurologic pathology, or general deconditioning can contribute to muscle performance impairment. The clinician must consider the possible mechanisms contributing to the more dramatic as well as subtle changes in muscle recruitment patterns to develop the appropriate exercise intervention. After the underlying mechanism(s) are identified, precise exercise can be prescribed to activate, restore, or improve muscle control and performance of the trunk muscles. The following section describes exercises to establish control over specific trunk muscles. Subsequent sections investigate the various causes of reduced muscle performance around the lumbar spine and recommend activities and techniques to alleviate individual causes of muscle performance impairment.

Exercise for Motor Control

Research has established a link between lumbar dysfunction and altered base (i.e., muscle performance) and modulator (i.e., neuromuscular control) function of the *intrinsic or deep trunk muscles* defined to include the TrA, LM, and pelvic floor.[110,116]

General strengthening programs for the trunk muscles may not adequately recruit or improve the muscle performance of the deep and often underused trunk muscles. Localized and specific exercise aimed at training neuromuscular control of the intrinsic spinal muscles may be critical to improving subtle patterns of muscle recruitment necessary for optimal segmental stability in the lumbar spine.[117–119] Similarly, specific exercises aimed at training neuromuscular control and muscle performance of the intrinsic spinal muscles plus the gluteus medius, gluteus maximus, biceps femoris, deep hip lateral rotators, and latissimus dorsi may be critical for optimal SIJ stability and load transference from the upper and lower quarter to the low back.[120,121] A pelvic floor contraction, in particular (see Chapter 18), is indicated for the chronic, unstable SIJ because of the shared muscle of the piriformis and obturator internus and the important supportive function of the pelvic floor to the pelvic girdle.[121]

Before presenting the exercise recommendations for the intrinsic spinal muscles, three additional concepts must be addressed:

1. Exercises chosen should promote optimal length-tension properties of the trunk and pelvic girdle muscles. The affected muscles should be trained at the length desired for function. Too often, the lumbar spinal muscles are strengthened in the lengthened range because of use of a Valsalva maneuver, resulting in abdominal distension or "pooching," lumbar flexion, and bearing down on the pelvic floor (see Fig. 17-12). A disadvantage to strengthening the muscles in a lengthened range is the contribution this may have toward altered length-tension properties. The lumbar spinal muscles muscles need to be of the right length to support the spine and pelvis in good static alignment and have the correct length-tension properties to continue to support the spine and pelvis during dynamic activities.

2. A second important principle is specificity of training or the principle of specific adaptation to imposed demands (SAID principle). For example, although a sit-up is a functional activity, it is not the primary function of all the abdominal muscles for ADLs and IADLs. It has been proposed that the intrinsic spinal muscles muscles are linked with the control of stability of the spine against the perturbation produced by movement of the limbs.[33] The primary role for the deep trunk muscles is to provide static stability to the trunk during movements of the extremities and dynamic stability during trunk movements. However, it is important to realize that all the trunk muscles play a role in static and dynamic control of the trunk dependent on the demand placed on the spine and the level of skill involved in performing the activity.

3. A third principle governs exercise progression. The stages of motor control (i.e., mobility, stability, controlled mobility, and skill) can be used to progress lumbopelvic exercise. Mobility and stability usually occur together in the lumbopelvic region. Stability is often a problem at the dysfunctional segmental level, and mobility is more likely to be a problem at an adjacent lumbar level or in some associated region (e.g., hip, thoracic spine, shoulder girdle). To be most effective, simultaneous reconciliation of mobility and stability impairments is desired. When developing a program focusing on stability, the chosen direction of force must be based on the directions in which the spine is

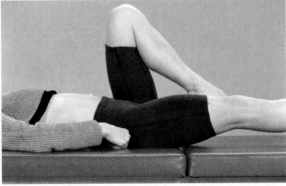

A

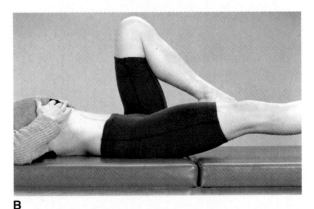

B

FIGURE 17-12. (A) Use of the abdominal muscles in a lengthened range. Note protrusion of the umbilicus. (B) Use of the oblique abdominal muscles and TrA in the short range.

most susceptible to motion and the directions most correlated with symptom reproduction.[8,122,123] After adequate mobility and stability are achieved, the patient is progressed to controlled mobility (BADLs) and then to skill-level activities (IADLs). According to a study by Richardson and Jull,[40] patients who followed a graded program of exercise to improve the muscle performance and neuromuscular control of the intrinsic spinal muscles experienced pain resolution within 4 weeks, with only a 29% recurrence rate at 9 months. These results were compared with a control group of LBP patients who exercised aerobically by jogging and swimming. They too were pain-free at 4 weeks, but they had a LBP recurrence rate of 79% at 9 months. Specificity seems to be the key to the proper prescription of the exercises that correspond with improved neuromuscular control and muscle performance of the deep trunk muscles. This treatment approach demands a high level of skill by the instructor in teaching the exercise and a high level of patient compliance and attention to detail. Continual reassessment of muscle recruitment capabilities and muscle performance is necessary to progress or modify the exercise for optimal results.

Patient-related instruction is the first step to establish awareness over the individual intrinsic spinal muscles. Display 17-4

DISPLAY 17-4
How to Teach the Components of the Intrinsic Spinal Muscle Group Synergy

- The clinician must first determine the presence or absence of the intrinsic spinal muscles synergy by palpating the TrA, LM, and external palpation of the pelvic floor if necessary (see Chapter 18). Although it is not necessary to facilitate the intrinsic spinal muscles in this manner, often the easiest component of the intrinsic spinal muscles to activate is the pelvic floor (see Chapter 18 and Patient-Related Instruction 17-1). After the patient has contracted the pelvic floor, the therapist can palpate the other components of the intrinsic spinal muscles.

- The **TrA** can be palpated medially and deep to the ASIS. Contraction of the TrA should feel like taut fascia under the fingertips, whereas contraction of the IO will push the fingertips out superficially. Toning down the force of contraction will assist in isolating the TrA. Another indication that the TrA has contracted is that the waist will pull inward laterally like the function of a girdle, and the umbilicus will be gently pulled in toward the spine. The umbilicus pulled upward toward the ribs coupled with rib cage depression indicates dominance of the RA and is a common mistake.

- The **LM** can be palpated best at the L5 level just medial and deep to the spinous process. If the LM is not contracting, the therapist can provide an explanation to the patient as to the function of this muscle with respect to sacral nutation, lumbar extension, and stabilization against rotational forces. Visually, show the patient models and pictures of the region and LM muscles. Cue for tactile input by palpating directly over the LM at the affected level. Key to isolation of the LM is to facilitate a submaximal isometric contraction. Patients often have initial difficulty in facilitating a LM contraction in a home exercise program. This is particularly true for patients with a chronic condition and for postoperative patients. Manual techniques can be used to help facilitate recruitment in the early stages of neuromuscular training. Figure A illustrates a manual technique for facilitating recruitment of LM musculature. Another technique is to use isometric hip lateral rotation (see Patient-Related Intervention 17-1). After a consistent LM contraction can be elicited, ask the patient to perform a body check and determine whether focusing on contraction of the LM facilitated a pelvic floor contraction. You as the clinician can palpate the TrA to determine whether it has contracted in synergy with the LM and pelvic floor. You can ask the patient to vary the initial muscle activation focus from the pelvic floor, to the LM, to the TrA to ensure the synergy is intact.

- Contraction of the intrinsic spinal muscles should occur in conjunction with good breathing habits. Ask the patient to perform a deep diaphragmatic breath and assess the quality of the inhalation and exhalation technique. If the quality is poor, teach the patient diaphragmatic breathing as discussed in Chapter 22. Next, ask the patient to take a deep diaphragmatic breath with a relaxed, not forced, exhalation. Before the next breath, ask the patient to slowly and gently contract the intrinsic spinal muscles synergy, then resume normal relaxed breathing. After relaxed breathing can be performed while sustaining an intrinsic spinal muscles contraction, the intrinsic spinal muscles supine progression (see Self-Management 17-1) and intrinsic spinal muscles series (Self-Management 17-2) can be prescribed.

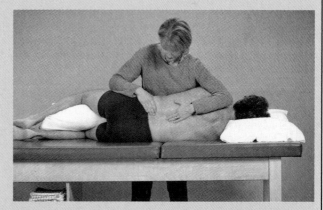

FIGURE A. Sidelying manually resisted lumbar multifidus exercise. Restoration of lumbar multifidus activity may need to begin by facilitating the muscle at the specific level of spinal pathology with a manual technique. Low-load rotary resistance is applied to the affected segment in a side lying position as if testing for passive physiologic intervertebral movement. The patient is encouraged to maintain the submaximal contraction against the therapist's resistance into rotation. The therapist palpates the segmental level to ensure multifidus activity. EMG reveals that the multifidus is active in rotation both ipsilateral and contralateral as a stabilizer.[24] The primary role of the multifidus is to oppose the flexion moment associated with rotation.

contains specific instruction for the clinician as to how to train the intrinsic spinal muscles. Patient-Related Instruction 17-1: How to Activate Your Intrinsic Spinal Muscles describes in patient terms, techniques to activate the intrinsic spinal muscles.

Self-Management 17-1: Supine Intrinsic Spinal Muscles Progression describes a series of exercises in the supine position to progressively challenge and load the local (intrinsic) spinal muscles and global spinal muscles. When prescribing the supine intrinsic spinal muscles progression (see Self-Management 17-1) the individual should be aware that isolated use of the intrinsic spinal muscles is not possible throughout all the levels of the exercise. Generally, beyond level I, most individuals will require recruitment of more global muscles for stabilization, such as internal and external

oblique abdominal muscles. The exercise is progressed from level I to level V through a combination of progressively longer lever arms in the form of hip and knee extensions and increased loads in the form of moving one limb advanced to moving both limbs simultaneously. The direction of forces imposed on the spine also must be considered in advancing the exercise, particularly from level III to level IV. Level III and level IV may be interchanged with respect to difficulty, depending on which direction of force the patient has most difficulty controlling. Level III combines sagittal- and transverse-plane forces because of the unilateral limb movement, whereas level IV induces a strong sagittal-plane force because of the bilateral limb movement. If an individual has difficulty controlling rotational forces, progression

---

Patient-Related Instruction 17-1

How to Activate Your Intrinsic Spinal Muscles

What are the intrinsic spinal muscles?
The intrinsic spinal muscles refers to a group of deep muscles that, under normal circumstances, work together to provide stability to the lower back and pelvis. In normal function they should contract automatically and simultaneously before any upper extremity, lower extremity, or trunk movement—in effect, before any movement you make. The intrinsic spinal muscles muscles include

- The diaphragm—your primary breathing muscle
- The pelvic floor—attached to the bony ring of the pelvis from the tailbone to the pubic bone
- The lumbar multifidus—the deepest layer of the back muscles
- The transversus abdominus—the deepest layer of the abdominal muscles

How do you activate them?
This section describes intrinsic spinal muscles awareness activities. These activities must be mastered before using the intrinsic spinal muscles with more advanced self management activities and activities of daily living. NOTE: Your physical therapist will work with you individually to identify the best strategy to initiate your intrinsic spinal muscles. You may only need to contract one of these muscles to get them all to activate.

- To contract the pelvic floor:
  Think of slowly and gently pulling the tip of your tailbone toward your pubic bone. Try not to contract the rectal portion of your pelvic floor, but rather more of the portion closer to your pubic bone. To see if you are using the correct muscles, the next time that you urinate, let out half the volume of your bladder and then stop the flow of urine with the least amount of effort possible. Be aware of which muscles you are using. NOTE: This *test* is not to be used as a daily exercise. It is simply a method for you to identify which muscles make up the pelvic floor. Another image is to think about an elastic cord anchored between your feet and extending up toward your umbilicus. Think about pulling the cord tight from the anchor point upward toward your umbilicus. Monitor your seat and inner thigh muscles to be sure you are relaxed in these muscle groups.

- To contract the lumbar multifidus
  Think of initiating a *very tiny* tilt of the sacrum (moving the tailbone away from your body as if to arch your back). The contraction should be isometric (the muscle contracts but the joint does not move). Another image is to think about an elastic cord running between your "dimples" in your low back. Think about tightening the cord between your dimples. This may help you to feel the contraction of the lumbar multifidii.
  Another method to begin to feel your lumbar multifidus is to lie on the floor with your knee bent and you heel pressing into the leg of a table (pictured). Press your heel *gently* (about 10% effort) into the leg of the table. Think about contracting your "dimple" muscle as you perform the push. Hold for 10 seconds. Repeat 4 times each leg.

- To contract the transversus abdominis
  Slowly and gently pull your lower abdomen inward. Imagine trying to "zip up" a slightly tight pair of pants. You can feel the tension in the muscle under a finger placed 1 in inward from the front pelvic bones. You should feel a tensing of the deep muscle, not a bulging of the more superficial muscles. Another image is to think about an elastic cord running between the two prominent pelvic bones (called the *ASIS*). Think about tightening the cord between these two bones. This may help you to isolate your transversus abdominis from the other abdominal muscles.

- To activate the intrinsic spinal muscles synergy
  Your physical therapist will help you to identify which intrinsic spinal muscles muscle best activates the entire intrinsic spinal muscles group. Next, take a deep diaphragmatic breath, allowing your ribs to expand to the front, sides, and back. Allow the air to exhale naturally. Before you take another breath, *slowly and gently* contract your intrinsic spinal muscles. Next, resume normal breathing while maintaining contraction of your intrinsic spinal muscles. Your physical therapist will instruct you how to proceed from this step.

- Positions to activate your intrinsic spinal muscles:
  ___ back lying   ___ stomach lying
  ___ sidelying   ___ quadruped
  ___ sitting   ___ standing
  ___ squatting   ___ walking

SELF-MANAGEMENT 17-1 *Supine Intrinsic Spinal Muscles Progression*

Purpose: A back lying activity to strengthen and improve muscle control over your deep trunk muscles including your lumbar multifidus (LM), transverse abdominus (TrA), and pelvic floor. Use of progressively more difficult leg movements challenge your intrinsic spinal muscles muscles. Higher levels will require use of more superficial muscles, but the intrinsic spinal muscles should still be activated as the local stabilization strategy. You can think of this progression as strengthening from the "inside out."

Starting Position: Lie on your back on a firm surface, such as the floor, with knees bent, feet flat on the floor, and shoes off. To feel the TrA, place your fingertips deep to the inside of your front pelvic bones (your physical therapist will show you the exact location). Refer to the Patient-Related Instruction sheet that teaches how to contract each muscle of the intrinsic spinal muscles. Take a deep diaphragmatic breath in (your physical therapist will teach you the correct technique for diaphragmatic breathing). Allow the exhalation to occur naturally, do not force the exhalation. Before you take your next breath, activate your intrinsic spinal muscles. Resume normal breathing. After normal breathing has been established, you can begin the prescribed level of this exercise.

TIP:
- The abdominal muscles must be pulled in, not *pooched* or distended. The pelvic floor must be pulled up, not pushed downward. These errors in strategy often occur as increased strain is placed on the abdominal and pelvic floor muscles from the progressively difficult leg movements.

- The lumbar spine must remain in a neutral position with a *slight* forward curve—just enough to fit your hand between your back and the floor—and not move into further forward curve or excessively flat. If needed, you may use a small hand towel rolled under the small of your back to provide feedback as to the position of your spine.

Movement Technique: Your physical therapist will check off the level(s) you are to perform with the appropriate dosage.

Level I: While keeping your intrinsic spinal muscles activated, *slowly* **slide** one leg down to a straight position followed by **sliding** the other leg down so that both are in a straight position. If your back is arched, you may need to limit your heel slide so that your pelvis is not pulled out of a neutral position. Next, **slide** one leg up the table to a flexed hip and knee position. After you have completed this movement, **slide** the same leg back to a straight position. Repeat with the opposite limb.

TIP: The pelvis must remain in neutral and not rotate. The spine must remain in neutral and not flatten, arch,

or rotate. To keep your spine and pelvis stable you must be sure to keep your intrinsic spinal muscles activated, especially during the initiation of the heel slide because this is the moment when the neutral position is often lost.

Dosage
Sets/repetitions _____
Frequency _____

Level II: Assume the start position. Lift one leg off the floor until your hip is at a 90-degree angle with the floor. Next, **slide** the other leg down to a fully extended position while keeping the opposite leg **elevated** off the floor. **Slide** the leg back to the same position as the nonmoving limb. Repeat with the other leg.

TIP: As soon as you are unable to stabilize the pelvis and lumbar spine with your intrinsic spinal muscles, stop and rest for a minute before continuing. If your hip flexors (front thigh muscles) are short, you will not be able to fully extend your leg without moving your spine or pelvis out of neutral. In this case, stop sliding your leg when you notice your spine or pelvis moving from the neutral position. Eventually, your hip flexor muscles will lengthen as your abdominal muscles shorten and become stronger.

Dosage
Sets/repetitions _____
Frequency _____

Level III: Repeat level II, but instead of sliding your leg down and back, **glide** your leg down and back. The nonmoving leg should remain in a flexed position **off** the floor.

TIP: It is easy to transition from a flat abdomen to a pooched abdomen and from keeping the pelvic floor pulled upward to pushing it downward at this level. Keep the intrinsic spinal muscles activated and continue to breathe.

Dosage
Sets/repetitions _____
Frequency _____

Level IV: Begin from the start position, and lift **both** legs off the floor at the same time to the 90-degree position. Return to the start position by lowering both legs at the same time. **Slide** both legs simultaneously to the fully extended position, and **slide** both legs back to the start position.

Dosage
Sets/repetitions _____
Frequency _____

Level V: Repeat level IV, but **glide** both legs down and back to the start position.

Dosage
Sets/repetitions _____
Frequency _____

TABLE 17-5	Neutral and Functional Spine Positions	
SPINE POSITION	**DEFINITION**	**CLINICAL JUDGMENT OF POSITION**
Neutral	Lumbar spine in slight extension. ASIS and pubic symphysis in the same vertical plane[a]	In supine, enough lumbar extension curve that the clinician can palpate the lumbar spinous processes, but not so much lumbar extension so as to pass hand through to the other side
Functional spine	Position of greatest stability, least stress, fewest symptoms for an individual for any given activity	Varies with pathology, activity, and symptoms

[a]Maitland GD. Vertebral Manipulation. 4th Ed. London: Butterworth, 1977.

SELF-MANAGEMENT 17-2 *Intrinsic Spinal Muscles Series*

Purpose: The purpose of this series of activities is to progressively recruit your intrinsic spinal muscles, aided by your more superficial trunk muscles as needed, in a variety of positions. Be sure to activate your intrinsic spinal muscles prior to and during these various activities to strengthen "from the inside out." Your physical therapist will check off the positions you are able to perform with good technique and will teach you appropriate variations and progressions of these activities.

Back Lying: You can perform the back lying intrinsic spinal muscles progression in this position. Refer to the back lying intrinsic spinal muscles progression handout.

Side Lying:

Start position: Lie on your side with your hips and knees bent about 45 degrees. Place one or two pillows between your knees. You may need to place a small towel under your waist.

Movement technique: Slowly rotate your hip so that your knee cap rotates slightly upward. Do not allow your pelvis to move.

TIP: You can advance this activity to a straighter hip position and add a lifting movement with your thigh. Your physical therapist will teach you this progression and provide you with a more detailed handout.

Dosage
Repetitions: _____
Frequency: _____

Stomach Lying:

Start position: Lie on your stomach with a pillow positioned vertically under your chest and hips. Bend your elbows and rest your hands on the back of your head.

Movement technique: Lift your elbows only about 1/2 in off the surface. Hold the position for 5 to 10 seconds. Return your elbows to the start position.

TIP: You can advance this exercise by changing your arm positions and movements or by adding leg movements. Your physical therapist will teach you the appropriate progression and provide you with a more detailed handout.

Dosage
Repetitions: _____
Frequency: _____

Quadruped:

Start position: Assume a position on your hands and knees, centering your hips over your knees and your shoulders over your hands. Rotate your pelvis so that your hips are at a 90-degree angle with your thigh, spine straight, and head in line with the rest of your spine.

TIP: Do not round your spine upward, drop your head, or arch your low back excessively.

Movement technique: Lift one arm off the table top surface. It is not important to lift the arm fully overhead. Return your hand to the supporting surface.

TIP: Do not let your spine and pelvis move from the start position when lifting your hand. Your physical therapist will teach you how to advance this exercise with variations in the start position or by adding arm and leg movements together.

Dosage
Repetitions: _____
Frequency: _____

Sitting:

Start position: Sit on a chair with a straight seat pan and straight back. Hips and pelvis should be at a right angle with the seat pan. Shoulders should be centered over hips.

Movement technique: Slowly straighten one leg as far as possible without letting your spine or pelvis move out of the start position. Return to the start position and repeat with the other leg.

TIP: Do not let your spine or pelvis move backward (slump) or rotate. Your physical therapist can advance this exercise with combined arm and leg movements.

Dosage
Repetitions: _____
Frequency: _____

Activities of Daily Living: Your physical therapist will teach you how to engage your intrinsic spinal muscles with various movements used in your daily activities such as squatting, stair stepping, lifting, reaching, or walking.

from level II to level IV may be easier than to level III. These factors, combined with patient skill at accomplishing the criteria described previously, can guide the clinician in advancing the exercise.

It is important that the exercise is not progressed to the next level unless the prescribed number of repetitions of the previous level can be achieved *and* the following criteria have been met:

- The lumbar spine should not deviate from the initial starting position, which should be in a neutral spine position (Table 17-5).
- The trunk muscles should be functioning at optimal lengths (i.e., not lengthened).
- The RA should not be dominating the synergy.
- Valsalva maneuver is discouraged.

Self-Management 17-2: Deep Trunk Muscle Series challenges the intrinsic spinal muscles muscles in a variety of positions and motor control levels. Similar to the supine progression, as the difficulty of the exercise is progressed, the intrinsic spinal muscles will not be sufficient for proper stabilization and more superficial muscles will need to assist in the stabilization process. However, the patient needs to be cautioned to continue to recruit the intrinsic spinal muscles, thereby strengthening "from the inside out."

Another exercise focusing on the ability of the intrinsic spinal muscles to stabilize the spine and pelvis is illustrated in Self-Management 17-3: Bent-Knee Fall-Out. Similar to level II and III illustrated in Self-Management 17-1, this exercise challenges the intrinsic spinal muscles ability to stabilize against extension and rotation torques. The introduction of rotational torques requires the synergy of abdominal obliques to control the rotational torques. For example, if the patient is having difficult controlling right pelvic rotation with a right hip abduction/extension/lateral rotation movement, the patient is cued to recruit the left external and right internal oblique to control the rotation.

An increased measure of difficulty can be introduced to any of these exercises by using half or full foam rolls or gym balls. An unstable surface is believed to facilitate recruitment of the deep trunk muscles and stimulate the proprioceptors and balance reactions that are necessary for function.[98,124–127] Care must be taken to introduce this variation when the patient is capable of using subtle recruitment patterns and does not use excessive superficial muscle co-contraction to balance on the roll or ball. Progression to a higher stage of motor control often suffices, unless the specific goal is to challenge balance and proprioception. If the latter is the goal, this progression should not "replace" an exercise designed to improve muscle performance, rather be another exercise prescribed to improve balance control.

As shown in the deep trunk muscle progressions, exercises emphasizing stability through increased neuromuscular control and muscle performance can be progressed to sitting or standing. In sitting, extremity movements can be used in much the same way as in supine positions to challenge the spine to stabilize against various directional forces, with the emphasis on using the entire lumbopelvic stabilizing system in a synergistic manner. For example, sitting while raising the arms in the sagittal plane can challenge the spine to stabilize against sagittal forces, and changing the movement to a unilateral arm raise or to a diagonal direction challenges the spine to stabilize against a transverse plane force. Sitting on a gym ball (Fig. 17-10) making the base of support unstable, can further challenge sitting. The patient is encouraged to use the appropriate intrinsic spinal muscles strategy learned in previous localized exercises by presetting the contraction before arm or leg movements. Stabilization progressions can also be developed in standing. Standing on a half or full foam roll can further challenge a standing progression (Fig. 17-11).

After neuromuscular control and adequate muscle performance are established to stabilize the spine against movements of the extremities and further strength is required

---

SELF-MANAGEMENT 17-3 *Bent-Knee Fall-out*

Purpose:	To train you to move your thigh independently of your pelvis, lengthen your inner thigh muscles, strengthen and shorten weak and overstretched abdominal muscles, and train your intrinsic spinal muscles to stabilize against rotational forces
Starting Position:	Back lying with one leg straight and the other hip and knee bent with the foot flat on the floor. Place your hands on your pelvis as indicated by your physical therapist to monitor pelvic motion. Your physical therapist may ask you to place ___ pillows under the outside of the bent knee to let the knee fall into something.
TIP:	Before beginning the movement, engage your intrinsic spinal muscles. Be sure to keep it engaged throughout the entire movement and continue to breathe in a relaxed manner.
Movement Technique:	Let the bent knee fall out to the side. Do not allow motion to occur in the pelvis. Relax the inner thigh muscles completely before returning to the start position.

Dosage
Repetitions: _____
Frequency: _____

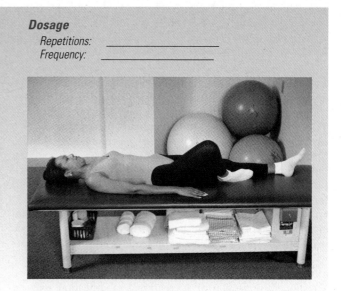

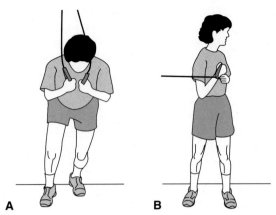

FIGURE 17-13. Tubing can be used to add isometric resistance to create an upright stability activity. The goal is to maintain the spine in neutral through isometric contractions of the trunk musculature while the upper quarter, trunk, or lower quarter is moving in sagittal or transverse planes. In this example, the primary motion is occurring at the hips in the (A) sagittal or (B) transverse plane while the trunk remains in neutral alignment via isometric contractions of the intrinsic spinal muscles and more superficial trunk muscles.

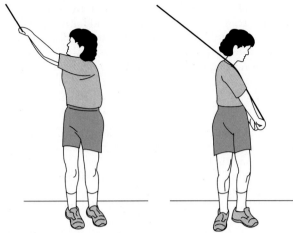

FIGURE 17-14. A progression from Figure 17-13 is controlled mobility. Instead of holding the trunk in neutral alignment, the lumbar spine is incorporated into combined movement patterns with the remainder of the spine, hips, knees, ankles, and feet. Controlled mobility activities can be performed about separate planes of movement (e.g., sagittal, transverse, frontal plane). Caution must be practiced when moving in multiple complex planes of movement (e.g., combined flexion/rotation) resulting from the potential injurious stress to the lumbar spine. Resistance can be applied through pulleys, elastic tubing, or weighted balls. The patient can perform these activities on an unstable surface such as foam rolls or high-density foam squares. With all controlled mobility drills, the motion can occur in the lumbar spine, but most of the motion should occur in the thoracic spine and hips, with the least occurring in the lumbar spine.

from an occupation or recreational activity to achieve a functional outcome, higher forces are required than can be supplied by the extremities alone. Dumbbells, weighted balls, ankle weights can be used to progress the previously described exercises. Pulleys or elastic tubing can also be used to increase the force requirements of the trunk musculature to stabilize the spine. For example, the patient can be challenged to maintain trunk stability with an isometric contraction while pulling the weight up or down (Fig. 17-13A), side to side or in a rotary motion. The emphasis initially is on dynamic motion at the hips, (Fig. 17-13B), while avoiding motion through the trunk (i.e., stability level of stages of motor control). This exercise requires effective stabilization of the trunk through the intrinsic spinal muscles muscles and active recruitment or more superficial trunk muscles and latissimus dorsi, gluteus maximus, gluteus medius, hamtrings, adductors, and hip rotators. All of these muscles are important in stabilization of the lumbar spine and pelvic girdle through the posterior, anterior, and oblique muscular systems. The load is increased as tolerated, and the speed is maintained at a low level.

Preparation for high-level functional return requires more advanced strength training that incorporates spine motion as part of the total movement pattern (i.e., controlled mobility and skill stages of motor control). Programs of this nature may include spine motions involving concentric and eccentric work with variable resistance in all planes, such as controlled mobility in the sagittal plane and in combined planes (Fig. 17-14). At this stage, the various isokinetic machines (e.g., MedX, MET (Medical Exercise Therapy) rotation trainer) and any pulley apparatus or elastic resistance can be useful. The chosen movement pattern should be tailored to those required for the patient's occupational or recreational activities.

Rotation is often not well tolerated by those with a true articular instability of the lumbar spine or SIJ, particularly when the pelvis is fixed in an apparatus or in sitting. Patients with true articular instability should avoid motion in the affected region and should train strictly in isometric modes. Vocational counseling or recreational modification may be necessary for those with true articular instability. Counseling focuses on choosing activities that avoid rotational movement patterns. In cases where lumbopelvic joint dysfunction fails to respond to physical therapy modes of stabilization, a trial of prolotherapy may be considered. Dorman and co-workers observed in vitro that injecting chemical irritants into ligamentous tissue incites collagen proliferation.[128] Theoretically, scarring and tightening of the ligaments results in stabilization of the joint. Present studies provide no evidence that prolotherapy injections alone have a beneficial role in the treatment of CLBP. However, repeated ligament injections, irrespective of the solution used, may give prolonged partial relief of pain and disability as part of a multimodal treatment program, including exercise.[129] If injury to specific structures, such as ligaments or fascia, can be related to a specific clinical presentation and subsequent loss of function associated with pain, a case could be made for the use of prolotherapy.

As with all resistive exercise, after the muscle performance has reached a functional level, functional activities must be added to the program. However, it is unnecessary to wait until the end of the rehabilitation program to train functional activities. These should be considered from the beginning in designing the plan of care. For example, a minimal expectation for a patient in acute pain is to perform hip and knee flexion (see Self-Management 17-1, Level I) and bent-knee fall-outs (see Self-Management 17-3) in a supine position without pain. These duplicate movements are necessary for pain free bed mobility.

The definition of a successful functional outcome varies. Success for one person may be to perform light housework; for another, success may mean resuming heavy lifting in a job, playing a racket sport, or running long distances. The ability to return to desired functional activities, regardless of the level, requires neuromuscular skill to control motion of the trunk and pelvic girdle in relation to the other extremities. This requires interactive stabilization and movement strategies during total-body movement patterns. Exercises addressing force or torque generation of the trunk muscles should be part of a comprehensive rehabilitation program addressing all related body functions and structures. To achieve the neuromuscular skills necessary to return to activity at any level, functional exercises must be practiced with precise movement and recruitment patterns and for many repetitions frequently throughout the day. This requires a high level of commitment on the part of the patient. The exercises used to progress to a functional outcome are based on the postures and movement patterns used during ADLs and occupational and recreational activities. No two functional retraining programs should be the same, because each program is tailored to the individual's functional goals. Examples of functional activities are provided in the "Posture and Movement Impairment" section.

Neurologic Impairment and Pathology Mechanical (e.g., compression, traction) and biochemical (e.g., inflammatory response) factors arising from lumbopelvic dysfunction can result in nerve root pathology. For example, a herniated nucleus pulposus (HNP) at the L5–S1 level can cause mechanical and biochemical irritation to the L5 nerve root and medial branch of the dorsal rami, resulting in weakness in the gluteus medius and same-level LM, respectively.[130] The underlying pathology or impairment causing the mechanical or biochemical irritation must be treated, if possible, to affect the efferent input into the corresponding musculature. Exercise to improve force or torque capability of the affected musculature without treating the underlying neurologic dysfunction will prove futile. Nonetheless, exercise may be a large part of the solution. For example, excessive mobility at a segmental level can lead to degenerative disk disease,[131] which can result in nerve root compression and reduce efferent input into the associated musculature. Exercises to improve the stability of the offending segment coupled with exercises to improve the mobility of other segments or regions (e.g., thoracic spine rotation, hip joint flexion) can reduce the mechanical stress on the nerve root, thereby contributing to restoration of neurologic input into the affected musculature. Appropriate strengthening exercises for the affected musculature (see Display 17-5) can be more effective after the neurologic compromise is resolved.

Another neurologic cause of impaired muscle performance is nerve injury resulting in muscle paresis or paralysis, which can occur as a complication of surgery or from a traction injury to the nerve. LM segmental atrophy at the surgical site has been reported in the CLBP population after surgical intervention.[132] It is thought to be the result of iatrogenic lesions of the dorsal rami and innervation failure of the low back muscles after surgery. This finding is highlighted as a possible cause of "postoperative failed back syndrome" and is supported by histologic evidence.[133] Other investigators have reported denervation of segmental paraspinal musculature in patients with the radiologic diagnosis of segmental hypermobility.[115] These changes were thought to result from traction injury of the posterior primary rami segmentally supplying the muscle at the hypermobile segment. The ability for exercise to reverse the effects of denervation is related

to the neurophysiologic recovery of the damaged nerve. Nonetheless, sustained mechanical stress from segmental instability delays or inhibits healing, and exercise targeted toward increasing segmental stability can reduce mechanical stress on the segment and augment healing. If nerve regeneration occurs, specific exercises focused on improving force or torque generation are necessary to "reeducate" the previously denervated muscle.[134] Specific exercise recommendations will be discussed subsequently.

Muscle Strain Muscle strain can result from a variety of mechanisms:

- Trauma (e.g., spinal extensors and LM after a motor vehicle accident)
- Overuse (e.g., one diagonal EO and IO muscles in a competitive rowing team member)
- Gradual continuous stretch (e.g., EOs in a swayback or lordotic posture)

Strain to lumbopelvic musculature, particularly if caused by trauma, is difficult to diagnose, because it often occurs with injury to other tissues in the motion segment. If a strain is suspected, the activity or technique, starting position, and dosage depend on the severity of the strain, the stage of healing, and the mechanism of injury. Severe strains in early stages of recovery and chronic strains with long-term disuse must start with low-intensity isometric exercises. Strains resulting from chronic stretch must be supported in a short range and exercised with low initial loads and gradual progressions with a focus on generating tension in the short range and avoiding the overstretch range. For example, in the case of an EO strain resulting from marked lordosis and anterior pelvic tilt, use of an abdominal binder combined with low-load exercises in a neutral spine and pelvis position may be indicated in the early stages of recovery (see Patient-Related Instruction 17-1 and Self-Managements 17-1 and 17-2).

If the strain is the result of overuse, ultimate recovery must involve improving the force or torque production and recruitment patterns of the underused synergist(s). For example, strain to one diagonal oblique abdominal muscle is a common injury among members on a rowing team. It is caused by repetitive flexion and unilateral rotation. Changing the movement pattern to greater flexion and rotation occurring at the hips, and improving the force and torque capability of the posterior spinal muscle group (to minimize the flexion component during unilateral rotation) and opposite oblique abdominal muscle group, may be indicated.

Rarely does a patient progress from a trunk muscle strain in the expected time frame, primarily because of frequent reinjury of the muscle. Reinjury is most likely a result of poor protection of the injured area during postures and movement patterns the patient is unaware he or she is performing. It is the responsibility of the therapist to educate the patient to avoid postures and movement patterns most likely contributing to delayed healing and to use improved postures and movement patterns to promote the healing process.

General Disuse and Deconditioning General disuse and deconditioning of the trunk and pelvic girdle muscles can result from the previously described causes. However, the trunk and pelvic girdle muscles also are susceptible to deconditioning as

DISPLAY 17-5
Resisted Exercises for the Lumbopelvic System

Stability Activities for the Anterior Aspect
- Intrinsic spinal muscles activation (see Patient-Related Instruction 17-1)
- Leg slides (see Self-Management 17-1)
- Prone knee bend (see Self-Management 17-5)
- Hip and knee flexion, hip abduction and lateral rotation (see Self-Management 17-3)

Stability Activities for the Posterior Aspect
- Intrinsic spinal muscles activation (see Patient Related Instruction 17-1)
- Manual lumbar multifidus facilitation (see Figure A in Display 17-4)
- Sidelying small-range hip abduction
- Prone small-range hip extension (see Self-Management 19-1: Stomach-Lying Hip Extension in Chapter 19)
- Prone neutral spine isometric

Stability Activities for Lumbopelvic Synergy
- Intrinsic spinal muscles activation (see Patient Related Instruction 17-1)
- Sitting upper extremity flexion, abduction, rotation (Figs. A and B)
- Quadruped arm lift (Fig. C)
- Intrinsic Spinal Muscle Series: Self Management 17-2

Controlled Mobility Activities for Lumbopelvic Synergy
- Trunk curl sit-up (see Self-Management 17-4)
- Trunk sagittal and transverse plane motion in standing (see Fig. 17-14)

Skill Activity for Lumbopelvic Synergy
- Monitor performance of recreational or occupational skills

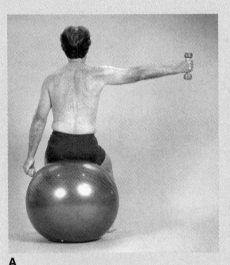

A

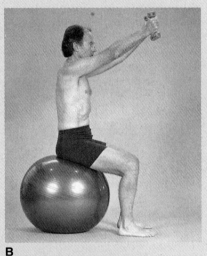

B

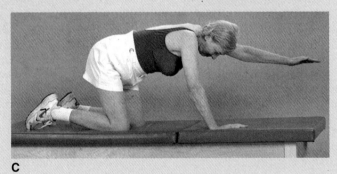

C

a result of general decreased activity level. Trunk and pelvic girdle deconditioning may be a leading cause of lumbopelvic syndromes and therefore are critical areas to address in prevention. Individuals with general deconditioning require a careful examination so that a graded conditioning program is focused on the specific muscles in need of strengthening and that the program is initiated at the appropriate level of difficulty. The dilemma with most trunk-strengthening exercises performed to improve fitness (e.g., bent-knee sit-ups, crunches, roman chair hyperextensions, abdominal or back strengthening machines) is that the exercise is often performed at a higher level than

that at which the muscles can safely and precisely execute the movement. When one synergist of a group is relatively weak, the other synergists often produce the necessary force or torque required to perform the desired movement, thereby reinforcing the muscle imbalance and increasing the risk of injury to the lumbopelvic region.

It is beyond the scope of this text to analyze all the common fitness exercises used to strengthen the trunk muscles. Because the ability to curl up to a sit-up should be considered a normal ADL and because various forms of the sit-up are still commonly performed, a concise analysis of this exercise is provided.

The sit-up can be considered as two distinct phases of one movement: trunk flexion followed by hip flexion (Fig. 17-15). The RA and IO produce the trunk flexion phase, as indicated by rib cage depression (RA) and rib angle widening (IO), and the hip flexors produce the hip-flexion phase.[60] The role of the EO is to offset the anterior force on the pelvis and lumbar spine exerted by the hip flexor muscles as evidenced by a narrowing of the rib angle during the sit-up phase.[60]

Although hip flexors may exhibit some weakness associated with postural problems (e.g., weak hip flexors in the swayback posture), it rarely interferes with performing the hip-flexion phase of the sit-up. The problem in accurately performing a straight leg sit-up is usually weakness of the abdominal muscles, specifically the RA and IO in completing the trunk curl phase and the EO during the hip-flexion phase. As a result, because of a premature hip flexion phase, the lower portions of the RA and IO do not get a dynamic stimulus and the lumbar spine is vulnerable to the extension forces exerted by the hip flexor muscles lifting a longer lever arm.

Instruction in proper execution of the sit-up requires a complex level of analysis and decision making considering the performance of the abdominal muscles in relation to the hip flexor muscles and structural factors. Self-Management 17-4: Sit-Up offers a detailed description of the sit-up. It is important to teach the client to complete the trunk-curl phase before the sit-up phase for proper execution of this exercise.

The lower extremities constitute about one third of the body weight.[135] This means that the force exerted by the trunk in the supine position is greater than that of the lower extremities, and the feet need to be held down during the hip-flexion phase. However, if the spine flexes sufficiently as the trunk raises and the center of mass moves downward toward the hips, the trunk, in many persons, can be raised in flexion without having the feet held down. Most adolescents and women can perform the sit-up without having their feet held down because of a combination of body proportion (e.g., upper body less mass relative to lower body) and segmental trunk flexion lowering the center of mass.

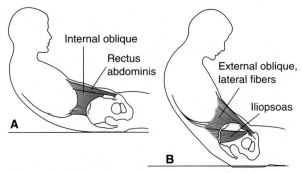

FIGURE 17-15. The sit-up can be considered a two-phase activity. (A) The first phase is the trunk curl. As trunk flexion is slowly initiated by raising the head and shoulders form a supine position, the rib cage depresses anteriorly (RA) and the ribs flare outward, increasing the infrasternal angle (internal oblique). The pelvis tilts posteriorly simultaneously with the head and shoulders raising. (B) As the trunk is raised in flexion on the thighs, the sit-up enters the second or hip-flexion phase. As the hip flexors exert a strong force to tilt the pelvis anteriorly, the EO maintains the spine in flexion and the pelvis in posterior rotation. The infrasternal angle decreases, as evidence of the EO activity. (Adapted from Kendall FP, McCreary EK, Provance PG. Muscles Testing and Function. 4th ed. Baltimore, MD: Williams & Wilkins, 1993.)

In contrast, many men may need to have some added force applied (usually very little) at the point where the trunk curl is completed and the hip flexion begins because mass of the upper body is greater than that of the lower body. This may also be true for women with a stiff trunk because of the inability to segmentally flex the spine, which creates a longer lever arm and may require the feet to be held down during hip flexion. If it is necessary to stabilize the feet during the hip-flexion phase, the feet should be held down *only during the hip-flexion phase* to ensure full trunk flexion before the hip-flexion phase begins. If the feet are held down prematurely or throughout the sit-up, the hip flexors are given fixation, and the trunk can be raised by hip flexion instead of trunk flexion.

Elevation of the feet during the sit-up can indicate abdominal muscle fatigue. For example, an individual may be able to curl the trunk through a specified arc of motion without requiring the feet to be held down (or held down only during hip flexion) for the first few sit-ups. However, in subsequent sit-ups, the feet begin to rise before the specified arc of motion is completed. With the onset of abdominal fatigue, the feet elevate when previously elevation was not observed or rise earlier in the range if fixation is required during the hip-flexion phase, because the abdominal muscles are no longer producing enough torque to flex the trunk through the specified arc of motion. Therefore, the hip flexors act earlier in the range to raise the trunk, with the feet rising as a result.

For many years, sit-ups were performed with the legs straight, but the emphasis has shifted to doing the exercise in the bent-knee position. For this reason, the bent-knee position is compared with the hip-extended position. The bent-knee sit-up has long been advocated as a means of minimizing or eliminating the action of the hip flexors, placing them "on slack" during the sit-up. This idea, which has persisted for many years among professionals and the public, is false and misleading. The abdominal muscles do not cross the hip joint and can therefore only flex the trunk. The sit-up, whether the hips are extended or flexed, is a strong hip flexor exercise; the difference is the arc of hip joint motion through which the hip flexors act (i.e., hips extended: 0 to 80 degrees flexion; hips flexed: 50 to 125 degrees flexion). Because the hip joint moves to completion of hip flexion ROM with the hips and knees flexed, high repetitions of this type of sit-up may be more conducive to the development of short hip flexors than the sit-up with the hips extended.

Although normal flexibility of the back is desired, excessive flexibility is not. A contraindication to performing a bent-knee sit-up is excessive flexibility of the lumbar spine. With the hips extended, the center of mass is slightly anterior to the first or second sacral segment. With the hips and knees bent, the center of mass moves cranially. The lower extremities exert less force in counterbalancing the trunk during the sit-up with the hips and knees flexed than with the hips extended. To sit up from the bent-knee position, the feet must be held down, or the trunk must flex excessively to move the center of mass downward. As the curl progresses, the center of mass moves distally toward the hip joint. In the hip-extended position, by the time the hip-flexion phase arrives, the center of mass has moved toward the hips, which encourages the hips (not the lumbar spine) to flex during the sit-up phase. With the hips flexed, the center of mass may not reach the axis of motion of the hips by the

SELF-MANAGEMENT 17-4 *Sit-Up*

Purpose: To strengthen the abdominal muscles and hip flexor muscles necessary to sit up from a supine position

Starting Position: Back lying with hips and knees straight. Your physical therapist will determine if you are to begin this exercise in a supine position with hips and knees straight or with pillows under your knees. Your physical therapist will also determine if you will require fixation of your feet during the sit-up phase of this exercise.

TIP: To perform this exercise with proper technique, follow the tips listed:

Start with an intrinsic spinal muscles contraction and hold this contraction throughout the entire sit-up and return to the start movement.

Do not push your abdomen out or your pelvic floor down.

Curl your trunk to the same spine level with the selected arm position.

Maintain lumbar flexion and posterior pelvic tilt during the hip flexion phase.

If you require fixation for your feet, do not use the fixation until the sit-up phase.

If you did not require fixation for level I, you should not require fixation at any level of the exercise. Ask your physical therapist if you have trouble keeping your feet down during the sit-up phase of level II or III. Premature lifting of your feet can be an indication of abdominal fatigue.

Movement Technique:

Level I: With your arms in front of your body, bring your chin to your chest, and slowly curl your trunk as you come to a full sitting position. Slowly reverse the curl and resume the start position.

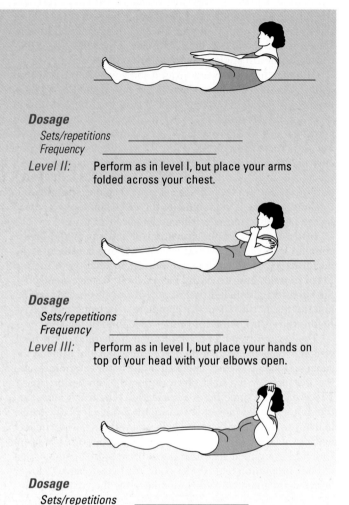

Dosage
Sets/repetitions _____
Frequency _____

Level II: Perform as in level I, but place your arms folded across your chest.

Dosage
Sets/repetitions _____
Frequency _____

Level III: Perform as in level I, but place your hands on top of your head with your elbows open.

Dosage
Sets/repetitions _____
Frequency _____

hip-flexion phase, thereby imposing a flexion moment on the lumbar spine versus the hip joints. The persons most in danger of being adversely affected by repeated bent-knee sit-ups are children and young adolescents because of their tendency toward excessive flexibility. Adults with LBP associated with excessive flexion flexibility of the low back may also be adversely affected by this exercise.

A precaution to performing a straight-leg sit-up is short hip flexors. In the supine position with the legs straight, a person with short hip flexors lies in anterior pelvic tilt and lumbar extension. The danger with performing the sit-up from this position is that the multijoint hip flexors (i.e., tensor fascia lata [TFL] and rectus femoris) pull the pelvis into more anterior pelvic tilt and subsequently the spine into further extension during the hip-flexion phase. The bent-knee position releases the downward pull of the short hip flexors, allowing the pelvis to tilt posteriorly and the lumbar spine to relatively flex. This relieves the extension stress on the low back. However, the hips and knees should be bent only as much as needed

to allow the pelvis to reach neutral in the supine position. This position should be maintained passively by using a large enough roll or pillow under the knees. Prescribing bent-knee sit-ups (even in a partially bent-knee position) to individuals with short hip flexors is not the final solution, and this position should not be used indefinitely. Short hip flexors often accompany lengthened EO muscles because of the anterior pelvic tilt posture induced by the short hip flexors. The bent-knee sit-up neither addresses the short hip flexors nor the lengthened EOs. Working toward a goal of being able to lie supine with the pelvis in neutral is accomplished by minimizing and gradually decreasing the amount of hip flexion permitted in the start position. Consequently, it is important to perform exercises to stretch the short hip flexors (see Self-Management 17-5: Prone Knee Bend), to strengthen and shorten the EO muscles (see Self-Management 17-1: Supine Intrinsic Spinal Muscles Progression), and to attend to undesirable postural habits (e.g., avoiding excessive anterior pelvic tilt and lumbar lordosis).

SELF-MANAGEMENT 17-5 *Prone Knee Bend*

Purpose: To lengthen the hip flexors and quadriceps, improve the strength of the intrinsic spinal muscles, and train the pelvis and spine to remain still during knee bending movements

Starting Position: Facelying with both lower limbs straight and knees together.

Options: You may need _____ pillows under your hips, as indicated by your physical therapist.

You may need to position your thigh out to the side.

Movement Technique: Before moving your legs, engage your intrinsic spinal muscles. Maintain this contraction as you bend one knee as far as possible *without movement in the pelvis or spine*

Options: Bend both knees at the same time while keeping knees and ankles together.

Correct: pelvis remains still
No motion

Incorrect: pelvis tilts
or rotates

Dosage
Repetitions: _____
Frequency: _____

A contraindication to either bent knee or straight leg sit-up techniques is concern about compressive loading of the spine. Lumbar compressive loads >3,000 N were predicted for both straight-leg and bent-knee sit-up techniques.[136] In the presence of an HNP, for example, the issue of using straight-leg or bent-knee sit-ups is not as important as the issue of whether or not to prescribe sit-ups at all.

A trend in abdominal strengthening is a trunk curl or "crunch" performed without the hip-flexion phase. If the EO muscle is weak, making the lumbar spine vulnerable during the hip-flexion phase of the sit-up, performance of only the trunk-curl phase should be safe and effective for strengthening the abdominal muscles. There is less intradiskal pressure in performing the trunk curl than in a full sit-up.[32] However, the trunk curl focuses primarily on producing torque for movement rather than force or torque for stabilization of lumbar segments. This preferentially recruits the RA and IO over the EO. Moreover, the trunk curl is contraindicated for any person with a thoracic kyphosis because of the stress thoracic flexion exerts on the kyphosis. Alternative exercises should be suggested for persons with poor lumbar stabilization and thoracic kyphosis (see Self-Managements 17-1 and 17-2).

If the trunk curl is chosen, the therapist should determine the position in which the patient should start—a small towel roll under the knees, a wedge-shaped pillow under the head and shoulder, or a pillow under the knees. Before any trunk movement, an intrinsic spinal muscles contraction should be initiated (see Patient-Related Instruction 17-1). With the arms extended forward, the patient should flex the chin toward the chest and continue to curl the upper trunk as far as the spine can flex (see Self-Management 17-4). If the subject cannot perform the curl to completion of his or her spine flexion because of abdominal weakness, a wedge-shaped pillow can be placed behind the head and shoulders to limit the range and decrease the effect of gravity. As abdominal muscle strength improves, sequentially, smaller pillows can be used. If the hip flexors are short, temporary use of a pillow under the knees can be used to decrease the pull of the hip flexors on the spine and allow the individual to lie in supine with the pelvis and spine in neutral. Table 17-6 summarizes features related to the prescription of the sit-up and its variations.

Range of Motion, Muscle Length, and Joint Mobility

Clinical decisions regarding exercise prescription for ROM, muscle length, and joint mobility must be considered in relation to other regions of the spine, upper quarter, and lower quarter.

TABLE 17-6 Summary of Indications, Contraindications, and Precautions in Prescribing Sit-ups and Sit-up Variations

EXERCISE	INDICATIONS	CONTRAINDICATION AND PRECAUTIONS
Bent knee sit-up	Lordosis	Short hip flexors, excessive trunk flexion ROM, thoracic kyphosis
Temporary use of pillows under knees for sit up	Short hip flexors	
Straight leg sit-up	At least 3+/5 strength of all abdominal muscles and hip flexors	Acute or subacute disc pathology
Trunk curl (only)	Weak EOs, acute or subacute disk pathology	Thoracic kyphosis
Temporary use of wedge under spine	<3/5 in lower fibers of abdominals, stiff lumbar region (restricted in flexion)	

Hypermobility

Diagnosis of hypermobility and true articular instability can be made from careful clinical examination.[72,87] The examiner should also seek to discover the impairments contributing to the hypermobility or articular instability.[8] Four factors can be responsible for the development of a hypermobile segment: trauma (e.g., motor vehicle accident resulting in an acceleration injury), pathology (e.g., rheumatoid arthritis, degenerative joint changes), structural impairment (spondylolisthesis, HNP, asymmetric tropic changes in the ZJ), or chronic repetitive movement patterns. With repetitive movement, hypermobility can develop within the lumbopelvic region in response to a relatively less mobile segment or region. Theoretically, in a multijoint system with common movement directions, any given movement follows the segments providing the least resistance, resulting in abnormal or excessive movement of segments with the least amount of stiffness.[8] With repeated movements over time, the least stiff segments increase in mobility, and the more stiff segments decrease in mobility.

Sahrmann has termed the site of abnormal or excessive motion *the site of relative stiffness or flexibility*.[8] The term *relative* is key to this concept. For example, the fifth lumbar vertebra, because of its biomechanical and anatomic properties, is more adapted to produce rotation than any other lumbar segment. It is therefore *relatively* more flexible in the direction of rotation. This becomes a clinical problem or impairment only if the segmental motion becomes excessive. A contributing factor is the relative stiffness at other spinal segments and regions in the upper and lower quarters that are designed for rotation. For example, playing golf involves a significant amount of total-body rotation to achieve a proper golf swing. If the hips or feet are relatively stiff in rotation, this pattern may impose excessive rotational stress on the spine. If the thoracic spine or upper lumbar segments are stiff in rotation, this pattern may impose excessive rotation on the L5 segment.

The cause-and-effect relationship of relative flexibility can be addressed through a comprehensive program of improving mobility at the relatively more stiff segments or regions and improving stiffness at the relatively more mobile segment. Stiffness should be increased at the site of relative flexibility by improving neuromuscular control, muscle performance (i.e., hypertrophic changes), and length-tension relationships of the stabilizing muscles (see the "Muscle Performance Impairment" section) around the site of relative flexibility coupled with educating the patient and training postures and movement patterns (see the "Posture and Movement Impairment" section) that improve the distribution of mobility between associated regions and the lumbopelvic region. According to a study by Shirley et al.,[137] voluntary submaximal contractions as low as 10% MVC demonstrated an increase in lumbar posterior to anterior (PA) stiffness. This conclusion points to the importance of motor control and simply teaching the patient to activate the spinal muscles at low levels to increase segmental stability.

Exercises to reduce hypermobility at a segmental level or within the pelvis can be progressed according to traditional stages of motor control: mobility, stability, controlled mobility, and skill. The stage of mobility can be thought of as improving mobility at relatively stiff or hypomobile segment(s) or region(s) in the specific direction(s) desired to reduce the stress at the associated hypermobile segment. Activities

and techniques to improve mobility are presented in the "Hypomobility" section.

The stage of stability can be thought of as improving motor control, muscle performance (particularly hypertrophic changes), and length-tension properties of the affected muscles to increase stiffness at the site of relative flexibility. Specific activities and techniques chosen to promote stiffness and stability at a site of relative flexibility should be based on the direction the segment is susceptible to motion. Sahrmann developed the term *direction susceptible to motion (DSM)* to describe this relationship.[8] To stimulate adaptive shortening in a lengthened muscle, exercises must be performed with the spine in neutral or functional positions with the muscles in the corresponding length. The patient must be educated to avoid habitual postures that place a lengthening stress on the muscle (e.g., avoid standing in a swayback in the presence of lengthened EO). In some cases, immobilization in the short range (e.g., use of an abdominal binder or taping) may be necessary to facilitate adaptive shortening. To stimulate hypertrophic changes that lead to increased muscle stiffness, prescribe exercises for specific muscles dosage levels for hypertrophy (i.e., 10 to 12 repetition max sets).

Controlled mobility focuses on the ability of the lumbopelvic region to move dynamically in all three planes with appropriate distribution of movement and torques within the lumbar region and between associated regions of the upper extremities, thoracic spine, SIJ, hip, knee, ankle, and foot. Skill is reached when the patterns of muscle activation become automatic and internalized by the patient during functional activities. Display 17-5 provides recommendations for exercises to develop stability through the stages of motor control.

To be most effective in reducing hypermobility with exercise, the therapist should educate each patient to use appropriate spine positions during all exercises and functional activities. There is no particular lumbopelvic functional position that is best for all patients and for all activities. Although the standard is the neutral position (see Table 17-5), it may not be achieved by all patients and for all activities, in which case the functional position of the spine should be used. The functional position (see Table 17-5) varies with physiologic status and stresses from ADLs and IADLs. It varies among individuals and circumstances. For example, to avert exacerbation of symptoms, patients with spinal stenosis must avoid extension. The functional position may vary with the patient's activity. For example, flexion should be avoided during heavy lifting from the floor to the waist. Some authorities argue that the spine should be held in end-range extension for maximal protection and efficiency of motion in lifting.[138] However, end-range extension should be avoided during lifting from waist level to overhead, and the functional position may be biased toward flexion to avoid injury to the spine with this activity. Functional spinal posture may vary with the patient's behavior of symptoms. The more severe, irritable, and acute the condition, the more limited the functional position of the spine becomes to avoid symptoms.

Hypomobility

To be most effective, activities or techniques to reduce hypermobility must occur simultaneously with activities or techniques to increase mobility in related regions that are relatively more stiff. Many activities or techniques can be used to increase mobility, such as manual techniques (e.g., articular joint mobilization, muscle energy techniques, soft-tissue mobilization); passive self-stretch or self-mobilization; or active assisted, active, and resisted exercise.

There are multiple justifications for the use of manual therapy including (see Chapter 7):

- Psychologic effects as a result of patient-therapist interaction[139]
- Mechanical effect (e.g., altering positional relationships or mobilizing joints through stretching or rupturing restrictive structures)[140]
- Neurophysiologic effect (e.g., activation of the gate control mechanism, reflexogenic decrease of muscle hypertonicity)[140]

Research does not support the use of rotatory manual techniques for reduction of herniations in contained or uncontained disks[141–143]; in fact, rotatory techniques seem contraindicated in diskogenic dysfunctions and tensile strain to annular fibers as a result of rotation may further weaken nuclear containment.[144] Research also does not support the rationale that manual therapy can affect the positional relationship in the SIJ and thus decrease complaints.[86] Neurophysiologic mechanisms may offer a better explanation of the effects of manual therapy. Clinical outcome studies demonstrate better results with manual therapy techniques when patients with nonspecific LBP are classified using clinical guideline indices.[145]

Passive intervention in the form of manual therapy or manual exercise without some form of active exercise is discouraged. One potential hazard in providing purely passive intervention is that the patient may not participate *actively* in the rehabilitation process. This may prevent the patient from achieving full recovery or contribute to recurrence, because the patient is unable to manage the condition independently. Whenever possible, active participation in the form of patient-related education and self-management exercise is encouraged.

Active assisted ROM, active ROM, proprioceptive neuromuscular facilitation techniques (see Chapter 13), and passive stretching can also be used to increase mobility (see Chapter 7). This discussion focuses on self-management exercises, emphasizing passive and active stretching.

Passive stretching may be necessary, particularly for muscle groups with adaptive shortness. Careful muscle length testing determines which trunk and pelvic girdle muscles require stretching. Superficial trunk muscles, such as the RA, quadratus lumborum, and lumbar erector spinae, and multijoint hip muscles, such as TFL/iliotibial band, semitendinosus or semimembranosus (medial HSs), biceps femoris (lateral HSs), hip adductors, and rectus femoris, are susceptible to adaptive shortening.

Care must be taken when stretching muscles crossing the hip joint in individuals with lumbopelvic dysfunction, because the SIJ or lumbar spine often becomes the site of relative flexibility when the hip becomes hypomobile. Stabilization of the pelvic attachment while the distal attachment moves requires special attention in lumbopelvic patients because the spine or SIJ becomes the path of least resistance and therefore easily moves before the feeling of a stretch.

An example of proper stabilization for a diarthrodial muscle with attachments on the pelvis is the supine passive HSs stretch. The HSs may be passively stretched in supine with one hip flexed and the ipsilateral knee extended (to the

BUILDING BLOCK 17-1

1. Provide specific criteria for positioning for the:
   - Contralateral limb
   - Spine and pelvis
   - Ipsilateral limb
2. How could you isolate medial versus lateral HSs?
3. Based on your knowledge of the dosage for stretching, prescribe specific duration and repetitions for an effective stretch.

point of mild HSs tension) and the foot against a wall while the contralateral hip and knee are extended. The lumbopelvic region is stabilized in part by the appropriate recruitment of the intrinsic spinal muscles muscles and by the underlying surface. The length of the HSs determines the distance from the wall and angle of SLR. Certain criteria are used for proper stabilization to facilitate the optimal stretch (see Building Block 17-1).

Neuromeningeal Hypomobility

Loss of mobility of the nervous system can occur as a result of congenital disorders, trauma, surgical complications, or degenerative changes.[6,73,146] There are two types of neuromeningeal hypomobility: the tethered cord syndrome and the nerve root and dural movement dysfunction. The tethered cord syndrome forms a contraindication to physical therapy intervention; however, nerve root and dural movement dysfunction can respond quite well to neural mobilization techniques.[73] Before intervention, neuromeningeal mobility should be assessed and its influence determined. Specific exercises may be prescribed that are designed to improve mobility of the neural system (see Self-Management 17-6: Neuromeningeal Mobilization). The related anatomy, physiology, and application principles must be well understood for the effective and safe use of this type of treatment. This topic is worthy of more extensive coverage. Detailed information is provided by Butler.[73]

Pain

LBP is the most common type of pain reported by adults in physician offices.[147] Of frustration to the clinician is the difficulty associated with identifying the pathoanatomical cause for most cases of LBP, leading many to consider LBP as a single "nonspecific" disorder. Most studies evaluating the treatment effectiveness of interventions for LBP have been based on this presumption and have generally demonstrated small to no treatment effects. However, most providers think of LBP as a more heterogeneous disorder, and the inability to more specifically match patients to interventions is one possible explanation for the lack of research evidence proving the effectiveness of treatments and the suboptimal outcomes of clinical care.

The difficulty in diagnosing the pathoanatomic cause of pain stems from the varied sources of nociceptive structures and the complex interaction of peripheral and central mechanisms responsible for the experience of pain. The physiologic and psychologic impact that lumbopelvic pain has on the

SELF-MANAGEMENT 17-6 *Neuromeningeal Mobilization*

Purpose: To improve the mobility of your sciatic nerve and its branches into the calf and foot and to reduce the pain coming from a loss of mobility in the sciatic nerve

Assessment: Before beginning this exercise, you must first assess the status of your neural mobility.

Slump in your low back and pelvis as far as possible.

Bring your chin toward your chest.

Flex your foot as far as possible.

Slowly extend the knee on the side of symptoms as far as possible.

Stop at the onset or worsening of symptoms.

Notice the angle of your knee. You will recheck this angle after performing the exercise. You should be able to extend your knee further if you are successful with mobilizing your nerve.

If the angle is less, you have exacerbated your nerve and should repeat the series, reducing the range of motion of each movement in the series. Recheck the knee angle. It should be back to the original assessment position or may be improved.

Starting Position: Slump in your low back, and roll your pelvis back as far as possible. *Slightly* flex your neck to take the stress off the forward head position the slumped posture placed your head in.

Movement Technique: Repeat each activity up to 15 times.

Knee mobilization: Keeping your ankle relaxed, extend your knee until you feel *mild* tension behind your knee. Relax back to the start position.

Ankle mobilization: Extend your knee about three fourths of the distance you found during the assessment. Flex and extend your ankle.

Neck mobilization: Extend your knee three fourths of the distance you found during the assessment. Flex your ankle toward your head about three fourths of the distance of its full range of motion. Actively flex your chin toward your chest and release to the start position.

Reassess after the first cycle. If you have been successful as described under the assessment, repeat the cycle ____ times.

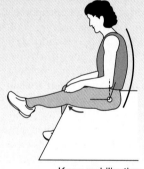
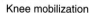
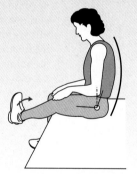
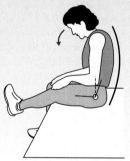

| Knee mobilization | Ankle mobilization | Neck mobilization |

person can create profound participation restriction. It is often difficult to determine the individual contribution of physiologic and psychologic impairment, necessitating treatment that deals with both categories of impairment. The experience of musculoskeletal origin pain is a complex process involving both the peripheral nervous system and the central nervous system and is beyond the scope of this chapter. The reader is referred to Chapter 10 and additional reading on the topic.[148–150] This section deals with the treatment of pain based solely on body function and structures.

Treatment of the physiologic musculoskeletal component of pain can include interventions along a vast spectrum of choices, ranging from pharmaceutical intervention in the form of oral medications, or injections to physical therapy, to surgery—applied individually or in any combination. The choice of intervention must be tailored to each case, ideally with input from all practitioners involved in the case.

This section discusses therapeutic exercise as one type of intervention for the treatment of musculoskeletal lumbopelvic pain. Although the exercises suggested in this section were chosen to demonstrate activities or techniques to treat different underlying causes of pain, many are used to treat associated impairments, such as those of mobility, muscle performance, posture, and motor control. Consequently, they may be referred to in other sections of this chapter, illustrating the complex interaction of impairments and the diversity and versatility of the exercises.

To make informed decisions about the exercises chosen to treat pain, the clinician should understand the physiologic impact that pain has on the structures of the lumbopelvic region. There is evidence of segmental changes within the deep low back muscles in the presence of LBP.[34,134,150–154] Atrophy has been found on the ipsilateral side and at the corresponding clinically determined level of symptoms in the LM, whose potential segmental stabilizing role in the lumbar spine is becoming increasingly well recognized.[34,155] Histologic changes have been found in the type I fibers of the LM in patients with herniated IVDs and CLBP.[152,156–159] The changes identified in the type I fibers may result from pain-provoked, low-tension muscle contraction, which is not strong enough to stimulate type II fibers.[35] Others have hypothesized that the atrophy is consistent with pain-induced disuse.[153] Although the physiologic changes are not well understood, they do occur and contribute to impairments in muscle performance and neuromuscular control, particularly in the LM.

A patient with CLBP and poor segmental control over the stabilizing and movement functions of the affected motion segment(s) is caught in a cycle of pain and dysfunction. Reducing the mechanical or chemical causes of pain is critical to breaking the cycle and allowing the structures affected by pain and inflammation to recover if provided with the appropriate stimulus.

Most structures in the lumbar spine can be a source of pain at some time under the right circumstances, making it difficult or impossible to diagnose a specific pathoanatomic cause of pain. The nerve root, disk annulus, facet joint, and muscle seem to be the most acceptable candidates for sources of pain.[160] The mechanisms of pain production are described as a combination of mechanical and chemical irritation of the nociceptive receptors within the tissues. It is not clear whether mechanical stresses lead to chemical irritation, which sensitizes the tissue, or chemical irritation makes tissue more sensitive to mechanical stress. The two mechanisms most likely coexist in the vast majority of cases.

In the spinal canal, the HNP is a strong candidate for the cause of inflammation and irritation of nerve roots and nerve endings. Because of the juxtaposition of disk and nerve roots in the spinal canal, sciatica (i.e., pain radiating from the low back into the buttock, posterior thigh, and leg) is likely to rise from compression of the dorsal root ganglion and inflamed nerve roots. When a painful condition is set in peripheral tissue, the consequent barrage of noxious signals into the spinal cord can sensitize somatosensory neurons in the dorsal horn. These sensitized neurons can contribute to a condition of CLBP.[161]

The physical therapist is most interested in the mechanical cause of pain as it relates to movement. A systematic physical examination can reveal postures, stabilization and movement strategies that contribute to the onset of pain, worsen existing pain, or conversely, reduce or abolish pain.[123,162]

One philosophical approach to treating mechanical causes of pain related to posture or movement is to teach the patient to modify postures or movements that are associated with the onset or worsening of pain.[8,12,123,162] Within the context of an examination based on tests used to determine postures and movements associated with pain, the therapist instructs the patient in strategies to modify posture and movement patterns associated with pain and treat the associated physiologic impairments contributing to the undesirable posture and movement strategies (e.g., ROM, joint mobility, muscle performance, neuromuscular control). This approach is believed to intervene mechanically by avoiding the postures and movements that are associated with pain, and chemically by allowing the painful structures to "rest" and reduce or halt the inflammatory process. For example, in the patient who reports worsening of pain during forward bending, the lumbar-pelvic relationship is faulty, with excessive motion in the low back relative to the hips.[163] If the pain is reduced or abolished when the patient is instructed to bend with a greater contribution of movement from the hips and less movement from the low back, this information can be used to devise an exercise intervention. Examples of exercises to include in such a program are listed in Display 17-6.

DISPLAY 17-6
Exercises to *Improve* Hip Flexion Mobility and *Decrease* Lumbar Flexion Mobility

- Exercises to improve hip flexion mobility
- Hand-knee rocking (see Self-Management 19-6: Hand-Knee Rocking in Chapter 19)
- Supine hip flexion without lumbar flexion or rotation (Fig. A)
- Exercises to reduce lumbar flexion mobility
- Seated knee extension (see Self-Management 19-7: Seated Knee Extension in Chapter 19)

- Standing hip flexion (Fig. B)
- Instruction to alter posture and movement patterns
- Corrected Sitting Posture (see Patient-Related Instruction 18-4: Proper Sitting Posture in Chapter 18)
- Improved lumbar pelvic movement (see Patient-Related Instruction 17-3)

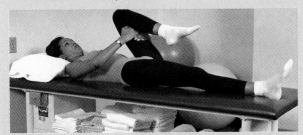

A

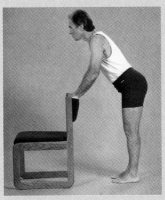

B

In many cases, reducing the mechanical stress on the affected structures by improving mobility in adjacent regions, improving stability in the affected region, and making associated changes in posture and movement patterns are sufficient steps to resolve the episode of pain without need for other interventions. In other instances, complementary interventions (e.g., joint mobilization or manipulation, traction, physical agents, pharmaceutical intervention, psychologic counseling) by the physical therapist or other practitioners involved in the case may be necessary to treat additional mechanical, chemical, or psychologic contributions to pain.

McKenzie developed another therapeutic exercise approach for the treatment of pain.[164,165] A simplified example of this approach is the use of movements that reduce or abolish symptoms. Self-reports of postures related to pain, observation of posture, and uniplanar movements (e.g., flexion, extension, lateral flexion) are used to assess the effect of posture and movement on symptoms. During the examination, each movement is rated according to terms used to describe a change in status (e.g., improve, worsen, status quo). After the movement, or repeated movements, the patient is asked to compare his or her symptoms with the baseline.

The concepts of *peripheralization* (i.e., pain or paresthesia that moves distally away from the spine) and *centralization* (i.e., pain or paresthesia that is abolished or moves from the periphery toward the lumbar spine) are used to determine which movements should be used in self-treatment. For example, if repeated forward bending peripheralizes symptoms and extension centralizes symptoms, extension-related exercises would be used in self-management to modulate symptoms (see Self-Management 17-7: Prone Press-Up Progression). This approach to the treatment of acute LBP has been effective in restoring function,[165] particularly if used in conjunction with a treatment-based classification approach to low back syndrome.[7] In a retrospective study of 87 patients with leg and LBP, Donnelson et al.[166] found that all patients with excellent outcomes of McKenzie-based diagnosis and treatment showed centralization during the initial evaluation.

SELF-MANAGEMENT 17-7 *Prone Press-Up Progression*

Purpose: To improve the mobility of your low back into backward bending, stretch the front trunk muscles, move your leg pain toward your back or abolish it completely, and/or progressively relieve the pressure on your lumbar disk.

TIP: Your physical therapist may ask you to perform special exercises to reduce any shift you exhibit in your spine before the execution of this exercise.

Starting Position: Face lying with legs straight.

Movement Technique: Your physical therapist will inform you of the levels of this exercise you are to perform and the duration of time you should spend at each level.

TIP: You should *not* progress to the next level if your pain does not change in intensity or position (i.e., does not move toward your spine) or moves further down your leg.

Level I: Remain on your stomach with your hands supporting your forehead.

Dosage
Repetitions: _____
Frequency: _____

Level II: Prop up onto your forearms. Be sure you relax the muscles in your back.

Dosage
Duration _____
Sets/repetitions _____
Frequency _____

Level III: Place your hands next to your shoulders. Press your upper trunk upward with your arms through the prescribed range of motion. Be sure the muscles in your back are fully relaxed.

Dosage
Range of motion _____
Sets/repetitions _____
Frequency _____

McKenzie's conceptual model for treatment of diskogenic dysfunctions theorizes that with annular fibers present to exert force on the NP, the NP will move posteriorly during flexion and anteriorly during extension.[6,82] Other rationales include effects related to activating gate control mechanisms, neural tissue relaxation, decreasing mechanical stimulation of nerve roots and other nociceptive tissues, and disk hydration.[82,167–171]

Positional techniques can also be used to modulate pain. For example, a patient can be taught to use positional traction if the goal is to separate joint surfaces to expedite relief of pain (Fig. 17-16). The theory behind positional traction is similar to that for other types of traction (see "Traction" in a later section of this chapter) in that the technique is used to affect the mechanical causes of pain.[172]

Self-mobilization or "prescriptive articular exercise," can be prescribed to correct articular dysfunction, particularly that which relates to the SIJ. For example, a patient who presents with recurrent sacroiliac articular dysfunction (e.g., anterior innominate rotation) that is mechanically contributing to his or her pain should be able to self-treat the articular dysfunction rather than relying solely on the therapist to restore articular function.[173] An example of a prescriptive articular exercise is illustrated in Self-Management 17-8: Self-Mobilization for an Anterior Innominate Dysfunction. For this type of technique to be successful, the patient must learn to evaluate his or her dysfunction and to perform the appropriate technique with precision only until correction is achieved. It also must be emphasized to the patient that these techniques are not considered part of the regular exercise regimen; they should be used only for articular dysfunction that contributes to the patient's symptoms. Although pain is the most common symptom, paresthesias and weakness are also symptoms related to articular dysfunction and should be used as indications for this treatment technique. A relative contraindication for this technique is a hip joint that is hypermobile in the posterior/inferior direction. Repeated use of this technique in the presence of a hypermobile hip may cause further increases in hip laxity and subsequent pain. Self-Management 17-9: Self-Mobilization for a Sacral Dysfunction can be used if the specific dysfunction is a sacral torsion in which the sacrum is rotated causing a unilateral counter-nutation. This technique activates both piriformis and LM to restore sacral nutation. From a sequencing standpoint, a technique to correct an articular dysfunction should be performed before any other exercise. Normalizing

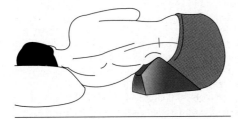

FIGURE 17-16. Positional traction. The use of a foam wedge allows maximal lateral flexion at a desired segmental level because of its sharp apex and ability to accommodate to the bony pelvis. The wedge easily can be made at a business that specializes in the manufacturing or design of foam products. The recommended density is CD-80. The preferred dimensions are 0 × 8 × 8 × 18 in (small) and 0 × 10 × 10 × 18 in (large).

SELF-MANAGEMENT 17-8 *Self-Mobilization for an Anterior Innominate Dysfunction*

Purpose: To normalize the position and motion of your pelvis

Starting Position: Backlying on a firm surface.

Movement Technique: Keep your ___ hip and knee straight. Pull your ___ knee toward your chest until you feel a mild barrier. Gently squeeze your ___ gluteal muscles against an unyielding force exerted by your hands keeping your knee to your chest. Hold your contraction for 8 to 10 seconds. On relaxation, flex your hip and rotate your pelvis posteriorly until you feel a new barrier. Repeat this process three to four times.

Dosage
Repetitions: _____
Frequency: _____

SELF-MANAGEMENT 17-9 *Self-Management for a Sacral Dysfunction*

Purpose: To restore normal position and movement of your sacrum

Starting Position: Lie on your stomach on the floor with your legs on either side of a table leg or door. Bend your ___ knee to 90 degrees and position your heel against the table leg or door.

Movement Technique: First, activate your pelvic floor muscles, transverse abdominus, and LM. *Gently* (about 10% maximum pressure) press your heel into the table leg or door. *Use your deep hip muscles (not your thigh muscles). Hold the contraction for 10 seconds.*

Dosage
Repetitions: _____
Frequency: _____

articular alignment and segmental mobility may normalize muslce tone and activation capabilities that will be necessary for subsequent exercises maximum effectiveness.

For patients with non-specific CLBP, there is compelling evidence that active rehabilitation that is directed toward return to normal activity and work can reduce absence from work more than did traditional care.[174] Examples are graded activity interventions that include physical exercise, application of operant-conditioning behavioral principals, and promotion of improved functioning and safe return to work even if pain persists.

In an acute onset of LBP, inflammation often dominates the clinical picture, and attempts at altering mechanical causes may not lessen the pain. The clinician must treat inflammation with the appropriate adjunctive modalities (e.g., cryotherapy, electrotherapy), protective measures (e.g., corset, SIJ belt), and controlled rest, but strict bed rest should be avoided (see Chapter 7). Moreover, the patient's physician should be alerted so that, if necessary, appropriate pharmacologic agents may be prescribed or modified.

Exercise is not contraindicated when an inflammatory response dominates the clinical picture. The primary goal is to reduce the inflammatory process, which is typically achieved in physical therapy by reducing mechanical stress in the region. The patient may be prescribed a lumbopelvic support or belt to reduce movement and redistribute spinal loads.[175] Exercises encouraging controlled rest are prescribed to enable the patient to perform basic movements without causing pain. To move without inducing an increase in baseline pain, motion must be prevented at the affected lumbar spine segment or SIJ. Patient education is critical to teach the patient what postures and movements to avoid to reduce mechanical stress. Exercise may involve low-intensity isometric recruitment of the stabilizing muscles of the lumbar spine and SIJs with simultaneous small-range movements of the extremities. Altering the length of lever arms, limiting the ROM, and adjusting the position of the exercise to a gravity-lessened position are examples of altering the exercise to reduce the stress on the inflamed segments. Prophylactic ROM exercises for associated regions and neuromeningeal mobility exercises[73] (see Self-Management 17-6) also may be used to prevent unnecessary loss of movement.

As the acute pain reduces in intensity and irritability and as functional movement improves, more advanced exercises may be introduced, focusing on impairments in muscle performance, ROM, muscle extensibility, joint mobility, balance, and relatively more advanced postures and movement patterns. Transition to more advanced stages of care is rarely simple; it is often necessary to revert to more specific treatment of acute pain because of the difficulty in prescribing the optimal dosage for more advanced exercise. The dosage often stresses any given element of the movement system beyond its tolerance, resulting in increased pain and inflammation. Exercise gradation should therefore err on the conservative side to avoid exacerbation of symptoms.

Patients should be educated about when to modify or stop exercise in light of increased symptoms (e.g., numbness, paresthesia, pain) beyond acceptable time frames (e.g., if symptoms are increased for more than 24 hours). Continuing to exercise when symptoms increase significantly or when increased symptoms exceed acceptable time frames can be counterproductive to progress. Educating the patient to heed the body's warning signs and to modify exercises appropriately

(e.g., decrease lever arms, work in gravity-lessened position, decrease repetitions, decrease frequency, longer rest periods) can prevent the complications of excessive stress on healing tissues.

The muscular changes that occurred as a result of lumbopelvic pain (e.g., muscle performance capabilities, cross-sectional area, neuromuscular control) may not improve naturally after the pain has ceased and the patient resumes functional activities.[35,105] Specific localized exercises as described in this chapter can restore the ideal lumbopelvic muscle control and performance (see Building Block 17-2).

An Earlier sections (see "Myology" and "Muscle Performance Impairment") discussed the role of the TrA, LM, and pelvic floor in the stabilization of the lumbopelvic region. Specific stabilization exercises aimed at improving motor control and muscle performance of the intrinsic spinal muscles muscles appear effective in reversing atrophic changes in the LM muscles in patients with acute LBP[105] and may reduce recurrence rates after first episode of acute LBP.[176] In a subgroup of patients with structural abnormalities predisposing them to segmental instability, specific stabilization exercises reduced long-term pain and disability levels when compared with general exercise.[177]

BUILDING BLOCK 17-2

1. A clinical example may provide insight into the complex relationships between pain and the development of hypermobility as well as other physiologic impairments in the lumbopelvic region. A 45-year-old male presents with LBP. He has a flat back, a slight pelvic shift in standing, and increased foot pronation and foot abduction on the right. During the examination, the physical therapist notices that the pelvis and lumbar spine rotate during the initiation of active hip flexion in the supine position and that this movement provokes LBP. When the patient is properly cued to recruit the intrinsic spinal muscles muscles; pelvis and spine rotation is reduced, and symptoms are eliminated. Other tests throughout the examination confirm that the L5–S1 segmental level is the site of relative flexibility in the direction of flexion and rotation. The examination should determine all contributing physiologic impairments. What examination findings would you expect in relation to key muscle testing, motor control over intrinsic spine muscles, and muscle flexibility?

2. To develop a program to improve the stability at the site of relative flexibility, each of the correlating impairments must be addressed. The program emphasizes achieving local spinal control over flexion and rotation stresses, addressing all correlated impairments, and improving quality of total-body movement and training kinesthetic awareness to control spinal postures and movements in the direction associated with symptoms. Given this case study, develop an exercise program that addresses all relevant impairments. Provide at least one exercise upgrade or functional transition for each exercise. Be sure to include dosage information.

Posture and Movement Impairment

Effective education in the area of posture and movement is essential to recover from and prevent recurrence of lumbopelvic syndromes. Education regarding posture and movement should be initiated at the time of the first visit. By the end of the initial examination, the clinician should be aware of the postures and movements that exacerbate symptoms[55] and therefore be able to instruct the patient in simple recommendations regarding sitting, standing, and recumbent postures. Basic movement patterns can be instructed, such as bed mobility (see Patient-Related Instruction 17-2: Bed Mobility), sit to stand, and bending (see Patient-Related Instruction 17-3: Lumbar-Pelvic Movement) and lifting maneuvers. The specific postures and movement patterns chosen to teach the patient should be based on the patient's pathology, impairments, activity limitations and participation restrictions. For example, a person with a diagnosed HNP at L4 may have different sitting recommendations than a person with spinal stenosis. The former is advised to avoid sustained end-range flexion, while the latter is advised to avoid sustained, end-range extension. The bottom line is that patients need to understand why, not just what to do, to facilitate empowerment and commitment to change.[178,179] They must play an active role in their treatment to obtain optimum benefit.[180–184]

In addition to education regarding posture and movement during ADLs, the clinician must consider specific posture and movement patterns for each prescribed exercise to be most effective. For example, allowing a patient with disk pathology to sit or move in lumbar flexion during a sitting knee extension exercise not only reduces the effectiveness of the HS stretch, but also places additional stress on the disk. The initial and ending posture of the spine and pelvis during the movement of knee extension must be emphasized. Similarly, allowing a patient with spondylolisthesis to move into segmental anterior translation of the affected spinal level during level II of the supine intrinsic spinal muscles progression (see Self-Management 17-1) can exacerbate symptoms related to the spine pathology. Attention to posture and movement during *all* exercises prescribed enhances their effectiveness. This requires a high level of supervision by the physical therapist. Research has shown that higher levels of supervision are associated with better outcomes with individuals with CLBP.[185]

The ultimate goal of each individual seeking treatment is to achieve a desired functional outcome. This involves skill in total-body posture and movement patterns that use optimal stabilization and dynamic recruitment patterns. The entire therapeutic exercise intervention plan is geared toward this final goal. To achieve skill in posture and movement, the individual must pay close attention to precision of movement during specific functional exercises (e.g., heel slides to improve bed mobility skills), during ADLs (e.g., squatting maneuvers), and during IADLs (e.g., playing golf). The clinician should teach or "coach" the patient in proper stabilization and movement strategies using the foundation of neuromuscular control, muscle performance, mobility, and proprioception that the impairment-based exercises have provided.

Aspects of posture and movement retraining can be incorporated into any stage of rehabilitation. Training begins by splitting complex movements into a number of simple component sequences. The choice of activity is determined by the functional requirements of the individual. At each progression of the program, more advanced posture and movement strategies are introduced. For example, an introductory postural strategy may be to teach the individual to sit properly in an ergonomic chair. Later, the patient may be progressed to sitting in a standard chair or on a soft surface such as a gym ball. The following are examples of movement patterns used in ADLs that require education and training for proper performance:

The more advanced the movement pattern, the more the task needs to be broken into simplified components to ensure that the proper amount of movement occurs in the segments where movement is desired and that stabilization occurs where no movement is desired. After skill is achieved at each component, simple movements are linked together to form the total activity sequence. Teaching skill in movement requires high levels of motivation and compliance from the patient and in-depth knowledge of concepts of motor learning and movement analysis by the clinician. Chapter 9 further addresses exercise prescription for the treatment of posture and movement impairments (see Building Block 17-3).

Specific exercises may be linked together in a circuit-training format. Examples of functional circuits include lifting circuits to retrain occupational functional outcomes and sport- or technique-specific circuits to retrain recreational activity functional outcomes. The lifting circuit may include a variety of manual handling procedures, such as single- and double-handed lifts with a variety of different shapes and weights, pushing and pulling activities, and reaching high and low levels.

Almost any piece of equipment, whether designed for a specific exercise, sport, or work activity, can be adapted to fit the principles of lumbopelvic functional movement retraining. Only imagination limits the exercise program after the principles are understood. Exercises can be adapted to meet

---

◆ Patient-Related Instruction 17-2

Bed Mobility

To reduce the stress on your low back, your physical therapist may ask you to get out of bed in a specific manner. The following instructions pertain to safe bed mobility.

- Activate your intrinsic spinal muscles and slide one foot at a time up the bed until your knees are flexed and your feet are flat on the bed. Be sure to prevent your back from arching or rotating by using your intrinsic spinal muscles.
- If you are not close to the side of the bed, you must bridge and slide until you are close to the side of the bed. Be sure to keep your intrinsic spinal muscles activated while bridging and sliding.
- Roll your body as one unit until you are lying on your side. Do not lead with your upper body or pelvis because this will result in a rotational stress on your spine that is detrimental to the healing process.
- Gently let your feet slide off the bed while simultaneously pushing yourself into the upright position with your hands.
- TIP: Be sure to maintain an intrinsic spinal muscles contraction during all components of this maneuver. You should be able to perform this skill without increase in symptoms. Talk to your physical therapist if you are unable to transfer from back lying to sitting without increased symptoms.

Patient-Related Instruction 17-3

Lumbar-Pelvic Movement

When you bend forward to pick up a light object, such as a shirt or a pencil, you can practice moving with the appropriate relationship between your low back and pelvis. The following are key points to keep in mind while bending forward:

Bending Forward (A to C)

- Leading with your head, slowly curl your spine as you bend forward.
- Think about relaxing at each vertebral segment.
- Try to keep your knees straight and minimize the backward shift of your hips.
- After you have reached the level of your low back in your forward bend, try to rotate your pelvis.
- Do not flex your low back further after your pelvis has stopped rotating.
- If you need to bend more to reach the desired distance, bend your hips and knees instead of flexing your low back beyond the rotation of your pelvis.
- At the end of the forward bend, relax your low back.

Return From Forward Bend (D to G)

- Lead with your hips and pelvis by contracting your gluteal muscles.
- Your low back should only extend after your pelvis has achieved its neutral position.
- At the end of the range, you may need to pull in with your abdominal muscles to achieve your neutral pelvic position.

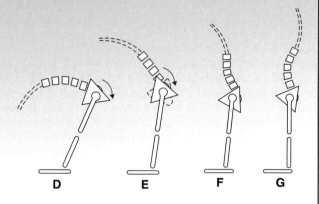

Adapted from Calliet R. Low Back Pain. 3rd Ed. Philadelphia, PA: FA Davis, 1981.

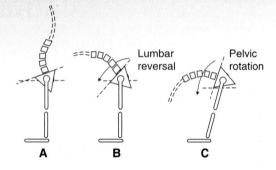

A   B   C

BUILDING BLOCK 17-3

The following are examples of movement patterns used in ADLs that require education and training in proper performance:

1. Simple bed mobility and sit-to-stand transfers
2. Small bends and squatting maneuvers
3. Gait (Fig. A) and stair stepping (Fig. B)
4. Occupational activities, such as lifting mechanics
5. Recreational activities, such as baseball (Fig. C)

Teach a partner safe patterns of movement during bed mobility, sit-to-stand transfers, small knee bends, and squatting maneuvers. Teach a partner how to lift from floor to waist, then from waist to shoulder height. Consider what region of the body you would teach a baseball pitcher to emphasize in movement during a pitch.

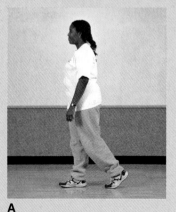

A

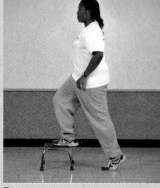

B

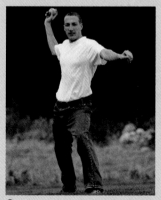

C

the demands of the patient's work and recreation. The clinician must be careful not to progress the patient faster than he or she can learn to control motion with the optimal strategies. Diligence displayed by the patient and clinician is rewarded with fewer setbacks and higher gains in functional return (see Building Block 17-4 and Case Study 17-1).

> **BUILDING BLOCK 17-4**
>
> Develop a sport-specific circuit for a soccer player with LBP.

 CASE STUDY 17-1

HISTORY

The patient was a 54-year-old female with a 10+ year history of LBP. The pain had an insidious onset, but has gotten worse in the past year. Pain intensity, using a numeric pain rating scale, is 5/10 on average and 7/10 at worst. Standing, lifting, and walking more than 20 minutes made symptoms worse; sitting and lying with a pillow under the knees alleviates the pain. She estimates her sleep is disrupted about 30% to 40% of the time. Associated symptoms included an intermittent ache along the paraspinal musculature and a throbbing pain radiating into the buttock and posterior thigh. The patient reported having no saddle paresthesia, change in bowel and bladder function, or generalized weakness or incoordination of her lower extremities.

Other medical history included an appendectomy, tonsillectomy, hysterectomy, hypertension, hypercholesterolemia, and depression. Her depressive symptoms were being treated with bupropion hydrochloride. Other current medications included lisinopril and hydrochlorothiazide for hypertension, metoclopramide for gastroesophageal reflux, and lamotrigine for stabilizing mood. The patient's work activities included lifting and carrying boxes of files and sitting at a computer. Her hobbies included gardening. The patient's goals were to garden and perform all work duties with a pain level of 4/10.

EXAMINATION

At intake, the patient's Oswestry Low Back Disability Questionnaire (ODQ) score was 18/50, her Beck Depression Index (BDI) was 8/63, indicating minimal depressive symptoms; and her Fear-Avoidance Belief Questionnaire (FABQ) work subscale score was 38/42, indicating high fear-avoidance behavior concerning work activities. However, her FABQ physical activity subscale score was 10/24, indicating minimal fear-avoidance behavior concerning physical activity outside of work.

Her posture included increased thoracic kyphosis and lumbar lordosis with anterior pelvic tilt and iliac crest asymmetry with right ilium high. During the stance phase of gait, it was observed that her lumbar spine moves excessively into extension and rotation instead of the stance hip moving into extension. Patellar reflexes were 1+ bilaterally, and Achilles reflexes could not be elicited. Dermatomal function was normal, but there was a slight reduction in anterior Tibialis force production on the right. Standing lumbar active range of motion revealed non-reversal of lumbar extension, but no pain during flexion. Slight pain was elicited upon return from extension. Passive range of motion (PROM) during a right

SLR, as measured with bubble inclinometry, was 52 degrees, with reproduction of right gluteal pain, but sensitizing using dorsiflexion was negative. Left SLR was positive at 60 degrees for familiar back pain, and sensitizing with dorsiflexion was negative also. Hip extension PROM during a Thomas test, as measured using bubble inclinometry with the knee flexed, revealed right hip extension lacking 18 degrees and left hip extension lacking 15 degrees. Manual muscle tests of the hip revealed right gluteus medius muscle strength was 3/5, left 3+/5, and gluteus maximus muscle strength was 3+/5 bilateral. Abdominal performance testing, which was conducted as described by Sahrmann, showed inability to perform level 1 correctly. Palpation assessment of transverse abdominus and LM demonstrated poor activation with verbal cueing. Passive intervertebral testing revealed guarding with posterior/anterior pressure at L4/L5 and a positional fault in extension and rotation.

EVALUATION

Based on the initial examination data, the mediators influencing the patient's chronic LBP were categorized using the WHO-ICF model (see Case Study Table 17-1). It is hypothesized that the listed impairments contribute to the relative flexibility of the lumbar spine in the DSM of extension and rotation include poor muscle performance of the intrinsic spinal muscles muscles combined with short hip flexors.

INTERVENTION

The patient was educated on her physical therapist's diagnosis, prognosis, and plan of care. She was seen for 10 visits over 12 weeks. Patient education, specific exercise for associated impairments, and graded exercise were used to address her avoidance of physical activity. Specifically, she was educated during the initial visit that pain did not signal harm, but that by moving with improved patterns of movement and using improved posture habits, it would be possible for her to perform more work related duties and leisure activities with less pain. It was explained, however, that she needed to maintain a consistent activity pace, and to stay as active as tolerable. This was reinforced during discussions in subsequent visits.

Two examples of exercises to address specific impairments in motor control and muscle performance are listed below.

Self-Management 17-1 demonstrates an exercise progression targeting the impairments in the intrinsic spinal muscles simultaneous with lengthening the hip flexors. While the intrinsic spinal muscles contract in the short range, the hip

(continued)

CASE STUDY 17-1 *(Continued)*

flexor muscles elongate. If the patient allows the hip flexors to pull the pelvis and spine out of alignment, the exercise becomes detrimental to altering the site of relative flexibility. In a patient with a hypermobile SIJ, the site of relative flexibility may be at the SIJ rather than the lumbar spine. The exercise must be monitored, focusing on stabilizing the iliosacral region rather than the lumbar spine by monitoring and preventing movement of the ASIS in an anterior inferior direction. The patient can be taught to control the specific spine stabilization strategy with targeted muscle activation patterns.

In conjunction with this exercise, the patient can work on the same relationship in other positions, such as prone (see Self-Management 17-5). The lumbopelvic region is stabilized through appropriate intrinsic spinal muscles recruitment, and the knee is flexed to the point of mild tension and before the loss of lumbopelvic stabilization. Emphasis is placed on relaxation of the rectus femoris and TFL simultaneously with stabilization of the spine against the extension force imposed by the short hip flexors. Eventually, the patient can progress to the closed chain and the walk stance progression (see Self-Mangement 19-2: Walk Stance Progression) with emphasis on controlling lumbopelvic position in relation to the extending hip. These active movements prepare the patient for the ultimate goal of stabilizing the lumbar spine during standing tasks and during the stance phase of gait. The therapist will most likely need to coach the patient in the proper stabilizing strategies during gait.

OUTCOME

At 12 weeks, the patient reported that she was able to bend and carry charts at work for a full day without increased pain. She regularly sat at stood at work for 30 minutes without pain. Her worst pain was reported as 3/10. Her ODQ score was 6/50. Hip flexion with the Thomas test was 6 degrees on the left and 10 degrees on the right. Abdominal strength was graded as level 2 and she could demonstrate activation control over transverse abdominus and LM at L4 and L5 levels. The patient canceled a follow-up appointment at 14 weeks and subsequently was contacted by telephone. Final questionnaires revealed an ODQ score of 2/50, a BDI of 4/63, an FABQ work subscale score of 0/42, and an FABQ physical activity subscale score of 0/24. Pain intensity, as measured with a numeric pain rating scale, was 2/10 at worst. The patient stated that she was "much improved."

CASE TABLE 17-1 **The World Health Organization's International Classification of Functioning, Disability and Health (WHO-ICF) Model Applied to the Evaluation of Patient with CLBP**

	BODY STRUCTURES AND FUNCTIONS	ACTIVITIES	PARTICIPATION
Patient's perspective	Pain in back and back of thigh	Standing	Unable to garden
		Lifting	Decreased work tolerance
		Walking 20 min	Interrupted sleep
Physical therapist's perspective	Reduced muscle power functions (b730)	Lifting and carrying objects (d430)	Remunerative employment (d850)
	Reduced mobility of joint functions (b710)	Maintaining body positions (d410)	Recreation and leisure (d920)
	Gait pattern functions (b770)		
	Neuromusculoskeletal and movement-related functions, other specified (b798)		
CONTEXTUAL FACTORS			

Personal

Temperament and personality functions: fear-avoidance behavior for physical activities and perceived ability to function in work activities and leisure activities.

Environmental

• Products and technology for employment (e135)
• Labor and employment, systems, and policies (e590)

THERAPEUTIC EXERCISE INTERVENTION FOR COMMON DIAGNOSES

The following section discusses three of the most common diagnoses of the lumbopelvic region. Although SIJ syndrome is not discussed, it should be evaluated and treated combining concepts related to both the lumbopelvic region and hip joint (see Chapter 19). The reader is challenged to develop a comprehensive lumbo-pelvic-hip therapeutic exercise prescription for each individual SIJ syndrome patient encountered.

Lumbar Disk Herniation

The peak incidence of herniated lumbar disks is in adults between the ages of 30 and 55 years.[186] Disk herniation without trauma can be thought of as one factor in a continuum of the spinal degenerative process. The degenerative process can progress from minor muscular or soft-tissue injuries to abnormal spinal biomechanics, which ultimately can break down the underlying joint structure and create facet arthritis, disk degeneration, herniated disk, spinal stenosis, neurologic entrapment, and severe permanent disability.[187] A patient who suffers a spinal annular tear could develop spinal stenosis years later. The primary role of physical therapists involved in the treatment of lumbopelvic syndromes is to assist in the diagnostic process early, treat the sources (if known) and causes of dysfunction appropriately, and prevent severe pathologic conditions from developing. Unfortunately, the initial low back injury is often thought of as a benign muscular or ligamentous injury and is not heralded as the first sign of a process that can lead to severe pathoanatomy and disability.

The beginning of the degenerative process is an annular tear resulting in a disk protrusion or annular bulge. With a disk protrusion, the NP does not herniate from the disk; it is confined by the annular fibers. This may be the typical "back sprain" that results from bending, lifting, and frequent twisting. It often gives a person LBP with little or no pain radiation into the legs. The pain is usually relieved quite rapidly with rest or curtailment of most bending or lifting activities for several days. Patients are usually fairly comfortable when on their feet, but when they change from a lying to a sitting position or from sitting to standing, the pain can be acute and disable them from fully standing. The probable cause of the pain is the flexion or torsion forces imposed on the disk during these movements. These episodes, if not treated appropriately, can recur and become more frequent as time progresses. Eventually, they can lead to the more disabling disk herniation.

If the annular tear progresses to full annular disruption, a HNP results. Penetration of the nuclear material into peripheral areas that are highly sensitive to mechanical and chemical stimulation may be the source of the disabling pain felt in disk herniation. Clinically, disk herniation can be divided into the following subsets:

- HNP without neurologic deficit
- HNP with nerve root irritation
- HNP with nerve root compression

HNP without neurologic deficit has signs and symptoms similar to those of an annular tear but is slower to recover and imparts slightly more disability. No encroachment on the nerve root has occurred with this condition. HNP with nerve root irritation has signs and symptoms, including sciatica, paresthesias, and positive SLR, but no neurologic deficit is diagnosed. HNP with nerve root compression has signs of nerve root irritation plus neuroconductivity changes. A massive midline disk herniation may cause spinal cord or cauda equina compression, requiring immediate surgical referral. Fortunately, the cauda equina syndrome occurs in only 1% to 2% of all lumbar disk herniations that result in surgery.[175]

Examination and Evaluation Findings

Sciatica is a symptom of nerve root irritation that could be caused by a HNP. Sciatica is defined as a sharp or burning pain radiating down the posterior or lateral aspect of the leg, usually to the foot or ankle, often associated with numbness or paresthesia. Coughing, sneezing, or the Valsalva maneuver often aggravates the pain. Sciatica caused by disk herniation is worsened by prolonged sitting and improved by walking, lying supine, lying prone, or sitting in a reclined position.[188] The absence of sciatica makes a clinically important lumbar disk herniation unlikely.[186,189–191] The estimated incidence of disk herniation in a patient without sciatica is 1 in 1,000.[21]

The SLR test can be used as a factor in diagnosing a HNP. A symptomatic disk herniation tethers the affected nerve root. Pain results from stretching the nerve by straight-leg raising from the supine or sitting position. In the supine SLR test, tension is transmitted to the nerve roots after the leg is raised beyond 30 degrees, but after 70 degrees, further movement of the nerve is negligible.[192] A typical SLR sign is one that reproduces the patient's sciatica between 30 and 60 degrees of elevation.[186,193,194] The lower the angle producing a positive result, the more specific the test becomes, and the larger is the disk protrusion found at surgery.[195,196] Care must be taken to differentiate HS tension from sciatica. Sensitizing techniques (e.g., neck flexion, ankle dorsiflexion) can be used to determine whether the pain experienced is originating from HS tension or nerve irritation.

Straight-leg raising is most appropriate for testing the lower lumbar nerve roots (L5 and S1), where most herniated disks occur.[186] Irritation of higher lumbar roots is tested with femoral nerve stretch (i.e., flexion of the knee with the patient prone).

About 98% of clinically important lumbar disk herniations occur at the L4–5 or L5–S1 intervertebral level,[186,196,197] causing neurologic impairments in the motor and sensory regions of the L5 and S1 nerve roots. The most common neurologic impairments are weakness of the ankle and great toe dorsiflexors (L5) or ankle and foot plantar flexors (S1), diminished ankle reflexes (S1), and sensory loss in the feet (L5 and S1).[186,196,197] In a patient with sciatica and suspected disk herniation, the neurologic examination can be concentrated on these functions. Among patients with LBP alone (no sciatica or neurologic symptoms), the prevalence of neurologic impairments is so low that extensive neurologic evaluation is usually unnecessary.[21]

Higher lumbar nerve roots account for only about 2% of lumbar disk herniations.[186,196,197] They are suspected when numbness or pain involves the anterior thigh more prominently than the calf. Testing includes patellar tendon reflexes, quadriceps strength, and psoas strength.[186,196,197] Quadriceps weakness is virtually always associated with impairment in the patellar tendon reflex.[198]

The most consistent finding with a low lumbar midline disk herniation, called *cauda equina syndrome*, is urinary retention.[21,198–202] Unilateral or bilateral sciatica, sensory and motor deficits, sexual dysfunction (i.e., decreased sensation during intercourse, decreased penile sensation and impotence), and abnormal SLR also are common examination findings.[200–202] The most common sensory deficit (i.e., hyperesthesia or anesthesia) occurs over the buttocks, posterosuperior thighs, and perineal regions.[199–202] Finally, decreased anal sphincter tone can be a neurologic sequelae of cauda equina syndrome.[200] Kostuik et al.[200] warns that a central disk lesion, especially at the L5–S1 disk, can pose a diagnostic challenge because it affects only the lower sacral roots and causes no motor or reflex changes in the legs.

There is a growing consensus that plain roentgenograms are unnecessary for every patient with LBP because of a low yield of useful findings, potentially misleading results, substantial gonadal irradiation, and common interpretive disagreements.[21] The Quebec Task Force on Spinal Disorders suggests that early roentgenography is necessary only under the following conditions:

- Neurologic deficits
- Patient older than 50 or younger than 20 years of age
- Fever
- Trauma
- Signs of neoplasm[203]

Magnetic resonance imaging and computed tomography can be used even more selectively, usually for surgical planning.[21] The finding of herniated disks and spinal stenosis in many asymptomatic individuals[204,205] indicates that imaging results alone can be misleading. Valid decision-making requires correlation with a comprehensive history and physical examination.

Treatment

There is no recipe approach toward the exercise management of LBP, even if a specific structural diagnosis, such as HNP with nerve root irritation, is offered. Determining which interventions to use depends on diagnostic information regarding the pathoanatomic process and the physiologic impairments contributing to the pathomechanical process and on the psychologic impairments, patient disability profile, including the desired "return to" activities and participations. The following concepts of care for specific stages of disk herniation can guide management of the degenerative disk process.

Acute Stage In the acute stages of any injury, the immediate goals are often to relieve pain and to reduce or halt the inflammatory process so that the healing process can occur unimpeded. Investigations into the biochemistry of disc degeneration and herniation indicate that intraspinal inflammation is a major cause of radicular pain.[206] A neurotoxic, inflammatory mediator phospholipase is contained within the disc nucleus and is released after annular injury. Early intervention and patient adherence to the recommendations addressing pain and inflammation in the case of HNP are essential for achieving a rapid recovery and for preventing chronic pain and disability.

Along with physical therapy intervention, the patient's physician usually prescribes steroidal or nonsteroidal anti-inflammatory medications and may suggest epidural steroid injection. Corticosteroids have powerful anti-inflammatory effects. The use of epidural steroid injection, performed by experienced physicians who have shown competence in the technical aspects of this procedure, has produced favorable outcomes, particularly if used in conjunction with physical therapy.[207] A systematic review utilizing the criteria established by the Agency for Healthcare Research and Quality

(AHRQ) for evaluation of randomized and non-randomized trials, and criteria of Cochrane Musculoskeletal Review Group for randomized trials was used to study the efficacy of epidural steroid injections.[206] In managing lumbar radicular pain with interlaminar lumbar epidural steroid injections, the level of evidence was strong for short-term relief and limited for long-term relief. The evidence for lumbar transforaminal epidural steroid injections in managing lumbar nerve root pain was strong with short-term and long-term improvement. A systematic review of randomized controlled studies determined that there is strong evidence that exercise therapy is not more effective for acute LBP (defined as pain for 12 or less weeks) than other active treatments with which it has been compared.[208] The primary role of the physical therapist may be to promote the concept of "controlled rest." This intervention may take the form of posture and activity modification (i.e., avoidance of flexed postures, sitting, and bending or lifting activities), pacing activity and rest, positions for pain relief, and most importantly, guiding the patient through this phase to avoid developing fear avoidance behaviors. It is important to teach the patient to avoid flexed and asymmetric postures, flexion and rotation movements, and sitting (which elevates disk pressures) to enhance healing and prevent reinjury to the healing disk. The clinician also can teach the patient how to use cryotherapy at home to control inflammation. Traction can be a useful adjunctive modality in the acute phase. Similar to the recommendations of Delitto et al.,[209] the most common examination criterion cited by clinicians as an indication for traction is the presence of signs of nerve root compression.[210] (see the "Adjunctive Interventions" section).

Exercise can play a vital role in the treatment of pain and inflammation. For example, careful prescription of exercises based on the McKenzie diagnostic classification system may be useful in the early treatment of disk-related signs and symptoms (see Examination and Evaluation: Range of Motion, Muscle Length, and Joint Mobility and Therapeutic Exercise Intervention for Common Physiologic Impairments: Pain and Self-Management 17-7).[161,164,211]

As with any mechanically induced injury, the causes of muscle or soft-tissue injury must be avoided. In the acute phase of disk herniation, due to altered movement patterns from the pain, it is often difficult to determine the postures and movements associated with the development of segmental dysfunction (see Building Block 17-5).

In the acute phase of disk herniation, the patient is often susceptible to the effects of immobilization as a result of the protective nature of this phase of care. Treatment to maintain or improve mobility of adjacent segments within the lumbar spine and thoracic spine and the extensibility of lower extremity muscles is vital for reducing stress on the

 BUILDING BLOCK 17-5

In the acute phase of managing a herniated disc, it is useful to teach the patient basic bed mobility movements. Name two exercises you have learned in this chapter that would help a patient move in bed with less pain.

BUILDING BLOCK 17-6

Devise a safe stretch to the piriformis that will not place torsional stress on the sacrum or lumbar spine.

injured segment and reducing the effects of immobilization that may play a role in recurrence of the condition. For example, joint mobilization of the thoracic spine and segments above and below the affected segmental level, along with soft-tissue mobilization of the erector spinae group, can maintain joint mobility during the acute phase. Piriformis spasm is a common secondary effect of lower lumbar disk herniation. Soft-tissue mobilization and passive stretching to this muscle can decrease pain associated with the spasm (see Building Block 17-6).

Treatment to maintain or improve mobility in the neural tissues also is critical in the acute stages. Adverse neural tension is a common sequel of HNP. It can affect muscle performance and lumbopelvic mobility. Neuromeningeal mobility should be assessed and its influence determined. Specific exercises may be prescribed that are designed to improve mobility of the neural system (see Self-Management 17-6). Initially, tolerance is usually very low, and neuromeningeal mobility exercises must be performed with caution, usually in recumbent positions to prevent exacerbating symptoms. Neuromeningeal mobility exercises performed during the acute stage may prevent chronic complications from increased neural tension. The related anatomy, physiology, and application principles must be well understood for the effective and safe use of this type of treatment. This topic is worthy of more extensive coverage; further guidance in prescribing these exercises has been provided by Butler.[73]

The clinician should encourage the patient to maintain some activity level, such as swimming or walking, during the acute stage. Swimming can be employed with the use of a kick board to minimize unwanted spinal motion while promoting aerobic fitness and lower extremity motion. Walking with a corset, wearing good shock-absorbing shoes, and walking on a soft surface (e.g., gravel) may reduce disk pressure enough to tolerate the stress of walking. In addition to the benefits of movement, the benefits of low-level aerobic exercise are gained.

Subacute and Chronic Stages   After the acute pain has subsided and the patient has more freedom of movement, the treatment should focus on altering postures and movements and the associated impairments that produce symptoms. The ultimate goal is the return to the highest possible level of function with the safest and most desirable postures and movement patterns possible.

Review the sections on treatment of impairments to understand the concept of exercise intervention for mobility, muscle performance, balance, coordination, posture, and movement impairments and the progression through traditional stages of motor control. This information provides the basis for developing a progressive program of intervention for a patient with disk pathology beyond the acute stages of care.

Education is considered to be the most important intervention to provide the patient with troubleshooting and decision-making tools to protect against developing chronic disability experienced by many persons with disk disease. The patient must be taught self-management techniques to gain control over the pathology and remain less reliant on the health care system for ongoing treatment. The clinician must teach the patient to temporarily manage acute exacerbations with cryotherapy, positional techniques, or repeated shift correction and extension movements.[161] Instruction in body mechanics, ergonomics, and ongoing fitness activities are equally important in preventing recurrence. Evaluation of the home and work environment, work-station ergonomics, and the development of fitness programs are preventive strategies the clinician may implement. Perhaps the most important outcome of patient education is the sense of confidence gained by the realization that back problems can be managed while the patient continues to function and lead a productive life.

Spinal Stenosis

Spinal stenosis is defined as an abnormal narrowing of the spinal canal (central) or the intervertebral foramen (lateral).[212] Central stenosis can result from osteophyte enlargement of the inferior articular process or vertebral bodies, congenitally decreased anteroposterior or mediolateral diameters of the spinal canal, hypertrophy of the ligamentum flavum, spondylolisthesis, or neoplasm that impinges on the cauda equina. Lateral stenosis is typically caused by subluxation of the facets as a result of disk narrowing. Extension and rotation positional faults of the segment produce further narrowing. Symptoms are usually segmental because of entrapment of the nerve root.

Examination and Evaluation Findings

The characteristic history of persons with spinal stenosis is that of neurogenic claudication (i.e., pain in the legs) and, occasionally, neurologic deficits that occur after walking. In contrast to arterial ischemic claudication, neurogenic claudication can occur on standing (without ambulation), may increase with cough or sneeze, is associated with normal arterial pulses,[213] and is relieved by flexion of the lumbar spine. One often-used test to discriminate between ischemic and neurogenic claudication is stationary biking. The patient is positioned in lumbar flexion and asked to pedal. This test will likely reproduce symptoms if the source is ischemic claudication, whereas with the spine positioned in flexion, neurogenic claudication is less likely.

Increased pain on spine extension is typical of stenosis. Although flexion is usually painful with herniated disks, it can be a position of relief for patients with spinal stenosis. Patients feel more comfortable walking in a stooped position, cycling, walking behind a shopping cart or lawn mower, or walking up an incline or stairs, rather than walking on a flat surface, down an incline, or downstairs.[214,215]

Treatment

Recently, the surgical literature published in this field is sending a message to look for new strategies in the field of rehabilitation and conservative treatments before considering decompressive, instrumented surgery, or minimally invasive techniques that are presently offered in the field of modem lumbar chronic pain treatment.[216] This is great news for physical therapists that can provide much insight and rehabilitative skill to conservative treatment of spinal stenosis. Treatment of spinal stenosis is based on symptoms related to postures and movements. If the patient has mild symptoms that fluctuate with mechanical, postural, and movement changes, he or she can be accommodated with appropriate patient-related education, exercise, external lumbar support, (i.e., corset), and nonsteroidal anti-inflammatory medication. Although nonoperative measures cannot reverse a true anatomic impairment, they can accommodate it by increasing the foraminal or spinal canal diameter.

Exercise should focus on physiologic impairments that may contribute to foraminal or spinal canal narrowing:

- Poor muscle performance from the intrinsic spinal muscles (TrA, LM, and pelvic floor) resulting in insufficient support to the lumbar spine
- Short hip flexors contributing to anterior pelvic tilt and lumbar lordosis
- Thoracic kyphosis with overstretched and weak thoracic erector spinae accompanying lumbar lordosis
- Asymmetry of pelvic girdle and lower extremity muscle length and strength resulting in lumbar scoliosis and lateral foraminal narrowing

Canal or foraminal narrowing is typically associated with spine extension, combined extension and rotation, or anterior translation. Postures associated with relative extension (i.e., kyphosis and lordosis), combined extension and rotation (i.e., kyphosis and lordosis and limb length discrepancy), or anterior translation (i.e., swayback) should be avoided, and the patient should be instructed in postural correction to remedy these postural habits.

The clinician should teach the patient to avoid movement patterns that require repeated extension, rotation, or shearing and to develop control over these forces when unavoidable (see Building Block 17-7).

Limited ambulation is a frequent functional limitation among patients with spinal stenosis. Harness-supported treadmill ambulation or use of a walker, crutches, or a cane for patients with leg pain brought on by walking can be used as a progressive return to walking without symptoms. The amount of unloaded force can be progressed until unloading force is no longer required to relieve pain during ambulation.[217]

Patients should be instructed in recreational activities that do not produce symptoms. Exercise biased toward flexion should be encouraged, such as walking on a treadmill with a slight incline, cycling, or walking while pushing a stroller. Exercise biased toward extension should be discouraged, such as walking on a flat surface, walking downhill, or swimming.

Spondylolysis and Spondylolisthesis

Spondylolysis, a bilateral defect in the pars interarticularis, occurs in 58% of adults.[218] Approximately 50% of those never progress to any degree of spondylolisthesis, a condition of forward subluxation of the body of one vertebrae on the vertebrae below it.[218] Spondylolisthesis is not limited to any specific segment of the spine. However, it occurs most commonly at the L5–S1 segmental level, primarily because of the angulation of the L5 segment with respect to the vertical plane. Defects or impairment of any of the supporting structures can lead to subluxation of the superior segment on the inferior segment. Spondylolisthesis has been classified[219] by cause into five types:

1. Type I, isthmic: A defect in the pars interarticularis may be caused by a fracture or by an elongation of the pars without separation.
2. Type II, congenital: The posterior elements are anatomically inadequate because of developmental deficiency. This occurs rarely.
3. Type III, degenerative: The facets or the supporting ligaments undergo degenerative changes, allowing listhesis. There is no pars defect, and the condition worsens with age.
4. Type IV, elongated pedicle: The length of the neural arch elongates to allow listhesis. This is essentially an isthmic type. Traction forces are apparently contributory.
5. Type V, destructive disease: Metastatic disease, tuberculosis, or other bone disease may change the structure of the supporting tissues.

Examination and Evaluation Findings

The patient may complain of backache, gluteal pain, lower limb pain or paresthesias, hyperesthesia, muscle weakness, intermittent claudication, or bladder and rectal disturbances. The physical examination may reveal that symptoms worsen on return from forward bending that is accompanied by lumbar extension. If the patient is cued to lead with the gluteal musculature and recruit the intrinsic spinal muscles, symptoms are reduced. The clinical diagnosis is suspected if this finding is accompanied by inspection and palpation of the spine in which a depression at the listhesis level is noticed. Percussion over the segment may elicit pain. Radiologic confirmation can be made by a lateral view of the lumbosacral region. A roentgenogram can diagnose spondylolysis or spondylolisthesis and the degree of subluxation, which can be graded.

Treatment

In general, treatment of spondylolysis or spondylolisthesis is nonsurgical.[220] Treatments include bracing, exercise, and nonsteroidal anti-inflammatory medications. In children and adolescents, immobilization in a thoracolumbosacral brace, activity modification, and exercise expedite healing of the defect.[221,222]

Exercise, posture and movement retraining, and activity modification are the cornerstones of the rehabilitation

BUILDING BLOCK 17-7

Name at least three ADLs that require movement into extension that you will examine and retrain if faulty or too stressful for your patient's spine.

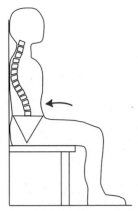

FIGURE 17-17. Sitting posterior pelvic tilt. This activity can be used by individuals with lordosis, anterior pelvic tilt, weak and overstretched abdominal muscles (particularly EO and TrA), and short hip flexors. The supine intrinsic spinal muscles progression is often contraindicated for this type of patient due to the anterior translation force exerted by the iliopsoas and anterior pelvic tilt force exerted by the TFL and rectus femoris. The patient sits with her back against a wall and is instructed to pull the umbilicus toward the spine to reduce the lordosis. Sitting takes the stretch off the hip flexors, and the pelvis should be able to move posteriorly with greater ease than in standing with the hip flexors on relative stretch. Use of a gluteal contraction over an abdominal contraction is discouraged. This exercise can be progressed to standing in slight hip and knee flexion (to release tension on the hip flexors) and then to standing upright once the abdominal muscles are strong enough and the hip flexor muscles are of sufficient length to attain a neutral pelvic position. The advantage of this exercise is that it can be performed frequently throughout the day.

program. As for the patient with spinal stenosis, lumbar extension and shearing forces should be avoided. Exercises focused on resolving the impairments associated with extension or shearing forces should be prescribed, and strong emphasis should be placed on intrinsic spinal muscles strengthening and posture and movement retraining. Figure 17-17 is a good position to activate the intrinsic spinal muscles without the anterior force from the hip flexors as in Self-Management 17-1. Self-Management 17-2 can provide initial exercises to stimulate the stability necessary for recovery from spondylolisthesis. If a brace is used in conjunction with physical therapy, the physical therapist should communicate with the physician regarding the prescribed immobilization period and weaning program. Most often, the patient can continue to participate in sports during the immobilization period and is encouraged to do so. However, activity modification also may be advised. Activities such as volleyball and gymnastics are associated with significant extension movements and shearing forces imposed on the lumbar spine. If movement patterns cannot be modified enough to reduce symptoms during these activities, the patient may need to be counseled to seek another form of recreation or athletic endeavor.

ADJUNCTIVE INTERVENTIONS

Bracing and traction are commonly used adjunctive interventions in the treatment of lumbopelvic pain syndromes. Refer to the website for a discussion of these interventions

KEY POINTS

- A thorough understanding of the anatomy and biomechanics of the lumbopelvic region is prerequisite to appropriate therapeutic exercise prescription for this region.
- Exercise must be based on a thoughtful and systematic examination process identifying the physiologic and psychologic impairments most closely related to the individual's activity limitations and participation restrictions.
- Therapeutic exercise intervention for common physiologic impairments must be coordinated to address associated impairments and prioritized to address those most closely related to activity limitations and participation restrictions.
- Exercise management of common pathoanatomic diagnoses must not follow a recipe approach, but rather be highly prescriptive and relate to the patient's unique impairments, activity and participation restrictions.

CRITICAL THINKING QUESTIONS

1. Prioritize postures from the most to the least stressful on the lumbar spine.
2. Describe the principles for the use of optimal body mechanics during lifting.
3. Describe the biomechanical differences between the bent-knee and straight-leg sit-up. What would be the best abdominal exercise for an individual with a HNP? Spinal stenosis or spondylolisthesis? How would you modify the sit-up for a person with a kyphosis/lordosis posture type?
4. How can exercise impact chemical causes of pain?
5. What postures place the EO in a lengthened position, making it susceptible to strain resulting from overstretch?
6. Given the following activities: flexion phase of forward bending, sidelying hip abduction, and seated rotation. Describe the optimal site and direction of relative flexibility during these movements. (Hint: during the return from forward bending, the optimal site of *relative* flexibility is the hip in the direction of extension versus the lumbar spine in the direction of extension.)
7. What is the conceptual basis for treatment of a relative flexibility or stiffness problem?
8. Define the anatomic injury that occurs with disk prolapse and the three subsets of disk herniation.
9. Define the three clinical categories of signs and symptoms associated with HNP.
10. Define the broad category of spinal stenosis and the two types of stenosis.
11. Discuss the difference between spondylolysis and spondylolisthesis.
12. What is the common posture and movement that a person with either stenosis or spondylolisthesis should avoid?
13. How would you instruct a patient with stenosis or spondylolisthesis in intrinsic spinal muscles strengthening? (Hint: you want to avoid forces that produce extension or anterior translation on the lumbar spine.)
14. Discuss the musculature involved in force closure of the SIJ.

15. Refer to Case Study No. 5 in Unit 7.

    a. Based on her history and physical examination findings, what is the likely medical diagnosis for this patient?

    b. What are the faulty posture and movement patterns associated with onset of her symptoms?

    c. What are the correlating physiologic impairments? List them under the headings used in this chapter (e.g., mobility, muscle performance).

    d. Develop an exercise program addressing all pertinent impairments related to her activity limitations and participation restrictions.

    e. Be sure to include patient-related instruction tips.

REFERENCES

1. Van Tulder MW, Koes BW, Bouter LM. Conservative treatment of acute and chronic nonspecific low back pain: a systematic review of randomized controlled trials of the most common interventions. Spine 1997;22:2128–2156.
2. Waller B, Lambeck J, Daly D. Therapeutic aquatic exercise in the treatment of low back pain: a systematic review. Clin Rehabil 2009;23:3–14.
3. Chou R, Huffman LH; American Pain Society; American College of Physicians. Nonpharmacologic therapies for acute and chronic low back pain: a review of the evidence for an American Pain Society/American College of Physicians clinical practice guideline. Ann Intern Med 2007;147:492–504. [Review. Erratum in: Ann Intern Med 2008;148:247–248. Summary for patients in: Ann Intern Med 2007;147:I45.]
4. Bouter LM, van Tulder MW, Koes BW. Methodologic issues in low back pain research in primary care. Spine 1998;23:2014–2020.
5. Hayden JA, van Tulder MW, Tomlinson G. Systematic review: strategies for using exercise therapy to improve outcomes in chronic low back pain. Ann Intern Med 2005;142:776–785.
6. McKenzie RA. The Lumbar Spine: Mechanical Diagnosis and Therapy. Lower Hutt, New Zealand: Spinal Publications, 1981.
7. Delitto A, Erhard RE, Bowling RW. A treatment-based classification approach to low back syndrome: identifying and staging patients for conservative treatment. Phys Ther 1995;75:470–498.
8. Sahrmann SA. Diagnosis and Management of Musculoskeletal Pain Syndromes. St. Louis, MO: Mosby, 1999.
9. Spitzer WO, Nachemson A. A scientific approach to the assessment and management of activity-related spinal disorders: a monograph for clinicians. Report of the Quebec Task Force on Spinal Disorders. Spine 1987;12:51.
10. Bernard TN, Kirkaldy-Willis WH. Recognizing specific characteristics of nonspecific low back pain. Clin Orthop 1987;217:266–280.
11. Mooney V. The syndromes of low back disease. Orthop Clin North Am 1983;14:505–515.
12. Bigos S, Bowyer O, Braen G, et al. Acute Low Back Problems in Adults. AHCPR Publications 95–0624. Rockville, MD: Agency for Health Care Policy and Research, Public Health Service, U.S. Department of Health and Human Services, 1994.
13. Roach KE, Brown MD, Albin RD, et al. The sensitivity and specificity of pain response to activity and position in categorizing patients with low back pain. Phys Ther 1997;77:730–738.
14. BenDebba M, Torgerson WS, Long DM. A validated, practical, classification procedure for many persistent low back pain patients. Pain 2000;87:89–97.
15. Fritz JM, Cleland JA, Childs JD. Subgrouping patients with low back pain: evolution of a classification approach to physical therapy. J Orthop Sports Phys Ther 2007 Jun;37:290–302.
16. Ferreira ML, Ferreira PH, Latimer J, et al. Comparison of general exercise, motor control exercise and spinal manipulative therapy for chronic low back pain: a randomized trial. Pain 2007;131:31–37.
17. Van Dillen LR, Sahrmann SA, Norton BJ, et al. Movement system impairment-based categories for low back pain: stage 1 validation. J Orthop Sports Phys Ther 2003;33:126–142.
18. Marras WS, Parnianpour M, Ferguson SA, et al. The classification of anatomic- and symptom-based low back disorders using motion measure models. Spine 1995 Dec;20:2531–2546.
19. O'Sullivan P. Diagnosis and classification of chronic low back pain disorders: maladaptive movement and motor control impairments as underlying mechanism. Man Ther 2005;10:242–255.
20. Abenhaim L, Rossignol M, Gobeille D, et al. The prognostic consequences in the making of the initial medical diagnosis of work-related back injuries. Spine 1995;20:791–795.
21. Deyo RA, Rainville J, Kent DL. What can the history and physical examination tell us about low back pain? JAMA 1992;268:760–765.
22. Twomey L, Taylor J. Spine update: exercise and spinal manipulation in the treatment of low back pain. Spine 1995;20:615–619.
23. Vleeming A, Snijders C, Stoeckart J, et al. A new light on low back pain. Proceedings from the Second Interdisciplinary World Congress on Low Back Pain and Its Relation to the Sacroiliac Joint. La Jolla, CA: November 9–11, 1995.
24. Bogduk N. Clinical Anatomy of the Lumbar Spine and Sacrum. 3rd Ed. New York, NY: Churchill Livingstone, 1997.
25. Pearcy MJ, Tibrewal SB. Three dimensional x-ray analysis of normal movement in the lumbar spine. Spine 1984;9:582–587.
26. Vicenzino G, Twomey L. Side flexion induced lumbar spine conjunct rotation and its influencing factors. Aust Physiother 1993;39:4.
27. Vleeming A, Pool Goudzard A, Stoeckart R, et al. The posterior layer of the thoracolumbar fascia: its function in load transfer from spine to legs. Spine 1995;20:753–758.
28. MacIntosh J, Bogduk N, Gracovetsky S. The biomechanics of the thoracolumbar fascia. Clin Biomech 1987;2:78–83.
29. Morris JM, Benner G, Lucas DB. An electromyographic study of the intrinsic muscles of the back in man. J Anat 1962;96:509.
30. Andersson GBJ, Ortengren R, Herberts P. Quantization electromyographic studies of back muscle activity related to posture and loading. Orthop Clin North Am 1977;8:85–96.
31. Porterfield JA, DeRosa C. Mechanical Low Back Pain: Perspectives in Functional Anatomy. 2nd Ed. Philadelphia, PA: WB Saunders, 1998.
32. Aspden RM. Review of the functional anatomy of the spinal ligaments and the lumbar erector spinae muscles. Clin Anat 1992;5:372–387.
33. Hodges PW, Richardson CA. Contraction of the abdominal muscles associated with movement of the lower limb. Phys Ther 1997;77:132–144.
34. Hides JA, Stokes MJ, Saide M, et al. Evidence of lumbar multifidus muscle wasting ipsilateral to symptoms in patients with acute/subacute low back pain. Spine 1994;19:165–172.
35. Rantanen J, Hurme M, Falck B, et al. The lumbar multifidus muscle five years after surgery for a lumbar intervertebral disc herniation. Spine 1993;18:568–574.
36. Valencia F, Munro R. An electromyographic study of the lumbar multifidus in man. Electromyogr Clin Neurophysiol 1085;15:205–221.
37. Moseley GL, Hodges PW, Gandevia SC. Deep and superficial fibers of the lumbar multifidus muscle are differentially active during voluntary arm movements. Spine 2002;27:E29–E36.
38. Williams P, Warwick R, Dyson M, et al., eds. Gray's Anatomy. Edinburgh: Churchill Livingstone, 1987.
39. Hodges PW, Richardson CA. Neuromotor dysfunction of the trunk musculature in low back pain patients. Proceedings of the World Confederation of Physical Therapists Congress. Washington DC, 1995.
40. Richardson CA, Jull GA. Muscle control, pain control. What exercises would you prescribe? Manual Ther 1995;1:1–2.
41. Jull G, Richardson C. Rehabilitation of active stabilization of the lumbar spine. In: Twomey L, Taylor J, eds. Physical Therapy of the Lumbar Spine. 2nd Ed. New York, NY: Churchill Livingstone, 1994.
42. Richardson CA, Jull GA. Concepts of assessment and rehabilitation for active lumbar stability. In: Boyling JD, Palastanga N, eds. Grieve's Modern Manual Therapy of the Vertebral Column. 2nd Ed. Edinburgh: Churchill Livingstone, 1994.
43. Wingarden JP, Vleeming A, Snidjers CJ, et al. A functional-anatomical approach to the spine-pelvis mechanism: interaction between the biceps femoris muscle and the sacrotuberous ligament. Eur Spine J 1993;2:140.
44. Hodges PW, Richardson CA. Dysfunction of transversus abdominis associated with chronic low back pain. Proceedings of the 9th Biennial Conference of the Manipulative Physiotherapists Association of Australia, Gold Coast, Queensland, 1995.
45. Beal MC. The sacroiliac problem: review of anatomy, mechanics and diagnosis. J Am Osteopath Assoc 1982;81:667–679.
46. Hodges PW, Cresswell A, Thorstensson A. Preparatory trunk motion accompanies rapid upper limb movement. Exp Brain Res 1999;124:69–79.
47. Hodges PW, Richardson. Transversus abdominus and the superficial abdominal muscles are controlled independently in a postural task. Neurosci Lett 1999;265:91–94.
48. Hodges PW, Richardson CA. Altered trunk muscle recruitment in people with low back pain with upper limb movement at different speeds. Arch Phys Med Rehabil 1999;80:1005–1012.
49. Snijders CJ, Vleeming A, Stoeckart R. Transfer of lumbosacral load to iliac bones and legs. Part 1: Biomechanics of self-bracing of the sacroiliac joints and its significance for treatment and exercise. Clin Biomech 1993;8:285–300.
50. Snijders CJ, Vleeming A, Stoeckart R, et al. Biomechanics of sacroiliac joint stability: validation experiments on the concept of self-locking. Proceedings from the Second World Congress on Low Back Pain, San Diego CA, 1995.
51. Sapsford RR, Hodges PW. Contraction of the pelvic floor muscles during abdominal maneuvers. Arch Phys Med Rehabil 2001;82:1081–1088.
52. Frymoyer JW. Back pain and sciatica. N Engl J Med 1988;318:291–298.
53. Saal J. The role of inflammation in lumbar pain. Spine 1995;20:1821–1827.
54. National Center for Health Statistics, Vital and Health Statistics. Detailed Diagnosis and Procedures, National Hospital Discharge Survey 1986, 1987. Washington, DC: U.S. Department of Health and Human Services, 1988–1989.
55. Maluf KS, Sahrmann SA, Van Dillen LR. Use of a Classification System to Guide Nonsurgical Management of a Patient With Chronic Low Back Pain. Phys Ther 2000;80:1097–1111.
56. Magee DJ. Orthopedic Physical Assessment. 3rd Ed. Philadelphia, PA: WB Saunders Co., 1997.
57. American Physical Therapy Association. Guide to Physical Therapist Practice. 2nd Ed. 2001;81:S43–S95.

58. Esola MA, McClure PW, Fitzgerald GK, et al. Analysis of lumbar spine and hip motion during forward bending in subjects with and without a history of low back pain. Spine 1996;1;21:71–78.
59. Lindström I, Ohlund C, Eek C, et al. The effect of graded activity on patients with subacute low back pain: a randomized prospective clinical study with an operant-conditioning behavioral approach. Phys Ther 1992;72:279–290.
60. Kendall FP, McCreary EK, Provance PG. Muscles Testing and Function. 4th Ed. Baltimore: Williams & Wilkins, 1993.
61. Addison R, Schultz A. Trunk strength in patients seeking hospitalization for chronic low back pain. Spine 1980;5:539–544.
62. Mayer TG, Smith SS, Keeley J, et al. Quantification of lumbar function. Part 2: sagittal plane trunk strength in chronic low-back pain patients. Spine 1985;10:765–772.
63. McNeil T, Warwick D, Andersson G, et al. Trunk strengths in attempted flexion, extension, and lateral bending in healthy subjects and patients with low back disorders. Spine 1980;5:529–537.
64. Pope MH, Bevins T, Wilder DG, et al. The relationship between anthropometric, postural, muscular, and mobility characteristics of males ages 18–55. Spine 1985;10:644–648.
65. Holmstrom E, Moritz U, Andersson M. Trunk muscle strength and back muscle endurance in construction workers with and without back pain disorders. Scand J Rehabil Med 1992;24:3–10.
66. Nicolaison T, Jorgensen K. Trunk strength, back muscle endurance and low back trouble. Scand J Rehabil Med 1985;17:121–127.
67. Cresswell A, Grundstrom H, Thorstensson A. Observations on intraabdominal pressure and patterns of intramuscular activity in man. Acta Physiol Scand 1992;144:409–418.
68. Wilke H, Wolf S, Claes L, et al. Stability increase of the lumbar spine with different muscle groups. Spine 1995;20:192–198.
69. Kirkaldy-Willis W, Farfan H. Instability of the lumbar spine. Clin Orthop 1982;165:110–123.
70. Paris S. Physical signs of instability. Spine 1985;10:277–279.
71. Richardson C, Jull G, Hodges P, et al. Therapeutic Exercise for Spinal Segmental Stabilization in Low Back Pain. Edinburgh: Churchill Livingstone, 1999.
72. Meadows J. The principles of the Canadian approach to the lumbar dysfunction patient. In: Wadsworth C, ed. Management of Lumbar Spine Dysfunction, Home Study Course 9.3. La Crosse, WI: Orthopaedic Section, American Physical Therapy Association Inc., 1999.
73. Butler DS. The Sensitive Nervous System. Adelaide, Australia: Noigroup Publications, 2000.
74. Ruta DA, Garratt AM, Wardlaw D, et al. Developing a valid and reliable measure of health outcome for patients with low back pain. Spine 1994;19:1887–1889.
75. Holt AE, Shaw NJ, Shetty A, et al. The reliability of the low back outcome score for back pain. Spine 2002;27:206–210.
76. Waddell G, Main CJ. Assessment of severity in low back disorders. Spine 1984;9:204–208.
77. Main CJ, Waddell G. Behavioral responses to examination. A reappraisal of the interpretation of "nonorganic signs." Spine 1998;23:2367–2371.
78. Waddell G, McCulloch JA, Kummel E, et al. Nonorganic physical signs in low back pain. Spine 1980;5:117–125.
79. Karas R, McIntosh G, Hall H, et al. The relationship between nonorganic signs and centralization of symptoms in the prediction of return to work for patients with low back pain. Phys Ther 1997;77:354–360.
80. Hayes B, Solyom CAE, Wing PC, et al. Use of psychometric measures and nonorganic signs testing in detecting nomogenic disorders in low back pain patients. Spine 1993;18:1254–1262.
81. McKenzie RA. The Lumbar Spine: Mechanical Diagnosis and Therapy. Waikanae, New Zealand: Spinal Publications, 1981.
82. Huijbregts PA. Lumbopelvic Region: Aging, Disease, Examination, Diagnosis, and Treatment. In: Wadsworth C, ed. Current Concepts in Orthopaedic Physical Therapy. Home Study Course 11.2. La Crosse, WI: Orthopaedic Section, American Physical Therapy Association Inc., 2001.
83. Maher CG, Adams R. Reliability of pain and stiffness assessments in clinical manual lumbar spine examination. Phys Ther 1994;74:801–811.
84. Maher CG, Latimer J, Adams R. An investigation of the reliability and validity of posteroanterior spinal stiffness judgments made using a reference-based protocol. Phys Ther 1998;78:829–837.
85. Phillips DR, Twomey LT. Comparison of manual diagnosis with a diagnosis established by a uni-level spinal block procedure. In: Singer KP, ed. Integrating Approaches. Proceedings of the Eighth Biennial Conference of the Manipulative Physiotherapists Association of Australia. Perth: 1993:55–61.
86. Cibulka MT, Delitto A, Koldehoff RM. Changes in innominate tilt after manipulation of the sacroiliac joint in patients with low back pain. Phys Ther 1988;69:1359–1363.
87. Lee D. The Pelvic Girdle. 2nd Ed. Edinburgh: Churchill Livingstone, 1999.
88. Fairbank JCT, Cooper J, Davies JB, et al. The Oswestry Low Back Disability Questionnaire. Physiotherapy 1980;66: 271–273.
89. Million R, Hall W, Nilsen KH, et al. Assessment of the progress of the back pain patient. Spine 1982;7:204–212.
90. Roland M, Morris R. A study of the natural history of back pain. Part I: development of a reliable and sensitive measure of disability in low back pain. Spine 1983;8:141–144.
91. Greenough CG, Fraser RD. Assessment of outcome in patients with low back pain. Spine 1992;17:403–412.
92. Bendebba M, Dizerega GS, Long DM. The Lumbar Spine Outcomes Questionnaire: its development and psychometric properties. Spine J 2007;7:118–132.
93. Jenkinson C. Measuring Health and Medical Outcomes. London: UCL Press, 1994.
94. Kopec JA, Esdaile JM. Spine update: functional disability scales for back pain. Spine 1995;1:1887–1896.
95. Chatzitheodorou D, Mavromoustakos S, Milioti S. The effect of exercise on adrenocortical responsiveness of patients with chronic low back pain, controlled for psychological strain. Clin Rehabil 2008;22:319–328.
96. Lewit K. Manipulative Therapy in Rehabilitation of the Locomotor System. 2nd Ed. Oxford: Butterworth Heinemann, 1991.
97. Nies-Byl N, Sinnott PL. Variations in balance and body sway in middle-aged adults: subjects with healthy backs compared with subjects with low-back dysfunction. Spine 1991;16:325–330.
98. Mok NW, Brauer SG, Hodges PW. Hip strategy for balance control in quiet standing is reduced in people with low back pain. Spine 2004;29:E107–E112.
99. Shirado O, Ito T, Kaneda K, et al. Flexion-relaxation phenomenon in the back muscles: comparative study between healthy subjects and patients with chronic low back pain. Am J Phys Med Rehabil 1995;74:139–144.
100. Watson PJ, Booker CK, Main CJ, et al. Surface electromyography in the identification of chronic low back pain patients: the development of the flexion relaxation ratio. Clin Biomech 1997;12:165–171.
101. Kaigle AM, Wessberg P, Hansson TH. Muscular and kinematic behavior of the lumbar spine during flexion-extension. J Spinal Disord 1998;11:163–174.
102. Sihvonen T, Partanen J, Hanninen O, et al. Electric behavior of low back muscles during lumbar pelvic rhythm in low back pain patients and healthy controls. Arch Phys Med Rehabil 1991;72:1080–1087.
103. Nouwen A, Van Akkerveeken PF, Versloot JM. Patterns of muscular activity during movement in patients with chronic low-back pain. Spine 1987;12:777–782.
104. Ng JK, Richardson CA, Parnianpour M, et al. EMG activity of trunk muscles and torque output during isometric axial rotation exertion: a comparison between back pain patients and matched controls. J Orthop Res 2002;20:112–121.
105. Hides JA, Richardson CA, Jull GA. Multifidus muscle recovery is not automatic after resolution of acute, first-episode low back pain. Spine 1996;21:2763–2769.
106. Hodges PW, Richardson CA. Inefficient muscular stabilization of the lumbar spine associated with low back pain: a motor control evaluation of transversus abdominis. Spine 1996;21:2640–2650.
107. O'Sullivan P, Twomey L, Allison G, et al. Altered patterns of abdominal muscle activation in patients with chronic low back pain. Aust J Physiother 1997;43:91–98.
108. Hodges PW, Richardson CA. Contraction of the abdominal muscles associated with movement of the lower limb. Phys Ther 1997;77:132–142; discussion 142–144.
109. Panjabi MM. The stabilizing system of the spine. Part I. Function, dysfunction, adaptation, and enhancement. J Spinal Disord 1992;5:383–389.
110. Grabiner M, Kohn T, Ghazawi AE. Decoupling of bilateral paraspinal excitation in subjects with low back pain. Spine 1992;17:1219–1223.
111. Roy S, DeLuca C, Casavant D. Lumbar muscle fatigue and chronic low back pain. Spine 1989;14:992–1001.
112. Roy S, DeLuca C, Snyder-Mackler L, et al. Fatigue, recovery, and low back pain in varsity rowers. Med Sci Sports Exerc 1990;22:463–469.
113. Haig A, Weismann G, Haugh L, et al. Prospective evidence for changes in paraspinal muscle activity after herniated nucleus pulposus. Spine 1993;17:926–929.
114. Suzuki N, Endo S. A quantitative study of trunk muscle strength and fatigability in the low back pain syndrome. Spine 1984;8:69–74.
115. Biederman HJ, Shanks GL, Forrest WJ, et al. Power spectrum analysis of electromyographic activity. Spine 1991;16:1179–1184.
116. Hodges P, Richardson C, Jull G. Evaluation of the relationship between laboratory and clinical tests of transversus abdominis function. Physiother Res Int 1996;1:30–40.
117. Stanford ME. Effectiveness of specific lumbar stabilization exercises: a single case study. J Manual Manipulative Ther 2002;10:40–46.
118. Hagins M, Adler K, Cash M, et al. Effects of practice on the ability to perform lumbar stabilization exercises. Ortho Sports Phys Ther 1999;29:546–555.
119. Barr KP, Griggs M, Cadby T. Lumbar stabilization: core concepts and current literature, Part 1. Am J Phys Med Rehabil 2005;84(6):473–480.
120. van Wingerden JP, Vleeming A, Buyruk HM, et al. Stabilization of the sacroiliac joint in vivo: verification of muscular contribution to force closure of the pelvis. Eur Spine J 2004 May;13:199–205.
121. Pel JJ, Spoor CW, Pool-Goudzwaard AL, et al. Biomechanical analysis of reducing sacroiliac joint shear load by optimization of pelvic muscle and ligament forces. Ann Biomed Eng 2008 Mar;36:415–424.
122. Van Dillen LR, Sahrmann SA, Norton BJ, et al. Effect of active limb movements on symptoms in patients with low back pain. J Orthop Sports Phys Ther 2001;31:402–413.
123. Van Dillen LR, Maluf KS, Sahrmann SA. Further examination of modifying patient-preferred movement and alignment strategies in patients with low back pain during symptomatic tests. Man Ther 2009 Feb;14:52–60.

124. Neumann P, Gill V. Pelvic floor and abdominal muscle interaction: EMG activity and intra-abdominal pressure. Int Urogynecol J Pelvic Floor Dysfunct 2002;13:125–132.

125. Bullock-Saxton JE, Janda V, et al. Reflex activation of gluteal muscles in walking. Spine 1993;18:704–708.

126. Anderson KG, Behm DG. Maintenance of EMG activity and loss of force output with instability. J Strength Cond Res 2004 Aug;18:637–640.

127. Norwood JT, Anderson GS, Gaetz MB, Twist PW. Electromyographic activity of the trunk stabilizers during stable and unstable bench press. J Strength Cond Res 2007 May;21:343–347.

128. Dorman T. Pelvic mechanics and prolotherapy. In: Vleeming A, Mooney V, Dorman T, Snijders C, Stoeckart R, eds, Movement, Stability, and Low Back Pain: The Essential Role of the Pelvis. New York, NY: Churchill Livingstone, 1997:501–522.

129. Yelland MJ, Del Mar C, Pirozzo S, et al. Prolotherapy injections for chronic low back pain: a systematic review. Spine 2004 Oct 1;29: 2126–2133.

130. Kelly JP. Reactions of neurons to injury. In: Kandel E, Schwartz J, eds. Principles of Neural Science. New York, NY: Elsevier, 1985.

131. Risk factors for back trouble [editorial]. Lancet 1989;8650:1305–1306.

132. Sihvonen T, Herno A, Paljarvi L, et al. Local denervation of paraspinal muscles in postoperative failed back syndrome. Spine 1993;18:575–581.

133. Kawaguchi Y, Matsui H, Tsui H. Back muscle injury after posterior lumbar surgery. Spine 1994;19:2598–2602.

134. Lindgren K, Sihvonen T, Leino E, et al. Exercise therapy effects on functional radiographic findings and segmental electromyographic activity in lumbar spine and instability. Arch Phys Med Rehabil 1993;74:933–939.

135. Boileau JC, Basmajian JV. Grant's Method of Anatomy. 7th Ed. Baltimore, MD: Williams & Wilkins, 1965.

136. McGill AM. The mechanics of torso flexion: situps and standing dynamic flexion manouevres. Clin Biomech 1995;10:184–192.

137. Shirley D, Ellis E, Lee M. The response of posteroanterior lumbar stiffness to repeated loading. Man Ther 2002;1:19–25.

138. Schipplein OD, Trafimow JH, Andersson GB, et al. Relationship between moments at the L5/S1 level, hip and knee joint when lifting. J Biomech 1990;23:907–912.

139. Paris SV. Loubert PV. Foundations of Clinical Orthopaedics. St. Augustine, FL: Institute Press, 1990.

140. Herzog W, Scheele D, Conway PJ. Electromyographic responses of back and limb muscles associated with spinal manipulative therapy. Spine 1999;24: 146–152.

141. Wilson JN, Ilfeld FW. Manipulation of the herniated intervertebral disc. Am J Surg 1952;173–175.

142. Zhao P, Feng TY. The biomechanical significance of herniated lumbar intervertebral disk: a clinical comparison analysis of 22 multiple and 39 single segments in patients with lumbar intervertebral disk herniation. J Manipulative Physiol Ther 1996;19:391–397.

143. Zhao P, Feng TY. Protruded lumbar intervertebral nucleus pulposus in a 12 year old girl who recovered after non-surgical treatment: a follow-up case report. J Manipulative Physiol Ther 1997;20;551–556.

144. Huijbregts PA. Fact or fiction of disc reduction: a literature review. J Manual Manipulative Ther 1998;6:137–143.

145. Delitto A, Cibulka MT, Erhard RE, Bowling RW, Tenhula JA. Evidence for the use of an extension-mobilization category in acute low back syndrome: a prescriptive validation pilot study. Phys Ther 1993;73:216–228.

146. Hinderer KA, Hinderer SR, Shurtleff DB. Myelodysplasia. In: Campbell SK, Vander Linden DW, Palisano RJ, eds. Physical Therapy for Children. 2nd Ed. Philadelphia, PA: WB Saunders Co., 2000.

147. Deyo RA, Mirza SK, Martin BI. Back pain prevalence and visit rates: estimates from U.S. national surveys, 2002. Spine 2006;31:2724–2727.

148. Melzack R, Coderre TJ, Katz J, et al. Central neuroplasticity and pathological pain. Ann N Y Acad Sci 2001 Mar;933:157–174.

149. Salter MW. Cellular neuroplasticity mechanisms mediating pain persistence. J Orofac Pain 2004;18:318–324.

150. Rainville P, Bushnell MC, Duncan GH. Representation of acute and persistent pain in the human CNS: potential implications for chemical intolerance. Ann N Y Acad Sci 2001;933:130–141.

151. Fisher M, Kaur D, Houchins J. Electrodiagnostic examination, back pain and entrapment of posterior rami. Electromyogr Clin Neurophysiol 1985;25: 183–189.

152. Mattila M, Hurme M, Alaranta H, et al. The multifidus muscle in patients with lumbar disc herniation: a histochemical and morphometric analysis of intraoperative biopsies. Spine 1986;11:733–738.

153. Stokes M, Cooper R, Jayson M. Selective changes in multifidus dimensions in patients with chronic low back pain. Eur Spine J 1992;1:38–42.

154. Macdonald D, Moseley GL, Hodges PW. Why do some patients keep hurting their back? Evidence of ongoing back muscle dysfunction during remission from recurrent back pain. Pain 2009;142:183–188.

155. Panjabi M, Abumi K, Duranceau J, et al. Spinal stability and intersegmental muscle forces: a biomechanical model. Spine 1989;14:194–199.

156. Fitzmaurice R, Cooper R, Freemont A. A histomorphometric comparison of muscle biopsies from normal subjects and patients with ankylosing spondylitis and severe mechanical low back pain. J Pathol 1991;163:182A.

157. Ford D, Bagall K, McFadden K, et al. Analysis of vertebral muscle obtained during surgery for correction of a lumbar disc disorder. Acta Anat 1983;116:152–157.

158. Lehto M, Hurme M, Alaranta H, et al. Connective tissue changes of the multifidus muscle in patients with lumbar disc herniation. Spine 1989;14:302–308.

159. Zhu XZ, Parnianpour M, Nordin M, et al. Histochemistry and morphology of erector spinae muscle in lumbar disc herniation. Spine 1989;14:391–397.

160. Cavanaugh JM. Neural mechanisms of lumbar pain. Spine 1995;20:1804–1809.

161. McKenzie R. The Lumbar Spine. Upper Hutt, New Zealand: Wright & Carmen, 1981.

162. Van Dillen LR, Sahrmann SA, Norton BJ, et al. The effect of modifying patient-preferred spinal movement and alignment during symptom testing in patients with low back pain: a preliminary report. Arch Phys Med Rehabil 2003;84:313–322.

163. Van Dillen LR, Sahrmann SA, Wagner JM. Classification, intervention, and outcomes for a person with lumbar rotation with flexion syndrome. Phys Ther 2005;85:336–351.

164. McKenzie R. Prophylaxis in recurrent low back pain. N Z Med J 1979;89: 22–23.

165. Erhard RE, Delitto A, Cibulka MT. Relative effectiveness of an extension program and a combined program of manipulation with flexion and extension exercises in patients with acute low back syndrome. Phys Ther 1994;74:1093–1100.

166. Donnelson R, Silva G, Murphy K. Centralization phenomenon. Spine 1990;15:211–213.

167. White AA, Panjabi MM. Clinical Biomechanics of the Spine. 2nd Ed. Philadelphia, PA: JB Lippincott Co, 1990.

168. Schnebel BE, Simmons JW, Chowning J, et al. A digitizing technique for the study of movement of intradiskal dye in response to flexion and extension of the lumbar spine. Spine 1988;13:309–312.

169. Schnebel BE, Watkins RG, Dillin W. The role of spinal flexion and extension in changing nerve root compression in disc herniations. Spine 1989;14: 835–837.

170. Magnusson ML, Pope MH, Hansson T. Does hyperextension have an unloading effect on the intervertebral disc? Scand J Rehabil Med 1995;27:5–9.

171. Adams MA, Dolan P, Hutton WC. The lumbar spine in backward bending. Spine 1988;13:1019–1026.

172. Saunders H. The use of spinal traction in the treatment of neck and back conditions. Clin Orthop Rel Res 1983;179:31–38.

173. Ellis JJ, Spagnoli R. The hip and sacroiliac joint: prescriptive home exercise program for dysfunction of the pelvic girdle and hip. In: Orthopedic Physical Therapy Home Study Course 971. LaCrosse, WI: Orthopedic Section, American Physical Therapy Association, 1997.

174. Staal JB, Hlobil H, Twisk JW, et al. Graded activity for low back pain in occupational health care: a randomized, controlled trial. Ann Intern Med 2004;140:77–84.

175. Pel JJ, Spoor CW, Goossens RH, Pool-Goudzwaard AL. Biomechanical model study of pelvic belt influence on muscle and ligament forces. J Biomech 2008;41:1878–1884.

176. Richardson C, Jull G, Hodges P, et al. Therapeutic Exercise for Spinal Segmental Stabilization in Low Back Pain. Edinburgh, Scotland: Churchill Livingstone, 1999.

177. O'Sullivan PB, Twomey LT, Allison GT. Evaluation of specific stabilizing exercise in the treatment of chronic low back pain with radiologic diagnosis of spondylolysis or spondylolisthesis. Spine 1997;22:2959–2967.

178. Pfingsten M. Functional restoration—it depends on an adequate mixture of treatment. Der Schmertz 2001;15:492–498.

179. Poulter D. Letters to the editor-in-chief; empower the patient. J Orthop Sports Phys Ther 1999;29:616–617.

180. Adams N, Ravey J, Bell J. Investigation of personality characteristics in chronic low back pain patients attending physiotherapy out-patient departments. Physiotherapy 1994;80:514–519.

181. Bigos SJ, McKee J, Holland JP, et al. Back pain, the uncomfortable truth—assurance and activity paradigm. Der Schmertz 2001;15:430–434.

182. Goodwin R, Goodwin N. An audit into a spinal rehabilitation programme. Br J Ther Rehabil 2000;7:275–281.

183. Lively M. Sports medicine approach to low back pain. South Med J 2002; 95:642–646.

184. Staal JB, Hlobil H, van Tulder MW, et al. Return-to-work interventions for low back pain: a descriptive review of contents and concepts of working mechanisms. Sports Med 2002;32:251–267.

185. Liddle SD, Baxter GD, Gracey JH. Exercise and chronic low back pain: what works? Pain 2004;107(1–2):176–190.

186. Spangfort EV. Lumbar disc herniation: a computer aided analysis of 2504 operations. Acta Orthop Scand 1972;142:1–93.

187. Yong Hing KHB, Kirkaldy-Willis WH. The pathophysiology of degenerative disease of the lumbar spine. Orthop Clin North Am 1983;14:491–504.

188. Nachemson A, Elfstrom G. Intradiskal dynamic pressure measurements in the lumbar discs. Scand J Rehabil Med 1970;51:10–40.

189. Alpers BJ. The neurological aspects of sciatica. Med Clin North Am 1953;37:503–510.

190. Andersson GBJ, Deyo RA. History and physical examination in patients with herniated lumbar discs. Spine 1996;21:10S–18S.

191. Van den Hoogen HMM, Koes BW, Van Eijk JTM, et al. On the accuracy of history, physical examination, and erythrocyte sedimentation rate in diagnosing low back pain in general practice. Spine 1995;20:318–327.
192. Brieg A, Troup JDG. Biomechanical consideration in the straight-leg-raising test: cadaveric and clinical studies of medial hip rotation. Spine 1979;4:242–250.
193. Charnley J. Orthopedic signs in the diagnosis of disc protrusion with special reference to the straight leg raising test. Lancet 1951;1:186–192.
194. Kosteljanetz M, Bang F, Schmidt-Olsen S. The clinical significance of straight-leg-raising (Lasegue's sign) in the diagnosis of prolapsed lumbar disc. Spine 1988;13:393–395.
195. Shoqing X, Quanzhi Z, Dehao F. Significance of straight-leg-raising test in the diagnosis and clinical evaluation of lower lumbar intervertebral disc protrusion. J Bone Joint Surg Am 1987;69:517–522.
196. Kortelainen P, Pruanen J, Koivisto E, et al. Symptoms and signs of sciatica and their relation to the localization of the lumbar disc herniation. Spine 1985;10:88–92.
197. Hakelius A, Hindmarsh J. The comparative reliability of preoperative diagnostic methods in lumbar disc surgery. Acta Orthop Scand 1972;43:234–238.
198. Blower PW. Neurologic patterns in unilateral sciatica. Spine 1981;6:175–179.
199. Aronson HA, Dunsmore RH. Herniated upper lumbar discs. J Bone Joint Surg Am 1963;45:311–317.
200. Kostuik JP, Harrington I, Alexander D, et al. Cauda equina syndrome and lumbar disc herniation. J Bone Joint Surg Am 1986;68:386–391.
201. O'Laoire SA, Crockard HA, Thomas DG. Prognosis for sphincter recovery after operation for cauda equina compression owing to lumbar disc prolapse. BMJ 1981;282:1852–1854.
202. Tay ECK, Chacha PB. Midline prolapse of a lumbar intervertebral disc with compression of the cauda equina. J Bone Joint Surg Br 1979;61:43–46.
203. Spitzer WO, LeBlanc FE, Dupuis M, et al. Scientific approach to the assessment and management of activity related spinal disorders: a monograph for clinicians: report of the Quebec Task Force on Spinal Disorders. Spine 1987;12(Suppl 7):S16–S21.
204. Weisel SE, Tsourmas N, Feffer H, et al. A study of computer-assisted tomography. I: the incidence of positive CAT scans in an asymptomatic group of patients. Spine 1984;9:549–551.
205. Boden SD, Davis DO, Dina TS, et al. Abnormal magnetic resonance scans of the lumbar spine in asymptomatic subjects. J Bone Joint Surg Am 1990;72:403–408.
206. Abdi S, Datta S, Trescot AM, et al. Epidural steroids in the management of chronic spinal pain: a systematic review. Pain Physician 2007;10:185–212.
207. Weinstein SM, Herring SA, Derby R. Contemporary concepts in spine care. Epidural steroid injections. Spine 1995;20:1842–1846.
208. van Tulder MW, Malmivaara A, Esmail R, et al. Exercise therapy for low back pain. Cochrane Database Syst Rev 2000:CD000335. [Review. Update in: Cochrane Database Syst Rev 2005:CD000335.]
209. Delitto A, Erhard RE, Bowling RW. A treatment based classification approach to low back syndrome: identifying and staging patients for conservative treatment. Phys Ther 1995;75:470–485; discussion 485–479.
210. Harte AA, Baxter GD, Gracey JH. The efficacy of traction for back pain: a systematic review of randomized controlled trials. Arch Phys Med Rehabil 2003;84:1542–1553.
211. Busanich BM, Verscheure SD. Does McKenzie therapy improve outcomes for back pain? J Athl Train 2006;41:117–119.
212. Dirckx JH, ed. Stedman's Concise Medical Dictionary for the Health Professional. 3rd Ed. Baltimore, MD: Williams & Wilkins, 1997.
213. Turner JA, Ersek M, Herron L, et al. Surgery for lumbar spinal stenosis: attempted metaanalysis of the literature. Spine 1986;11:436–439.
214. Dong GX, Porter RW. Walking and cycling tests in neurogenic and intermittent claudication. Spine 1989;14:965–969.
215. Porter RW. Spinal stenosis. Semin Orthop 1989;1:97–111.
216. Robaina-Padrón FJ. Controversies about instrumented surgery and pain relief in degenerative lumbar spine pain. Results of scientific evidence. Neurocirugia (Astur) 2007;18:406–413.
217. Fritz JM, Erhard RE, Vignovic M. A nonsurgical treatment approach for patients with lumbar spinal stenosis. Phys Ther 1997;77:962–973.
218. Admundson GM, Wenger DR. Spondylolisthesis: natural history and treatment. Spine 1987;1:323–328.
219. Caillet R. Low Back Pain Syndrome. Philadelphia, PA: FA Davis, 1981.
220. Majid K, Fischgrund JS. Degenerative lumbar spondylolisthesis: trends in management. J Am Acad Orthop Surg 2008;16:208–215.
221. Frymoyer JW, Krag MH. Spinal stability and instability: definitions, classification, and general principles of management. In: Dunsker SB, Schmidek HH, Frymoyer JW, et al., eds. The Unstable Spine (Thoracic, Lumbar, and Sacral Regions). Orlando, FL: Grune & Stratton, 1986.
222. Frymoyer JW, Akeson W, Brandt K, et al. Clinical perspectives. In: Frymoyer JW, Gordon SL, eds. New Perspectives on Low Back Pain. Park Ridge, IL: American Academy of Orthopedic Surgeons, 1989.

chapter 18

The Pelvic Floor

ELIZABETH SHELLY

Physiologic impairments of the gynecologic, urinary, and gastrointestinal systems are often treated with medications or surgery. However, physical therapists have become increasingly involved in the rehabilitation of these patients. Pelvic floor dysfunction refers to dysfunction of the entire pelvis including bladder, bowel, intestines, bones, joints, and muscles and includes such diagnosis as urinary and fecal incontinence, pelvic organ prolapse, urinary retention, and painful penetration. The *pelvic floor muscles* (PFMs) refers collectively to muscles that span from the pubic bone to the coccyx. This area includes skeletal muscles under voluntary control, which responds to the same training techniques as other skeletal muscles in the body. PFM rehabilitation addresses the skeletal muscles of the pelvic floor and can prevent or reverse pelvic floor dysfunction.[1] Clinical audit in the United Kingdom showed that 79% of patients receiving PFM training improved sufficiently to avoid urological surgery.[2]

This chapter introduces students to the *anatomy and kinesiology* of the PFMs, physiology of micturition, and anatomic and physiologic impairments of the pelvic floor. Management of common physiologic impairments of the PFM, pelvic floor–related diagnoses, and their impact on other areas of the body are described, and clinical applications are provided.

All physical therapists should screen patients for pelvic floor impairments and provide basic instruction in strengthening these skeletal muscles. This chapter provides screening and evaluation tools that do not require internal vaginal evaluation or surface electromyography (EMG) of the pelvic floor and explains how to teach pelvic floor exercises (PFEs), which strengthen the PFMs and specifically address impaired muscle performance. Arnold Kegel was an obstetrician who pioneered PFM strengthening in the 1940s.[3] The Kegel (pronounced "kagel") exercise, as it is commonly known, is a contraction of the PFMs around an object, preferably a pressure biofeedback device. Patients often use Kegel exercises and PFE synonymously. This chapter also discusses pelvic pain associated with PFM impairment. A working knowledge of normal function of the lumbopelvic and hip structures is necessary to accurately treat PFM spasm (see Chapters 17 and 19).

Postgraduate study is recommended for therapists interested in directly treating the PFMs.

The specialized therapist must know how to examine and evaluate all of the structures of the pelvic floor to understand the medical diagnoses and treatment interventions for PFM dysfunction. A complete evaluation of this area often requires intravaginal palpation and surface EMG evaluation. These evaluation skills are usually not considered entry-level skills.

REVIEW OF ANATOMY AND KINESIOLOGY

The many inconsistencies in labeling the structures of the pelvic floor found in the medical literature can make the study of these muscles confusing. This section outlines the terminology used by most clinicians.[4,5] Because most patients with PFM dysfunction are female, female anatomy is discussed in this chapter, but the pelvic diaphragm layers and intrapelvic hip rotators are essentially the same in both sexes.

Skeletal Muscles

Currently, the term "pelvic floor" refers to all the structures of the lower pelvis including the boney pelvis, viscera, fascia and ligaments, and PFMs. The skeletal muscles of the pelvic floor (Fig. 18-1) are specifically called "pelvic floor muscles"[4] and can be divided into four layers, from superficial to deep: (a) the anal sphincter, (b) superficial genital muscles, (c) Perineal membrane, and (d) the pelvic diaphragm.[5]

The *anal sphincter* (Fig. 18-2) is the most superficial skeletal muscle. The anal sphincter includes the internal anal sphincter (i.e., smooth muscle) and the external anal sphincter (i.e., skeletal muscle). These sphincters fuse superiorly with the puborectalis component of the pelvic diaphragm muscle. These three muscles function together to provide fecal continence. Neurologic innervation is provided from the fourth sacral nerve and the inferior branch of the pudendal nerve.

The *superficial genital muscles* (Fig. 18-3) aid in sexual functioning of the pelvic floor, and the perineal membrane (Fig. 18-4) is part of the continence mechanism. The three superficial genital muscles are the bulbocavernosus, the ischiocavernosus, and the superficial transverse perineal. The three muscles of the perineal membrane are the urethrovaginal sphincter, the compressor urethrae (formerly known together as the deep transverse perineal), and the sphincter urethrae (Table 18-1).[6–9]

Pelvic Diaphragm Muscles

The pelvic diaphragm (Fig. 18-5) contains the largest skeletal muscle group in the pelvic floor, the levator ani muscles. The four muscles of the levator ani are the coccygeus, the iliococcygeus, the puborectalis, and the pubococcygeus muscle.

The coccygeus muscle originates at the spine of the ischium and inserts on the anterior portion of the coccyx and S4. In other mammals, this muscle controls the tail movement. In humans, the coccygeus flexes the coccyx and may help stabilize the sacrum through its sacrococcygeal attachments.[9] The iliococcygeus originates from the pubic

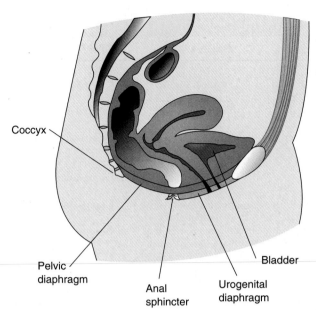

Coccyx

Pelvic diaphragm

Anal sphincter

Urogenital diaphragm

Bladder

FIGURE 18-1. PFM layers.

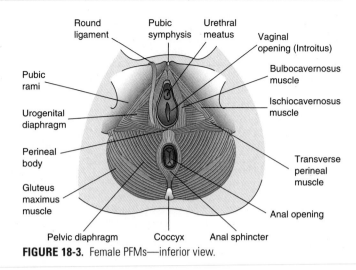

Round ligament

Pubic symphysis

Urethral meatus

Vaginal opening (Introitus)

Bulbocavernosus muscle

Ischiocavernosus muscle

Pubic rami

Urogenital diaphragm

Perineal body

Gluteus maximus muscle

Transverse perineal muscle

Anal opening

Pelvic diaphragm   Coccyx   Anal sphincter

FIGURE 18-3. Female PFMs—inferior view.

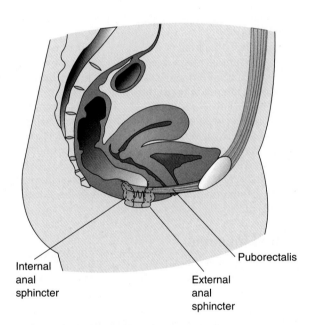

Internal anal sphincter

External anal sphincter

Puborectalis

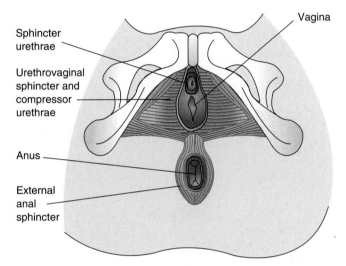

Sphincter urethrae

Urethrovaginal sphincter and compressor urethrae

Anus

External anal sphincter

Vagina

A

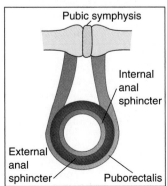

Pubic symphysis

Internal anal sphincter

External anal sphincter

Puborectalis

Transverse section

FIGURE 18-2. Anal sphincter.

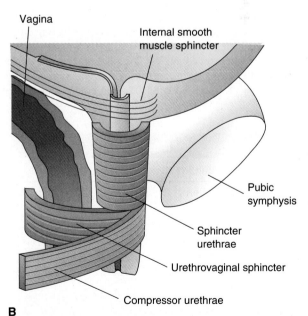

Vagina

Internal smooth muscle sphincter

Pubic symphysis

Sphincter urethrae

Urethrovaginal sphincter

Compressor urethrae

B

FIGURE 18-4. Female urogenital diaphragm—(A) Inferior view. (B) Side view. (Schussler B, Laycock J, Norton P, Stanton S, eds. Pelvic Floor Re-education Principles and Practice. New York, NY: Springer-Verlag, 1994.)

TABLE 18-1	**Muscles of the Urogenital Triangle**			
MUSCLE	**ORIGIN**	**INSERTION**	**INNERVATION**	**FUNCTION**
Superficial Perineal				
Bulbocavernosus	Corpus cavernosum of the clitoris	Perineal body	Perineal branch of pudendal S2–4	Clitoral erection
Ischiocavernosus	Ischial tuberosity and pubic rami	Crus of the clitoris	Perineal branch of pudendal S2–4	Clitoral erection
Superficial transverse	Ischial tuberosity	Central perineal tendon	Perineal branch of pudendal S2–4	Stabilizes perineal body
Perineal Membrane				
Urethrovaginal sphincter	Vaginal wall	Urethra	Perineal branch of pudendal S2–4	Compression of urethra
Sphincter urethra	Upper two thirds of urethra	Trigone ring	Perineal branch of pudendal S2–4	Compression of urethra
Compressor urethra	Ischiopubic rami	Urethra	Perineal branch of pudendal S2–4	Compression of urethra

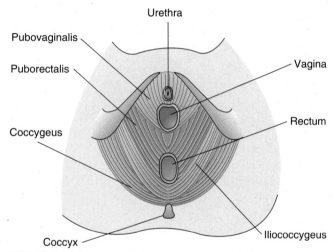

FIGURE 18-5. Female pelvic diaphragm—superior view.

ramus and arcus tendentious levator ani (an extension of the obturator internus fascia) and inserts onto the coccyx. The pubococcygeus originates at the posterior aspect of the os pubis and inserts on the perineal body and vaginal walls, forming a sling around the vagina. The puborectalis originates from the pubic bone and obturator internus fascia and inserts onto the coccyx and lateral walls of the rectum, similarly forming a sling around the rectum and increasing rectal continence.[10] The innervation of the levator ani muscles is from the ventral rami of S2 through S4 and possibly the pudendal nerve of S2 through S4[11,12] (Table 18-2). The function of the levator ani muscles is to support the pelvic viscera and close the pelvic floor.[13]

The pelvic diaphragm muscles are approximately 70% slow-twitch muscle fibers (type 1) and 30% fast-twitch muscle fibers (type 2).[7] Both types of muscle fibers have specific functions in the pelvic floor, and a complete exercise program should train both types of muscle fibers. The physiology of these muscles is similar to that of other skeletal muscles. Sensation in the region is limited and may be decreased with surgery or childbirth. The PFM responds to quick stretch and has extensive fascia throughout the muscle layers (see Table 18-2). The PFMs contract as a unit to achieve various functions. Impairments can occur in a single layer or throughout the entire skeletal muscle layers.

Related Muscles

Hip function may need to be considered with PFM dysfunction and PFM dysfunction with hip dysfunction.

TABLE 18-2	**Levator Ani Muscles**			
MUSCLE	**ORIGIN**	**INSERTION**	**INNERVATION**	**FUNCTION**
Coccygeus	Spine of the ischium	Anterior portion of the coccyx and S4	Ventral rami, S4, and S5	Flex the coccyx
Pubococcygeus	Posterior os pubis	Perineal body, vaginal walls	Inferior rectal branch of the pudendal nerve, S2–4, and ventral rami, S2–4	Support of the pelvic viscera Compression of the vagina
Puborectalis	Pubic bone, arcus tendineus	Anterior coccyx, lateral rectum	Inferior rectal branch of the pudendal nerve, S2–4, and ventral rami, S2–4	Support of the pelvic viscera Compression of the rectum
Iliococcygeus	Pubic rami, arcus tendineus	Coccyx	Inferior rectal branch of the pudendal nerve, S2–4, and ventral rami, S2–4	Support of the pelvic viscera

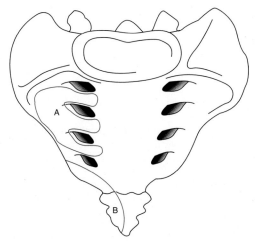

FIGURE 18-6. The anterior sacrum. Origin of the piriformis (A) and coccygeus (B).

(Fig. 18-6).[14,15] The inferior border of the piriformis is close to the superior border of the coccygeus muscle (Fig. 18-7). The levator ani muscles attach to an extension of the obturator internus fascia (i.e., the arcus tendinous levator ani). Clinically, it appears that impairments in length, strength, endurance, and patterns of recruitment of the piriformis and obturator internus muscles can contribute to PFM impairments and vice versa.[16]

The adductor muscle group also may participate in PFM pain syndromes and overactive bladder. Adductor fascia at the pubic rami is in close proximity to the superficial perineal muscle fascia. The psoas minor and major muscles, iliacus, and quadratus lumborum are key muscles to treat in lumbopelvic dysfunctions including PFM pain syndromes.

Pelvic Floor Function

Organ Support Function

The PFMs provide support to the pelvic organs. Wei stated that normal pelvic organ support is achieved by ligamentous support from above, PFMs function from below, and the structural geometry achieved by normal function of both.[5] Recovery of organ support requires attention to restoring PFM function (i.e., PFM rehabilitation) firstly and in some cases restoring ligament support (i.e., surgery).[17] Women with pelvic organ prolapse more often have defects in the levator ani and generate less vaginal closure force than women with good organ support.[18] At rest, the PFMs maintain a minimal resting tone. The forces of gravity and increased intra-abdominal pressure (e.g., laugh, cough, sneeze, vomit, lift, strain) encourage prolapse or protrusion of the pelvic organs. Strong PFMs help to support the organs against increased intra-abdominal pressure and enhance normal functioning. The supportive function is primarily performed by the tonic, slow-twitch muscle fibers.

Trunk Support Function

PFM and transversus abdominis muscles have been shown to co-contract.[19] This co-contraction along with contraction

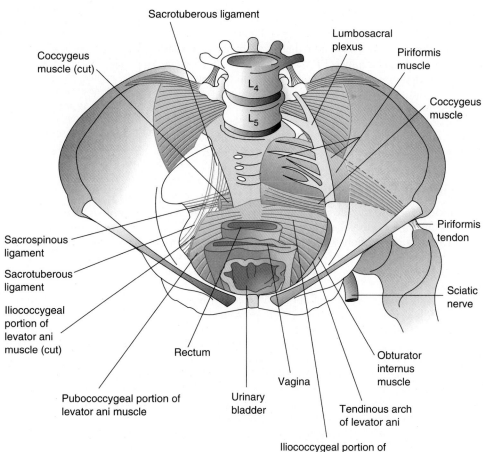

FIGURE 18-7. Piriformis and pelvic area—superior view.

of the deep multifidus muscles appears to enhance trunk stability. In addition, the PFMs have been shown to increase muscle activation before movement as a precontraction to assist the abdominals in stabilizing the trunk.[20] Many studies have documented bladder dysfunction in association with low back pain (LBP).[21] One study showed 78% of 200 women reporting to a physical therapy (PT) clinic with a chief complaint of LBP had urinary incontinence (UI).[22] Smith et al.[23] have documented decreased balance ability in women with stress urinary incontinence (a condition related to PFM weakness) compared to continent women. Current research results are supporting the role of the PFM in orthopedic conditions. It is essential that all physical therapists understand the role of the PFM, symptoms, and possible treatments.

Sphincteric Function

The PFMs provide closure of the urethra and rectum for continence. During normal function, quick closure of the orifices is provided by the phasic, fast-twitch fibers. Closure during rest (i.e., static resting tone) is provided by the slow-twitch muscle fibers. Continence is preserved when the pressure in the urethra (provided by several structures including the PFMs) is higher than the pressure in the bladder. Loss of sphincteric function may lead to incontinence. The medical literature commonly points out that incontinence is a symptom and not a disease; based on the terminology used in this book, incontinence results from impairments not a pathologic condition. Intervention should be aimed at the impairments that contribute to the syndrome of incontinence.

Sexual Function

The vagina has very few sensory nerve fibers.[24] The PFMs provide proprioceptive sensation that contributes to sexual appreciation. Hypertrophied PFMs provide a smaller vagina and more friction against the penis during intercourse. This results in the stimulation of more nerve endings and provides pleasurable sensation during intercourse. Strong PFM contractions occur during orgasm. Patients with weak PFMs often cannot achieve orgasms.[24] In men, the PFMs assist in achieving and maintaining an erection.[25,26]

Physiology of Micturition

Micturition refers to the physiologic process of urination and involves a complex set of somatic and autonomic reflexes. An explanation of micturition is provided in Display 18-1. This information is included so the therapist can explain the basics of normal bladder function to the patient and assist with basic bladder retraining.

Urine is produced steadily at about 15 drops per minute. Bladder filling is constant, except in the presence of bladder irritants, which increase urine production. There is always urine in the bladder. Urine continues to collect, and the bladder passively expands until approximately 150 mL of fluid is collected. Stretch receptors in the bladder then signal the brain that it may be necessary to get to the bathroom soon. This is called the first sensation to void. The detrusor muscle (i.e., muscle of the bladder) remains quiet, and the PFMs maintain normal resting tone. Filling continues until 200 to 300 mL, when a stronger sensation of urgency is felt from increased activation of stretch

receptors. The detrusor and PFMs remain unchanged. A severe urge to void usually occurs at 400 to 550 mL.[9,27] The brain eventually directs the person to a toilet, clothes are removed, and the person either sits on or stands over the toilet to void. The PFMs relax, the detrusor contracts, and urine flows out.[28] The PFMs return to resting tone when the urine flow stops. Postvoid residual studies show how much urine is left in the bladder after urination. Normative values vary, but most practitioners consider it normal to have 5 to 50 mL of urine left in the bladder after a normal urination. It is neither necessary nor desirable to increase intra-abdominal pressure (i.e., bear down) at any time during urination.[29]

Dysfunctions of micturition are complex. The screening questionnaire in Display 18–5 can help identify patients with dysfunctions of micturition who may need further medical intervention and who should be referred to the physician.

DISPLAY 18-1
Micturition Facts

- The bladder's job is to store urine and empty fully at the appropriate time and place.
- It is necessary to allow normal filling of the bladder for normal bladder function. A person should not go to the bathroom "just in case."
- It is important to drink six to eight 8-oz glasses of fluid per day. Decreasing fluids does not decrease incontinence and may make urgency worse because concentrated urine is a bladder irritant.[107]
- It is normal to urinate six to eight times in a 24-hour period with normal fluid intake. More than eight times per day is called *urinary frequency*. In rare cases, the physician instructs patients to empty more frequently.
- The normal voiding interval is 2 to 5 hours.
- Normal nocturnal voiding frequency (after the patient has gone to bed for the evening) is zero to one time per night for children and adults younger than 65 years of age and one to two times per night for adults older than 65 years of age.
- Each urination should be 8 to 10 oz. If urination is completed in 2 to 3 seconds, the voided volume is usually small and the voiding interval could have been longer.
- Hovering over the toilet may result in incomplete emptying of the bladder. Overflow from the adductors and gluteals to the PFM results in increased tone in the PFM and decreased urine flowing out.
- Many fluids can irritate the bladder, causing urgency and increasing urine production. The most common *bladder irritants* are caffeine (e.g., coffee, tea, cola, medications, chocolate), alcohol, carbonated beverages, and nicotine. Many other substances can be irritants, including artificial sweeteners, acid-containing foods (citrus, tomatoes, coffee, soda), and some over-the-counter and prescription medications. Eliminating or limiting bladder irritants decreases symptoms of urgency and urge incontinence.
- Women should always clean well after using the toilet by reaching around behind and wiping from front to back. This ensures that fecal matter is not introduced into the urethra and decreases the incidence of infection.

IMPAIRMENTS OF BODY STRUCTURES

Many factors contribute to normal function of the PFMs. Some of these factors cannot be changed by physical therapy interventions. The two major causes of structural impairments are birth injury and neurologic dysfunction.

Birth Injury

Vaginal delivery may result in tears, overstretching, or crush injury of the PFMs (i.e., between the baby's head and the pubic rami) or may cause complete or partial denervation of unilateral or bilateral pudendal nerves (i.e., stretch injury or avulsion of the nerve).

Dollan found 80% of vaginal deliveries showed evidence of pudendal nerve reinnervation indicating trauma to the nerve. This occurrence was associated with longer pushing and larger babies.[30] Mild and moderate injuries can be effectively treated with behavioral interventions (see the "Impaired Muscle Performance" section). However, severe trauma may result in severe muscle damage (usually unilateral) and decreased sensory or motor innervation sufficient to render the muscle ineffective. This type of trauma occurs in a very small percentage of births. Very fast deliveries do not allow time for tissue stretch and may result in a "burst" effect, extensively tearing the tissue. Deliveries with a pushing phase longer than 2 hours may result in stretch injury to nerves and muscles. Use of forceps to assist delivery may result in increased trauma to the muscles.[31] Many other factors during delivery may influence PFM outcomes, including the woman's position, leg position, size of the baby, medical interventions, medications given, and the use of an episiotomy.[32,33] However, most women with vaginal deliveries sustain only minor, temporary dysfunctions and recover fully. To maximize birth recovery, all women of childbearing age should receive accurate preventative education on PFM health.[34]

Neurologic Dysfunction

Many central and peripheral nervous system (PNS) dysfunctions affect PFM function.[35] PNS conditions, such as disk herniation and spinal cord injury, may result in sensory or motor denervation of the PFMs. Diabetes may result in sensory or motor denervation of the PFMs and autonomic neuropathy with disruption of bladder function. The pelvic plexus includes many small nerves that are often not visible during surgery. These nerves are not located in a consistent pattern in all patients. Radical pelvic operations, such as total hysterectomy[36] and radical prostatectomy,[37] may result in inadvertent disruption of the sensory and motor nerves to the bladder and PFMs. Patients may be able to strengthen the remaining innervated muscles to achieve full supportive and sphincteric function. Central nervous system (CNS) diseases such as cerebrovascular accidents,[38] multiple sclerosis,[39] and Parkinson disease may affect cognitive control of the bladder and PFMs. These conditions may also affect the patient's ability to get to the toilet or to recognize the toilet and may affect the patient's social awareness of continence. In these patients, urinary incontinence is associated with eventual functional dependence and poor survival.[40] Maintaining functional independence should include treatment of PFM dysfunction and continence.

IMPAIRMENTS OF MENTAL FUNCTIONS

Motivation

PFM strengthening requires motivation and persistence. Adherence to PFM exercise programs has been shown to be predictive of positive outcomes.[41,42] Several factors limiting full participation in PFM exercises have been identified. These include lack of time and motivation, inconvenience, poor social support, and cultural beliefs.[43] Improvement in muscle function with PFM therapy can be quick and dramatic, but it is more often slow and gradual. Some patients do not have enough motivation to complete therapy and find it easier to wear incontinence pads. Incontinence affects patients' lives differently. Some patients are devastated and severely limited by a small amount of urine leaking two or three times per week. Other patients view large leaks two or three times per day as a mild inconvenience. The perceived severity of the condition helps determine motivation. Ask the patient, "On a scale of 0 to 10, how severely does your condition affect your life (0 = no effect; 10 = severely limiting)." Therapists must strongly encourage patients throughout the therapy to maintain motivation. Depression and poor motivation may limit a patient's progress with PME.

Sexual Abuse

An estimated one of three girls has been abused before the age of 14. Only one of five cases is reported. Some studies show that there is a higher incidence of gynecological problems among sexual abuse survivors.[44] All therapists should be aware of symptoms of sexual abuse (Display 18-2) and should have some exposure to techniques to facilitate rehabilitation of these patients (Display 18-3). It is especially important to be sensitive to these issues when treating PFM dysfunction and pelvic pain (see Building Block 18-1). Therapists are encouraged to seek additional information on sexual abuse survivors (see the "Recommended Reading" section).

EXAMINATION/EVALUATION

All patients could benefit from screening for PFM dysfunction. Understanding the risk factors for PFM dysfunction helps the therapist identify patients who may benefit from

---

DISPLAY 18-2
Symptoms of Sexual Abuse

- Low self-esteem, feelings of loss of control
- Poor body awareness, often not trusting their own physical or emotional feelings
- Difficulty with anger and violence
- Difficulty with sexuality and intimacy; may avoid sex completely or compulsively seek sex
- Denies and forgets instructions or appointments
- Self-mutilating or addictive behaviors
- Controlling of environment, treatment, or your time
- Multiple personalities
- Dissociation (i.e., avoidance of eye contact, distant look), an unconscious defense mechanism to separate the mind from the body and protect the mind from impending trauma; may occur during the treatment sessions

DISPLAY 18-3
Guidelines for Therapy with Known or Suspected Sexual Abuse Survivors

- Give the patient control over as much as you can in the environment and in therapy.
- Offer names of community support services and psychologists skilled in the treatment of sexual abuse survivors.
- Do not touch the patient without permission, and avoid hugging or other nonessential physical contact.
- Never allow the patient to disassociate.
- Be honest with the patient about your ability and knowledge (or lack of) in this area.

in-depth questioning. Screening tools are provided to identify PFM impairments and dysfunctions. Therapists are cautioned that questionnaires can be misleading[45] and full urologic workup is indicated if conservative treatment is not successful. This section also outlines the information that is gathered by specialized therapists from internal vaginal examinations and from patient self-evaluations. Other examination tools used by the specialized therapists include external observation, EMG and pressure biofeedback, and real-time ultrasound imaging.

Risk Factors

A brief screening questionnaire should be given to all patients. Patients with medical histories that include many risk factors may be screened using a more detailed form. Risk factors are related to the causes of various dysfunctions (see Display 18-4 and Case Study 18-1).

Screening Questionnaires

Two types of screening questionnaires can be used to determine whether patients have dysfunctions of the pelvic floor. Questions should be clear and direct. A broad question such as "Are you incontinent?" usually results in a false-negative response.

BUILDING BLOCK 18-1

Another therapist is working in the gym with a 15-year-old male with Osgood Schlatter. You notice this patient moves away when the therapist touches his thigh and appears uncomfortable when the therapist is standing close to him. Your college has expressed frustration with this patient's lack of coordination and body awareness making accurate exercises very difficult in the clinic and at home. In addition, the patient is very particular about the time of his appointment, which plinth he wants to work on, how the Thera-Band is arranged, and always cleans the mat before he sits on it. Discuss how you might share your concerns of possible sexual abuse history in this patient with your college and what steps might be taken to make his therapy more tolerable for him and more effective.

DISPLAY 18-4
Risk Factors for Underactive and Overactive PFM

Underactive PFM[46–49]
- Vaginal childbirth, pregnancy.
- Increased body mass index (BMI), increased waist line.
- Chronic or prolonged coughing, as with pulmonary diseases, smoking.
- Arthritis, functional impairments, hip fracture, falls.
- Long-term incorrect lifting or straining with a Valsalva maneuver (i.e., increased intra-abdominal pressure with bearing down), including incorrect straining with exercise.
- Chronic constipation.
- Menopause and estrogen use.
- Neurologic dysfunctions that may affect peripheral nerves of the pelvis and many central nervous system (CNS) diseases including dementia.
- Medical comorbidities such as diabetes mellitus (DM), peripheral vascular disease (PVD), congestive heart failure (CHF), thyroid problems.
- Decreased awareness of PFMs with disuse atrophy.
- Pelvic surgery, previous hysterectomy.
- Urinary incontinence is associated with LBP in both sexes.[21] 78% of 200 women reporting to a PT clinic with chief complaint of LBP had UI.[22]
- Age—although UI increased with age, it is not a significant factor after adjustment for confounding conditions. UI does occur in young women especially athletes.[50–52]

Overactive PFM
- Back and pelvic pain with joint dysfunction, especially if related to a direct fall on the buttock or pubic bone[53]
- Muscle imbalance of the hip muscles, abdomen or pelvis, or lumbar spine, including shortened muscles or connective tissue in the trunk and pelvis[53]
- Habitual PFM holding (e.g., excessive emotional stress, or fighting the urge to urinate)[54]
- Abdominal adhesions and adhered scars in the pelvic region[55]
- Deep episiotomy or perineal tearing with childbirth
- Pelvic surgery[56]
- Pelvic conditions, such as endometriosis, irritable bowel syndrome, or interstitial cystitis[57,58]
- History of or current fissures or fistulas
- Connective tissue disease such as fibromyalgia
- History of sexual abuse, 40% to 50% of women with CPP have a history of abuse[59–62]
- History of or current sexually transmitted disease or recurrent perineal infections, including yeast infections
- Dermatologic conditions such as lichen sclerosis and lichen planus

Brief Screening Questionnaire
Evaluation of all patients, especially those with the risk factors listed in Display 18-4, should include three questions:

- Do you ever leak urine or feces?
- Do you ever wear a pad because of leaking urine?
- Do you have pain during intercourse?

Detailed Screening Questionnaire
Therapists must understand the dysfunctions of the PFM and their diagnostic classifications and the types of incontinence

CASE STUDY 18-1

Mary Smith is a 50-year-old mother of two with LBP. She works in a busy office and does not exercise often. List

Ms. Smith's risk factors for underactive and overactive PFMs.

DISPLAY 18-5
Detailed PFM Questionnaire

The patient should respond with *never, sometimes,* or *often* to the following questions:

1. Do you leak urine when you cough, laugh, or sneeze?
2. Do you lose urine when you lift heavy objects such as a basket of wet clothes or furniture?
3. Do you lose urine when you run, jump, or exercise?
4. Do you ever have such an uncomfortable, strong need to urinate that you leak if you do not reach the toilet? Do you sometimes leak with this strong urge?
5. Do you develop an urgent need to urinate when you hear running water?
6. Do you develop an urgent need to urinate when you are nervous, under stress, or in a hurry?
7. When you are coming home, can you usually make it to the door but then lose urine just as you put the key in the lock?
8. Do you have an urge to urinate when your hands are in cold water?
9. Do you find it necessary to wear a pad at any time because of leakage?
10. Does your bladder awaken you from sleep? How many times each night?
11. How often do you leak urine or feces?
12. How often do you inadvertently leak gas?
13. Do you ever feel as though you are "sitting on a ball" or that there is something "in the way" when you are sitting?
14. Do you ever feel as though something is "falling out" of your perineal area?
15. Do you find it hard to begin urination?
16. Do you have a slow urinary stream?
17. Do you strain to pass urine?
18. Do you have pain during vaginal penetration, including intercourse, insertion of a tampon, or vaginal examination?
19. Do you have pelvic pain with sitting, wearing jeans, or bike riding?

---

to fully understand the interpretation of the results of this screening tool. A detailed screening questionnaire should be given if the patient responds affirmatively to the questions of the brief screening questionnaire. The longer version should be administered to a patient with pelvic, trunk, or back pain who is recovering slower than expected (see Display 18-5).

Questions 1 through 14 (see Display 18-5) may indicate an underactive PFM or urgency that may be treated using

PFEs. A positive response to questions 1 through 3 indicates symptoms of stress incontinence. A positive response to questions 4 through 8 indicates symptoms of urge incontinence. A positive response to questions 13 and 14 may indicate organ prolapse. Questions 13 through 19 may indicate overactive PFM, incoordination, obstruction, or urinary retention. The PFM should relax during urination. Poor relaxation or incoordination may result in symptoms of obstruction (i.e., positive responses only to questions 15 through 17). These patients may also need evaluation by a physician to rule out mechanical obstruction. If the patient has symptoms of overactive PFM (i.e., positive response to questions 13 through 19), proceed with full evaluation of the sacroiliac, hip girdle, and pelvic fascia (see Case Study 18-2).

Results of the Internal Examination

A complete PFM evaluation is necessary to prescribe an appropriate exercise program for the PFMs. It includes an extensive history, symptom documentation, identification of associated factors, and internal vaginal or rectal examinations. Surface EMG or pressure biofeedback evaluation may also be added. The specialized therapist obtains the following information from the internal examination of the PFMs[28]:

Muscle performance is assessed in the form of power and endurance. *Power* is defined as the ability to contract (manual muscle grade of 0 through 5). This grade provides information on how much lift (i.e., supportive function) and closure (i.e., sphincteric function) the PFMs have. The muscle bulk of the PFMs can be palpated to help determine possible duration of rehabilitation and rehabilitation potential. Patients with a small, thin PFM require a longer rehabilitation time and generally have less rehabilitation potential than those with good PFM bulk. *Endurance* is defined as the ability to hold a slow-twitch muscle contraction and repeat the contraction. Clinicians also determine how many fast-twitch muscle contractions can be done. The quality of the contractions is also evaluated.

Resting tone between contractions is assessed, looking specifically for altered tone impairments.

Coordination of the PFMs and the relationship with associated muscles are assessed. Muscle dominance patterns or inappropriate contractions of the gluteal muscles, adductor group, and abdominal muscles are assessed.

CASE STUDY 18-2

You have asked Ms. Smith the PFM screening questions. She does report urine leakage with sneezing but does not wear pads. She denies pain with intercourse. Create a list

of follow-up questions to ask Ms. Smith to determine more about her condition.

DISPLAY 18-6
Contraindications or Precautions to Internal Evaluation of the PFM

- Pregnancy
- Within 6 weeks of vaginal or cesarean delivery
- Within 6 weeks after pelvic surgery
- Atrophic vaginitis, a condition of fragile skin seen in cases of estrogen deficiency
- Active pelvic infection
- Severe pelvic or vaginal pain, especially pain during penetration or intercourse
- Children and presexual adolescents
- Lack of informed consent
- Lack of therapist's training (The therapist should obtain specialized training in performing internal evaluations of the PFM. Training can be obtained in postgraduate courses or through individual instruction from a midwife, physician, nurse, or trained physical therapist.)

Other impairments, such as pelvic floor trigger points, decreased sensation, and scars or myofascial adhesions, may limit strengthening.

Internal examination of the PFMs is the gold standard for determining if the patient is performing a PFM contraction correctly.[63,64] However, internal examinations cannot or should not be performed in some cases (see Display 18-6). At which time, the specialized therapists would choose one of the alternative examination techniques.

Patient Self-Assessment Tests

When an internal evaluation cannot be performed, self-assessment tests can help patients and the therapist identify some of the impairments of the PFMs. Therapists can use the results of self-assessment tests to prescribe PFEs with some accuracy.

A possible evaluation tool used when the therapist cannot perform an internal evaluation is the digital vaginal self-examination (i.e., finger in the vagina test). Begin with patient education, as outlined later in the Active Pelvic Floor Exercises. This section also includes information about verbal cues for the proper contraction of PFMs. After a brief introduction to the PFMs and the exercise, the patient should be instructed in the digital vaginal self-examination test (see Patient-Related Instruction 18-1: Testing Your PFM by Performing the Digital Vaginal Self-Examination [Finger in the Vagina Test]). Digital vaginal self-examination is often accepted by female patients and can be taught to male patients (i.e., finger in the rectum test) in the same manner if they are having trouble learning the correct contraction with other methods. Many factors influence continence and PFM function. Some practitioners use the stop urine test to determine PFM function. Current literature does not support the value of this test.[65]

The finger in the vagina test cannot evaluate all aspects of muscle function but can give some indication of the muscles' abilities and provide guidance in prescribing exercises. Patient progress should be judged by reexamination of the PFM function; however, if this is not possible, it may be judged by decreasing symptoms. Patients can perform the

Patient-Related Instruction 18-1

Testing Your PFM by Performing the Digital Vaginal Self-Examination

The following test can help you determine your current ability and monitor your recovery. Perform this test before beginning your PFM exercise program and then periodically throughout the training period, approximately every 2 weeks. Fluctuations in muscle ability occur in response to fatigue, medications, hormones, and other factors. The PFMs are more likely to be weak at the end of the day, when you are sick, and just before menstruation.[24] For an accurate comparison, repeat the test at the same time of the day and the same time of the monthly menstrual cycle as the original test. Any exercise program takes time and dedication. As with other muscles, the PFMs may take 4 to 6 months to strengthen. After you have performed the test, report the following information to your therapist: how many seconds you can hold the contraction, how many of these long-hold contractions you can do, and how many quick contractions you can do.

Digital Vaginal Self-Examination (Finger in Vagina or Rectum)

Place your finger into the vagina or rectum up to the level of the second knuckle. Palpate the muscle on either side of the vagina or rectum while you contract the PFM, pulling the muscles up and in. You should feel the muscles contract around your finger and pull your finger up and in. If you feel tissues pushing out of your body or bulging, ask your health care professional to evaluate the area. Determine how long you can hold the PFM contraction and how many times you can repeat that contraction. Then perform quick maximal contractions (1-second hold). Count the number of quick contractions you can perform before the muscle tires.

test at home and report to the therapist, or the test can be done in the clinic if sufficient privacy is available (i.e., closed-door treatment room with a plinth or recliner is suggested). In the clinic, the therapist can briefly step out of the room while the patient performs the test or can remain in the treatment room with the patient adequately draped. The patient should provide the following information:

- Duration (in seconds) of PFM endurance contraction
- Number of repetitions of PFM endurance contractions
- Number of repetitions of quick muscle contractions

A second self-assessment test, the jumping jack test, is a test of advanced strength (see Patient-Related Instruction 18-2: Jumping Jack Test). It is usually not given to sedentary, incontinent patients. It is helpful for athletes and other active individuals who know how to do the PFE well. Patients may use this test to judge continued progress after active therapy has ended (see Building Block 18-2).

Ultrasound Imaging for PFM Dysfunction

Over the past 5 years, the interest and availability of ultrasound imaging in physical therapy have increased. Imaging of the PFM gives the general physical therapist a valid tool to objectively measure the PFM without internal palpation.[66] This modality can also be used to provide biofeedback to the

Patient-Related Instruction 18-2

Jumping Jack Test

This test is used only to evaluate PFM ability under physical stress. To begin, empty your bladder, and then perform five jumping jacks. If no urine leaks out, wait 1½ hours, and do five more jumping jacks. If no leakage occurs, wait 1½ hours, and repeat the five jumping jacks. The test proceeds until leakage occurs. Make a note of how long after urination and how many jumping jacks you could do before urine leakage occurs. It is important to continue drinking as usual during the test. There are no normative values for this test, but some therapists feel a patient should be able to do 5 to 10 jumping jacks 2 to 3 hours after urination without leaking.

Circle the number of jumping jack at which urine leakage occurs

Immediately—1 2 3 4 5
½ hour—1 2 3 4 5
1 hour—1 2 3 4 5
1½ hours—1 2 3 4 5
2 hours—1 2 3 4 5
2½ hours—1 2 3 4 5
3 hours—1 2 3 4 5
3½ hours—1 2 3 4 5
4 hours—1 2 3 4 5

BUILDING BLOCK 18-2

Your patient is a 24-year-old female 2 month post–surgical repair of an anterior cruciate ligament. She has been progressing nicely in her recovery and is now returning to jumping practice in preparation for return to volleyball. During one of her therapy sessions, she suddenly stops and excuses her self to the bathroom. Upon her return, she is not as aggressive with her jumping and appears self-conscious. During one of her exercises, you notice a small wetness in the perineal area. Describe how you might approach this patient's apparent urinary leakage during therapy. Describe how to perform the patient self-assessment tests.

patient and enhance PFM contraction learning. The ultrasound probe is placed transverse or sagittal in the suprapubic region with the sound waves directed caudal into the pelvis. Ultrasound imaging has been shown to be an effective assessment tool for PFM volume, anatomy, and movement.[67,68]

Sample patient goals

- The patient will have decreased number of nighttime voids from ___ no. to___ no.; allowing improved sleep and decreased fall risk.
- The patient will be able to participate in _____ (sport, housework, and work) with ___% decrease in urinary leakage.
- The patient verbalizes understanding of independent home exercise program to increase PFM function.
- The patient achieves increased time between voids to ___ no. of hours for work and social activities.
- Activities of daily living (ADLs) are not limited by urgency urinary incontinence or frequency (see Case Study 18-3).

THERAPEUTIC EXERCISE INTERVENTIONS FOR COMMON PHYSIOLOGIC IMPAIRMENTS

This section outlines the physiologic impairments and possible treatments of the PFMs and related structures. Several types of impaired PFM functions are possible:

- Impaired muscle performance of the PFMs, abdominal muscles, and hip muscles
- Pain and altered tone of the PFMs, hip muscles, and trunk muscles
- Mobility impairments causing PFM dysfunction as a result of adhesions, scar tissue, and connective tissue disorders
- Posture impairments
- Coordination impairments of the PFMs, PFMs during ADLs, PFMs with the abdominal muscles, and abdominal muscles alone

Impaired Muscle Performance

Pelvic Floor Muscles

Impaired muscle performance (impairment in strength, power, or endurance) is the most commonly treated impairment of the PFMs. PFM performance may be impaired by trauma during vaginal delivery, CNS or PNS neurologic dysfunction, surgical procedures, decreased awareness of PFMs, disuse, prolonged increased intra-abdominal pressure, pelvic congestion or swelling, and back or pelvic pain. Impaired muscle performance is usually the primary impairment in the underactive PFM diagnostic classification.

The PFMs are 70% slow-twitch muscle fibers with the critical role of providing support to pelvic organs against gravity in all upright positions. PFMs are postural muscles

CASE STUDY 18-3

Ms. Smith states that she does not exercise partly because of fear of leaking and has had to leave the movie theater during a movie to urinate. You have both decided it is important to address this dysfunction. You explained the self-assessment tests last week, and the patient has performed them as you requested and is reporting the results.

Results of jumping jack test—1½ hours first jumping jack
The number of repetitions and amount of hold time per contraction—5-second hold 10 times
The number of quick contractions—20
List three goals specific to urinary incontinence for this patient.

and must be able to maintain some baseline tone for long periods. Weak, easily fatigued, saggy muscles do not support the pelvic organs. Lengthened muscles may result in pain and pressure in the perineum because structures "hang" on the ligamentous supports and stretch the nerves. Poor endurance of the PFMs is a common finding in many women without symptoms of PFM dysfunction. Most women probably have endurance impairment of the PFMs long before functional impairments of leaking urine or prolapse occur. Teaching PFEs to *all* adults may help to prevent PFM dysfunctions in the future.[1] This is especially true with prenatal and postpartum women and women after menopause or gynecologic surgery.

The treatment for impaired muscle performance is active PFEs.[69–72] These strengthening exercises are explained later in the "Active Pelvic Floor Exercises" section.

Abdominal Muscles

Impaired abdominal muscle performance often results in a pendulous abdomen and can contribute to PFM dysfunction, especially incontinence. Restoring abdominal wall length and strength and avoiding Valsalva maneuvers are the goals of PFM dysfunction treatment.

Treatment of impaired abdominal muscle performance is described in detail in Chapter 17. Patients with PFM dysfunction should be taught not to bear down (i.e., Valsalva maneuver) during exercises and ADLs. Valsalva maneuvers can contribute to incontinence and may increase the chance of pelvic organ prolapse.

Hip Muscles

Hip impairments (see Chapter 19) are often underlying causes of overactive PFM. The piriformis, obturator internus, and adductors are the most likely muscles involved because of their proximity to the PFMs. Any muscle impairment affecting the sacroiliac joint may also contribute to overactive PFM (see Chapter 17).

Active Pelvic Floor Exercises

PFEs specifically address impaired muscle performance of the PFMs. Many patients know these exercises as Kegel exercises. Proper contraction and relaxation of the PFMs are necessary for normal function and are the focus of treatment for most PFM impairments. A correct technique is essential and should ideally be confirmed with vaginal or rectal palpation. If this is not possible, use patient self-assessment described above or rehabilitative imaging ultrasound. Teaching PFE without internal palpation or biofeedback is difficult for the therapist and the patient. However, this section gives the therapist a comprehensive plan for teaching effective PFE, including patient education, verbal cues for proper PFM contraction, home exercise programs, and methods for putting the exercise program together. Therapists use the treatment dosage information in conjunction with the patient's self-assessment and awareness exercises to prescribe an individualized PFE program.

Dosage

The therapist uses the results from the patient's self-evaluation test (i.e., digital vaginal self-examination test) to prescribe an individualized exercise program for PFM strengthening.

The therapist also should consider the following parameters, even when prescribing PFE without the benefit of an internal examination. The therapist should remember the basic principles of overload (i.e., the muscle must be challenged to its fullest capacity to improve strength) and specificity (i.e., patients should exercise the muscle correctly in isolation). Patients can be taught these ideas and can learn to progress in their own programs.[63] PFEs must be individualized for the patient to reach his or her full rehabilitation potential. Many well-intentioned publications give "cookbook" exercise programs that are too hard for the average incontinent patient (e.g., hold for 10 seconds and repeat 10 to 15 times). Patients try to follow these instructions, realize that their symptoms are not changing, and ultimately abandon the exercises. These same patients have achieved good results with careful instructions and individualized programs.

Duration How many seconds should the patient hold the endurance muscle contraction? If the evaluation reveals that the patient can hold the contraction for 3 seconds (not uncommon for weak muscles), the therapist asks the patient to hold the PFM contraction (i.e., Kegel contraction) for 3 to 4 seconds before resting and repeating the exercise. Sustained PFM contractions are progressed to a maximum of 8 to 12 seconds.[64,72] This parameter shows the endurance of the muscles. Endurance impairments of PFMs are common.

Rest How long should the patient rest between endurance muscle contractions? Increased resting tone (i.e., overactive PFM) and weak muscles require longer rest times. Twice as much rest time as hold time is advised for a weak muscle (e.g., 3-second hold, 6-second rest, and repeat). Rest time is decreased as strength increases (e.g., 10-second hold, 10-second rest, and repeat). A quality PFM contraction requires complete relaxation at the end of each exercise.[73] Incomplete relaxation does not train a muscle in its full range of motion and may result in spasm and pain. Complete relaxation between contractions produces a more functional muscle.

Endurance Contraction Repetitions How many endurance contractions should the patient do in one set before fatigue? For the patient previously described, the therapist would determine how many 3-second contractions the patient can complete. The average patient with endurance impairment is able to perform only 5 to 10 repetitions before fatiguing. The exercise program must be individualized for maximum benefit.

Quick Contraction Repetitions How many quick contractions should the patient do in one set? A complete PFE program includes quick endurance muscle contractions. The therapist prescribes the number of quick contractions based on how many can be done at the initial evaluation. Quick contractions involve quick, maximal recruitment of the PFMs, followed by quick relaxation. These contractions are usually held for <2 seconds. Quick contraction of the PFM is necessary to avoid leaking during quick movements such as sneezing, jumping, and running.

Sets How many sets should the patient do in 1 day? Patients with weak PFMs should do a set of contractions (as determined previously) several times during the day. The sets should be spaced throughout the day and performed up to three to four times per day, with a total of 30 to 80 pelvic floor contractions per day.[64] A meta-analysis of PFE and symptom reduction shows that as little as 24 contractions per day can be beneficial.[74]

Activity

Posture Gravity pulls down on the pelvic floor in upright positions. Patients with very weak PFMs should therefore do their exercises in the horizontal position (i.e., gravity neutral). Patients with moderately strong PFMs can perform exercises in the sitting position (i.e., against gravity) and advance to the standing position as they feel stronger. Results of the manual muscle test (MMT) using an internal examination of the PFMs provide the basis for prescribing exercise positions accurately. All patients should eventually progress to doing PFEs while standing, because it is necessary for the muscles to function well in this position (i.e., most incontinence occurs while standing). Some publications recommend that women practice PFEs while driving or waiting in line. However, initially, patients should learn these exercises in a quiet place so they can concentrate and perform the exercises correctly. After the exercises are learned well, patients can do them while waiting in line or watching TV.

Accessory Muscle Use Contraction of the abdominal, adductor, and gluteal muscles can result in an overflow to the PFMs.[75] The principles of overflow are used to facilitate strengthening of weak PFMs. Simply stated, overflow is the intentional contraction of associated muscles to increase recruitment of very weak muscles. This technique is usually reserved for patients with an MMT result of 1/5 or 0/5. Some patients with 2/5 results need facilitation, but most therapists begin treatment without facilitation and add it later if the patient is not progressing as expected. Conversely, if the patient has an MMT result of 3/5 or higher, the therapist discourages the use of accessory muscles. Eventually, all patients should learn to contract the PFMs without accessory muscles. Several studies[76,77] have shown the close synergy of the abdominal muscles (particularly the transversus) and the PFM (see Chapter 17). Therefore, it is neither necessary nor desirable to keep the abdominal muscles completely silent during a PFM contract. However, an abdominal contract with bearing down is never desirable and will result in poor results.

Patient Education Before teaching patients how to do the PFEs, they should be educated about the location and function of the PFMs, and the importance of normal PFM function should be explained.

There are many commercially available charts, posters, and handouts that give a two-dimensional view of the location of the PFMs. However, many patients find three-dimensional models more helpful. Pelvic models that have the PFMs and obturator internus muscles in place help in explaining the proximity of the PFMs to the muscles of the buttocks and hips. Alternatively, the therapist can use a standard pelvic bone model and place her hand from the coccyx to the pubic bone to signify the muscles. The patient should understand that the PFMs are internal (approximately 2 in into the vagina) and are in close proximity to the hip muscles. However, it is neither necessary nor desirable to contract the hip muscles while exercising the PFM, unless the therapist is using overflow principles.

An explanation of Kegel's three functions of the PFMs (the three Ss) is usually sufficient for the patient:

- Supportive: They hold the pelvic organs in.
- Sphincteric: They stop urine, feces, and gas from escaping until the person reaches the toilet.
- Sexual: They help women grip the penis and increase sexual feelings. They help men form and maintain an erection.

The therapist should teach the differences in function between quick and endurance contractions. The analogy of sprinters and marathoners helps to explain the quick and endurance properties of the muscle. Sprinters depend on the quick muscle fibers, which are mainly responsible for the sphincteric function. The quick fibers contract quickly before a sneeze or cough. Marathon runners depend on the endurance muscle fibers, which provide the supportive function and hold up the organs. A combination of quick and endurance fibers assists in sexual function.

The following points are examples of the importance of normal muscle function. The information can be individualized for each patient:

A well-exercised muscle has a good blood supply and may recover better from trauma such as childbirth or surgery. PFEs started during pregnancy result in less incontinence and pain after delivery.[78,79]

It is easier to learn these exercises before changes occur from surgery, pregnancy, childbirth, or aging. All women should have a basic knowledge of the PFMs and how they should be exercised (especially if they have any of the risk factors revealed by the screening questionnaires). PFEs should be a part of a woman's basic self-care, such as brushing her teeth and showering.

As stated earlier, incontinence is a symptom not a disease. It is not an inevitable sequel of pregnancy, surgery, or aging, and 87% of patients can significantly reduce or eliminate incontinence with PFEs.[64]

Exercising these muscles before and after bladder suspension surgery may enhance the operative results.[80] Some patients still have symptoms after bladder surgery or become incontinent several years later. Strengthening the PFMs may reduce the likelihood of recurring symptoms.

The normal PFM function is helpful in the treatment of low back and pelvic pain.[81] Weakness or spasm in this muscle group may result in stress to adjacent hip muscles and perpetuate activity limitations. Hip, buttock, and leg pain may not resolve unless this muscle group is functioning normally.

About 49% of patients verbally instructed in PFEs are doing them incorrectly.[82] Approximately 25% are pushing down on the pelvic floor.[82] This makes the dysfunction worse. The therapist must describe the exercises correctly and encourage patients to use the home exercises described in the next section. Display 18-7 provides verbal cues that can be used to instruct a patient how to perform a PFM contraction.

Home exercises are an essential aspect of PFM strengthening. Before patients begin to perform these exercises on their own at home, they must have a complete understanding of their muscles and how to exercise them. The therapist should be aware of a patient's comprehension of the following exercises. Many patients nod and agree just to end the discussion of an embarrassing subject. The therapist should

> ### DISPLAY 18-7
> ### Verbal Cues Used to Teach Pelvic Floor Contractions
>
> - Tighten and lift the muscles around your vagina, and pull them up and inward, as if to stop urine flow.
> - Tighten the muscles that you would use to stop gas from escaping at an embarrassing time.
> - Pull your muscles up and in, as if you had the urge to urinate and could not stop to use the toilet.
> - Gently push out, as if to pass gas, and then quickly pull the muscles back up and in.

address this form of exercise with the same professionalism and completeness as she does for any other exercise. This approach can place the patient at ease, and it emphasizes the importance of the exercises.

Follow-up of the home exercise program is important. At subsequent sessions, ask patients how many, how long, and in what position they are doing the exercises; if they feel the contraction; if the muscles are getting stronger; and if the symptoms are decreasing. To improve compliance, it may be helpful for patients to keep a diary of the exercise routine and list how many times per day incontinence occurs.

These home exercises are used in conjunction with the self-assessment test described in the evaluation section of this chapter (see Self-Management 18-1: Home Awareness Exercises). After going over the self-assessment test and home awareness exercises with the patient, this information may be copied and given to the patient to take home with her.

The patient should perform the tests and awareness exercises at home and then report to the therapist for documentation of results and development of an individualized PFE program.

Putting It All Together—The Exercise Program
The exercises described in Self-Management 18-1: Home Awareness Exercises are designed to help the patient identify and effectively contract the PFMs. However, it is important to create an exercise program that challenges the PFMs of each patient.

For example, if a patient's self-assessment test (e.g., digital self-examination) shows that the PFM contraction was held for 5 seconds and repeated five times and that 10 quick contractions were performed, her evaluation results would be as follows:

- Duration of endurance contraction hold: 5 seconds
- Repetitions of endurance contractions: five times
- Repetitions of quick contractions: 10 times

With this information, the therapist could prescribe the following exercise prescription (see Display 18-8). Five PFM contractions are held for 5 seconds with a 10-second rest in between (double rest is given to patients with poor PFM function). Remind the patient to relax completely in between contractions. Ten quick PFM contractions are done to train the quick function of the muscle. Repeat the set four to six times per day; weak muscles need to be exercised in short sessions many times during the day. Exercises should be performed lying down. The patient should contract the PFMs before and during stressful activities, such as coughing, sneezing, lifting, and straining. All patients should be given functional training activities such as "squeeze before you sneeze."[73]

SELF-MANAGEMENT 18-1 *Home Awareness Exercises*

These exercises are used to help you understand what you should be doing during the Kegel or pelvic muscle exercise. Try the exercises at home, and report the results to your physical therapist. Remember that this is an internal muscle, and you should try not to contract the leg or buttock muscles. During these exercises try to identify

1. If you are doing the exercises correctly
2. How long you can hold the contraction (in seconds) up to 10 seconds
3. How many repetitions you can perform holding the contraction for the previous length of time
4. How many quick contractions you can perform

Index finger on perineal body:

Place your index finger on the perineal body (i.e., the skin between the vagina or penis and the rectum) or lightly over the anus. This can be done over your underpants in some cases. Contract the PFMs, and feel the perineal tissue moving away from your finger, up and into the pelvic cavity. If the PFM is very weak, you may not feel much movement. However, you should never feel the anus or perineal tissue moving toward your finger or bulging. If you feel tissues moving toward your finger, stop exercising, and ask your physician, midwife, physical therapist, or other health professionals to instruct you in the proper PFM contraction.

Finger into vagina or rectum:

Place your index finger into the vagina or rectum up to the level of the second knuckle. Palpate the muscle on either side of the vagina or rectum while you contract the PFMs, pulling them in and up. You should feel the muscles contract around your finger and pull your finger up and in. If you feel tissues pushing out of your body or bulging, ask your health care professional to examine the area.

Visual exercise:

Women Lie on your back with your knees bent and your head resting on several pillows. Hold a mirror so that you can see your perineal body and rectum. Contract the PFMs up and in, and watch the perineal tissues moving up into the body. It may be difficult to see the movement if the muscles are very weak. Seek further professional instruction if any tissue comes toward the mirror or bulges outward.

Men Stand in front of a long mirror, and watch the penis as you contract the PFM up and in. The penis should move slightly upward during the contraction.

Sexercise—(for women):

Contract the PFMs around the penis during intercourse.

Self-assessment and modification of the exercise program continue periodically throughout rehabilitation. Remember to ask the patient how often and how many PFM exercises she can do (see Case Study 18-4). Ask if her symptoms are improving (i.e., decreasing incontinence).

Pain

Pelvic Floor Muscles

PFM spasm with or without muscle shortening occurs in response to many situations outlined in the "Overactive PFM" section of this chapter. Pain and altered tone impairments may be caused by lumbopelvic or hip impairments, tonic holding patterns of the PFMs, abdominal adhesions and adhered scars in the trunk and perineum, fissures, and fistulas. Pain and altered tone impairments are usually the primary impairments of overactive PFM.[83] Coccyx pain is rarely a result of sacrococcygeal joint mobility impairment, but it usually is caused by referred pain from spasm and trigger points in the surrounding muscles. The PFMs, obturator internus, gluteus maximus, and piriformis can refer pain to the coccyx (Fig. 18-8).

Treatment of PFM spasm includes manual soft tissue manipulation of the PFM vaginally, rectally, or externally around the ischial tuberosities and coccyx. Surface EMG biofeedback and PFEs may also help restore the normal tone of the PFMs. In some cases, the PFMs become "frozen" and cannot relax or contract effectively (see Patient-Related Instruction 18-3: Importance of Relaxing the PFMs). Modalities such as electrical stimulation, ultrasound, hot, and cold are being used on the perineum to treat the spasm. The therapist should learn the logistics of applying the modality onto the perineum.[84] Modality parameters and other treatment considerations are the same as those used for spasm in other areas of the body.

Hip Muscles

Any muscle imbalance at the hip and trunk may contribute to overactive PFM through sacroiliac joint impairments.[81] It is often difficult to pinpoint the origin of pain in the lower pelvic region. Muscle spasm and trigger points are common causes of pain in the perineum, groin, and coccyx areas. Travell and Simon[14] described referred pain patterns originating from trigger points in the adductors, PFMs, obturator internus, and piriformis (Figs. 18-8 and 18-9). Spasm and trigger points in these muscles may be primary or secondary impairments and should be treated in all patients with PFM dysfunction. The treatment for hip muscle spasms includes soft tissue manipulation, modalities (i.e., ultrasound, electrical stimulation, hot or cold packs), therapeutic exercises for stretching and strengthening, and patient education about body mechanics and postures.

Trunk Muscles

Iliopsoas and abdominal trigger points and spasm may be the primary muscular impairment in pelvic pain conditions. Iliopsoas spasm may irritate the pelvic organs that overlie them and vice versa, making iliopsoas altered tone impairments an important condition to treat in cases of visceral dysfunction. Treatment of these muscles is essential to full recovery.

Joint Mobility and Range of Motion (Including Muscle Length) Impairments

Spasms of the PFMs are often related to sacroiliac, sacrococcygeal, pubic symphysis, and lumbar joint mobility impairments. These impairments may be primary or secondary and include hypomobility or hypermobility (see Chapter 7). Mobility restriction of the scar tissue and connective tissue in the perineum and groin can also affect PFM's function greatly.

Joint Integrity and Mobility Impairments of the Lumbopelvic Region Resulting in PFM Dysfunction

Hypomobility or hypermobility of the sacroiliac joint, pubic symphysis, or sacrococcygeal joint may cause the secondary impairment of PFM altered tone (i.e., spasm).[81,85] Pain from lumbopelvic–hip joint integrity or mobility may lead to a tonic holding pattern of the PFMs similar to that seen in the cervical muscles after an acceleration injury (i.e., whiplash).

CASE STUDY 18-4

Develop a PFE program for Ms. Smith using the self-assessment information provided earlier.

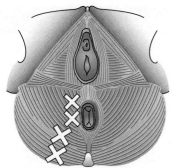
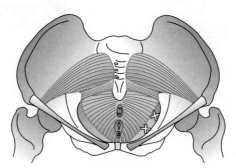

Sphincter ani, levator ani, and coccygeus (view from below)

Obturator internus

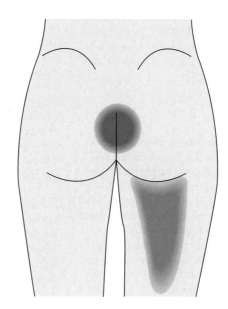

FIGURE 18-8. Trigger points (x) and their referral pain patterns *(shaded areas).*

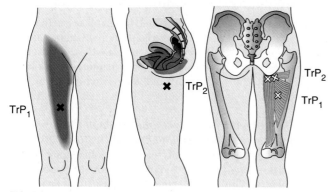

FIGURE 18-9. Trigger points (TrP) of the hip adductors (x) and their referral pain patterns *(shaded areas).*

Sacroiliac mobility impairments may also cause pain-induced PFM weakness. Any malalignment of the pelvis can alter the origin and insertion alignment of the PFMs and impair function by causing spasm or weakness. Significant joint integrity and mobility impairments in all PFM dysfunctions should be treated to achieve full healing. Joint mobilization, positioning, soft tissue mobilizations, therapeutic exercise, and other modalities treat joint integrity and mobility impairments.

The hypogastric plexus (T10 through L2) provides sympathetic innervation to the pelvic and perineal areas. Normal joint mobility in the T10 through L2 region may normalize sympathetic nerve output to the perineum and decrease pelvic pain symptoms. This hypothesis is based on clinical findings and has not been researched in experimental trials (see Case Study 18-5).

CASE STUDY 18-5

During the pelvic examination, you identify signs of sacroiliac dysfunction. Explain to Ms. Smith how her urinary leakage may be related to her LBP.

Lumbopelvic Joint Mobility Impairments Resulting from PFM Dysfunction

Unilateral PFM spasms may contribute to and perpetuate pelvic joint mobility impairments. In some cases, untreated PFM spasm may be the reason for continued mobility impairments. This is seen commonly in the sacroiliac joint and less frequently in the sacrococcygeal joint. Because of PFM attachment onto the sacrum, unilateral PFM spasms can result in torque of the sacrum similar to the torque created by a unilateral piriformis spasm. Unilateral PFM spasms can occur as a result of trauma, such as adductor strain with insertion injury, birth injury, or a fall on the pubic rami. PFM spasm can be caused by sacroiliac joint mobility impairment and then become the reason for continued joint dysfunction. Whether it is the primary or secondary impairment, release of the PFM spasm is needed to restore and maintain normal sacroiliac joint mobility in these cases.

Lumbopelvic Joint Mobility Impairments Resulting from Adhesions

Visceral adhesions may cause sacroiliac joint mobility impairments, especially if unilateral adhesions from the organ to the sacrum are severe. Specialized therapists use visceral mobilization techniques to manipulate organs and abdominal fascial tissue. These techniques are used to stretch adhesions and restore normal movement of lumbopelvic joints and pelvic organs. For example, in endometriosis, endometrial tissue implants in the abdominopelvic cavity outside the uterus. As with the tissue inside the uterus, the explanted tissue responds to hormones during the menstrual cycle causing irritation, inflammation, and eventually scars and adhesions. Adhesions from endometriosis can be extensive throughout the abdomen and are often treated with laparoscopic laser surgery. Adhesions can pull on the ilium, coccyx, or sacrum and constrict bowels or fallopian tubes, altering joint and organ function. Bowel adhesion to the pelvic side wall is found in 14 out of 15 patients with chronic pelvic pain.[86] Soft tissue mobilizations of abdominal adhesions and organs can enhance organ function and may be the necessary link in maintaining normal mobility in the pelvic joints.

Scar Mobility Restrictions

Episiotomy is a common obstetric procedure that involves making a cut in the perineal body immediately before vaginal delivery, usually to ease delivery (Fig. 18-10). Vaginal

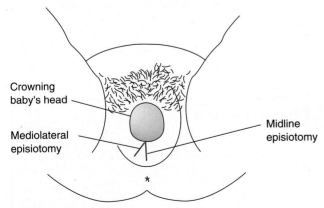

FIGURE 18-10. Possible sites of episiotomy.

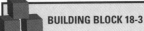

BUILDING BLOCK 18-3

A 40-year-old female with thoracic pain recently underwent a tummy tuck. She has limited trunk extension and weakness in the upper back. What measurements would be important to collect in the abdominal region? List three abdominal treatments that may decrease her thoracic pain.

tissue may tear as an extension of an episiotomy or in lieu of an episiotomy at the time of delivery. Episiotomies and tears may result in adhesions and pain wherever the scar tissue occurs—at the perineal body, tissue inside the vagina, and even toward or into the rectum. Adhesion pain usually occurs in the immediate postpartum stage and abates in most women after 4 to 6 weeks. However, this pain persists in some women and can be so severe that intercourse is impossible and every bowel movement hurts. Sitting may be impossible, or sitting tolerance may be limited. Muscle spasm and adhesions are the most common impairments. Conversely, some patients demonstrate pain-inhibited PFM weakness. Treatment includes soft tissue manipulation and friction massage of scars externally and internally. Modalities, such as ultrasound, hot packs, and cold packs, also are used. PFEs and biofeedback are important in restoring the normal contraction and relaxation of muscles (see Building Block 18-3).

Connective Tissue Mobility Restrictions

Muscle strains often result in irritation to connective tissues and shortening of fascia and tendons. Groin injuries commonly traumatize the adductor muscle group. This is a very large muscle group that inserts onto the pubic ramus and ischial tuberosity. Physical therapists often treat the distal adductor muscle and fascia, whereas restrictions in connective tissue mobility and muscle spasms of the proximal adductor muscles are often left untreated. Tissue at the insertion of the adductor muscles to the pubic arch should be evaluated and treated in patients with persistent groin pain. A similar condition may occur in the hamstring muscles. The hamstring tendon sends a slip of connective tissue to the sacrotuberous ligament, which eventually fuses with the posterior sacroiliac ligaments. Impaired mobility of connective tissue at the proximal hamstring muscle may be related to persistent sacroiliac joint dysfunction. These conditions may occur with spasm of the PFMs. Treatment of connective tissue mobility impairment includes soft tissue mobilization, therapeutic exercise, and modalities (i.e., ultrasound, electrical stimulation, and hot packs).

Posture Impairment

Poor posture and body mechanics are commonly associated with joint mobility impairments. Education about proper posture and body mechanics is included in the treatment of all patients with joint dysfunction of the lumbopelvic area. Sitting posture demands special attention in patients with overactive PFM (see Patient-Related Instruction 18-4: Proper Sitting Posture).

Patient-Related Instruction 18-4

Proper Sitting Posture

- Proper sitting posture is essential for relief of perineal and tail bone pain.
- Weight should be shifted forward on the two "sit bones" and thighs.
- There should be no pressure on the tail bone.
- Push your buttocks back in the chair so there is no space between your very low back and the chair.
- Use a small towel roll at your waist to maintain the inward curve if needed.
- A firmer chair can support your posture better and decrease pressure on the tail bone.
- Poor sitting posture places weight on the coccyx.

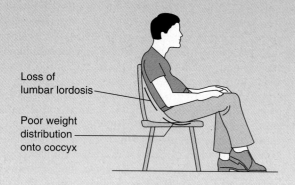

Loss of lumbar lordosis

Poor weight distribution onto coccyx

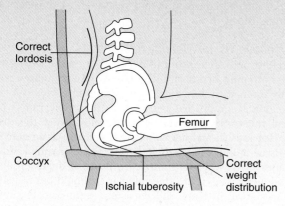

Correct lordosis

Femur

Coccyx

Correct weight distribution

Ischial tuberosity

Proper sitting posture places weight on the ischial tuberosities and posterior thigh.

Coordination Impairment

Coordination impairment is related to inappropriate patterns of timing and recruitment of the PFMs and abdominal muscles. This impairment includes incoordination of the PFM contraction, incoordination of the abdominal contraction, incoordination of the PFMs during ADLs, and incoordination of the PFMs with the abdominals.

Pelvic Floor Muscles

Coordination impairment of the PFMs is the inability of all of PFMs to contract and relax at the appropriate times. Manual evaluation of the PFMs and biofeedback training may

Patient-Related Instruction 18-5

Squeeze Before You Sneeze

Practice contracting the PFMs immediately before sneezing, coughing, laughing, lifting, or straining. This is similar to training yourself to bring your hand to your mouth before you sneeze. By voluntarily contracting the PFMs before increases in abdominal pressure, you will eventually create a habit, and the PFM will contract automatically.

reveal the patient's inability to create and hold a synchronous contraction. This problem is usually related to decreased awareness of the PFMs. In nonneurologic conditions, the patient can usually learn the correct sequencing and timing of contraction through some form of biofeedback (e.g., surface EMG; pressure; contracting around a finger, penis, or similar object).

Pelvic Floor Muscles During Activities of Daily Living

Coordination impairment of the PFMs during ADLs is observed in stress incontinence, with urine leaking during lifting, coughing, and sneezing. In some cases, leaking results from impaired performance of the PFMs. However, some patients have fairly good PFM strength but do not contract the PFMs at the proper time during the activity. All patients must learn to contract the PFMs before and during increased intra-abdominal pressure (e.g., cough, lift, sneeze) (see Patient-Related Instruction 18-5: Squeeze Before You Sneeze). One study showed that this type of training alone can decrease urine leakage up to 70%.[73,87] In addition, it is necessary to relax the PFM during activities such as micturition and defecation. Inability to relax during these activities may result in obstructed voiding and defecation in which the bowel and bladder are unable to empty completely (see Building Block 18-4). Inability to relax during intercourse may result in painful penetration (also know as dyspareunia).

Pelvic Floor Muscles with Abdominal Muscles

Needle EMG studies show that the abdominal muscles participate in a synergy with the PFMs.[76,77] The therapist should understand proper contraction of the PFMs with the abdominal muscles to correctly instruct the patient. An exercise to experience this can help the student to understand the relationship of the PFM and abdominal muscles. Start by sitting up tall in a chair and pouching the abdominal muscles outward. Keep the abdomen pouched out and contract the PFMs, notice the amount of effort needed and the force

BUILDING BLOCK 18-4

A 34-year-old tennis player is having stress urinary incontinence during the serving maneuver of her game. What might be the pathophysiology of this condition? What could you suggest she do to decrease her leakage?

TABLE 18-3 **Coordination of the PFM**

ACTIVITY	NORMAL PFM ACTION	NORMAL ABDOMINAL ACTION	DYSFUNCTIONAL PFM ACTION	RESULT OF DYSFUNCTIONAL ACTION
Lifting	Contraction	Inward contraction by obliques	Relaxation or weak contraction	Leaking urine
Bowel movement	Relaxation	Bulging contraction by rectus abdominis with Valsalva maneuver	Contraction	Difficulty passing feces, constipation, pain

generated by the PFMs. Next, sit up in the chair and pull the abdominals inward, supporting the abdominal contents and the back. While holding the abdominal contraction gently and contracting the PFMs, notice the effort needed and the force generated by the PFMs.

Most persons feel a stronger PFM contraction when the abdominals are pulled inward properly. This is especially evident in the presence of PFM weakness. The PFMs cannot contract effectively when the abdominals pouch out, while bearing down, or during a Valsalva maneuver. In PFM training, it is especially important not to bear down and bulge the abdominals outward with the PFM contraction.

Bearing down is associated with PFM relaxation during bowel movement. PFM contraction during defecation is an example of PFM coordination impairment. This results in difficulty passing feces and often causes constipation and pain, which may be diagnosed as obstructed defecation. The patient must learn how to relax the PFMs at the proper time in association with the proper abdominal contraction for defecation (Table 18-3).

Abdominal Muscles

Coordination impairment of the abdominal muscles results in an inability to pull the muscles inward. These impairments must be treated before considering PFM timing with the abdominals. See Chapter 17 for specific training techniques.

CLINICAL CLASSIFICATIONS OF PELVIC FLOOR MUSCLE DYSFUNCTION

PFM dysfunctions have two clinical classifications, which are used internationally by specialized physical therapists, nurses, and physicians.[4] Two additional classifications are presented for a complete view of pelvic physical therapy. Clinical classifications are intended to guide the therapist in treatment planning. However, the type and severity of physiologic impairments within the dysfunction vary, and treatments must be individualized. Each classification has a brief description of the syndrome and a discussion of the cause, common impairments, and activity limitations. There are many possible causes for these dysfunctions, which often result from a combination of pathologic conditions and comorbidities. In many cases, the primary cause is unknown. Therapists should have some understanding of the causes and comorbidities of the dysfunction they are treating, although it is not always necessary to pinpoint the cause for effective treatment. It is necessary to identify the correct impairment for effective treatment.

Much of the information on PFM dysfunctions is based on the clinical observations of gynecologic physical therapists around the country. Unfortunately, few studies have been performed on the physical therapy treatment of these patients. All four clinical classifications are presented to provide a complete view of the dysfunctions treated by physical therapists. The medical diagnoses associated with supportive and overactive PFMs are discussed later in this chapter.

There are two internationally accepted clinical classifications:

1. Underactive PFM
2. Overactive PFM

Other classifications are

3. Incoordination dysfunction
4. Visceral dysfunction

Underactive PFM

Underactive PFM results from the loss of strength and integrity of contractile tissues; this dysfunction is weakness and sagging of the PFMs. Common medical diagnoses often associated with underactive PFM are stress incontinence, mixed incontinence, and pelvic organ prolapse (see Patient-Related Instruction 18-6: Boat at the Dock—Role of PFMs in Organ Prolapse). The supportive role of the PFMs in continence was discussed earlier in this chapter.

Etiology and Comorbidities

Severe birth injury may result in anatomic impairments of the PFMs and nerves in the area. More commonly, the trauma of vaginal delivery results in moderate or mild muscle impairments. Altered muscle length or tension may occur with stretch during delivery. Stretching of connective tissue or muscle beyond its elastic capacity renders the tissue permanently long. The increased length of connective tissue means that the muscle must generate more force to accomplish the same function. Functional weakness and impaired muscle performance result. Hypertrophy of the remaining muscles often produces the desired effect of improved support of the PFMs.

Muscle atrophy can result from central and PNS dysfunction, including nerve damage from pelvic surgery. Temporary neurologic dysfunction, such as mild stretch to the pudendal nerve during delivery, often responds well to PFE. In conditions of mild or incomplete nerve damage, the remaining PFMs often become hypertrophied and produce good functional outcomes. One study reported 15% to 20%

Patient-Related Instruction 18-6

Boat at the Dock—Role of PFMs in Organ Prolapse

- Imagine there is a boat tied to a dock (A). The pelvic organs (i.e., bladder, uterus, and rectum) are the boat. The ropes holding the boat to the dock are the ligaments that support the organs from above. The water is the PFM.
- If the water level drops (B) (i.e., loss of support or weakness of the PFMs), the boat (organs) hangs on the ropes (ligaments). Eventually, the ropes stretch out and break, resulting in the boat (organs) falling down (i.e., prolapse).
- If you pull the boat back up by replacing the ropes (i.e., organ suspension surgery) without raising the water level (i.e., PFMs strengthening) (C), the boat will continue to hang on the ropes and eventually falls down again (i.e., prolapse). Falling happens quicker if you jump on the boat (i.e., increase pressure in the abdomen from cough, sneeze, lift, or improper exercise).
- Long-lasting results are more likely if you raise the water level (i.e., PFMs strengthening) and stop jumping on the boat (i.e., reduce unnecessary increases in abdominal pressure). In this case, the ropes (ligaments) may or may not need to be replaced (i.e., ligament and pelvic organ surgery).

Pelvic organs   Pelvic ligaments

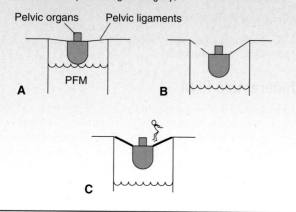

PFM

A   B

C

straining with Valsalva maneuvers and chronic or prolonged coughing or vomiting perpetuate incontinence and prolapse symptoms and slows recovery of PFM strength. These chronic increases in intra-abdominal pressure may initiate PFM impairment. Pregnancy and abdominal obesity increase intra-abdominal pressure. Obesity correlates with increased incontinence.[89–91]

Hormones released during pregnancy loosen the connective tissue of PFM tendons, which causes the muscles to sag. Because pregnancy is a temporary condition, most physicians and therapists are not concerned about symptoms of underactive PFM during pregnancy. However, 9 months of prolonged intra-abdominal pressure, especially with improper lifting at work, during exercise and ADLs, or in lifting another child, and prolonged, hormone-induced lengthening may result in significant postpartum supportive PFM dysfunction, even with a cesarean delivery.[92]

Common Impairments

The most common physiologic impairments of underactive PFM are impaired PFM performance, including PFM weakness, increased PFM length, increased connective tissue length, and muscle atrophy; endurance impairment of the PFMs; and impaired abdominal muscle performance, including weakness and increased length of the abdominals.

The less common physiologic impairments associated with underactive PFM should also be treated for full recovery. Coordination impairment of the PFMs during ADLs often exists to some degree in underactive PFMs; coordination impairments of the abdominal muscles also occur with underactive PFM. When the PFMs are fairly strong and incoordination is significant, the patient is given the diagnosis of incoordination dysfunction. Pain impairments of the PFMs may be a concurrent problem that may lead to pain-induced weakness. In this case, the origin of pain must be treated to reach maximum muscle strength. Joint mobility impairment of the lumbopelvic region may also affect the PFMs. A summary of impairments and suggested interventions for underactive PFM is provided in Display 18-9.

of patients undergoing radical pelvic surgery had permanent voiding dysfunctions.[88] Pelvic surgery may result in complex anatomic changes that affect PFM function.[89]

Many young children are taught not to touch or look at the perineum. In some cases, this early training results in adults with decreased awareness of the PFMs. Decreased awareness does not necessarily result in PFM weakness, but disuse atrophy may occur when decreased awareness is combined with other risk factors, such as menopause and bed rest. Decreased awareness of PFM contraction often exists concurrently with other impairments and makes rehabilitation more challenging. Many patients with severely decreased awareness can benefit from biofeedback instruction to identify the correct muscle contraction. The PFMs are used less when a Foley catheter is in place and while patients are on prolonged bed rest. These restrictions may result in disuse atrophy and impairment of PFM performance.

Prolonged increased intra-abdominal pressure may result in stretching of the PFMs or their tendons and may contribute to pelvic organ prolapse. Repeated, incorrect lifting or

---

DISPLAY 18-9

Summary of Impairments and Suggested Interventions for Underactive PFMs

- Impaired performance and endurance of the PFM: weakness, increased length, atrophy
  - PFE with facilitation, overflow, biofeedback or vaginal weights
  - Neuromuscular electrical stimulation (NMES)
- Coordination impairment of the PFM: decreased awareness of how to contract correctly
  - PFE with biofeedback and during ADLs
- Coordination and impaired performance of the abdominals
  - Therapeutic exercise for the abdominals
  - Proper contraction of abdominals with function
- Pain in PFM and mobility of pelvic joints
  - Soft tissue mobilization, scar mobilization
  - Joint mobilization, muscle energy techniques
  - Modalities such as heat, cold, ultrasound, and electrical stimulation

Activity Limitations

Patients may exhibit symptoms of stress incontinence, mixed incontinence, and organ prolapse. Loss of urine with coughing, sneezing, laughing, lifting, or exercising often requires the use of absorbent products (i.e., incontinence pads or diapers). Some patients limit or modify activities for fear of leaking urine.[93] Patients may avoid shopping trips, overnight vacations, outdoor activities, and sports because of incontinence. Urinary frequency is urination more than seven times in a 24-hour period, and urination sometimes occurs as often as every 30 to 40 minutes. Frequency in conjunction with urinary urgency may require modification of ADLs, because patients usually do not venture far from the toilet. Lack of PFM support may be painful and result in decreased ability to ambulate or exercise.

Overactive PFM

Overactive PFM is a complex category related to pain and spasm of the PFMs. Common medical diagnoses associated with overactive PFM include levator ani syndrome, pelvic floor tension myalgia, coccygodynia, vulvodynia, vestibulitis, vaginismus, animus, chronic pelvic pain, and dyspareunia. Overactive PFM may result from pelvic joint dysfunctions, hip muscle imbalance, and abdominopelvic adhesions and scars affecting the PFM function.

Etiology and Comorbidities

The cause of overactive PFMs is often more difficult to identify than the cause of other dysfunctions. Lumbopelvic joint mobility impairments or pathology is one of the most common impairments found in patients with overactive PFM. Injuries, such as a fall onto the coccyx or pubic ramus, are common for these patients. Lumbopelvic joint dysfunction may result from PFM dysfunction or may directly or indirectly cause PFM spasm. Tonic holding patterns and spasm may result from the proximity of muscles to traumatized pelvic joints.

Hip joint integrity and mobility, pain, and muscle performance impairments contribute to overactive PFM through its effect on the pelvic joints. Spasm of the associated muscles, particularly the obturator internus and piriformis, can directly irritate the PFMs, causing holding and spasm.

Abdominal or perineal adhesions and scars can cause overactive PFM. Pelvic organs must slide freely during physiologic functions such as peristalsis, bowel movement, or vaginal penetration during intercourse. Abdominal adhesions can restrict pelvic organ movement and cause pain and spasm of PFMs during bowel movement or intercourse. Severe adhesions of the uterosacral ligaments may restrict sacroiliac joint mobility. Adhesions may be a result of pelvic or abdominal surgery or an inflammatory condition of the abdomen, such as endometriosis. Perineal scars (often found in third- or fourth-degree episiotomies) can cause adhesions to the rectum and vaginal walls. These scars can be so painful that patients dread every bowel movement. Other painful conditions such as interstitial cystitis, endometriosis, fissures, and fistulas may also cause holding patterns in response to pain. Holding patterns of the PFMs may occur as a response to excessive generalized stress or reflect an emotional connection to the perineum.[94] Excessive holding of the PFMs because of pain or stress often leads to trigger points, ischemic changes, and tissue shortening.

Connective tissue diseases such as fibromyalgia are associated with overactive PFMs, particularly vulvodynia. Pelvic pain, as discussed earlier, may be a problem for sexually abused individuals. The exact connection is unknown, but emotional holding of the PFMs and physical trauma to the perineum may play a part in the eventual development of overactive PFM.

Common Impairments

There are many possible primary physiologic impairments in overactive PFM. Careful evaluation is necessary to determine the most significant impairments in each patient. The most common impairments of overactive PFM are altered tone of the PFMs, including spasm and trigger points; altered tone (e.g., trigger points, spasm) of associated muscles of the hip, buttock, and trunk; impaired muscle performance and coordination impairments of the hip, leading to muscle imbalance around the hip; joint mobility impairments of lumbopelvic joints, particularly the sacroiliac, pubic symphysis, and lower lumbar facet joints; mobility impairments of scar and connective tissue; and posture impairment, contributing to pelvic joint dysfunction. Pain impairment because of hypersensitivity of the perineal skin is common in vulvodynia, but it is not typical of other overactive PFMs. A summary of impairments and suggested interventions are provided in Display 18-10.

Activity Limitations

Overactive PFMs have activity limitations similar to other pelvic pain syndromes, such as low back and pelvic girdle pain. The ability to work (e.g., lift, sit, push, drive, and clean house), recreate, ambulate, sleep, and perform ADLs may be limited. Activity limitations unique to overactive PFM may result in a decreased ability or inability to sit because of severe perineal pain. Some patients cannot wear jeans or ride a bike. Routine Pap smears can be painful or impossible. The affected woman often has a decreased ability or an inability to have sexual intercourse or sexual contact of any kind.

Many women and men are embarrassed to talk to their doctors, family, and friends about pelvic, perineal, or genital pain. It is difficult to explain the reasons for activity limitations if you are unable to tell someone the location or the nature of the pain. This creates emotional stress. Chronic pelvic pain patients often suffer in silence for many years before they find a medical professional who is able to treat them effectively.

Incoordination Dysfunction

Incoordination dysfunction can be divided into neurologic and nonneurologic syndromes. Detrusor sphincter dyssynergia is a type of incoordination resulting from a neurologic lesion in the spinal cord between the brain stem and T10. The PFMs and smooth muscle internal sphincter contract during a bladder contraction so that urine is unable to be expelled. This condition should be monitored by a physician. Symptoms of neurologic incoordination are similar to the obstructed voiding symptoms listed in the screening evaluation questionnaire. The therapist should refer the patient to the physician if neurologic incoordination or obstructed voiding is suspected.

Incoordination dysfunction may be a minor dysfunction with underactive or overactive PFMs, or it may occur as the

DISPLAY 18-10
Summary of Impairments and Suggested Interventions for Overactive PFM

- Altered tone of the PFM: muscle spasm and trigger points
  - Biofeedback for training the PFM to relax
  - Rhythmic contract and relax of the PFM (quick PFE)
  - Soft tissue mobilization, vaginally or rectally
  - Electrical stimulation on the perineum, vaginally or rectally
  - Relaxation training, autonomic nervous system balancing
  - Vaginal or rectal dilators
  - Ultrasound at the insertion of the PFM at the coccyx
  - Heat or cold over the perineum
- Altered tone of the associated muscles of the hip, buttock, and trunk-muscle spasm
  - Soft tissue mobilization
  - Therapeutic exercises for stretching
  - Modalities such as ultrasound, electrical stimulation, heat, and cold
- Muscle impairments and coordination impairments of the associated muscles of the hip, buttocks, and trunk: muscle imbalances around the trunk and hip joint
  - Therapeutic exercises for strengthening and stretching
  - Coordination training of muscles around a joint (i.e., around the hip) or between several areas (hip and abdominals)
- Mobility impairment of scar and connective tissue of the perineum, inner thighs, buttocks, and abdominals
  - Soft tissue mobilization, scar mobilization
  - Visceral mobilization
  - Modalities such as ultrasound, heat, and microcurrent
- Mobility impairments (e.g., hypermobility, hypomobility) of pelvic joints: sacroiliac, pubic, lumbar, hip, and sacrococcygeal
  - Joint mobilization, muscle energy techniques, positional release, craniosacral therapy
  - Posture and body mechanics education
  - Therapeutic exercises for muscle imbalances
  - Modalities such as ultrasound, heat, cold, electrical stimulation, and TENS
- Faulty posture leading to undue stress on the pelvic structures
  - Instruction in proper sitting and standing posture and body mechanics
  - Use of cushions, lumbar rolls, and modified chairs
- Pain in the perineum with hypersensitivity of the skin and mucosa
  - Modalities such as cold, heat, ultrasound, and electrical stimulation
  - Education on avoiding perineal irritants

PFE, pelvic floor exercise; PFM, pelvic floor muscle; TENS, transcutaneous electrical nerve stimulation.

BUILDING BLOCK 18-5

You have been working with a 20-year-old female with LBP and poor trunk stability for 3 weeks. Her symptoms are somewhat better but she continues to have pain. You suspect she would benefit from PFM training. How can you measure her PFM ability? How would you explain to her why it is important to do these exercises?

this dysfunction. Decreased awareness may reflect an emotional condition or a social conditioning. Pain in the pelvic or abdominal area may disrupt recruitment patterns. Surgical intervention may result in inhibition of the muscles—the muscles forget what to do, when to do it, and how it should be done. Some patients have never been aware of the PFMs and have developed poor recruitment patterns.

Common Impairments of Nonneurologic Incoordination Dysfunctions

PFM weakness may be a minor impairment. Most of these patients are found to have good PFM strength on the MMT. Coordination impairment is the primary physiologic impairment. Coordination impairment of the PFMs was discussed previously in the "Coordination Impairment" section.

Activity Limitations of Nonneurologic Dysfunctions

The most common activity limitation of incoordination dysfunction is stress incontinence with urine leaking during increased intra-abdominal pressure, such as during coughing, sneezing, or lifting. Patients also may have obstructed defecation with constipation and rectal pain (see Building Block 18-5).

Visceral Dysfunction

Visceral dysfunction is a pseudo-PFM dysfunction. It is a disease or abnormality in mobility or motility of the abdominopelvic visceral tissues that leads to pain and musculoskeletal impairments. Detrusor instability, often found in patients with urge incontinence, is the most widely seen visceral dysfunction directly related to the PFMs. It is characterized by irritated detrusor contractions and is often related to PFM impairments. Urge incontinence responds well to underactive PFM treatments. The causes, impairments, and treatment of urge incontinence are discussed later in Therapeutic Exercise Intervention for Common Diagnoses.

Etiology and Comorbidities

Visceral dysfunction encompasses several medical diagnoses: urge incontinence, endometriosis, pelvic inflammatory disease, dysmenorrhea, surgical scars, irritable bowel syndrome, and interstitial cystitis. These conditions may result in impairments whose primary origin is abdominopelvic pain or adhesions caused by organ disease. Knowledge of the causes and medical management of these diseases are necessary to treat the resulting impairments. A multidisciplinary approach is optimal when dealing with visceral dysfunction. Treatment of comorbid musculoskeletal impairments often results in decreased pain and increased function.

primary dysfunction. Nonneurologic incoordination dysfunction is characterized by absent or inappropriate patterns of timing and recruitment of the PFMs. Common medical diagnoses associated with incoordination dysfunction include stress incontinence, constipation with obstructed defecation, and pelvic pain.

Etiology and Comorbidities of Nonneurologic Incoordination Dysfunctions

The cause of pure nonneurologic incoordination dysfunction is often related to disuse and decreased awareness of the PFMs and abdominals. Muscle atrophy is not significant in

Common Impairments

Weakness of the abdominal muscles, especially the oblique and transversus layers, may occur in response to pain in the abdomen, causing a pendulous abdomen with poor visceral and lumbar support. Secondary lumbopelvic joint mobility impairment and posture impairments may result. Altered tone (e.g., spasm) or impaired muscle performance (e.g., weakness) of the PFMs may also occur as a result of pain in the lower pelvic organs. Chronic pelvic pain postures often occur with long-standing abdominopelvic pain.[95] These postures result in posture impairment; mobility impairments of pelvic and lumbar joints; altered tone, pain, and trigger points in trunk and lower extremity muscles; and impaired performance of the hip muscles with length and tension changes. Abdominal adhesions and scar mobility restrictions may result in decreased mobility or motility of abdominal and pelvic organs and pelvic joints. When organ mobility is restricted, cramping, pain, and altered organ function may result. For example, abdominal adhesions may form around parts of the bowel, constricting the bowel lumen and making passage of feces painful.

Mobility impairments play a major role in visceral dysfunctions. Visceral mobilization techniques are used by physical therapists to restore normal mobility of organs.

Activity Limitations

Activity limitations vary greatly in cases of visceral dysfunction. In the case of dysmenorrhea (i.e., painful menstruation), patients may have 2 to 3 days each month of intense abdominal pain that confines them to bed. Other conditions result in constant abdominopelvic pain and cause activity limitations such as those of patients with trunk or back pain, who have a decreased ability to work, sit, walk, lift, have intercourse, play sports, exercise, or perform ADLs. Activity limitations may be directly related to organ dysfunction. For example, interstitial cystitis causes the person to urinate as often as every 15 minutes. Irritable bowel syndrome may result in alternating diarrhea and constipation, with many patients experiencing abdominal pain and bloating. These functions are unpredictable and often force patients to remain near the toilet for fear of severe cramping or incontinence of feces.

THERAPEUTIC EXERCISE INTERVENTIONS FOR COMMON DIAGNOSES

This section describes the most common medical diagnoses for the pelvic floor region and suggests physical therapy interventions. The diagnostic classifications group impairments of body functions into common syndromes. The medical community uses a different classification system, and physical therapists should be aware of the medical classifications, testing, and medical treatment of these conditions to enhance their ability to provide effective physical therapy intervention.

The associated medical diagnoses discussed here are commonly associated with underactive and overactive PFMs. Medical diagnoses associated with underactive PFM usually fall into two categories—incontinence and organ prolapse. Both can be extremely complex conditions with many associated impairments and comorbidities. Some conditions associated with underactive PFMs are impairments of body structures and cannot be changed with physical therapy intervention.

The most common medical diagnoses associated with overactive PFM include chronic pelvic pain, levator ani syndrome, coccygodynia, vulvodynia, vaginismus, anismus, and dyspareunia. The most common impairments of body functions for each diagnosis are discussed with the diagnosis. Any impairment may be significant, and failure to address all significant impairments may limit the patient's progress. Any and all combinations of impairments listed for overactive PFM can be associated with these diagnoses. Each patient should be evaluated thoroughly, impairments identified, and treatment plans developed based on the severity and significance of each impairment.

Incontinence

Incontinence is defined as the complaint of any involuntary leakage of urine, feces, or gas.[96] More than 13,000,000 persons in the United States have urinary incontinence. This figure includes approximately 50% of nursing home patients. Several large studies have found overall urinary incontinence prevalence of 13% to 25%.[1,52] Careful evaluation of these patients often reveals PFM weakness and treatable comorbidities. Approximately 80% of these incontinent patients can be significantly helped with noninvasive behavioral techniques used by physical therapists, occupational therapists, and registered nurses.[64]

Incontinence can be a limiting condition. It may occur during sports activities and cause embarrassment.[97] Nygaard[93] conducted a questionnaire study of women who exercised. She found that 47% had incontinence during exercise. Twenty percent of those women modified their exercise routines solely because of incontinence. Some women even stop exercising because of incontinence. This disruption in exercise ability may have a significant effect on physical therapy for other areas of the body. The therapist may encounter poor compliance with exercises that cause incontinence. The instructions included in this chapter may be enough to correct or minimize symptoms so that the patient can return to active exercises.

Incontinence also may limit elderly persons' activity levels. In some cases, incontinence causes embarrassment and may result in seclusion from social activities, family functions, and work.[98] PFM strengthening can help these patients return to an active lifestyle without fear of embarrassing leakage.[99] Incontinence also may result in secondary conditions such as skin breakdown, which can be a serious medical consequence for the elderly patient. All physical therapy patients should be questioned about leakage, and, if appropriate, instructions should be given to help remedy the situation. Women with urge UI and nocturia are three times more likely to fall.[100-101]

Understanding the most common types of incontinence assists therapists in developing treatment plans. Physicians broadly categorize bladder dysfunctions as the failure to store urine and the failure to empty urine. Stress, urge, and mixed incontinence are examples of a failure to store urine. Overflow incontinence is the failure to empty urine. The full screening questionnaire provided earlier helps to identify the type of incontinence. Stress and mixed incontinence are the two types directly related to underactive PFMs. Urge incontinence is a visceral dysfunction. Overflow and functional incontinence are usually not related to underactive PFM of the PFMs (see Table 18-4). The pathophysiology

TABLE 18-4 **Types of Incontinences, Symptoms, Diagnosis Classification, and Possible Treatments**

TYPES OF INCONTINENCES	SYMPTOMS	DIAGNOSIS CLASSIFICATION	POSSIBLE TREATMENT
Stress incontinence	Small urine leak with cough, sneeze, exercise	Underactive PFM, PFM weakness	PFEs, biofeedback, vaginal cones, electrical stimulation
Urge incontinence	Moderate or large urine leaks with strong urge to urinate	Visceral dysfunction, may have PFM weakness also	Bladder training, PFEs if needed, biofeedback, electrical stimulation
Mixed incontinence	Symptoms of stress and urge incontinence	Underactive PFM, PFM weakness, visceral dysfunction	Bladder training, PFE biofeedback vaginal cones, electrical stimulation
Overflow incontinence	Small amounts of urine leaking constantly with cough and sneeze, straining to start urination, feeling of incomplete emptying	Possible incoordination dysfunction (PFM contraction during urination), visceral dysfunction (atonic bladder), overactive PFM (PFM spasm or pain)	Medical evaluation may be needed, advanced PFM rehabilitation with biofeedback, electrical stimulation, MFR, PFE, bladder training
Functional incontinence	Long or difficult trip to the toilet with leaking on the way	Mobility impairment of decreased ambulation ability, poor transfer ability, decreased finger coordination	Gait training, strengthening exercises for lower and upper extremities, environmental modifications

MFR, myofascial release; PFEs, pelvic floor exercises; PFM, pelvic floor muscle.

of incontinence is complex. Recent research into this complexity is beyond the scope of this chapter. A simplified explanation of incontinence is provided here and should give the beginner practitioner a good basis for general clinical assessments.

Stress Incontinence

Stress incontinence is defined as involuntary leaking of urine on effort or exertion such as during coughing, laughing, sneezing, and lifting.[96] Continence is maintained when the pressure in the urethra is higher than the pressure in the bladder. Strong PFMs help to increase the pressure in the urethra.[103] The perineal membrane and the sphincter urethrae muscles play a large role in the closure of the urethra (see Fig. 18-4).

In stress incontinence, the patient coughs, and pressure in the abdominal cavity is increased, pressing down on the bladder. If urethral pressure is low (usually because the PFMs are not strong enough), the urethra is forced open slightly, and a small amount of urine leaks out (Fig. 18-11).

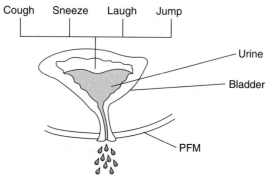

FIGURE 18-11. Stress incontinence.

The causes of stress incontinence are similar to the causes of underactive PFM. Impairments of body functions include impaired PFM performance, shortened endurance, and coordination impairments. The treatment for pure stress incontinence includes PFM exercises, vaginal weights, and electrical stimulation.[70,71]

Urge Incontinence

Urge incontinence is defined as leaking urine associated with a strong urge to urinate.[96] The normal urge to urinate is a result of activation of stretch receptors in the detrusor muscle. During this urge, the detrusor remains stable and does not contract. In some patients, a very strong urge to urinate is associated with inappropriate detrusor contractions. Unstable detrusor contractions are contractions of the bladder muscle at incorrect times (e.g., when not positioned over the toilet to void). Strong, unstable detrusor contractions, as seen in overactive bladder or detrusor instability, increase bladder pressure and may result in incontinence. The volume of urine leaked is usually larger than that with stress incontinence and may include the entire contents of the bladder. In some cases, urge incontinence may occur without unstable detrusor contractions (i.e., sensory urgency).

The underlying cause of urge incontinence is often unclear and may include PNS or CNS nerve damage. It is suspected that poor bladder habits (especially going to the bathroom too frequently) and bladder irritants (such as caffeine, nicotine, and alcohol) contribute to the condition. PFM weakness with impaired muscle performance and endurance impairment is often found in patients with urge incontinence. Coordination impairment of the PFMs during detrusor contraction may also be present. In this situation, the PFMs do not contract in response to the urge to urinate, and a small increase in bladder pressure may cause urine leakage. Primary treatment for urge incontinence can include bladder retraining, avoiding

BUILDING BLOCK 18-6

Your new patient is a 75-year-old male with Parkinson disease and difficulty walking. He is currently using a walker in the house and has poor balance. During an intake interview with your new patient, he admits that he has some urine leakage and gets up three to four times during the night. Discuss why nocturnal urination is of concern in this patient. List four ideas to address this concern.

---

bladder irritants, PFE, low-frequency electrical stimulation, and medications.

Mixed Incontinence

Mixed incontinence is a combination of stress and urge incontinence symptoms and is thought to be a progression of incontinence symptoms over time. These patients report leaking urine with increases in intra-abdominal pressure and with a strong urge to urinate. The causes of mixed incontinence are similar to the causes of underactive PFMs. The PFMs are usually weak. Treatment of this condition is similar to the treatment for urge incontinence: bladder training, avoiding bladder irritants, PFM exercises, electrical stimulation, vaginal weights, and, in some cases, medications.

Overflow Incontinence

Overflow incontinence results from a failure to empty the bladder fully. Obstruction of the urethra by tumor, scar tissue around the urethra, an enlarged prostate, overactive PFM, or other mechanical blockage may prevent the bladder from emptying. Decreased contractility of the bladder from a neurologic deficit, such as peripheral nerve injury associated with radical pelvic surgery, cauda equina injury, or diabetes, also may contribute to overflow incontinence.

In overflow incontinence, the bladder does not empty fully, and high volumes of urine are maintained in the bladder. When the bladder pressure is higher than the urethral pressure, small amounts of urine "spill out." This small but constant leaking may or may not be related to increased intra-abdominal pressure and is characteristic of overflow incontinence. Physical therapy impairments may include pain and altered tone from spasm of the PFMs. Mobility impairment may be caused by adhered scars. Many cases involve neurologic incoordination of the PFMs or primary visceral dysfunction and require medical intervention. A full medical evaluation is essential. Therapists should refer the patient to the doctor if overflow incontinence is suspected. Physical therapy treatment by pelvic floor specialists may include biofeedback, electrical stimulation, myofascial release, PFEs, and bladder training (see Building Block 18-6).

Functional Incontinence

Functional incontinence is defined as the loss of urine because of gait and locomotion impairment. Incontinence is a secondary condition in pure functional incontinence; the primary impairment is a gait and locomotion impairment—an inability to get to the toilet quickly enough. It is not unusual for an elderly or disabled patient to require 5 to 10 minutes to rise

DISPLAY 18-11
Helping Patients with Functional Incontinence

- Improve the speed of the sit-to-stand transfers by raising the height of the chair, providing a chair with arms, improving shoulder depression and elbow extension strength, and improving lower extremity strength in the quadriceps and gluteals.
- Improve the speed of ambulation to the bathroom by providing appropriate assistive devices, clearing obstacles from the pathway to the toilet, bringing the patient's chair closer to the toilet (e.g., move the sitting room to the side of the house nearest the toilet) or bringing the toilet closer to the patient (e.g., place a commode or urinal near the bed or sitting room), and improving balance and coordination, strength, and endurance of the lower extremities.
- Improve the speed of ambulation in the bathroom by clearing obstacles (especially rugs) and providing grab bars for ambulation without assistive devices if the bathroom is too small for the device to fit easily.
- Improve speed of lowering clothes by providing patient with Velcro-open pants, suggesting that women wear skirts and dresses, and improving finger coordination and dexterity to manage buttons and zipper more quickly.
- Improve stand-to-sit transfer onto the toilet by providing a raised toilet seat and handrails and by improving lower extremity function.
- Consider impairments of mental function in a patient's ability to recognize the bathroom. It may be helpful to place a picture of a toilet on or near the door or to leave the door open. In severe cases, even when patients are brought to the toilet, they may still not understand what to do.
- Absorbent garments (i.e., diapers and pads) are available for men and women in a variety of sizes. Helping patients and caregivers to choose appropriate garments may allow increased participation in work, social, and recreational activities. Always make sure that the physician has been informed of the patient's incontinence and that conservative treatments have been tried.

---

from a chair, ambulate with a walker to the toilet, maneuver in front of the toilet, lower his or her clothes, and sit down. Elderly patients often have less ability to store urine because of PFM weakness and less ability to defer the urge to urinate than younger persons. The mobility-impaired patient may leak urine on the long journey to the toilet. Patients may also have PFM dysfunction or impairments of body structures. However, treatment of gait and locomotion impairments and adjustments to the environment can improve function, and physical therapists are well suited to help these patients. Some ideas for helping these patients are detailed in Display 18-11.

Pelvic Organ Prolapse

Pelvic organ prolapse is the second largest category of medical diagnosis associated with underactive PFMs. The cause of prolapse may be complex and is often associated with underactive PFM and prolonged increases in intra-abdominal pressure. A simple explanation of prolapse and PFM function is presented in the Patient-Related Instruction 18-6. The most common types of organ prolapses (Fig. 18-12) are cystocele (i.e., protrusion of the bladder into the anterior

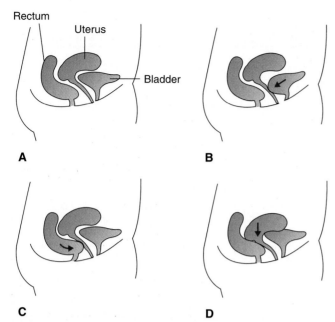

FIGURE 18-12. Common types of organ prolapses. (A) Normal organ positions. (B) Cystocele. (C) Rectocele. (D) Uterine prolapse.

vaginal vault), uterine prolapse (i.e., displacement of the uterus into the vaginal canal), and rectocele (i.e., protrusion of the rectum into the posterior vaginal vault).

Common symptoms include a sensation of organs "falling out," feelings of pain or pressure in the perineum[96] that may limit functional activities in standing, feeling that there is something bulging in the vagina, sensations of sitting on a ball, difficulty defecating (i.e., rectocele), difficulty urinating (i.e., cystocele), or painful intercourse (i.e., uterine prolapse). All patients should learn how to protect the PFMs from undue stress. However, it is essential that patients with pelvic organ prolapse learn how to avoid increased intra-abdominal pressure. Physical therapy treatment involves educating patients on decreasing intra-abdominal pressure (see Patient-Related Instruction 18-7: Decreasing Intra-abdominal Pressure) and PFM exercises.

Chronic Pelvic Pain

Chronic pelvic pain is the most widely seen diagnosis associated with overactive PFM. It is analogous to the diagnosis of low back pain—it does not give specific information about what type of impairment may be present. The most common impairments are altered tone and performance impairments of the associated muscles of the trunk and hips, poor posture, and mobility impairments of the pelvic and lumbar joints. Therapists should remember the roll of the PFMs in sacroiliac dysfunctions. All patients with chronic pelvic pain should be screened for PFM dysfunction, evaluated, and treated if needed (see Building Block 18-7).

Levator Ani Syndrome

Levator ani syndrome is another diagnosis that may be used universally for patients with vaginal or rectal pain. Patients report pain in the coccyx, sacrum, or thigh. Levator ani syndrome refers to spasm and trigger points in the pelvic

---

Patient-Related Instruction 18-7

Decreasing Intra-abdominal Pressure

- Avoid constipation, and do not strain with defecation (i.e., bowel movement). Drink lots of fluids to help avoid constipation and soften stools. Consult with a dietitian or physician about dietary changes and medications to avoid constipation.
- If you have difficulty getting out of the chair, scoot to the edge of the chair, lean forward, and push up with the arms. Avoid bearing down and breath holding. Instead, contract the abdominals inwardly, breathe out, and contract the PFMs while you stand up.
- Lift properly with inward contraction of abdominals and outward breath on effort. Avoid bulging the abdominals outward and bearing down.
- Exercise correctly using an inward abdominal contraction. Avoid bearing down and pouching the abdominal muscles outward. Unnecessary increases in intra-abdominal pressure may occur while lifting weights that are too heavy and with abdominal exercises that are too advanced. Curl-ups or sit-ups commonly cause the abdominals to bulge. Avoid curl-ups if you have organ prolapse. You should advance to weight lifting, advanced abdominal exercises, and jogging slowly and carefully if you have PFM weakness.
- If you are a postpartum woman, it is especially important to restore adequate PFM strength before returning to high-impact aerobics, jogging, and advanced weight lifting. The jumping jack test (see Patient-Related Instruction 18-2: Testing Your Pelvic Floor Muscle by Performing the Digital Vaginal Self-Examination) can be used to determine the ability of the PFM to withstand stress. It is important to continue active rehabilitation of the PFM during your return to vigorous exercise. If incontinence persists or worsens, you may have to delay the return to vigorous exercises until more strength of the PFM is gained.
- It is important to seek medical treatment for chronic coughing or vomiting and to contract the PFM during coughing or vomiting. You can counterbrace the PFM by contracting during coughing and vomiting. Support the perineal tissue with gentle upward pressure of the hand over the perineum during coughing and vomiting spells.

---

diaphragm layer of the PFMs. Patients often report pain with defecation and increased pain with sitting. Some patients say they feel like they are "sitting on a ball" (this can also be a symptom of organ prolapse).

BUILDING BLOCK 18-7

Your new patient is a 45-year-old female with primary complaint of left buttocks and posterior leg pain. List five risk factors for overactive PFM that might be present in this patient. What finding would lead you to consider a PFM dysfunction and how would you address it?

Pelvic floor tension myalgia is pain in the PFMs, which is usually associated with spasm or chronic tension. This diagnosis is similar to levator ani syndrome, and many practitioners use the two names interchangeably.

Coccygodynia

Coccygodynia indicates pain at the coccyx bone. Pain at the coccyx is usually not related to the sacrococcygeal joint. More often, it is related to trigger points of the PFMs, obturator internus, gluteus maximus, or piriformis. Patients often have sacroiliac joint mobility impairments and less frequently have sacrococcygeal joint mobility impairments. Coccygodynia is a common sequel of falls directly on the buttocks. Patients report pain with sit-to-stand transfers, possibly because of gluteal muscle contraction or sacroiliac dysfunction. Coccygodynia patients have pain that limits sitting.

The most common impairments associated with levator ani, tension myalgia, and coccygodynia include altered tone of the PFMs and associated muscles; mobility impairments of scars, connective tissues, and pelvic joints; and faulty posture, especially in sitting. All patients with this diagnosis must learn to sit with their weight balanced on the ischial tuberosities and not on the tail bone (see Patient-Related Instruction 18-4). Some patients need to use a special cushion to relieve pressure on the coccyx. The most effective cushion is a seat wedge approximately 2.5 in tall with a small cutout in the posterior aspect (Fig. 18-13). A typical donut-shaped cushion places direct pressure on the coccyx and is therefore not recommended.

Vulvodynia

Vulvodynia is a broad diagnosis of pain in the external genitalia, perineum, and vestibule. It can be a severe, often idiopathic condition that may or may not be associated with PFM dysfunctions. It is categorized as localized (involving only one area) or generalized (symptoms in many areas of the perineum). It is also categorized as provoked (only occurring with palpation or penetration) or unprovoked (pain is present at all times even without contact).[104] Patients report stabbing pain in the vagina and less commonly the rectum. Many patients are completely unable to have vaginal penetration of any kind (e.g., intercourse, speculum evaluation, tampon insertion). Symptoms are increased with sitting and by wearing tight pants.

The causes of vulvodynia are complex and can include overactive PFM, environmental irritants or reactions, alteration in the vaginal mucosal properties and nerve inputs in the area, or a complication of pelvic surgery. Infection by bacterial and viral organisms (i.e., yeast infections are common) commonly precede the onset of vulvodynia but their relationship to the condition is not understood.[105] Vulvodynia is a difficult condition to treat. A multidisciplinary approach is best. All impairments should be considered, especially mobility impairments of the pelvic and lumbar joints, mobility impairments of scars, and altered tone of the PFMs and associated muscles. These patients need special instructions in avoiding perineal irritants (see Patient-Related Instruction 18-8: Avoiding Perineal Irritants) and may benefit from pain-reducing modalities such as transcutaneous electrical nerve stimulation at the sacral nerve roots.

Vaginismus

Vaginismus is defined as a spasm of muscle around the vagina, the superficial muscle layer, or pelvic diaphragm layer. Patients report symptoms similar to those of vulvodynia,

Patient-Related Instruction 18-8

Avoiding Perineal Irritants

Avoid unnecessary irritation to the vaginal tissue to encourage healing of the area. The vaginal tissue is like the tissue in your mouth. It needs to stay moist and should not be vigorously cleaned with harsh soaps. Here are some suggestions to decrease the irritation of the vaginal tissue:

Clothing
Avoid tight clothes, especially jeans and pantyhose. It is also helpful to avoid bike riding, because pressure and rubbing on the perineum can increase irritations.
Wear 100% cotton white underpants that are washed separately in hot water with a mild detergent; avoid bleach and fabric softeners.

Hygiene
Use white, unscented toilet tissue and pat dry after urination. Some women spray the vaginal area with a fine mist of plain water then pat dry.
Wash the vaginal area gently with mild soap (i.e., natural glycerin-based soaps without deodorants or fragrances).
Do not douche unless it is suggested by your doctor.
Avoid dripping shampoo or other soaps on the vaginal area while in the shower.
Soak in the tub with clear water—no bubble bath, bath beads, or other fragrance additives. Do not wash yourself in the tub; wash in the shower.

Menstruation
Avoid tampons if possible.
Avoid pads with fragrances. Consider trying cotton washable menstrual pads.
Do not douche, unless suggested by your doctor.

Medications
Speak to your doctor before using any prescription or over-the-counter cream on the perineum. Many creams can be irritating and make the situation worse.
Do not self-medicate for yeast infections.
Some contraceptive creams or jellies and lubricants can irritate. Speak to your doctor about an appropriate contraceptive method. Pure vegetable oil can be used as a vaginal lubricant without irritation by many women.

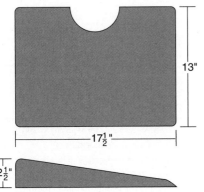

FIGURE 18-13. Coccygodynia seat cushion.

although to a lesser degree. Dyspareunia (i.e., painful intercourse) is a common symptom of vaginismus. Muscle spasms may be a secondary impairment in response to a medical condition, such as atrophic vaginismus or fistula (i.e., a small opening in the skin similar to a small cut at the corner of the mouth). Primary dyspareunia may occur with vaginismus as a result of fear of penetration.

Nonrelaxing Puborectalis Syndrome

Nonrelaxing puborectalis syndrome or anismus is a spasm of the anal sphincters. It is similar to vaginismus in that it may be a secondary impairment caused by trauma, fissure, fistula, or hemorrhoids at the anal opening. Patients report severe pain with defecation, which often leads to constipation because patients delay defecation. Other PFMs may or may not spasm.

Dyspareunia

Dyspareunia is the symptom of painful penetration and can be associated with all of the diagnoses previously described. It can be divided into two categories: pain at initial penetration or pain with deep penetration. Pain with initial penetration may be caused by superficial muscle spasm (i.e., vaginismus), skin irritation (i.e., vulvodynia), or adhered, painful episiotomy. Deep penetration dyspareunia may be related to spasm of the PFMs (e.g., levator ani syndrome, tension myalgia) or organ prolapse with visceral adhesions. The most common impairments found in vaginismus, anismus, and dyspareunia are altered tone of the PFMs and associated muscles and mobility impairment of scars and connective tissue.

ADJUNCTIVE INTERVENTIONS

Many patient-related instructions have been included throughout this chapter. Education is essential for this patient population. When was the last time someone talked with you about how to urinate? Take time and make sure your patients understand anatomy and good bladder health, because they are often too embarrassed to admit that they do not know.

Physical therapy for the PFMs applies the same principles of treatment used for other weak and painful muscles. Therapeutic exercise principles are the same, and modalities are used for the same reasons. This section lists the modalities used in underactive and overactive PFMs. Several techniques are explored in more detail to enhance the therapist's ability to treat PFM impairments.

The skilled practitioner can employ various modalities and techniques to enhance the effect of active PFE for the treatment of underactive PFMs, including the diagnosis of incontinence. Modalities and techniques are chosen based on the patient's degree of muscle weakness. For a manual muscle grade of 0 to 2, the practitioner can include the following modalities or techniques:

- Facilitation with muscle tapping of the PFMs
- Overflow exercises of the buttocks, adductors, and lower abdominals
- Biofeedback with pressure or a surface EMG device
- Electrical stimulation
- Bladder training
- Coordination of PFMs during ADLs

For manual muscle grade of 3 to 5, the practitioner can include weighted cones inserted into the vagina and PFEs in more stressful activities, such as weight lifting. These patients continue to benefit from bladder training and biofeedback but should be weaned away from facilitation, overflow, and electrical stimulation.

Many other interventions are used in conjunction with exercises for the treatment of overactive PFMs (see Display 18-10). Interventions used for muscle spasms in other areas of the body can be used with PFM spasms as well. Later sections describe perineal scar mobilization and a method for externally palpating the PFMs.

Biofeedback

It is necessary to give all patients some form of feedback, whether it is with the finger in the vagina, a mirror, or biofeedback machines during PFEs. Some practitioners use biofeedback machine evaluation and treatment with all PFM dysfunction patients. Surface EMG and pressure biofeedback are two methods of machine biofeedback. This type of biofeedback is especially helpful if the patient has decreased sensation or decreased motivation.

Pressure biofeedback involves an air chamber connected to a manometer, which records pressure changes. The air chamber is inserted into the vagina, and the patient contracts the PFMs around it. The PFM contraction creates an increase in pressure in the vagina that is recorded and displayed for the patient and therapist. Some pressure devices collect specific data on pressure changes; others are used only for immediate feedback to the patient. Therapists must be careful to instruct PFE correctly, because bearing down increases pressure and may be misinterpreted as proper PFM contractions.

Surface EMG can provide even more information about the muscle contraction, patterns of recruitment, and resting tone. It is a powerful tool in treating PFM dysfunction.[106] An internal vaginal or rectal probe or surface electrodes are used to pick up the electrical muscle activity of the PFMs so that it can be displayed. Stand-alone surface EMG units provide feedback in the form of a bar graph or line of lights. This gives information about one part of the contraction at a time. The units are helpful for home training. Computer-assisted surface EMG units can show the electrical muscle activity of the entire PFM contraction or several contractions in a row on one screen (Fig. 18-14). This allows the therapist to

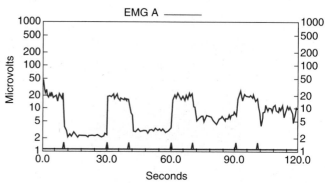

FIGURE 18-14. Print out of computer-assisted surface electromyographic treatment showing elevating baseline. (From Shelly B, Herman H, Jenkins T. Methodology for Evaluation and Treatment of Pelvic Floor Dysfunction. Dover, NH: The Prometheus Group, 1994.)

Column # Directions

  1 Urination in toilet: check, measure, or count # of seconds.
  2 Make a check if a urine leak occurs, note small or large.
  3 Note the reason for the accident (jump, sneeze, lift, water, urge).
  4 Note type and amount of fluid intake.

Fill in the day and date at the top of each column.

Name_____   Acct.#_____

DAY												
	toilet	leak	reason	fluid	toilet	leak	reason	fluid	toilet	leak	reason	fluid
6 am												
7 am												
8 am												
9 am												
10am												
11am												
12am												
1pm												
2pm												
3pm												
4pm												
5pm												
6pm												
7pm												
8pm												
9pm												
10pm												
11pm												
12pm												
1am												
2am												
3am												
4am												
5am												
TOTAL												
# of pads												

Stop Test Results_____   **Patient's Signature**_____

Type of pad used_____

FIGURE 18-15. Bladder diary.

TABLE 18-5 Features Determined from a Bladder Diary	
MEASURE	**PURPOSE**
Average voiding interval	Determine bladder schedule
Frequency of voids in 24 hours	Bladder habits and outcome data
Nocturnal voiding frequency	Bladder habits and outcome data
Number of incontinence episodes in 24 hours	Outcome data
Cause of accidents	Stress or urge symptoms
Total fluid intake	Counsel on normal fluid intake
Number of bladder irritants per day	Counsel on decreasing bladder irritants

Abrams P, Cardozo L, Fall M, et al. The standardization of terminology of lower urinary tract function: report from the standardization sub-committee of the International Continence Society. Am J Obstet Gynecol 2002;21:167–178.

compare recruitment at different times in the contraction. Surface EMG is the ideal method of feedback in down training (i.e., relaxation training) for patients with overactive PFM. Biofeedback therapy for patients with stress, urge, or mixed incontinence is given an A rating by the Agency for Health Care Policy and Research guidelines on the management of urinary incontinence.[64] This means that properly designed research studies support the effectiveness of biofeedback for the treatment of these patients.

Basic Bladder Training

Bladder training is scheduled voiding to regain normal voiding patterns. It is used in cases of urgency, frequency, urge incontinence, or mixed incontinence. Have the patient record the time of day he or she urinates in the toilet, the time of urine leakage (i.e., incontinence), and why urine leaked (e.g., cough, sneeze, lift). It is also helpful for the patient to record the amount and type of fluid intake. Information should be collected for 3 to 6 days. This type of record is called a bladder diary (see Fig. 18-15). Bladder diaries can be simple or complex. The purpose of the simple bladder diary is to determine the features shown in Table 18-5.

The cause of the accidents helps identify the type of incontinence. Total fluid intake and the number of bladder irritants can be used to counsel patients on appropriate fluid intake. Bladder irritants must be limited for successful treatment of urge incontinence. However, limiting overall fluid intake does not decrease incontinence either.[107] Patients should be encouraged to drink 6 to 8 cups of fluid per day.

The average voiding interval (i.e., average time between urinations) is the most important piece of information gained from the bladder diary for bladder retraining. Ask the patient to urinate in the toilet at the average voiding interval you determined from the bladder diary, whether they need to urinate or not. For example, if the average voiding interval was 1 hour, ask the patient to void in the toilet every 60 minutes—no sooner and no later. The bladder eventually becomes accustomed to the schedule, and urgency decreases. Most patients can increase the voiding interval by 0.5 hour every week. Do not increase the voiding interval if incontinence or urgency is worse or unchanged. Patients do not follow the bladder training schedule at night. Nocturnal voiding gradually improves as the daytime voiding interval increases. The goal is a voiding interval of 2 to 5 hours, with seven or fewer voids per day.

Urge deferment is taught to allow patients to maintain the voiding interval. If the urge arrives before the prescribed voiding interval, patients are encouraged to use the techniques in the Patient-Related Instruction 18-9: Urge Deferment. Patients need to practice several different techniques to find the most effective technique for them. After the urge has passed, patients should try to wait until the correct time to urinate. Patients unable to complete a bladder diary have been shown to have less success with behavioral therapy for urinary incontinence.[70]

Scar Mobilization

Adhesion of perineal scars can cause pain with intercourse (i.e., dyspareunia), pain with bowel movement, and weakness or spasm of the PFMs. The goal of scar mobilization is to lengthen connective tissue and scar adhesions, allowing fascial layers to slide easily over one another. Complete scar

Patient-Related Instruction 18-9

Urge Deferment

- Sit down; pressure on the perineum helps calm the bladder.
- Relax and breathe; nervousness and anxiety contribute to urgency.
- Small PFM contractions help to reflexively relax the bladder.
- Keep the mind busy; attend to a task involving a lot of attention. Tell yourself you cannot stop to go to the bathroom, count backwards, or pretend you are in the car and there is no bathroom available.
- Practice mind over matter; the mind has great influence over the bladder. For example, you are on a 2- or 3-hour car ride, and you feel the urge to urinate. If you say to your bladder, "Not now; calm down; I'll go later," the urge goes away. The bladder may become conditioned to produce the sensation of urgency and bladder contractions with certain activities (e.g., before leaving home, before a speech, walking past the bathroom, arriving home, while unlocking the door). It is important to break these habits and establish control over the bladder. (Rather than the bladder controlling your actions.)

Patient-Related Instruction 18-10

Self-Mobilization of Scar Tissue

- Wash your hands thoroughly before beginning
- Choose one of the following positions:
  - Lying on the bed with pillows to prop the head up
  - Sidelying on the bed
  - In the tub
- Use your index finger to reach around from the back while sidelying, or use your thumb to reach the vagina from the front.
- Apply firm, downward pressure on the scar, usually located on the posterior vaginal wall. This probably feels uncomfortable but should not be extremely painful. Constantly holding pressure results in softening of tissue, similar to the feeling of your thumb sinking into a stick of butter.
- Maintain downward pressure for 1 to 3 minutes; then begin gentle oscillations in all directions. Do not allow your finger or thumb to slide over the skin; take the skin with you as your thumb oscillates. Continue these oscillations for several more minutes.

- Move on to another area of the scar, or finish the session.
- Use a hot towel on the perineum or soak in a hot tub to help dissipate any residual soreness.

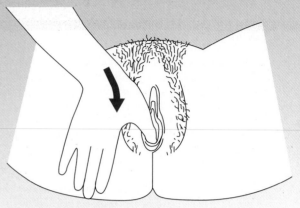

Episiotomy scar massage.

management includes internal myofascial release of scars, mobilization of scars by patients or their partners, ultrasound, PFE, and heat if needed. One method for teaching mobilization of scar tissue is described in Patient-Related Instruction 18-10: Self-Mobilization of Scar Tissue.

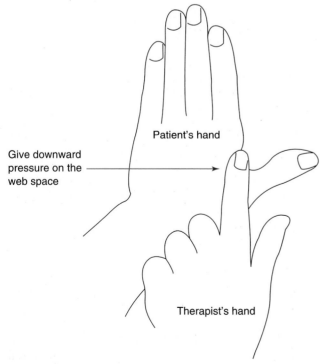

FIGURE 18-16. Describing self-mobilization of a vaginal scar using the patient web space.

The therapist can describe the technique using the patient's web space between the thumb and the first finger as the posterior vagina (Fig. 18-16). This allows the therapist to give the patient the experience of the amount of pressure that is appropriate and to show how to perform the oscillations. Oscillations are similar to friction massage in that the goal is to slide the skin over the second layer of fascia, thereby breaking adhesions and restoring mobility.

Tolerance to scar mobilization varies with the severity of adhesions. Most women find that pain with deep myofascial release of scars decreases as the adhesions loosen. Dyspareunia usually decreases as scars loosen. Some women find it difficult to effectively massage their own vaginal scars. It may be difficult to reach the vagina, or it may be difficult to cause self-inflicted pain. In this case, partners can be trained in a similar manner to assist with treatment. Scar mobilization before intercourse can help decrease dyspareunia. Scar mobilization should not be performed in the presence of open wounds, rash, or infection. Postpartum women should wait at least 6 to 8 weeks after delivery and should check with the physician if questions arise.

Externally Palpating the Pelvic Floor Muscles

It is possible to palpate the PFMs externally at the insertion to the coccyx and along the length of the muscle at the medial ischial tuberosity. The benefits of this palpation are limited, but it is helpful in palpating and treating trigger points in some parts of the levator ani and obturator internus muscles. This method does not give access to all areas of the PFM. This palpation requires skilled instruction and practice to perfect. Patient position, therapist preparation, therapist position, hand positions, and technique are described in Display 18-12.

DISPLAY 18-12
Externally Palpating the PFMs

- Patient position: Place the patient in sidelying with the top leg in approximately 60 to 80 degrees of hip flexion and the knee comfortably bent. Put two or three pillows under the top leg to provide stability in neutral abduction or adduction, and allow the patient to relax the leg fully. Total patient relaxation is necessary for deep PFM palpation.
- Therapist's position: The therapist is positioned behind the patient and finds the tip of the ischial tuberosity on the uppermost ilium.
- Therapist's preparation: This palpation may be done through underpants but is more effective if the fingers are on bare skin. The therapist should wear a vinyl glove on the palpating hand because it will be close to the anus and perineum.
- Hand position: The most effective hand position is supination, with all four fingers adducted in full finger extension. Keep the hand parallel to the table, and place the fingertips on the skin between the ischial tuberosity and the anus (just medial to the ischial tuberosity).
- Technique: Apply gentle inward pressure, directing your fingertips toward the anterior-superior iliac spine (ASIS) of the top ilium. Closeness to the ischial tuberosity results in the skin pulling taught and restricting deep palpation. In this case, reposition the fingers more medial toward the rectum, taking up some skin slack (see figure). The levator ani muscles are rather deep, being the third layer in the pelvic floor. Depth from the skin varies greatly and can be more than 1.5 in. When a firm resistance is felt, ask the patient to contract the PFMs. You should feel a firm PFM contraction pushing your fingers outward.
- With the PFMs at rest, assess for pain, spasm, and connective tissue restriction in the usual manner. Angling the fingers anteriorly and posteriorly can give information about different areas of the levator ani muscle group. The obturator internus is a little more difficult to palpate. A review of anatomy is necessary to orient yourself to the location of the muscle in

the sidelying position. Keep the palpating hand in the position described previously, and gently change the angle of the hand so that the wrist and elbow drops and the fingers move upward into the tissue above. The obturator internus is located in this area. The muscle should feel somewhat soft. Have the patient contract the muscle to ensure correct location. External rotation can be tested by asking the patient to lift the top knee upward toward the ceiling while keeping the foot on the supporting surface. The therapist resists this motion with a hand on top of the knee. A small isometric contraction should result in palpable muscle tension. The palpation depth is important. Shallow palpation results in palpation of the medial ischial tuberosity. In this case, continue straight, inward pressure until the tissue releases to a deeper level, and then angle the wrist down and the fingers upward. Myofascial release of the muscle or connective tissue can be carried out in this position if impairments are identified.

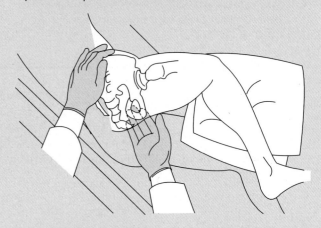

External palpation of PFMs. (Adapted from Hoppenfeld S. Physical Examination of the Spine and Extremities. New York, NY: Appleton-Century-Crofts. 1976.)

KEY POINTS

- The PFMs include four skeletal muscle layers: anal sphincter (continence), superficial genital muscles (sexual functioning), perineal membrane (continence), and pelvic diaphragm (continence, pelvic support).
- The pelvic diaphragm includes the levator ani which is made up of the coccygeus, pubococcygeus, puborectalis, and iliococcygeus and is the largest muscle group in the pelvic floor. These muscles are skeletal muscles under voluntary control and have 70% slow-twitch and 30% fast-twitch muscle fibers. They span from the pubic bone to the tail bone and between the ischial tuberosities. The PFM is close to many hip muscles (i.e., obturator internus and piriformis), but it is neither necessary nor desirable to move the legs while contracting the PFMs.
- The three functions of the PFM are supportive (i.e., prevents pelvic organs from prolapsing), sphincteric (i.e., prevents involuntary loss of urine, feces, and gas from the urethra and rectum), and sexual (i.e., increases sexual appreciation and maintains erection).

- All patients should be screened for PFM dysfunction with these simple questions. Do you ever leak urine or feces? Do you ever wear a pad because of leaking urine? Do you have pain during intercourse? If indicated, a more comprehensive questionnaire can be given to attempt to identify the type of incontinence and other limiting factors.
- Patients can be given self-assessment tests and taught self-awareness exercises: jumping jack test, digital self-examination (finger in the vagina), index finger on the perineal body, visual exercise, sexercise, and squeezing around an object. These home exercises help to develop the exercise program and ensure the patient is contracting the PFM correctly.
- Through home self-assessment, the patient reports the number of seconds a PFM contraction can be held, repetitions of endurance contractions, and repetitions of quick contractions.
- Impairments that affect PFM function include performance impairments of the PFMs, abdominals, and hip muscles; pain and altered tone of the PFMs, hip muscles, and trunk muscles; lumbopelvic joint mobility impairments; posture impairments; and coordination impairments of the PFMs and the abdominal muscles.

- PFM dysfunctions have two clinical classifications that are used by pelvic physical therapists internationaly: underactive PFM (i.e., loss of support usually as a result of impaired PFM performance) and overactive PFM (i.e., pain and altered tone impairment in the PFMs). Two additional classifications include incoordination dysfunction (i.e., coordination impairment with poor timing and recruitment of PFMs) and visceral dysfunction (i.e., dysfunctions of the pelvic viscera with possible PFM involvement). PFM dysfunctions can result in significant activity limitations and affect the quality of life.
- Incontinence is the most common result of underactive PFM. The most common types of incontinence are stress incontinence (i.e., loss of urine and increased intra-abdominal pressure with a cough, sneeze, laugh, or lift), urge incontinence (i.e., very strong urge to urinate, usually associated with a bladder contraction, which results in leaking urine), mixed incontinence (i.e., combined stress and urge incontinence), overflow incontinence (i.e., obstruction at the urethra or a flaccid bladder that allows high volumes of urine to collect in the bladder and spill over), and functional incontinence (i.e., leaking of urine because of an inability to ambulate to toilet quickly).
- Pelvic organ prolapse is another common diagnosis resulting from PFM weakness. Forms include cystocele (i.e., bladder prolapse into the vagina), uterine prolapse (i.e., uterine displacement into the vagina), and rectocele (i.e., rectal prolapse into the vagina).
- The PFMs contribute greatly to the stability of the trunk, and impairments of the PFMs are present in many orthopedic dysfunctions including low back pain and chronic pelvic pain. Treatment of PFM dysfunction will greatly enhance outcomes of orthopedic treatment in this area.
- With the results of screening questionnaires, the physical therapist should be able to develop an exercise program, including the duration of endurance contraction, rest between endurance contractions, repetitions of endurance contractions, repetitions of quick contractions, number of sets per day, exercise position, need for overflow facilitation from accessory muscle, and other treatments that may be helpful.

- All physical therapists should be aware of the PFMs and be prepared to give generalized strengthening instructions.
- Teaching PFEs involves educating the patient on the location and function of the PFMs and the importance of normal PFM function, providing accurate verbal clues, and teaching home assessment and awareness exercises. The most effective verbal cue seems to be "Pull your sphincter muscles up and in as if you do not want gas to come out." Many patients become discouraged and abandon PFEs. Therapists must continue to monitor the patient's progress and to actively encourage participation in the PFE program.

CRITICAL THINKING QUESTIONS

1. Imagine you have urge urinary incontinence and are being sent to physical therapy for shoulder pain. For some reason the therapist always puts you on the plinth farthest from the bathroom near the kitchen where someone always seems to be washing dishes during your therapy time. Your therapist is a very attractive younger person of the opposite sex and you are embarrassed to share your dilemma. Describe how you would feel about your situation. Describe the impact on your life (i.e., work, family, social interactions, emotions). List some things you might change because of your condition.
2. You are treating a 30-year-old man who fell off a ladder onto his right buttock. After 3 weeks of quality treatment, he has experienced significant decrease in low back and sacroiliac pain, but he can only sit for 1 1/2 hours and experiences pain with sit to stand transfers and when going up stairs. He finally admits that his tail bone hurts and that it feels as though he is "sitting on a ball." Your evaluation shows no dysfunction in the lumbar spine and persistent hypomobility of the right sacroiliac. Which muscles should you assess for dysfunction, and how would you treat them? Think about how you would explain to the patient that his pain may be related to the PFMs.

 LAB ACTIVITIES

1. Work in groups of two. One person pretends to be the patient. Pick a scenario from the list below or make up your own.
   Possible patient scenarios—add details as needed
   A 24-year-old female 4 months after vaginal delivery of her third child with buttocks pain and stress incontinence
   A 61-year-old male with urgency and LBP
   A 55-year-old male sp a fall on the tailbone during roller-skating. Now with coccyx pain
   An 81-year-old female with diabetes mellitis (DM), rheumatoid arthritis (RA), chronic obstructive pulmonary disease (COPD), mild dementia, and limitated ambulation
   An 18-year-old gymnast with LBP, dysmenorrhea, and occasional urine leakage

A 44-year-old female with endometriosis and abdominal pain
A 70-year-old male status post prostatectomy with mixed incontinence symptoms, LBP, and abdominal weakness
   A. Practice administering the screening and long questionnaires.
   B. Practice explaining the location and function of the PFMs and the importance of PFEs using words, posters, and models. Write down layman's terms used to describe the area.
   C. Practice explaining the appropriate self-assessment test and home awareness exercises to the patient.
2. Bladder diary interpretation—two examples given (see additional files)

(continued)

LAB ACTIVITIES *(Continued)*

3. Develop a PFE program—two examples given (see additonal files)
4. Perform the self-assessment test and self-awareness exercises at home, and develop an appropriate exercise program for yourself. Exercise programs should include the following:
   a. Results of jumping jack test
   b. The number of repetitions and amount of hold time per contraction
   c. The amount of rest that should be taken between contractions
   d. The number of quick contractions per set
   e. The number of sets per day
   f. Suggested position of exercises (i.e., lying down or upright)
   g. Other methods of strengthening that should be considered

5. Practice palpating the PFMs externally at the ischial tuberosity. Evaluate for pain, trigger points, spasm, and connective tissue tension. Make sure you are on the correct muscle by having the patient contract that muscle.
6. Sit up tall in the chair, and push your abdominal muscles outward. Keep the abdomen distended, and contract the PFMs. Notice the amount of effort needed and the force generated by the PFMs. Next, sit up in the chair, and pull the abdominals inward, supporting the abdominal contents and the back. Hold the abdominal contraction gently and contract the PFMs. Notice the effort needed and the force generated by the PFMs. Next, try to contract the PFMs and bear down, pouching out the abdominals. Try to contract the PFMs and then pull the abdominals inward correctly.

REFERENCES

1. Landefeld CS, Bowers BJ, Feld AD, et al. National institutes of health state-of-the-science statement: Prevention of fecal and urinary incontince in adults. Ann Intern Med 2008;148(6):449–458.
2. Bond E, Dorey G, Eckford S, et al. The role of pelvic floor muscle exercise in reducing surgical management of women with stress incontinence: a clinical audit. J Assoc Chartered Physiother Women's Health 2004; 95: 66–70.
3. Kegel A. Progressive resistance exercises in the functional restoration of the perineal muscles. Am J Obstet Gynecol 1948;56:238.
4. Messelink B, Benson T, Bergham B, et al. Standardization of terminology of pelvic floor muscle function and dysfunction: report from the pelvic floor clinical assessment group of the International Continence Society. Neurourol Urodynam 2005;24:374–380.
5. Wei JT, DeLancey JO. Functional anatomy of the pelvic floor and lower urinary tract. Clin Obstet Gynecol 2004;47:3–17.
6. Stein TA, DeLancey JOL. Structure of the perineal membrane in females. Obstet Gynecol 2008;111:686–693.
7. Schussler B, Laycock J, Norton P, Stanton S, eds. Pelvic Floor Re-education Principals and Practice. New York, NY: Springer-Verlag, 1994.
8. DeLancey J, Richardson A. Anatomy of genital support. In: Benson T, ed. Female Pelvic Floor Disorders. New York, NY: Norton Medical Books, 1992.
9. Walters M, Karram M. Clinical Urogynecology. St. Louis, MO: Mosby-Year Book, 1993.
10. Kerney R, Sawhney R, DeLancey J. Levator ani muscle anatomy evaluated by origin-insertion pairs. Obstet Gynecol 2004;104:168–173.
11. Barber M, Bremer R, Thor K, et al. Innervation of the female levator ani muscles. Am J Obstet Gynecol 2002;187:64–71.
12. Grigorescu BA, Lazarou G, Olson TR, et al. Innervation of the levator ani muscles: description of the nerve branches to the pubococcygeus, iliococcygeus, and puborectalis muscles. Int Urogynecol J Pelvic Floor Dysfunct 2007.
13. Ashton-Miller JA, Howard D, DeLancey JO. The functional anatomy of the female pelvic floor and stress continence control system. Scand J Urol Nephrol Suppl 2001;207:1–125.
14. Travell J, Simons D. Myofascial Pain and Dysfunction: The Trigger Point Manual. Vol 2. Baltimore, MD: Williams & Wilkins, 1992.
15. Mcminn R, Hutchings R. Color Atlas of Human Anatomy. Chicago: Year Book Medical Publishers. 1977.
16. Hulme J. Beyond Kegels. Missoula, Mont: Phoenix Publishing Co; 1997.
17. Jarvis SK, Hallam TK, Lujic S, et al. Peri-operative physiotherapy improves outcomes for women undergoing incontinence and or prolapse surgery: results of a randomized controlled trail. Aust NZJ Obstet Gynecol 2005;45(4):300–3003.
18. DeLancey JOL, Morgan DM, Fenner DE, et al. Comparison of levator ani muscle defects and function in women with and without pelvic organ prolapse. Obstet Gynecol 2007;109:295–302.
19. Sapsford RR, Hodges PW, Richardson C. Co-activation of the abdominal and pelvic floor muscles during voluntary exercises. Neurourol Urodyn 2001;20:31–42.
20. Critchley D. 2002. Instructing pelvic floor contraction facilitates transversus abdominis thickness increase during low-abdominal hollowing. Physiother Res Int 2002;7(2):65–75.
21. Finkelstein MM. Medical conditions, medications and urinary incontinence. Analysis of a population based survey. Can Fam Phys 2002;48:96–101.
22. Eliasson K, Elfving B, Nordgren B, et al. Urinary incontinence in women with low back pain. Man Ther 2008;13(3):206–212.
23. Smith MD, Coppieters MW, Hodges PW. Is balance different in women with and without stress urinary continence? Neurourol Urodynam 2008;27:71–78.
24. Chiarelli P. Women's Waterworks—Curing Incontinence. Snohomish, WA: Khera Publications, 1995.
25. Dorey G, Speakman M, Feneley R, et al. Randomized controlled trial of pelvic floor muscle exercises and manometric biofeedback for erectile dysfunction. Br J Gen Pract 2004;54:819–825.
26. Van Kampen M, De Weerdt W, Claes H, et al. Treatment of erectile dysfunction by perineal exercise, electromyographic, biofeedback, and electrical stimulation. Phys Ther 2003;83:536–543.
27. Sapsford RR. The pelvic floor and its related organs. In: Sapsford R, Bullock-Saxton J, Markwell S, eds. Women's Health. Philadelphia, PA: WB Saunders Co; 1998:56–86.
28. Haslam J, Laycock J ed. Therapeutic Management of Incontinence and Pelvic Pain. 2nd Ed. London: Springer-Verlag, 2008.
29. DeLancey J, Richardson A. Anatomy of genital support. In: Benson T, ed. Female Pelvic Floor Disorders. New York, NY: Norton Medical Books, 1992.
30. Dolan LM, Hosker GL, Mallett VT, et al. Stress incontinence and pelvic floor neurophysiology 15 years after the first delivery. BJOG 2003;110:1107–1114.
31. Sultan AH, Kamm MA, Hudson CN, et al. Anal-sphincter disruption during vaginal delivery. New Engl J Med 1993;329:1905–1911.
32. Goldberg J, Purfield P, Roberts N, Lupinacci P, Fagan M, Hyslop T. The Philadelphia Episiotomy Intervention Study. J Reprod Med 2006;51:603–609.
33. Weber AM, Meyn L. Episiotomy use in the United States: 1979–1997. Obstet Gynecol 2002;100:1177–1182.
34. Meyer S, Hohlfeld P, Achtari C, et al. Pelvic floor education after vaginal delivery. Obstet Gynecol 2001;97:673–677.
35. Wein AJ. Neuromuscular dysfunction of the lower urinary tract and its management. In: Walsh PC, Retik AB, Vaughan ED, Wein AJ, eds. Campbell's Urology. Philadelphia, PA: WB Saunders, 2002:931–1026.
36. Swinn MJ, Fowler CJ. Bladder dysfunction in neurological disorders. In: Pemberton JH, Swash M, Henry MM, eds. The Pelvic Floor: Its Function and Disorders. London: WB Saunders; 2002:296–312.
37. McCallum TJ, Moore KN, Griffiths D. Urinary incontinence after radical prostatectomy: implications and urodynamics. Urol Nurs 2001;21:113–124.
38. Sakaibara R, Hattori T, Yasuda K, et al. Micturitional disturbance after acute hemispheric stroke: analysis of the lesion site by CT and MRI. J Neurol Sci 1996;137:47–56.
39. de Seze, Ruffion A, Denys P, et al. The neurogenic bladder in MS, a review of the literature and proposal of management guidelines. Mult Scler 2007;13:915.
40. Wade D, Langton HR. Outlook after an acute stroke: urinary incontinence and loss of consciousness compared in 532 patients. Q J Med 1985;56:601–608.

41. Bo K, Talseth T. Long-term effect of pelvic floor muscle exercises 5 years after cessation of organized training. Obstet Gynecol 1996;87:261–265.
42. Lagro-Jenssen T, Van Weel C. Long-term effect of treatment of female incontinence in general practice. Brit J Gen Pract 1998;48:1735–1738.
43. Paddison K. Complying with pelvic floor exercises: a literature review. Nursing Standard 2002;16(39):33–38.
44. Sachs-Ericsson N, Blazer D, Plant EA, et al. Childhood sexual and physical abuse and the 1-year prevalence of medical problems in the National Comorbidity Survey. Health Psychol 2005;24(suppl 1):32–40.
45. James M, Jackson S, Shepherd A, et al. Pure stress leakage symptomatology: is it safe to discount detrussor instability? Br J Obstet Gynecol 1999;106:1255–1258.
46. Wagg A, Majumdar A, Toozs-Hobsob P, et al. Current and future trends in the management of overactive bladder. Int Urogynecol J 2007;18:81–94.
47. Fonda D, DeBeau CE. Incontinence in the frail elderly. In: Abrams P, Cardozo L, Khoury S, Wein A, eds. Third International Consultation on Incontinence. Plymouth, UK: Health Publication Ltd, 2005.
48. Jackson RA, Vittinghoff E, Kanaya AM, et al. Urinary incontinence in elderly women: findings from the Health, Aging, and Body Composition Study. Obstet Gynecol 2004;104:301–307.
49. Minassian VA, Stewart WF, Wood GC. Urinary incontinence in women: variation in prevalence estimates and risk factors. Obstet Gynecol 2008 Feb;111(2 Pt 1):324–331.
50. Figuers CC, Boyle KL, Caprio KM. Pelvic floor muscle activity and urinary incontinence in weight-bearing female athletes vs. non-athletes. JWHPT 2008; 32:7–11.
51. Dockter M, Kolstad AM, Martin KA, et al. Prevalence of urinary incontinence: a comparative study of collegiate female athletes and non-athletic controls. JWHPT 2007;31:12–17.
52. Lawrence JM, Lukacz ES, Nager CW, et al. Prevalence and co-occurrence of pelvic floor disorders in community-dwelling women. Obstet Gynecol 2008;111:678–685.
53. Neville CE, Fitzgerald CM, Mallinson T, et al. Musculoskeletal dysfunction in female chronic pelvic pain: A blinded study of examination findings. Clinical Research Poster Presentation, clinical research World Congress of Physical Therapy, Vancouver, Canada June 4, 2007.
54. Lilius HG, Valtonen EJ. The levator ani spasm syndrome: a clinical analysis of 31 cases. Ann Chir Gynaecol Fenn 1973;62:93–97.
55. Fitzgerald MP, Kotarinos R. Rehabilitation of the short pelvic floor. II: Treatment of the patient with the short pelvic floor. Int Urogynecol J 2003;14:269–275.
56. Kjerulff KH, Langenberg PW, Rhodes JC, et al. Effectiveness of hysterectomy. Obstet Gynecol 2000;95:319–326.
57. Lukban JC, Parkin JV, Holzberg AS, et al. Interstitial cystitis and pelvic floor dysfunction: a comprehensive review. Pain Med 2001;2:60–71.
58. Ness RB, Soper DE, Holley RL, et al. Effectiveness of inpatient and outpatient treatment strategies for women with pelvic inflammatory disease: results from the Pelvic Inflammatory Disease Evaluation and Clinical Health (PEACH) Randomized Trial. Am J Obstet Gynecol 2002;186:929–937.
59. Rapkin AJ, Kames LD, Darke LL, et al. History of physical and sexual abuse in women with chronic pelvic pain. Obstet Gynecol 1990;76:92–96.
60. Collett BJ, Cordle CJ, Stewart CR, et al. A comparative study of women with chronic pelvic pain, chronic nonpelvic pain and those with no history of pain attending general practitioners. Br J Obstet Gynaecol 1998;105:87–92.
61. Lampe A, Solder E, Ennemoser A, et al. Chronic pelvic pain and previous sexual abuse. Obstet Gynecol 2000;96:929–933.
62. Latthe P, Mignini L, Gray R, et al. Factors predisposing women to chronic pelvic pain systematic review. BMJ 2006;332:749–755.
63. Woman's Hospital Physical Therapy Department. The Bottom Line on Kegels. Baton Rouge, LA: A Woman's Hospital Publication, 1997.
64. Urinary Incontinence Guidelines Panel. Urinary Incontinence in Adults: Clinical Practice Guideline. AHCPR Pub. No. 92–0038. Rockville, MD: Agency for Health Care Policy and Research, Public Health Service, U.S. Department of Health and Human Services, March 1996.
65. Sampselle C, DeLancey J. The urine stream interruption test and pelvic muscle function. Nurs Res 1992;41:73–77.
66. Whittaker JL. Ultrasound Imaging for Rehabilitation of the Lumbopelvic Region. Edinburgh: Churchill Livingstone, 2007.
67. Dietz HP, Jarvis SK, Vancaille TG. The assessment of levator muscle strength: a validation of three ultrasound techniques. Int Urogyn J 2002;13:156–159.
68. Bo K, Sherburn M, Allen T. Transabdominal ultrasound measurement of pelvic floor muscle activity when activated directly or via transversus abdominis muscle contraction. Neurourol Urodyn 2003;22:582–588.
69. Pages I, Jahr S, Schaufele MK, et al. Comparative analysis of biofeedback and physical therapy for treatment of urinary incontinence in women. Am J Phys Med Rehabil 2001;80:494–502.
70. Bo K, Talseth T, Hulme I. Single blind, randomized controlled trail of pelvic floor exercise, electrical stimulation, vaginal cones and no treatment in management of genuine stress incontinence in women. BMJ 1999;318:487–493.
71. Arvonen T, Fianu-Johnson A, Tyni-Lenne R. Effectiveness of two conservative modes of physical therapy in women with urinary stress incontinence. Neurourol Urodyn 2001;20:591–599.
72. Bo K. Pelvic floor muscle training. In: Bo K, Berghmans B, Morkved S, Kampen MV, eds. Evidence-based Physical Therapy for the Pelvic Floor. Philadelphia: Elsevier, 2007.

73. Miller JM, Ashton-Miller JA, Delancey J. A pelvic muscle pre-contraction can reduce couch-related urine loss in selected women with mild stress urinary incontinence. J Am Geriatric Soc 1998;46:870–874.
74. Choi H, Palmer MH, Park J. Meta-analysis of pelvic floor training: randomized controlled trials in incontinent women. Nursing Res 2007;56:226–234.
75. Bo K, Stien R. Needle EMG registration of striated urethral wall and pelvic floor muscle activity patterns during cough, Valsalva, abdominal, hip adductor and gluteal contractions in nulliparous healthy females. Neurourol Urodyn 1994;13:35–41.
76. Neumann P, Gill V. Pelvic floor and abdominal muscle interaction: EMG activity and intra-abdominal pressure. Int Urogynecol J 2002;13:125–132.
77. Sapsford RR, Hodges PW, Richardson CA, et al. Co-contraction of the abdominal and pelvic floor muscles during voluntary exercise. Neurourol Urodyn 2001;20:31–42.
78. Nielsen C, Sigsgaard I, Olsen M, et al. Trainability of the pelvic floor—a prospective study during pregnancy and after delivery. Acta Obstet Gynecol Scand 1988;67:437–440.
79. Sampselle C. Changes in pelvic muscle strength and stress urinary incontinence associated with childbirth. J Obstet Gynecol Neonatal Nurs 1990;19:5: 371–377.
80. Sueppel C, Kreder K, See W. Improved continence outcomes with preoperative pelvic floor muscle strengthening exercise. Urol Nurs 2001;21: 201–210.
81. Lee D. The Pelvic Girdle. 2nd Ed. Edinburgh: Churchill Livingstone, 2004.
82. Bump R, Hurt G, Fantl A, et al. Assessment of Kegel pelvic muscle exercises performed after brief verbal instruction. Am J Obstet Gynecol 1991;165:322–329.
83. Tu FF, As-Sanie S, Steege JF. Musculoskeletal causes of chronic pelvic pain: a systematic review of existing therapies. Part II. Obstet Gynecol Surv 2005;60:474–483.
84. American Physical Therapy Association. Women's Health Gynecological Physical Therapy Manual. Alexandria, VA: APTA, 1997. 1-800-999-APTA, ext. 3237.
85. Herman H. Conservative management of female patients with pelvic pain. Urol Nurs 2001;20:393–417.
86. Keltz MD, Peck L, Liu S, et al. Large bowel to pelvic sidewall adhesions associated with chronic pelvic pain. J Am Assoc Gynecol Laparosc 1995;3:55–59.
87. Miller JM, Perucchini D, Carchidi LT, et al. Pelvic floor muscle contraction during a cough and decreased vesical neck mobility. Obstet Gynecol 2001;97:255–260.
88. Weih AJ, Barret DM. Voiding Function and Dysfunction: A Logical and Practical Approach. Chicago: Year Book Medical Publishers, 1988.
89. Sherburn M, Guthri JR, Dudley EC, et al. Is incontinence associated with menopause? Obstet Gynecol 2001;98:628–633.
90. Elia G, Dye TD, Scarlati PD. Body mass index and urinary incontinence symptoms in women. Int Urogynecol J 2001;12:366–369.
91. Subak LL, Johnson C, Whitcomb E, et al. Does weight loss improve incontinence in moderately obese women? Int Urogynecol J 2002;13:40–43.
92. Rortvent G, Hannestad YS, Daltveit AK, et al. Age-and type- dependent effects of parity on urinary incontinence: the Norwegian EPINCONT study. Obstet Gynecol 2001;98:1004–1010.
93. Nygaard I, DeLancey J, Arnsdorf L, et al. Exercises and incontinence. Obstet Gynecol 1990;75:848–851.
94. Van der Velde J, Laan E, Everaerd W. Vaginismus, a component of a general defense reaction. An investigation of pelvic floor muscle activity during exposure to emotional-inducing film excerpts in women with and without symptoms of vaginismus. Int Urogynecol J 2001;12:328–331.
95. King PM, Ling FW, Rosenthal RH. Musculoskeletal factors in chronic pelvic pain. J Psychosom Obstet Gynaecol 1991;12(suppl):87–98.
96. Abrams P, Cardozo L, Fall M, et al. The standardization of terminology of lower urinary tract function: report from the standardization sub-committee of the International Continence Society. Am J Obstet Gynecol 2002;21: 167–178.
97. Bo K, Sundgot Borgen J. Prevalence of stress urinary incontinence among physically active and sedentary female students. Scand J Sports Sci 1989;11:113–116.
98. Meade-D'Alisera P, Merriweather T, Wentland M, et al. Depressive symptoms in women with urinary incontinence: a prospective study. Urol Nurs 2001;21:397–399.
99. Burgio KL, Locher JL, Roth DL, et al. Psychological impairments associated with behavioral and drug treatment of urge incontinence in older women. J Gerontol B Psychol Sci Soc Sci 2001;56:46–51.
100. Brown JS, McGhan WF, Chokroverty S. Comorbidities associated with over-active bladder. Am J Manage Care 2000;6(11 Suppl):S574–S579.
101. Takazawa K, Arisawa K. Relationship between the type of urinary incontinence and falls among frail elderly women in Japan. J Med Invest 2005;52(3–4): 165–171.
102. Teo JS, Briffa NK, Devine A, et al. Do sleep problems or urinary incontinence predict falls in elderly women? Aust J Physiother 2006;52(1):19–24.
103. McCrush D, Robinson D, Fantl J, et al. Relationship between urethral pressure and vaginal pressures during pelvic floor muscle contraction. Neurourol Urodynam 1997;16:553–558.
104. Bachmann GA, Rosen R, Pinn VW, et al. Vulvodynia: a state-of the art consensus on definitions, diagnosis and management. J Reprod Med 2006;51:447–456.

105. Zolnoun D, Hartmann K, Lamvu G, et al. A conceptual model for the pathophysiology of vulvar vestibulitis syndrome. Obstet Gynecol Survey 2006;61:395–401.

106. Herndon A, Decambre M, McKenna PH. Interactive computer games for treatment of pelvic floor dysfunction. J Urol 2001;166:1893–1898.

107. Pearson B. Liquidate a myth: reducing liquid intake is not advisable for elderly with urine control problems. Urol Nurs 1993;13:86–87.

Kegel A. Sexual function of the pubococcygeus muscle. West J Surg Obstet Gynecol 1952;10:521.

Urinary incontinence—the management of urinary incontinence in women. Royal College of Obstetrics and Gynaecologists, London UK, 2006.

Clinical guidelines for physiotherapy management of females aged 16–65 years with stress urinary incontinence. The Chartered Society of Physiotherapy. London, UK, 2004.

RECOMMENDED READINGS

PATIENT EDUCATION

Bass E, Davis L. The Courage to Heal: A Guide for Women Survivors of Child Sexual Abuse. 3rd Ed. New York, NY: Harper & Row, 1994.

Burgio K. Staying Dry. Baltimore, MD: John Hopkins University Press, 1989.

Wise D, Anderson R. A Headache in the Pelvis. Occidental, CA: National Center for Pelvic Pain Research, 2003.

PHYSICAL THERAPY BOOKS

Haslam J, Laycock J, ed. Therapeutic Management of Incontinence and Pelvic Pain. 2nd Ed. London: Springer-Verlag, 2008.

Bo K, Berghmans B, Morkved S, Kampen MV, eds. Evidence-based Physical Therapy for the Pelvic Floor. Philadelphia, PA: Elsevier, 2007.

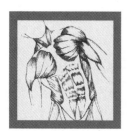

chapter 19
The Hip

CARRIE M. HALL

WITH CONTRIBUTIONS BY ANDREW STARSKY

The primary roles of the hip joint are to support the weight of the head, arms, and trunk during erect standing postures and dynamic weight-bearing activities such as walking, running, and stair climbing and to provide a pathway for transmission of forces between the lower extremities and pelvis. The structure and function of the hip affect the function of the entire lower kinetic chain and the upper quadrants through its articulation with the pelvis proximally and the femur distally.

Neither structure nor function of the hip joint can be examined without considering the weight-bearing function of the joint and the interdependence with the other joints of the lower extremity and lumbopelvic (LP) region. These issues are examined in this chapter. Anatomy and kinesiology review can be found on the website. Common anatomic impairments and the evidence-based components of examination and evaluation of the hip joint also are described. Therapeutic exercise interventions are suggested for the treatment of physiologic impairments and selected diagnoses of the hip joint.

IMPAIRMENTS OF BODY STRUCTURES

Five impairments of body structures (or anatomic impairments) of the hip joint are worthy of consideration because of the impact they have on hip function: angle of torsion, angle of inclination, center edge angle, leg length discrepancy (LLD), and femoral acetabular impingement (FAI). Each impairment of body structure, independently or in combination with other impairments (body structure or function), warrants careful consideration about the impact on hip joint function and the function of joints proximal or distal to the hip.

Angles of Inclination and Torsion

Angle of Inclination

As discussed earlier, angles of inclination and torsion are normal anatomic relationships of the femur. However, the degree of inclination or torsion can become abnormal when the values are greater or less than normal. Abnormal angulations of the femur are considered impairments of body structures. These anatomic impairments of the femur can significantly alter hip joint mechanics, which can alter the mechanics of adjacent segments proximally and distally in the kinetic chain.

In early infancy, the angle of inclination is about 150 degrees because of the abducted position of the femur in utero. The angle decreases with age to the normal adult value of 125 degrees, with further decreases to the normal older adult angle of 119 degrees.[1,2] The angle is somewhat smaller in females and somewhat larger in males.[2] A pathologic increase in the angle is called coxa valga (Fig. 19-1A), and a pathologic decrease is called coxa vara (Fig. 19-1B).[2]

The position of the greater trochanter influences the mechanical stress of the hip joint, the extent of contraction of the gluteus medius and minimus muscles, and the mechanical stress of the femoral neck.[3] A normal neck-shaft angle appears to achieve a maximum lever arm of the abductor muscles and the best compromise between articular pressure and bending stress on the femoral neck. A very high position of the greater trochanter (coxa vara) can result in shortening of the lever arm of the abductor muscles, resulting in lower articular pressure, but high bending stress of the femoral neck. Conversely, in a valgus hip, bending stress is lower, but hip abductor moment arm is greater and articular pressure is higher.

Angle of Torsion

The newborn infant has a maximum angle of torsion of approximately 40 degrees. This decreases to an average of 32 degrees at the age of 1 year and further decreases to 16 degrees by the age of 16 years.[4] The angle is normally about 12 to 15 degrees in the adult, but it may range from 8 to 30 degrees and, as with the angle of inclination, varies between sexes and among persons.[1,5] A pathologic increase in the angle of torsion is called anteversion (Fig. 19-2A), and a decrease is called retroversion (Fig. 19-2B). Anteversion and retroversion can be screened for during a clinical examination (see Examination/Evaluation).

Because the hip joint can only tolerate a limited amount of torsion (12 to 15 degrees) without jeopardizing its congruence, a pathologic increase (>15 degrees) or decrease (<12 degrees) in the angle of torsion is manifested distally at the femoral condyles. In the standing position, the femoral condyles of an individual with femoral anteversion are oriented medially, and in femoral retroversion, they are oriented laterally when the femoral head is in a position of maximum congruence. The individual with femoral anteversion functioning with the femoral condyles facing laterally risks losing congruence of the femoral head in the acetabulum. Similarly, the individual with femoral retroversion functioning with the femoral condyles facing medially also risks losing congruence of the femoral head in the acetabulum. As these impairments are anatomical and cannot be directly treated therapeutically, the practitioner must be aware of these impairments of body structures when guiding femoral alignment during exercise and function.

Center Edge Angle or Angle of Wiberg

A line connecting the lateral rim of the acetabulum and the center of the femoral head forms an angle with the vertical known as the center edge angle, also called the angle of Wiberg (Fig. 19-3). The center edge angle for the average adult is 22 to 42 degrees.[5] Although this is a normal angle,

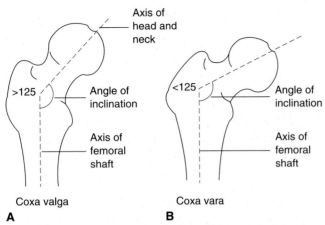

FIGURE 19-1. Abnormal angles of inclination. (A) A pathologic increase in the angle of inclination is called coxa valga. (B) A pathologic decrease in the angle of inclination is called coxa vara.

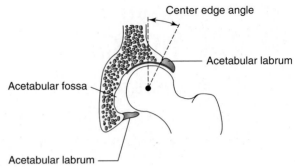

FIGURE 19-3. The center edge angle or angle of Wiberg.

variations in the angle can lead to altered stability of the femoral head, in which case it would be considered an anatomic impairment.

A smaller center edge angle (i.e., more vertical orientation) of the acetabulum may result in decreased congruency of the head of the femur and the acetabulum, placing the head of the femur at increased risk of superior dislocation of the head of the femur. Children are at greater risk for this type of dislocation than adults, because the center edge angle normally increases with age.[6] It may be for this reason that congenital dislocation is more common at the hip than any other joint in the body.[7]

Leg Length Discrepancy

LLD, when measured from one common bilateral point of reference proximally to another common bilateral point of reference distally, is a unilateral difference in the total length of one leg compared with the other. LLD is commonly thought of as resulting from a structural fault in the anatomic length of the long bones, hemipelvis, or asymmetric structural development of the spine (i.e., scoliosis), in which case it would be considered an impairment of body structures. However, LLD often is the result of the

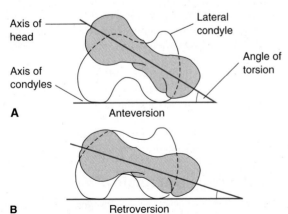

FIGURE 19-2. (A) A pathologic increase in the angle of torsion is called anteversion. (B) A pathologic decrease in the angle of torsion is called retroversion. (From Norkin CC, Levangie PK. Joint Structure and Function: A Comprehensive Analysis. 2nd Ed. Philadelphia, PA: FA Davis, 1992.)

functional relationships of the spine, pelvis, long bones, and bones of the feet about all three axes of motion. For example, an individual standing in a neutral subtalar position, measured bilaterally from the tip of the medial malleolus to the horizontal plane (i.e., flat surface), should have equal measurements of both limbs. If the individual is allowed to pronate one foot, the medial malleolus of the pronated foot moves closer to the ground. The difference in height may be as much as ¼ to ¾ of an inch. This would be considered an impairment of body function as opposed to body structure, resulting in LLD. Structural and functional LLDs are common clinical terms used to describe the two types of LLDs.[8,9] Table 19-1 summarizes definitions of the clinical terms used to describe LLD.

LLD has been associated with hip pain, knee pain, LBP, and with lower extremity stress fractures.[10–13] Studies have shown increased hip joint forces of up to 12% in the relatively short and long limbs with LLDs of 3.5 to 6.5 cm.[14] In general, an LLD of more than 2.0 cm results in asymmetry in contact time, first and second force peaks, and loading and unloading rates of the vertical ground reaction force in gait.[15] The most common mechanism for dealing with minor degrees of limb length discrepancy is the induction of pelvic tilting in the coronal plane. In normal individuals, pelvic obliquity of 6.1 degrees can totally accommodate for a LLD of 2.2 cm.[16] With LLD > 2 cm, the coronal plane mechanism is necessarily augmented by changes in the sagittal plane, which occur at the ankle and knee in standing. The knee responds with flexion of the long limb, whereas the long leg ankle demonstrates increased dorsiflexion at terminal stance and the short leg ankle produces early heel rise and greater degrees of plantar flexion during stance.[16] The combination of these changes have the effect of shortening the functional length of the long limb both in the stance and swing phases while lengthening the shorter limb during the stance phase. Because of the changes in forces incurred at the hip and gait asymmetries, it appears that more than 2 cm of LLD can significantly affect kinetics and kinematics throughout the kinetic chain and therefore should be addressed. LLD of <2 cm affect pelvic alignment and may need to be addressed depending on the associated impairments and pathology. Evaluation and treatment of LLD is addressed in later sections.

Femoral Acetabular Impingement

FAI can result for abnormalities in the shape of the femoral head (known as cam impingement; Fig. 19-4B) or the acetabulum (known as pincer impingement; Fig. 19-4C). Either of these abnormalities or a combination of the two (Fig. 19-4D) can

TABLE 19-1	Definitions of Structural and Functional Leg Length Discrepancies		
TERM	**TYPE OF IMPAIRMENT**	**DEFINITION**	**MEASUREMENT TECHNIQUE**
Structural	Body Structure or Anatomic	Actual osseous length difference between the hemipelvis, femur, and tibia	Standing anteroposterior x-ray film or ultrasound imaging[15]
Functional	Body Function or Physiologic	Position of osseous structures as they relate to each other and to the environment during weight-bearing function	Actual difference between two pairs of identical reference points (e.g., greater trochanter and medial malleolus)

result in decreased space between the femoral head/neck and the acetabulum and subsequent impingement. This impingement typically occurs with the combined movement of hip flexion, adduction, and internal rotation.[17] The cause of the problem is under considerable debate. It is possible that overload of the joint can cause changes to the bone and cartilage due to abnormal arthrokinematic motions during ADLs and sport.

EXAMINATION AND EVALUATION

Examination and evaluation of the hip can be isolated to the hip in the case of specific hip pathology (e.g., rheumatoid arthritis, osteoarthritis [OA], avascular necrosis of the femoral head, labral pathology). However, even for a diagnosis isolated to the hip, evaluation of the knee, ankle-foot, and LP regions may provide useful information (e.g., rigid, supinated foot contributing to reduced shock absorption to the arthritic hip). Similarly, the hip is commonly included in the examination and evaluation of other regions to assess impairments of body structures or function of the hip that may be contributing to dysfunction in the affected region (e.g., a stiff hip contributing to lumbar hypermobility).

The descriptive examination and evaluation information presented in this section is not intended to be comprehensive or reflect any specific philosophical approach; it simply serves as a general review of pertinent tests performed in most hip examinations.

History

In addition to the general data generated from a patient/client history as defined in Chapter 2, the following information is important to obtain from a patient with impairment, activity limitation or participation restriction, or disability involving the hip joint. Of particular importance is a history of congenital hip dysfunction (e.g., congenital hip dysplasia), childhood hip conditions (e.g., slipped capital epiphysis, severe anteversion treated with bracing), previous hip joint injury, or a family history of OA or rheumatoid arthritis. These conditions along with age and gender received an evidence grade of Level I in a recently published clinical practice guideline.[18] Although the hip can become injured as a result of trauma, the clinician is more likely to encounter hip dysfunction as a result of cumulative microtrauma. In the latter case, it is important for the practitioner to gain an understanding of the activities of daily living (ADLs), recreational, and occupational activities with which the patient is involved on a repetitive basis and which activities seem to provoke symptoms. Of particular interest is a history of intense sport before skeletal maturity. Much of this information can be obtained through self-report forms (Display 19-1) and the formal interview can clarify subjective information.

Lumbar Spine Clearing Examination

The prevalence of LP conditions in the general population, combined with the fact that pathology in the LP region can manifest in referred pain patterns into the hip (e.g., posterior buttock) and cause neurologically mediated weakness of hip joint musculature (particularly the gluteal musculature), supports routine lumbar screening during any hip examination. A typical lumbar clearing examination is outlined in Chapter 17. Although this scan may seem extensive, excluding or diagnosing lumbar or sacroiliac joint involvement is critical

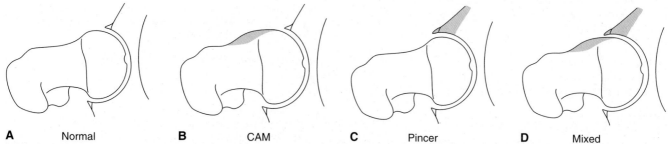

A Normal   **B** CAM   **C** Pincer   **D** Mixed

FIGURE 19-4. (A) Normal femoral head, neck, and acetabular labral anatomy, (B) Femoral sided impingement got its name, "CAM," from the Dutch word meaning "cog" describing the femoral head and neck relationship as aspherical or not perfectly round. During motions such as hyperflexion and internal rotation of the hip, the Cam lesion is able to fully engage within the joint. This results in cartilage loss over the femoral head and corresponding acetabulum, as well as labral tears. CAM lesions predominately affect the cartilage within the hip joint, resulting in a characteristic peeling of the cartilage off the bone. Cartilage wear is the definition of arthritis; therefore, this type of impingement is considered a pre arthritic condition. (C) The second category of FAI is the "pincer" type lesion, referring to the "over coverage" of the acetabulum in respect to the femoral head. Pincer comes from the French word meaning "to pinch." The "extra" bone of the acetabulum repetitively hits upon the femoral neck resulting in the pinching of the labrum in between. (D) CAM lesions often coexist with pincer lesions. CAM lesions are believed to lead to articular cartilage injury first, whereas pincer lesions are believed to crush and tear the labrum first.

DISPLAY 19-1
Self-Report Form

Functional Index

Walking
- ❑ Pain does not prevent me walking any distance.
- ❑ Pain prevents me walking more than 1 mi.
- ❑ Pain prevents me walking more than $1/2$ mi.
- ❑ Pain prevents me walking more than $1/4$ mi.
- ❑ I can only walk using a stick or crutches.
- ❑ I am in bed most of the time and have to crawl to the toilet.

Work (applies to work in home and outside)
- ❑ I can do as much work as I want to.
- ❑ I can only do my usual work, but no more.
- ❑ I can do most of my usual work, but no more.
- ❑ I cannot do my usual work.
- ❑ I can hardly do any work at all (only light duty).
- ❑ I cannot do any work at all.

Personal Care (washing, dressing, etc.)
- ❑ I can manage all personal care without symptoms.
- ❑ I can manage all personal care with some increased symptoms.
- ❑ Personal care requires slow, concise movements because of increased symptoms.
- ❑ I need help to manage some personal care.
- ❑ I need help to manage all personal care.
- ❑ I cannot manage any personal care.

Sleeping
- ❑ I have no trouble sleeping.
- ❑ My sleep is mildly disturbed (<1 hour sleepless).
- ❑ My sleep is mildly disturbed (1 to 2 hours sleepless).
- ❑ My sleep is moderately disturbed (2 to 3 hours sleepless).
- ❑ My sleep is greatly disturbed (3 to 5 hours sleepless).
- ❑ My sleep is completely disturbed (5 to 7 hours sleepless).

Recreation/Sports (Indicate Sport If Appropriate
_____)
- ❑ I am able to engage in all my recreational/sports activities without increased symptoms.
- ❑ I am able to engage in all my recreational/sports activities with some increased symptoms.
- ❑ I am able to engage in most, but not all of my usual recreational/sports activities because of increased symptoms.
- ❑ I am able to engage in a few of my usual recreational/sports activities because of my increased symptoms.
- ❑ I can hardly do any recreational/sports activities because of increased symptoms.
- ❑ I cannot do any recreational/sports activities at all.

Acuity
(answer on initial visit)
- ❑ How many days ago did onset/injury occur? ____ days

Stairs
- ❑ I can walk stairs comfortably without a rail.
- ❑ I can walk stairs comfortably, but with a crutch, cane, or rail.
- ❑ I can walk more than one flight of stairs, but with pain or weakness.
- ❑ I can walk less than one flight of stairs.
- ❑ I can manage only a single step or curb.
- ❑ I am unable to manage even a step or curb.

Uneven Ground
- ❑ I can walk normally on uneven ground without loss of balance or using a cane or crutches.
- ❑ I can walk on uneven ground, but with loss of balance or with the use of a cane or crutches.
- ❑ I have to walk very carefully on uneven ground without using a cane or crutches.
- ❑ I have to walk very carefully on uneven ground even when using a cane or crutches.
- ❑ I have to walk very carefully on uneven ground and require physical assistance to manage it.
- ❑ I am unable to walk on uneven ground.

Standing
- ❑ I can stand as long as I want without pain.
- ❑ I can stand as long as I want, but it gives me extra pain.
- ❑ Pain prevents me from standing for more than 1 hour.
- ❑ Pain prevents me from standing for more than 30 minutes.
- ❑ Pain prevents me from standing for more than 10 minutes.
- ❑ Pain prevents me from standing at all.

Squatting
- ❑ I can squat fully without the use of my arms for support.
- ❑ I can squat fully, but with pain or using my arms for support.
- ❑ I can squat $3/4$ of my normal depth, but less than fully.
- ❑ I can squat $1/2$ of my normal depth, but < $3/4$.
- ❑ I can squat $1/4$ of my normal depth, but < $1/2$.
- ❑ I am unable to squat any distance due to pain or weakness.

Sitting
- ❑ I can sit in any chair as long as I like.
- ❑ I can only sit in my favorite chair as long as I like.
- ❑ Pain prevents me sitting more than 1 hour.
- ❑ Pain prevents me sitting more than $1/2$ hour.
- ❑ Pain prevents me sitting more than 10 minutes.
- ❑ Pain prevents me from sitting at all.

Pain Index
Please indicate how much pain you feel at this time on the scale below

|_____|
No Pain   Worst Pain Imaginable

——— **PLEASE COMPLETE ON LAST VISIT ONLY** ———

Improvement Index ***Please indicate the amount of improvement you have made since the beginning of your physical therapy treatment on the scale below.***

|_____|
No Improvement   Complete Recovery

Work Status
1. No lost work time
2. Return to work without restriction
3. Return to work with modification
4. Have not returned to work
5. Not employed outside the home
Work days lost because of condition: ____ days

Adapted from Therapeutic Associates Outcome System. Therapeutic Associates, Inc. 15060 Ventura Blvd., Suite 240, Sherman Oaks, CA 91403-2426.

to accurate diagnosis of lower quadrant symptoms. Positive test results for the lumbar clearing examination can indicate a need for a more thorough lumbar or sacroiliac joint examination. It is not unusual to have symptoms from both the lumbar and hip region complicating the examination and treatment of patients with LQ dysfunction.

Other Clearing Tests

The practitioner should examine and evaluate associated regions. Although the hip may be the source of symptoms, it is common for multiple regions to be involved, particularly in patients with long-standing impairments, activity limitations and participation restrictions. A thorough examination of all involved regions permits the clinician to develop an integrated and comprehensive plan of care. For example, impairments of the pelvic floor may affect function of the hip. Screening for pelvic floor dysfunction can alert the practitioner to any associated pelvic floor conditions (see Chapter 18).

Visceral involvement or serious disease or disorders should be excluded. Pain in the hip and pelvic region can also result from visceral sources (see Appendix 1). A thorough history and physical examination and evaluation can alert the practitioner to visceral involvement or serious disease or pathology.

The hip must be excluded as the source of symptoms experienced in other regions. Because the hip is largely innervated at the L3–L4 level, hip pathology occasionally causes pain to be referred to the knee.[19,20] This is well documented in children, in whom any examination for knee pain must include a hip examination,[21] but this must not be forgotten as a source of knee pain in the adult. A patient of any age complaining of knee pain without apparent knee pathology or impairments should have the hip examined as a potential source of pain.

Gait and Balance

Gait evaluation is an essential component of the examination of a person with a hip dysfunction. Analysis of gait should include observation of the hip along with the rest of the kinetic chain about all three planes of motion during each critical event in gait (e.g., initial contact, loading response, midstance, terminal stance, and swing). Of particular importance are the relationship of pelvic and hip motion (i.e., amount of lateral pelvic tilt and hip adduction [Trendelenburg sign; see Fig. 19-5]) and the relationship of

hip and lower extremity motion (i.e., hip medial rotation, tibial medial rotation, and foot pronation). Because the hip functions interdependently with other regions in the body, the relationship of distal and proximal segments to the hip must also be evaluated.

Video analysis can assist in this complex examination procedure, because the video can be taken from any angle and can be viewed in slow motion to allow precise observation of the components of gait. Hypotheses can be generated about the cause of any observed gait deviation that can be confirmed or negated as a result of the additional data collected.

Balance tests are often included in hip examinations because of the high incidence of falls resulting in hip injury and fracture. Balance testing should identify intrinsic (i.e., related to the individual) and extrinsic (i.e., associated with environmental factors) factors related to the risk of falling.

Low-tech balance assessments can identify risk factors for falls.[22] Strong correlations have been found among performance-based measures and fall risk, as well as between performance-based measures and self-report measures. Five variables are significantly related to fall risk[22]:

1. Berg Balance Scale score[23]
2. Dynamic Gait Index score[24]
3. Balance Self-Perceptions Test score[25]
4. History of imbalance
5. Type of assistive device used for ambulation

High-tech, computerized, force-platform balance devices commonly measure the ability to maintain the center of pressure within the base of support against progressive perturbations. This information is highly objective and is often used to track progress in developing postural balance.

Joint Mobility and Integrity

Arthrokinematic motions are relatively limited at the hip joint in comparison to osteokinematic motions. Arthrokinematic tests of the hip should include: lateral/medial translation, distraction and compression, and anteroposterior/posteroanterior glides.[26] The quantity of motion, the end feel, and the presence/location of pain should be noted. Tests for joint integrity should assess for joint stability and pain provocation. Lee has developed arthrokinetic tests for joint stability at the hip. These tests are described in Table 19-2.[26]

Muscle Performance

Impairments in muscle performance can result from numerous sources, and tests of muscle performance combined with results of other tests should attempt to determine the presence and cause of reduced muscle performance. The following discussion highlights specific types of muscle performance testing procedures used to diagnose the presence and source of impairment of muscle performance.

Specific *manual muscle testing* (MMT) of muscles surrounding the hip joint can provide information regarding muscle performance capability of each muscle or fiber direction of a single muscle (e.g., anterior versus posterior gluteus medius).[27,28] Comprehensive MMT of the hip musculature also can determine the relationship of muscle performance capability of synergist and antagonist musculature around the

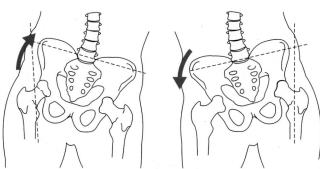

A Trendelenburg   **B** Compensated Trendelenburg

FIGURE 19-5. Trendelenburg sign. (A) Positive Trendelenburg sign with lateral pelvic tilt and hip adduction. (B) Compensated Trendelenburg sign with lateral pelvic tilt and hip abduction.

TABLE 19-2 Hip Arthrokinetic Tests of Stability

TEST	INDICATION	DESCRIPTION
Proprioception/ arthrokinetic stability	Tests integrated neuromuscular function	Patient standing in front of plumb line, shifts weight to stand on one leg with eyes closed. Examiner observes the degree of lateral shift of the center of gravity from the plumb line. Bilateral comparison is made.
Torque test	Global tests of passive stability and pain provocation. Intends to stress all the ligaments simultaneously.	Patient in supine, ipsilateral femur is extended until anterior rotation of the inominate begins. The femur is medially rotated to end range. Apply a slow steady posterolateral force along the line of the neck of the femur.*
Inferior band of the iliofemoral ligament	Differentiates inferior band of iliofemoral ligament	If passive femoral extension elicits pain, this ligament may be the etiologic factor.
Iliotrochanteric band of the iliofemoral ligament	Differentiates iliofemoral ligament	Patient is positioned as in the torque test, but the femur is adducted and laterally rotated. The same force is applied as in the torque test.**
Pubofemoral ligament	Differentiates the pubofemoral ligament	Patient is positioned as in the torque test, but the femur is abducted and fully laterally rotated. The same force is applied as in the torque test.**
Ischiofemoral ligament	Differentiates the ischiofemoral ligament	With the patient in supine, the ipsilateral femur is slightly extended, abducted, and fully medially rotated. The same force is applied as in the torque test.**

*If this test is painless, the subsequent differentiating tests are not required.

**If pain is elicited, this ligament may be an etiological factor.

Adapted from Lee D. The Pelvic Girdle. Churchill Livingstone, 1999:103–104.

---

hip (e.g., posterior gluteus medius versus tensor fascia lata (TFL) as hip abductors). Essential muscles to test include:

1. Gluteus medius
2. Gluteus minimus
3. Psoas
4. Deep hip lateral rotators
5. Gluteus maximus
6. Hamstrings
7. Quadriceps
8. Tensor fascia lata

Positional strength testing can determine the length-tension properties of the relevant muscle (see Chapter 5). It is often of interest to the examiner to determine length-associated changes in muscles within a synergy. Management of a muscle functioning weakly resulting from length-associated changes is different from a weak muscle resulting from strain or disuse. For example, a lengthened posterior gluteus medius with positional weakness should be carefully strengthened in the short range (i.e., abduction, extension, lateral rotation) and isolated from the relatively short and strong tensor fascia lata (abduction, flexion, medial rotaton). Stretching of the antagonist may be recommended,[29] but is often accomplished with specific strengthening of the affected muscle. In this case, strengthening the gluteus medius in extension and lateral rotation will elongate the anterior portion of the TFL.

Selective tissue tension tests combine active and passive range of motion (ROM) with resisted tests of muscles around the hip joint complex. Results of these tests can assist the examiner in the differential diagnosis of a contractile versus non-contractile lesion.[30] The major muscle groups (i.e., hip flexion, extension, abduction, adduction, and rotation) should be tested one by one if a contractile lesion is suspected. Careful positioning of additional resisted tests can identify which synergist is at fault. For example, if the hip flexor group is implicated, it is possible through careful positioning to further differentiate the TFL from iliopsoas.

If a selective tissue tension test is positive, interpretation of the *resisted test* can indicate the severity of tissue lesion. Table 25-1 in Chapter 25 explains diagnostic findings with respect to resisted tests.

Resisted tests can also screen for a neurologic cause of reduced force production, particularly in reference to the fatigability of the muscle being tested. Hip musculature is innervated by the lumbar and sacral plexus; consequently, low back dysfunction often results in neurologic weakness around the hip. In addition, numerous peripheral nerves can be involved in nerve entrapment syndromes around the hip, which can result in motor changes (see Table 19-3 for an overview of these syndromes). This topic will be discussed in more detail in a subsequent section of this chapter). Careful neuroconductive screening can diagnose peripheral versus spinal nerve-mediated weakness.

Pain and Inflammation

Examination for pain and inflammation is done concurrently with other tests to determine the source. Inflammation is difficult to examine in the hip joint, because it is deep within the pelvis and cannot be readily palpated. Positive findings for a capsular pattern[30] (defined in Display 19-2) of hip mobility and end-feel assessment (i.e., pain before limitation of motion is reached) indicate former or active inflammation.

Examination of the pain level should be incorporated into the subjective and objective portion of the examination. The patient should answer questions regarding pain level by using a visual, numeric, or verbal analog scale over a 24-hour cycle in relation to specific activities and in general.[31] During the physical examination, the patient should be questioned about the onset, location, and intensity of pain with respect to each test performed.

The specific source of symptoms may not be diagnosed without additional tests that are beyond the scope of physical therapy practice (i.e., radiologic, electrodiagnostic, and laboratory studies). However, the mechanical contribution to the

TABLE 19-3 **Regional Approach to Nerve Entrapment Syndromes**

REGION	SUBREGION	NERVE
Anterior	Inguinal	Ilioinguinal nerve
		Genitofemoral nerve
		Iliohypogastric nerve
		T11/T12/L1 nerve root
	Suprapubic	Genitofemoral nerve
		Iliohypogastric nerve
		T11/T12/L1 nerve root
	Thigh	Lateral femoral cutaneous nerve of thigh
		Genitofemoral nerve
		Femoral nerve
		Obturator nerve
Lateral	Buttock	Ilioinguinal nerve
		Iliohypogastric nerve
		Lateral cutaneous nerve of thigh
		T12 nerve root
	Thigh	Lateral cutaneous nerve of thigh
		Posterior cutaneous nerve of thigh
Posterior	Buttock	Posterior rami of the lumbar, sacral, and coccygeal nerves
		Iliohypogastric nerve
		Lateral cutaneous nerve of thigh
		Posterior cutaneous nerve of thigh
		T12
	Thigh	Lateral cutaneous nerve of thigh
		Inferior medial and lateral cutaneous nerves
		Posterior cutaneous nerve of thigh

development or fortitude of the symptoms can be diagnosed through careful examination and evaluation of the impairments that contribute to increased biomechanical stress to the hip joint.

Posture and Movement

Specific LP and lower quadrant alignment should be examined in all three planes. Hypotheses can be developed regarding the contribution of faulty alignments at the ankle, foot, knee, and LP regions to the alignment of the hip. The practitioner can also create hypothesis regarding muscles that are too long based on joint position, but muscle length testing is indicated to determine whether muscles are too short and the extent to which muscles are lenghtened. Initial screening for LLD should be performed by evaluating:

1. iliac crest heights
2. spine, pelvic, femur, tibia, and foot alignments
3. bony landmarks of the pelvis, knee, and ankle

In addition, the specific alignment about all three planes of motion, of the spine, pelvis, hip, tibia, and foot/ankle complex should be noted during simple ADLs such as squatting,

ascending and descending stairs, and sit-to-stand transfers. Hypothesis regarding the interrelationships of the lower limb segments can be generated (i.e., foot pronation, genu valgum, femur medial rotation, and lateral pelvic tilt on the short side).

Range of Motion and Muscle Length

ROM testing of the hip joint includes several assessments. *Quick tests* are functional movements that are used to ascertain the patient's willingness and ability to move and the requisite extent of the examination to follow. Such tests for the hip include flexing the hip and knee while putting the foot on a standard step height, forward bending, squatting, and sitting with one leg crossed over the other.

Active and passive open chain osteokinematic ROM should be carefully measured. It is important to determine osteokinetic mobility of the hip joint along the continuum of hypermobility to hypomobility about all three axes of motion by carefully stabilizing the spine and pelvis during passive ROM examination techniques.

Qualitative assessment of active and passive ROM combined with clinical reasoning can supply specific diagnostic information:

- A firm overpressure applied to a motion is used to exclude or diagnose joint pathology. Overpressure can also be used to determine the hip end-feel and therefore the structures providing the barrier to further motion.
- Assessment of the sequence of pain and limitation can grade the irritability of the condition and guide the intensity of treatment.[30]
- The pattern of restriction indicates the presence of a capsular pattern (see Display 19-2). This is an indication of joint inflammation.[30]

DISPLAY 19-2
Established Capsular Pattern[30]

1. 50 to 55 degrees of limitation of femoral abduction
2. 0 degrees of femoral medial rotation from neutral
3. 90 degrees of limitation of femoral flexion
4. 10 to 30 degrees of limitation of femoral extension
5. Femoral lateral rotation and adduction are fully maintained

- The combined results of passive and active movement testing can implicate a contractile or inert structure.[30] For example, the findings of passive movement painful in one direction and active movement painful in another implicate a contractile structure.

Tests of muscular extensibility are also important in assessing ROM of the hip. Common extensibility tests include determining the length of several muscles:

- Medial and lateral hamstrings (hamstring length should be examined as a group and individually as medial and lateral hamstrings)
- Hip flexors (hip flexor length should be assessed individually for the iliopsoas, rectus femoris, and TFL)
- Hip adductors/abductors (particularly TFL)
- Hip rotators

The examiner should assess for a lack of extensibility and for excessive extensibility. A hypothesis should be developed regarding what impact a lack of extensibility or excessive extensibility will have on the function of the hip and related regions.

Work (Job/School/Play), Community, and Leisure Integration or Reintegration (Including Instrumental Activities of Daily Living)

Although measures of physiologic impairments are important for diagnosis, prognosis, and treatment planning, functional ability and quality of life are better indicators of outcome.[32] Functional ability can be measured directly through observation of functional tasks or by the use of self-report measures. Display 19-1 illustrates a general self-report measure with a specific section devoted to the hip. The Harris Hip Function Scale is another, but it is specific to degenerative conditions of the hip (Display 19-3). The Harris Hip Function Scale was originally designed to assess patient status after the onset of traumatic arthritis of the hip.[33] This scale combines a patient's report of pain and his or her capacity for ambulation and self-care. These tasks account for 91% of the score, and deformity and hip ROM account for 9% of the score. The advantages of this scale are that it is heavily weighted toward function, is easy to administer, and is familiar to most clinicians. The Harris Hip Function Scale has been used as the gold standard in a number of studies and has been shown to be reliable with an ICC of 0.82 to 0.91. Other measures include the Hip Osteoarthitis Outcomes Scale and the Lower Extremity Functional Scale (LEFS). These measures are examined in more detail by Binkley et al.[34]

Special Tests

Numerous special tests are used to confirm or negate symptoms or suspected diagnoses of the hip. For the commonly used special tests discussed in this section, specific information regarding the technique of application can be found in the related references.

The Trendelenburg test is used to evaluate the functional force or torque capability of the hip abductor muscle group. During gait, the patient may exhibit a positive Trendelenburg sign (see Fig. 19-6C) or compensated Trendelenburg sign (see Fig. 19-6B).[25] However, other gait deviations of the hip indicate hip abductor torque impairment, such as excessive hip medial rotation, pelvic counter-rotation, or excessive lateral pelvic shift. These other gait deviations, although not traditionally called Trendelenburg signs, are also indicators of reduced hip abductor muscle performance and are particularly related to positional weakness of the gluteus medius.

If the examiner suspects that one of a patient's legs may be shorter than the other, specific tests are indicated to determine whether a structural or functional LLD exists. Radiographs or other imaging techniques should be used when accuracy is critical. Ultrasound measurement of LLD offers a reliable, noninvasive, and easily performed method.[35] This technique is superior to clinical measuring methods and radiologic examinations.[36] In general, although imaging techniques are considered to be the most accurate method for determining LLD, they are costly, time consuming, and, in the case of radiographs and computed tomography (CT), the patient is exposed to radiation. As a result, alternative clinical methods have been developed. Two methods have emerged over the years: (a) an "indirect method" performed in standing using lift blocks under the short leg and visually examining the level pelvis, termed the "iliac crest palpation and book correction" method (ICPBC)[37,38] and (b) a "direct method" done in supine measuring the distance of fixed bony landmarks with a measuring tape. Two commonly used tape measure methods include measuring the distance between (a) the anterior inferior iliac spine (ASIS) and the lateral malleolus[37] and (b) the ASIS and the medial malleolus.[39] There is still disagreement regarding the validity and reliability of both the clinical methods. The average of two measures between the ASIS and the medial malleolus and the ICPBC method both appear to have acceptable validity and reliability when used as a screening tool.[38,40]

The clinical determination of the angle of torsion is commonly called the Trochanteric Prominence Angle Test (TPAT) (Fig. 19-7).[41] The developers of this test demonstrated that this measurement correlates well with intraoperative measurements, and it is considered to be more accurate than radiographic techniques.[41] Yet, a more recent study concluded that clinical application of the TPAT is limited by both the variable anatomy of the proximal femur and examiner difficulties related to the soft tissues surrounding the hip joint.[42] In the hands of a single, experienced clinician, the TPAT performed poorly, underestimating or overestimating the femoral anteversion by more than 5 to 10 degrees.[42] Nonetheless, this method may be acceptable if the goal of the test is to screen for the presence of abnormal angles of torsion. If accuracy is desired, two- or three-dimensional CT imaging is thought to be the most precise method for determining femoral anteversion.[43] Differences in hip rotation ROM can also indicate abnormal femoral torsion. To predict an abnormally high anteversion angle (above mean +2 standard deviations [SD]), the difference between medial and lateral rotation (measured in hip extension) must be 45 degrees or more, whereas an abnormally low anteversion angle (lower than mean −2 SD) could be predicted when lateral rotation is at least 50-degrees higher than medial rotation.[44] Other clinical diagnostic tests have been studied as well. The FABER or Patrick test, where the patient is supine with the tested leg in flexion, abduction, and external rotation. The FABER test has been discussed as an appropriate test to detect intra-articular injuries in the athletic population. The FADIR (flexion, adduction, forced internal rotation in 90 degrees of hip flexion) is a commonly used test for FAI. A review of common special tests for the hip can be found in the text by Konin et al.[45]

DISPLAY 19-3
Harris Hip Function Scale

(*Circle one in each group*)

Pain (44 points maximum)

None/ignores	44
Slight, occasional, no compromise in activity	40
Mild, no effect on ordinary activity, pain after unusual activity, uses aspirin	30
Moderate, tolerable, makes concessions, occasional codeine	20
Marked, serious limitations	10
Totally disabled	0

Function (47 points maximum)

Gait (*walking maximum distance*) (33 points maximum)

1. Limp:

None	11
Slight	8
Moderate	5
Unable to walk	0

2. Support:

None	11
Cane, long walks	7
Cane, full time	5
Crutch	4
Two canes	2
Two crutches	0
Unable to walk	0

3. Distance walked:

Unlimited	11
Six blocks	8
Two to three blocks	5
Indoors only	2
Bed and chair	0

Functional Activities (14 points maximum)

1. Stairs:

Normally	4
Normally with banister	2
Any method	1
Not able	0

2. Socks and tie shoes:

With ease	4
With difficulty	2
Unable	0

3. Sitting:

Any chair, 1 hour	5
High chair, ½ hour	3
Unable to sit ½ hour any chair	0

4. Enter public transport

Able to use public transportation	1
Not able to use public transportation	0

Absence of Deformity (*requires all four*) (4 points maximum)

1. Fixed adduction <10	4
2. Fixed internal rotation in extension <10	0
3. Leg length discrepancy <1¼ in	
4. Pelvic flexion contracture <30	

Range of Motion (5 points maximum)

Instructions

Record 10 degrees of fixed adduction as "–10 degrees abduction, adduction to 10 degrees"

Similarly, 10 degrees of fixed external rotation as "–10 degrees internal rotation, external rotation to 10 degrees"

Similarly, 10 degrees of fixed external rotation with 10 degrees further external rotation as "–10 degrees internal rotation, external rotation to 20 degrees"

	Range	Index Factor	Index Value*
Permanent flexion			
A. Flexion to	____°		
(0–45 degrees)		1.0	
(45–90 degrees)		0.6	
(90–120 degrees)		0.3	
(120–140 degrees)		0.0	
B. Abduction to	____°		
(0–15 degrees)		0.8	
(15–30 degrees)		0.3	
(30–60 degrees)		0.0	
C. Adduction to	____°		
(0–15 degrees)		0.2	
(15–60 degrees)		0.0	
D. External rotation in extension to	____°		
(0–30 degrees)		0.4	
(30–60 degrees)		0.0	
E. Internal rotation in extension to	____°		
(0–60 degrees)		0.0	

*Index value = range × index factor

Total index value (A + B + C + D + E)	_____
Total range of motion points (multiply total index value × 0.05)	_____
Pain points:	_____
Function points:	_____
Absence of Deformity points:	_____
Range of Motion points:	_____
Total points (100 points maximum)	_____

<70 = poor, 70–80 = fair, 80–90 = good, 90–100 = excellent

Harris WH. Traumatic arthritis of the hip after dislocation and acetabular fractures: Treatment by mold arthroplasty. J Bone Jt Surg 1969;51A:737–755.

THERAPEUTIC EXERCISE INTERVENTIONS FOR COMMON PHYSIOLOGIC IMPAIRMENTS

After examination and evaluation of the hip and all related regions, the clinician should have a thorough understanding of the activity limitations affecting the patient and the related impairments. The diagnosis and prognosis are formulated, and an intervention is planned.

The decision to treat any impairment lies in its relationship to the activity limitation and participation restriction. Prioritization of impairments is critical to effective and efficient intervention. Exercise intervention should be kept as functional as possible. However, if the impairment is profound, specific exercise may be necessary to improve the level of performance and motor control until it can be incorporated into a functional activity. Specific exercise and functional activity examples are provided in the discussion of exercise intervention for common impairments of body functions affecting the hip.

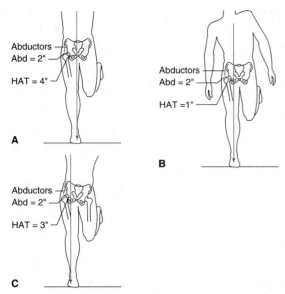

FIGURE 19-6. (A) In right unilateral stance, the weight of the head, arms, and trunk (HAT) act 4 in from the right hip, producing an adduction torque around the right hip joint. The abductors, acting 2 in. from the right hip joint, generate a large force to produce an abduction torque sufficient to counterbalance the torque produced by HAT. (B) When the trunk is laterally flexed toward a stance limb, the moment arm of the HAT is substantially reduced, whereas that of the abductors remains unchanged. The result is a substantially diminished torque from the HAT and a corresponding decreased hip abductor force to counterbalance the HAT torque. This is called a **compensated Trendelenburg sign**. Patients will use this gait pattern to reduce the joint reaction force and thus alleviate pain. (C) The pelvis drops on the opposite side of the stance limb when the abductor force cannot counterbalance the torque produced by HAT. This is called a **positive Trendelenburg sign**, and is used as a compensation for hip abductor weakness.

IMPAIRED MUSCLE PERFORMANCE

The section on kinetics describes the powerful forces required from the musculature surrounding the hip joint for accomplishing ADLs. The force-generating capability of any muscle around the hip joint may be compromised for one of the following reasons:

- Neurologic pathology (e.g., peripheral nerve, nerve root, neuromuscular disease)
- Muscle strain

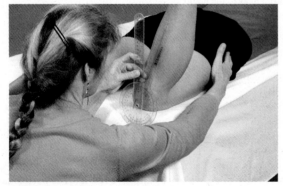

FIGURE 19-7. TPAT test. The TPAT presumes that when the subject is prone, with the hip in extension, and the most prominent portion of the greater trochanter is rotated into maximum lateral position, the femoral neck will be parallel to the floor. The angle of rotation of the shank segment relative to vertical at this point reflects the overall angle of torsion.

- Altered length-tension relationships (either resulting from anatomic or physiologic impairments)
- General weakness from disuse resulting from muscle imbalance, general deconditioning, or reduced muscle torque production for a specific performance level (e.g., high-level athlete in training)
- Pain and inflammation

Endurance impairments at the hip must be thought of in light of the tremendous force-generating requirements of the gluteal musculature during functional activities. Endurance is required to meet the repetitious demands of walking, jogging, running, and so on. Proper synergy among all muscles involved in the gait cycle keeps the intensity of muscle action at an aerobic level. When one muscle in a synergy group reduces its function, it imposes greater demands on other muscles, potentially rendering them anaerobic and therefore far less energy efficient,[46] or causes compensatory strategies, such as reliance on the iliotibial band (ITB) for stability or a compensatory Trendelenburg pattern to reduce the need for muscle force to keep the center of mass within the base of support. Dosage parameters depend on the performance level desired by the individual (e.g., walking 50 ft without pain, running a marathon in the best time possible), with an emphasis on high repetitions instead of maximal force production.

Neurologic Pathology

To develop the appropriate plan of care, it must be determined whether the source of the neurologically-induced weakness is a lower motor neuron lesion which affects nerve fibers traveling from the anterior horn of the spinal cord to the relevant muscle(s) (e.g., nerve root, peripheral nerve) or upper motor neuron lesion which affects the neural pathway above the anterior horn cell or motor nuclei of the cranial nerves (e.g., primary lateral sclerosis).

If the clinician has determined that the cause is lower motor neuron in origin, it must then be determined whether the pathology is at the level of the nerve root or in a peripheral nerve. A dysfunction at the level of the lumbar spine can induce nerve root pathology that can manifest as weakness of the muscles innervated by the affected segmental levels.[47] The clinician must thoroughly screen the LP region to confirm or negate the hypothesis of spinal influence on the reduced force-generating capability of muscles surrounding the pelvic girdle.

Numerous peripheral nerves surround the hip. The section on Nerve Entrapment Syndromes will discuss the potential peripheral nerve injuries affecting the hip region.

After a thorough examination and evaluation process, the neurologically-induced hip joint weakness must be treated. Whether the source of the neurologic involvement is from the nerve root or peripheral nerve, the origin of the problem must be treated appropriately for the affected muscle torque production to improve.

Despite alleviation of neurologic factors, weakness contributing to activity limitation may still exist. The level of weakness depends on the degree and duration of neurologic involvement. Display 19-4 provides a clinical example to illustrate this point.

Muscle Strain

Force-generating capability may be compromised by an injury to the muscle in the form of muscle strain.

DISPLAY 19-4
Case Example of Neurologic Factors Contributing to Weakness at the Hip

Case presentation:
A 13-year-old gymnast has had a 5-month complaint of postero-lateral hip pain. At the time of her initial evaluation, she was diagnosed with a gluteus medius strain. Appropriate treatment of her gluteus medius strain did not improve her condition after 3 months. At that time, her physician performed a thorough lumbar screen. Radiologic reports indicated a grade II L5–S1 spondylolisthesis with slight L5 nerve root compression occurring with end-range lumbar extension. As a result of the additional diagnosis of spondylolisthesis, she was treated with lumbosacral bracing and exercise to correct impairments related to the spine instability. During the next 3 months, her hip pain began to resolve, although only after a dual program was developed for treatment of the spondylolisthesis and gluteus medius strain.

Explanation of outcome:
the L5 nerve root innervates the gluteal musculature. Irritation of the nerve root at the unstable spinal level could interrupt the motor function of the L5 nerve root, resulting in neurologically induced weakness of the gluteus medius.[47] Without full afferent input into the gluteus medius, it may be vulnerable to strain,

especially at the level of this patient's activity. Effective healing could not occur until afferent input into the gluteus medius was fully restored, which could not occur until the stability of L5–S1 segmental level was sufficient for her activity level. After the L5–S1 level became more stable and normal afferent input was restored to the affected musculature, a gradual conditioning program for the gluteus medius muscle was necessary to restore muscle performance to the functional level desired by this patient.

Sample exercise program:
An example of a progressive strengthening program for the gluteus medius is illustrated in Self-Management 19-1: Gluteus Medius Strength Progression. This progression begins in prone for the muscle with a 3/5 or lower MMT grade[27] and progresses to sidelying with increasing lever arms to increase the load on the muscle. As muscle performance improves, transition to functional positions and movements can be introduced. Self-Management 19-2: Walk Stance Progression can be progressed to a leap, with the focus on controlling frontal and transverse plane forces at the hip on landing.

Hamstring muscle strains are among the most common muscle injuries in athletes.[48,49] Factors causing hamstring strain include poor flexibility, inadequate muscle strength or endurance, dyssynergic contraction, inadequate warm-up, and return to activity before complete recovery.[48,50–52] Sahrmann proposes hamstring overuse as another etiology for hamstring strain.[53] The hamstrings participate in force couples around the lumbopelvic-hip complex, contributing to posterior pelvic rotation, hip extension, and, indirectly, hip medial and lateral rotation. During gait, all portions of the hamstring are active from midswing to early loading response (see Table 19-4 in website). From midswing to initial contact, the role of the hamstrings is to decelerate flexion of the hip. At initial contact and loading response, the biceps femoris is thought to decelerate tibial medial rotation that occurs with foot pronation.[46] Because of the multiple roles of the hamstrings, it is

quite possible to sustain an overuse injury. Display 19-5 describes possible mechanisms of hamstring overuse.

Treatment of a hamstring strain should follow the guidelines for tissue healing outlined in Chapter 11. However, for the hamstrings to fully recover, treatment must be focused on the *cause* of the strain. If the cause of the strain is overuse, the load must be reduced on the hamstrings during meaning-

SELF-MANAGEMENT 19-1 *Stomach-Lying Hip Extension*

Purpose:	To strengthen the seat muscles, train you to move your hip independent of your pelvis and spine, and stretch the muscles on the front of your hip
Start Position:	Lie on your stomach on a firm surface, and place ____ pillows under your torso.
Movement Technique:	• Preset your spine and pelvic position by activating your inner core, abdominals, and gently squeezing your seat muscle. Try to keep your thigh muscles relaxed.
	• Use your abdominal muscles to control the position of the pelvis. Think of keeping your pubic bone rotated toward your ribs.
	• Use your seat muscles to *barely* lift your thigh off the floor.
	• Return your thigh to the floor and repeat the lift with the other leg.

Dosage
Sets/repetitions _____
Frequency _____

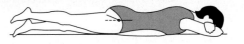

DISPLAY 19-5
Mechanisms of Hamstring Overuse

- Subtle imbalances in force or torque production and endurance between the hamstrings and gluteus maximus may lead to excess demand on the hamstrings to decelerate hip flexion during late midswing and hip medial rotation at initial contact.
- Significant forefoot varus (see Chapter 21), combined with length-tension alterations and reduced force or torque production of the deep hip lateral rotators, may lead to overuse of the biceps femoris. Without optimal foot mechanics and hip lateral rotator function, the biceps femoris load is exaggerated because of the increased role it must play in decelerating femoral and tibial medial rotation at initial contact through the midstance phase of gait.
- Underuse of the oblique abdominal muscles may lead to overuse of the hamstrings because of the increased role they must play to exert a posterior rotational force on the lumbopelvic region.

ful functional activities. Improving the muscle performance and neuromuscular control of the *underused synergists* and correcting for any biomechanical factors (e.g., foot orthotic to correct for forefoot varus) constitute a recommended course of action.

Two commonly underused synergists involved in the cause of hamstring overuse strain are the gluteus maximus and deep hip lateral rotators. Examples of therapeutic intervention for progressive strengthening of the gluteus maximus and deep hip lateral rotators are shown in Self-Management 19-1: Stomach-Lying Hip Extension and Figure 19-14. The exercises illustrated are considered specific, nonfunctional exercises. There are two reasons to prescribe this type of exercise instead of more functionally relevant exercise. First, the force-generating capability of the muscle is inadequate to allow it to fully participate in a functional task. Second, the kinesthetic awareness of the muscle may be such that the patient's ability to selectively recruit it during a functional task may be insufficient.

After force-generating capability and kinesthetic awareness of the proximal posterior hip musculature are improved sufficiently, graded functional activities can be initiated. Self-Management 19-2: Walk Stance Progression and Self-Management 19-3: Step-Up, Step-Down illustrate functional progressions of specific exercises that use the gluteus maximus, quadriceps, deep hip lateral rotators in sagittal-plane kinetic chain activities. Other functional exercises shown to activate this musculature to at least 40% of MVC include single limb squat and the lunge (forward, sideways).[54] The clinician must be concerned with the recruitment of the underused synergists during each exercise. Subtle changes in lower quarter kinematics can affect muscle recruitment strategies.[55] For example, keeping the trunk more vertical during a step activity can diminish the use of gluteus maximus relative to the quadriceps (Figure 19-8A) versus inclination of the trunk toward a more horizontal position can increase the use of gluteus maximus relative to the quadriceps (Fig. 19-8B)[56]. Display 19-6 describes the role of various muscles during these exercises.

Overstretch can also be a contributing factor to muscle strain. For example, the gluteus medius muscle is susceptible to strain resulting from length-associated changes, which can occur in an individual with an apparent LLD and resulting iliac crest height asymmetry.[53] On the side of the high iliac crest, the hip is adducted, and the gluteus medius is in a chronically lengthened position. As a result, this muscle is at risk for strain. Treatment of this type of strain must involve exercises that resolve the contributing factors to the LLD in conjunction with treatment to improve the length-tension properties, muscle performance, and neuromuscular control of the gluteus medius. In the early stages of recovery, taping (Fig. 19-9) can unload the muscle and support it at an appropriate length, providing a positive environment for healing.

 SELF-MANAGEMENT 19-2 *Walk Stance Progression*

Purpose:	To teach the correct pattern to move your body over your hip, teach a good strategy to balance on one leg, and strengthen your hip and other lower extremity muscles to support your lower extremities in good alignment for activities you perform in standing.

Level I

Start Position:
- Stand in a staggered stance position with your involved leg in front of your uninvolved leg.
- Check the position of your feet, knees, hips, and pelvis.
- Feet should be facing straight ahead with arches in neutral.
- Knees should be facing straight ahead without turning in or out excessively (if you have anteverted or retroverted hips, the knee position may be modified).
- Hips and pelvis should be facing forward and level.

Movement Technique:
- Slowly bend your front hip and knee while leaning slightly toward your front leg.
- Pivot at your hips and lean your trunk forward so that it is parallel to the line of your lower leg. Do not round or arch your back.
- Do not bend your knee further than the length of your foot. Hold this position for 10 seconds.
- Activate your inner core (Note: activate your inner core in preparation for all the levels of this exercise).

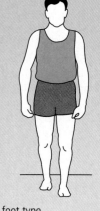

- Turn on your deep hip lateral rotators by keeping your knee centered over your feet (do not let your knee turn inward).
- If your arch drops excessively, hold the arch of your foot up while you keep your big toe down. If your arch remains high and rigid, allow it to roll inward slightly. Your PT will clarify the movement of your foot based on your foot type.

Level 1

Dosage
Sets/repetitions _____
Frequency_____

Level II: Single limb stance

Start Position:
- The start position for this exercise is the end position of level I.

Movement Technique
- Progress from the walk stance position by lifting your back heel upward as you straighten your front knee and hip (A).

(continued)

SELF-MANAGEMENT 19-2 *Walk Stance Progression (Continued)*

- Be sure your feet, knees, hips, pelvis, and spine are in good alignment.
- Hold this position for 3 seconds.
- Slowly bring your back thigh forward by bending the hip and knee (as if to take a step forward) (B).
- Balance for up to 30 seconds.

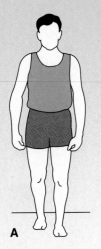

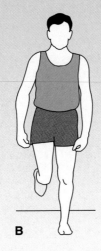

A   **B**

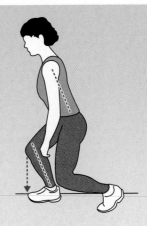

Level III

Dosage
   Sets/repetitions _____
   Frequency _____

Level IV: Lunge

Start Position

- Stand with both feet on the floor and weight equally distributed between both limbs.
- Take a step forward and watch your pelvis, hip, knee, ankle, and foot position as in level I. Do not let your back arch.
- This is a ballistic exercise. Be extra careful about your position.

Level II

Dosage
   Sets/repetitions _____
   Duration _____
   Frequency _____

Level III: Split Squat

Start Position
- Position yourself in a staggered stance with your involved leg forward.
- Lean toward your front limb as in Level I.
- Keeping your spine, pelvis, hips, knees, and ankles steady, slowly lower yourself until you see or feel your pelvis tilting or rotating out of the start position.
- The movement should be occurring at your hip and knee. Your front knee should only bend as far as the length of your foot. (Note: a good rule of thumb is to keep your lower leg bone parallel to your torso throughout the entire maneuver.)
- Most of your weight should be over your front limb; if you feel your back limb straining, shift your weight onto your front limb.
- Slowly rise upward while keeping your weight shifted forward.
- Repeat up and down while remaining in a forward position over your front foot.

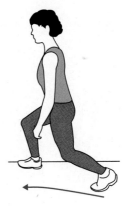

Level IV

Dosage
   Sets/repetitions _____
   Frequency _____

Severe strains may require use of a cane in the contralateral hand to unload the muscle enough to induce healing. Exercises to progressively strengthen the gluteus medius are depicted in Self-Management 19-4: Gluteus Medius Strength Progression and Self-Management 19-2. Other exercises shown to activate the Gluteus Medius include the lateral band walk (Fig. 19-10 A1, A2), single limb squat (Fig. 19-10B), single limb dead lift (Fig. 19-10C), hop (forward, sideways), and lunge (forward and sidways), though these are high level progressions and require 4–4+/5 gluteus medius strength.[54] When prescribing closed chain exercises, caution must be taken in ensuring proper kinematics. Of particular concern

SELF-MANAGEMENT 19-3 *Step-Up, Step-Down*

Purpose: To strengthen your spine, hip, knee, ankle, and foot muscles and to improve your balance in single limb stance

Step-Up

Start Position: Stand facing a step.

Movement Technique

- Lift your leg onto the step, keeping your thigh in midline and your pelvis level. Do not hike your pelvis while lifting your leg onto the step. This movment should take place only at the hip and knee.
- After your foot is on the step, check its position. The arch should be up with the big toe down.
- Lean toward the step, being sure that your knee is in line with your foot (note: this may vary if you have anteverted or retroverted hips) and your pelvis is level.
- Looking at your body from the side, a good rule of thumb is to flex your knee no further past the length of your foot and to keep your lower leg bone parallel to your torso throughout the entire step up and down maneuver.
- Step-up while keeping your pelvis level, knee over toes, and arch up. Be sure to lean into your hip, but do not let your pelvis tilt.
- Variation: You can stand to the side of a step and step-up sideways. This variation places more stress on your outside hip muscles. Be sure to keep your pelvis level.

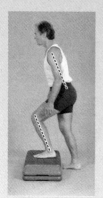 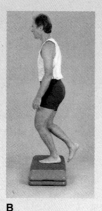

A   **B**

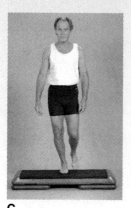

C

- Variation: You can step off the back of the step. Do not step down fully, but merely touch your toe on the floor and step back up again so as not to fully unload the weight of your body through the stance leg. This makes the stepping leg work harder. This variation places more stress on your quadriceps.

Dosage
Sets/repetitions _____
Resistance (step height) _____
Frequency _____

Step-Down

Start Position: Stand on a step that is higher than you can control during a step-down movement.

Movement

- Flex the foot of the leg you are stepping down with.
- Bend the hip and knee of the foot remaining on the step as you lower your flexed foot toward the floor.
- Lean forward so as to bend at your hip. Do not let your knee bend further than the length of your foot.
- Do not completely step down, but stop just short of the floor and hold this position for up to 10 seconds.
- Be sure that your pelvis is level, your knee over your toes (Note: this may vary if you have anteverted or retroverted hips), and your arch up as you lower your leg. Do not deviate from this position.
- Variation: You may need to use an external device to assist you in your balance

  ___ Hold a ski pole, dowel rod, or upside down broom in each hand.
  ___ Hold a ski pole, dowel rod, or upside down broom in the opposite hand from which you are balancing.
  ___ Hold a weight in the hand of the hip on which you are balancing.

- Variation: After you can balance well during the lowering phase, you can further challenge your balance by using arm movements. When you have lowered yourself as far as you can control, raise the arm on the same side or opposite side of the leg on which you are balancing.

  ___ Raise it up and down to the side.
  ___ Raise it up and down to the front.
  ___ Raise it toward and away from the midline of your body.

Dosage
Sets/repetitions _____
Assistance (amount of weight in hand) _____
Resistance (step height) _____
Frequency _____

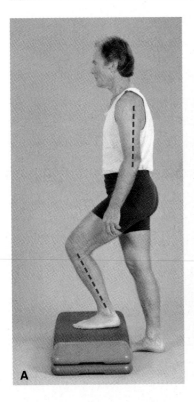 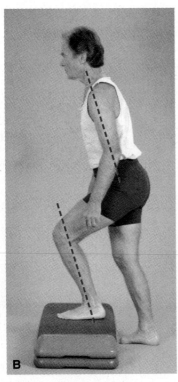

FIGURE 19-8. (A) Side view of step-up exercise with vertical trunk orientation, decreased hip flexion, and center of mass posterior to the axis of rotation of the hip and knee. Step-up from this start position promotes use of a hamstring and soleus strategy to pull the hip and knee into extension to raise the center of mass upward. Relative to the quadriceps and gluteus maximus recruitment, this position favors use of the quadriceps primarily because of the lack of hip flexion. (B) Side view of step-up exercise with good spine, hip, knee, and ankle/foot relationships. Note the forward inclination of the trunk. A good rule of thumb is to teach the exerciser to keep the trunk parallel to the tibia during the entire phase of vertical to lowering and the return motion. This will best ensure proper balance between the gluteus maximus, hamstrings, and quadriceps during closed chain activities.

are pelvic, femur, tibia, ankle/foot alignment and movement patterns to prevent further stretch to the gluteus medius (i.e., pelvic lateral tilt, femur adduction, femur medial rotation, excessive tibia medial rotation or foot pronation with knee and hip flexion).

Disuse and Deconditioning

Disuse and deconditioning of the hip joint musculature, particularly of the abductor muscles, is quite common. Disuse or deconditioning can result from injury or pathology affecting the hip and surrounding structures or from acquired movement patterns that promote disuse. For example, weakness in the gluteal musculature in hip joint OA is a common finding, but research has not determined whether it is the cause or the result of hip joint pathology.[57] Atrophy and pain both contribute to the decrease of muscle strength in hip OA.[58] Because hip muscles participate in gait, sit to stand, squatting, and ascending/descending stairs, weakness of hip muscles can affect the performance of basic ADLs.

It is reasonable to consider that acquired posture and movement habits can contribute to altered length-tension properties and disuse of the hip musculature. For example, a slightly high iliac crest, as commonly occurs in a handedness

---

DISPLAY 19-6
Role of Lower Extremity Muscles During Closed Chain Exercises

- The gluteus maximus muscle decelerates hip flexion in the lowering phase of the split squat, lunge, and step-down and accelerates hip extension during the rising phase of the split squat, lunge, and step-up.
- The quadriceps muscle decelerates knee flexion during the lowering phase of the split squat, lunge, and the step-down and accelerates knee extension during the rising phase.
- The deep hip lateral rotators are recruited to control hip medial rotation during all phases of each exercise.
- The posterior tibialis and peroneus longus muscles control foot pronation during the stance phase of each exercise, which assists in controlling tibial and femur medial rotation up the kinetic chain.

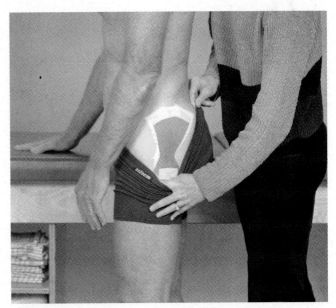

FIGURE 19-9. Taping to support a strained gluteus medius. This tape is best applied with the hip is biased in abduction and lateral rotation to prevent strain to the glutues medius.

SELF-MANAGEMENT 19-4 *Gluteus Medius Strength Progression*

Purpose: To strengthen the hip muscles that keep your hip and pelvis in good alignment when you walk (highest level of this exercise [level V] helps to stretch the band on the outside of the thigh)

Level I: Prone Hip Lift

Start position
- Lie on your stomach on a firm surface. Place ___ pillows under your torso as indicated in the illustration.
- Your legs should be in line with your hips and rotated *slightly* outward.

Movement Technique
- First you must activate your inner core plus abdominal muscles to stabilize your pelvis. Contract your abdominal muscles so that your pubic bone moves toward your ribs.
- Squeeze your buttock muscle.
- *Slightly* lift your leg and move it sideways through as much range as your hip allows. The indication that your hip has moved through its full available range is that your pelvis begins to tilt sideways and your spine sidebends. Do not move your hip any further after you feel your pelvis or spine move. Hold this position for 10 seconds.
- Return your hip to a start position.

Dosage
Sets/repetitions _____
Frequency _____

Level II: Prone Hip Lift With Elastic

Perform as in level I, but attach a ___ piece of elastic around your ankles.

Dosage
Sets/repetitions _____
Frequency _____

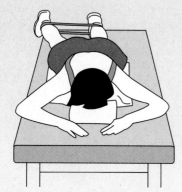

Level II: Prone hip abduction with elastic

Level III: Sidelying Hip Rotation

Start Position
- Lie on your uninvolved side, with your hips in full extension and knees bent to 90 degrees, Place ___ pillows between your knees.
- Be sure you are on your side, with your head and neck in line with your spine and your spine in neutral, not rotated forward or backward.

Movement Technique
- Keep your trunk still by activating your inner core and abdominal muscles. Slowly roll your hip backward (like opening a clam shell). This movement is very small. Your Physical therapist (PT) will assist you in feeling how subtle this movement is. Hold this position for 10 seconds.
- Slowly teturn to the start position.

Dosage
Sets/repetitions _____
Frequency _____

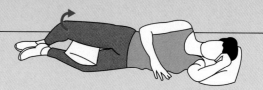

Level III: Sidelying hip lateral rotation

Level IV: Sidelying Knee Extension

Start Position
- As in level III.

Movement Technique
- Turn out your hip without letting your pelvis or spine tilt backward or forward by activating your inner core and abdominal muscles.
- Extend your knee fully. Hold this position for 10 seconds.
- Keeping your hip turned outward, slowly return your thigh to the start position.
- You can progress this position by using ankle weights.

Dosage
Resistance _____
Sets/repetitions _____
Frequency _____

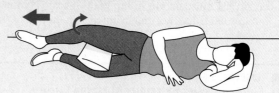

Level IV: Sidelying leg extension

Level V: Sidelying Concentric/Eccentric Contractions

Start Position
- You can now begin to work on concentric (shortening) and eccentric (lengthening) contractions.
- As in Level IV, move to fully extended position.

Movement Technique
- Slowly lower your leg about 10 degrees, hold bottom position for 10 seconds.
- Slowly lift your leg about 10 degrees above neutral, hold top position for 10 seconds.
- Relax your leg onto the pillow before you begin the next repetition.

(continued)

SELF-MANAGEMENT 19-4 *Gluteus Medius Strength Progression (Continued)*

- *Variation*: You can also perform this level from a fully hip-extended position. It is helpful to lie against a wall, positioning your pelvis such that your pelvis is against the wall and both "cheeks" are touching the wall. In addition, your therapist may ask you to position a small towel behind your upper buttock to ensure your hip is in extension when it slides up the wall. Slide your heel up the wall through a full hip range of motion. Do not compensate by tilting your pelvis or sidebending your spine. Hold this position for 10 seconds.
- Keeping your hip turned outward, slowly lower your leg to the start position.

Dosage
Sets/repetitions _____
Frequency _____

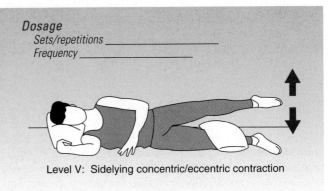

Level V: Sidelying concentric/eccentric contraction

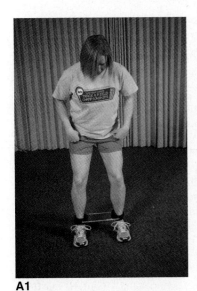

A1

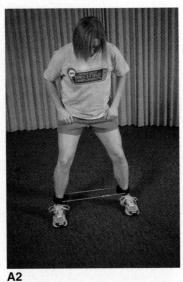

A2

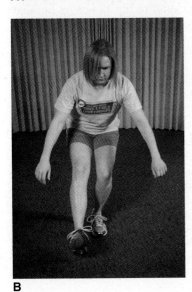

B

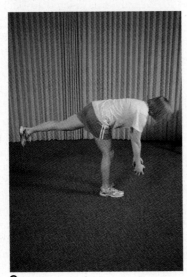

C

FIGURE 19-10. Exercises shown to Lateral band walk (A1, A2), single limb squat (B), single limb dead lift (C).

pattern on the dominant side, contributes to lengthening of the ipsilateral gluteus medius,[27] which affects its force-generating capability during function.[59] The muscle tends to function at its relatively lengthened state during gait (with the hip adducted).[60] Eventually, this movement pattern may become more exaggerated, contributing to excessive hip adduction during the stance phase of gait and further reliance on stability from passive tension of the ITB.[61] As the hip increases its use of the ITB for passive stability, gluteus medius participation may decrease. Subsequently, the gluteus medius is subject to further deconditioning. This imbalance has been demonstrated in distance runners with iliotibial band syndrome (ITBS).[62] Long-distance runners with ITBS have weaker hip abduction strength in the affected leg compared with their unaffected leg. After 6 weeks of training with special attention directed to specifically strengthen the gluteus medius, hip abductor torque increased 34% to 51% and 22 of 24 athletes were pain-free and able to return to running.

The iliopsoas is active in the initial swing phase and terminal stance phase of gait; and presumably in ascending stairs.[62] Its activity probably is related to the lateral rotation and hip flexion, which accompanies the initial swing phase of gait. Faulty patterns of hip flexion can indicate underuse of the iliopsoas and overuse of another synergist. The following examples describe faulty hip flexion patterns:

- Hip hike during the swing phase of gait or stair climbing suggests recruitment of lateral trunk musculature to hike the hip instead of using the iliopsoas to flex the hip (Fig. 19-11).
- Hip flexion with medial rotation (Fig. 19-12) suggests use of TFL as the predominant hip flexor instead of the iliopsoas.

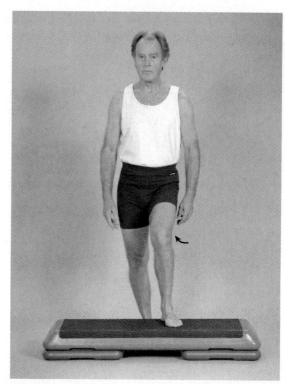

FIGURE 19-12. Medial femoral rotation versus neutral hip rotation of the left femur accompanying hip flexion during stair climbing.

Sahrmann states that repetitive alteration in the optimal path of instant center of rotation of the hip during flexion and the resulting compensatory hip and LP movement patterns predispose the hip and LP region to further impairments and pathologic conditions.[53] Specific exercises to improve the force-generating capability of the iliopsoas (see Self-Management 19-5: Iliopsoas Strengthening) and gradual movement reeducation in hip flexion patterns during function (i.e., swing phase of gait and stair climbing) are indicated to improve iliopsoas muscle performance and participation in the hip flexion force couple.

Reduced participation of the gluteus maximus profoundly affects gait and the ability to ascend stairs.[46] Gluteus maximus activity is related to deceleration of hip flexion at terminal swing and isometric extensor support of the flexed hip at initial contact and during the loading response phases of gait.[46] Squatting, step-ups, step-downs, and sit-to-stand exercises are functional methods for improving the gluteus maximus force-generating capability and its recruitment during functional movement patterns, provided the proper kinematics are promoted (see Fig. 19-13).

Hip lateral rotators are active from the initial contact to midstance of gait, presumably to decelerate the medial femoral rotation occurring as a result of foot pronation. Signs of excessive hip medial rotation during weight acceptance and the single-limb support phases of gait need to be examined to determine the contributing impairments (e.g., hip anteversion, genuvalgum, foot pronation, hip medial rotation). Use of orthotic support as the exclusive remedy for hip medial rotation should be avoided. There is evidence that the kinematic effects of orthotic intervention are small and not systematic.[63] Instead, specific exercise and functional retraining of the

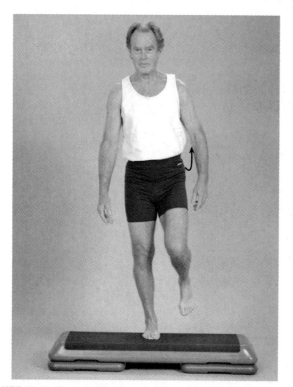

FIGURE 19-11. Use of a hip-hike strategy versus independent hip flexion on the left to ascend the stairs.

SELF-MANAGEMENT 19-5 *Iliopsoas Strengthening*

Purpose: To strengthen the muscle deep in the front of your pelvis that lifts your leg and controls the forward rotation of your hip joint

Start Position: Sit with your feet flat on a firm surface, back straight, pelvis erect, and arms resting at your sides.

Movement Technique

Level I—Passive lift, hold, lower

- Use your hands to lift your knee toward your chest as far as possible without letting your lower back round or "slump" backward.
- Hold this position for the prescribed number of seconds.
- Lower your leg to the start position.

Level II—Resisted hip flexion

- Perform as in Level I, but push against your knee in a down and slightly outward direction for the prescribed number of seconds.
- Lower your leg to the start position.

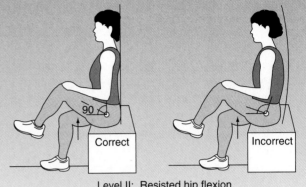

Level II: Resisted hip flexion

Dosage
Sets/repetitions _____
Duration _____
Frequency _____

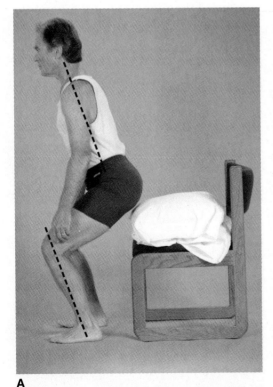

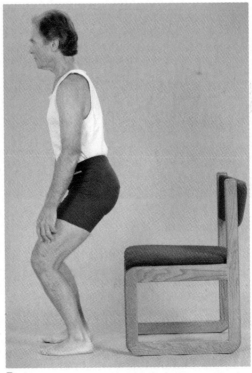

A   **B**

FIGURE 19-13. Chair squats. Note the forward inclination of the trunk and parallel lines of the trunk and tibia. (A) Chair squats can be made easier with the use of pillows. (B) Gradually taking away the pillows can make the exercise more difficult.

hip lateral rotator functional control should be emphasized (Figs. 19-14 and 19-15; see Self-Management 19-2). Even in the presence of foot and ankle related impairments and orthotic intervention, isolated hip lateral rotator muscle strengthening is indicated to assist in pronation control (see Building Block 19-1).

Range of Motion, Muscle Length, Joint Mobility, and Integrity Impairments

ROM and joint mobility impairments of the hip can span the continuum of hypomobility to hypermobility. The extreme clinical manifestation of hypomobility is the arthritic hip

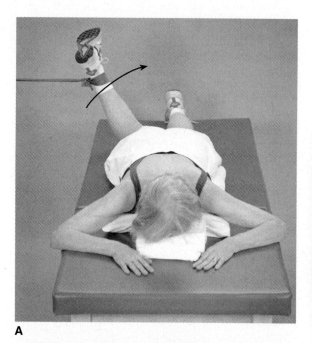

A

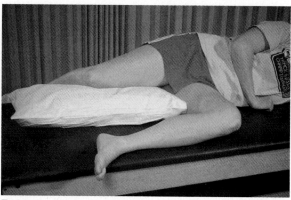

B

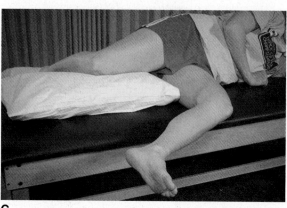

C

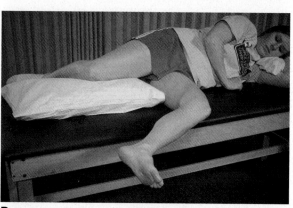

D

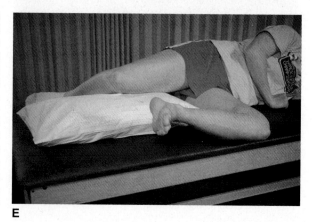

E

FIGURE 19-14. (A) Prone hip lateral rotation with elastic. The patient is instructed to stabilize the pelvis in the sagittal and transverse planes with inner core recruitment while rotating the hip from medial rotation to midline or slight lateral rotation. The slow release back to medial rotation emphasizes eccentric control of the lateral rotators. The hip extended position favors all hip lateral rotators, including lateral hamstrings and gluteus maximus. (B) The sidelying position at 90 degrees of hip flexion provides better isolation of the deep hip lateral rotators from the gluteals and hamstrings. (C) This illustration shows an isometric contraction by slightly extending the knee so that the hip rotators are holding the tibia against gravity. Be careful of adductor recruitment by ensuring the pelvis is perpendicular to the ground. (D) This diagram shows an eccentric contraction. (E) This diagram shows a concentric contraction. All types of contractions can be trained for various purposes as they relate to function of the deep hip lateral rotators.

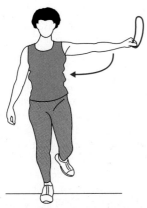

FIGURE 19-15. Single-limb balance challenges hip lateral rotators in a more functional position by adding torsional destabilizing stress through resisted movement of the upper extremities into horizontal adduction.

with a capsular pattern of limitation. The extreme clinical manifestation of hypermobility is congenital dysplasia of the hip, creating chronic instability in the hip joint. Between these extreme conditions, more subtle mobility impairments can affect the function of the hip.

Hypermobility

Because of the inherent stability of the hip, hypermobility is not commonly thought of as an impairment in the adult hip, but rather as an impairment in the developing hip[64] or complication in total hip arthroplasty.[65]

With the increasing use of arthroscopy at the hip, surgeons have discovered labral tears to be more common than thought.[66,67] Observations in the study reported by McCarthy et al.[66] suggest that acetabular labral lesions may be a contributory factor to the evolution and progression of OA of the hip. The working hypothesis is that a primary anterior labral tear disrupts the stability of the hip, especially at the extremes of joint motion. This leads to abnormal gliding of the articular surfaces under dynamic torsional loading conditions. In this sense, it is plausible that loss of the presumed stabilizing and weight-bearing roles of the labrum at the extremes of motion (where the labrum would be anticipated to exert its most significant effect) could predispose the hip to additional degeneration. Alternatively, lesions of the anterior labrum may represent a final common pathway of deterioration in hips with a wide variety of primary disorders.

BUILDING BLOCK 19-1

Consider a 57-year-old female with positive a Trendelenburg sign on the left side and bilateral weakness in the hip abductors and lateral rotators. She shows some mild osteoarthritis bilaterally but does not want to have surgery. She presents with slow gait speed, poor control of the core musculature, and bilateral pronation. Develop three exercises that would be appropriate for this patient to maximize her function.

Hip joint hypermobility has been shown to be associated with OA in numerous studies and warrants careful attention for the prevention of hip degenerative joint disease.[68–70] Treatment of the unstable developing hip usually consists of positioning, bracing, or surgery,[71,72] whereas treatment of the hypermobile (rarely unstable) adult hip usually consists of therapeutic exercise and posture and movement retraining.[53]

The etiology of hypermobility can be either arthrokinematic or osteokinematic. Arthrokinematic hypermobility is defined as linear translation that is excessive, whereas osteokinematic hypermobility is angular translation that is considered excessive. These two types of hypermobility can exist separately or together. Sahrmann[53] describes a syndrome in the hip (femoral anterior glide syndrome) in which abnormal anterior translation of the hip accompanies hip flexion resulting from stiffness in the posterior capsule and/or excessive extensibility of the anterior capsule, yet hip flexion ROM may be normal or restricted. Another syndrome (femoral adduction with medial rotation) is described in which excessive hip adduction and medial rotation occur in combination, without the presence of excessive linear translation of the hip joint.[53] Femoral adduction syndrome can become exaggerated to the point that lateral glide mobility becomes excessive, thus involving both osteokinematic and arthrokinematic hypermobility (femoral lateral glide syndrome).[53] A person with femoral adduction or lateral glide syndrome may have a broad pelvis, an apparent LLD (the high side being symptomatic), femur medial rotation, genu valgum, and foot pronation as predisposing risk factors. These alignment faults contribute to stretch to the abductor and lateral rotator muscle groups and lateral capsuloligamentous structures allowing excessive adduction, medial rotation, and lateral glide to occur during ADLs and sports. Patterns of sustained postures and repetitive movements can predispose an individual to a variety of syndromes because of soft-tissue extensibility changes in the myofascial or periarticular tissues leading to hypermobility in osteokinematic or arthrokinematic patterns.

Careful examination should distinguish between osteokinematic and arthrokinematic hypermobility; the diagnosis of the latter being more difficult to resolve than the former. The primary objective of any therapeutic exercise intervention for the treatment of hypermobility, regardless of etiology, is to promote joint stability and prevent continued stress on the overstretched or torn tissues (myofascial or periarticular) via postural and movement pattern changes and improving length-tension properties and muscle performance of all muscles involved. Given the example of the person with a femoral adduction syndrome, correction of postural habits such as sitting with his or her legs crossed, or standing with the affected leg in adduction, is indicated. Protecting the lateral structures from excessive stretch in the sidelying position with pillows between the legs is imperative. All movements should be performed with the focus on avoiding femur adduction and medial rotation patterns. Hip adductor stretching may be indicated to reduce the adductor moment on the hip joint (see Fig. 19-16). Strengthening both gluteus medius (Self-Management 19-4: Gluteus Medius Strength Progression) and glutues minimus (Fig. 19-17) can be valuable to improving stability against adductor moments. Dosage for strengthening hip abductor and lateral rotators should prioritize muscle hypertrophic changes to enhance joint stiffness.

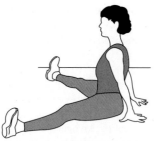

FIGURE 19-16. A method of stretching hip adductors. The patient is instructed in maintaining a neutral pelvis (sitting with the back against the wall can help prevent posterior pelvic tilt) and increasing the range of hip abduction versus trunk forward bend (as is commonly depicted in adductor stretches).

Whenever excessive medial rotation ROM is measured, care must be taken to screen for anteversion. A common associated finding with hip anteversion is weakness of the hip lateral rotators (i.e., deep hip rotators, gluteus maximus, posterior fibers of gluteus medius). In the presence of excessive medial rotation ROM, with or without anteversion, exercise to improve muscle performance of the lateral rotators is indicated. Lateral rotator strengthening exercises, to be most effective, should be coupled with education about altering postural habits (e.g., reduce the incidence of standing with the femur in excessive medial rotation) and movement training to improve recruitment of lateral rotators during closed chain function. See Patient-Related Instruction 19-1: Standing Knees Over Toes and Patient-Related Instruction 19-2: Walking With Knees Over Toes for examples of posture and gait education and training. Caution must be taken when strengthening hip lateral rotators in the presence of anteversion so as not to push the individual into too much lateral rotation, which will induce arthrokinematic hypermobility (see the following section for further explanation).

Individuals with hip anteversion can present with two unique hypermobility problems related to attempts to compensate for the anatomic impairment. Persons with hip anteversion may engage in activities that promote extreme hip lateral rotation, such as ballet or soccer. The anteverted hip is forced to function in extreme lateral rotation for accurate performance of the activity. The head of the femur can be forced to translate excessively anteriorly and laterally to achieve the laterally rotated femur position,[73] often resulting in anterior groin pain. Hip joint hypermobility subsequently develops in an anterior and lateral direction.[73] Mounting evidence suggests a link between increased anteversion angles and OA.[74–79] It is possible that the anterolateral hypermobility may be a predisposing factor in the development of OA. To prevent or alleviate this impairment, the patient should be educated about his or her unique lower extremity biomechanics and lateral rotation ROM limitations. The therapist may need to counsel the individual to seek a recreational activity that does not require significant lateral rotation ROM.

Another common movement impairment that develops in the individual with anteverted hips is to achieve lateral rotation ROM by laterally rotating the tibia on the femur (see Fig. 19-18).[80] The person with this compensatory alignment should also be educated about his or her unique lower extremity biomechanics and hip lateral rotation ROM limitations to prevent rotational hypermobility problems at the tibiofemoral joint and potential knee joint pathology (see Building Block 19-2).[74,81,82]

Hypomobility

Hypomobility impairments, particularly in the direction of flexion and medial rotation, can be found in the young, middle-age, and elderly adult hip joint. Subtle losses in flexion and medial rotation may indicate early arthritic changes[30] or hypomobility caused by chronic lack of use as a result of altered movement patterns. A fully established capsular pattern (see Display 19-2) can be a hallmark finding for the arthritic hip.[30]

Pain need not be an essential component of early arthritic changes and hypomobility findings. For example, OA (confirmed radiologically) leading to considerable restriction of

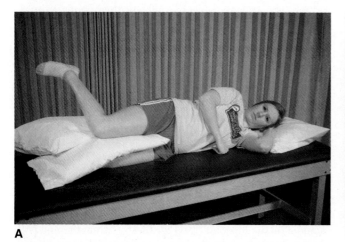

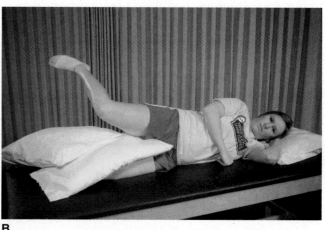

A **B**

FIGURE 19-17. Gluteus Minimus strengthening is also important when stabilizing against adduction moments. (A) The patient is positioned in sidelying with hip extended, knees bent to 90 degrees, and one to two pillows between the knees to keep femur in neutral with respect to the frontal plane. The patient is instructed to turn the knee inward and lift the foot upward (engaging the medial rotators). (B) The next step to better isolate the gluteus minimus is to slightly abduct the femur while it remains in extension and medial rotation. To make this exercise more difficult, cuff weights can be added to the ankle.

Patient-Related Instruction 19-1
Standing Knees Over Toes

Your neutral hip position may vary depending on the structure of your hips. Your physical therapist will instruct you as to your neutral position if you have a structural variation in your hips.

From the front
- Your weight should be distributed equally between both feet.
- Your pelvis should be level from side to side
- The left side of your pelvis should be in line with the right side of your pelvis (i.e., one side of your pelvis should not be in front of the other side)
- Your knees should be in line with your feet; if you bend your knees, your knees would be directed over the midline of your feet.
- Your feet should be hip-width apart and *slightly* turned outward.
- The arch of your foot should be *slightly* elevated, with your big toe down.

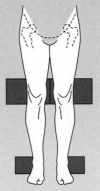

Ideal alignment

From the side
- Your pelvis should be in neutral, with the front pelvis bones in the same plane as your pubic bone.
- Your knees should not be bent or locked.
- Your ankle should fall below your knee, with your lower leg at a 90-degree angle with respect to your foot.

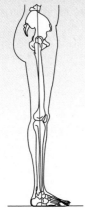

Patient-Related Instruction 19-2
Walking With Knees Over Toes

When you walk

- Your knee should be fully extended at the instant of heel strike, then immediately bend slightly to absorb shock. Do not let your knee lock back as you bring your weight over your foot. This hyperextension reduces your shock absorption and places undesirable stress on the ligaments and joint surfaces on your knees.
- Though your hip should turn inward slightly at heel strike, think of activating your deep hip lateral rotators to slow down this rotation and prevent your knee from turning in excessively as your body weight moves over your foot.
- Though your arch must drop a slight amount (pronation) at the time of heel strike in order to absorb shock, think of using your foot muscles to prevent your arch from dropping too low as your body weight moves over your foot.
- Keep your inner core and abdominal muscles activated to prevent your pelvis from tilting forward. This is particularly important as your body weight moves in front of your foot and your hip must extend. If you do not hold your abdominal muscles tight, your pelvis may tilt or rotate instead of your hip extending.
- Be sure to roll through your foot to a full toe-off phase of gait. If someone were behind you, they could see the backs of your toes if you achieve full toe-off phase. This re-supinates your foot and prepares you for the next step.

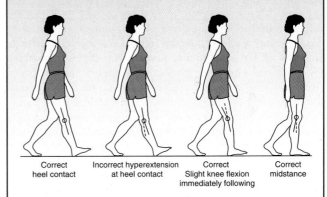

| Correct heel contact | Incorrect hyperextension at heel contact | Correct Slight knee flexion immediately following | Correct midstance |

activity limitation, but they may complain of LBP because of the movement imposed on the back as a result of decreased hip mobility.

Hip joint hypomobility may result from altered LP movement patterns because of a combination of anthropometric (e.g., high center of mass), occupational, and environmental (e.g., sports, recreation, hobbies) factors. It is hypothesized that, ultimately, as hip mobility decreases, lumbar mobility increases. This finding has been demonstrated in measuring LP rhythm during forward bending,[83–87] particularly in the early phase of forward bending. The investigators of these studies found a significant relationship between a relative loss of hip flexion mobility and relative increased lumbar flexion mobility. Knowledge of this relationship is critical for the clinician prescribing exercise and retraining movement patterns. Functional

range in the capsular pattern may not cause pain, even when the capsule is stretched quite hard.[30] This is a typical finding in middle-age men with a capsular pattern of restriction at the hip. Commonly, they have no complaints of hip pain or related

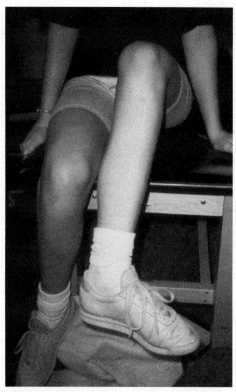

FIGURE 19-18. Excessive tibiofemoral rotation associated with hip anteversion in an individual who has participated extensively in ballet. Picture shows individual voluntarily laterally rotating the tibia. (From Sahrmann. Diagnosis and Treatment of Movement Impairment Syndromes. St. Louis: Mosby, 2002.)

activities such as bending forward to brush one's teeth, making the bed, and reaching into the refrigerator involve moderate amounts of hip and lumbar flexion. Hip stiffness resulting from reduced extensibility in capsule, ligament, or myofascial structures may impose excessive motion on the lumbar spine during forward-bending activities, which may ultimately lead to microtrauma and macrotrauma of the lumbar spine. Exercises to increase hip flexion mobility and lumbar stability, combined with retraining LP rhythm during forward-bending activities, are important to mitigate impairments associated with the cause of LBP in this particular patient subset. A useful exercise to retrain hip and lumbar movement is illustrated in Self-Management 19-6: Hand-Knee Rocking.

BUILDING BLOCK 19-2

Consider the 15-year-old female with general hypermobility. The patient is enrolled in ballet and tap dance classes. She complains of anterior and lateral hip pain which gets worse after dance. She presents with weakness of the gluteus medius and gluteus minimus, deep hip lateral rotators, poor transverse plane control with a squat, and no evidence of retro/anteversion. Develop three specific exercise interventions, one closed chain exercises, and one taping technique for this patient to decrease her pain and increase her stability.

Another source of hypomobility may be the presence of FAI (Fig. 19-4) described earlier. The malformation of either the femoral head/neck and/or the acetabulum can lead to decreased ROM secondary to pain from the structural impingement. In lieu of surgery, this type of pathology may respond well to exercise intervention aimed at reduction and controlling hip internal rotation and adduction during activities. A commercially available orthotic, the S.E.R.F. (Stability thru External Rotation of the Femur) strap, provides tactile feedback during activity to help meet this goal (Fig. 19-19).

The hamstrings have been implicated as a potential source of hip stiffness.[87] A common stretch for the hamstrings is illustrated in Figure 19-20. A selective medial or lateral hamstring stretch can be induced by rotating the hip in the medial direction to stretch the lateral hamstrings and lateral direction to stretch the medial hamstrings. Because the hamstrings are a

---

◉ **SELF-MANAGEMENT 19-6 Hand-Knee Rocking**

Purpose: To improve the range of motion of your hips, stretch the posterior hip muscles, and train independent movement between your hips, pelvis, and spine

Start Position
- Position yourself on your hands and knees so that your hips are directly over your knees and hands are directly under your shoulders.
- Knees and ankles should be hip-width apart with feet pointing straight back
- Your spine should be flat with a slight curve downward in your low back and your pelvis tilted so that your hip joint is at a 90-degree angle.

Movement Technique: Rock backward at the hip joint only. Stop at any sensation of movement in your back.
Variation: Your PT may ask you to gently squeeze a ball or towel roll between your heels to activate your deep hip lateral rotators. This will help to stabilize your hip in the socket and prevent excessive flexion at the hip joint.

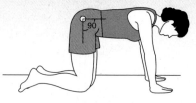

Rock backward slightly

Back stays straight

Hip joint angle decreases

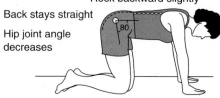

Dosage
  Sets/repetitions _____
  Frequency _____

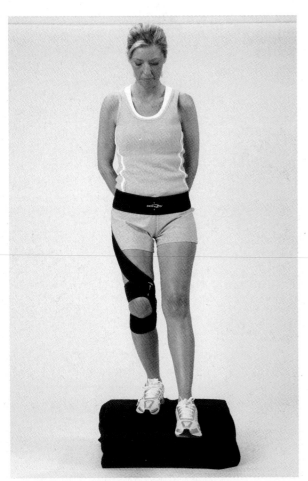

FIGURE 19-19. The S.E.R.F. Strap consists of thin, elastic material that is secured to the proximal tibia, wraps around the distal thigh, and is anchored around the pelvis or shown here. The line of action S.E.R.F strap pulls the hip into external rotation (with permission from JOSPT.)

diarthrodial muscle, knee extension must be maintained while the hip flexes to ensure optimal stretch stimulus. After the hamstrings have been stretched passively, an active exercise should be performed to ensure the new length is used during function. One exercise that uses hamstring length during an active movement pattern is illustrated in Self-Management 19-7: Seated Knee Extension.

Another joint in the kinetic chain that may become stressed because of a relative loss of mobility in the hip joint is the knee. During squatting movements, loss of hip flexion ROM may impose increased motion on the lumbar spine (Fig. 19-21A) and the knee joint (Fig. 19-21B). Loss of hip joint mobility is a common finding in persons complaining of overuse-related knee conditions such as patellofemoral dysfunction and patellar tendinitis or tendinosis. Improved hip joint ROM and muscle performance of the gluteus maximus coupled with improved squatting movement patterns can reduce the stress on the knee joint. Progressive squatting exercises with optimal kinematics at the hip and knee are recommended to decrease excessive forces at the low back and knee (see Self-Management 19-8: Progressive Squat).

Emphasis has been placed on hip flexion and medial rotation hypomobility impairments, but loss of hip extension ROM is another common finding, particularly in patients with

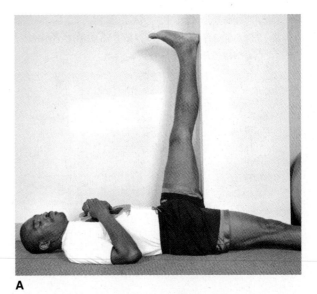

A

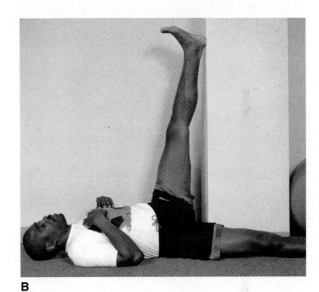

B

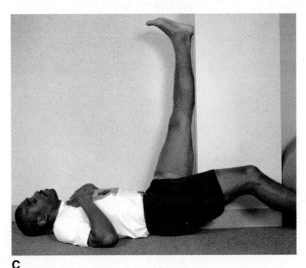

C

FIGURE 19-20. (A) Supine passive hamstring stretch with proper proximal stabilization (B) pelvic rotation is a common faulty technique during this stretch (C) Posterior pelvic tilt is another common faulty technique associated with this stretch.

SELF-MANAGEMENT 19-7 *Seated Knee Extension*

Purpose: To stretch the hamstring and calf muscles and train independent movement between your low back and pelvis and your hip and lower leg

Start Position: Sit with your back straight, pelvis erect, and arms resting at your sides.

Movement Technique:
- Activate your inner core with particular attention to the lumbar multifidus.
- Slowly straighten your knee, being sure not to let your pelvis rock backward. Stop when you feel tension developing behind your knee. Hold this position for the prescribed number of seconds.

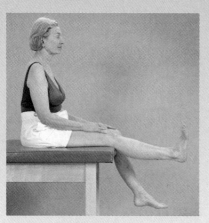

- Variations
  ___ After your knee has moved as far as possible, move your ankle so that your foot points upward toward your knee.
  ___ Rotate your hip and knee outward before you begin the stretch.
  ___ Rotate your hip and knee inward before you begin the stretch.

Dosage
  Sets/repetitions _____
  Duration _____
  Frequency _____

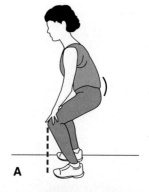

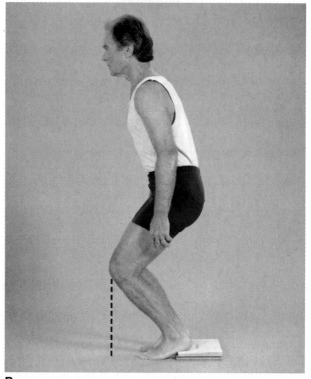

B

FIGURE 19-21. Squat. (A) Faulty squat technique performed with increased lumbar flexion as compensation for decreased hip flexion. (B) Faulty squat technique performed with increased knee flexion as compensation for decreased hip flexion.

end-stage hip arthritis. With myofascial or periarticular stiffness across the anterior hip, the pelvis may rest in a relative anterior tilt in relaxed standing. This posture may contribute to a relative increase in anterior pelvic tilt and lumbar extension to achieve an upright position (see Fig. 19-22A). During gait, hip extension is unable to be achieved, which may result in excessive lumbar extension or rotation. On return from the forward bend, the patient leads with lumbar extension versus hip extension (Fig. 19-22B) the pelvis does not achieve a neutral position, and excessive lumbar extension is imposed on the lumbar spine to achieve an upright position (Fig. 19-22C).

A common finding associated with loss of hip extension ROM is positional weakness in the external oblique muscles, lower rectus abdominis, and transversus abdominis because of the chronically anterior tilted pelvis. Treatment of this

impairment requires careful stretching of the affected hip flexor muscles concurrent with positional strengthening of the appropriate abdominal muscle groups (see Chapter 18).

Specific muscle length tests reveal which hip flexor muscles are contributing to the lack of hip extension ROM. Often, the diarthrodial hip flexors (i.e., rectus femoris and TFL/ITB) are stiff or short. Traditional stretches for the diarthrodial hip flexors do not follow the basic guidelines for optimal stretching because proximal stability is often not maintained (Fig. 19-23). Alternative stretches are recommended for optimal results. Self-Management 19-9: Hip Flexor Stretch illustrates an isolated passive diarthrodial hip flexor stretch. For maximal efficiency with this stretch, it is critical to maintain the stability of the pelvis and spine while maintaining the femur and tibia in a neutral position during knee flexion. To isolate the stretch to the TFL, slight lateral rotation and adduction of the femur at end-range is

SELF-MANAGEMENT 19-8 *Progressive Squat*

Purpose: To progressively strengthen your hip girdle muscles and train independent movement between your hips and spine

Start Position: Stand with weight equally distributed between both feet with your pelvis and spine in neutral. Your neutral hip position may vary depending on the structure of your hips. Ask your physical therapist for instructions on your neutral hip position.

Movement Technique:

Level I: Small Knee Bend

- Slowly bend your hips and knees.
- Do not bend your knees farther than the length of your feet. Think of sitting back slightly.
- Be sure that your feet are facing ahead, with knees over toes and pelvis level as you bend.
- A good rule of thumb is to keep your lower legs parallel to your torso during the lowering and raising phase of this, and subsequent levels, of this maneuver.
- Return to the upright position by using your seat and front thigh muscles. Be sure to complete the rising phase by returning to the neutral spine and pelvic position.

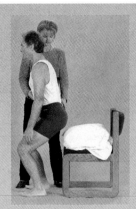

Level II

Level III: Partial Squat

- Perform as in Level II, but do not use a chair as a stopping point; instead, lower yourself as far as is comfortable.
- As you move deeper into the squat, you will need to bend your hips more (remember that your knees should not bend further forward than the length of your feet) to keep your balance.
- Be sure that your low back does not arch during this movement. Your spine should remain neutral to a slight amount of flexion, depending on your start position. Your PT will advise you on the posture of your spine during this exercise.

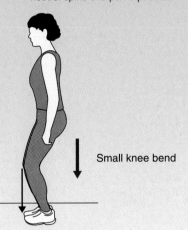

Small knee bend

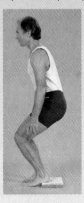

Level I

Level II: Chair Squat

- Perform as in Level I, but lower yourself to a chair with ___ pillows.
- Try not to collapse into the chair, but rather slowly lower yourself. A good challenge is to hover over the seat just before you sit down.
- Return to the upright position by using your seat and front thigh muscles. Be sure to complete the rising phase by returning to the neutral spine and pelvic position.

Level III

- Variation

Perform Level III with a dumbbell in each hand.

Perform Level III in a squat rack with a barbell.

Dosage

Sets/repetitions _____

Frequency _____

Weight _____

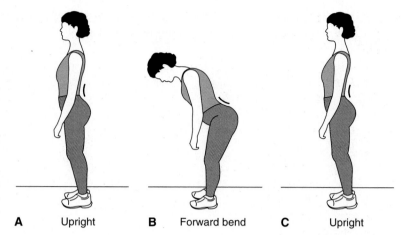

FIGURE 19-22. (A) Anterior pelvic tilt and lumbar lordosis. (B) On the return from forward bend the patient leads with lumbar extension versus pelvic extension. (C) If the pelvis stops rotating posterior before it reaches a neutral position, excessive lumbar extension is imposed on the spine to achieve an upright posture.

A Upright   **B** Forward bend   **C** Upright

suggested. Compensatory tibia lateral rotation may occur as the ITB is stretched. The patient must be cautioned to maintain tibiofemoral alignment by medially rotating the tibia during the stretch.

Self-Management 17-5: Prone Knee Bend in Chapter 17 illustrates an active diarthrodial hip flexor stretch. This stretch uses active movement of knee flexion in an extended hip position to place repeated stretch on the diarthrodial hip flexors while contracting the abdominal muscles to stabilize the pelvis. As the abdominal muscles are recruited to stabilize the pelvis in this stretch, simultaneous elongation of the

diarthrodial hip flexors and abdominal strengthening in the shortened range occurs.

To ensure that gains in hip extension mobility are used in a functional context, the clinician must confirm that proper

FIGURE 19-23. Traditional standing hip flexor stretches do not effectively stabilize the spine and pelvis. Note the anterior pelvic tilt and hip flexion in this individual attempting to perform this commonly used hip flexor stretch.

◉ **SELF-MANAGEMENT 19-9** *Hip Flexor Stretch*

Purpose:	To stretch the front thigh muscles
Start Position	• Sit on the edge of a table so that your thigh is halfway off.
	• Lie back while bringing both knees toward your chest.
	• Pull your knees toward your chest until your low back just touches the tabletop surface.
Movement Technique	• While grasping behind your knee, lower your other leg toward the floor, keeping your knee bent to 90 degrees.
	• Keep your thigh in the midline; do not let it drift to the side.
	• Do not let your thigh rotate inward

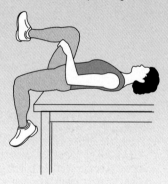

• Variation: Let your thigh drop out to the side instead. Turn your lower leg inward. Gently pull your thigh toward midline until you feel slight tension in your iliotibial band.
• Hold for 15 to 30 seconds.

Dosage
Sets/repetitions _____
Frequency _____

movement patterns are being used during functional activities. Precise performance of functional movement patterns requires hip extension mobility and abdominal control to prevent anterior pelvic rotation and to achieve full hip joint extension.

Achieving control over hip extension and pelvic position during functional activities such as the late stance phase of gait (see Patient-Related Instruction 19-2: Walking With Knees Over Toes), sit to stand, hip extension phase of squatting, and the return from forward bending (see Patient-Related Instruction 19-3: Return From Forward Bending With a

Neutral Pelvis) is necessary to ensure the specific ROM improvements are carried into ADLs.

Balance

Approximately 25% to 35% of persons older than 65 years experience one or more falls each year.[88–90] Falls are a leading cause of morbidity and mortality of persons older than 65 years,[91,92] and many of the falls result in hip fractures which are a leading cause of mortality and morbidity among older people in the United States.[93] In 1995, hip fracture was the tenth leading reason for hospitalization for Medicare beneficiaries,[94] and the prevalence and costs of hip fracture are expected to grow as the older population increases.[95,96] The hip fracture rate in the United States is about twice as high for women as for men,[97,98] and residents of nursing homes have been reported to have a three to eleven times greater risk than nonnursing home residents of hip fracture in the United States,[99] Netherlands,[100] France,[101] and Finland.[102] Hip fracture has a high impact on patients' health and medical costs. A high risk for hip fracture is predicted by low bone density, prior fragility fractures, and a high risk of falling.[103–105] Improved postural stability and balance can improve fear of falling and delay the onset of fall events for older adults.[106–109]

T'ai chi has been valuable in promoting posture stability and balance control in the well elderly.[110–113] The T'ai chi progression (i.e., bipedal weight shifting to uniped positions) focuses less on centering the center of mass within the base of support and more on learning corrective strategies for instability. The advanced forms serve the purposes of destabilizing the individual in a controlled fashion, engaging new movement strategies and facilitating the confidence level of the participant.

Force-platform biofeedback systems can also be used to train posture stability and balance control. However, the focus of force-platform biofeedback systems is different than that of T'ai chi balance training. The former is typically concerned with learning to enhance center of mass or center of pressure movement within the limits of stability, and the latter is concerned with learning controlled motions as those limits are passed. Furthermore, the force platform based systems utilize visual feedback to the patient, which may not be as effective as other types of intrinsic feedback, such as proprioception.[114] Controlled clinical studies have not demonstrated a reduction in falls or delays in fall occurrences among older persons using force-platform biofeedback systems.[115] This may be because the ability to control the center of pressure during quiet standing or with the added provision of random but moderate perturbations, used during typical machine-based postural training, may not translate well into a functional situation, thereby not resulting in decreased fear of falling or delayed onset of fall events for older adults.

The ability to effectively treat patients with balance disorders can be enhanced by a clearer understanding of the problems underlying balance. Treatment of impaired balance must focus on the intrinsic and extrinsic factors related to the balance disorder. This requires extensive examination and evaluation of muscle performance, ROM, joint mobility, vestibular function, balance reactions, and environmental factors. Clinicians trained in balance-related rehabilitation have shown

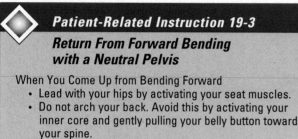

Patient-Related Instruction 19-3

Return From Forward Bending with a Neutral Pelvis

When You Come Up from Bending Forward
- Lead with your hips by activating your seat muscles.
- Do not arch your back. Avoid this by activating your inner core and gently pulling your belly button toward your spine.
- Complete the motion by bringing your pelvis back to neutral before finishing the spine movement.
- At the bottom of the motion, be sure your spine, buttock, and thigh muscles are fully relaxed before you reverse the motion.

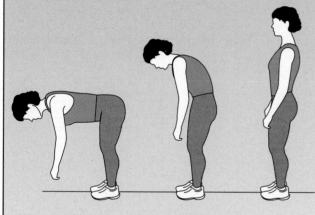

When You Rise Upward From a Squatting Motion
- Be sure to complete the motion by fully extending your hips until your pelvis reaches neutral. Finish the motion with spine extension.
- Activate your inner core and abdominal muscles as you rise to ensure your pelvis remains in neutral. Your back extensors finish the motion.

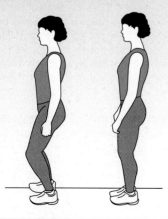

that compliance with a multidimensional, individualized exercise program that addresses the impairments and activity limitations associated with balance deficits can improve balance and mobility function and reduce the likelihood of falls.[25]

Display 19-7 lists general guidelines that can assist the practitioner in developing balance training activities for the hip, and Display 19-8 describes a sample progression of balance tasks (see Building Block 19-3).

Pain

Pain is undoubtedly the most common reason persons seek physical therapy for hip-related dysfunction. The prevalence of hip pain in the elderly is 14.3% for those 60 years of age and older.[117]

The most important aspect of therapeutic exercise intervention for hip pain is the differential diagnosis of the etiology as well as the mechanical cause of the pain. Traumatic and overuse soft-tissue injuries include muscular, bursal, tendinous, or ligamentous inflammation, contusions, strains, and sprains. Skeletal injuries can involve the physis or apophysis in children, and skeletal disorders include fractures, subluxations, dislocations, stress injuries, infections, and avulsions. Patients with nontraumatic hip pain from systemic conditions such as rheumatoid arthritis, juvenile arthritis, ankylosing spondylitis, tumors, and metabolic bone disease should be suspected when the severity or course of the injury is atypical. Persistent hip pain can originate from intraarticular disorders such as avascular necrosis, OA, loose bodies, labral tears, or pyarthrosis. Hip pain also may be secondary to a lumbar spine disorder. Nerve entrapment syndromes involving the ilioinguinal, genitofemoral, and lateral femoral cutaneous nerve of the thigh may present as hip pain or paresthesias (to be discussed in more detail under Nerve Entrapment Syndromes).

Pain from the hip joint can be referred anteriorly to the groin, referred laterally in the region of the greater trochanter, or radiate down the anterior and medial thigh to the knee. Occasionally, referred knee pain can occur with little or no pain in the hip.

Pain posterior to the hip or in the buttock is frequently associated with lumbar spine pathology, but it can also arise from the hip. Pain from the spine commonly radiates down the posterior thigh, occasionally to below the knee, but hip pain rarely radiates below the knee. Severe synovitis or acute arthritis can produce pain in the entire hemipelvis. Pain related to ITB fascitis is experienced in the lateral thigh and can be mistaken for lumbar radiculopathy. Because this condition occurs commonly in the elderly, spinal stenosis can be incorrectly implicated as the source of the lateral thigh pain.

Whether or not the source of the pain is diagnosed, the biomechanical cause should be established. Treatment must work toward alleviating impairments related to the source and cause of pain and inflammation for long-term resolution. Treatment of the cause of the pain and inflammation often relieves symptoms without specific treatment of the source. Several examples of treatment of the cause of pain and inflammation are presented throughout this chapter. Treatment of potential sources of hip pain and possible contributing factors can follow the general guidelines illustrated in Display 19-9 (see Building Block 19-4).

DISPLAY 19-7
Guidelines for Balance Training Activities

- In treating balance impairments with training programs, including T'ai chi, progressive drills, and computerized balance devices, the specific demands of compensatory stepping or grasping reactions that are found to cause difficulty (e.g., lateral weight transfer, rapid foot or arm movement, crossover steps) should be addressed. These skills can be addressed through unpredictable exercise conditions, such as the use of dense foam or having an outside perturbation such as a partner pushing or pulling the patient off balance. Cautious progression toward uniped motions is indicated, especially because this position is experienced by most older persons before falling.

- When training balance control, stepping and grasping reactions are not just strategies of last resort. These strategies can be initiated very early, well before the center of mass is near the stability limits of the base of support.[115] One goal of balance training may be to reduce the incidence of stepping and grasping strategies as posture stability and balance are increasingly challenged. Display 19-8 provides examples of progressive uniped balance tasks. The goal of the exercise would be to balance on one limb, with the progressive self-induced perturbations (e.g., arm movements), without using a grasping or stepping strategy to prevent a fall.

- For anteroposterior perturbations, the fixed-support ankle strategy (i.e., ankle muscular response to arrest the motion of the center of mass) may provide an early defense against destabilization, followed by a stepping or grasping strategy.[115]

- When using an anteroposterior destabilizing force (e.g., uniped with sagittal arm movements), expect the ankles to provide the stabilizing force to maintain postural stability.

- A fixed-support hip strategy (i.e., hip muscular response to arrest the motion of the center of mass) may be limited to a special task condition that precludes the option of stepping or grasping.[115] Use of a fixed-support hip strategy would be inappropriate under normal conditions.

- Lateral destabilization complicates the control of compensatory stepping because of anatomic or physiologic restrictions on the lateral lower extremity movement and the associated prolonged uniped balance demand. Aging appears to be associated with increased difficulty in controlling lateral postural stability, which may be of specific relevance to the problem of lateral falls associated with hip fractures.[107] Exercises designed to provide frontal-plane destabilizing forces (e.g., uniped with frontal-plane arm movements) would especially be indicated in the aging population. Side-stepping strategies for recovery to prevent a fall are important skills for this population to learn.

- Assistive devices can aid the individual in balance control before developing functional balance control through a comprehensive training program. Use of a cane in the nondominant hand has reduced the rate of falls by up to fourfold.[116] Cutaneous information from fingertip contact, through a cane, and from a stable surface is more powerful than vision in stabilizing sway in stance.[116]

DISPLAY 19-8
Examples of Progressive Balance Tasks

- Balance on one leg on a firm surface is progressed to an unstable surface such as dense foam.
- Balance on one leg while rotating the head on a firm surface is progressed to dense foam.
- Balance on one leg with frontal, sagittal, or transverse plane arm movements on a firm surface is progressed to dense foam.
- Perform the previous balance task, but follow the arm movements with the eyes and head.
- Balance on one leg and move the trunk and upper body into contralateral flexion and rotation (i.e., reach for inside of ipsilateral ankle and foot) and ipsilateral extension and rotation (i.e., reach for object superior, lateral, and posterior to the head), and follow the arm movements with the eyes and head.
- Perform the previous three exercises while holding a weighted ball.

BUILDING BLOCK 19-3

An 81-year-old male is referred to your clinical with a diagnosis of "poor balance" and orders to "evaluate and treat." The patient ambulates very slowly, with short step length, flexed, rigid posture, and no assistive device. The patient can only stand on one leg for 1 to 2 seconds and presents with increased sway even during quiet standing. The patient also presents with decreased flexibility of the hip flexors and adductors. Develop three interventions to improve this patient's safety and maximize his function.

Posture and Movement Impairment

Posture and movement training of the hip is used to optimize kinetics and kinematics at the hip joint as well as to influence the kinetics and kinematics of other joints in the kinetic chain. Similarly, posture and movement training of other joints in the kinetic chain can influence the kinetics and kinematics of the hip. Intervention focusing on posture and movement is pivotal to all therapeutic exercise interventions. Exercise should be taught with careful attention to details of posture and movement. All patients should be provided with instruction in avoiding posture and movement habits that contribute to the cause of symptoms and in developing alternative habits that will reduce or eliminate symptoms.

With respect to hip alignment, it is important to understand that pelvic tilt is not always an accurate measure of hip joint angle. Knee joint angle can also affect hip joint angle. For example, when the knees are flexed, the hips are flexed, even if the pelvic tilt is near neutral, and when the knees are hyperextended, the hips will be extended, even if the pelvic tilt is slightly anterior (Fig. 19-24). Be sure to correct for pelvic tilt *and* knee joint angle when treating posture impairments at the hip. This holds true for transverse and frontal plane posture impairments as well.

Movement impairments at the hip, as with posture impairments, can be affected by impairments at other segments. The cause of any given hip movement impairment must be diagnosed from the data collected during the examination of the patient. For example, limited hip flexion during a step-up activity may result from a loss of hip flexion ROM, reduced joint mobility, weakness in the hip flexors, or poor trunk stabilization. Only a thorough examination can reveal the cause of the movement impairment. Once the

DISPLAY 19-9
Guidelines for Pain Relief Involving the Hip Joint

- *Activity modification*: Initially, the clinician should encourage patients to maintain muscle performance and ROM of the hip while avoiding risk activities, such as running, carrying heavy loads (especially contralateral to the painful hip[118]), or prolonged standing.
- *Physical agents or electrotherapeutic modalities*: The use of cryotherapy, moist heat, or electrotherapeutic modalities may help modulate pain or decrease inflammation. Because of the anatomic position of the hip, these modalities may have limited effectiveness in treating intraarticular inflammation or sources of pain.
- *Manual therapy*: Appropriate use of joint and soft-tissue mobilization can improve physiologic impairments related to pain and inflammation, such as joint mobility and tissue extensibility. Joint mobilization can also be used to modulate pain (see Chapter 7).[119]
- *Therapeutic exercise intervention*: Gentle active ROM exercises in the pain-free range can be used to modulate pain, similar to the grade III joint mobilizations described by Maitland.[119]
- *Assistive devices*: When a person has a limp caused by pain, use of an assistive device in the contralateral hand is neces-

sary to reduce the load on the hip. A cane in the contralateral hand of a patient can reduce the joint reaction force by as much as 30%.[129] Patients often are reluctant to use an assistive device for fear of "giving in to the condition." Patient-related instruction must include an explanation that temporary use of an assistive device will reduce the load at the hip and allow the pain and inflammation to resolve. Exercise to improve mobility and force- or torque-generating capability of the appropriate musculature is required to discontinue use of the assistive device without risk of recurrence of symptoms.
- *Weight loss*: Overweight persons must work diligently on weight loss through proper nutritional counseling and aerobic activity tolerated by a painful hip, including non–weight-bearing activity such as aquatic activities or cycling. It is possible that cumulative exposure to excessive body mass may increase the risk of developing hip OA[120,121] and the worsening of the disease.[122,123]
- *Biomechanical support*: Carefully prescribed foot orthotics can improve skeletal alignment and potentially influence contact forces at the hip.[124]

> ### BUILDING BLOCK 19-4
>
> Consider a 71-year-old male post open reduction internal fixation (ORIF) of the left femur secondary to a fall. The patient complains of 8/10 pain in the anterior and lateral aspect of the left hip. The patient is now to be ambulating weight bearing as tolerated (WBAT) per the doctor's orders. The patient presents with 3/5 strength of the hip flexors, extensors, and abductors as well as limited ROM into hip extension. The patient still needs moderate assistance to stand and for ambulation. Develop a treatment plan for this patient to accelerate his rehabilitation and recovery.

underlying cause(s) are established, an appropriate intervention can be developed to manage the associated impairments (i.e., muscle stretching, joint mobilization, muscle strengthening).

Although posture and movement retraining are ultimate goals in most physical therapy interventions, changes in posture and movement patterns require basic skills in mobility, muscle performance, and motor control. To affect a posture or movement change, mobility, length-tension properties, and muscle performance must be at functional levels, and kinesthetic awareness about joint position, joint motion, or a specific muscle recruitment pattern must be developed.

The initial focus of any intervention should be on improving impairments of body functions to a functional level. After these impairments have achieved a functional level of capac-

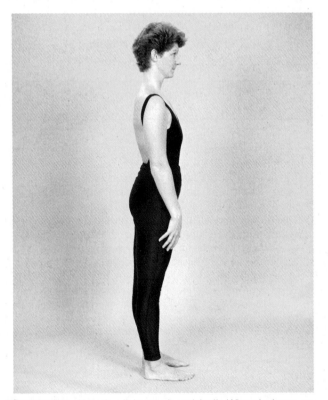

FIGURE 19-24. Note the slight anterior pelvic tilt. When the knees are hyperextended, the hips will be extended, even if the pelvic tilt is slightly anterior.

ity, gradual transition from specific exercises addressing physiologic impairments to greater emphasis on posture and movement patterns used during functional exercise, and activities should occur until the primary emphasis is on functional retraining. Examples of exercises to improve posture and movement of the hip joint are presented throughout this chapter.

Limb Length Discrepancy

Although LLD is not considered a postural impairment isolated to the hip, it is discussed here because of its functional implication at the hip as the transmitter of forces from the ground and lower extremities to the trunk and upper extremities. Functional LLD is the most difficult form to diagnose and treat. Nearly any movement of an osseous segment out of its normal plane of reference in relation to other bones can create a shorter or longer distance between proximal and distal reference points. Altered osseous positions can occur about any axis of motion and in any segment. Minor alterations in position in any one segment, when added to minor alterations in position of other segments, can lead to a substantial LLD.

To further complicate matters, functional LLD can coexist with structural LLD—sometimes exaggerating the LLD and sometimes compensating for the LLD. For example, a structurally longer limb may compensate for its length with lateral pelvic tilt, knee flexion, or foot pronation. After the type of LLD and the segments involved are accurately diagnosed as functional, structural, or combined LLD, appropriate intervention must be determined.

Treatment of LLD ranges from posture and movement training to shoe inserts to various surgical techniques including limb lengthening and shortening and epiphysiodesis. After it has been determined that the LLD is not completely amenable to posture and movement training, other nonsurgical or surgical interventions are indicated. There is disagreement regarding the correct treatment in regards to magnitude of LLD. Reid and Smith[125] suggest dividing LLD into three categories, mild (0 to 30 mm), moderate (30 to 60 mm), and severe (>60 mm), in which mild cases should either go untreated or treated nonsurgically, moderate cases should be dealt with on a case-by-case basis and some should be dealt with surgically, and severe cases should be corrected surgically. Moseley suggests a similar breakdown: 0 to 20 mm requiring no treatment, 20 to 60 mm requiring a shoe lift, epiphysiodesis, or shortening, 60 to 200 mm requiring lengthening that may or may not be combined with other procedures, and >200 mm prosthetic fitting.[126]

Structural Leg Length Discrepancy The most common treatment for mild structural LLD is the use of shoe lifts, which consists of a heel lift, shoe insert, or building up the sole of the shoe on the shorter leg. In general, up to 20 mm of correction can be made with an insert, whereas further corrections should be done on the sole of the shoe.[127,128] If an equinus anatomic impairment exists, a heel lift is more appropriate than a full-sole lift. The amount of lift prescribed depends on the limb length difference and the patient's physiologic tolerance to change. Individuals with long-standing, significant structural discrepancies generally do not tolerate significant, rapid change because of the osseous and soft-tissue adaptations that have developed over time. Minimal height adjustments at infrequent intervals should be made until the maximal necessary change has occurred.

Functional Limb Length Discrepancy   Treatment of functional LLD should consider the physiologic impairments at each involved segment and the interactions between levels. For example, a functionally short limb caused by femoral and tibial medial rotation and by foot pronation could have associated impairments of:

- Lengthened or weak posterior gluteus medius and deep hip lateral rotators
- Lengthened or weak foot supinators
- Forefoot or rearfoot varus

Appropriate exercises, biomechanical support, and posture and movement training are necessary to alleviate the related impairments.

Patients with functional LLD related to lower extremity kinetic chain pronation (i.e., femur medial rotation, genu valgum, and foot pronation) may benefit from temporary or permanent foot orthotics to assist in controlling pronation throughout the kinetic chain. However, caution must be used in prescribing orthotics to remedy physiologic impairments up the kinetic chain. Exercises to alleviate impairments of body functions contributing to pronation should be attempted first. If performance demands exceed the ability to control pronation, use of orthotics may be a useful adjunct.

Cautious use of sole or heel lifts to compensate for a functional LLD is recommended. The faulty strategy of displacing the center of mass over the base of support used by a patient with a functional LLD does not necessarily alter with a lift. The more common scenario is for the individual to continue with the same faulty strategy, thereby enhancing the functional LLD. For example, during initial contact phase of gait, the short limb may be functionally short as a result of positioning the hip in adduction with minimal displacement of the center of mass over the base of support. After adding a lift, a similar gait strategy may continue to be used, causing further exaggeration of the LLD. Often, training the patient to properly position the hip and accurately displace the center of mass over the base of support alleviates the LLD without the need for orthotic correction (see Self-Management 19-2, levels I and II).

THERAPEUTIC EXERCISE INTERVENTIONS FOR COMMON DIAGNOSES

Although it is beyond the scope of this text to present a comprehensive description and intervention plan for all diagnoses affecting the hip joint, a few selected diagnostic categories are presented. A brief overview of the etiology, examination/evaluation findings, and proposed intervention, with emphasis on therapeutic exercise, is presented for each diagnosis.

Osteoarthritis

OA is the most common form of arthritis, affecting millions of people in the United States. Among US adults 30 years of age or older, symptomatic disease in the hip occurs in approximately 3%.[129] OA increases with age- and sex-specific

differences are evident.[130–133] Other risk factors for hip OA include developmental disorders (Legg-Calve-Perthes disease, congenital hip dislocation, slipped capital femoral epiphysis), genetics, previous injury, sports exposure, and leg length disparity.[18] Because OA is a disease whose prevalence increases with age, it will become even more prevalent in the future as the bulging cohort of baby boomers grows older.

OA is a complex disease whose etiology bridges biomechanics and biochemistry. Evidence is growing for the role of systemic factors (such as genetics, dietary intake, estrogen use, and bone density) and of local biomechanical factors (such as muscle weakness, obesity, and joint laxity). These risk factors are particularly important in weight-bearing joints, and modifying them may present opportunities for prevention of OA-related pain and disability. The reader is referred to Chapter 12 for an in-depth discussion of the etiology of OA.

Diagnosis
Proper diagnosis of a patient with hip OA requires a careful history, physical examination, and review of appropriate radiographic and laboratory studies. The presence of radiographic changes (e.g., joint space narrowing, moderate malalignment, osteophytes at the marginal aspects of the joint) should correlate with positive examination findings at the hip joint to arrive at a diagnosis of hip OA. A positive radiographic finding alone does not indicate that the hip OA is the source of symptoms, because many other musculoskeletal and nonmusculoskeletal sources can mimic hip joint pain. Hip OA is a common sequelae of aging and is not always symptomatic. Many people with pathologic and radiographic evidence of OA have no symptoms.[134]

Laboratory tests may not detect serum abnormalities unless their presence is related to another disease process. The rheumatoid factor test is generally negative. If the rheumatoid factor is found in the serum of older patients, its presence may be unrelated to the arthritis because false-positive results for rheumatoid factor increase with age in the normal population.[135]

Gradual, progressive, chronic pain can be associated with OA. Intraarticular pain is usually described as deep, aching pain and can be experienced in the groin, around the greater trochanter, medial knee, and posterior buttock. The patient may induce or aggravate pain with moderate to vigorous activity and experience relief of pain with rest. Long periods of rest, however, may result in joint stiffness. The stiffness of OA is not as severe as that of rheumatoid arthritis. Mild activity usually dissipates the stiffness. A clinical prediction rule for the diagnosis of OA is described in Display 19-10.

DISPLAY 19-10
Clinical Prediction Rule for Diagnosing Hip Osteoarthritis[136]

If at least 4 of 5 variables were present, the positive likelihood ratio was equal to 24.3 (95% confidence interval: 4.4–142.1), increasing the probability of hip OA to 91%.

Variables
- Self reported squatting as an aggravating factor
- Active hip flexion causing lateral hip pain
- Scour test with adduction causing lateral hip or groin pain
- Active hip extension causing pain
- Passive internal rotation of less than or equal to 25 degrees

Treatment

Major advances in management of OA to reduce pain and disability are yielding an impressive array of available treatments ranging from acupuncture to chondrocyte transplantation, new oral anti-inflammatory medications, and patient-related instruction. Evidence for the efficacy of commonly used oral therapies, alternative therapies, biomechanical interventions, such as exercise, and behavioral interventions directed toward enhancing self-management is mounting (see Display 19-11). In the vast majority of cases, surgical treatment of OA is considered only after failure of nonsurgical treatments.[127] Recently, biologic approaches to the surgical treatment of OA have been explored.[128,137]

The following sections will review concepts related to therapeutic exercise intervention for the treatment of impairments related to hip OA.

Pain and Inflammation Management of pain and inflammation for hip OA can follow the general guidelines discussed in a previous section (see Display 19-9). Activity modification may be one of the most significant aspects of treatment for pain and inflammation. The changes may include modification of basic and instrumental ADLs. The patient should be instructed in joint protection techniques during prolonged postures (i.e., standing with equal weight bearing on both feet, using an assistive device) and common movement patterns (i.e., carrying heavy loads in the hand on the involved side or in both hands equally).[129] The patient can convert vigorous weight-bearing activities (e.g., running, tennis) to non–weight-bearing activities (e.g., biking, swimming, water aerobics).

Specific to hip OA, treatment addressing the cause of the pain should focus on altering the biomechanics of the hip. The degeneration in OA is caused by a breakdown of chondrocytes, which are an essential element of articular cartilage. This breakdown may be initiated by biomechanical stress. A primary goal of the intervention should be to alter biomechanical forces acting on the joint. Restoring joint ROM and tissue extensibility in flexion, extension, medial rotation, and abduction and restoring dynamic muscle performance of gluteus medius, minimus, deep hip lateral rotators, and maximus enables the joint to function in improved alignment and movement patterns. This in turn can reduce the biomechanical stress to the focal area of degenerative joint disease (DJD) and result in decreased pain.

Range of Motion and Joint Mobility Specific exercises to improve ROM and joint mobility may include passive (Figs. 19-25 and 19-26) and active stretching (Self-Management 19-6), and mobilization in the affected directions (see Chapter 7). When performing passive stretching, care must be taken to stabilize the pelvis, sacroiliac joint (SIJ), and lumbar region, and guide the hip in the acetabulum to prevent impingement. Active exercises should be employed whenever possible. Active exercises improve ROM and joint mobility with the added bonus of recruitment of the muscles necessary to move the joint in the desired direction during function. Examples of active exercises to improve hip mobility in persons with hip OA are shown in Self-Management 19-4 and Self-Management 19-8. Another useful technique to teach the patient with OA in the hip is self-traction (Fig. 19-27).

Muscle Performance The patient can be instructed in specific exercises to improve muscle performance (see Self-Managements 19-1 and 19-4). Whenever possible, functional exercises should be employed. For example, standing on the involved hip in neutral hip joint alignment and lifting the uninvolved hip onto a step can stimulate hip abductor recruitment on the weight-bearing side. However, weight-bearing exercises on a hip with OA may exacerbate symptoms, particularly if the alignment is faulty. Adjunctive use of a cane, walking stick, ski pole, or dowel rod in the contralateral hand during weight-bearing exercise can reduce the amount of work necessary for the ipsilateral hip abductors. This approach reduces the joint reaction force and joint pain and increases tolerance to weight-bearing exercise.

Another method to reduce the joint reaction force enough to allow weight-bearing exercise is to hold a weight in the hand on the involved side.[129] The amount of weight can be graded to use the least amount necessary to reduce pain and allow optimal alignment during the step-up activity.

Regardless of the method used to unload the hip, the appropriate strategy for unilateral balance must be reinforced. The gluteus medius and TFL are synergist hip abductors. It is common for the TFL to dominate the stance recruitment pattern, particularly if the hip is in flexion or medial rotation. Education regarding the neutral position of the hip and gluteus medius recruitment is critical to the optimal outcome of this exercise. This may require additional activity from the inner core muscles to control anterior pelvic tilt.

Step-up activities stimulate hip extensor recruitment of the stance limb[57] and facilitate hip flexion mobility, particularly if emphasis is placed on hip flexion during the step-up (Fig. 19-28), and step-down activities stimulate gluteus medius recruitment.[57] Care must be taken during stepping activities to prevent Trendelenburg patterns and to reinforce proper length-tension properties of the gluteus medius (i.e., hip should not adduct more than 5 to 8 degrees, and femoral medial rotation should be kept to a minimum). All stepping activities can be graded by altering the step height or adding weight. A small step height (4 in) and carrying a weight in the involved side hand reduces the force-generating requirements of the hip extensors and abductors. Conversely, larger step heights (8 to 12 in) and carrying a weight in the contralateral hand increase the force-generating requirements.

Dosage parameters regarding repetition for these exercises depend on whether the goal is to improve force/torque or endurance capabilities. Higher repetitions with a decreased load focus on endurance, and lower repetitions with a higher load focus on force production.

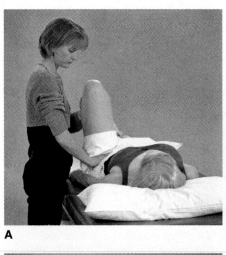
A

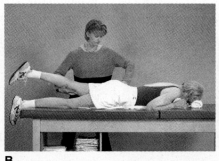
B

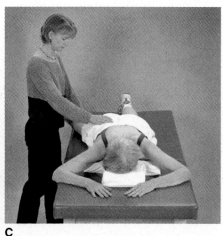
C

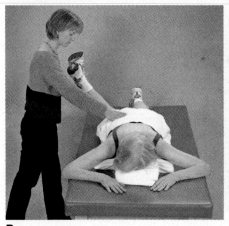
D

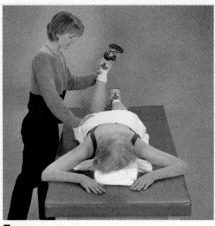
E

FIGURE 19-25. Passive range of motion to the hip in (A) flexion, (B) extension, (C) abduction, (D) medial rotation, and (E) lateral rotation. Note the stabilization of the pelvis to make certain that movement occurs at the hip in isolation. In the case of hip flexion, a simultaneous posterior-inferior glide of the head of the femur can reduce anterior hip impingement that occurs with a stiff posterior joint.

Balance   Injury to a joint and musculotendinous structures, as in hip OA, probably results in altered somatosensory information that can adversely affect motor control.[158] Progressive balance training can have a positive effect on function of the arthritic hip. Self-Management 19-2, levels I and II can be useful in training an individual to balance on one limb with correct form. After the patient is able to stand on one limb with appropriate muscle recruitment and joint

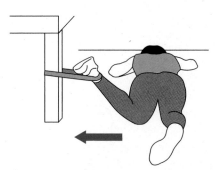

FIGURE 19-26. Prone hip medial rotation stretch with elastic. The patient is instructed to stabilize the pelvis in sagittal and transverse planes via inner core contraction. It is important to keep the femur in contact with the floor to ensure a precise rotational stretch. If the hip flexors are short, use of a pillow under the hips can allow the knee to flex 90 degrees with minimal compensatory hip flexion. This exercise is contraindicated in the presence of knee pathology.

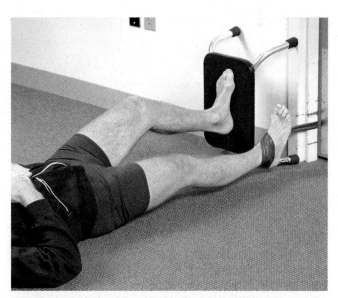

FIGURE 19-27. Self-traction of the hip. The involved limb is given traction by the use of a belt or other stiff material around the ankle which is secured in a door jam, whereas the contralateral limb pushes off a surface as shown. This technique can provide a decompression stress to the joint and stretch the joint capsule.

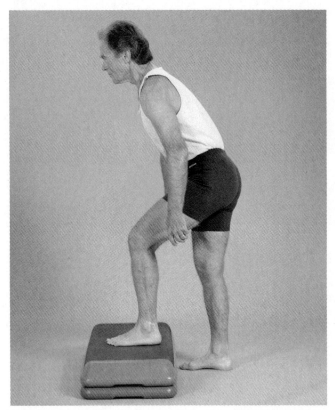

FIGURE 19-28. Side view of a step-up exercise with exaggerated hip flexion to focus on hip flexion mobility and gluteus maximus recruitment.

loading strategies with reduced pain, balance activities can be added to the program. Progression should be taken slowly to prevent an inflammatory reaction in the hip, which would be counterproductive to improved function.

Posture and Movement Patient-related instructions regarding improved weight-bearing habits are critical to the long-term effectiveness of therapeutic exercise. The person with hip OA must be cautioned to avoid positioning the involved limb in the capsular pattern (i.e., hip flexion and lateral rotation). Instruction in use of the inner core should not be overlooked because of its effect on improving pelvic position. Small ROM wall squats can be useful to provide a stretch to the anterior myofascial structures simultaneous with inner core strengthening (see Fig. 13-4). During function, use of assistive devices such as canes, crutches, or walkers can be quite effective in reducing joint stress during ambulation, and consequently decrease antalgic gait patterns. Problem solving to develop improved posture and movement patterns to allow continued participation in social and occupational activities is time well spent with a patient.

Adjunctive Interventions Because the hip is a weight-bearing joint, it is important that the individual maintains optimal weight through proper nutrition and aerobic activity. Non–weight-bearing aerobic activities are recommended for persons with hip OA.[159]

Use of a stationary bike with the seat relatively high can serve as means of maintaining aerobic activity with minimal weight-bearing stress on the joint. Aquatic exercise programs have been shown to be effective for the treatment of OA of the knee and hip, with 75% of subjects reporting improvement in pain and function after a 6 week bout of aquatic PT.[160,161] Swimming, non–weight-bearing exercise with inflatable supports, or weight-bearing exercises in a pool (see Chapter 16) minimize stress on the hip joint.

Manual therapy has been used to improve hip ROM and decrease OA pain, especially in patients without signs of severe OA. Manual therapy; consisting of stretching, manual traction, and long axis manipulation; was found to be superior to exercise in some studies. The combination of manual therapy and exercise yeilded improvement in six of seven patients with hip OA.[162]

Iliotibial Band–Related Diagnoses

The extensive deep fascia that covers the gluteal region and the thigh like a sleeve is called the fascia lata. It is attached proximally to the external lip of the iliac crest, the sacrum and coccyx, the sacrotuberous ligament, the ischial tuberosity, the ischiopubic rami, and the inguinal ligament. Distally, it is attached to the patella, the tibial condyles, and the head of the fibula. The dense portion of the fascia lata situated laterally is designated the ITB. The TFL and three fourths of the gluteus maximus insert into the ITB so that its distal attachment serves as a conjoint tendon of these muscles. The TFL can be functionally differentiated into anteromedial (Fig. 19-29A) and posterolateral fibers (Fig. 19-29B and C). The anteromedial fibers have a greater mechanical advantage for hip flexion (Fig. 19-29A), and the posterolateral fibers have a greater mechanical advantage for hip abduction (Fig. 19-29B) and medial rotation (Fig. 19-29C).[163]

During normal walking, the anteromedial fibers generally are quiet, whereas the posterolateral fibers are active near initial contact.[163] With sequentially increased locomotor velocity, anteromedial fiber activity increases near preswing and initial swing, presumably to decelerate the extending hip and accelerate flexion of the thigh, and posterolateral activity increases at initial contact, presumably to decelerate the

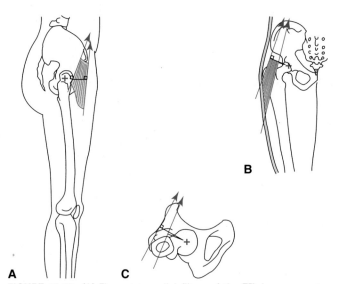

FIGURE 19-29. (A) The anteromedial fibers of the TFL have a greater mechanical advantage for hip flexion. (B) The posterolateral fibers of the TFL have a greater mechanical advantage for hip abduction and (C) medial rotation. (From Pare EB, Stern JT, Schwartz JM. Functional differentiation within the tensor fascia latae. J Bone Joint Surg Am 1981;63A:1457.)

DISPLAY 19-12
ITB-Related Diagnoses

- *ITB fascitis*: Inflammation of the ITB resulting from overuse of ITB for stability.
- *Trochanteric bursitis*: In trochanter bursitis, the bursa becomes inflamed because of the pressure exerted by a short ITB moving back and forth over the greater trochanter during movement.
- *ITB friction syndrome (also known as ITB syndrome)*: In ITB friction syndrome, pain and tenderness are localized to the lateral femoral condyle because of a short ITB exerting pressure over the lateral femoral condyle.
- *Patellofemoral dysfunction*: Shortness of the ITB can contribute to patellofemoral dysfunction because of its insertion into the lateral retinaculum of the patellofemoral joint and its tendency to dominate over the quadriceps for knee stability (see Chapter 20).
- *TFL strain*: TFL strain can occur from overuse of a short TFL/ITB or a stretched TFL/ITB complex. The former is more common, but there are instances of strain of the stretched TFL/ITB. The TFL/ITB on the side of the adducted hip (usually the high iliac crest), if there are no associated hip medial rotation or hip flexion alignment or movement faults, is subject to continuous tension and therefore strain.
- *Faulty movement patterns at the hip and tibiofemoral joints*: Faulty movement patterns of the hip and tibiofemoral joints related to the TFL/ITB are critical to understanding the effect of muscle imbalance on the function of these joints. Sahrmann provides more information on this subject.[53]

DISPLAY 19-13
Key Tests for Differential Diagnosis of Iliotibial Band Fascitis from Sciatica

Key Tests

- Palpation over the length of the fascia lata may elicit tenderness, especially over the greater trochanter or near the point of insertion lateral to the patella.
- Hip flexion, abduction, and medial rotation (TFL manual muscle test) may test painful.
- The Ober test (test for ITB length) reveals shortness of the TFL/ITB, and further stretch may elicit pain. Paresthesias along the peroneal nerve distribution may worsen with ankle inversion.
- Lumbar spine clearing test results are negative for reproduction of the patient's symptoms.

Associated Findings

- Hip rotation ROM may reveal excessive medial rotation relative to lateral rotation ROM.
- Positional weakness of the synergistic muscles of the gluteus medius, gluteus maximus, iliopsoas, and quadriceps.
- Hip anteversion.
- Excessive medial rotation, positive Trendelenburg sign, or limited hip extension in gait.

adduction moment.[163] The posterolateral fibers of the TFL/ITB complex have also been implicated in providing stability against varus stress at the knee.[164] The anteromedial fibers are active during the hip flexion phase of the step-up, and the posterolateral fibers are active during the loading phase of the step-up.

Because of the vast functional roles of the TFL/ITB complex, it is prone to overuse injuries (see Display 19-12).[53] The following sections provide etiologic and treatment information for the most common ITB-related diagnoses.

Iliotibial Band Fascitis

A condition, sometimes mistakenly diagnosed as sciatica, is that of pain associated with inflammation of the fascial band from overuse of the TFL, commonly called ITB fascitis.[53] Pain may be limited to the area covered by the fascia along the lateral surface of the thigh or may extend upward over the buttocks and involve the gluteal fascia. Painful symptoms may extend below the knee, with associated symptoms of paresthesia in the region of the lateral calf.

A review of the anatomy of the lateral aspect of the knee demonstrates the relationship of the peroneal nerve to the muscles and fascia in this area. Peroneal nerve irritation can result from pressure from rigid bands of fascia in a short ITB or from the effect of traction from taut bands of fascia in an overstretched ITB. Peroneal nerve irritation can manifest as symptoms in the lateral calf.[27]

Symptoms are similar to plantar fascitis; often worse in the morning and improve with minimal weight bearing, but they then worsen with continued weight bearing. Tests

to differentiate ITB fascitis from sciatica are summarized in Display 19-13. Presumably, this condition results from overuse of the TFL/ITB. Concurrent with any overuse syndrome is underuse of the related synergists about any axis of motion in which the affected muscle functions. The more deconditioned the underused synergists become, the greater the force-producing requirements become for the TFL/ITB complex, until finally the force-producing requirements exceed the muscle and fascial capability, and inflammation results. Display 19-14 summarizes the synergist relationships that may become imbalanced, leading to TFL/ITB overuse.

Iliotibial Band Friction Syndrome

Although iliotibial band friction syndrome (also known as iliotibial band syndrome) manifests at the knee, it is presented here because therapeutic exercise intervention is focused at

DISPLAY 19-14
Potential Synergist Relationships with TFL/ITB Overuse

- The anteromedial TFL can dominate the hip flexion force couple, contributing to underuse of the iliopsoas.
- The posterolateral TFL can dominate the hip abduction and medial rotation force couples, contributing to underuse of the gluteus medius, upper fibers of the gluteus maximus, and gluteus minimus.
- Because the ITB can provide stability to the knee, overuse of the ITB may contribute to underuse of the quadriceps.
- The hip tends to function in medial rotation patterns, thereby contributing to underuse of the hip lateral rotator force couple, including the deep hip rotators, posterior fibers of the gluteus medius, and lower fibers of the gluteus maximus.

the imbalances in flexibility and muscle performance at the hip. ITB syndrome is an overuse syndrome first described by Olson and Armour.[164] The ITB lies anterior to the lateral femoral condyle with the knee in extension and moves posterior to the lateral epicondylar prominence with knee flexion. Biomechanical research of ITB syndrome has demonstrated that friction occurs near footstrike, predominantly in the foot contact phase, between the posterior edge of the ITB and the underlying lateral femoral epicondyle.[165] The posterior fibers of the ITB are more problematic in this syndrome than the anterior fibers. This is supported by the surgically known fact that the posterior fibers of the ITB are tighter against the lateral epicondyle than the anterior fibers.[166] Repetitive knee flexion and extension causes the posterior edge of the ITB to rub across the lateral epicondyle, which gives rise to an inflammatory reaction in the tissue deep to the ITB.

ITB syndrome is quite common in long distance runners, cited as the second most common injury, with a sex discrepancy prevalence of 38% male and 62% female.[167] ITB syndrome in runners results from a complex of training errors, muscle imbalances in performance and flexibility, inappropriate surface and terrain, lower extremity alignment, and inappropriate footwear.

The clinical symptoms of ITB syndrome include lateral knee pain and occasional snapping laterally. The area is tender over the lateral condyle and pain can be provoked by exerting pressure over the lateral epicondyle during active knee flexion, particularly at 30-degree flexion.[168] It is not uncommon for this syndrome to be misdiagnosed as another condition that causes lateral knee pain such as lateral meniscal tear, lateral collateral ligament sprain, or popliteal tendinitis.[166] Coronal magnetic resonance imaging can be useful to determine a differential diagnosis.[167]

Other ITB-Related Syndromes

Similar causes exist for the remaining ITB diagnoses, although with slightly different symptoms. Although some of these diagnoses manifest at the knee, treatment must focus on the cause of the condition, which is TFL/ITB overuse at the hip.

Treatment

Therapeutic exercise intervention for each of the ITB-related diagnoses should take into consideration the biomechanical factors causing the syndrome and the related anatomic and physiologic impairments.

Pain and Inflammation   In the acute phase, treatment should be directed toward alleviating the pain and inflammation with medication (i.e., nonsteroidal anti-inflammatory drugs), physical agents (i.e., cryotherapy), electrotherapeutic modalities, and unloading (e.g., use of a cane, taping, proper positioning at night with pillows between knees if sidelying).[53,168] As acute symptoms subside, succeeding treatments should be directed toward resolving the impairments and activity limitations associated with the condition.

Range of Motion   ROM impairments are most often associated with a stiff or short TFL/ITB complex.[169] Stretching the TFL/ITB complex is indicated but can pose a challenge to the clinician and patient. The TFL/ITB has many actions at the hip. For an optimal stretch, the TFL/ITB must be elongated simultaneously in all directions opposite its actions.

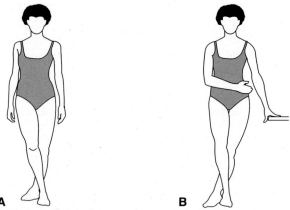

FIGURE 19-30. Commonly prescribed TFL/ITB stretch that does not stretch the TFL/ITB in all directions opposite its actions. (A) Crossing the legs commonly places the hip joint in medial rotation. (B) Swaying laterally, with the hip medially rotated, stretches the gluteus medius and lateral capsule more than the TFL/ITB.

It is critical that the stretching be specifically directed to the area in need of stretch, and some commonly prescribed TFL/ITB stretches do not meet these criteria (Fig. 19-30).

An assisted stretch emphasizing the posterolateral fibers is shown in Figure 19-31. This stretch ensures the most precise positioning for the best outcome. The obvious disadvantage of this stretch is that rarely can an individual self-stretch in this position. Over time, he or she may be able to master the control required after a series of hip abduction exercises with the emphasis on eccentric control of the gluteus medius (see Self-Management 19-4). This exercise also emphasizes improving the force-generating capability and kinesthetic awareness of the gluteus medius—a critical, underused synergist. A self-stretch exercise for the TFL/ITB is shown in Figure 19-32. This stretch is directed more toward the anterolateral fibers and is considered an active stretch because of the activation of the abdominal muscle group and gluteus maximus to rotate the pelvis posteriorly.

TFL/ITB stretching should not be used in isolation with the hope that the stretch will permanently improve the length. The clinician must seek the related impairments and activity limitations that perpetuate the shortness. For example, short

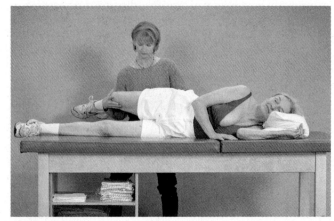

FIGURE 19-31.   Assisted Ober stretch position. The hip must be in concurrent hip extension, lateral rotation, and adduction without lateral pelvic tilt. This is difficult to perform without assistance.

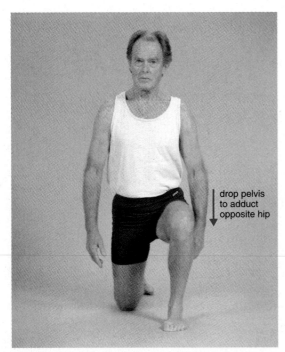

FIGURE 19-32. ITB stretch to the extended hip. In the half-kneel stretch position, the patient is asked to maximally drop the contralateral pelvis to adduct the ipsilateral hip. The patient also is asked to extend the hip by means of posterior pelvic tilt (using the gluteus maximus and abdominal muscles). A slight hip lateral rotation can be added to stretch the PL fibers. This technique is best used for hip conditions as weightbearing on the knee can be uncomfortable in patients with knee conditions.

posterolateral fibers of the TFL/ITB do not remain stretched if the person stands and moves with the hip in excessive medial rotation. Improvements in muscle performance of

the underused synergists coupled with education regarding postural habits and neuromuscular training of new movement patterns are essential to restoring length to the ITB on a more permanent basis.

Muscle Performance   Correction of muscle performance deficits of the hip abductor muscles has been shown to be correlated with recovery from ITB syndrome.[62] Perhaps progressive strengthening of additional underused synergists such as the iliopsoas, gluteus maximus, and quadriceps can further assist in reducing the physiologic and biomechanical requirements of the TFL/ITB. After functional muscle performance is achieved, attention to biomechanical elements to ensure recruitment of these synergists/antagonists during function is essential to full recovery.

The initial exercise prescription depends on the positional strength of these muscles. For example, the iliopsoas may require active assist initially, progressing to active holding, resistive holding, and finally functional exercises (see Self-Management 19-5 and the swing phase of Self-Management 19-3). The emphasis initially is on end-range isometrics, followed by eccentric, and finally concentric contractions to ensure the improvement of the positional strength of the iliopsoas at end range. The goal with this approach is to improve the length-tension relationships of the relatively lengthened, weaker synergist to the TFL/ITB in hip flexion. An example of a functional movement recruiting the iliopsoas may include repeated swing phase of a step-up with avoidance of hip medial rotation or hip hike accompanying the hip flexion pattern.

Adjunctive Intervention   For a strained TFL/ITB due to continuous tension, use of taping as illustrated by Kendall et al.[27] (Fig. 19-33A) can unload the strained structure. Because the femur must not function in excessive medial rotation, taping the hip in a slight amount of lateral rotation

FIGURE 19-33. Taping techniques to unload the ITB. (A) Unloading the TFL/ITB with lateral longitudinal taping using a technique developed by Florence Kendall. (B) Unloading the TFL/ITB with anterior to posterior strips positioned proximally over the TFL and placed every 2 to 3 in distally. The patellofemoral joint may need to be taped medially to prevent lateral displacement from the stretch placed on the ITB distally.

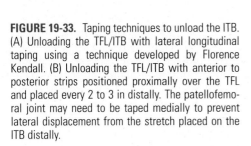

A

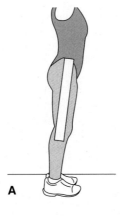

B

BUILDING BLOCK 19-5

Consider a 19-year-old female track runner who presents with pain 6/10 on the lateral aspect of the right hip, worse with running. The patient presents with weakness of the gluteus medius and deep hip lateral rotators. You analyze her running and notice pronation at initial contact with subsequent excessive femoral adduction and internal rotation with knee valgus during loading. Develop a prioritized treatment plan for this patient to return to running with less pain.

may be indicated. An alternative taping technique is illustrated in Figure 19-33B. Applying firm pressure over the TFL while applying tape over this area may unload the TFL and therefore encourage more gluteus medius participation during functional activities (see Building Block 19-5).

Nerve Entrapment Syndromes

Although nerve entrapment syndromes represent a relatively small group of conditions causing hip, groin, or buttock pain, an understanding of the etiology of these syndromes can facilitate a precise diagnosis and promote efficient management of the condition. Display 19-15 lists the possible nerve entrapment syndromes that can be a source of hip, groin, or buttock pain.

The anatomic possibilities for nerve entrapment syndromes in this region arise from the lumbosacral plexus and its branches (Fig. 19-34). Unless nerve entrapment syndromes produce "hard" neurologic signs of motor weakness, sensory loss, or change in tendon reflexes, specific diagnosis may be difficult. This is particularly true of nerve entrapments around the pelvis where the cutaneous sensory dermatomes overlap considerably and many of the nerves have no motor innervation that can be easily tested, resulting in nonspecific and poorly localized pain or paresthesia complaints. A thorough knowledge of the anatomy of the region is necessary to diagnose nerve entrapment syndromes at the hip. Table 19-3 assists the reader with differential diagnosis by providing a regional approach to the diagnosis of nerve entrapment syndromes.

DISPLAY 19-15
Specific Nerve Entrapment Syndromes as a Cause of Pain in the Hip, Groin, and Buttock

- Iliohypogastric nerve
- Ilioinguinal nerve
- Genitofemoral nerve
- Obturator nerve
- Lateral cutaneous nerve of the thigh
- Femoral nerve
- Pudendal nerve
- Posterior cutaneous nerve of the thigh
- Superior and inferior gluteal nerves
- Sciatic nerve

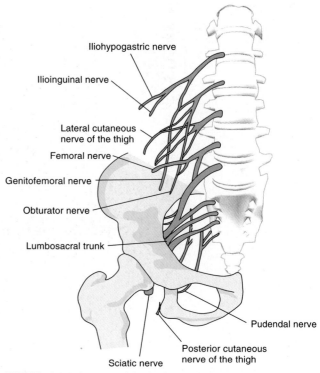

FIGURE 19-34. Anatomy of the lumbosacral plexus.

For the purposes of this text, the discussion of entrapment syndromes will be focused on symptoms in the region of the buttock and posterior thigh. The piriformis syndrome has been described as a form of sciatic nerve entrapment causing buttock and posterior thigh pain and the piriformis muscle has been implicated as a potential source of sciatica symptoms.[170] The original description of this condition dates from 1928 when Yeoman[171] stated that insufficient attention had been paid to the piriformis muscle as a potential cause of sciatica.

Although there may be numerous cases in which sciatic pain is associated with a short piriformis, Kendall[27] and Sahrmann[53] describe a variation of this syndrome in which the piriformis is lengthened.

The length of the piriformis must be carefully assessed before planning an intervention for this syndrome. For example, in a faulty standing position with the femur in adduction and medial rotation and the pelvis in anterior pelvic tilt, the piriformis muscle is placed on stretch. The piriformis muscle is pulled taut, potentially entrapping the sciatic nerve. Pressure on the sciatic nerve may result from tension from the adjacent taut piriformis muscle. If the nerve pierces through the piriformis, an injurious tension may be imposed on the sciatic nerve along with the stretched muscle. Because the piriformis is actively used during gait, abnormal gait patterns can impose stress on the piriformis and related sciatic nerve. With a stretched piriformis, repetitive movements of the hip in medial rotation and adduction and movements of the pelvis in anterior pelvic tilt can impose friction on the nerve, resulting in inflammation of the neural tissue. Strain of the piriformis can ensue as a result of the muscle functioning in a chronically stretched position.

| TABLE 19-4 | **Differential Diagnosis of Stretched Piriformis Syndrome** |

Key tests
Standing alignment
Selective tissue tension tests
Range of motion
Palpation
Positional strength
Functional tests
Lumbar clearing examination

Signs
Lordosis and anterior pelvic tilt
Hip flexion and medial rotation
High iliac crest on involved side
<90 degrees of hip flexion, with adduction and medial rotation reproduces symptoms
Passive or active lateral rotation and abduction reduces symptoms
Resisted knee flexion is negative
Excessive hip medial rotation relative to lateral rotation within the involved side
Excessive medial rotation of the involved side relative to the uninvolved side
Tenderness elicited in region of the sciatic notch
Weakness in hip lateral rotators and posterior gluteus medius
Tendency to function in hip medial rotation, hip adduction, and anterior pelvic tilt during functional activities
Repetitive movements in medial rotation and/or adduction, with the pelvis in anterior tilt, reproduce symptoms
Lateral rotation, abduction, and neutral pelvic alignment relieves symptoms
Symptoms diminish or disappear when not bearing weight

Diagnosis

Differential diagnosis of buttock and posterior thigh pain can be quite complex. One has to consider the potential causes of symptoms including; piriformis (lengthened, shortened, strained, or hypertrophied), obturator internus/gemelli complex, lumbosacral radiculopathy, or referred pain. Given the anatomic relationship of the piriformis to the various nerves in the deep gluteal region, it is possible that the buttock pain represents entrapment of the gluteal nerves. Pain caused by piriformis strain can also be felt deep in the buttock. Posterior thigh pain can be caused by the posterior cutaneous nerve of the thigh, which would explain the absence of distal sciatic neurologic signs in some cases. It is possible that the obturator internus/gemelli complex is an alternative cause of neural compression. For this reason, "deep gluteal syndrome" may be a more appropriate term for symptoms isolated to the buttock.[172] Symptoms of sciatica related to a stretched, short, or hypertrophied piriformis can be experienced from the posterior buttock extending inferiorly as far as the toes. Symptoms of pain or tingling may appear in the cutaneous areas below the knee supplied by branches of the peroneal or posterior tibial nerve before symptoms of numbness or signs of weakness become apparent.

Key tests used in making a differential diagnosis that includes a stretched piriformis, a shortened piriformis, lumbar radiculopathy, or referred pain are summarized in Table 19-4.

Treatment

For the purposes of this text, this discussion will be isolated to the piriformis syndrome. Therapeutic exercise intervention is based on the physiologic and morphologic status of the piriformis. Careful differential diagnosis of whether the muscle is strained, lengthened, shortened, or hypertrophied is necessary to develop the appropriate therapeutic exercise intervention. For example, a short piriformis must be stretched, whereas this would aggravate a lengthened piriformis syndrome. Periodic ROM measures combined with positional strength testing and dynamic functional testing can indicate the status of recovery of the strain and length-tension properties. The following sections provide guidelines for the therapeutic exercise intervention for all forms of the piriformis syndrome.

Pain Patients should be instructed in positions that relieve nerve pain and which positions to avoid to prevent further nerve irritation. Regardless of the length of the piriformis, relief may be achieved by placing the involved leg in lateral rotation and abduction in lying and standing positions. Sitting with the hips in lateral rotation (i.e., legs crossed at the ankles), avoiding extreme hip flexion, or sitting on a firm surface to support the femoral head in the acetabulum can alleviate symptoms while sitting.

Posture and Movement Permanent changes with respect to postural habits are encouraged to help alter the length-tension properties of the muscle. The patient should be instructed to position the limb to take the muscle off stretch (i.e., hip adduction, medial rotation, or extreme flexion). Limb position should be monitored during ADLs such as transitioning from sit to stand, squatting, and during stance phase of gait. Cues to maintain neutral transverse and frontal plane alignment can reduce repetitive stretch to the piriformis.

Muscle Performance In the case of a strained or lengthened piriformis, gradual progressive strengthening is indicated. Often the muscle is quite weak initially due to the strain or shifted length-tension properties. Caution must be used with dosage parameters so as not to exceed the muscle's physiologic capabilities. Exercise in the short range is indicated for the lengthened piriformis. Strengthening exercises should be avoided for the short or hypertrophied

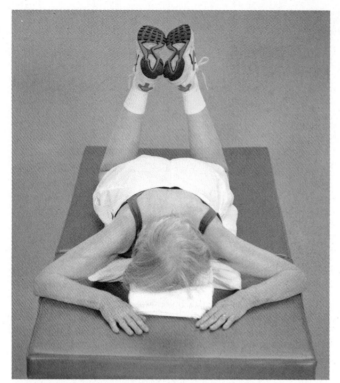

FIGURE 19-35. Prone foot pushes strengthen the piriformis isometrically in the short range. The patient positions the hip in abduction and lateral rotation. The patient pushes the heels together with a submaximal contraction. Submaximal contraction is desired over maximal to reduce the amount of accessory muscle recruitment (i.e., lateral hamstrings and adductors). Duration and repetitions are determined based upon the goal of the exercise (i.e., strength versus endurance).

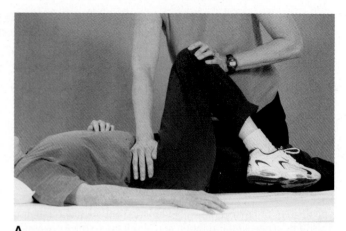

A

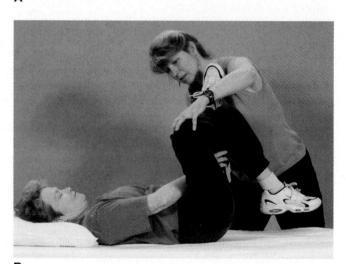

B

FIGURE 19-36. Piriformis stretch. (A) Passive stretch for the piriformis muscle. With the patient lying supine, the lower extremity is grasped at the flexed knee. The lateral aspect of the iliac crest and the ASIS are stabilized by the cranial hand while the caudal hand flexes the femur to 60 degrees and guides the femur into adduction. (B) Self-stretch of the piriformis and other deep hip rotators. After 60-degree hip flexion, the piriformis medially rotates the femur. To stretch the right deep hip lateral rotators, the patient lies supine and the right femur is flexed and laterally rotated such that the right ankle rests on the posterior aspect of the distal left thigh. From this position, the left hip is flexed until tension is perceived in the right buttock.

piriformis. Exercises that can target hip lateral rotator strength and length-tension properties include; prone foot pushes (Fig. 19-35), prone hip extension with pelvic stabilization (Self-Management 19-1), sidelying hip abduction with emphasis on lateral rotation (Self-Management 19-4), and hip lateral rotation strengthening in the short range (Fig. 19-14).

Strengthening the abdominal muscles (see Chapter 18) in the short range may be necessary to address an associated anterior pelvic tilt in the strained or lengthened piriformis syndrome. Strengthening the ipsilateral gluteus medius (Self-Management 19-4) may be necessary to reduce adduction patterns that will add further stress to a strained or lengthened piriformis.

After the muscle performance of the piriformis has improved to maintain the femur in neutral while bearing weight, exercises can be progressed to standing. In the lengthened or strained piriformis, the focus is to train the femur to function in less medial rotation and adduction and the pelvis in less anterior tilt, without promoting excessive hip flexion. In the short or hypertrophied piriformis syndrome, the focus is to train the femur to function in less lateral rotation and abduction and encourage the hip to function in more flexion (see Self-Managements 19-2, 19-3, and 19-8; and Fig. 19-8.)

Range of Motion Stretching the piriformis is contraindicated for the strained or lengthened piriformis. However, stretching the opposing medial rotators may be necessary if the stiffness or shortness contributes to the hip functioning in

medial rotation, imposing undue tension on the lengthened piriformis. Stretching the medial rotators (e.g., posterolateral fibers of the TFL, gluteus minimus, anterior gluteus medius) can be difficult to perform unassisted. Assisted stretching with the patient in a prone position into lateral rotation, with careful stabilization of the pelvis and the tibia, ensures optimal stretch to the medial rotators (see Fig. 19-25E). The pelvis must be stabilized actively or passively to prevent anterior pelvic tilt and lumbar extension while stretching the TFL/ITB complex.

Stretching the piriformis is indicated in the short or hypertrophied piriformis syndrome. Passive stretches for the piriformis are shown in Figure 19-36.

Stretching the low back muscles (see Self-Management 19-6) may be necessary to reduce forces contributing to anterior pelvic tilt. This same stretch can be used to stretch the piriformis. Caution must be heeded when stretching the low back

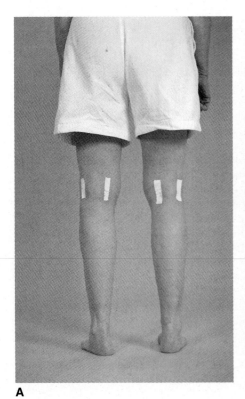

A

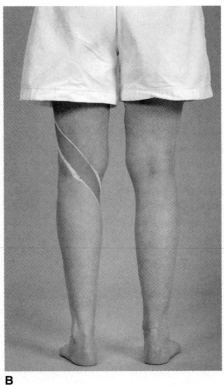

B

FIGURE 19-37. Excessive medial rotation of the femur in standing as shown by (A) tape on the hamstring tendons. (B) Corrective taping posterior to the knee. To encourage hip lateral rotation and tibia medial rotation, the tape is applied from the lateral femur distally to the medial tibia and from the medial tibia proximally toward the lateral femur. NOTE: Because this taping procedure does not anchor the tape to any bony prominence, its ability to prevent unwanted tibiofemoral movement is questionable. At best, it can provide temporary feedback to the patient until the tape has sufficiently stretched.

muscles in the lengthened piriformis syndrome so as not to place further tension on the sciatic nerve while moving into hip flexion, the emphasis should be on achieving a flat low back and not on hip flexion.

Stretching the ipsilateral hip adductors (Fig. 19-16) or abductors (Figs. 19-31 and 19-32) may be necessary to improve frontal plane alignment of the hip depending on the initial length of the piriformis.

Adjunctive Interventions   Support to a strained piriformis is indicated for rapid recovery. The lengthened piriformis should also be supported to relieve tension and allow for length-tension changes to occur. The combination of taping, posture, and exercise providing this support can be determined on a case by case basis, but it must be addressed in some fashion and for a period sufficient to allow recovery.

Taping techniques to support the limb in more neutral positions and provide feedback to avoid medial rotation and adduction are indicated for the stretched or strained piriformis. McConnell[173] has developed a taping technique for

the buttock that can support a strained piriformis and assist in unloading neural tissues. Taping behind the knee can serve as "biofeedback" to prevent excessive medial rotation tendencies during standing exercises and function (Fig. 19-37B; see Building Block 19-6).

KEY POINTS

- The structure of the hip joint is designed for stability and to withstand high kinetic forces.
- The angles of inclination and torsion are critical to ideal functioning of the hip joint.
- The ligaments of the hip provide significant stability to the hip, particularly in hip extension, adduction, and medial rotation.
- The tension of the ligaments correspond to positions of stability and instability of the hip.
- Hip osteokinematic ROM is closely linked to the LP region. Limitation in hip mobility may manifest in compensatory LP mobility and at the knee, ankle, and foot, although to a lesser degree.
- Hip arthrokinematic motions follow convex moving on concave rules with rolling and translation (minimal as it may be) moving opposite in direction to the distal end of the femur.
- It is important to understand the function of the muscles that cross the hip and the relationships they have with the LP region and the knee joint.
- In vivo loads acting at the hip joint have demonstrated the average patient loads the hip joint with 238% body weight (BW) when walking at about 4 km per hour, while climbing upstairs increases joint contact force to 251% BW going downstairs to 260% BW.

BUILDING BLOCK 19-6

Consider a patient presenting with left sided gluteal pain that radiates down the posterior aspect of the left leg. The patient demonstrates decreased tolerance to sitting, weakness in the deep hip lateral rotators, increased medial rotation ROM of the left hip, and increased adduction and medial rotation patterns with sit to stand/stand to sit, step-ups/downs, and during loading phase of gait. Develop a treatment plan for this patient to address her pain.

LAB ACTIVITIES

1. How would you progress a patient with OA in standing exercises to improve weight acceptance and single-limb support phases of gait? Would you use any assistive devices?
2. With respect to Critical Thinking Question 4, develop a program of exercises that improve the mobility and associated force or torque impairment for each scenario. Teach this program to your partner. Assume that all manual muscle test grades are 3+/5. Progress specific nonfunctional exercises to functional exercises.
3. With respect to Critical Thinking Question 6, how would you begin to improve the force or torque production of a gluteus medius underused synergist with a positional strength grade of 3–/5. How would you progress this exercise as the positional strength improved? Teach your partner these exercises. Can you feel the TFL trying to dominate the exercise movement pattern? What is the associated pattern of movement with TFL dominance? Progress this exercise to standing functional exercises. How does the foot alignment contribute to the hip position in closed chain positions and movements?

4. Your partner has been diagnosed with ITBS. List synergists that may be underused and therefore, contribute to this diagnosis. Develop an exercise to improve muscle performance for each underused synergist. Consider each underused synergist has a 3+/5 muscle test grade.
5. Practice the balance progression described in Display 19-8. What type of balance strategy are you using? Develop balance drills that stress the frontal plane and crossover stepping strategies.
6. With respect to Critical Thinking Question 7, progress hip lateral rotator exercises from specific, nonfunctional exercises to functional exercises. How would you stress the lateral rotators in a single-limb balance drill (be creative)?
7. Refer to Case Study No. #9 in Unit 7. Develop a complete therapeutic exercise intervention plan using the intervention model developed in Chapter 2.
8. Refer to Case Study No. #10 in Unit 7. Develop a complete therapeutic exercise intervention plan using the intervention model developed in Chapter 2.

- A thorough hip examination is necessary to understand the anatomic and physiologic impairments in the hip and those in related regions that affect the patient's activity limitations and disability.
- Impairments in muscle performance, gait and balance, posture and movement, ROM, and joint mobility commonly occur together in hip-related conditions. Treatment must focus on the impairments most related to the presenting activity limitations and participation restrictions. The initial focus should be on restoring functional capacity of each relevant impairment and gradual progression toward functional activity.
- The primary focus of treatment of hip OA is to improve joint loading by increasing contact area for loading. Restoring proper joint mobility and soft tissue extensibility are pre-requisite to building force or torque related to optimal joint loading. Improving posture and movment patterns are critical to transition improved physiologic impairments into function. Balance skills are the final element to restoring more optimal movement patterns and joint loading.
- Numerous ITB-related syndromes exist. The focus of treatment is to improve the force or torque and functional recruitment of the underused synergists in meaningful functional movement patterns.
- The stretched piriformis syndrome can mimic lumbar radiculopathy. Correct differential diagnosis from lumbar radiculopathy, short piriformis syndrome, and hamstrings strain is mandatory for a successful outcome. Treatment focuses on improving the movement patterns and associated physiologic impairments that contribute to femur medial rotation and adduction and on anterior pelvic tilt, all of which can contribute to stress on the piriformis and the sciatic nerve.

CRITICAL THINKING QUESTIONS

1. To which type of knee alignment does coxa vara and coxa valga contribute?
2. What direction are the femoral condyles oriented in femoral anteversion versus retroversion? If a patient with femoral anteversion participates in ballet, what type of mobility problem could he or she develop? If a patient with femoral anteversion participates in soccer, what type of mobility could he or she develop? What are your recommendations for the alignment of the anteverted femur during sport activities?
3. What would be the compensatory lumbar motions and what phases of the gait cycle would be involved if right hip mobility were restricted in (a) flexion, (b) extension, or (c) medial rotation?
4. If the hip were restricted in flexion, what are the postural patterns at the pelvis and lumbar spine contributing to this hip flexion restriction? What movement patterns would you retrain to improve hip flexion mobility? What muscle force or torque impairments at the LP region would you be concerned about that could help perpetuate the hip flexion restriction? Answer these same questions with respect to restrictions in hip extension and medial rotation. What is this pattern of restriction (i.e., restricted hip flexion, medial rotation, extension) called?
5. Describe the Trendelenburg pattern of gait. Can you describe other hip joint movement patterns that could indicate hip abductor weakness?
6. In TFL/ITB overuse diagnoses, why is the hip the focus of treatment? What are the common underused synergists that contribute to TFL/ITB overuse?
7. How would you differentially diagnose a stretched piriformis syndrome from a short piriformis syndrome, lumbar radiculopathy, or strained hamstrings?

REFERENCES

1. Singleton MC, LeVeau BF. The hip joint: stability and stress: a review. Phys Ther 1975;55:957–973.
2. Frankel VH, Nordin M. Basic Biomechanics of the Skeletal System. Philadelphia, PA: Lea & Febiger, 1980.
3. Maquet P. Importance of the position of the greater trochanter. Acta Orthop Belg 1990;56:307–322.
4. Fabray G, MacEwen GD, Shands AR. Torsion of the femur: a follow-up study in normal and abnormal conditions. J Bone Joint Surg Am 1973;55:17–26.
5. Anda S, Svenningson S, Dale LG, et al. The acetabular sector angle of the adult hip determined by computed tomography. Acta Radiol Diagn 1986;27:443–447.
6. Svenningsen S, Apalset K, Terjesen T, et al. Regression of femoral anteversion. Acta Orthop Scand 1989;60:170–173.
7. Williams PL, Warwick R, eds. Gray's Anatomy. 37th Ed. Philadelphia, PA: WB Saunders, 1985.
8. Danbert RJ. Clinical assessment and treatment of leg length inequalities. J Manip Phys Ther 1988;11:290–295.
9. Baylis WJ, Rzonca EC. Functional and structural limb length discrepancies: evaluation and treatment. Clin Pediatr Med Surg 1988;5:509–520.
10. McCaw ST. Leg length inequality: implications for running injury prevention. Sports Med 1992;14:422–429.
11. Rothenberg RJ. Rheumatic disease aspects of leg length inequality. Semin Arthritis Rheum 1988;17:196–205.
12. Tjernstrom B, Olerud S, Karlstrom G. Direct leg lengthening. J Orthop Trauma 1993;7:543–551.
13. Knutson GA. Incidence of foot rotation, pelvic crest unleveling, and supine leg length alignment asymmetry and their relationship to self-reported back pain. J Manipulative Physiol Ther 2002;25:110E.
14. Brand RA, Yack HJ. Effects of leg length discrepancies on the forces at the hip joint. Clin Orthop 1996;333:172–180.
15. Kaufman KR, Miller LS, Sutherland DH. Gait asymmetry in patients with limb length inequality. J Pediatr Orthop 1996;16:144–150.
16. Walsh M, Connolly P, Jenkinson A, et al. Leg length discrepancy—an experimental study of compensatory changes in three dimensions using gait analysis. Gait Posture 2000;12:156–161.
17. Martin RL, Eneski KR, Draovitch R, et al. Acetabular labral tears of the hip: examination and diagnostic challenges. Journ Ortho Sports Phys Ther 2006;36(7):503–515.
18. Cibulka MT, White DM, Woehrle J, et al. Hip pain and mobility deficits—hip osteoarthritis. J Orthop Sports Phys Ther 2009;39(4):A1–A25.
19. Collier J, Longmore J, Hodgetts T. Oxford Handbook of Clinical Specialties. 4th Ed. Oxford: Oxford University Press, 1995.
20. Emms H, O'Connor M, Montgomery S. Hip pathology can masquerade as knee pain in adults. Age Ageing 2002;31:67–69.
21. Dee R, Hurst L, Gruber M, et al. Principles of Orthopedic Practice. 2nd Ed. London: McGraw-Hill, 1997.
22. Shumway-Cook A, Galdwin M, Polissar NL, et al. Predicting the probability for falls in community-dwelling older adults. Phys Ther 1997;77:812–819.
23. Berg KO, Wood Daphinee SL, Williams JT, et al. Measuring balance in the elderly: validation of an instrument. Can J Public Health 1989;41:302–311.
24. Shumway-Cook A, Woollacott MH. Motor Control: Theory and Practical Applications. Baltimore, MD: Williams & Wilkins, 1995.
25. Shumway-Cook A, Gruber W, Baldwin M, et al. The effect of multidimensional exercise on balance, mobility, and fall risk in community-dwelling older adults. Phys Ther 1997;77:46–57.
26. Lee D. The Pelvic Girdle. Edinburgh: Churchill Livingstone, 1999.
27. Kendall FP, McCreary EK, Provance PG. Muscles Testing and Function. 4th Ed. Baltimore, MD: Williams & Wilkins, 1993.
28. Daniels L, Worthingham C. Muscle Testing: Techniques of Manual Examination. 4th Ed. Philadelphia, PA: WB Saunders, 1980.
29. Bandy WD, Sanders B. Therapeutic Exercise for Physical Therapy Assistants. 2nd Ed. Philadelphia, PA: Lippincott Williams & Wilkins, 2007.
30. Cyriax J. Textbook of Orthopedic Medicine. Vol 1. 7th Ed. London: Bailliere Tindall, 1978.
31. Duncan GH, Bushnell MC, Lavigne GJ. Comparison of verbal and visual analogue scales for measuring the intensity and unpleasantness of experimental pain. Pain 1989;37:295–303.
32. Jette AM. Using health-related quality of life measures in physical therapy outcomes research. Phys Ther 1993;73:528–537.
33. Harris WH. Traumatic arthritis of the hip after dislocation and acetabular fracture: treatment by mold arthroplasty. J Bone Joint Surg Am 1969;51:737–755.
34. Binkley JM, Stratford PW, Lott SA, et al. The lower extremity functional scale (LEFS): scale development, measurement properties, and clinical application. Phys Ther 1999;79:371–383.
35. Konermann W, Gruber G. Ultrasound determination of leg length. Orthopade 2002;31:300–305.
36. Krettek C, Koch T, Henzler D, et al. A new procedure for determining leg length and LLD inequality using ultrasound. Unfallchirug 1996;99:43–51.
37. Woerman AL, Binder-MacLeod SA. Leg length discrepancy assessment: accuracy and precision in five clinical methods of evaluation. J Orthop Sports Phys Ther 1984;5:230–238.
38. Hanada E, Kirby RL, Mitchell M, et al. Measuring leg length discrepancy by the "iliac crest palpation and book correction" method: reliability and validity. Arch Phys Med Rehabil 2001;82:938–942.
39. Beattie P, Isaacson K, Riddle DL, et al. Validity of derived measurements of leg-length differences obtained by use of a tape measure. Phys Ther 1990;70:150–157.
40. Gogia PP, Braatz JH. Validity and reliability of leg length measurements. J Orthop Sports Phys Ther 1986;8:185–188.
41. Ruwe PA, Gage JR, Ozonoff MB, et al. Clinical determination of femoral anteversion. A comparison with established techniques. J Bone Joint Surg Am 1992;74:820–830.
42. Benfanti P, Blackhurst DW, Allen BL. Assessment of femoral anteversion in children with cerebral palsy: accuracy of the trochanteric prominence angle test. J Pediatr Orthop 2002;22:173–178.
43. Sugano N, Noble PC, Kamaric E. A comparison of alternative methods of measuring femoral anteversion. J Comput Assist Tomogr 1998;22:610–640.
44. Kozic S, Gulan G, Matovinovic D, et al. Femoral anteversion related to side differences in hip rotation. Passive rotation in 1,140 children aged 8–9 years. Acta Orthop Scand 1997;68:533–536.
45. Konin JG, Wiksten D, Isear JA, et al. Special Tests for orthopedic examination. 3rd Ed, Thorofare, NJ: Slack, 2006.
46. Lyons K, Perry J, Gronley JK, et al. Timing and relative intensity of hip extensor and abductor muscle action during level and stair ambulation. Phys Ther 1983;63:1597–1605.
47. Kelly JP. Reactions of neurons to injury. In: Kandel E, Schwartz J, eds. Principles of Neural Science. New York: Elsevier, 1985.
48. Agre JC. Hamstring injuries. Proposed aetiological factors, prevention, and treatment. Sports Med 1985;2:21–33.
49. Clanton TO, Coupe KJ. Hamstring strains in athletes: diagnosis and treatment. J Am Acad Orthop Surg 1998;6:237–248.
50. Grace TG. Muscle imbalance and extremity injury. A perplexing relationship. Sports Med 1985;2:77–82.
51. Mair J, Mayr M, Muller E, et al. Rapid adaptation to eccentric exercise-induced muscle damage. Int J Sports Med 1995;16:352–356.
52. Mair SD, Seaber AV, Glisson RR, et al. The role of fatigue in susceptibility to acute muscle strain injury. Am J Sports Med 1996;24:137–143.
53. Sahrmann SA. Diagnosis and Treatment of Movement Impairment Syndromes. St. Louis, MD: Mosby, 2002.
54. Distefano LJ, Blackburn JT, Marshall SW, et al. Gluteal muscle activation during common therapeutic exercises. J Orthop Sports Phys Ther 2009;39:532–540.
55. Abelbeck KG. Biomechanical model and evaluation of a linear motion squat type exercise. J Strength Cond Res 2002;16:516–524.
56. Yu B, Holly-Crichlow N, Brichta P, et al. The effects of the lower extremity joint motions on the total body motion in sit to stand movement. Clin Biomech 2000;15;449–455.
57. Long WT, Dorr LD, Healy B, et al. Functional recovery of noncemented total hip arthroplasty. Clin Orthop Rel Res 1993;288:73–77.
58. Arokoski MH, Arokoski JP, Haara M, et al. Hip muscle strength and muscle cross sectional area in men with and without hip OA. J Rheumatol 2002;29;2187–2195.
59. Neumann DA, Soderberg GL, Cook TM. Electromyographic analysis of hip abductor musculature in healthy right-handed persons. Phys Ther 1989;69:431–440.
60. Inman VT. Functional aspects of the abductor muscles of the hip. J Bone Joint Surg 1947;29:607–612.
61. Fredericson M, Cookingham CL, Caudhari AM. Hip abductor weakness in distance runners with iliotibial band syndrome. Clin J Sport Med 2000;10:169–175.
62. LaBan MM, Raptou AD, Johnson EW. Electromyographic study of function of iliopsoas muscle. Arch Phys Med Rehabil 1965;676–679.
63. Nigg BM, Stergiou G, Cole D. Effect of shoe inserts on kinematics, center of pressure, and leg joint moments during running. Med Sci Sports Exerc 2003;35:314–319.
64. Paton RW, Hossain S, Eccles K. Eight-year prospective targeted ultrasound screening program for instability and at-risk hip joints in developmental dysplasia of the hip. J Pediatr Orthop 2002;22:338–341.
65. Lachiewicz PF, Soileau ES. Stability of total hip arthroplasty in patients 75 years or older. Clin Orthop 2002;405:65–69.
66. McCarthy J, Noble P, Schuck M, et al. The role of labral lesions to the development of early degenerative hip disease. Clin Orthop 2001;393:25–37.
67. Andrews JR: Current concepts in sports medicine: the use of COX-2 specific inhibitors and the emerging trends in arthroscopic surgery. Orthopedics 2000;23(Suppl):769–772.
68. Teitz CC, Kicoyne RF. Premature osteoarthrosis in professional dancers. Clin J Sport Med 1998;8:255–259.
69. vanDijk CN, Lim LS, Poortman A, et al. Degenerative joint disease in female ballet dancers. Am J Sports Med 1995;23:295–300.
70. Andersson S, Nilsson B, Hessel T, et al. Degenerative joint disease in ballet dancers. Clin Orthop 1989;238:233–236.
71. Mubarak SJ, Leach JK, Wenger DR. Management of congenital dislocation of the hip in the infant. Contemp Orthop 1987;15:29–44.
72. Pemberton PA. Osteotomy of the ilium with rotation of the acetabular roof for congenital dislocation of the hip. J Bone Joint Surg Am 1958;40:724.

73. Reikeras O, Bjerkreim I, Kolbenstvedt A. Anteversion of the acetabulum in patients with idiopathic increased anteversion of the femoral neck. Acta Orthop Scand 1982;53:847–852.

74. Gulan G, Matovinovic D. Nemec B, et al. Femoral neck anteversion: values, development, measurement, common problems. Coll Antropol 2000;24:521–527.

75. Reikeras O, Hoiseth A. Femoral neck angles in OA of the hip. Acta Orthop Scand 1982;53:781–784.

76. Reikeras O, Bjerkreim I, Kolbenstvedt A. Anteversion of the acetabulum and femoral neck in normals and in patients with OA of the hip. Acta Orthop Scand 1983;54:18–23.

77. Terjesen T, Benum P, Anda S, et al. Increased femoral anteversion and OA of the hip joint. Acta Orthop Scand 1982;53:571–575.

78. Guinti A, Morone A, Olmi R, Rimondi E, et al. The importance of the angle of anteversion in the development of arthritis of the hip. Ital J Orthop Trauma 1985;11:23–27.

79. Tonnis D, Heinecke A. Current concepts review—acetabular and femoral anteversion: relationship with OA of the hip. J Bone Joint Surg 1999;81:1747–1770.

80. Fabry G, Cheng LX, Molenaers G. Normal and abnormal torsional development in children. Clin Orthop 1994;302:22–26.

81. Eckhoff DG. Femoral anteversion in arthritis of the knee [letter]. J Pediat Orthop 1995;15:700.

82. Eckhoff DG, Montgomery WK, Kilcoyne RF, et al. Femoral morphometry and anterior knee pain. Clin Orthop 1994;302:64–68.

83. Mellin G. Correlations of hip mobility with degree of back pain and lumbar spinal mobility in chronic low back pain patients. Spine 1988;13:668–670.

84. Thurston AJ. Spinal and pelvic kinematics in osteoarthrosis of the hip joint. Spine 1985;10:467–471.

85. Offerski CM, Macnab I. Hip-spine syndrome. Spine 1983;8:316–321.

86. Esola MA, McClure PW, Fitzgerald GK, et al. Analysis of lumbar spine and hip motion during forward bending in subjects with and without a history of significant low back pain. Spine 1996;21:71–78.

87. Li Y, McClure PW, Pratt N. The effect of hamstring muscle stretching on standing posture and on lumbar and hip motions during forward bending. Phys Ther 1996;76:836–849.

88. Tinetti ME, Ginter SF. Identifying mobility dysfunctions in elderly patients; standard neuromuscular examination or direct assessment. JAMA 1988;259:1190–1193.

89. Tinetti ME, Speechly M, Ginter SF. Risk factors for falls among elderly persons living in the community. N Engl J Med 1988;319:1701–1707.

90. Nevitt MC, Cummings SR. Risk factors for recurrent non-syncopal falls: a prospective study. JAMA 1989;261:2663–2668.

91. Kanten DN, Mulrow CD, Gerety MB, et al. Falls: an examination of three reporting methods in nursing homes. J Am Geriatr Soc 1993;41:662–666.

92. National Safety Council. Accident Facts and Figures. Chicago: National Safety Council, 1987.

93. Thapa PB, Gideon P, Cost TW et al. Antidepressants and the risk of falls among nursing home residents. N Engl J Med 1998;339:875–882.

94. Health Care Financing Administration. Quality Resume. HCFA's Medicare Quality of Care Report of Surveillance Measures. Baltimore, MD: Health Care Financing Administration, 1998.

95. Rose S, Maffulli N. Hip fractures: an epidemiological review. Hosp Joint Dis 1999;58:197–201.

96. Youm T, Koval KJ, Zuckerman JD. The economic impact of geriatric hip fractures. Am J Orthop 1999;28:423–428.

97. Gallagher JC, Melton LJ, Riggs BL, et al. Epidemiology of fractures of the proximal femur in Rochester, Minnesota. Clin Orthop 1980;150:163–171.

98. Cummings SR, Black DM, Rubin SM. Lifetime risks of hip, Colles', or vertebral fracture and coronary heart disease among white post-menopausal women. Arch Intern Med 1989;149:2445–2448.

99. Rudman IW, Rudman D. High rate of fractures for men in nursing homes. Am J Phys Med Rehab 1989;68:2–5.

100. Ooms ME, Vlasman P, Lips P, et al. The incidence of hip fractures in independent and institutionalized elderly people. Osteoporos Int 1994;4:6–10.

101. Miravet L, Chaumet-Riffaud P, Ranstam J. Residential care and risk of proximal femur fracture. Bone 1993;14:S73–S75.

102. Lüthje P. Incidence of hip fracture in Finland: a forecast for 1990. Acta Orthop Scand 1985;56:223–225.

103. Cummings SR, Nevitt MC, Browner WS, et al. Risk factors for hip fracture in white women: study of Osteoporotic Fractures Research Group. N Engl J Med 1995;332:767–773.

104. Stewart A, Walker L, Porter RW, et al. Predicting a second hip fracture: the potential role of dual x-ray absorptiometry, ultrasound, and other risk factors in targeting of preventive therapy. J Clin Densitom 1999;2:363–370.

105. Colon-Emeric CS, Sloane R, Hawkes WG, et al. The risk of subsequent fractures in community-dwelling men and male veterans with hip fracture. Am J Med 2000;109:324–326.

106. Rose DJ, Clark S. Can the control of bodily orientation be significantly improved in a group of older adults with a history of falls? J Am Geriatr Soc 2000;48:275–282.

107. Perrin PP, Gauchard GC, Perrot C, et al. Effects of physical and sporting activities on balance control in elderly people. Br J Sports Med 1999;33:121–126.

108. Brooke-Wavell K, Athersmith LE, Jones PR. Brisk walking and postural stability: a cross-sectional study in postmenopausal women. Gerontology 1998;44:288–292.

109. Brooke-Wavell K, Prelevic GM, Bakridan C, et al. Effects of physical activity and menopausal hormone replacement therapy on postural stability in post-menopausal women-a cross-sectional study. Maturitas 2001;31:167–172.

110. Tse S, Baily DM. T'ai chi and postural control in the well elderly. Am J Occup Ther 1992;46:295–300.

111. Wolf SL, Barnhart HX, Ellison GL, et al. The effect of t'ai chi quan and computerized balance training on postural stability in older subjects. Phys Ther 1997;77:371–384.

112. Wong AM, Lin YC, Chou SW, et al. Coordination exercise and postural stability in elderly people: effect of Tai Chi Chuan. Arch Phys Med Rehabil 2001;82:608–612.

113. Zwick D. Rochell A, Choski A, et al. Evaluation and treatment of balance in the elderly: a review of the efficacy of the berg balance test and tai chi quan. Neuro Rehabil 2000;15:49–56.

114. Boudrahem S, Rougier PR. Relation between postural control assessment with eyes open and center of pressure visual feedback effects in healthy individuals. Exp Brain Res 2009;195:145–153.

115. Maki BE, McIlroy WE. The role of limb movements in maintaining upright stance: the "change in support" strategy. Phys Ther 1997;77:488–507.

116. Jeka JJ, Lackner JR. Fingertip contact influences human postural control. Exp Brain Res 1994;100:495–502.

117. Christmas C, Crespo CJ, Franckowiak SC, et al. How common is hip pain among older adults? Results from the Third National Health and Nutrition Examination Survey. J Fam Pract 2002;51:345–348.

118. Neumann DA, Cook TM, Sholty RL, et al. An electromyographic analysis of hip abductor muscle activity when subjects are carrying loads in one or both hands. Phys Ther 1992;72:207–217.

119. Maitland GD. Peripheral Manipulation. 2nd Ed. London: Butterworths, 1977.

120. Felson DT. Preventing knee and hip OA. Bull Rheum Dis 1998;47:1–4.

121. Gelber AC, Hochberg MC, Mead LA, et al. Body mass index in young men and the risk of subsequent knee and hip OA. Am J Med 1999;107:542–548.

122. Heliovaara M, Makela M, Impivaara O, et al. Association of overweight, trauma, and workload with coxarthrosis: a health survey of 7217 persons. Acta Orthop Scand 1993;64:513–518.

123. Okama-Keulen P, Hopman-Rock M. The onset of generalized OA in older women: a qualitative approach. Arthritis Care Res 2001;45:183–190.

124. Mundermann A, Nigg BM, Humble RN, et al. Foot orthotics affect lower extremity kinematics and kinetics during running. Clin Biomech 2003;18:254–262.

125. Reid DC, Smith B. Leg length inequality: a review of etiology and management. Physiother Can 1984;36:177–182.

126. Moseley CF. Leg length discrepancy and angular deformity of the lower limbs. In: Lovell and Winter's Pediatric Orthopaedics. 4th Ed. Philadelphia, PA: Lippincott-Raven, 1996.

127. Felson DT, Lawrence RC, Hochberg MC, et al. Osteoarthritis: new insights. Part 2: treatment approaches. Ann Intern Med 2000;133:726–737.

128. Goldberg V, Caplan AI. Biological Restoration of Articular Surfaces. American Academy of Orthopaedic Surgeons Instructional Course Lectures. Rosemont, IL: American Academy of Orthopaedic Surgeons, 1999.

129. Felson DT, Lawrence RC, Dieppe PA, et al. Osteoarthritis: new insights. Part 1: the disease and its risk factors. Ann Intern Med 2000;133:635–646.

130. van Saase, van Romunde LK, Cats A, et al. Epidemiology of OA: Zoetermeer survey. Comparison of radiological OA in a Dutch population with that in 10 other populations. Ann Rheum Dis 1989;48:271–280.

131. Mikkelsen WM, Dodge HJ, Duff IF, et al. Estimates of the prevalence of rheumatic diseases in the population of Tecumseh, Michigan, 1959–60. J Chronic Dis 1967;20:351–369.

132. Cunningham LS, Kelsey JL. Epidemiology of musculoskeletal impairments and associated disability. Am J Public Health 1984;74:574–579.

133. Felson DT, Naimark A, Anderson J, et al. The prevalence of knee OA in the elderly. The Framingham OA Study. Arthritis Rheum 1987;30:914–918.

134. Dieppe P. What is the relationship between pain and OA? Rheumatol Eur 1998;27:55–56.

135. Price SA, Wilson LM. Pathophysiology: Clinical Concepts of Disease Processes. 2nd Ed. New York: McGraw-Hill, 1982.

136. Sultive TG, Lopez HP, Schnitker DE, et al. Development of a clinical prediction rule for diagnosing hip osteoarthritis in individuals with unilateral hip pain. J Orthop Sports Phys Ther 2008;38:542–550.

137. Buckwalter JA, Mankin HJ. Articular Cartilage: Degeneration and OA, Repair, Regeneration and Transplantation. Rosemont, IL: American Academy of Orthopaedic Surgeons, 1998.

138. Bradley JD, Brandt KD, Katz BP, et al. Comparison of an anti-inflammatory dose of ibuprofen, an analgesic dose of ibuprofen, and acetaminophen in the treatment of patients with OA of the knee. N Engl J Med 1991;325:87–91.

139. Williams HJ, Ward JR, Egger MJ, et al. Comparison of naproxen and acetaminophen in a two-year study of treatment of OA of the knee. Arthritis Rheum 1993;36:1196–1206.

140. Towheed TE, Hochberg MC. A systematic review of randomized controlled trials of pharmacological therapy in patients with OA of the hip. J Rheumatol 1997;24:349–357.

141. Eccles M, Freemantle N, Mason J. North of England evidence based guideline development project: summary guideline for non-steroidal anti-inflammatory drugs versus basic analgesia in treating the pain of degenerative arthritis. The North of England Non-Steroidal Anti-Inflammatory Drug Guideline Development Group. BMJ 1998;317:526–530.

142. The management of chronic pain in older persons. AGS Panel on Chronic Pain in Older Persons. American Geriatrics Society. Geriatrics 1998;53(Suppl 3): S8–S24.

143. Ronca F, Palmieri L, Panicucci P, et al. Anti-inflammatory activity of chondroitin sulfate. OA Cartilage 1998;6(Suppl A):14–21.

144. Deal CL, Schnitzer TJ, Lipstein E, et al. Treatment of arthritis with topical capsaicin: a double-blind trial. Clin Ther 1991;13:383–395.

145. Ernst E. Acupuncture as a symptomatic treatment of OA. A systematic review. Scand J Rheumatol 1997;26:444–447.

146. Berman BM, Singh BB, Lao L, et al. A randomized trial of acupuncture as an adjunctive therapy in OA of the knee. Rheumatology (Oxford) 1999;38: 346–354.

147. Ayral X. Injections in the treatment of OA. Best Practices Res Clin Rheumatol 2001;15:609–626.

148. Creamer P. Intra-articular corticosteroid treatment in OA. Curr Opin Rheumatol 1999;11:417–421.

149. Conrozier T, Vignon E. Is there evidence to support the inclusion of viscosupplementation in the treatment paradigm for patients with hip osteoarthritis? Clin Exp Rheumatol 2005;23:711–716.

150. McGibbon CA, Krebs DE, Mann RW. In vivo hip pressures during cane and load-carrying gait. Arthritis Care Res 1997;10:300–307.

151. Neumann DA. An electromyographic study of the hip abductor muscles as subjects with a hip prosthesis walked with different methods of using a cane and carrying a load. Phys Ther 1999;79:1163–1173.

152. Lorig KR, Mazonson PD, Holman HR. Evidence suggesting that health education for self-management in patients with chronic arthritis has sustained health benefits while reducing health care costs. Arthritis Rheum 1993;36:439–446.

153. Superio-Cabuslay E, Ward MM, Lorig KR. Patient education interventions in OA and rheumatoid arthritis: a meta-analytic comparison with nonsteroidal antiinflammatory drug treatment. Arthritis Care Res 1996;9:292–301.

154. Cronan TA, Groessl E, Kaplan RM. The effects of social support and education interventions on health care costs. Arthritis Care Res 1997;10: 99–110.

155. Minor MA, Hewett JE, Webel RR, et al. Efficacy of physical conditioning exercise in patients with rheumatoid arthritis or OA. Arthritis Rheum 1989;32:1397–1405.

156. Ettinger WH Jr, Burns R, Messier SP, et al. A randomized trial comparing aerobic exercise and resistance exercise with a health education program in older adults with knee OA. The Fitness Arthritis and Seniors Trial (FAST). JAMA 1997;277:25–31.

157. van Baar ME, Assendelft WJ, Dekker J, et al. Effectiveness of exercise therapy in patients with OA of the hip or knee: a systematic review of randomized clinical trials. Arthritis Rheum 1999;42:1361–1369.

158. National Institutes of Health. Total Hip Replacement: NIH Consensus Statement. Bethesda, MD: US Department of Health and Human Services, 1994.

159. McAlindon TE, LaValley MP, Gulin JP, et al. Glucosamine and chondroitin for treatment of OA: a systematic quality assessment and meta-analysis. JAMA 2000;283:1469–1475.

160. Wyatt FB, Milan S, Manske R, et al. The effects of aquatic and traditional exercise programs on persons with knee OA. J Strength Cond Res 2001;15:337–340.

161. Hinman RS, Heywood SE, Day AR. Aquatic physical therapy for hip and knee osteoarthritis: results of a single blind randomized controlled trial. Phys Therapy 2007;87:32–43.

162. MacDonald CW, Whitman JM, Cleland JA, et al. Clincial outcomes following manual physical therapy and exercise for hip osteoarthritis: a case series. J Orthop Sports Phys Ther 2006;36:588–599.

163. Pare EB, Stern JT, Schwartz JM. Functional differentiation within the tensor fascia latae. J Bone Joint Surg Am 1981;63:1457–1471.

164. Olson JH, Armour WJ. Sports injuries and their treatment. Philadelphia, PA: Lippincott, 1975.

165. Orchard JW, Fricker PA, Abud AT, et al. Biomechanics of iliotibial band friction syndrome in runners. Am J Sports Med 1996;24:375–379.

166. Nishimura G, Yamato M, Tamai K, et al. MR findings in iliotibial band syndrome. Skeletal Radiol 1997;26:533–537.

167. Taunten JE, Clement DB, McKenzie DC, et al. A retrospective case-control analysis of 2002 running injuries. Br J Sports Med 2002;36:95–101.

168. Nobel CA. The treatment of iliotibial band friction syndrome. Br J Sports Med 1979;13:51–54.

169. Winslow J, Yoder E. Patellofemoral pain in female ballet dancers: correlation with iliotibial band tightness and tibial external rotation. J Orthop Sports Phys Ther 1995;22:18–21.

170. Freiburg AH, Vinke TH. Sciatica and sacroiliac joint. J Bone Joint Surg 1934;16:126–136.

171. Yeoman W. The relationship of arthritis of the sacro-iliac joint to sciatica. Lancet 1928;11:1119–1122.

172. McCrory P, Simon B. Nerve entrapment syndromes as a cause of pain in the hip, groin, and buttock. Sports Med 1999;27:261–274.

173. McConnell J. Recalcitrant chronic low back and leg pain—a new theory and different approach to management. Man Ther 2002;7:183–192.

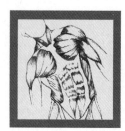

chapter 20
The Knee

LORI THEIN BRODY AND ROBERT LANDEL

The knee is one of the most frequently injured joints in the body. The quadriceps muscle spans the anterior thigh and crosses the tibiofemoral joint, producing knee extension when tensed. The patella enhances muscle performance across the longest lever arm of the body. Impairments at the knee joint can produce significant activity limitations and performance restrictions. The closed chain demands of daily activities such as walking, standing, and rising from a chair require smooth, coordinated action of the lower extremity neuromuscular system.[1-5] When considering impairments around the knee joint, the impact of these impairments on the related joints in the kinetic chain also must be addressed.

REVIEW OF ANATOMY AND KINESIOLOGY

A thorough understanding of the anatomy and kinesiology of the knee joint is necessary to comprehend the impact of impairments on function of the kinetic chain. The unique kinematic relationships of lower extremity joints depend on the local anatomic structures. A brief review of key aspects follows, with further information available on the website.

Anatomy

The osteology of the knee joint consists of the convex medial and lateral femoral condyles articulating with the concave proximal tibial plateau.[6] The medial condyle extends further distally than the wider lateral condyle, contributing to the quadriceps angle (Q-angle) and knee valgus posture commonly seen.[7] The triangular shaped patella, with its concave undersurface, articulates with the convex femoral condyles (Fig. 20-1).

Key aspects of the knee osteology include:

- condylar asymmetry contributes to the screw home mechanism (femoral internal rotation coupled with tibial external rotation during terminal extension)[8]
- lateral tibial plateau is small, more circular, and concave compared with the oval-shaped, flatter medial tibial plateau
- patella has two convex surfaces divided into three facets each, plus an additional "odd" facet

The tibiofemoral joint is comprised of fibrous capsule lines with a synovial membrane. The capsule is supported by several ligaments including the medial (MCL) and lateral collateral ligaments (LCL), *respectively*, the oblique popliteal ligament and the arcuate complex. The primary anterior-posterior stability is provided by the anterior (ACL) and posterior (PCL) cruciate ligaments.[9,10] The patella is stabilized by the quadriceps muscles and the multiple fascial layers surrounding and enveloping this sesmoid bone[11,12] (Fig. 20-2). The medial and lateral menisci are crescent-shaped fibrocartilaginous structures interposed between the tibia and femur, adding congruity to seemingly incompatible surfaces. The medial meniscus is semilunar and attached peripherally to the coronary ligament, while the lateral meniscus is nearly circular and only loosely attached peripherally[13] (see Table 20-1).

The complex interaction among joints from the pelvis and hips through the feet make discussion of myology at the knee more complicated. For the purposes of anatomy, only the muscles crossing the knee joint proper will be discussed. Review of muscles at adjacent joints can be found in their respective chapters (Chapters 19 and 21). The primary anterior muscles are the quadriceps femoris, consisting of the rectus femoris, vastus lateralis (VL), vastus intermedius, and vastus medialis (VM). These muscles serve as the primary knee extensors. The posteriorly located hamstring muscles are comprised of the biceps femoris, semimembranosus, and semitendinosus and serve as the primary knee flexors. These muscles also assist hip extension and rotation. Medially, the gracilis, adductor magnus, and adductor brevis function to adduct the hip but also serve to stabilize the medial aspect of the knee joint. The lateral musculature (gluteus maximus, tensor fasciae latae, and iliotibial tract) functions primarily at the hip but can be symptomatic at the knee as well.[14]

Kinematics

Although the knee joint is classified as a simple hinge joint, the kinematics of this joint are the result of the complex interplay of bony and soft tissue anatomy. Key aspects of tibiofemoral kinematics are as follows, and further information can be found on the website:

- The tibiofemoral has six degrees of freedom including three rotations: flexion and extension medial and lateral, and valgus and vaurs; and three translations: anterior and posterior, medial and lateral, and distraction and compression.[8]
- Normal range of motion (ROM) is from 0 degrees (full extension) to 140 degrees of flexion.
- Flexion is limited by the cruciate ligaments and posterior horns of the menisci.[15,16]
- Extension is limited by the cruciate ligaments, posterior capsule, and anterior horns of the menisci
- Differential size of femoral condyles plus soft tissues contribute to the screw home mechanism

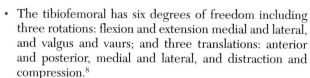

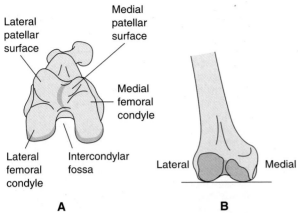

FIGURE 20-1. (A) View of the femoral surface from the inferior articulating surface. Note the more anterior prominence of the lateral femoral condyle. (B) The medial femoral condyle is longer than the lateral, and the lateral femoral condyle lies more directly in line with the shaft than the medial. However, the prominence of the medial femoral condyle results in a horizontal articulating surface. (Adapted from Norkin CC, Levangie PK. Joint Structure and Function: a Comprehensive Analysis. 2nd Ed. Philadelphia, PA: FA Davis, 1992:340.)

- Varus or valgus stress is likely to damage respective collateral ligament and cruciate ligaments
- The instant center of rotation changes throughout the ROM. Alterations in the instant center of rotation following injury can produce areas of increased loading on articular cartilage[15,16] (see Fig. 20-3).

Understanding the kinematics of the patellofemoral joint helps guide intervention choices for problems such as patellofemoral pain, discussed in detail later in the chapter. As the knee flexes from the fully extended position, the inferior pole first contacts the femur at approximately 20 degrees. As flexion proceeds to 90 degrees, the contact area includes more of the central portion of the patella, and it is not until 135 degrees that the medial odd facet contacts the medial femoral condyle.[17] This habitual noncontact and secondary cartilage underloading may contribute to the degeneration seen at the odd facet.

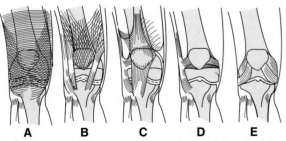

FIGURE 20-2. The multiple soft tissue layers affect the patellofemoral joint: (A) the superficial arciform layers with transverse fibers over patella and patellar tendon; (B) the intermediate oblique layer with chevron-oriented fibers from the rectus femoris, VL, and VM; (C) the deep longitudinal layers, which are extremely adherent to the anterior surface of the patella; (D) the deep transverse layer blending with fibers of the ITB; and (E) the deep capsular layer composed of the medial and lateral patellomeniscal ligaments. (Adapted from Dye SF. Patellofemoral anatomy. In: Fox JM, Del Pizzo W, eds. The Patellofemoral Joint. New York, NY: McGraw-Hill, 1993:5.)

TABLE 20-1	**Arthrology Key Concepts at the Knee**

- Posteriorly, capsule reinforced by the oblique popliteal ligament
- Medially, capsule reinforced by three layers of the MCL (superficial, middle deep layers)
- Laterally, capsule extends to tibial margin and fibular head, and is reinforced by LCL
- Anteriorly, capsule blends with expansion of VL and VM muscles to attach to patella and patellar tendon
- Anterior expansion continues medially and laterally to collateral ligaments and tibial condyles
  - Known as medial and lateral patellar retinacula or
  - Extensor retinaculum
  - Multiple layers implicated in patellofemoral pathology (Fig. 20-2)
- Capsule reinforced by patellar tendon
- Synovial plicae are embryonic remnants of synovial septa remaining into adulthood that may cause symptoms.

In ideal static alignment, the patella is situated slightly laterally because of the screw home mechanism that lateralizes the tibial tubercle. As the knee flexes and the tibia derotates, the patella is drawn into the trochlear groove. The patella remains in the trochlear groove until approximately 90 degrees of flexion. With continued flexion, the patella moves laterally and completes a lateral C-shaped curve. This motion occurs passively as the knee flexes through a ROM. However, this tracking changes during active knee extension, and the patella moves superiorly along the line of the femur if the vastus medialis obliquus (VMO) and the VL are in balance.

Kinematics of Gait
A ROM of 0 to 60 degrees at the knee is necessary for normal gait. However, this presumes normal mobility at the pelvis, hip, ankle, and foot. Any limitations at adjacent joints may require additional motion at the knee. When the foot makes initial contact with the ground, the knee is fully extended. The knee then flexes to 15 degrees during the loading response of gait. After this initial flexion, the knee begins to extend until it reaches full extension at midstance. As the body weight passes over the limb, the knee passively flexes to 40 degrees. As the knee moves into the initial swing phase, the knee

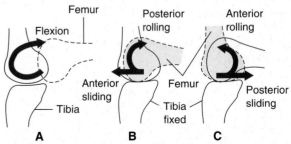

FIGURE 20-3. (A) Pure rolling of the femur on the tibia. The femur would roll off the tibia if no gliding occurred. (B) Posterior rolling and anterior gliding occur with flexion, while (C) anterior rolling and posterior gliding occur with extension. (Adapted from Norkin CC, Levangie PK. Joint Structure and Function: A Comprehensive Analysis. 2nd Ed. Philadelphia, PA: FA Davis, 1992:355.)

TABLE 20-2 Kinetics and Kinematics of the Gait Cycle at the Knee

PHASE OF THE GAIT CYCLE	ROM (DEGREES)	MOMENT	MUSCLE ACTIVITY	MUSCLE CONTRACTION TYPE
Initial contact	0	Flexion	Quadriceps	Isometric
			Hamstrings	At hip, isometric
Loading response	Flexes 0–15	Flexion	Quadriceps	Eccentric
Midstance	Extends to 5 flexion	Flexion moving toward extension	Quadriceps	Concentric
Terminal stance	Extends to 0	Extension	Minimal	
Preswing	Flexes to 40	Flexion	Minimal	
Initial swing	Flexes from 40 to 60		Hamstrings	Concentric
Midswing	Extends from 60 to 30		Mostly passive with some hamstrings	Eccentric
Terminal swing	Extends from 30 to 0		Hamstrings	Eccentric
			Quadriceps	Concentric

further flexes to 60 degrees to assist the foot clearing the floor. The knee then continues to extend through the midswing and terminal swing phases, achieving full extension before initial contact (Table 20-2).

Kinetics

Tibiofemoral Joint
Ground reaction forces and muscle activation combine to create significant forces about the knee joint. Malalignment in any plane can result in considerable focal increases in force. Motions occurring in the sagittal plane result primarily in activation of the knee flexors and extensors. During the loading response phase of the gait cycle, a flexion moment requires quadriceps activation isometrically and eccentrically to counteract the moment. As the knee approaches midstance, the flexion moment is moving toward an extension moment, and the quadriceps muscles are active until the knee is fully extended. Subsequently, muscle activity about the knee is minimal because of the passive nature of the terminal stance and preswing phases despite the respective extension and flexion moments. As the leg enters the swing phase, the hamstrings are active to flex the knee in initial swing and to decelerate the leg in terminal swing, whereas the quadriceps are active only in terminal swing to extend the leg (see Table 20-2).

Ground reaction forces, muscular forces, and the normal lower extremity alignment combine to produce important loads in the frontal plane. During the stance phase, the varus moment produces a relative compression in the medial compartment and distraction in the lateral compartment of the knee. This puts greater loads on the medial articular structures (e.g., articular cartilage, meniscus) and on the lateral stabilizing structures (e.g., LCL, joint capsule). Force plate analysis demonstrates that ground reaction vertical force rarely exceeds 115% to 120% of body weight during normal ambulation. However, during jogging and running, ground reaction forces approach 275% of body weight.[15]

Patellofemoral Joint
In addition to ground reaction forces, joint reaction forces are created at the patellofemoral joint by tension in the quadriceps and the patellar tendon. As the knee flexes in a weight-bearing position, greater quadriceps torque is required, and joint reaction force increases. For example, the quadriceps

torque during level walking is one-half of the body weight, stair climbing is three to four times the body weight, and squatting is seven to eight times the body weight.[18] These compressive forces can be minimized by a properly aligned patella, which disperses the force over a large surface area. Patellar subchondral bone with a strong, well-organized trabecular arrangement also minimizes joint reaction forces. Pathology, such as degeneration of patellar or femoral chondral surfaces, further reduces the capability of responding to PFJRFs.

The balance between the VMO and VL appears to be important for maintaining normal patellar tracking, although the precise recommendations are unclear. Results of surface electromyography (EMG) have suggested an approximately 1:1 ratio of VMO to VL input in normal individuals and <1:1 in those with patellofemoral pain.[19,20] This issue will be discussed further in the "Patellofemoral Pain" section. Small amounts of swelling (as little as 20 mL fluid) may inhibit the VMO.[21]

IMPAIRMENTS OF BODY STRUCTURES

The primary anatomic impairments at the knee occur in the frontal plane. Alignments of the hip, knee, and ankle combine to form an integrated kinetic chain, which must be considered in its entirety. The position of the hip affects the position of the knee, and the position of the knee dictates foot position. The anatomic impairments at the knee must be evaluated in light of the posture of the lumbopelvic, hip, ankle, and foot joints.

Genu Valgum
The femur descends obliquely from the hip in a distal and medial direction. This medial angulation with a vertical tibia results in a valgus angle at the knee, or genu valgum (Fig. 20-4A). This medial angle is 5 to 10 degrees. Any angle greater than this is considered to be excessive genu valgum. This valgus position places greater load on the lateral compartment of the knee and relatively unloads the medial compartment. Over time, development of degenerative joint disease in the lateral compartment produces physiologic lengthening of the MCL as the lateral compartment collapses and the medial compartment is unloaded. Increases in the angulation increase the lateral pull of the quadriceps, placing excessive

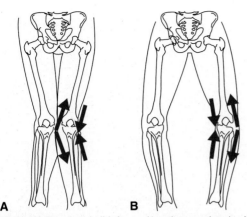

FIGURE 20-4. (A) Decreased tibiofemoral angle associated with coxa vara results in genu valgum. (B) Increased tibiofemoral angle associated with coxa valga results in genu varum. (Adapted from Norkin CC, Levangie PK. Joint Structure and Function: A Comprehensive Analysis. 2nd Ed. Philadelphia, PA: FA Davis, 1992:344.)

loads on the patellofemoral joint and increasing the risk of patellar dislocation. Genu valgus is associated with coxa varum at the hip and excessive pronation at the subtalar joint.

Genu Varum

When the angulation of the femur and tibia is vertical (0 degrees) or laterally oriented, the condition is referred to as genu varum (Fig. 20-4B). Genu varum increases the loads in the medial compartment of the knee and relatively unloads the lateral compartment. Genu varum is associated with coxa valgum, and because the heel contact occurs in a calcaneal varus position, excessive pronation occurs to orient the calcaneus vertically.

EXAMINATION AND EVALUATION

As with all the joints of the lower extremity, a comprehensive knee examination includes the adjacent joints and the lumbopelvic region. The choice of specific tests and measures for the examination depend on the situation. The following sections discuss key aspects of knee joint examination.

Patient/Client History

The most important data to be gathered first are subjective information, which guides the objective examination and provides the clinician with important information about activity limitations and participation restriction. Key questions focus on which symptoms are most disabling for the patient, who may experience pain, instability, mobility loss, weakness, catching, or other aggravating symptoms. From this information, the clinician chooses tests to match the patient's symptoms and designs a treatment program to address the activity limitations and participation restrictions described by the patient. At the knee, symptoms of giving way, catching, or locking may be present in addition to complaints of pain. The examination must clarify the source of the symptoms through thorough questioning and appropriate test and measure choices. For example, a history of a deceleration injury along with complaints of the knee giving way, would lead the clinician to tests such as a Lachman's to assess the integrity of the ACL.

Tests and Measures

The objective examination should begin with observation of posture and the position of the limb. Basic tests for the lumbopelvic and hip regions should be performed. Any of these areas may refer pain to the thigh, knee, or calf. See Magee's *Orthopedic Physical Assessment*[22] for a more complete description of examination techniques.

THERAPEUTIC EXERCISE INTERVENTION FOR BODY FUNCTION IMPAIRMENTS

After a thorough examination and determination of the diagnosis and prognosis, the treatment plan is implemented. Any impairments found must be correlated with an activity limitation or participation restriction, with this aspect of the patient's care treated concurrently. However, some impairments must be improved before their associated activity limitation or participation restriction can be addressed.

Mobility Impairment: Mobility of Joint Functions (ICF: b710)

The first step in treating decreased mobility of the knee is determining the cause. Mobility can be decreased because of any type of connective tissue (i.e., musculotendinous, capsular) shortening. Mobility can be diminished by iatrogenic or pathologic abnormalities such as an incorrectly placed ligament graft, a hypertrophic fat pad, or disuse. Examining the pattern of limitation and the patient's location of pain can clarify the cause of mobility impairment. Hypomobility at the knee joint results in compensation at adjacent joints. For example, squatting down with limited knee motion requires additional motion at the hip, ankle, and low back, and these joints are at risk for injury from the excessive demands placed on them. Thus adjacent joints must be examined simultaneously.

Mobilization Techniques

Capsular restriction is common after total knee arthroplasties, multiple operations, or immobilization for any reason. Capsular limitations can occur at the tibiofemoral joint, patellofemoral joint, or both, and the source of the limitation must be ascertained. Full knee extension requires superior glide of the patella and anterior glide of the tibia on the femur. Knee flexion requires inferior glide of the patella along with posterior glide of the tibia on the femur. Capsular restrictions are treated with the respective glides and joint distraction techniques (Fig. 20-5). Traction techniques are often helpful for increasing knee ROM. To increase knee flexion ROM, the therapist should apply distal traction to the knee flexed over the edge of the table while gently moving the knee into further flexion. A cable weight system works well for applying traction to increase knee extension ROM. Using a figure-of-eight strapping technique around the foot and ankle, attach the strap to the cable of a weight stack. A small bolster or towel roll should be placed under the ankle. The patient moves away from the weight stack enough to lift it, applying longitudinal traction to the leg. Additional weight can be placed on top of the knee to push it into further extension (Fig. 20-6).

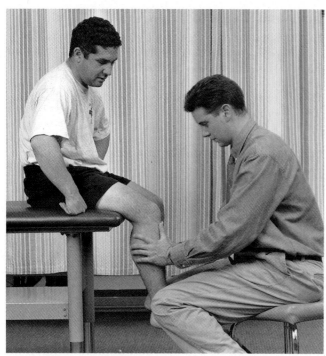

FIGURE 20-5. Joint distraction and posterior glide of the tibia on the femur can be performed simultaneously to increase knee joint flexion mobility.

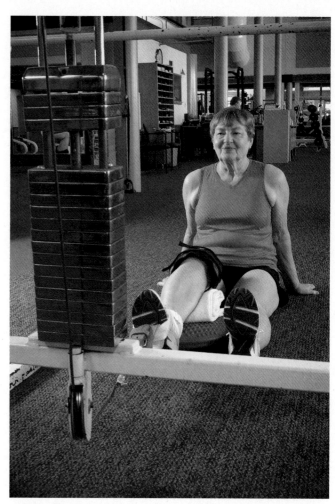

FIGURE 20-6. Knee extension with longitudinal distraction applied by a stack weight.

Self-stretching exercises work well to increase knee flexion ROM. A gravity assisted supine wall slide works well to facilitate knee flexion. Starting with the buttocks approximately 18 in. from the wall, place the feet up on the wall. Slowly slide the affected knee down until a stretch if felt. The position can be modified by bringing the buttocks closer or further from the wall (Fig. 20-7). The knee can be easily stretched while sitting in a chair at work or school. Slide the foot of the involved knee as far back as possible, then slide forward in the chair, keeping the foot planted, further flexing the knee. Self stretching is also effective in prone, using a strap or an ankle weight, if at least 90 degrees of flexion is available.

Self stretching for extension can be more challenging. Prone hangs work well, with the patient lying prone with the knee at the edge of the table and the leg hanging off the end. An ankle weight can be added to increase the force into extension. A similar activity can be performed in supine with a small bolster under the ankle, letting gravity and/or additional weight on the knee press the knee into extension.

Quadriceps setting is an excellent exercise to increase and maintain superior patellar glide (see Self-Management 20-1: Quadriceps Setting Exercise). However, if adhesions in the suprapatellar pouch limit the excursion of patellar glide, these exercises may increase patellar pain. Patellar mobilization in the direction of limitation can be performed by the therapist or by the patient in a home program (see Self-Management 20-2: Patellar Mobilization Performed by the Patient).

Stretching Techniques

Limitations caused by muscle shortening usually are treated with stretching exercises. The quadriceps and hamstring muscles may be lengthened in several positions, but care must be taken to ensure proper positioning of the spine, pelvis, and hip. Incorrect positioning can increase the stress in these areas and decrease the effectiveness of the stretch. The quadriceps may be stretched across the knee only or, with the addition of rectus femoris stretching, across the hip (Fig. 20-8). The pelvis must be prevented from tilting anteriorly, increasing lumbar extension during this stretch (see Self-Management 20-3: Quadriceps Stretching While Avoiding Lumbar Extension). Stretching the quadriceps at the knee may also be performed in prone with an abdominal support to prevent excessive lumbar extension.

The hamstrings are easily stretched in a sitting position with the knee extended and the lumbar spine held in neutral. Avoid posteriorly tilting the pelvis or flexing the lumbar spine. This exercise can be performed throughout the day at a variety of workstations (Fig. 20-9). The medial hamstrings may be emphasized by laterally rotating the leg, and the lateral hamstrings may be emphasized by medially rotating the leg. Horizontally adducting the hip with internal rotation of the hip enhances stretching of the iliotibial band (ITB) and its associated lateral structures (Fig. 20-10).

In addition to the major muscle groups acting at the knee, the closed chain nature of the lower extremity necessitates assessment at adjacent joints. For example, shortening of the medial rotators of the hip or the gastroc-soleus can contribute to patellofemoral pain at the knee. These tissues must be examined over all the appropriate joints.

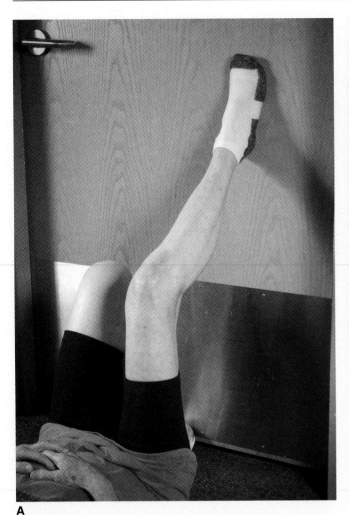
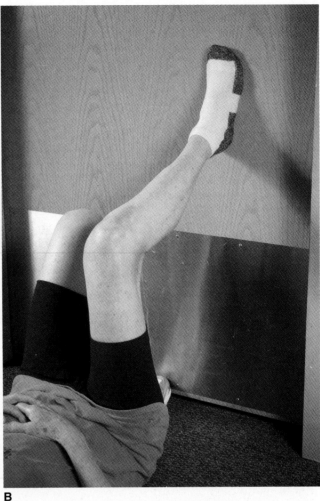

A   **B**

FIGURE 20-7. Wall slide for knee flexion ROM. (A) Starting position. (B) Slide the foot down the wall until a gentle stretch is felt.

◆ *SELF-MANAGEMENT 20-1* **Quadriceps Setting Exercise**

Purpose:	To strengthen quadriceps muscle, mobilize patella superiorly, stretch tight tissues behind the knee, and reeducate the quadriceps how to work
Position:	Sitting with the legs straight out, toes pointed up to the ceiling; a small towel may be placed behind the knee
Movement Technique:	
Level 1.	Tighten the quadriceps muscle on top of your thigh. You should see your kneecap move up toward your hip. Your knee may push down toward the floor, and your foot may come up off the floor. You should be unable to manually move your kneecap when doing a quadriceps set correctly. If you are having difficulty, try doing a quadriceps set on the other leg at the same time. Be sure your hip muscles stay relaxed.

Level 2.   Perform the same quadriceps set in a standing position.

Repetitions: ____ times

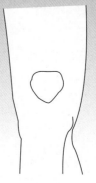

Relaxed muscle

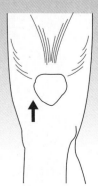

Tightened muscle

SELF-MANAGEMENT 20-2 *Patellar Mobilization Performed by the Patient*

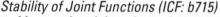

Purpose:	To increase the mobility of the kneecap in all directions
Position:	Sitting with the legs straight out, toes pointed up to the ceiling
Movement Technique:	Using your fingers or the heel of your hand, push your kneecap (A) down toward your foot, (B) toward the outside, (C) toward the inside, and (D) up toward your hip. Hold each position for a count of five. These movements should not be painful.

Repetitions: ___ *times*

Stability of Joint Functions (ICF: b715)

Problems with stability of joint functions are associated with instability. At the knee joint stability function are related to patellar instability and tibiofemoral instability.[23] Hypermobility is associated with clinical signs such as knee recurvatum and subtalar joint pronation. This combination may predispose individuals to patellofemoral pain at the knee.

Treatment of hypermobility at the knee joint requires postural education and retraining. This education is foc-

used at all lower extremity joints and the lumbopelvic area. Good posture requires an integrated approach throughout the entire kinetic chain. Any further training must be superimposed on correct postural mechanics. After this posture is achieved, closed chain activities emphasizing cocontraction of lower extremity musculature enhance postural stability (Fig. 20-11). High-repetition, low-resistance activity is used to enhance stability (Display 20.1).

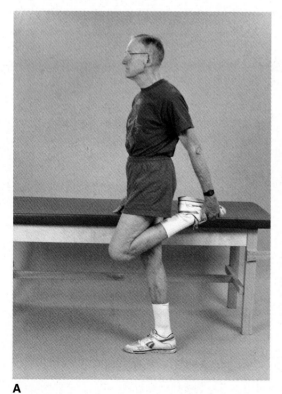

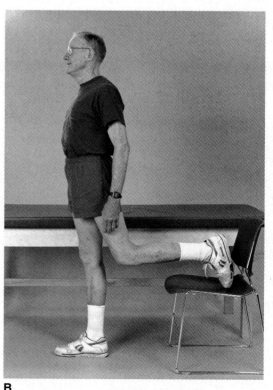

A **B**

FIGURE 20-8. Quadriceps stretching while standing. (A) Across the knee only. (B) Across the hip and knee.

SELF-MANAGEMENT 20-3 *Quadriceps Stretching While Avoiding Lumbar Extension*

Purpose: To increase flexibility of the quadriceps muscles

Position: This exercise can be performed in several positions. Pick a position that is comfortable or convenient for you, but avoid arching your back when stretching; tighten your abdominal muscles to keep your back steady.

1. In a sidelying position, with abdominal muscles tightened (A)
2. In a standing position, with some support, abdominal muscles tightened, and knees close together (B)
3. On your stomach, with a small pillow or towel under your hips and abdominal muscles tightened (C)

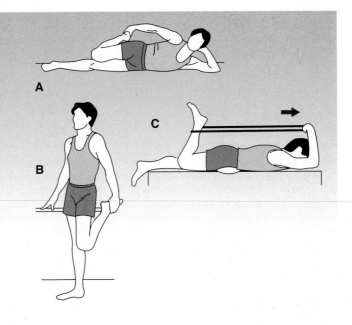

Movement Technique: Grasp your ankle or a strap attached to your ankle, pulling it toward your buttocks until you feel a gentle stretch in the front of your thigh. Hold each stretch for 15 to 30 seconds.

Repetitions: ___ times

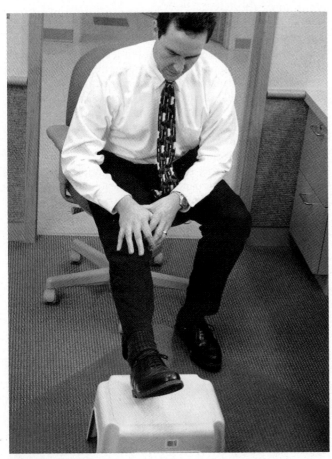

FIGURE 20-9. Hamstring stretch while seated at a workstation.

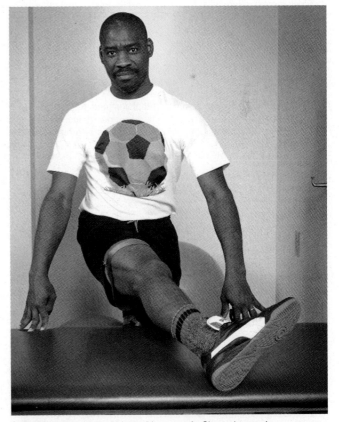

FIGURE 20-10. Lateral hip and leg stretch. Close observation prevents trunk rotation substitution for hip adduction.

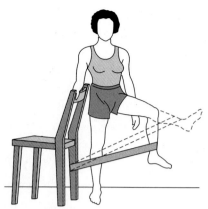

FIGURE 20-11. Knee extension exercise using tubing and with a focus on posture. This is a closed chain exercise on the weight-bearing side, and an open chain exercise on the non–weight-bearing side. It requires considerable balance and postural control.

DISPLAY 20-1

Impaired Muscle Performance Associated with Neurologic Condition

Patient Case Study No. 1: Patient is a 54-year-old woman diagnosed with post anoxic Parkinsonism 10 years earlier. She has managed well until the past year when she experienced a progressive increase in her symptoms. She notes a decrease in her walking ability as well as lower extremity weakness and occasional falling. Patient reports three falls in the last 6 months, each time landing on her knees. She now has constant knee pain which compounds her gait dysfunction. Pain rated at 5 on 0 to 10 scale, location in knees and low back

PMH: a medication error during a hospitalization produced an anoxic brain injury 12 years earlier. One year after the injury the patient began developing symptoms of Parkinsonism. Pt also has a history of chronic low back pain. Patient has history of meniscectomy in left knee.

Obs: Patient has resting tremor B with low amplitude; no rigidity in UE with cogwheeling in right arm; finger tapping movements markedly bradykinetic; gait markedly impaired with the following characteristics: difficulty initiating gait; small shuffling steps; marked bradykinesia during attempts to turn; significant and prolonged freezing; patient is 1+ effusion in left knee

Examination

MMT: strength testing limited by parkinsonism; quadriceps and hip flexor muscle strength grossly 4/5; hip abductor and hip extensor 4/5

ROM: decreased mobility in hip rotation; decreased trunk ROM in all directions 25% to 30%. Knee flexion ROM from 5 to 110 degrees because of decreased use.

Flexibility: decreased flexibility in hamstring muscles, quadriceps, and hip flexor muscles

Activity limitations:

1. Unable to walk more than ¼ mi; requires use of walker
2. Unable to do most household chores
3. Unable to walk a full flight of stairs
4. Unable to squat ¼ normal distance
5. Unable to stand for more than 20 minutes

Participation restrictions:

1. Unable to work outside the home or participate in her usual volunteer activities.
2. Limited socialization secondary to inability to walk any distance or to stand for more than 20 minutes

---

Muscle Performance Impairments (ICF: b730, b740)

Impaired muscle performance about the knee includes decreases in strength, power, and endurance of major muscle groups such as the quadriceps and hamstrings. The quadriceps are essential for controlling the motion and joint reaction forces across the knee joint, and as such, are critical for maintaining the long-term health of the joint surfaces. The muscles controlling the knee joint require, at a minimum, both strength and endurance. For many individuals, power is critical as well. Strength is necessary to raise the body up out of a chair or up the stairs. Endurance is necessary for walking any distance. Common non–weight-bearing exercises for increasing quadriceps and hamstring strength can be found in Table 20-3.

Many persons also need power for performing work or recreational activities that require generating a great deal of strength in a short period of time (as in jumping activities, or lifting very heavy objects). Chapter 5 describes a variety of strength, endurance, and power training activities. Plyometric exercises are commonly used to build power in the muscles surrounding the knee joint. Be sure that the individual is ready for such vigorous, impactful activities, or an overuse injury may occur. Also be sure that activities of this level are necessary for the patient. Not all patients are candidates for plyometric exercises. Common weight-bearing exercises for the lower extremity can be found in Table 20-4.

Neurologic Causes

Neurological disorders can produce impairments in muscle performance in muscles surrounding and supporting the knee joint. The most common cause is a lumbar spine injury or disease. In addition to directly affecting the quadriceps or hamstring musculature, lumbar spine pathology affecting proximal or distal musculature necessarily affects gait and other movement patterns. Altered movement patterns affect knee joint mechanics and ultimately the joint itself. Any complaints of knee joint impairments should prompt examinations of the spine and proximal and distal joints.

Other neurologic disorders, such as multiple sclerosis or Parkinson disease, profoundly affect the ability to produce torque about the knee. Each of these situations must be evaluated within the context of the disease process. Because many muscles and movement patterns are affected, a more global examination is necessary to determine the treatment strategy.

Some authorities have suggested there is a neurologic component to patellofemoral pain. Studies of different quadriceps activation patterns in response to a patellar tendon tap have suggested timing differences in those with or without patellofemoral pain.[19,24,25]

The key consideration when designing interventions for those with neurologically mediated impaired muscle performance is ensuring use of the desired muscle. Neurologic weakness produces alterations in firing patterns to accomplish movement in the most efficient manner possible. Synergists may accommodate for weakness, or biomechanical modifications may enhance the activity of other muscles as compensation for the weakness. For example, a forward lean during stair ascent allows the hip extensors to compensate for weak

TABLE 20-3 **Quadriceps and Hamstring Strengthening Non–Weight Bearing**

EXERCISE	GOAL	POSITION	PATIENT CUES	KEY POINTS
Quadriceps setting	1. Quadriceps strength 2. Dynamic knee control 3. Patellar mobility 4. Muscle reeducation	Any position with knee extended	"Tighten knee, push knee down, push from front of thigh, lock kneecap"	Ensure that quadriceps are firing and that the patient is not substituting with hip extension. Patella should be locked down and unable to be moved by therapist; cue patient that activation should be comfortable and does not need to be maximal
Straight leg raise (SLR)	1. Quadriceps and hip flexor strength 2. Dynamic knee control 3. Muscle reeducation 4. Core muscle strengthening	Supine with knee extended	"Breathe, tighten quadriceps, lift leg to 60 degree angle, lower slowly, relax quadriceps, exhale"; if performed in standing, cue patient to "tighten knee then lift leg as in a soldier march"	Make sure patient has full control of knee via quadriceps set; if patient is unable to perform in supine, decrease lever arm length relative to gravity; i.e., perform closer to a vertical standing position
Short arc quad	1. Quadriceps strengthening 2. Muscle reeducation 3. Eccentrics for tendinopathies	1. Supine or long sitting with knee flexed over a bolster or short sitting with block for knee flexion 2. Standing	"Tighten quadriceps, lift foot until knee is extended, lower slowly" or "pretend you are trying to gently kick a ball"	1. If for eccentrics only, have patient lift leg to full extension with contralateral leg, then quadriceps set and lower involved leg slowly; work only in painfree range; this may be any portion of the knee extension ROM 2. The shorter lever arm in standing often makes this an easier exercise
Multi-angle isometrics	1. Quadriceps strengthening 2. Muscle reeducation	Short sitting with knee flexed	"Push and hold for 6 seconds, then relax." Repeat approximately every 15 degrees or in positions as dictated by injury or surgery	Can use manual resistance from another person, isometric against opposite leg, isometric against resistive bands, or with an ankle weight, using the contralateral limb to move the involved knee to the appropriate angle and hold
Knee extension: isotonic concentric and/or eccentric contractions	1. Quadriceps strengthening 2. Muscle reeducation	Short sitting	"Straighten out your knee, hold and lower slowly"	Verbal cues will change depending upon type of muscle contraction
Hamstring isometrics	1. Hamstring strengthening 2. Muscle reeducation	Short sitting, long sitting or supine	"Tighten and hold your hamstrings as if you were trying to pull your heel back toward your buttocks"	Can be done at any angle or at multiple angles, as with multiple angle isometrics for the quadriceps
Hamstring curls	1. Hamstring strengthening 2. Muscle reeducation	Nearly any position depending upon how resistance is applied: standing, sitting, prone, supine, etc.	"Bend your knee pulling your heel toward your buttocks"	Ankle weights: best lever against gravity is in standing; in prone exercise will become gravity assisted, making it an eccentric quadriceps exercise Resistive bands: any position Isokinetics: any position

TABLE 20-4 **Common Weight-Bearing Exercises for the Lower Extremity**

EXERCISE	POSITION	PATIENT CUES	KEY POINTS
Wall sits/slides	Feet away from wall so that tibia remains vertical at lowest point of sit	"Squeeze your buttocks together and tighten your quadriceps. Slowly slide down the wall"	Core tight and stabilized; hips, knees, feet in alignment, avoiding valgus at knees
Weight-bearing terminal knee extension (TKE)	Standing facing therapist or stationary object with tubing attached; tubing around posterior aspect of knee	"Keeping your foot fixed on the floor, extend your knee against the resistance of the tubing"	Tighten quadriceps with gluteals as a secondary agonist
Squat	Feet shoulder width apart, hips, knees and feet in line; may modify depending upon patient situation	"Sit back like sitting on a chair; keep trunk upright, slight curve in low back; hips and knees in line"	Avoid forward lean; can be performed, full (to 90 degree flexion), partial, or mini; can be advanced by adding resistive tubing under the feet, weights in hands or weight bar across shoulders
Split squat	Feet in stride with pelvis level	"Squat down keeping	Keep tibia in front vertical; tighten pelvis and keep neutral spine
Lunge	Normal stance with one foot stepping out	"Step forward and squat down"	Can be performed stepping forward, backward or to side
Step ups/downs	Facing step	"Tighten quadriceps and hip muscles, then step"	Can be performed stepping forward, backward or to side; keep good alignment of hip, knee and foot

quadriceps (Fig. 20-12). Close monitoring of exercise quality is necessary to ensure training of the desired muscle. See Building Block 20-1.

Muscular Strain

The ability to produce torque at the knee can be affected by muscular strain injuries. The quadriceps and hamstring muscle groups are the most commonly injured, often the result of sudden decelerative forces. The quadriceps decelerate the flexing knee during the loading response of the gait cycle, and the hamstrings decelerate the forward swinging shank during the terminal swing phase. These eccentric muscle contractions may produce macrotraumatic or microtraumatic injury.

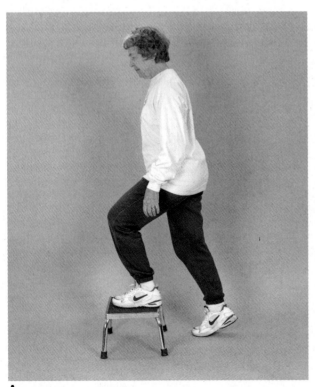
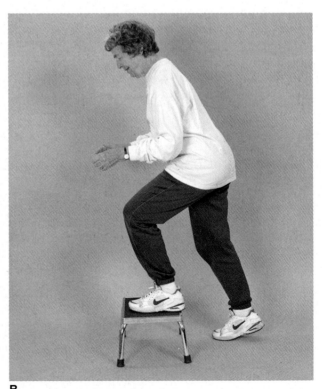

A   **B**

FIGURE 20-12. (A) Ascending stairs using proper mechanics. (B) Ascending stairs with the hip extensor muscle substituting for a weak quadriceps muscle.

BUILDING BLOCK 20-1

Consider the patient in Display 20-1, Case Study No. 1.

1. Given the history and examination findings, what are the likely compensations this patient is making in order to maintain her functional abilities.
2. How might your treatment program reflect these compensations? What exercises or components might be emphasized?
3. Write some possible short- and long-term goals for this patient.

The quadriceps may be injured as the result of a contusion. A blow from an object such as a ball or hockey puck can produce a deep muscle contusion that requires special rehabilitation consideration. Initially bleeding within the muscle must be controlled, followed by progressive mobility and strengthening. When returning the patient to function, the role of the affected muscle in should be retrained to fit the expected activity. For example, the runner with a hamstring strain injury as a result of the swing phase of gait should be trained in an open chain, decelerative function. Inertial exercise or other forms of repetitive decelerative exercise also can be used (Fig. 20-13). Research has shown that athletes who completed a trunk stabilization and progressive agility program had a significantly lower reinjury rate than those who completed a traditional static stretching and progressive resistive hamstring strengthening program.[26] For those returning to sports, plyometric exercises are an excellent choice for retraining the lower extremity muscles.

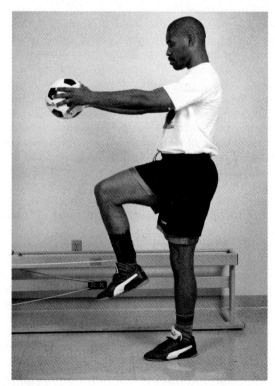

FIGURE 20-13. Hamstring muscle training with inertial exercise for high-repetition, low-resistance acceleration and deceleration training.

Disuse and Deconditioning

Disuse of the knee musculature occurs primarily in the quadriceps and may occur as a result of an injury at the knee or from any other joint in the kinetic chain, including the low back. An injury at an associated joint can prevent participation in usual activities, leading to disuse of musculature throughout the kinetic chain. Disuse of the quadriceps affects the loading and midstance phases of the gait cycle, during which the quadriceps decelerate the flexing knee, followed by a change of direction and acceleration into knee extension. This quadriceps action decreases loads on the joint surfaces and is critical in maintaining the health of the knee joint (Display 20.2).

The quadriceps muscles work to decelerate the body when descending stairs and, along with the hip musculature, to ascend stairs and arise from a sitting position. Disuse can lead to profound changes in how activities of daily living (ADLs) are performed. Failure to perform these activities efficiently

DISPLAY 20-2
Impaired Muscle Performance Due to Disuse and Deconditioning

Patient Case Study No. 2: Patient is a 78-year-old male who c/o increased leg tiredness with walking and inability to walk as far as he could previously; having difficulty getting in and out of chairs and ascending stairs; knees "feel weak." Patient has moderate to severe osteoarthritis in both knees.

PMH: Chronic asthma; stable ventricular tachycardia with right bundle branch block since 1988; Renal cancer status post radical nephrectomy in 2001; left flank gunshot wound 62 years ago with continuous problems with abdominal hernias; bilateral hand tremor, left greater than right, getting worse per patient report.

Obs: patient has bilateral trendelenberg pattern, truncal obesity and B LE atrophy; walks with short steps, DOE after walking into treatment room from waiting area

6 minute walk test: at rest: HR 49, O_2 sat 96%; distance walked 885 without assistive device with 1 rest period; post-walk vitals: HR 116, recovers in 3 minutes; O_2 sat 96%

BERG Balance Scale: 47/56 total score. Indicates a low risk of falls with standing tasks without upper extremity support. vWith no history of falls in the last 6 months indicates 22% probability of future falls. Dynamic Gait Index: 21/24 total score, without an assistive device.

Score indicates a low risk of falls with walking

MMT: normal throughout except: hip abd 4/5 B; hip ext 4-/5 B; knee extension 4/5 B

ROM: normal throughout with the exception of decreased hip external rotation

Functional strength: requires extensive UE use for transfers in and out of chair

Activity limitations:

1. Patient unable to walk more than 400 feet without stopping to rest
2. Unable to walk more than one flight of stairs
3. Inability to walk on uneven ground.
4. Able to squat only ¼ of normal depth

Participation restrictions:

1. Patient unable to maintain household and yard due to LE weakness and fatigue.
2. Unable to participate in his usual walking group, a primary social outlet for him.

BUILDING BLOCK 20-2

Consider the patient in Display 20-2, Case Study No. 2 to answer the following questions:

1. Do you think the patient's activity limitations and participation restrictions are related to underlying impairments? If so, how might you evaluate this theory?
2. If you are unable to determine the underlying cause of his functional loss, or if you believe it to be a combination of multiple factors, please suggest three exercises that might address multi-factorial nature of the problem.
3. Write some possible short- and long-term goals for this patient.

and continuously places additional loads on adjacent joints. Treatment should focus on the primary cause of the disuse as well as strengthening activities for the quadriceps muscle. See Building Block 20-2.

THERAPEUTIC EXERCISE INTERVENTION FOR COMMON DIAGNOSES

Ligament Injuries

Anterior Cruciate Ligament

The ACL is one of the most commonly injured ligaments in the knee. The short- and long-term morbidity associated with an ACL injury with or without reconstructive surgery has made this injury the nemesis of many athletes. Fortunately, the ACL injury has become better understood and better managed, resulting in significant decreases in morbidity. The ACL tear usually occurs as the result of a quick deceleration, hyperextension, or rotational injury and does not involve contact with another individual. Injury to the ACL is frequently associated with injuries to the MCL, the medial meniscus, and the lateral meniscus. In the adolescent, the ACL may avulse from the tibial spine rather than tear in the midsubstance, and it should be surgically repaired with bone-to-bone fixation.

Although functioning independently, the ACL and PCL guide the instant center of rotation of the knee, thereby controlling the joint arthrokinematics. Any alteration in normal kinematics can produce focal areas of increased articular cartilage and other soft tissue loading. Sequelae such as degenerative joint disease and tendinitis must be considered when determining prognosis and treatment approach. Injury to the ACL can result in significant activity limitations and potential participation restrictions because of its role as the primary restraint against anterior tibial translation. Patients with ACL-deficient knees were found to have altered joint arthrokinematics in the transverse plane during walking.[27] The authors suggest that the repeated rotational instability may play a role in the development of meniscus tears or osteoarthritis. Rupture of the ACL results in substantially increased anterior translation, with the maximum occurring between 15 and 45 degrees of flexion.[15] The posterior horn

of the medial meniscus provides secondary restraint against anterior tibial translation and is at risk for injury after an ACL rupture. The ACL provides stability against tibial medial and lateral rotation and against varus and valgus stresses.

Because of its role in controlling the instant center of rotation, some individuals experience episodes of instability after ACL injury and subsequently fail conservative treatment. They may have surgery using static restraints to reconstruct the ACL. These tissues include the central one third of the patellar tendon or the hamstring tendon.[28] Those involved in high-demand sports usually have more difficulty returning to activities without symptoms. Preinjury hours of sports participation, age, and arthrometer testing were correlated with a need for surgery 90 days or more post-injury.[29] Continued vigorous activity with an unstable knee can lead to meniscal tears, especially at the posterior horn of the medial meniscus.

Significant impairments, activity limitations, and participation restrictions occur after ACL tears. These can be found outlined in Table 20-5.

Persons may become disabled because these limitations prevent return to work, leisure activities, or basic or instrumental ADLs.

Rehabilitation issues of concern when treating the individual after ACL injury include the impairments, activity limitations, and participation restrictions identified during the evaluation and any concomitant injuries. Associated injury to the MCL or meniscus affects the rehabilitation program. The arthrokinematic changes and potential for secondary injury guide rehabilitation. Resistive open chain quadriceps exercises between 15 and 45 degrees are often avoided because of the increased anterior tibial translation found with this type of exercise. This translation is minimized in a closed chain exercise, a good choice after ACL injury or reconstruction. Because of the difficulty in returning to deceleration and cutting maneuvers, the rehabilitation program should include these types of movements along with resistive, balance, and coordination activities in multiple planes. Exercises may include resisted lateral movements, resisted rotational movements, and activities on unstable surfaces. Individuals returning to high demand athletics frequently participate in a plyometric program as well. See Building Block 20-3.

Because of the high incidence of ACL injuries in athletes, particularly female athletes, clinicians have been searching for factors predisposing females to these injuries, and for interventions to prevent their occurrence.[30–33] A number of factors have been considered, including muscle flexibility, joint laxity, postural factors (i.e., genu recurvatum, excessive foot pronation), notch width, neuromuscular coordination, hormone levels, training and conditioning, and position. Sorting out the contributions of these factors has been a challenge, particularly because there is overlap among many of the factors. Factors such as increased knee laxity measures and increased dynamic knee valgus and high abduction loads during landing from a jump seem to be predictive of future ACL injuries.[31] However, a large body of evidence is accumulating supporting the success of neuromuscular training programs on the biomechanics of jumping, neuromuscular performance and on the subsequent incidence of ACL injuries.[30–36] These studies have found that neuromuscular training can improve neuromuscular performance as measured by a crossover hop test.[36] Such training improved the biomechanics of landing from a

TABLE 20-5 Common Impairments, Activity Limitations, and Participation Restrictions Following Knee Ligament Injuries

LIGAMENT INJURY	EXAMINATION FINDINGS	ACTIVITY LIMITATIONS	PARTICIPATION RESTRICTIONS	REHABILITATION ISSUES
ACL tear: acute	Effusion + Lachman test + Arthrometer testing Pain, instability, loss of motion, limited WB	Need for assistive device ADL, IADLs limited Difficulty with stairs	Inability to participate in work, sports, leisure activities requiring any physical exertion, full WB or lifting or carrying objects	Concomitant injuries (MCL, meniscus, etc.) Avoid open chain quadriceps exercises from 15 to 45 degrees due to increased anterior shear Restore full motion, prepare for surgery if planned
ACL tear: chronic (symptomatic)	Chronic low grade effusion + Lachman's, pivot shift tests Instability + Arthrometer testing	Inability to participate in usual activities due to instability	Inability to participate in usual activities due to instability	Protection of secondary stabilizers such as medial meniscus Joint protection perspective
PCL tear	+ Posterior drawer, posterior sag tests Effusion, LOM, limited WB	Need for assistive device ADL, IADLs limited Difficulty with stairs Difficulty walking down ramps/inclines	Inability to participate in work, sports, leisure activities requiring any physical exertion, full WB or lifting or carrying objects	Protection of structures in medial and anterior compartments History of osteoarthritis, varus alignment, patellofemoral pain
MCL tear	Loss of full extension, flexion + Valgus stress test at 30 degrees Tender over MCL History of valgus stress Local swelling but no joint effusion	Difficulty with frontal & transverse plane movements Difficulty walking on uneven surfaces	Inability to participate in work, sports, leisure activities requiring walking on uneven surfaces, frontal plane movements, etc.	Structural properties of ligament may lag behind clinical testing ability
LCL tear	History of varus, hyperextension stress Loss of full extension + Varus stress test at 30 degrees Tender over LCL Local swelling but no joint effusion	Minimal limitations unless combined with posterior-lateral corner injury Difficulty with frontal plane movements	Limitations in high demand physical activities especially those involving quick direction changes	Prolonged course of ligament remodeling

jump, decreasing knee adduction moments, and peak landing forces.[35] More importantly, neuromuscular retraining programs have significantly reduced the incidence of ACL injuries.[32,33,36] The neuromuscular training programs should include

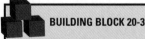

BUILDING BLOCK 20-3

Consider a 22-year-old male recreational basketball player who tore his ACL 2.5 weeks ago and will be undergoing surgical ACL reconstruction in a few weeks if he continues to experience instability. He also has a first degree MCL injury.

1. Describe three exercises you might use to strengthen his quadriceps in preparation for surgery. Include rationale for your choices.
2. What criteria might be used for initiating frontal or transverse plane activities. Provide examples of low level frontal and/or transverse plane activities.

education on the proper mechanics of landing, jumping, and changing direction. See Patient-Related Instruction 20-1: Proper Landing, Cutting and Direction Change Techniques for prevention of ACL Injuries. It is difficult to know which component resulted in the decreased incidence of injury: the education, strength increases, neuromuscular coordination improvement, or changes in biomechanics/posture. However, the combination of these factors in the neuromuscular training program has been effective in decreasing ACL injuries in female athletes (see Display 20-3).

For individuals involved in sports requiring deceleration, cutting and jumping, reconstruction of the ACL may be necessary to allow return to the previous competitive level. A new ligament is comprised of either the mid-1/3 of the patellar tendon or a looped hamstring tendon. The ligament is placed within the knee arthroscopically and is fixated in bony tunnels. A sample protocol for rehabilitation following ACL reconstruction can be found in Table 20-6. A similar program can be followed for non-operative treatment of ACL injuries, keeping in mind any complications of continued instability.

Patient-Related Instruction 20-1

Proper Landing, Cutting, and Direction Change Techniques for Prevention of ACL Injuries

- land softly on both feet
- land on the forefoot and roll to the rearfoot
- keep knees over toes, avoiding knees rolling in
- activate and tighten hip and thigh muscles to stiffen and stabilize knees
- take several small steps to slow down and change direction, rather than a plant and twist

DISPLAY 20-3

Neuromuscular Training for Injury Prevention

- Warm-up: any large muscle group activity
  - jogging
  - bicycling
  - calisthenics
- Flexibility: stretching hip and leg muscle groups
  - quadriceps and hamstring muscles
  - hip flexors, extensors, rotators, abductors, adductors
  - calf musculature
  - low back
- Dynamic balance: teaching proper landing techniques
  - weight on ball of foot
  - hop with knees bent
  - land with knees in flexion
  - knees under hips avoiding internal rotation and adduction
- Dynamic balance: impact activities
  - front-back and side-to-side hopping
  - hop and stick the landing
  - cone hopping: with and without turns
  - agility drills including direction changes
  - vertical box hops: single and multiple, with and without turns

Posterior Cruciate Ligament

The PCL injuries represent an estimated 1% to 30% of all knee ligament injuries.[37] Most injuries occur as the result of a trauma such as a motor vehicle accident, with fewer PCL injuries occurring in sports.[37] The mechanism producing a PCL injury is most often a blow to the anterior aspect of the tibia, forcing it posteriorly. Less commonly, the PCL is

TABLE 20-6 Rehabilitation Following an ACL Reconstruction

	PHASE 1	PHASE 2	PHASE 3	PHASE 4
Goals	1. Full active knee extension comparable to contralateral knee and flexion to 125 degrees 2. No swelling 3. Knee control weight bearing and non–weight bearing 4. Normalize gait	1. Restore posture and control with basic movements 2. Increased lower extremity and core strength 3. Increased static and dynamic balance 4. ROM equal to contralateral leg	1. Performance of multi-plane strengthening and functional exercises 2. Effective eccentric control for impact loading 3. Functional dynamic mobility	1. Single leg control during impact 2. Effective posture and eccentric control with direction change 3. Efficient performance of skill activities
ROM and mobility	Knee extension with bolster under ankle Prone hang Supine wall slides Heel slides Seated knee flexion Patellar mobilization	Continue phase 1 until goal achieved Stationary bike with seat lowered for gentle stretch Prone knee flexion Stretching for other lower extremity muscle groups	Continue previous exercises as needed Add dynamic warm-up and dynamic mobility activities (i.e., skipping all directions, carioca, shuffles, etc.)	Continue dynamic warm-up
Muscle performance and proprioception	Quadricep and hamstring sets Standing leg lifts Weight shifts Double leg minisquats Toe raises Core strength (abdominals, crunches, etc.)	Squats Step backs down off a step Stationary lunge Single leg balance with arm and weight shift perturbation Core strength (advanced crunches and bridges)	Squat with knee lift Squat and reach Retro-step up Lunge walk (forward, back, side, diagonal) Take off and landing drills Advanced balance exercises Core strength (continue to advance)	Landing control: Jump rotations Fast feet and lunge Multi-plane leap and land Stop and go Hopping Cutting and pivoting drills Lunge with resistance Advanced core activities
Gait and cardiovascular	Diagonal weight shifts Backward stepping Step over 4 in obstacle	High knee walking all directions Hurdler walk with hip circles Diagonal stride and hold forward and back	Progress to appropriate cardiovascular activity	Progress to sport or activity specific cardiovascular training

injured as a result of hyperflexion, hyperextension, or a varus or valgus injury. In the case of hyperextension, the ACL is usually injured first. In the varus or valgus injury, the respective collateral ligament is injured, and in some cases, the ACL is injured before the PCL injury.

The PCL is the primary restraint to posterior subluxation of the tibia on the femur, providing approximately 95% of the resistance against posterotibial translation.[38] A tear of the PCL results in significant increases in posterior tibial translation, with the greatest occurring between 70 and 90 degrees.[39] The PCL resists varus or valgus translation and is a secondary restraint to lateral tibial rotation.[37] Along with the ACL, the PCL helps control the instant center of rotation at the knee and joint arthrokinematics. The alteration in joint arthrokinematics after PCL rupture can result in significant problems. Articular cartilage contact pressures in the medial and anterior compartments are increased after PCL rupture, with peak medial pressures at 60 degrees and peak anterior compartment pressures at 90 degrees of flexion.[37] The individual with a PCL rupture generally complains of pain related to these changes, rather than frank instability.

The natural history of the PCL-deficient knee is difficult to assess because of the heterogeneity of most populations studied. Many patients remain asymptomatic and are able to return to their preinjury activity levels, but others develop osteoarthritic changes in the medial and anterior compartments.[40] The clinician must consider the possibility of these changes and modify the rehabilitation program appropriately. Some persons with multiple ligament or soft tissue injuries undergo reconstruction of the PCL using static restraints such as the central one third of the patellar tendon, Achilles tendon, or allograft.

The extent of impairments, activity limitations, and participation restrictions after PCL rupture depends on associated injuries (see Table 20-5). When patients are seen for chronic activity limitations because of PCL deficiency, the subjective complaints usually are related to medial and anterior compartment pain and difficulty ambulating down a decline or stairs.

The issues affecting the rehabilitation approach are related to the potential medial and anterior compartment changes. Any additional ligament injuries that could further alter arthrokinematics or medial meniscal damage that could modify articular cartilage pressures have the potential to exacerbate compartmental changes. Comorbidities such as underlying osteoarthritic changes, a varus alignment, or history of patellofemoral pain negatively alter the prognosis. These issues should be the framework from which the rehabilitation program is designed. As in treating the ACL-deficient knee, open chain resistive exercise (knee flexion in this case) can increase posterior tibial translation, and closed chain activities are an important therapeutic exercise mode. A sample program following PCL reconstruction can be found on the website

Medial Collateral Ligament

The MCL consists of the tibial collateral ligament and the middle one third of the medial capsule (deep portion), which is subdivided into a thin anterior third, a strong middle third, and a moderately strong posterior third.[41] The incidence of MCL injuries is significantly higher than that of LCL injuries,

and the MCL has been reported to be the most frequently injured ligament of the knee.[42] Damage to the MCL occurs less frequently at the femoral insertion compared with the tibial insertion because of differences in the insertion site structures. The MCL is usually torn as a result of a valgus stress by a lateral blow or by forced abduction of the tibia, as occurs when catching the inside edge of a ski. Associated injuries may include the ACL and medial meniscus. In the adolescent, injury to the femoral or tibial growth plate often precedes injury to the MCL and should be considered in the differential diagnosis.

The MCL is the primary restraint against valgus loads, and it resists tibial medial rotation. Unlike the cruciate ligaments, the MCL has the capacity for repair without surgical intervention. Most MCL injuries heal well without any long-term damage to the knee, despite some residual valgus laxity.[43,44] For this reason, most MCL injuries are usually treated conservatively. In the individual with a combined MCL and ACL injury, a short period of recovery usually is allowed, followed by reconstruction of the ACL. Injuries to the MCL in the presence of ACL ruptures do not heal as well as isolated MCL sprains.[45] Repairing the MCL or ACL risks the loss of extension ROM. The effects of lengthy immobilization on the ligament substance and insertion sites have been studied.[45] In dogs, surgical repair followed by 6 weeks of immobilization of MCLs resulted in inferior mechanical and structural properties, even at 48 weeks. Woo et al.[45] reported that a remobilization period six times longer than the time of immobilization might be required for recovery. However, individuals with surgical stabilization of bony avulsions have an excellent prognosis.

The impairments, activity limitations, and participation restrictions seen after acute MCL sprains are similar to those of cruciate ligament sprains (see Table 20-5). The prognosis after isolated MCL sprain is generally good because of the ligament's ability to heal well. Some individuals may experience difficulties with lateral and rotational movements or with activities on uneven surfaces. Persons returning to physical work or recreation are most at risk for limitations in these areas. Although the clinical examination may be benign after 6 to 8 weeks of rehabilitation, the lengthy ligament remodeling process may limit the MCL's tolerance for high-demand loading.

The most significant rehabilitation issues in the isolated MCL injury are the fact that the remodeling process lags behind the clinical examination findings and the need for frontal and transverse plane rehabilitation techniques. Traditional clinical examination procedures are not sensitive enough to determine readiness to return to high demand activities. Frequently, the individual has full ROM, symmetric strength, minimal or no valgus laxity, no effusion, and no tenderness to palpation after a few weeks of rehabilitation. However, the MCL is not stressed much in ordinary daily activities or even in sagittal plane activities such as straight-ahead running. The ligament must be loaded and trained just like muscle tissue to ensure adequate remodeling for high-demand activities. Loading in the frontal and transverse planes must occur to strengthen the ligament and its bony attachments and to ensure a safe return to physical activities (Figs. 20-14 and 20-15). A sample program for rehabilitation following a grade II MCL injury can be found in on the website. See Building Block 20-4.

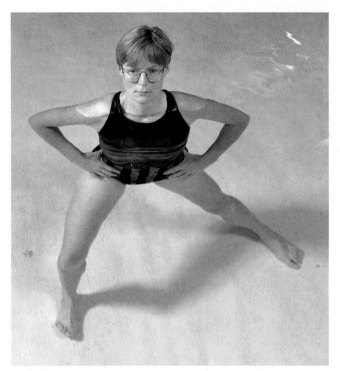

FIGURE 20-14. Side stepping in the pool is an early lateral movement activity.

Lateral Collateral Ligament

Injuries to the LCL are much less common than injuries to the MCL, and like MCL injuries, they heal well and without significant long-term disability. The LCL is the primary restraint to varus stress, and because of its location in the posterior one third, it also resists hyperextension, especially

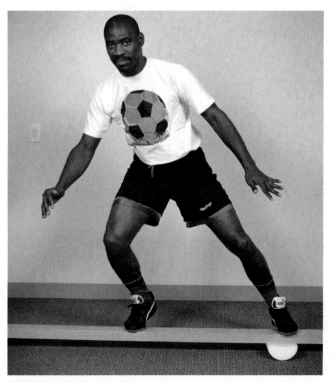

FIGURE 20-15. More challenging lateral movements include side stepping on a balance beam on foam rollers.

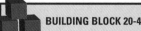

> **BUILDING BLOCK 20-4**
>
> Consider a 35-year-old patient with a second degree MCL injury who desires to return to skateboarding.
>
> 1. Describe three frontal plane and three transverse plane exercises that you would use once the patient tolerated exercise in this plane (early phase)
> 2. Progress these same exercises to an advanced level to prepare this patient to return to activity.

in the presence of a varus stress.[41] LCL injuries usually result from hyperextension varus forces, with or without contact with another individual. Complete tears occur in the ligament midsubstance or at the fibular insertion. Associated injuries may occur to the posterolateral structures, including the joint capsule, arcuate ligament, biceps femoris or popliteus tendons, or cruciate ligaments. In the adolescent, injury to the growth plate usually precedes ligament injury and should be considered in the differential diagnosis.

The natural history of the LCL injury rarely includes long-term disability because of its healing potential. Surgical repair of the isolated LCL is rarely performed. Individuals with significant varus deformities may experience instability after this injury and may require surgical stabilization. A bony avulsion should be surgically reattached. More extensive posterolateral corner injuries typically are reconstructed using static restraints or biceps femoris tenodesis.

The activity limitations and participation restrictions seen after a LCL injury are fewer than those seen with an MCL injury. Most individuals are minimally limited after this injury, except in the case of a third-degree tear or concomitant ligament or capsular injury (see Table 20-5).

Rehabilitation issues are similar to those for MCL injuries. The prolonged course of ligament remodeling must be considered, along with the importance of retraining the individual and loading the ligament in the frontal and sagittal planes.

Treatment of Ligament Injuries

Interventions should be aimed at achieving specific goals related to impairments, activity limitations, and participation restrictions. Impairments should be addressed if they are associated with an activity limitation or participation restriction or if continued impairment could lead to participation restriction in the future. Pain and effusion can be managed in the short term with physical agents, mechanical and electrotherapeutic modalities, and gentle therapeutic exercise. Cold packs, ice massage, compression therapies, and electrical stimulation are commonly used to minimize pain and effusion. Therapeutic exercise such as active and passive ROM activities within a comfortable range can provide lubrication to joint surfaces and can assist resorption of excessive joint fluid. The patient should receive instruction in the application of these procedures at home and guidance in modifying activities to minimize pain and effusion.

Traditional physiologic stretching and active and passive ROM activities facilitate restoration of preinjury joint

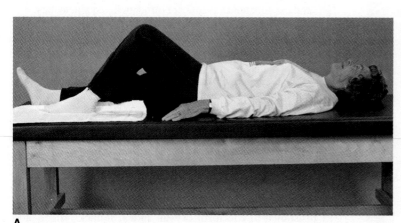

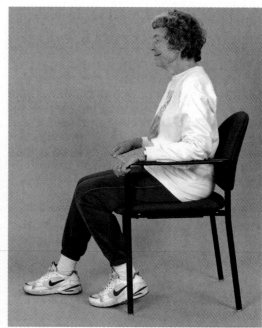

A   **B**

FIGURE 20-16. Active ROM for knee flexion. (A) Heel slides. (B) Seated knee flexion on a chair.

motion. Occasionally, joint mobilization techniques may be necessary, although ligamentous injury generally results in too much mobility rather than too little. However, lengthy immobilization or an inability to fire the quadriceps may result in a loss of knee extension ROM. Neuromuscular reeducation exercises such as quadriceps setting, hamstring setting, and other muscle activation techniques can restore the ability to fire muscles, which is a prerequisite for normalization of movement patterns. The home program should include exercises to facilitate ROM increases and neuromuscular reeducation exercises to advance gains made in the clinic (Fig. 20-16) (see Self-Management 20-4: Performing Flexion and Extension Mobility Exercises During the *Day*).

The pool is an excellent environment for performing mobility, normalizing gait, and initiating balance and gentle strengthening exercises. The water's buoyancy minimizes weight bearing while the hydrostatic pressure controls effusion. Walking, physiologic stretching, leg kicks, toe raises, single-leg balance, and squats can be easily accomplished in the pool (Fig. 20-17).

As the patient progresses out of the acute phase, more vigorous exercises may be initiated. Continuation of ambulation training and progression to ambulation without an assistive device are primary considerations for the return to normal activities. Land-based, closed chain exercises such as wall slides, minisquats, step-ups, stair stepping, and leg presses can facilitate functional activities such as stair climbing, rising from a chair, and getting in and out of a car (Fig. 20-18). Balance and coordination exercises such as step-ups, wobble board, single-leg pulleys, and toe raises without support can retrain balance reactions. Any motion loss, impaired muscle performance, pain, or effusion that are related to activity limitations should be addressed concurrently. Traditional progressive resistive exercises can be incorporated, keeping in mind the arthrokinematic issues. Weight machines, free weights, isokinetic devices, pulleys, and body weight

are means to accomplish increases in the ability to produce torque. See Building Block 20-5. The clinician must be aware of the loads placed on the knee ligaments with various

---

◆ **SELF-MANAGEMENT 20-4** *Performing Flexion and Extension Mobility Exercises During the Day*

Purpose:	To increase mobility in the knee
Position:	Sitting or in another position of comfort
Movement Technique:	Actively extend the leg as far as possible and then bend it back as far as possible. You may use your other leg to help lift it the last little bit or to push it back a little farther.

Repetitions: ___ times

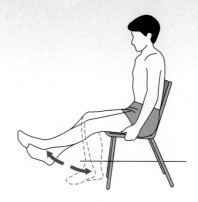

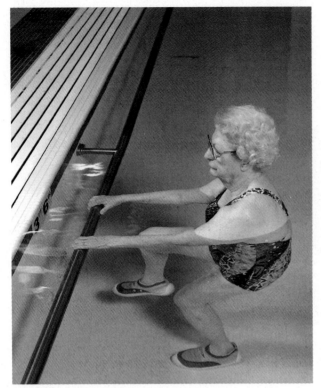

FIGURE 20-17. Single-leg minisquats in the pool are performed to increase mobility and strength.

exercises and use caution to avoid overstressing a healing ligament. For example, resistive hip adduction using a resistive band around the ankle places a significant load on the

MCL, which may be fine in the late stages but too much in the early stages (Fig. 20-19). At home, the use of body weight as resistance in the form of wall slides, squats, lunges, and step-ups is convenient and cost effective (see Patient-Related Instruction 20-2: Performing Weight-Bearing Exercises.

The final phase of rehabilitation helps return the patient to her premorbid level of function in ADLs, work, or recreation. Because the activity level and functional goals are different for each patient, the rehabilitation program must be tailored to individual needs. For the individual returning to sedentary work and recreational walking, discharge to an independent program may be considered after motion, strength, endurance, and impairments and activity limitations have been

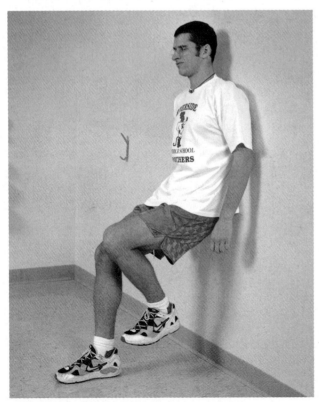

FIGURE 20-18. Single-leg wall slides.

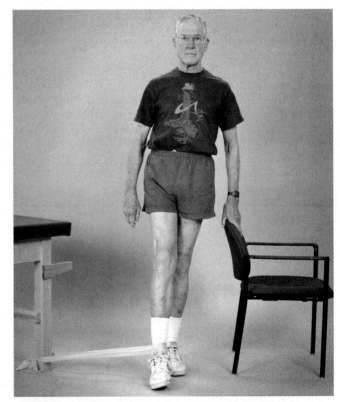

FIGURE 20-19. Resisted hip adduction using a resistive band.

Patient-Related Instruction 20-2

Performing Weight-Bearing Exercises

When performing exercises in weight bearing, the following important points should be reviewed:

1. Place only the amount of weight on your leg as allowed. This may be only part of your body weight.
2. Be sure that your knee is at the correct angle, as directed by your clinician.
3. Avoid hyperextending your knee (bending it backward).
4. Keep your knee in line with your toes and your hips. Avoid letting your knees "roll in" (i.e., being "knock-kneed").
5. Tighten your buttocks muscles together, and use the muscles in the front of your thigh, as directed by your clinician.
6. Hold each exercise for the amount of time specified by your clinician. Be sure to breathe in and out slowly while performing each exercise.

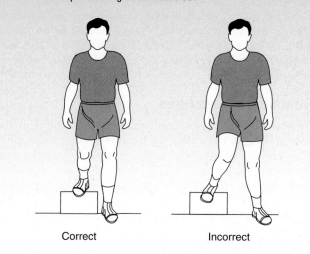

Correct   Incorrect

normalized. The patient should demonstrate a thorough understanding of the home management of impairments, including inflammation, pain, ROM, and strength. For individuals returning to a higher level of physical functioning, such as physical labor or sports activities, reconditioning to that level is necessary. This may require advanced work-related activities such as lifting, pushing, pulling, and carrying objects over uneven surfaces. A functional capacity evaluation may be performed to determine restrictions or precautions affecting a return to work.

Running, cutting, jumping, and sports skill activities can help ensure a safe return to sporting activities (Fig. 20-20). A running program or sport-specific drills may be used to test readiness to return to play. Completion of an appropriate functional progression can ensure a safe return to sports. Although this program does not need to be under the direct supervision of the physical therapist, it should be constructed with and guided by the clinician in conjunction with the patient. Any deficits in movement patterns should have been corrected by the clinician in the earlier therapy stages and should not be an issue at the functional progression stage.

Fractures

Knee fractures can involve the patella, distal femur, or proximal tibia. These fractures generally occur as a result of trauma such as a fall or motor vehicle accident but can also result from osteoporosis.

The rehabilitation issues associated with knee fractures include the effects of the original trauma, surgical procedures, and immobilization. A trauma significant enough to fracture a bone also causes substantial soft tissue damage, which is frequently overlooked. Damage to articular cartilage and fractures extending through the articular cartilage to the joint surface have the potential to affect the long-term health of the joint, and these issues should be considered in the rehabilitation program.

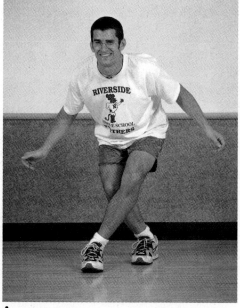
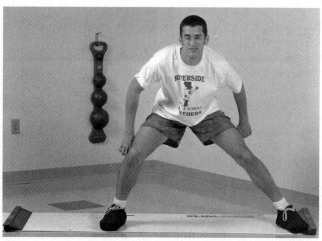

A   **B**

FIGURE 20-20. (A) Lateral crossover running in the late stage of rehabilitation. (B) Slide board lateral movements.

Patellar Fractures

Patellar fractures account for approximately 1% of all skeletal injuries and occur most frequently in persons between the ages of 40 and 50 years.[46] Falls account for the greatest percentage of patellar fractures, followed by motor vehicle accidents. Fractures can occur as a result of a forceful quadriceps contraction. Traumatic fractures usually produce comminuted fractures, while forceful quadriceps contraction cause transverse fractures. However, the degree of knee flexion, the patient's age, presence of osteoporosis, and the velocity of injury can affect the type and location of fracture.[46]

Treatment of patellar fractures can be conservative with immobilization and rehabilitation, or surgical, such as open reduction with internal fixation (ORIF) or partial patellectomy. Because of the morbidity associated with immobilization, ORIF is often the treatment of choice for medically sound candidates. A transverse fracture is distracted by quadriceps activation and is best treated by fixation. Tension cerclage wiring is frequently used, particularly for comminuted and transverse fractures. Because of the superficial nature of the patella, the hardware is frequently removed after healing is ensured. Occasionally, a small fragment or fragments are removed rather than fixated (i.e., partial patellectomy). The prognosis after patellar fracture is good if patellofemoral pain, muscular atrophy, and loss of motion are addressed. These impairments occur regardless of treatment method. With conservative management, the clinician must also be aware of the effects of immobilization on the soft tissues.

Distal Femur Fractures

Distal femur fractures are the consequence of trauma in most cases, although spiral fractures may occur in the elderly as the result of a twisting injury. Associated fractures are common and include the patella, tibial plateau, foot, ankle, and hip. Distal femur fractures can be classified as pure supracondylar, supracondylar and intercondylar, or monocondylar, each with subclassifications.[46] Fractures through the growth plate occur in children and adolescents and are classified as Salter types I through V.[47]

Treatment of distal femur fractures is categorized as conservative or surgical. Nondisplaced, minimally displaced, stable, or impacted fractures or fractures in individuals who are not surgical candidates may be treated with immobilization. Because of the morbidity associated with lengthy immobilization, surgical ORIF is the treatment of choice in most cases. Reduction of distal femur fractures requires restoration of the anatomic alignment and mechanical axes in the sagittal, frontal, and transverse planes. The specific surgical procedure and fixation choice depend on factors such as the type and location of fracture, quality of bone, associated injuries, and the patient's age and lifestyle. Complications after ORIF include deep vein thrombosis, infection, and delayed union or nonunion.

Tibial Plateau Fractures

Tibial plateau fractures occur almost exclusively as the result of trauma such as motor vehicle accidents, pedestrians hit by cars, accidental falls, or twists or direct blows to the knee. Fractures are produced by a varus, valgus, or compressive force, resulting in lateral plateau, medial plateau, or bicondylar fractures. Tibial plateau fractures are classified morphologically[46]:

1. Split fracture, in which the margin of the tibial plateau is separated from the rest of the plateau
2. Compression fracture, in which the subchondral bone is crushed but the margins are spared
3. Combination split-compression fracture

Compression fractures are the most difficult to diagnose, because the depressed fragments are often missed on standard radiographs. These fractures also are the most difficult to treat, because adequate reduction requires the elevation and stabilization of depressed fragments. Compression fractures are seen most commonly after falls from heights and in elderly individuals with osteoporosis.

Treatment of tibial plateau fractures depends on the location and type of fracture. Compression fractures with depressed fragments require surgical elevation and stabilization of the fragments. These fragments usually are supported with bone grafts, and split fractures are stabilized with screws, wires, or plates and lag screws. Conservative management with or without traction and immobilization is an option that must be considered in light of the deleterious effects of immobilization. Postoperative or postimmobilization rehabilitation depends on the numerous factors outlined previously.

Treatment of Fractures

Treatment programs for individuals with fractures at the knee may begin early after the fracture or after healing has taken place. Persons with fractures surgically fixated generally begin mobility and strengthening exercises soon after the operation (see Self-Managements 20-5: Prone Hang

SELF-MANAGEMENT 20-5 *Prone Hang for Knee Extension*

Purpose:	To increase mobility in knee extension and stretch tight tissues behind the knee
Position:	On your stomach, with your knee just over the edge of the table; a towel under your thigh may be more comfortable.
Movement Technique:	Let your knee straighten by hanging over the table's edge. Your clinician may want you to put weight on your ankle or to use your other leg to increase the stretch. Hold for 1 to 2 minutes.

Repetitions: ___ times

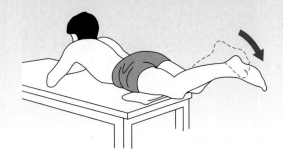

for Knee Extension and 20-6: Straight-Leg Raises). Active and passive ROM for flexion and extension and functional mobility exercises for the entire kinetic chain are initiated early. Quadriceps setting and hamstring setting exercises are started early to retrain these muscle groups. When permitted, closed chain weight-bearing exercises should be initiated, even if only partially weight bearing (see Patient-Related Instruction 20-3: Walking with Crutches. This will be determined by the physician based upon the fracture site and healing, as well as by the patient's ability to control the knee. Before beginning any weight-bearing exercise, the patient should demonstrate a good quadriceps set and the ability to dynamically control the knee. These activities can enhance articular cartilage nutrition throughout the kinetic chain and provide a stimulus for muscle activation. An exercise bicycle with little or no resistance can enhance nutrition and muscle activity in the area while improving mobility.

Pool exercise is excellent for the individual with a knee fracture. Weight bearing may be limited while muscle activation and mobility exercises are performed with assistance from buoyancy. Passive motion assisted by buoyancy or active motion can improve ROM about the knee (Fig. 20-21). Gait can be normalized with or without railing assistance.

Meniscal Injuries

The menisci were originally thought to be useless remains of leg muscles.[48] The importance of the meniscus to the long-term health of the knee has resulted in efforts to preserve the meniscus following injury. The menisci are composed primarily of type I collagen and are more fibrous than articular cartilage. The herringbone arrangement on the surface allows for shear forces that occur with normal joint arthrokinematics; the deeper major fiber orientation is circumferential. The menisci receive their blood supply from the medial and lateral superior and inferior geniculate arteries and have

SELF-MANAGEMENT 20-6 *Straight-Leg Raises*

Purpose:	To increase the strength of the quadriceps and hip flexor muscles and to improve control of the knee
Position:	Lying on your back, with your opposite knee bent and foot flat on the floor; stomach muscles are tightened.
Movement Technique:	This is a four step process.

1. Perform a quadriceps set, tightening the quadriceps muscles.
2. Slowly raise the leg until it is even with the opposite thigh.
3. Slowly lower the leg back to the floor.
4. Relax the quadriceps set. Be sure to relax the quadriceps muscle between each repetition.

Repetitions: ___ times

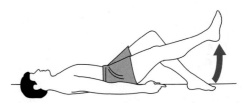

variable vascularity. The vascular supply penetrates 10% to 30% of the width of the medial meniscus and 10% to 25% of the width of the lateral meniscus. The peripheral one third is often called the red zone, the middle one third is the red-white zone, and the central one third is the white (avascular) zone. The meniscus receives its nutrition by diffusion, and it

---

Patient-Related Instruction 20-3

Walking with Crutches

When walking with crutches and some of your weight on the involved knee, several guidelines should be followed:

1. Make sure your weight is on your hands, not under your arms. Your arms should be slightly bent when your crutches fit properly.
2. When walking, place your crutches out first, followed by your involved leg and then your uninvolved leg.
3. Place your involved heel down first, let your knee bend slightly, and allow your foot to roll toward your toes as you begin to bring your uninvolved leg forward.
4. As you bring your uninvolved foot through, bend your involved knee, and pick it up behind you. Straighten the involved knee as you bring it past your crutches to place it on the floor in front of you. Your knee should be straight just before your heel contacts the ground.
5. When using a single crutch, be sure to use it on the side *opposite* your injured knee.

6. Check with your clinician to ensure that your gait with crutches is correct.

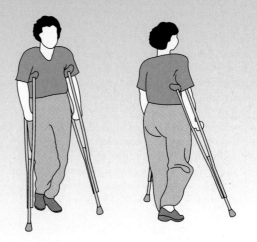

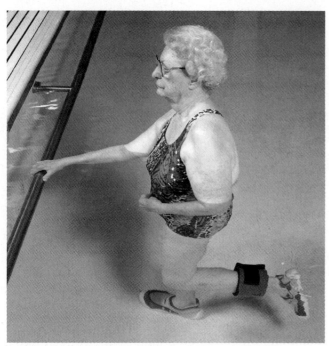

FIGURE 20-21. Buoyancy-assisted knee flexion using a buoyant strap. The return motion (to extension) is buoyancy resisted, eliciting a concentric quadriceps muscle contraction.

has a low metabolic rate and a low reparative response. Repair of the meniscus considers this low reparative response and often uses the peripheral blood supply to assist the healing process.

The menisci have many functions, underscoring the importance of maintaining their structure. In addition to enhancing joint congruity and stability, the menisci also function to transmit load across the knee joint, with approximately 40% to 50% of the compressive load transmitted through the meniscus in full extension and 85% at 90 degrees of flexion.[13,49] Partial meniscectomy with a 10% decrease in contact area increases peak local stresses by 65%, whereas total meniscectomy decreases the contact area by 75% and increases peak local stresses by 235%.[50] Total meniscectomy is no longer routinely performed because of the Fairbanks changes seen postoperatively. These changes include marginal femoral osteophyte ridging, flattening of the medial femoral condyle, and narrowing of the joint space.[51] The menisci also work as shock absorbers, although the subchondral bone is the main static shock absorber at the knee. Some of the most important functions of the menisci are joint lubrication and articular cartilage nutrition. The biphasic properties of the meniscus assist in providing a lubricant film across the joint surface with loading and unloading of the knee.[48]

The meniscus is most often injured traumatically, although degenerative tears are also common. Traumatic tears usually occur in individuals between the ages of 13 and 40 who are involved in physical activities or in those who sustain trauma in a fall or motor vehicle accident. Degenerative tears occur with increasing frequency with advancing age and are often complex tears. A degenerative tear can be precipitated by a specific stress, although it may seem to be minor, such as turning to walk a different direction.

Treatment

Degenerative tears associated with articular cartilage lesions often require surgery to remove loose fragments and to stimulate a healing response in the articular cartilage. Acute traumatic tears may heal without intervention if the tear is longitudinal and peripheral. Some tears may not heal but remain asymptomatic.[52] Tears producing mechanical symptoms such as catching, locking, and effusion are treated by partial meniscectomy or by meniscal repair. The treatment of choice depends on the type and location of the tear and on the associated injuries. For example, a meniscal repair in the posterior horn of the medial meniscus in an ACL-deficient knee does not heal well. However, if the ACL is reconstructed simultaneously, the meniscal repair has an opportunity to heal if provided a blood supply. Complex degenerative tears are nearly impossible to repair and probably will fail in the presence of articular cartilage degeneration.

The interventions chosen for patients with partial meniscectomy correlate with the changes in load distribution and increases in peak local stresses associated with this procedure. The knee has been distributing and dispersing loads during normal activities based on the patient's anatomy for many years. Suddenly, the load distribution is changed, and other structures must shoulder the burden of the load previously carried by the intact meniscus. The joint's ability to adapt to this change in loading pattern depends on many factors, including lower extremity alignment, quadriceps function, comorbidities, and the response to the stresses placed on it (i.e., Wolff law). The body must have time to adapt to the changing loading pattern, and although some individuals adapt quickly, others may develop symptoms of overload such as inflammation, effusion, or pain. Any activity that produces significant shear forces with compressive loading (e.g., squatting, steps) may overwhelm the load-bearing capabilities in some knees. Individuals with suboptimal alignment, degenerative joint disease, poor quadriceps function or neuromuscular control, or limited ROM probably will have the most difficulty.

Issues associated with meniscal repair are related to the normal meniscal motion during knee flexion and extension, the shear forces across the repair, and the location and type of tear repaired. The meniscus moves posteriorly up to 12 mm during knee extension to flexion, with most motion occurring between 0 and 15 degrees and beyond 45 degrees.[16,53] Although motion up to 80 to 90 degrees is permitted in the early phase actively and passively, weight-bearing activities through a large range should be avoided. Early partial weight bearing or weight bearing as tolerated is often permitted depending on the tear size, type, and location. The knee goes through a limited ROM in a weight-bearing position during normal gait. Repairs in the white zone, repairs with additional vascular access, or repairs of complex or radial tears are protected longer, and progression is dictated by the procedure. A sample program for intervention following meniscal repair can be found in Table 20-7.

DEGENERATIVE ARTHRITIS PROBLEMS
Articular Cartilage Lesions

Articular cartilage is a unique tissue that has remarkable properties, including an ability to be deformed and regain

TABLE 20-7	**Rehabilitation Guidelines Following Meniscal Repair**		
	PHASE 1	**PHASE 2**	**PHASE 3**
Goals	1. Post-op knee protection 2. Restore extension ROM 3. Eliminate effusion 4. Restore leg control	1. Single leg stance control 2. Normalize gait 3. Good control and no pain with functional movements, including step up/down, squat, partial lunge at <60 degrees flexion	1. Good control and no pain with sport and work specific movements, including impact
ROM exercises	Knee extension on bolster Prone hangs Supine wall slides to 90 degrees Heel slides to 90 degrees	Stretching for patient specific imbalances	Stretching for patient specific imbalances
Strength exercise	Quad sets SLRs Standing 4 way leg lifts with brace	Non-impact balance and proprioceptive drills Gait drills Hip and core strengthening Quadriceps strengthening: closed chain 0–60 degrees flexion	Strength and control drills related to sport or work movements Sport/work specific balance and proprioceptive drills Hip and core strengthening Movement control exercises beginning with low velocity, single plane progressive to higher velocity, multiplane Impact control exercises beginning 2 feet to 2 feet and progressing to single foot
Cardiovascular exercise	Upper body circuit training or UBE	Non-impact endurance training: Stationary bike	Sport and work specific energy demands
Precautions	1. Gradually wean from 2 to 1 to 0 crutches as long as the knee is in the locked brace and there is no increase in pain or swelling 2. Keep brace locked for all weight-bearing activities for 4 weeks 3. No flexion past 90 degrees	No forced flexion past 60 degrees flexion Avoid post-activity swelling No impact activities	Post-activity soreness should resolve in 24 hours Avoid post-activity swelling Avoid posterior knee pain with flexion
Progression criteria	1. Pain-free gait with locked brace without crutches 2. No effusion 3. Knee flexion to 90 degrees	1. Normal gait on all surfaces 2. Able to carry out functional movements without pain or unloading affected leg 3. Demonstrates good control 4. Single leg balance >15 seconds	Return to work/sport when patient achieves dynamic neuromuscular control with multi-plane activities without pain or swelling

its original shape, exceptional durability, and an unparalleled low-friction surface.[54] These are just a few of the properties that make articular cartilage so difficult to reproduce. Despite the prevalence of artificial joint replacements, the average life of an artificial joint is much shorter than that of native articular cartilage. This comparison highlights the unique characteristics of this material, which functions optimally in the presence of adequate ROM, joint stability, and an equitable load distribution.[48]

Articular cartilage is composed primarily of water, type II collagen, and proteoglycans.[54,55] Water is approximately 60% to 85% of the weight of articular cartilage and is responsible for its biphasic properties.[48,54,55] The water content decreases with age, increasing the stiffness and deformation of cartilage and decreasing its biphasic material properties. This decrease contributes to the changes seen in the normal aging process. Every joint has its own pattern or "footprint" on the surface,

reflecting the specific shear forces across that joint.[48] Articular cartilage in adults receives its nutrition by diffusion, and the cartilage in children receives some nutrition from the underlying subchondral bone.[55]

Articular cartilage responds to loads in a time-dependent manner like any other viscoelastic material; it creeps under a constant applied load and relaxes under a constant deformation. When an external load is applied to the cartilage surface, an instantaneous deformation occurs, and approximately 70% of the water within the cartilage may be moved, until the compressive stress within the articular cartilage matches the applied stress, and equilibrium is reached. Stress and relaxation also occur, depending on the length of time the cartilage is loaded. Cartilage also increases the congruity of the surfaces, distributing loads over a greater surface area.[54] The ability to withstand compressive loads (based on these properties) varies from joint to joint and within the same articular surface.[55]

From a mechanical perspective, the requirements for a healthy joint include freedom of motion, stability, and an equitable load distribution.[48] These necessities form the basis for some of the treatments for articular cartilage lesions. Adequate lower extremity strength to absorb loads during the loading response of the gait cycle, and normal movement patterns help minimize excessive loads on the articular cartilage. Partial-thickness articular cartilage lesions in adults do not heal, but they may not get any worse in a joint with good mobility, stability, and an equitable load distribution. However, in an ACL-deficient knee or a knee with a significant varus alignment, the lesion may progress from partial to full-thickness. When this lesion degrades far enough, bleeding occurs, and the healing process begins. This is the rationale for the microfracture technique, one of the marrow stimulation techniques. The microfracture technique uses an awl to place multiple small holes in the lesion to stimulate a healing response. However, the replacement tissue is fibrocartilage, which is a lesser-quality tissue than the original articular cartilage. The fibrocartilage may be adequate in the presence of adequate motion, joint stability, and equitable load distribution.

The rehabilitation program must consider the fundamental requirements for a healthy joint when determining the appropriate mode and progression of therapeutic exercise. Activities that minimize shearing forces while increasing stability and mobility provide the foundation for the therapeutic exercise program (see Patient-Related Instruction 20-4: Tips to Maintain the Long-Term Health of Your Knee). See Building Block 20-6. Additionally, the therapist must consider the importance of adjacent joints on knee function. Interventions directed toward the hip such as strengthening and mobilization have been shown to improve symptoms at the knee.[56,57]

Surgical Procedures

A variety of surgical procedures are used to improve function in patients with articular cartilage lesions. They can be classified as marrow stimulation techniques, resurfacing procedures, realignment procedures, and arthroplasty. The marrow stimulation techniques use bleeding at the joint surface in an attempt to initiate a healing response. Abrasion arthroplasty, drilling and microfractures are all techniques to stimulate bleeding and initiate healing. These procedures result in the deposition of fibrocartilage, which mechanically does not withstand the test of time. It may provide some temporary relief until the fibrocartilage fails. Resurfacing procedures include techniques such as osteoarticular transplants and autologous chondrocytes implantation. Discussion of these procedures can be found in Chapter 11.

Osteotomy

The high tibial osteotomy or tibial varus osteotomy is performed in cases of unicompartmental osteoarthritis and varus alignment; the supracondylar (femoral) osteotomy is used to treat unicompartmental osteoarthritis and valgus alignment.[58,59] The rationale behind high tibial osteotomy for varus alignment is that the alignment excessively loads the medial tibiofemoral compartment, which promotes osteoarthritis.[60] Conversely, the valgus alignment loads the lateral tibiofemoral compartment, leading to subchondral sclerosis, loss of cartilage space, and osteophyte formation, indicative of osteoarthritis. The tibial osteotomy is generally performed on patients wishing to delay total joint replacement. Despite the short-term success of tibial osteotomy, most results can be expected to deteriorate over time.[61]

The technique of tibial osteotomy includes making a wedge cut in the tibia at least 1.5 cm distal to the joint line. For a varus alignment, the lateral osteotomy is inclined medially and distally, and the tibia is fixated with hardware. A fibular osteotomy is performed as well. The results of this procedure depend on proper patient selection, accurate measurements, and adequate correction. Patients who

---

Patient-Related Instruction 20-4

Tips to Maintain the Long-Term Health of Your Knee

The following tips can help you maintain the long-term health of your knee:

1. Maintain the mobility of your knee. With your clinician's help, choose a couple of simple exercises to be done daily to maintain your ability to fully bend and straighten your knee.
2. Keep the muscles around your knee strong, especially the muscles in the front of your thigh and your hip muscles. With your clinician's help, choose a couple of simple exercises to be done daily to maintain the strength of your leg.
3. Maintain a healthy body weight.
4. Wear good supportive shoes that provide some shock absorption.
5. Use a supportive device (e.g., cane, crutch) when walking long distances.

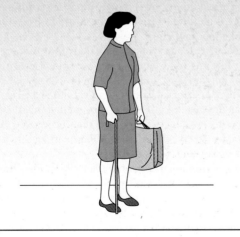

BUILDING BLOCK 20-6

Consider the 78-year-old patient with knee osteoarthritis in Display 20-2, Case Study No. 2. You have determined that the patient's sense of weakness in the knees is due to a combination of weak hip extensor muscles and weak quadriceps muscles. For each muscle group, describe three exercises that would isolate and focus strengthening on that group.

are poor candidates for this procedure include those with tricompartmental degeneration, significant ligamentous laxity, or markedly restricted motion.[62] Correction of varus deformities to at least 5 degrees of valgus produce the best results.[63-65] Two-plateau weight bearing is the ultimate goal, and excessive bone loss, inaccurate measurements, or inadequate correction can interfere with achieving this goal. Patients with preoperative low adduction moment at the knee maintained better clinical results that those with high adduction moment, suggesting that adaptive gait mechanics play a role in outcome.[66] Complications include infection, nonunion, patella baja, infrapatellar scarring, peroneal nerve palsy, and lateral ligament laxity.

Rehabilitation after tibial osteotomy is guided by the requirements for a healthy joint and the sudden change in loading patterns across the joint. The change in weight-bearing distribution may overload a previously underloaded compartment. The bony and soft tissues need adequate time to remodel and adapt to the change. How well the tissues adapt varies significantly from individual to individual, accounting for the variation in intervention choices, treatment frequency, and treatment duration. Restoration of normal ROM is essential to ensure distribution of loads over as large a range as possible. Normalization of movement patterns to minimize impact loads and excessive compartmental loading can prolong the life of the osteotomy. Quadriceps strengthening for shock absorption during the loading response of the gait cycle can minimize loads on the articular cartilage and subchondral bone.

Total Knee Arthroplasty

Individuals with significant bicompartmental (medial and lateral) or tricompartmental (medial, lateral, and anterior) osteoarthritis and associated impairments, activity limitations, and participation restriction are candidates for total knee arthroplasty (TKA). These individuals may have undergone previous osteotomies that subsequently deteriorated and may present with impairments such as pain, joint instability, or loss of motion. Pain is one of the chief indications for TKA; stability, bone integrity, and age are additional considerations. Patients generally seek medical attention when the pain becomes disabling, affecting their ability to participate in community, work, leisure, or basic ADLs. The materials and techniques used in TKA have advanced significantly, thereby increasing the patient pool, minimizing complications, and decreasing participation restriction.

The prostheses used are classified in many ways, including the number of compartments replaced (i.e., unicompartmental, bicompartmental, or tricompartmental), the degree of constraint (i.e., unconstrained, partially constrained, or fully constrained), and the type of fixation (i.e., cemented, cementless, or hybrid). The prosthesis choice depends on the status of the bone and any soft tissue deformities (e.g., ligament laxity, absence of PCL). Most prostheses are tricompartmental and partially constrained with hybrid fixation. Hybrid fixation usually includes a cemented tibial component and cementless femoral component. The design can presume that the PCL is intact (PCL retention) or absent (PCL substitution/posterior stabilized). Other prostheses are used in special cases, and this information should be obtained before initiating treatment.

Each design has its strengths and weaknesses and should be matched to the specific needs of the patient.

Cemented fixation allows for earlier weight bearing than biologic ingrowth, but loosening at the bone-cement interface has been a problem. The uncemented femoral component decreases operative time, reduces polyethylene wear from cement debris and avoids an adverse reaction to the materials, but is more costly and requires a more precise fit. The tibial component is the most problematic in both cemented and uncemented designs, with difficulty achieving fixation resulting in micromotion and failure. Specific design features are incorporated to assist in balancing soft tissues in three planes to avoid instability problems.

Complication of TKA includes loosening, infection, peroneal nerve palsy, patellar instability, fracture, instability and osteolysis. Bone ingrowth is negatively affected by nonsteroidal anti-inflammatory medication and oopherectomy. Other complications include polyethylene wear reactions, with pain, effusion and loss of motion developing about 5 years after surgery. Most complications are on the medial side, and the component may sink into the tibia on the medial side.

Several factors affect the rehabilitation approach after TKA. The type of prosthesis provides an indication of the underlying stability, bone quality, and ultimately the prognosis. Fixation choice also affects rehabilitation, with noncemented components protected longer to allow biologic ingrowth. Patellar instability is a problem in 5% to 30% of TKAs, and the clinician should be alert to signs of patellar subluxation or dislocation.[67] Ligamentous stability, particularly varus and valgus stability should be assessed after TKA. Most prosthetic designs assume that no ACL exists and that the PCL is variably intact. The medial and lateral ligaments and joint capsule provide most of the stability. The overall status of the patient's condition and the lower extremity can affect rehabilitation. Individuals with osteoarthritis at the knee may have concurrent changes in other lower extremity joints. Limitations in ROM at the hip and ankle can affect the function and prognosis at the knee. It is reasonable to attempt knee flexion ROM from 0 to 120 degrees or more. Patients with <120 degrees of flexion after TKA use compensatory movements of the hip, trunk, and ankle during daily activities.[68] See Table 20-8 for a sample rehabilitation program following TKA.

Interventions for Degenerative Arthritis Problems

Interventions used by physical therapists should address the impairments, activity limitations, and participation restrictions identified during the initial and subsequent evaluations. Impairments should be treated if they are associated with an activity limitation or participation restriction or if continued impairment could lead to participation restriction in the future. For example, limited ROM after abrasion arthroplasty may not be immediately disabling, but it could lead to future activity limitations or participation restriction by overloading focal areas of articular cartilage or by damaging other joints because of compensatory movements. Individuals with articular cartilage damage cannot expect to be cured of their problem, but they must learn to manage their symptoms and maintain the long-term health of their joint. Individuals with joint surface damage must demonstrate an understanding of the home management of impairments, including inflammation, pain, and mobility and strength loss.

TABLE 20-8 Rehabilitation Following TKA

	PHASE 1: INPATIENT	PHASE 2: EARLY OUTPATIENT	PHASE 3: MID- TO LATE OUTPATIENT
Goals	Pain control Independent in bed mobility Independent in transfers Stair function Safe use of assistive device ROM 5–90 degrees	Pain and swelling control Independent in mobility, transfers, stairs, and ambulation ROM 0–100 degrees Strength 3/5 to 4/5	Return to previous activities Gait 300 feet without assistive device ROM 0–120 degrees Effective home exercise maintenance program
Mobility	Tibiofemoral joint: AROM, AAROM, PROM into flexion and extension Joint mobilization: patellar mobilization, tibiofemoral distraction and mobilization CPM (continuous passive motion) Heel slides	Patellar mobilization AROM of all LE joints Stretching of major muscle groups Tibiofemoral mobilization	Mobilization as needed Contract-relax, other stretching activities as needed
Muscle performance	Quadriceps, hamstring, gluteal setting Active knee extension Straight leg raises TKE Hip abduction	Resisted knee extension Leg raises in all directions Mini-squats Toe raises Hamstring curls Leg press Isokinetics Lunges	Progressive resistive exercises Lower extremity and core strengthening exercises Activity-specific strengthening
Functional activities	Transfers Bed mobility Assistive device use; ambulation with walker or crutches Stair negotiation	Gait training with or without assistive device Up and down from chair Stair negotiation Balance activities	Work or activity-related activities ADL, IADL activities
Cardiorespiratory	N/A	Bicycle as tolerated Water walking	Per patient preference
Other	Ankle pumps for circulation Ice, compression for pain and swelling	Ice, compression as necessary to control swelling Community mobility	
Progression criteria	Independent in bed mobility Independent in transfers Ability to ambulate 150 feet with standby assistance Ability to negotiate stairs safely	ROM 0–115 degrees Strength 4/5 or 75% of contralateral side Full weight bearing although may still use assistive device Ambulation 300 feet Stairs using alternate pattern	

After surgery, physical therapy interventions are generally aimed at the immediate impairments of pain, effusion, and loss of motion and neuromuscular control. Physical agents, mechanical and electrotherapeutic modalities, and gentle mobility can minimize pain and facilitate resorption of an effusion. Therapeutic exercise in the form of active and passive motion, physiologic stretching, or joint mobilization facilitate normal osteokinematics and arthrokinematics. After the surgical incisions are healed or with the use of a bioclusive dressing, many of these impairments can be treated in the pool. The hydrostatic pressure of the water minimizes effusion, and the water's buoyancy limits weight bearing to a comfortable level. If progressive loading of the joint surface is the goal, gradually decreasing the water's depth can slowly increase the joint load.[69–71] Isometric setting exercises for the quadriceps, hamstrings, and gluteal muscles help reeducate these muscles while facilitating circulation.

In the subacute phase, rehabilitation continues to focus on residual impairments, activity limitations, and participation restrictions identified during reexamination. Ambulation training and progressive weight bearing advance according to the specific injury and therapeutic procedure. The rehabilitation should continue to focus on restoring full mobility, normalizing gait, and reestablishing full function to the individual. Mobility activities should emphasize activities that enhance articular cartilage nutrition, such as gentle active and passive ROM or compressive loading and unloading. Combining these two modes should be approached with caution to avoid overloading developing or remodeling fibrocartilage or articular cartilage. Closed kinetic chain exercises with significant weight bearing through a ROM should be incorporated judiciously (Fig. 20-22). Strengthening exercises must respect the changes in loading patterns after some surgical procedures. Eccentric strengthening of the quadriceps and gluteals facilitates shock absorption during the loading response phase of gait, stair and

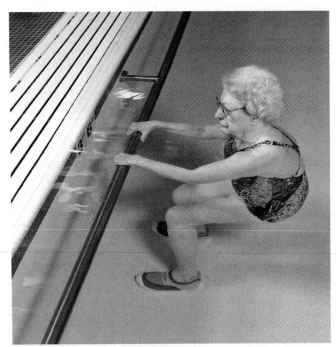

FIGURE 20-22. Squats are performed in the pool to increase flexion and ROM with minimal weight bearing.

incline descent, and lowering into a chair. Strengthening can be initiated in an open kinetic chain and progressed to a closed kinetic chain as the joint allows. Similar exercises must be performed on a daily basis as part of the home exercise program to continue the advances made in the clinic.

The final rehabilitation phase emphasizes return to the previous activity level or higher. For the individual undergoing a tibial osteotomy the expectation is return to a higher level of function because of a decrease in pain. Each person should be provided with a functional retraining program tailored to the activities to which she will be returning. Moreover, the importance of continuing an exercise program incorporating activities to maintain the long-term health of the joint must be emphasized. Demonstration of the ability to home manage an exacerbation of symptoms is fundamental to safe and cost-effective long-term management of articular cartilage lesions. Patient education to manage lifestyle factors such as walking distances, floor surfaces, time spent standing, maintenance of appropriate body weight, shoewear, and use of assistive devices is also a critical intervention.

TENDINOPATHIES

Tendinopathies about the knee occur most frequently in the patellar tendon but can also be found in the hamstring tendons and pes anserine tendon. ITB friction syndrome can be considered a type of tendinopathy. Although tendinopathies can result from an acute injury, they usually are caused by microtrauma or overuse. Repetitive loading without adequate recovery time prevents the normal adaptations to occur. Although single loads do not exceed the strength of the tendon, the cumulative loads exceed the reparative capabilities. Intrinsic factors contributing to tendinopathies include malalignment, limb length discrepancies, and muscular imbalance or insufficiency. Aging tissue has a lower reparative

capability, diminishing it ability to recover from overuse. Extrinsic factors include training errors, surfaces, environmental conditions, and footwear.[72]

Patellar Tendinopathy

Patellar tendinopathy occurs at the distal pole of the patella, and is distinct from Sinding-Larsen-Johanssen disease, which is apophysitis of the distal patellar pole, and from Osgood-Schlatter disease, which is apophysitis at the tibial tubercle. Both of these syndromes occur in adolescents before closure of the growth plates. Patellar tendinopathy has also been called *jumper's knee* because of its high prevalence in jumping and impact sports. The eccentric nature of jumping places tremendous loads on the patellar tendon, often resulting in overuse. The patellar tendon attaches one of the strongest muscle groups in the body, the quadriceps femoris, to its insertion using the patella as a "balance." The loads generated by the quadriceps mechanism are transmitted through the tendon to its bony attachments. Areas of increased stress such as transitional zones are susceptible to overuse. In the adult with closed epiphyses, the transition zone on the undersurface of the patella's distal pole is the most vulnerable area.

Tendinopathies of the patellar tendon can take various forms. Tendinopathies tend to demonstrate a normal macroscopic appearance, but microscopic abnormalities at the bone-tendon junction most always exist.[73] Necrosis and fragmented tissues with mucoid degeneration usually involve the deep central fibers at the tendinous insertion and can be palpated at the undersurface of the patella's distal pole.[74]

Individuals with patellar tendinopathies present with various degrees of impairments, activity limitations, and participation restrictions. The person often reports a history of pain and stiffness in the anterior knee that improves as the knee is warmed, gets sore as the activity continues, and gets stiff and sore after completion of the activity. Point tenderness is experienced on the undersurface of the distal pole of the patella and is best palpated by tipping the inferior border anteriorly to allow access to the undersurface. Activity limitations may include abnormal walking or running gait, pain with jumping or kneeling, or pain when ascending and descending stairs. Participation restrictions can include an inability to participate in community, work, or leisure activities, depending on the individual's lifestyle and activity limitations. Blazina et al.[75] categorized patellar tendinitis in athletes in four stages, based on the pain history (Display 20-4). Poor postural habit, such

DISPLAY 20-4
The Blazina Classification for Activity limitations Associated with Patellar Tendinitis

Stage 1: Pain after sports activity

Stage 2: Pain at the beginning of sports activity, disappearing with warm-up, and sometimes reappearing with fatigue

Stage 3: Pain at rest and during activity; inability to participate in sports

Stage 4: Rupture of the patellar tendon

Blazina ME, Kerlan RK, Jobe FW. Jumper's knee. Orthop Clin North Am 1973;4: 665–678.

as standing with the knees hyperextended, can contribute to patellar tendinitis because of a shortening of the quadriceps and patellar tendon.

Treatment

Rehabilitation for the individual with patellar tendinopathies focuses on the patellar tendon's role in decelerating knee flexion in gait, jumping, descending stairs, and many other functional activities. The role of tendon length and speed relative to deceleration activities forms the foundation for the rehabilitation program. Stretching exercises to ensure adequate tendon length are combined with eccentric quadriceps contractions of progressively increasing velocity up to the speeds used in daily activities. Before an individual can perform an eccentric muscle contraction, she must be able to preset isometric tension in the muscle. The rehabilitation program may begin with isometric contractions before progressing to eccentric contractions. Eccentric contractions can be performed in an open or a closed chain, recognizing that substitution may occur in a closed chain exercise. However, this may provide enough assistance to the injured tendon to allow pain-free exercise performance. A vigorous eccentric program is recommended prior to any surgical intervention.[76] Eccentric squats performed on a decline board (a board declined approximately 25 degrees) have been shown to be effective in treating patients with patellar tendinopathy.[76-78] In most research, patients performed exercises with external resistance on a decline board for 3 sets of 15 repetitions twice daily for up to 12 weeks. It has been suggested that the eccentric exercise results in decreased neovascularization at the tendon and resultant decreases in pain and improvements in function.[79] To create an optimal healing environment, adjuncts to the therapeutic exercise program are used and typically include forms of cryotherapy. The long-term prognosis for this problem in male athletes is only fair. A 15-year prospective study found that 53% of these athletes had quit sports because of this problem.[80]

Iliotibial Band Syndrome

Iliotibial band syndrome (ITBS) is the most common cause of lateral knee pain in individuals who regularly jog, bicycle, or walk for exercise.[81,82] Postural problems such as anterior pelvic tilt or knee hyperextension along with poor mechanics such as decreased gluteus medius or VMO activity can be predisposing factors. Biomechanical analysis of patients with ITBS showed greater hip adduction and knee internal rotation compared with those without symptoms.[81,82] Increases in these motions causes increased ITB strain at the lateral femoral condyle. It has been suggested that the *rate* of strain is more important than the *magnitude* of the strain.[83] While ITBS has traditionally been considered to be the result of friction over a bursa as the band passes anterior and posteriorly over the lateral femoral condyle, biomechanical and anatomical studies suggest that few people actually have a bursa in this area.[84,85] Moreover, it has been suggested that the band does not move across the epicondyle, but that the appearance of movement is the result of tensioning of the anterior and posterior bands of the ITB.[84]

The individual presenting with ITBS often complains of a sharp, stabbing pain at the lateral epicondyle that begins with the onset of activity and worsens as the activity progresses. Palpable tenderness over the lateral epicondyle can confirm the diagnosis. Predisposing factors such as poor postural habit or muscle imbalance should be identified during the examination. Hamstring, gluteal, quadriceps, and ITB flexibility and strength should be assessed. Any impairments or activity limitations identified during the examination should form the basis for the rehabilitation program. In many cases, a combination of predisposing factors, activity choices, and impairments converge to produce ITBS.

Treatment

Rehabilitation focuses on the identification and treatment of predisposing factors, impairments, and activity limitations. Patient education regarding these factors and conscientious participation in self-managing this problem contribute to a successful outcome. Postural education and identification of the underlying impairments (e.g., hip rotator weakness) provide the foundation for appropriate stretching or strengthening exercises. Stretching for the hip and knee musculature with emphasis on good posture is the mainstay of treatment. These stretches may be performed on land or in the pool (see Figs. 20-7 through 20-10). Ice may be used to treat pain and inflammation associated with this problem. Self-mobilization or massage is commonly used to decrease the pain associated with ITB symptoms. Foam rollers or other firm materials can be rolled along the ITB to self-massage this tissue.

Patellofemoral Pain Syndrome

The typical patient with patellofemoral pain syndrome (PFPS) is a young female who complains of pain in the anterior aspect of the knee.[25] The pain is aggravated by knee extension activities such as ascending or descending stairs, squatting, rising from a chair, or jumping. A wide variety of interventions for PFPS have gained widespread acceptance in the clinical community, including general and specific hip and knee strengthening using both open and closed kinetic chain exercises, providing surface EMG biofeedback, stretching, acupuncture, low level laser, patellar mobilization, corrective foot orthoses, patellar taping, and external patellar bracing.[86,87] Unfortunately, experimental evidence to support the use of many of these approaches is lacking, and conventional clinical practice often flies in the face of what little evidence does exist. An understanding of what is known about the efficacy of various interventions, and, where the research lags behind clinical practice, a thorough understanding of the etiology of the condition should guide the intelligent choice of management strategies for the patient with PFPS.

Cause: Etiology

The causes of PFPS can range from subluxation and dislocation to patellar malalignment. Frank dislocation resulting from a blow to the knee is simple to determine through history. Recurrent subluxation is suggested when the patient reports that her knee gives way with a sharp pain, usually when the knee is partially flexed in weight bearing. Rates of patellofemoral dislocations are highest during adolescence.[88] Patients with acute traumatic patellar instability will experience chronic instability or PF pain. Age at initial dislocation, anatomical abnormalities, and activity level may predispose a patient to a poor outcome.[89] This should be associated with radiographic evidence of a shallow intercondylar groove, hypermobility of the patella, and tenderness of both the patellar borders and femoral condyles. Patella alta increases the risk for patellar instability. Other causes of knee buckling (e.g., ligament tears) should be ruled out.

It is important not to overlook overuse as a causative factor. Not all patients with PFP demonstrate lateral subluxation or tracking.[90] This suggests other reasons must exist, and one should look for an increase in usage patterns associated with the onset of the anterior knee pain. Again, the patient's history will provide the clues, with repetitive work or recreational activities that stress the knee being key factors, such as an increase in running distance, an increase in workload demands, or a change in shoe wear.

It is generally accepted that PFPS results from a cascade of events. Poor alignment of the patella in the trochlear groove, typically with the patella tracking laterally, results in poor distribution of the patellofemoral joint reaction forces (PFJRF) on the posterior aspect of the patella.[91] The PFJRF is the amount of pressure on the joint surfaces of the patellofemoral joint, and is a function of the flexion angle of the knee and the amount of tension developed by the quadriceps muscle. As the knee flexes and as the quadriceps become more active, the PFJRFs increase. Under normal circumstances the pressure is distributed to both the medial and lateral facets, and with near end-range flexion, to the odd facet. When the patella tracks poorly, the PFJRFs will be concentrated into a smaller contact area, resulting in increased shear on the articular surfaces, leading to tissue breakdown, pain, and impaired function.[87,92,93] There is some evidence that runners who develop PFP have an increased impact shock during heel strike and during the propulsion phase than runners without PFP.[94] These authors also reported no association between excessively pro-needed or soup donated foot posture in the development of PFP.

The possible causes of patellar malalignment are generally separated into two basic categories. The first includes problems with the static structures such as the shape of the osseous surfaces or length of the fascia. The second category of patellar malalignment etiology includes issues related to the dynamic structures about the knee. In particular, there has been much discussion about the role of the vastus medialis longus (VML), vastus medialis obliquus (VMO), and the VL muscles' function in the development of PFPS. The thought is that an imbalance in the amount of pull or the timing of the contraction of these muscles will either cause or allow the patella to track laterally in the trochlear groove and produce a concentration of force to the retropatellar surface. In addition, poor alignment of the knee due to hip, foot or ankle dysfunction can cause a change in the angle of pull of these muscles and lead to altered patellar tracking. As the discussion that follows suggests, there is a lack of consensus in the research literature with regard to the etiology of PFPS, although the search continues. In the meantime, clinical experience and outcome studies demonstrate the effectiveness of conservative treatment for this disorder, although the relative effectiveness of any individual intervention has yet to be shown.

The Role of Static Structures

Messier et al.[95] reported that Q-angle appears to discriminate between runners with and without PFP. The Q-angle is formed by a line drawn from the anterior superior iliac spine to the middle of the patella, and from the middle of the patella to the tibial tuberosity. A greater Q-angle is thought to be associated with increased lateral forces on the patella and therefore associated with lateral patellar tracking. Increased genu valgus, internal rotation of the femur relative to the tibia, and a wide pelvis (as seen on average in women) all increase the Q-angle. While the latter cannot be changed, hip rotation and genu valgus can both be influenced by hip, foot and ankle mechanics. This underscores the need for the whole lower kinetic chain to be evaluated in the patient with PFPS.

Powers[96] found a difference in the depth of the trochlear groove between young women with and without PFP. Subjects with a shallower trochlear groove had a laterally tilted patella in terminal extension (30 to 0 degrees) and a laterally displaced patella in the last 9 degrees of extension. The patients with PFP had a greater degree of lateral patellar tilt than did the asymptomatic control subjects. This suggests that at terminal extension the osseous structures that prevent lateral tilt and displacement may be less than adequate. Herrington[97] found a significant difference in the lateral position of the patella in individuals with PFP compared to a control group using a highly reliable measurement method. In this method tape is placed over the patient's knee and the medial and lateral femoral epicondyles are marked. The distance from the medial and lateral epicondylar marks are measured. The lateral distance is subtracted from the medial distance, with a positive value indicating a lateral position of the patella and a negative value a medial position.

The effect of tibiofemoral rotation alignment and patellar alignment on patellofemoral joint contact area in individuals with and without PFP was studied using magnetic resonance imaging with the knee in full extension and the quadriceps contracted. In the PFP group, the patellar width and tibiofemoral rotation angle explained 46% of the variance in the contact area, whereas in the pain-free subjects patellar width was the only predictor of contact area. This suggests that tibiofemoral rotation may be one of the factors leading to a decrease in contact area in the patellofemoral joint, which then leads to anterior knee pain.[98]

There have been suggestions that controlling over-pronation at the foot would help alleviate PFPS by positively affecting the Q-angle. Pronation of the foot causes internal rotation of the tibia, which if carried into late midstance and terminal stance when the knee is extended will cause internal rotation of the hip as well. This shifts the patella medially relative to the ASIS and theoretically increases the lateral forces on the patella. One study suggests that foot motion is not associated with PFPS,[95] however there is evidence that foot orthoses can reduce PFPS symptoms.[86] Clearly more work needs to be done to discover the underlying mechanism of this relief.

The Role of Dynamic Structures

There is a school of thought which suggests that an imbalance between the VMO, pulling the patella medially, and the VL, pulling the patella laterally, in terms of timing or magnitude of contraction, was at least partly responsible for the onset of PFP.[99] Early studies suggested that painful joint distension could inhibit quadriceps function in the knee.[21,100] Other studies suggested a difference in reflex response times in patients with PFPS,[25,101] but their methods have been called into question.[102] There appeared to be support for a neural explanation for PFPS by some studies on patients with PFPS,[103–106] one of which had methodological problems in that the EMG was not normalized.[104] Other research has found no differences between symptomatic and asymptomatic subjects in either amount of VMO:VL EMG activity[107,108] or the timing of the onset of the two heads of the quadriceps[57,108,109] or in the reflex response times of the VMO relative to the VL.[102,109] Whether or not there is reduced timing or intensity of the VMO relative to the VL in patients with PFPS, it is not known if altered patellofemoral joint mechanics results. Early evidence suggests an *increase* in VML muscle EMG is associated with greater lateral patellar displacement and tilt.[110]

While the controversy about VMO/VL ratios and function continues, what seems to be clear is that improving quadriceps strength and endurance is an integral part of any rehabilitation program for PFPS. Poor knee extensor muscle endurance as measured by isokinetic dynamometry discriminates between symptomatic and asymptomatic runners.[95] Significant correlations have been found between measures of cross-sectional areas of the VMO muscle and the amount of patellar tilt at 0 and 30 degrees of flexion. This was most apparent in a subgroup of patients with extreme patellar tilt and lateral shift malalignments.[44]

Differential Diagnoses

It is important to differentiate patellofemoral pain from other disorders of the knee. Generally, PFPS will manifest in the anterior aspect of the knee as a diffuse ache, with the pain aggravated with activity such as ascending or descending stairs. Other pathologies, however, will also cause anterior knee pain and so general questions about the location of the pain will not be helpful in making the differential diagnosis. In addition, one or more disorders can coexist, further complicating the picture. Other causes of anterior knee pain include: irritation of the infrapatellar fat pad, patellar tendinopathy, Osgood-Schlatter disease, pes anserine bursitis or chondromalacia.

Patients with patellofemoral pain may complain of the knee locking and giving way. Giving way can be confused with cruciate ligament injury, and symptoms of locking can be confused with meniscal injuries. This type of complaint warrants further investigation during the physical examination.

Examination

History   Questions to the patient should explore whether the etiology appears to be due to trauma, congenital structural problems, or overuse. Questions regarding painful patellar movements (subluxations), limp, pain, running, climbing stairs, and prolonged sitting with the knees flexed may help differentiate between asymptomatic women, and subjects with anterior knee pain, patellar subluxation, and patellar dislocation.[30–33] Particular attention should be paid to determining what activities reproduce the patient's pain, as these motions can be used to monitor the patient's progress and the efficacy of an applied intervention.

Posture   An assessment of the patient's static alignment will provide clues as to the presence of abnormal mechanical stress being placed on the knee, which might be remediated with therapeutic exercise. Alignment problems may be caused by structural deformities (e.g., femoral anteversion

causing a toe-in stance), habitual usage patterns (e.g., tending to stand on one leg versus the other), impaired motor control or performance (e.g., weak hip abductors allowing hip abduction during stair descent), or ROM limitations (e.g., lack of hip external rotation).

Asymmetry or excessive lateral weight shift when assuming a single limb stance posture may signal weakness of the hip abductors or lack of hip control. This will result in a relative hip adduction on the stance limb, again biasing the knee toward an increase in Q-angle, an increase in the lateral forces acting on the patella and lateral patellar tracking. In addition, over time the hip adductors may become shortened.

Resisted Tests   As mentioned previously, habitual usage patterns and postural deviations can result in changes in the normal length-strength relationships of the muscles. It is important to perform a careful assessment of muscle function in the entire lower kinetic chain. Particular attention should be paid to the interactions of the pelvis, hip, foot, and ankle. A useful assessment of function that incorporates the entire lower extremity is the step down task. In performing this task the patient should maintain the knee aligned over the second toe. The hip should remain in the same alignment as during double limb stance, with allowance made for slight weight shift over the weight-bearing leg as the non–weight-bearing leg is lifted. Excessive lateral shift suggests hip weakness, particularly in the abductors and extensors. A drop of the non–weight-bearing pelvis occurring concurrently with the weight shift should increase suspicion of abductor weakness. If the knee moves medially over the foot during the step-down, besides hip abductor and extensor weakness one can suspect hip external rotation weakness. Suspicion can also be place on poor muscular control of foot pronation, particularly the posterior tibialis and gastrocnemius/soleus complex. This movement pattern will result in relative hip adduction and increase the lateral pull on the patella. When this pattern of movement is observed assessment of muscle strength (manual muscle testing at minimum) in these muscles is mandatory. The results of the strength tests will guide the choice of exercises.

Intervention

An appropriate management plan for PFPS should be based on the evaluation of all the collected data, which is distilled into a diagnosis. Issues related to impairments of body structures are not appropriate for physical therapy intervention. Habitual movement patterns can be corrected with movement reeducation. ROM impairments and motor deficits can be addressed through strengthening, stretching and manual interventions. Once pain has been reduced and as ROM impairments are being addressed, rehabilitation of the extensor mechanism and control of proper lower extremity alignment are the foundation of managing PFPS.

VMO Misconceptions   Much has been made about the imbalance between the VL and the vastus medialis obliquus (VMO) as a causative factor in PFPS. The VMO was first described as a separate functional component of the VM by Lieb and Perry[111] based on the orientation of the muscle fibers at their attachment to the patella. They concluded that the VMO was primarily responsible for stabilizing the patella medially. This led to the theory that poor VMO function would result in lateral tracking of the patella and cause

PFPS.[99] It followed that training the VMO and improving its function would be an important component of any intervention strategy aimed at decreasing the lateral tracking of the patella. Despite multiple investigations there does not seem to be a consensus about whether there is reduced VMO activity in patients with PFPS.[87,103–105,107–110,112–116] The discrepancy between study results may be due to the fact that the relative timing between the portions of the quadriceps muscles may be task specific.[117]

A common mistake made when interpreting EMG data is the misconception that a difference in EMG activity between two muscles, even when both are normalized, signifies a difference in muscle action on the joint. Unfortunately this misconception has led to the common clinical practice of using surface EMG biofeedback to "train" the patient to recruit the VMO to a greater degree than the VL.[118,119] The problem with this approach is fundamental: there is no way to assess VMO force production in vivo, and using EMG activity to reflect patellar stability is fraught with problems. EMG is a measure of the electrical activity of the muscle and not the amount of force or tension the muscle can produce. Physiologic and biomechanical factors, such as muscle cross sectional area and the orientation of the muscle's fibers relative to the joint motion, determine the effect the muscle has on the joint. In addition, in order to compare the activity of two different muscles the EMG signals must be normalized, or stated as a percent of the signal generated by a maximal contraction.

Another problem with designing intervention programs to improve VMO function is the assumption that training can improve VMO/VL timing. In addition, certain exercises are purported to selectively target and strengthen the VMO and thereby improve the VMO/VL strength ratio. These include exercises such as isometric quadriceps contractions, straight leg raises, and short arc quad exercises either alone or combined with resisted hip adduction and/or internal tibial rotation. As noted above, surface EMG is often used for biofeedback to assist in the process. The basis for choosing these exercises is the thought that the VMO is primarily responsible for terminal knee extension, or that the VMO has as part of it's origin a slip from the adductor magnus, or that internal tibial rotation improves the Q-angle and therefore the pull of the VMO. Isolated contraction of the VMO separate from the rest of the heads of the quadriceps, however, has never been demonstrated.[87] In the absence of selective recruitment of the VMO, it is unlikely that the VMO can be strengthened without the VL and indeed the rest of the quadriceps also being strengthened. A recent study supports this hypothesis, reporting improved torque and decreased pain regardless of whether or not EMG visual feedback was used.[120] If timing differences do exist, then at least one study showed that these differences disappear after exercises that focused on strengthening the quadriceps and hip abductors, without specific training for the VMO.[121] Indeed, studies which purport to change the timing onset of the VMO to the VL include training programs that exercise the entire quadriceps, making it difficult to ascribe the timing improvements to the techniques aimed at specifically changing the timing (e.g., EMG feedback).[114,122]

The amount of time, effort and attention paid to training the VMO is made further interesting in light of convincing evidence that general quadriceps strengthening results in positive outcomes, as discussed below.[123]

Evidence for PFP Interventions   There are many studies on the biomechanics of the syndrome, suggesting that the underlying assumption driving intervention choice is that by altering abnormal biomechanics one can improve the condition. However, there are relatively few studies of the direct clinical benefit of any particular management approach.[86,87,93,123] None of the studies are randomized controlled clinical trials and few investigate the efficacy of any single conservative intervention.

It is important to address the symptoms experienced during knee extension. Pain will inhibit muscle recruitment and therefore interfere with any attempt at muscle strengthening. The one single intervention that consistently appears to be of benefit is the use of patellar taping to reduce anterior knee pain during provocative activities such as ascending or descending stairs. Several studies have shown that patellar taping decreases the pain.[109,124–128] Successful application of patellar tape can provide immediate relief of symptoms experienced with performing the provocative activity. It is thought that patellar tape improves patella alignment, quadriceps function, and knee function in gait.[127–133] While the exact mechanism of the pain relief is unknown, it appears that taping alters neither the amplitude nor the timing of the vasti muscles.[129,131] In general, the tape is applied to the patella in a lateral to medial direction, pulling the patella medially with the idea that lateral patellar tracking is diminished.[125] It may be that the direction of the tape application does not matter, however: neutral, medial, and lateral glide taping techniques all decrease pain over non-taped conditions.[127] With improved tracking, the PFJRFs are more evenly distributed on the posterior surface of the patella. While the precise mechanism is not well understood, functional measures improve after the application of patellar tape.[108,129,133,134]

Bracing helped improve alignment of the patella as measured by kinematic MRI while the knee was under load.[135] Unfortunately, no attempt was made in this study to assess the effect of the brace on the subjects' symptoms, so the association between improved patellar alignment and positive outcomes was not clarified. There is some evidence that the use of a dynamic patellofemoral brace may prevent anterior knee pain in persons undergoing a strenuous training program.[136] Patellofemoral braces may be effective in reducing pain and increasing patellofemoral contact area.[137–140] While there is no evidence that supports the use of knee orthoses in all patients, it may be that a trial use of an orthosis will benefit certain patients.

A second goal of the rehabilitation process is improving static and dynamic alignment of the entire lower extremity. The presence of structural deformities may be addressed using compensatory measures. For example, over-pronation of the foot may be addressed using foot orthotics. However, the efficacy of this intervention as a primary method of treating PFPS has not yet been shown.[126] More recently, foot orthoses have been shown to be better than flat inserts in the short term, but they do not improve outcomes when added to typical physical therapy interventions.[141]

Other than structural deformities, the main impairments associated with poor alignment are limitations in the ROM, and motor function, which encompasses both strength and control. Patients with PFPS demonstrate significantly less flexibility of the gastrocnemius, soleus, quadriceps, and

TABLE 20-9 Stretching Exercises to Address Hip Soft Tissue Mobility Impairments		
IMPAIRMENT—LACK OF:	**PATIENT POSITION**	**KEY POINTS**
Hip extension	Half-kneel Supine, leg off table Sidelying Prone	• Stabilize pelvis to isolate femoral-pelvic movement
Hip flexion	Supine straight leg raise Knee extension with hip maintained in flexion	• Stabilize pelvis to isolate femoral-pelvic movement
Hip adduction	Half-kneel	• Maximize stretch to tensor fascia latae, minimize lateral trunk stretch
Hip external rotation	Half-knee on a chair	• Stabilize pelvis
Knee flexion with hip extended	Half-kneel Sidelying Prone	• Stabilize pelvis to isolate femoral-pelvic movement
Ankle dorsiflexion	Standing	• Prevent foot pronation to isolate ankle dorsiflexion • Address both gastrocnemius and soleus

hamstrings compared to healthy control subjects.[142] ROM limitations can be generally categorized as either being due to joint mobility restrictions or to soft tissue shortness. Appropriate joint mobilization techniques should be used to improve hip, tibiofemoral, patellofemoral, tibiofibular (both inferior and superior), talocrural, intercarpal, and metatarsal-phalangeal joint motion, as indicated by examination findings (see Chapter 7). Soft tissue restrictions can be addressed using soft tissue mobilization techniques that address specific areas of hypomobility, through longitudinal stretching either done manually by the therapist or done by the patient independently, or both. Hold-relax techniques work well in improving overall length of muscle. With regard to PFPS, key areas that need to be addressed include improving hip adduction (indicated by a positive Ober test), hip extension (Thomas test), external hip rotation, knee flexion with the hip extended (Thomas test), and ankle dorsiflexion (see Table 20-9). There is evidence that a 3-week program of quadriceps stretching improves flexibility, pain, and knee function.[143] Poor ankle dorsiflexion can lead to compensatory pronation at the subtalar joint, which causes internal rotation of the tibia. As noted earlier, this may adversely affect patellar alignment. ITB stretching has been advocated as part of an overall intervention program, with positive outcomes reported.[144] Based on the structure, tissue makeup and tensile properties of the ITB, it is unlikely that a stretching or soft tissue mobilization program will significantly lengthen it. It is more probable that length is gained in the proximal attachments of the ITB, likely the tensor fascia lata.

A simple active hamstring and gastrocnemius exercise that can be performed in sitting is appropriate and convenient for most patients. In a sitting position, the patient should support the low back with a firm hand support to maintain the lumbar lordosis. She slowly extends the lower leg while maintaining this lumbar lordosis. At the end of the comfortable ROM, she dorsiflexes the foot and holds for 15 to 30 seconds. This exercise can be performed frequently throughout the day (see Self-Management 20-7: Hamstring and Gastrocnemius Stretching While Maintaining a Lumbar Neutral Position).

Once pain has been addressed, the cornerstone of management of PFPS is improving strength and control of the lower extremity.[142,145–148] Interventions aimed at improving limited

ROM can proceed concurrently. Although emphasizing VMO recruitment currently has little evidence to support it, even should one choose this form of intervention the extensor mechanism will be positively affected and thus positive outcomes will be achieved. General quadriceps strengthening exercises are effective in treating the condition.[123]

SELF-MANAGEMENT 20-7 *Hamstring and Gastrocnemius Stretching While Maintaining a Lumbar Neutral Position*

Purpose:	To increase the flexibility of the hamstring and calf muscles
Position:	In a sitting position, place one hand behind your back to maintain the proper position of your lower back.
Movement Technique:	Maintaining this position, slowly straighten the knee until you feel a gentle stretch behind your thigh. While holding this position, pull your toes up, flexing your ankle until you feel a gentle stretch behind your calf. Hold for 15 to 30 seconds.

Repetitions: ____ times

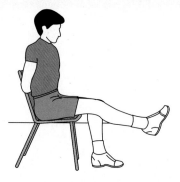

All resistance exercises should be performed in the pain-free ROM. It may be that only isometric exercise is tolerated in a highly irritated condition. If this is the case, multi-angle isometrics should be employed. There is no reason to emphasize terminal knee extension over exercise in greater amounts of flexion. Avoidance of patellofemoral joint compression forces can be counter-productive, considering that cartilage nutrition is dependent in large part on weight bearing. The guiding principle should be dispersing the PFJRF by increasing the patellofemoral contact area by improving patellar tracking. As the patient progresses to closed chain exercises, examples of controlling the ROM include altering the depth of squat, height of the step (step ups or downs), or height of the chair (stand to sit exercise).

A review of the available literature showed strong evidence that both open and kinetic chain exercises are at least equally effective exercise in reducing pain and improving function.[149] In one study, there appeared to be only a slight advantage to using only closed kinetic chain exercises over using only open kinetic chain exercises, but both modes result in improved function and decreased pain up to 3 months after concluding the exercise program.[150] In another study comparing leg press to open chain knee extension to no treatment, both types of exercise significantly decreased their pain and improved muscle strength and function.[151] Since all intervention should be directed at improving activityl limitations and participation restrictions, given the principle of specificity of exercise closed chain exercises may be a better choice for certain patients.

Performing all exercises with excellent lower extremity and trunk alignment is essential to addressing the dynamic mal-alignment issues. For example, step-down exercises are important, as stairs are a problem for most individuals with patellofemoral pain. In performing a step-down exercise the patient should maintain the knee aligned over the second toe.

Exercise difficulty should be adjusted to allow motion through the total target ROM while the alignment remains good. This may affect the choice of open versus closed chain exercise. For example, many individuals with PFPS have poor eccentric control during stair descent and drop off the step, catching their body weight with the uninvolved leg. When asked to control the step-down motion, many are unable to do so because of pain or inadequate muscle control. In this case, the step-down exercise is too demanding of the patient and is not yet indicated, because the patient cannot maintain optimal alignment. Open chain strengthening of the specific muscles may prove beneficial at this point, as specific muscles can be targeted for strengthening and the appropriate amount of resistance applied. In addition, taking into consideration the functional task required, emphasizing eccentric exercises would begin the training necessary for control of lowering the body weight during the step down task. For example, sidelying hip abduction with weight applied to the knee or ankle will selectively strengthen the primary movers. Eccentric contractions can be accomplished by assisting in the concentric lifting of the leg. One way to accomplish this is to simply have the patient flex the knee while raising the leg (shortening the lever arm and therefore decreasing the resistance to the abductors), and extending the knee during lowering (increasing the resistance during the eccentric phase of the movement). Alternatively, it may be that closed chain exercises can be performed using appropriate equipment, such as a leg press or inclined squat machine. These machines and others like them allow the amount of resistance to be adjusted to proper levels, as opposed to full weight-bearing exercises that demand control of body weight. Should open chain exercises be used at first, a progression toward closed chain exercises may improve the functional outcome.

The speed of the movement is an important exercise variable to consider. As the patient's control of the movement improves at slower speeds, the speed of movement should be increased to approximate normal function. Good alignment and form are still paramount goals regardless of the speed of movement. The individual should move slowly enough to be able to stop at any point during the motion to correct malalignment. Close observation can detect poor alignment of the hip, knee, and ankle or substitution at the hip (Fig. 20-23). For example, Willson et al.[152] reported that during a single leg hopping activity, women with patellofemoral

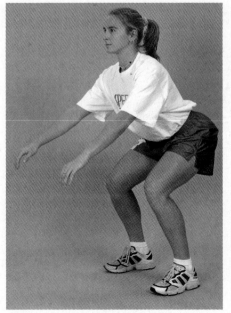 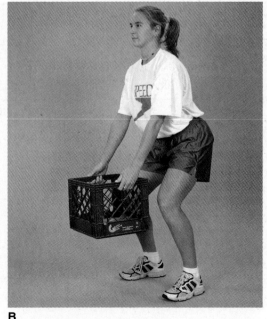

A   **B**

FIGURE 20-23. (A) Patient performing a squat exercise. (B) Progressing to a lifting exercise.

pain demonstrated increased hip abduction angle, flexion angle, abduction angular impulse, and decreased hip internal rotation angles as compared to a healthy control group. The use of bracing or taping may offer increased control during activities such as an eccentric step descent.[153] The foot position can also influence the lower extremity alignment and should be observed during the exercise program. Foot muscle training requires the individual to improve the alignment of the foot in relation to the leg and subtalar joint. This approach includes educating and training the individual to recognize a position close to the neutral position of the foot for all standing activities. As the individual lifts the arch, it is important to observe for and discourage anterior tibialis substitution. The tibialis posterior should lift the subtalar joint while the peroneus longus stabilizes the first ray. Pressing down (plantar flexing) through the first metatarsal head is often a beneficial cue to facilitate correct alignment and appropriate muscle recruitment. Recruitment of the foot intrinsic muscles to maintain a shortened arch should be encouraged.

Postoperative Rehabilitation

The three common types of surgical procedures for the patellofemoral joint are chondroplasties for debridement of patellar or femoral chondral degeneration, lateral retinacular release for the severely restricted lateral retinaculum, and realignment procedures for those with more complicated biomechanical problems. Surgery for PFP may become less common, as recent work suggests outcomes are no better than exercise alone.[154] Rehabilitation after any of these procedures should follow the program as previously outlined. With simple chondroplasties, the program should progress without problems unless significant pain or swelling exists. If more progressive chondral damage has occurred, more caution should be placed on gradual and careful reintroduction of activity and exercise to allow the accommodation of the chondral surfaces. With lateral retinacular releases, care should be taken to ensure the lateral retinaculum does not adhere to surrounding soft tissues. Aggressive releases must be progressed much more slowly than conservative releases, because postoperative pain and large amounts of edema are common. The time for recovery and the length of rehabilitation may also be prolonged as a result of aggressive surgery.

Prognosis

The prognosis for PFPS is generally good.[155] In one study, a regimented program of quadriceps, hamstrings and "ITB" stretching, 15 minutes of quadriceps electrical stimulation, isometric quadriceps setting, progressive straight leg raises and short arc quad exercises, ice after treatment, and Non-steroidal anti-inflammatory medication (NSAIDs) improved symptoms immediately after the physical therapy program in 87% of the patients studied.[156] Two-thirds thought their symptoms remained improved an average of 16 months after completion. The program consisted of treatment sessions three times per week for four to six weeks and progressed to resistance of 0.5 to 5.0 kg, increasing from 0 to 20 repetitions to three sets of ten repetitions. Unfortunately, there was no control group to compare with the intervention subjects, and there is no way to tell the efficacy of the individual interventions applied.

When only closed kinetic chain exercises are employed, the duration of symptoms and the reflex response time of the VMO are the only predictive factors of a positive outcome. The shorter the duration of symptoms or the faster the response of the VMO, the better the outcome was.[157] Otherwise, there is strong evidence that open and closed kinetic chain exercises are equally effective.[149]

KEY POINTS

- The relationships among the lumbopelvic, hip, knee, ankle, and foot necessitate a thorough examination and an integrated approach to treatment. This includes hip and core muscle strengthening for distal problems.
- Impairments of body structures, including femoral anteversion, coax valgum and varum, genu valgum and genu

▼ LAB ACTIVITIES

1. Demonstrate the likely gait pattern if your quadriceps strength was 3/5.
2. Demonstrate three strengthening exercises to treat quadriceps strength impairment, given a strength grade of 3/5.
3. Demonstrate two exercises to treat the activity limitations seen in the gait pattern.
4. Is an assistive device necessary? If so, what would you choose for this patient if she had no other impairments? Fit and instruct the patient in use of the device.
5. Demonstrate the likely gait pattern if the patient's quadriceps strength was 2/5.
6. Demonstrate three strengthening exercises to treat the quadriceps strength impairment, given a strength grade of 2/5.
7. Refer to Case Study No. 2 in Unit 7. Instruct your patient in the first phase of the exercise program. Have your patient demonstrate all exercises.

8. Create five exercises for a patient with subacute patellar tendonitis.
9. Determine your patient's 10 repetition maximum for a straight-leg raise with the weight.
   a. At the ankle
   b. Above the knee
10. Teach your patient how to check VMO firing during the following activities:
    a. Isometric quadriceps contraction while
       i. Sitting with the knee at 90 degrees
       ii. Sitting with the knee at 70 degrees
       iii. Sitting with the knee at 45 degrees
       iv. Sitting with the knee at 30 degrees
       vi. Sitting with the knee at 0 degrees
    b. Wall slide
    c. Sit to stand
    d. Lunge
    e. Gait

varum, a shallow trochlear groove, and foot pronation can predispose the patellofemoral joint to poor tracking and therefore to excessive loads.

- Impairments of body functions such as mobility or muscle performance loss at the hip, ankle, or foot can be manifested as symptoms in the anterior knee.
- Because of these compensations and the relationships among joints, therapeutic exercises may be performed incorrectly, allowing substitution to occur.
- Examination of the patellofemoral joint must include muscle length and joint mobility at the hip, knee, and ankle, and assessment of patellar position and motion relative to medial and lateral glide and patella alta.
- Examination of key functional movements such as stairs or a step down task will reveal lower kinetic chain strength and control impairments, in the form of poor alignment and performance.
- Improvements, within the entire lower kinetic chain, in impaired joint and soft tissue mobility, muscle performance and motor control, and general quadriceps strengthening result in positive outcomes with PFPS.
- The existence of problems with the timing of onset or the magnitude of VMO EMG signal remains controversial but appears to be non-existent. In any case no evidence exists to support specific recruitment of the VMO separate from the rest of the quadriceps. Attempts to do so probably serve to improve overall quadriceps function.
- The major impairments of body structures at the knee are genu valgum and genu varum. These postures predispose the lateral and medial compartments, respectively, to excessive loads.
- Impairments of body functions such as mobility loss at the knee can be compensated by motion at other joints. For example, increased ankle, hip, or lumbar motion can compensate for decreased knee flexion.
- Palpation, education, and biofeedback are techniques to ensure proper muscle firing patterns without substitution during rehabilitative exercises.
- Loss of the meniscus can lead to degenerative joint disease. Treatment after meniscectomy should focus on preservation of articular cartilage and joint protection techniques.
- The major function of the quadriceps muscle in the long-term health of the knee is its ability to absorb shock eccentrically in the loading phase of the gait cycle. A focus on eccentric, closed chain quadriceps exercise in the first 0 to 15 degrees of flexion is essential to maintain the health of articular cartilage.
- Patellar tendinitis results from the tendon's inability to withstand eccentric forces during impact activities. The rehabilitation program must eventually progress to eccentric impact activities if the patient is to return to this type of activity.

CRITICAL THINKING QUESTIONS

1. Read Case Study No. 6 in Unit 7.
   a. List the patient's impairments and activity limitations.
   b. Describe the relationship between this patient's impairments and activity limitations.
   c. Describe the relationship between this patient's impairments, activity limitations, and any participation restriction.
   d. Identify and prioritize short- and long-term goals.
   e. Choose a specific goal, and describe five different exercises used to achieve that goal. Include posture, mode, and movement.
   f. This patient is returning to work as a delivery truck driver. Describe three functional exercises that can prepare him for this activity.
   g. Presume that this same patient is returning to work as a basketball referee. Describe three functional exercises that can prepare him for this activity.
2. Read Case Study No. 3 in Unit 7.
   a. Describe three exercises to address her difficulty with stairs. Include posture, mode, movement, and precautions.
   b. Given her history, describe three exercises to increase the endurance of her quadriceps muscles. Include posture, mode, movement, and precautions.
   c. Describe three exercises to increase the endurance of her calf muscles. Include posture, mode, movement, and precautions.
   d. The patient no longer feels any muscle fatigue when performing the exercises outlined in questions b and c. Describe how you would progress each of these exercises. Include dosage parameters.

REFERENCES

1. Beynnon BD, Fleming BC, Johnson RJ, et al. Anterior cruciate ligament strain behavior during rehabilitation exercises in vivo. Am J Sports Med 1995;23:24.
2. Yack HJ. Comparison of closed and open kinetic chain exercise in the ACL-deficient knee. Am J Sports Med 1993;21:49.
3. Yack HJ. Anterior tibial translation during progressive loading of the ACL-deficient knee during weight bearing and non-weight-bearing exercise. J Orthop Sports Phys Ther 1994;20:247.
4. Parker MG. Biomechanical and histological concepts in the rehabilitation of patients with anterior cruciate ligament reconstructions. J Orthop Sports Phys Ther 1994;20:44–50.
5. Ciccotti MG, Kerlan RK, Perry J, et al. An electromyographic analysis of the knee during functional activities: the normal profile. Am J Sports Med 1994;22:645–650.
6. Moore KL. Clinically Oriented Anatomy. Baltimore, MD: Williams & Wilkins, 1980.
7. Pratt NE. Clinical Musculoskeletal Anatomy. Philadelphia, PA: JB Lippincott, 1991.
8. Norkin CC, Levangie PK. Joint Structure and Function: A Comprehensive Analysis. 2nd Ed. Philadelphia, PA: FA Davis, 1992.
9. Insall JN. Anatomy of the knee. In: Insall JN, ed. Surgery of the Knee. New York, NY: Churchill Livingstone, 1984:1–20.
10. Williams PL, Warwick R, Dyson M, et al., eds. Gray's Anatomy. 37th Ed. New York, NY: Churchill Livingstone, 1989.
11. Fulkerson J, Hungerford D. Disorders of the Patellofemoral Joint. 2nd Ed. Baltimore, MD: Williams & Wilkins, 1990.
12. Dye SF. Patellofemoral anatomy. In: Fox JM, Del Pizzo W, eds. The Patellofemoral Joint. New York, NY: McGraw-Hill, 1993:1–13.
13. Fu F, Thompson WO. Biomechanics and kinematics of meniscus. In: Finerman GAM, Noyes FR, eds. Biology and Biomechanics of the Traumatized Synovial Joint: The Knee as Model. Rosemont, IL: American Academy of Orthopaedic Surgeons, 1992:153–184.
14. Kendall FP, McCreary EK, Provance PG. Muscles Testing and Function. 4th Ed. Baltimore, MD: Williams & Wilkins, 1993.
15. Torzilli PA. Biomechanical analysis of knee stability. In: Nicholas JA, Hershman EB, eds. The Lower Extremity and Spine in Sportsmedicine. St. Louis, MO: CV Mosby, 1986:728–764.
16. Peterson L, Frankel VH. Biomechanics of the knee in athletes. In: Nicholas JA, Hershman EB, eds. The Lower Extremity and Spine in Sportsmedicine. St. Louis, MO: CV Mosby, 1986:695–727.
17. Hungerford DS, Barry M. Biomechanics of the patellofemoral joint. Clin Orthop 1979;144:11.
18. Reilly DT, Martens M. Experimental analysis of the quadriceps muscle force for various activities. Acta Orthop Scand 1972;43:126–137.

19. Voight ML, Weider DL. Comparative reflex response times of vastus medialis obliquus and vastus lateralis in normal subjects with extensor mechanism dysfunction. Am J Sports Med 1991;19:131–137.
20. Mariani P, Caruso I. An electromyographic investigation of subluxation of the patella. J Bone Joint Surg 1979;61:169–171.
21. Spencer JD, Hayes KC, Alexander IJ. Knee joint effusion and quadriceps reflex inhibition in man. Arch Phys Med Rehabil 1984;65:171–177.
22. Magee D. Orthopedic Physical Assessment. 3rd Ed. Philadelphia, PA: WB Saunders, 1997.
23. Hutchinson MR, Ireland ML. Knee injuries in female athletes. Sports Med 1995;19:222–236.
24. Karst G, Willett G. Onset timing of electromyographic activity in the vastus medialis oblique and vastus lateralis muscle in subjects with and without patellofemoral pain syndrome. Phys Ther 1995;75:813–823.
25. Witvrouw E, Sneyers C, Lysens R, et al. Reflex response times of vastus medialis oblique and vastus lateralis in normal subjects and in subjects with patellofemoral pain syndrome. J Orthop Sports Phys Ther 1996;24:160–165.
26. Sherry MA, Best TA. A comparison of two rehabilitation programs in the treatment of acute hamstring strains. J Orthop Sports Phys Ther 2004;34(3):116–125.
27. Georgoulis AD, Papadonikolakis A, Papageorgiou CD, et al. Three-dimensional tibiofemoral kinematics of the anterior cruciate ligament-deficient and reconstructed knee during walking. Am J Sports Med 2003;31(1):75–79.
28. Freedman KB, D'Amato MJ, Nedeff DD, et al. Arthroscopic anterior cruciate ligament reconstruction: a metaanalysis comparing patellar tendon and hamstring tendon autografts. Am J Sports Med 2003;31(1):2–11.
29. Daniel DM, Stone ML, Dobson BE, et al. Fate of the ACL-injured patient: a prospective outcome study. Am J Sports Med 1995;23(3):632–644.
30. Renstrom P, Ljungqvist A, Arendt E, et al. Non-contact ACL injuries in female athletes: an International Olympic Committee current concepts statement. Br J Sports Med 2008;42(6):394–412.
31. Hewett TE, Myer GD, Ford KR. Reducing knee and anterior cruciate ligament injuries in female athletes: a systematic review of neuromuscular training interventions. J Knee Surg 2005;18(1):82–88.
32. Gilchrist J, Mandelbaum BR, Melancon H, et al. A randomized controlled trial to prevent noncontact anterior cruciate ligament injury in female soccer players. Am J Sports Med 2008;36(8):1476–1483.
33. Silvers HJ, Mandelbaum BR. Prevention of anterior cruciate ligament injury in the female athlete. Br J Sports Med 2007;41(Suppl 1):i52–i59.
34. Hewett TE, Stroupe AL, Nance TA, et al. Plyometric training in female athletes: decreased impact forces and increased hamstring torques. Am J Sprots Med 1996;24:765–773.
35. Hewett TE, Lindenfeld TN, Riccobene JV, et al. The effect of neuromuscular training on the incidence of knee injury in female athletes. Am J Sports Med 1999;27:699–705.
36. Amundson FM. The effectiveness of a prevent injury enhance performance program on improving the neuromuscular performance of 14 to 18 year old high school female basketball players. Doctoral Dissertation, Rocky Mountain University of Health Professions, Provo, UT, 2003.
37. Galloway MT, Grood ED. Posterior cruciate ligament insufficiency and reconstruction. In: Finerman GAM, Noyes FR, eds. Biology and Biomechanics of the Traumatized Synovial Joint: The Knee as Model. Rosemont, IL: American Academy of Orthopaedic Surgeons, 1992:531–550.
38. Butler DL, Noyes FR, Grood ES. Ligamentous restraints to anterior-posterior drawer in the human knee: a biomechanical study. J Bone Joint Surg Am 1980;62:259–270.
39. Fukubayashi T, Torzilli PA, Sherman MF, et al. An in vitro biomechanical evaluation of anterior-posterior motion of the knee: tibial displacement, rotation, and torque. J Bone Joint Surg Am 1982;64:258–264.
40. Clancy WG, Shelbourne KD, Zoellner GB, et al. Treatment of knee joint instability secondary to rupture of the posterior cruciate ligament: report of a new procedure. J Bone Joint Surg Am 1983;65:310–322.
41. Zarins B, Boyle J. Knee ligament injuries. In: Nicholas JA, Hershman EB, eds. The Lower Extremity and Spine in Sportsmedicine. St. Louis, MO: CV Mosby, 1986:929–982.
42. Fetto JF, Marshall JL. Medial collateral ligament injuries of the knee: a rationale for treatment. Clin Orthop 1978;132:206–218.
43. Woo SL-Y, Newton PO, MacKenna DA, et al. A comparative evaluation of the mechanical properties of the rabbit medial collateral and anterior cruciate ligaments. J Biomech 1992;25:377–386.
44. Woo SL-Y, Inoue M, McGurk-Burleson E, et al. Treatment of the medial collateral ligament injury: II. Structure and function of canine knees in response to differing treatment regimens. Am J Sports Med 1987;15:22–29.
45. Woo SL-Y, Ohland KJ, McMahon PJ. Biology, healing and repair of ligaments. In: Finerman GAM, Noyes FR, eds. Biology and Biomechanics of the Traumatized Synovial Joint: The Knee as Model. Rosemont, IL: American Academy of Orthopaedic Surgeons, 1992:241–274.
46. Aglietti P, Chambat P. Fractures of the knee. In: Insall JN, ed. Surgery of the Knee. New York, NY: Churchill Livingstone, 1984:395–412.
47. Salter RB. Textbook of Disorders and Injuries of the Musculoskeletal System. 2nd Ed. Baltimore, MD: Williams & Wilkins, 1983.
48. Arnoczky S, Adams M, DeHaven K, et al. Meniscus. In: Woo SL-Y, Buckwalter JA, eds. Injury and Repair of the Musculoskeletal Soft Tissues. Park Ridge, IL: American Academy of Orthopaedic Surgeons, 1988:487–537.
49. Ahmed AM, Burke DL. In vitro measurement of static pressure distribution in synovial joints: part I. Tibial surface of the knee. J Biomech Eng 1983;105:216–225.
50. Baratz ME, Fu FH, Mengato R. Meniscal tears: the effect of meniscectomy and of repair on intraarticular contact areas and stress in the human knee. Am J Sports Med 1986;14:270–275.
51. Fairbank TJ. Knee joint changes after meniscectomy. J Bone Joint Surg Br 1948;30:664–670.
52. Fitzgibbons RE, Shelbourne KD. "Aggressive" nontreatment of lateral meniscal tears seen during anterior cruciate ligament reconstruction. Am J Sports Med 1995;23:156–165.
53. DeHaven KE, Arnoczky SP. Meniscal repair. In: Finerman GAM, Noyes FR, eds. Biology and Biomechanics of the Traumatized Synovial Joint: The Knee as Model. Rosemont, IL: American Academy of Orthopaedic Surgeons, 1992:185–202.
54. Buckwalter J, Hunziker E, Rosenberg L, et al. Articular cartilage: composition and structure. In: Woo SL-Y, Buckwalter JA, eds. Injury and Repair of the Musculoskeletal Soft Tissues. Park Ridge, IL: American Academy of Orthopaedic Surgeons, 1988:405–426.
55. Mow V, Rosenwasser M. Articular cartilage: biomechanics. In: Woo SL-Y, Buckwalter JA, eds. Injury and Repair of the Musculoskeletal Soft Tissues. Park Ridge, IL: American Academy of Orthopaedic Surgeons, 1988:427–463.
56. Currier LL, Froehlich PH, Carow SC, et al. Development of a clinical prediction rule to identify patients with knee pain and clinical evidence of knee osteoarthritis who demonstrate favorable short-term response to hip mobilization. Phys Ther 2007;87(10):1106–1119.
57. Cliborne AV, Wainner RS, Rhon DI, et al. Clinical hip test and a functional squat test in patients with knee osteoarthritis: reliability, prevalence of positive test findings, and short-term response to hip mobilization. J Orthop Sports Phys Ther 2004;34(11):676–685.
58. Coventry MB. Proximal tibial varus osteotomy for osteoarthritis of the lateral compartment of the knee. J Bone Joint Surg Am 1987;69:32–38.
59. Coventry MB. Proximal tibial osteotomy. Orthop Rev 1988;17:456–458.
60. Noyes FR, Barber SD, Simon R. High tibial osteotomy and ligament reconstruction in varus angulated, anterior cruciate ligament-deficient knees. Am J Sports Med 1993;21:2–12.
61. Hernigou P, Medeviell D, Deberyre J, et al. Proximal tibial osteotomy for osteoarthritis with varus deformity. J Bone Joint Surg Am 1987;69:332–354.
62. Kettelkamp DB, Leach RE, Nasca R. Pitfalls of proximal tibial osteotomy. Clin Orthop 1975;106:232–241.
63. Kettelkamp DB, Wenger DR, Chao EYS, et al. Results of proximal tibial osteotomy. J Bone Joint Surg Am 1976;58:952–960.
64. Keene JS, Dyreby JR. High tibial osteotomy in the treatment of osteoarthritis of the knee. J Bone Joint Surg Am 1983;65:36–42.
65. Insall JN, Joseph DM, Msika C. High tibial osteotomy for varus gonarthrosis. J Bone Joint Surg Am 1984;66:1040–1047.
66. Wang JW, Kuo KN, Andriacchi TP, et al. The influence of walking mechanics and time on the results of proximal tibial osteotomy. J Bone Joint Surg Am 1990;72:905–909.
67. Menkow RL, Soudry M, Insall JN. Patella dislocation following knee replacement. J Bone Joint Surg Am 1985;67:1321–1327.
68. Keays S, Mason M. The benefit of increased range of motion following total knee replacement. Platform presentation at the 12th International Congress of the World Confederation for Physical Therapy; June 25–30, 1995; Washington, DC.
69. Wang TJ, Belza B, Elaine Thompson F, et al. Effects of aquatic exercise on flexibility, strength and aerobic fitness in adults with osteoarthritis of the hip or knee. J Adv Nurs 2007;57(2):141–152.
70. Hinman RS, Heywood SE, Day AR. Aquatic physical therapy for hip and knee osteoarthritis; results of a single-blind randomized controlled trial. Phys Ther 2007;87(1):32–43.
71. Bartels EM, Lund H, Hagen KB, et al. Aquatic exercise for the treatment of knee and hip osteoarthritis. Cochrane Database Syst Rev 2007 Oct 17(4):CD005523.
72. Jarvinen M. Epidemiology of tendon injuries in sports. Clin Sports Med 1992;11:493–504.
73. Puddu G, Cipolla M, Cerullo G, et al. Non-osseous lesions. In: Fox JM, Del Pizzo W, eds. The Patellofemoral Joint. New York, NY: McGraw-Hill, 1993:177–192.
74. Leadbetter WB. Cell-matrix response in tendon injury. Clin Sports Med 1992;11:533–578.
75. Blazina ME, Kerlan RK, Jobe FW. Jumper's knee. Orthop Clin North Am 1973;4:665–678.
76. Bahr R, Fossan B, Loken S, et al. Surgical treatment compared with eccentric training for patellar tendinopathy (jumper's knee). A randomized, controlled trial. J Bone Joint Surg Am 2006;88(8):1689–1698.
77. Johsson P, Alfredson H. Superior results with eccentric compared to concentric quadriceps training in patients with jumper's knee: a prospective randomized study. Br J Sports Med 2005;39(11):847–850.
78. Young MA, Cook JL, Purdham CR, et al. Eccentric decline squat protocol offers a superior results at 12 months compared with traditional eccentric protocol for patella tendinopathy in volleyball players. Br J Sports Med 2005;39:102–105.

79. Ohberg L, Alfredson H. Effects on neovascularisation are behind the good results with eccentric training in chronic mid-portion Achilles tendinosis? Knee Surg Sports Traumatol Arthrosc 2004;12:465–470.

80. Kettunen JA, Kvist M, Alanen E, et al. Long-term prognosis for jumper's knee in male athletes: a prospective follow-up study. Am J Sports Med 2002;30(5):689–692.

81. Miller RH, Lowry JL, Meardon SA, et al. Lower extremity mechanics of iliotibial band syndrome during an exhaustive run. Gait Posture 2007;26(3):407–413.

82. Noehren B, Davis I, Hamill J. ASB clinical biomechanics award winner 2006 prospective study of the biomechanical factors associated with iliotibial band syndrome. Clin Biomech 2007;22(9):951–956.

83. Hamill J, Miller R, Noehren B, et al. A prospective study of iliotibial band strain in runners. Clin Biomech 2008;23(8):1018–1025.

84. Fairclough J, Hayashi K, Toumi H, et al. The functional anatomy of the iliotibial band during flexion and extension of the knee: implications for understanding iliotibial band syndrome. J Anat 2006;208(3):309–316.

85. Fairclough J, Hayashi K, Toumi H, et al. Is iliotibial band syndrome really a friction syndrome? J Sci Med Sport 2007;10(2):74–76.

86. Crossley K, Bennel K, Green S, et al. A systematic review of physical interventions for patellofemoral pain syndrome. Clin J Sports Med 2001;11(2):103–110.

87. Powers CM. Rehabilitation of patellofemoral joint disorders: a critical review. J Orthop Sports Phys Ther 1998;28(5):345–354.

88. Hinton RY, Sharma KM. Acute and recurrent patellar instability in the young athlete. Orthop Clin N Am 2003;34:385–396.

89. Beasely LS, Vidal AF. Traumatic patellar dislocation in children and adolescents: treatment update and literature review. Curr Opin Pediatr 2004;16:29–36.

90. Shellock FG, Mink JH, Deutsch AL, et al. Kinematic MRimaging of the patellofemoral joint: comparison of passive positioning and active movement techniques. Radiology 1992;184:574–577.

91. Kramer P. Patellar malignment syndrome; rationale to reduce excessive lateral pressure. J Orthop Sports Phys Ther 1986;8(6):301–309.

92. Fulkerson JP, Shea KP. Mechanical basis for patellofemoral pain and cartilage breakdown. In: Ewing JW, ed. Articular Cartilage and Knee Joint Function: Basic Science And Arthroscopy. New York, NY: Raven Press, 1990:93–101.

93. Papagelopoulos PJ, Sim FH. Patellofemoral pain syndrome: diagnosis and management. Orthopedics 1997;20(2):148–157; quiz 158–149.

94. Thijs Y, De Clercq D, Roosen P, et al. Gait-related intrinsic risk factors for patellofemoral pain in novice recreational runners. Br J Sports Med 2008;42(6):466–471.

95. Messier SP, Davis SE, Curl WW, et al. Etiologic factors associated with patellofemoral pain in runners [published erratum appears in Med Sci Sports Exerc 1991 Nov;23(11):1233]. Med Sci Sports Exerc 1991;23(9):1008–1015.

96. Powers CM. Patellar kinematics, part II: the influence of the depth of the trochlear groove in subjects with and without patellofemoral pain. Phys Ther 2000;80(10):965–973.

97. Herrington L. The difference in a clinical measure of patella lateral position between individuals with patellofemoral pain and matched controls. J Orthop Sports Phys Ther 2008;38(2):59–62.

98. Salsich GB, Perman WH. Patellofemoral joint contact area is influenced by tibiofemoral rotation alignment in individuals who have patellofemoral pain. J Orthop Sports Phys Ther 2007;37(9):521–528.

99. McConnell J. The management of chondromalacia patellae: a long term solution. J Aust Physiother 1986;32(4):215–222.

100. de Andrade JR, Grant C, Dixon AS. Joint distention and reflex muscle inhibition in the knee. J Bone Joint Surg 1965;47A:313–323.

101. Voight ML, Weider DL. Comparative reflex response times of vastus obliquis and vastus lateralis in normal subjects and subjects with extensor mechanism dysfunction. An electromyographic study. Am J Sports Med 1991;19:131–137.

102. Karst GM, Willett GM. Reflex response times of vastus medialis oblique and vastus lateralis in normal subjects and in subjects with patellofemoral pain [comment]. J Orthop Sports Phys Ther 1997;26(2):108–110.

103. Boucher JP, King MA, Lefebvre R, et al. Quadriceps femoris muscle activity in patellofemoral pain syndrome. Am J Sports Med 1992;20(5):527–532.

104. Souza DR, Gross MT. Comparison of vastus medialis obliquus: vastus lateralis muscle integrated electromyographic ratios between healthy subjects and patients with patellofemoral pain. Phys Ther 1991;71:310–316.

105. Gilleard W, McConnell J, Parsons D. The effect of patellar taping on the onset of vastus medialis obliquus and vastus lateralis muscle activity in persons with patellofemoral pain. Phys Ther 1998;78(1):25–32.

106. Hanten WP, Schulthies S. Exercise effect on electromyographic activity of the vastus medialis oblique and vastus lateralis muscles. Phys Ther 1990;70:561–565.

107. MacIntyre DL, Robertson DG. Quadriceps muscle activity in women runners with and without patellofemoral pain syndrome. Arch Phys Med Rehabil 1992;73(1):10–14.

108. Powers CM, Landel RF, Perry J. Timing and intensity of vasti muscle activity during functional activities in subjects with and without patellofemoral pain. Phys Ther 1996;76(9):946–955.

109. Karst GM, Willett GM. Onset timing of electromyographic activity in the vastus medialis oblique and vastus lateralis muscles in subjects with and without patellofemoral pain syndrome. Phys Ther 1995;75(9):813–823.

110. Powers CM. Patellar kinematics, part I: the influence of vastus muscle activity in subjects with and without patellofemoral pain. Phys Ther 2000;80(10):956–964.

111. Lieb FJ, Perry J. Quadriceps function: an anatomical and mechanical study using amputated limbs. J Bone Joint Surg Am 1968;50:1535–1548.

112. McClinton S, Donatell G, Weir J, et al. Influence of step height on quadriceps onset timing and activation during stair ascent in individuals with patellofemoral pain syndrome. J Orthop Sports Phys Ther 2007;37(5):239–244.

113. Stensdotter A-K, Hodges P, Ohberg F, et al. Quadriceps EMG in open and closed kinetic chain tasks in women with patellofemoral pain. J Mot Behav 2007;39(3):194–202.

114. Cowan SM, Bennell KL, Crossley KM, et al. Physical therapy alters recruitment of the vasti in patellofemoral pain syndrome. Med Sci Sports Exerc 2002;34(12):1879–1885.

115. Cowan SM, Bennell KL, Hodges PW. Therapeutic patellar taping changes the timing of vasti muscle activation in people with patellofemoral pain syndrome. Clin J Sport Med 2002;12(6):339–347.

116. Cowan SM, Bennell KL, Hodges PW, et al. Delayed onset of electromyographic activity of vastus medialis obliquus relative to vastus lateralis in subjects with patellofemoral pain syndrome. Arch Phys Med Rehabil 2001;82(2):183–189.

117. Stensdotter AK, Grip H, Hodges PW, et al. Quadriceps activity and movement reactions in response to unpredictable sagittal support-surface translations in women with patellofemoral pain. J Electromyogr Kinesiol 2008;18(2):298–307.

118. Ng GYF, Zhang AQ, Li CK. Biofeedback exercise improved the EMG activity ratio of the medial and lateral vasti muscles in subjects with patellofemoral pain syndrome. J Electromyogr Kinesiol 2008;18(1):128–133.

119. O'Sullivan SP, Popelas CA. Activation of vastus medialis obliquus among individuals with patellofemoral pain syndrome. J Strength Cond Res 2005;19(2):302–304.

120. Yip SLM, Ng GYF. Biofeedback supplementation to physiotherapy exercise programme for rehabilitation of patellofemoral pain syndrome: a randomized controlled pilot study. Clin Rehabil 2006;20(12):1050–1057.

121. Boling MC, Bolgla LA, Mattacola CG, et al. Outcomes of a weight-bearing rehabilitation program for patients diagnosed with patellofemoral pain syndrome. Arch Phys Med Rehabil 2006;87(11):1428–1435.

122. Cowan SM, Bennell KL, Hodges PW, et al. Simultaneous feedforward recruitment of the vasti in untrained postural tasks can be restored by physical therapy. J Orthop Res 2003;21(3):553–558.

123. Arroll B, Ellis-Pegler E, Edwards A, et al. Patellofemoral pain syndrome. A critical review of the clinical trials on nonoperative therapy. Am J Sports Med 1997;25(2):207–212.

124. Bockrath K, Wooden C, Worrell T, et al. Effects of patella taping on patella position and perceived pain. Med Sci Sports Exerc 1993;25(9):989–992.

125. Cushnaghan J, McCarthy C, Dieppe P. Taping the patella medially: a new treatment for osteoarthritis of the knee joint? BMJ 1994;308(6931):753–755.

126. D'Hondt NE, Struijs PA, Kerkhoffs GM, et al. Orthotic devices for treating patellofemoral pain syndrome. Cochrane Database Syst Rev 2002;(2):CD002267.

127. Wilson T, Carter N, Thomas G. A multicenter, single-masked study of medial, neutral, and lateral patellar taping in individuals with patellofemoral pain syndrome. J Orthop Sports Phys Ther 2003;33(8):437–443; discussion 444–438.

128. Whittingham M, Palmer S, Macmillan F. Effects of taping on pain and function in patellofemoral pain syndrome: a randomized controlled trial. J Orthop Sports Phys Ther 2004;34(9):504–510.

129. Bennell K, Duncan M, Cowan S. Effect of patellar taping on vasti onset timing, knee kinematics, and kinetics in asymptomatic individuals with a delayed onset of vastus medialis oblique. J Orthop Res 2006;24(9):1854–1860.

130. Callaghan MJ, Selfe J, McHenry A, et al. Effects of patellar taping on knee joint proprioception in patients with patellofemoral pain syndrome. Man Ther 2008;13(3):192–199.

131. Cowan SM, Hodges PW, Crossley KM, et al. Patellar taping does not change the amplitude of electromyographic activity of the vasti in a stair stepping task. Br J Sports Med 2006;40(1):30–34.

132. Ryan CG, Rowe PJ. An electromyographical study to investigate the effects of patellar taping on the vastus medialis/vastus lateralis ratio in asymptomatic participants. Physiother Theory Pract 2006;22(6):309–315.

133. Crossley KM, Cowan SM, McConnell J, et al. Physical therapy improves knee flexion during stair ambulation in patellofemoral pain. Med Sci Sports Exerc 2005;37(2):176–183.

134. Powers CM, Landel R, Sosnick T, et al. The effects of patellar taping on stride characteristics and joint motion in subjects with patellofemoral pain. J Orthop Sports Phys Ther 1997;26(6):286–291.

135. Shellock FG, Mink JH, Deutsch AL, et al. Effect of a patellar realignment brace on patellofemoral relationships: evaluation with kinematic MR imaging. J Magn Reson Imaging 1994;4(4):590–594.

136. Van Tiggelen D, Witvrouw E, Roget P, et al. Effect of bracing on the prevention of anterior knee pain—a prospective randomized study. Knee Surg Sports Traumatol Arthrosc 2004;12(5):434–439.

137. Powers CM, Ward SR, Chan L-D, et al. The effect of bracing on patella alignment and patellofemoral joint contact area. Med Sci Sports Exerc 2004;36(7):1226–1232.

138. Powers CM, Ward SR, Chen Y-J, et al. Effect of bracing on patellofemoral joint stress while ascending and descending stairs. Clin J Sport Med 2004;14(4):206–214.

139. Powers CM, Ward SR, Chen Y-J, et al. The effect of bracing on patellofemoral joint stress during free and fast walking. Am J Sports Med 2004;32(1): 224–231.

140. Lun VMY, Wiley JP, Meeuwisse WH, et al. Effectiveness of patellar bracing for treatment of patellofemoral pain syndrome [see comment]. Clin J Sport Med 2005;15(4):235–240.

141. Collins N, Crossley K, Beller E, et al. Foot orthoses and physiotherapy in the treatment of patellofemoral pain syndrome: randomised clinical trial [see comment]. BMJ 2008;337:a1735.

142. Piva SR, Goodnite EA, Childs JD. Strength around the hip and flexibility of soft tissues in individuals with and without patellofemoral pain syndrome. J Orthop Sports Phys Ther 2005;35(12):793–801.

143. Peeler J, Anderson JE. Effectiveness of static quadriceps stretching in individuals with patellofemoral joint pain. Clin J Sport Med 2007;17(4): 234–241.

144. Doucette SA, Goble EM. The effects of exercise on patellar tracking in lateral patellar compression syndrome. Am J Sports Med 1992;20(4):434–440.

145. Bolgla LA, Malone TR, Umberger BR, et al. Hip strength and hip and knee kinematics during stair descent in females with and without patellofemoral pain syndrome. J Orthop Sports Phys Ther 2008;38(1):12–18.

146. Bily W, Trimmel L, Modlin M, et al. Training program and additional electric muscle stimulation for patellofemoral pain syndrome: a pilot study. Arch Phys Med Rehabil 2008;89(7):1230–1236.

147. Robinson RL, Nee RJ. Analysis of hip strength in females seeking physical therapy treatment for unilateral patellofemoral pain syndrome. J Orthop Sports Phys Ther 2007;37(5):232–238.

148. Ireland ML, Willson JD, Ballantyne BT, et al. Hip strength in females with and without patellofemoral pain. J Orthop Sports Phys Ther 2003;33(11):671–676.

149. Heintjes E, Berger MY, Bierma-Zeinstra SMA, et al. Exercise therapy for patellofemoral pain syndrome. Cochrane Database Syst Rev 2003;(4): CD003472.

150. Witvrouw E, Lysens R, Bellemans J, et al. Open versus closed kinetic chain exercises for patellofemoral pain. A prospective, randomized study. Am J Sports Med 2000;28(5):687–694.

151. Herrington L, Al-Sherhi A. A controlled trial of weight-bearing versus non-weight-bearing exercises for patellofemoral pain. J Orthop Sports Phys Ther 2007;37(4):155–160.

152. Willson JD, Binder-Macleod S, Davis IS. Lower extremity jumping mechanics of female athletes with and without patellofemoral pain before and after exertion. Am J Sports Med 2008;36(8):1587–1596.

153. Selfe J, Richards J, Thewlis D, et al. The biomechanics of step descent under different treatment modalities used in patellofemoral pain. Gait Posture 2008;27(2):258–263.

154. Kettunen JA, Harilainen A, Sandelin J, et al. Knee arthroscopy and exercise versus exercise only for chronic patellofemoral pain syndrome: a randomized controlled trial. BMC Med 2007;5:38.

155. Baker MM, Juhn MS. Patellofemoral pain syndrome in the female athlete. Clin Sports Med 2000;19(2):315–329.

156. Whitelaw GP, Rullo DJ, Markowitz HD, et al. A conservative approach to anterior knee pain. Clin Ortho Relat Res 1989;246(Sept):234–237.

157. Witvrouw E, Lysens R, Bellemans J, et al. Which factors predict outcome in the treatment program of anterior knee pain? Scand J Med Sci Sports 2002;12(1):40–46.

chapter 21

The Ankle and Foot

JILL MCVEY, CARRIE M. HALL, JOHN P. MONAHAN, AND RYAN HARTLEY

The ankle and foot interact with the knee, hip, and spine to produce smooth, coordinated movement throughout the entire limb. Understanding these relationships is key to developing a successful therapeutic exercise program for the ankle and foot. Anatomic impairments (e.g., coxa vara, hip anteversion, forefoot varus), physiologic impairments (e.g., hypomobility, hypermobility, diminished muscle performance, loss of balance), or trauma at one joint can lead to dysfunction at other joints in the kinetic chain. Appropriately addressing the complex interplay of impairments throughout the kinetic chain typically results in improved function in the lower extremity. Effective examination, diagnosis, and exercise interventions are essential for long-term resolution of symptoms, impairments, functional loss, and disability.

IMPAIRMENTS OF BODY STRUCTURES

Impairments of body structures, or anatomic impairments, throughout the lower extremity can lead to abnormal alignment and movement patterns of the foot and ankle. Conversely, anatomic impairments of the foot and ankle can lead to abnormal alignment and movement patterns up the kinetic chain at the knee, hip, pelvis, and spine. Abnormal alignment and movement patterns (see Chapter 9) can result in excessive stress and strain on soft tissue and bony structures, leading to cumulative microtrauma and musculoskeletal pain. If left untreated, this microtrauma can result in musculoskeletal system pathology that can affect function and limit participation in meaningful activities.

When optimal alignment is lacking, the clinician must decide whether the alignment fault results from an impairment of body structure or function. An anatomic impairment cannot be altered with manual therapy or exercise intervention because it is a fixed structural abnormality. However, it can be treated with orthotic therapy and exercise to prevent the development of associated impairment of body function. An impairment of body function can be altered with appropriate intervention, such as joint mobilization, soft-tissue mobilization and stretching, and muscle strengthening.

The following impairments are described as structural and are therefore listed as anatomic impairments. Impairment of body functions are discussed in the context of therapeutic exercise intervention.

First Ray Hypermobility

First ray hypermobility is defined as dorsal translation of the first metatarsal and medial cuneiform with a soft endpoint. The structures responsible for first ray stability are plantar ligaments, extrinsic muscles inserting onto the first ray, and the plantar aponeurosis. Any changes in these structures can lead to abnormal function and progressive deformity of the first ray. If deformity develops in the first ray, functional stability is often compromised.[1] For example, during the stance phase of gait, vertical ground reaction forces will excessively dorsiflex the first ray, transferring the load to the other metatarsals.[2] This may lead to acquired pes planus, metatarsalgia, and metatarsal stress fractures.

Subtalar Varus

Subtalar varus is defined as an inverted twist within the body of the calcaneus.[3] While the foot is held in the subtalar neutral position, the bisection of the posterior calcaneus is inverted relative to the bisection of the distal tibia and fibula (Fig. 21-1). Subtalar varus may result in excessive pronation during loading response and midstance. The subtalar joint may resupinate in midstance; however, if the excessive pronation is significant, the subtalar joint may not reach the ideally neutral to slightly supinated position before heel rise. This may result in decreased midtarsal joint stability and increased forefoot shearing during propulsion, potentially straining supportive soft-tissue structures.

Forefoot Varus

Forefoot varus is an inversion deviation of the forefoot relative to the bisection of the posterior calcaneus (Fig. 21-2).[4] A forefoot varus posture may result in excessive pronation during midstance. As with subtalar varus, excessive pronation results in excessive forefoot mobility during push off. Supporting structures of the foot are strained, and lower extremity medial rotation takes place when lateral rotation

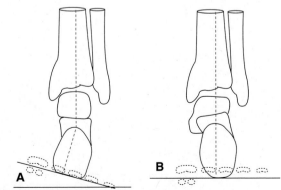

FIGURE 21-1. Posterior view of right foot subtalar varus. (A) Uncompensated subtalar varus. (B) Compensation for this impairment is usually excessive pronation. (From Gould JA. Orthopaedic and Sports Physical Therapy. 2nd Ed. St. Louis, MO: C.V. Mosby, 1990.)

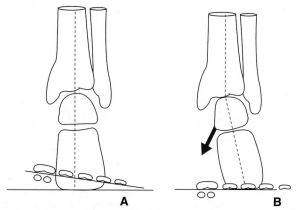

FIGURE 21-2. Posterior view of right foot forefoot varus. (A) Uncompensated forefoot varus. (B) Compensation for this impairment is usually excessive pronation. (From Gould JA. Orthopaedic and Sports Physical Therapy. 2nd Ed. St. Louis, MO: C.V. Mosby, 1990.)

should be normally occurring. This rotational fault can contribute to symptoms up the kinetic chain in the knee, hip, pelvis, and lumbar spine.

Forefoot Valgus

Forefoot valgus is an eversion deviation of the forefoot relative to the bisection of the posterior calcaneus (Fig. 21-3).[4] A forefoot valgus posture may result in early and excessive supination in midstance phase. Functionally, this compensation creates a rigid lever, and may compromise terrain adaptation and shock absorption. This may also cause a lateral weight shift, creating greater forces at the fifth metatarsal and potential lateral instability. Upon propulsion, the subtalar joint is likely to pronate to shift body weight from the lateral stance foot to the contralateral limb. The altered loading and subsequent instability increases the vertical ground reaction forces and may increase the risk for developing plantar pathology.[5]

Ankle Equinus

Ankle equinus is a structural abnormality of the talocrural joint whereby the 10 degrees of talocrural dorsiflexion necessary for gait is absent.[5] If ankle equinus is compensated, the forward progression of the tibia during stance phase forces significantly increased subtalar and midtarsal pronation; this may lead to a

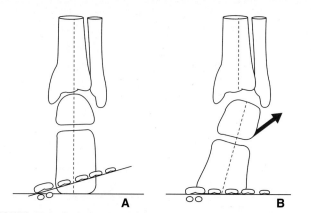

FIGURE 21-3. Posterior view of right foot forefoot valgus. (A) Uncompensated forefoot valgus. (B) Compensation for this impairment is usually excessive supination. (From Gould JA. Orthopaedic and Sports Physical Therapy. 2nd Ed. St. Louis, MO: C.V. Mosby, 1990.)

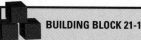

BUILDING BLOCK 21-1

Name one possible deviation in body structures and functions you would expect to see in an individual with:

1. Forefoot varus
2. Ankle equinus

variety of lower limb pathologies including Achilles tendonosis, plantar fasciitis, and digital neuritis.[5,6] If uncompensated, the patient may manifest a "bouncy," or apropulsive, gait secondary to early heel rise, which results in excessive pressures translated to the forefoot.[6] During the examination, the clinician must determine if the patient presents with a true osseous deformity versus limited talocrural dorsiflexion due to short or stiff extrinsic musculature, or stiff talucrural joint (see Building Block 21-1).

EXAMINATION AND EVALUATION

Examination and evaluation of the foot and ankle must consider the findings related to the foot and ankle and their relationships to the knee, hip, pelvis, and spine. The tests described in this section are primarily for the ankle and foot and should be considered in any foot and ankle examination. Note that examination of the knee and hip is also essential.

Patient/Client History

The patient's history guides the overall examination and provides the clinician with important information about activity limitations and participation restrictions. In addition to standard history and subjective examination questions, the clinician should inquire about usual footwear and daily activities, as these extrinsic factors can affect (or cause) symptoms.[7] The clinician uses this information to choose tests according to the patient's symptoms and designs a treatment program to address the impairments, activity limitations and participation restrictions described by the patient.

Balance

Balance is important to assess when a patient presents with foot and ankle dysfunction. See Chapter 8 for details.

Joint Integrity and Mobility

Several special tests are used to assess the integrity of foot and ankle structures. Many of these tests are used to closely assess the mechanics of the foot and ankle. Magee[8] provides a complete listing and description of special tests, the most common of which include varus and valgus stress testing of the ankle and the anterior drawer test.

Muscle Performance

Muscle function of the hip, knee, foot, and ankle should be tested in a logical order and based on patient history information and clinician's impression. All ankle and foot muscle function should be tested. Any proximal muscles in the back, hip, and knee that may affect the foot and ankle should be tested as well, as their weakness can compound distal mechanical faults.

Pain

Examination of the patient's pain and inflammation is performed as part of the subjective examination and is further clarified during the objective examination. Reports of warmth, swelling, and local tenderness indicate pain and inflammation. Palpable tenderness and warmth over specific anatomic structures are objective indications of pain or inflammation. The subjective and objective information are then correlated to guide the remaining examination and treatment planning.

Posture

Observation of posture and position of the lower extremity, including the lumbopelvic and hip regions, is an important aspect of the examination.[8–10] A detailed discussion of foot and ankle alignment may be found in the online supplement to this text.

Range of Motion and Muscle Length

Range of motion (ROM) and muscle length examination for this region should include both the foot and the ankle as well as the knee, hip, and spine. The following tests of ROM and muscle length should be performed:

- Hip and knee ROM and muscle length
- Calcaneal inversion and eversion ROM
- Midtarsal joint supination and pronation ROM
- First ray position and mobility
- Hallux dorsiflexion ROM
- First to fifth ray mobility
- Ankle dorsiflexion and plantar flexion ROM with the knee flexed and extended

Other Examination Procedures

A variety of additional examination procedures may be used depending on the specific patient situation. For example, patients with diabetes should have sensory testing and assessment of pulses. Anthropometric measurements such as circumferential measures are important in patients with swelling of the foot or ankle. Callous patterns on the foot suggest excessive shearing and load transfer. Footwear and orthotic assessment is necessary to evaluate proper fit, noting locations of excessive wear and tear. Most patients should undergo a gait examination to determine the kinetics and kinematics of their foot and ankle. Finally, the implementation of standardized functional testing establishes objective baseline measures and may identify underlying instabilities.[11]

THERAPEUTIC EXERCISE INTERVENTION FOR COMMON IMPAIRMENTS OF BODY FUNCTIONS

Therapeutic exercise is an invaluable clinical tool for treatment of body structure and function impairments of the ankle and foot. This section provides examples of therapeutic exercise for the treatment of impairments in balance, muscle performance, pain, posture and movement, ROM, muscle length, joint mobility, and integrity.

The clinician may need to make appropriate modifications based on individual signs and symptoms. Exercise recommendations for specific diagnoses of the ankle and foot are addressed in a later section.

Balance Impairment

The specific adaptations to imposed demands (SAID) principle indicates that the involved body structures must be sufficiently prepared to assume the loads required for the patient's chosen activities. Moreover, the patient must be able to control the ankle through extremes of motion while performing simultaneous actions with other extremities. Only a well-conditioned and neurologically trained ankle can facilitate balance and function in a variety of directions as the center of gravity fluctuates. The array of training surfaces and conditions is vast, allowing ample opportunity to offer fresh challenges throughout a patient's rehabilitation.[12] The clinician should take care to vary the speed and intensity of training as appropriate to enable maximal functional carry-over and to prevent reinjury.

The level of activity (e.g., walking to the mailbox versus playing competitive basketball) should be considered when designing proprioceptive training activities (see Patient-Related Instruction 21-1: Ideal Alignment During Walking). An average person recovering from an ankle or foot injury/condition should be able to balance on one leg for 30 seconds with eyes closed and mild external perturbation (i.e., with a balance board, foam, a balance machine, or another person providing an external force). This prepares the person to regain balance through improved neurological input to the ankle and foot musculature.

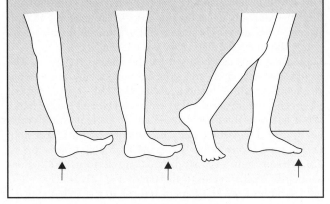

 Patient-Related Instruction 21-1

Ideal Alignment During Walking

You should attain ideal alignment during walking. The most difficult phase to control is during the weight-bearing period of the step. Place the heel, ball of the foot, and toes down on the floor as three distinct areas. The heel should hit slightly on the outside border without turning the entire foot out. The weight line should progress from the outside of the foot toward the big toe. Attempt to maintain the knee over the toes, with the foot progressing straight ahead and the long arch of the foot held upward. If these alignments are maintained throughout the weight-bearing period, the foot should feel stable for push-off.

SELF-MANAGEMENT 21-1 *Balance Activities*

Purpose: Increased balance on a single leg

Position: Standing on one leg, near a counter or in a doorway to provide a surface to stabilize if necessary

Movement Technique:

Level 1: Practice standing on a single leg with your eyes open for 30-second periods

Level 2: Eyes closed

Level 3: Standing on a pillow with your eyes open

Level 4: Standing on a pillow with your eyes closed

Dosage

Repetitions: _____

Frequency: _____

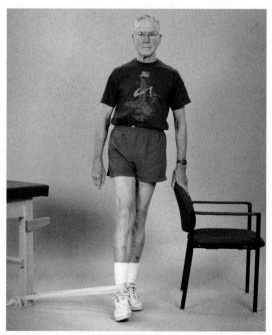

Another patient may need to return to high-level gymnastics; in this case, sport-specific drills implemented on a low balance beam are appropriate. Plyometric exercises in the form of progressive height jump-down activities prepare the ankle/foot to balance during high-impact activities.

Restoration of balance and coordination requires position sense, or proprioception. With an ankle sprain or muscle strain, proprioceptive nerve fibers are often injured. Just as muscles can become deconditioned after a period of immobilization, so too can proprioception. The proprioceptors should be retrained in a controlled, progressive manner starting as soon as possible. Use of a balance board can provide proportionate and progressive stress. The following exercise progression can be used at home without special equipment:

- Balancing on one leg with eyes open; progress to eyes closed standing in a door frame with hands close to the door jam for safety.
- Standing on one leg on a pillow or couch cushion with eyes open; progress to eyes closed.
- Controlled weight shifts to the limits of stability while standing on one leg with eyes open; progress to eyes closed, standing on a pillow, or both.

Single-leg balance can also be progressed by swinging the uninvolved lower extremity first in flexion and extension and then in abduction and adduction (see Self-Management 21-1: Balance Activities). The faster and greater excursion of the swing, the more the static stance is challenged.

Elastic bands can be used for the advanced patient. The band is tied in a circle and looped around a table leg or similar secure structure. Standing facing the table leg, the patient places their uninvolved ankle inside the circled elastic band. While balancing on the involved foot, the patient extends their hip against the elastic band. The patient performs extension-flexion oscillations before returning to double-limb support. The patient then turns 90 degrees and performs adduction-abduction oscillations into the band (Fig. 21-4). The rotating continues until the patient returns to the initial starting position. The exercise can be progressed by increasing oscillation repetitions, oscillation speed, moving the uninvolved limb through noncardinal planes, upgrading the tension of the elastic band, or adding foam or a balance board with single-limb support.

The importance of removing the visual system during balance training cannot be overemphasized. Individuals with a history of multiple ankle sprains present with impaired postural control as a result of repeated trauma to articular and ligamentous joint receptors. These individuals must rely heavily on visual cues to maintain equilibrium during dynamic

FIGURE 21-4. Resisted hip adduction retrains balance and proprioception on the weight-bearing limb. A chair or other stable surface must be available to ensure patient safety.

BUILDING BLOCK 21-2

How might balance programs differ for the following individuals:

- A 21-year-old college basketball player recovering from a mild ankle sprain
- A 75-year-old woman with osteopenia recovering from a fall

SELF-MANAGEMENT 21-2 *Resisted Toe Flexion*

Purpose:	Increased strength in toe flexor and intrinsic foot muscles
Position:	Standing with your foot along the length of the resisted band and with the band in one hand, pull up to pull toes up
Movement Technique:	Holding the band in this position, curl your toes down against the resistance of the band

Dosage
   Repetitions: _____
   Frequency: _____

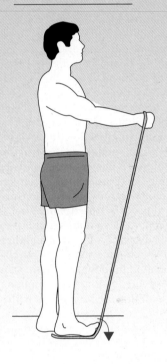

activities.[11] Forcing the somatosensory system to reorganize is only possible when it is trained independent of the visual system (see Building Block 21-2).

Muscle Performance

Resisted exercise is used to restore muscle performance because of muscle strain, neurologic deficit, or disuse. Although open chain exercise is useful to improve physiologic strength parameters and patient awareness of muscle function (i.e., muscle reeducation), it is critical to progress the exercise to funtional weight-bearing activities as soon as tolerated. In many cases, closed chain activity can be broken into simple steps and serve as a starting point for exercise prescription.

Intrinsic Muscles

Intrinsic muscle strengthening can be performed in a sitting position with the patient's feet placed on the end of a towel lying on the floor. The patient flexes their toes, attempting to draw the towel under the foot. Toe flexion should occur first at the MTP joints followed by the more distal IP joints, similar to the motion of catching a ball with the hand. An alternate technique with the same positioning is to make an arch with the tarsal and metatarsals by pressing the first MTP into the floor while rolling the arch upward. The patient should be cued to keep their heel and first MTP in contract with the ground. Repeat this process holding for 6 seconds (see Fig. 21-5). Using the toes to pick up marbles and other small objects also exercises the intrinsic musculature. Standing with a resistive band along

the bottom of the foot which draws the toes into extension can be used to resist toe flexion (see Self-Management 21-2: Resisted Toe Flexion). These exercises are of low intensity and may require high repetitions to achieve a training effect. Maintenance of the longitudinal and transverse arches during closed chain exercises such as small knee bends, the walk stance position, stair-stepping, and gait use the intrinsic musculature in a functional manner. The clinician must observe patient performance carefully to prevent unwanted hammer or claw toe positions during functional training drills (see Building Block 21-3).

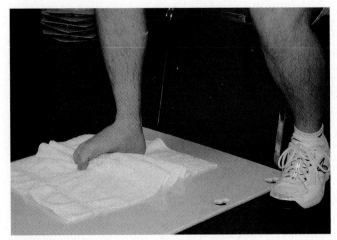

FIGURE 21-5. Intrinsic muscle strengthening of the foot.

BUILDING BLOCK 21-3

How might you instruct foot intrinsic strengthening so as to maximize appropriate form?

Extrinsic Muscles

The ankle musculature is vulnerable to neurologic weakness at the peripheral or nerve root level (see "Functional Nerve Disorders" later in this chapter). As always, careful examination and evaluation will diagnose the underlying etiology of the weakness. Optimal strengthening effects cannot be realized until neurologic sources of weakness are resolved.

Once it is determined that the musculatrue could benefit from progressive strengthening, open chain strengthening exercises for extrinsic musculature can be performed with elastic bands, tubing, or manual resistance. Care must be taken not to overload weak muscle groups, which may cause unwanted substitution patterns, abnormal joint shearing, and pain. Muscles must be recruited in isolation before they can be strengthened in functional exercises to avoid substitution patterns.

Resisted talocrural plantar flexion can be performed in a long-sitting position with the elastic band wrapped around the plantar surface of the forefoot. While holding the opposite end of the band, the patient plantar flexes against the resistance of the band (Fig. 21-6). A towel roll or small pillow placed under the leg proximal to the talocrural joint provides heel clearance. Resisted talocrural dorsiflexion (Fig. 21-7) and subtalar joint pronation and supination (Fig. 21-8) can be completed with an elastic band looped around a table leg or similar secure structure. The patient performs the intended movement against the resistance of the band. During these pronation and supination activities, the clinician should ensure the motion originates at the subtalar joint and not at the tibiofemoral or hip joint. A pulley and weight stack system can also be used for resistance.[12] For all extrinsic muscle strengthening activities, slow eccentric lengthening should be emphasized because of the deceleration function of these structures during gait. In the active population, it is common to see athletes perform a high volume of repetitions with various grades of exercise tubing, yet the musculature hardly fatigues.[12] For these individuals, manual resistance applied for 3 to 5 seconds for 10 to 12 repetitions may be a more appropriate challenge.

Closed chain, weight-bearing exercises are a natural progression toward functional activity recovery. Talocrural joint plantar flexors can be strengthened by performing double-leg toe stands off the end of a stair step, eccentrically controlling descent to end-range talocrural dorsiflexion without excessive pronation or eversion (Fig. 21-9). This is followed by concentric contraction to a neutral or slightly plantar-flexed position without excessive supination or inversion. The exercise is progressed by shifting weight toward the involved extremity and eventually performing a single-heel rise.

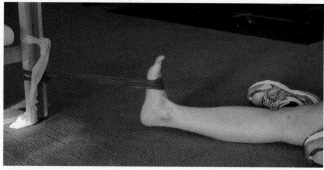

FIGURE 21-7. Talocrural dorsiflexion with a resistive band. A patient may require a high volume of repetitions to drive strength changes given the tibialis anterior's role during gait.

Dynamic ankle strengthening and stabilization can be performed in a sitting position with the knee at 90 degrees with the foot in contact of a small physioball (Fig. 21-10). This can be progressed to closed chain activities such as step-ups or lunges on a Both Sides Up (BOSU) device (Fig. 21-11). The latter exercises improve dynamic joint stabilization in a potentially safer context than with a wobble or balance board due to the wide and flat base of support of the BOSU device.[13]

Subtalar joint supinators can be strengthened by performing double-leg arch lifts. In a standing position, the patient is instructed to lift both arches, thereby rocking outward to the lateral portion of the feet. The clinician should ensure the patient's great toe remains in contact with the floor in order to promote the peroneus longus' role in stabilizing the first ray. Slow, controlled lowering to a neutral position is emphasized. Exercise intensity is increased by progressing body weight toward the involved extremity.

Pain

Prescription of appropriate exercise intensity is key when addressing pain. The severity, irritability, and nature of the patient's pain must be assessed and considered when developing and progressing exercise. For example, exercise for the involved joint should be initiated in the pain-free range during the acute stage, just up to the painful range in the subacute stage, and slightly into the painful range in the chronic stage. Active-assisted exercise may be required if the patient demonstrates poor active control. Exercise for the involved limb's hip and knee may be indicated to prevent disuse weakness, improve proximal control, and decrease pain. In many situations, stationary biking

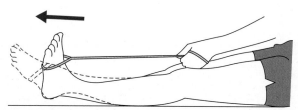

FIGURE 21-6. Resisted plantar flexion with a resistive band should emphasize plantar flexor–controlled eccentric dorsiflexion.

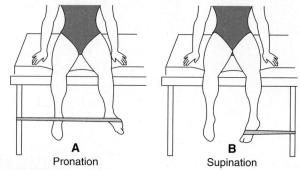

A Pronation   **B** Supination

FIGURE 21-8. Resisted supination and pronation with the knee flexed. Flexing the knee minimizes hip rotation substitution. (A) Resisted pronation. (B) Resisted supination.

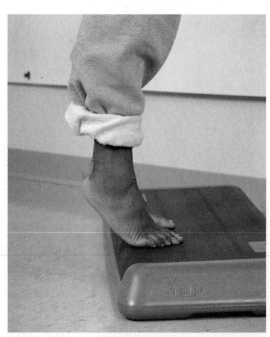

FIGURE 21-9. A standing toe raise will strengthen a number of muscles throughout the foot and ankle as medial, lateral, and intrinsic muscles stabilize the foot and ankle while the gastrocnemius and soleus muscles plantar flex the ankle.

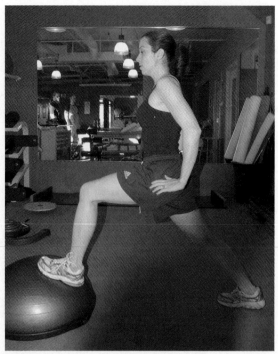

FIGURE 21-11. BOSU ball lunge. This device provides stability challenges to the ankle in a safe context when the flat side faces the floor.

is tolerated well and can maintain or improve cardiovascular and musculoskeletal health. Soft-tissue mobilization, taping and wrapping, cryotherapy, electrical stimulation, and a variety of other therapeutic modalities may be beneficial in conjunction with exercise for the control of pain and swelling.

Treating pain requires the clinician to determine its biomechanical cause. This chapter provides the reader with

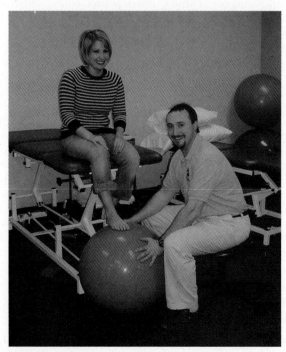

FIGURE 21-10. The therapist provides perturbations to the physioball while the patient maintains a neutral position of the knee and foot. To increase difficulty, start with predicted patterns and move to unpredicted patterns or close the eyes for an additional challenge with perturbations.

the theoretical framework and sample exercise options to diagnose and treat the underlying cause of pain.

Posture and Movement Impairment

Posture and movement impairments are often treated simultaneously with the foot and ankle. Ideal alignment and movement should be emphasized, regardless of which impairments are addressed.

The most common faulty movement patterns affecting the ankle and foot complex are excessive pronation and supination and should not be reinforced in prescribed exercise. The impairments responsible for excessive pronation (e.g., short gastrocnemius, stiff talocrural joint, forefoot varus, weak posterior tibialis) or supination (e.g., hypomobile first ray, hypomobile supinated talus post immobilization, forefoot valgus, short posterior tibialis) must be treated specifically and addressed during functional activity performance.

Numerous repetitions of exercise derived from gait components (e.g., walk stance, single-limb stance, step-through) should be employed frequently throughout the day to shape neuromuscular function and change a habitual faulty movement pattern (Fig. 21-12).

Functional exercise can begin early in the rehabilitation process with consideration of the nature of the injury. The aim of a functional exercise progression is to control a variety of motions into and out of a static position at varying speeds, to further reinforce ideal posture and movement habits. The program should also be consistent with the patient's activity level and functional goals. Trunk and lower extremity alignment, strength, mobility, and movement patterns must be assessed and treated during a functional exercise program.

Ambulating on a painful foot without an assistive device results in compensations and abnormal gait biomechanics. These abnormal biomechanics can create cumulative stress

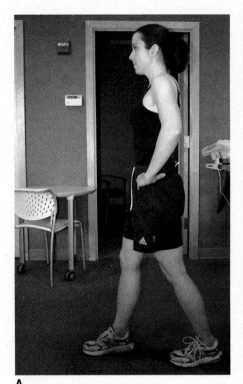
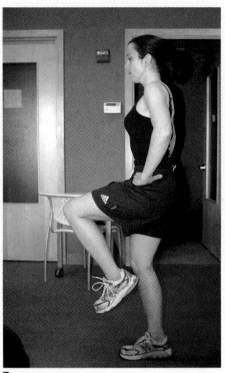

A   **B**

FIGURE 21-12. Walk-stance progression. Keeping the pelvis in neutral and minimizing rotation at the knee, the patient shifts their weight toward the front leg (A) and then flexes the back hip to 90 degrees (B). The patient may balance here for as long as able before returning their flexed leg back to the start position.

which affects both lower extremities and the trunk. These compensations can develop into habits that are difficult to alter.[14] Since gait is a primary functional goal, the patient is encouraged to use a four-point gait pattern with walker or two axillary crutches in conjunction with controlled partial weight bearing and a near-normal gait pattern (i.e., heel-to-toe pattern). Assistive devices are valuable when performing static and dynamic weight-shifting drills in preparation for weight bearing. Static weight-shifting drills consist of progressively shifting weight toward the involved foot. A bathroom scale under each foot, indicating the relative proportion of weight bearing, can be used for objectivity, control, and motivation. Dynamic weight-shifting drills may include the patient's involved foot on the floor and the uninvolved extremity stepping forward and backward. This drill can increase weight-bearing tolerance, promote heel to toe weight transfer, and facilitate controlled talocrural dorsiflexion.

Medial-lateral weight shifting can be facilitated through a circular weight-shifting drill. The patient uses an assistive device for balance and stands with weight equally distributed between their feet. The patient shifts their weight in a slow circular pattern beginning at the fifth metatarsal head. The patient then progresses posteriorly to the lateral heel, medially to the medial heel, and anteriorly to the first metatarsal head. The drill can be performed clockwise and counterclockwise and may be easier for the patient to perform with both lower extremities simultaneously. As weight-bearing tolerance improves, the drill can be progressed by increasing body weight toward a single-leg stance.

Functional exercises such as retrowalking, side-stepping, cross-over stepping, and resisted walking are also beneficial

for upgrading the patient's level of function. These drills are progressed by distance, speed, and resistance through elastic tubing or a pulley and weight-stack system. Exercise must be progressed to higher levels of function (e.g., stair stepping, running, jumping, cutting, sidestep over cones, slideboard, clock step) that are appropriate for each patient's goals (see Self-Management 21-3: Clock Step). Jumping down may be a critical functional demand for athletes and persons returning to moderate- and high-intensity occupations. This task can be initiated bilaterally on a 2- to 4-in box. Ideal alignment and movement patterns must be reinforced with each repetition of any drill. Orthotic prescription or counseling about proper footwear may be necessary to promote ideal function (see Patient-Related Instruction 21-2: Purchasing Footwear). If the patient requires a shoe to control excessive pronation, they may benefit from learning how to stress test potential footwear (Display 21-1).[15] However, exercise in bare feet may be appropriate during low- to mid-level activities to ensure foot muscle function is providing the ideal alignment and movement patterns instead of the orthotic or footwear providing external support. An exception is a severe anatomic impairment (e.g., significant forefoot varus), for which the use of a custom orthotic during all exercise is recommended.

Range of Motion, Muscle Length, Joint Integrity, and Mobility

The talocrural, subtalar, and midtarsal joints have triplane axes and therefore demonstrate triplane motion. Passive and active-assisted ROM exercise for treatment of hypomobility should follow the triplane concept. Accessory joint mobility should be assessed with initiation of joint mobilization

SELF-MANAGEMENT 21-3 *Clock Step*

Purpose: Improve dynamic stability, control, coordination and proprioception of the lower extremity

Position: Standing on involved lower extremity in the center of a circle with markers at each hour (i.e., like a clock)

Movement Technique: Single-leg squat with involved lower extremity while reaching out in a clock hour type pattern with opposite lower extremity. Toe touch with the out stretched lower extremity. Do this in clockwise and counterclockwise directions.

Dosage

Repetitions: __ times __ seconds
Frequency: _____

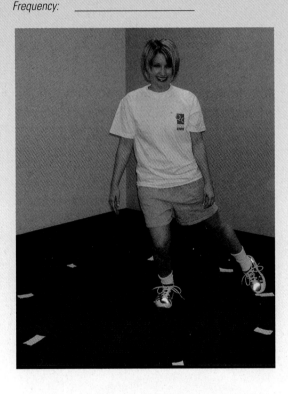

Patient-Related Instruction 21-2

Purchasing Footwear

Know your foot type. Your shoe size and width give a two-dimensional picture of your foot, but your foot is a three-dimensional object. Your foot's arch height affects the fit of your shoe. You can gauge your foot's arch height with a "wet test." Wet the soles of your feet, and then stand on a dry surface, such as a piece of cardboard, to leave an imprint of your foot. The imprint shows whether you have a flat (pronated), normal, or high-arched (supinated) foot. Match the bottoms of the shoes you're considering with your foot type.

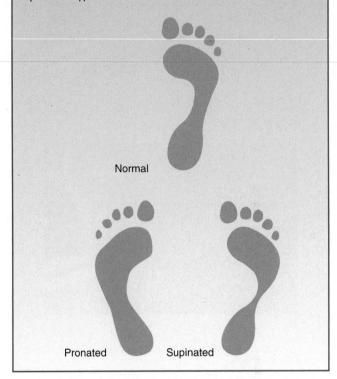

Normal

Pronated   Supinated

---

techniques if indicated. Open chain active stretch can be progressed to passive stretch and eventually progressed to utilize the new mobility during function.

Certain guidelines should be followed in addressing hypermobility impairments:

- In the acute phase, the hypermobile segment must be protected from excessive motion by taping, bracing, casting, or more stable footwear.
- Adjacent hypomobile segments should be mobilized with manual therapy or mobility exercise to prevent excessive motion from transferring to the hypermobile segment.
- Dynamic stabilization exercise should be initiated at the hypermobile segment.

At the foot and ankle, dynamic stabilization exercise can be in the form of proprioception training (see the "Balance Impairment" section) and functional retraining (see the "Posture and Movement Impairment" section).

Talocrural Joint

Talocrural joint dorsiflexion is a common limitation after injury or immobilization of the foot and ankle. This limitation can result from a short or stiff gastrocnemius or soleus muscle, from talocrural joint hypomobility, or both. The clinician must rely on the examination to determine the source of hypomobility. Complaints of anterior ankle discomfort during dorsiflexion may suggest talocrural joint hypomobility, anterior talocrural impingement, posterior compartment soft-tissue restrictions, and/or extensor weakness. Manual therapy techniques can be used to treat talocrural joint hypomobility. Gastrocnemius and soleus stretching are depicted in Figure 21-13. Carefully observe the patient during this activity to prevent subtalar pronation or excessive forefoot stretching while dorsiflexing at the talocrural joint. If the patient is using the long-sitting position, the clinician must ensure proper patient positioning by preventing posterior pelvic tilt and lumbar flexion due to short

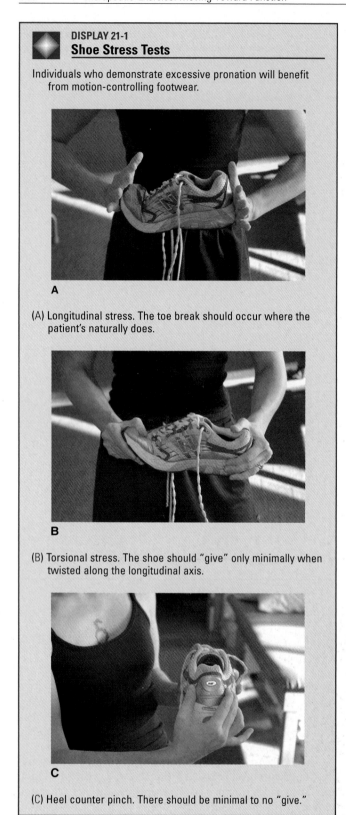

Individuals who demonstrate excessive pronation will benefit from motion-controlling footwear.

(A) Longitudinal stress. The toe break should occur where the patient's naturally does.

(B) Torsional stress. The shoe should "give" only minimally when twisted along the longitudinal axis.

(C) Heel counter pinch. There should be minimal to no "give."

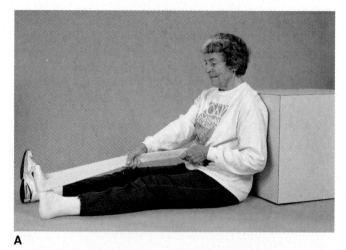

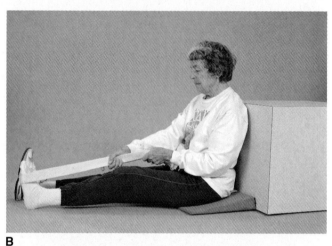

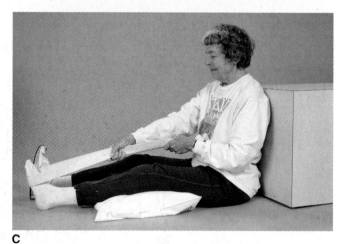

FIGURE 21-13. Increasing dorsiflexion mobility of the ankle. (A) Long-sitting gastrocnemius muscle stretch using a towel. (B) A cushion under the pelvis relieves some hamstring tension, allowing proper lumbopelvic posture. (C) Talocrural joint and soleus muscle stretching is emphasized by placing a pillow under the knees.

hamstrings. A cushion under the pelvis releases tension in the hamstrings and improves the patient's position (Fig. 21-13B). Talocrural joint dorsiflexion ROM can also be performed in a long-sitting position, but a pillow is placed under the knee to minimize the gastrocnemius and hamstring stretch. The soleus is stretched in this position if the talocrural joint has adequate dorsiflexion mobility (Fig. 21-13C).

The supine position is an alternative to the long-sitting position and can accommodate short hamstrings, maintaining better lumbopelvic alignment. It has the added benefit of stretching the hamstrings without overstretching the lumbar spine.

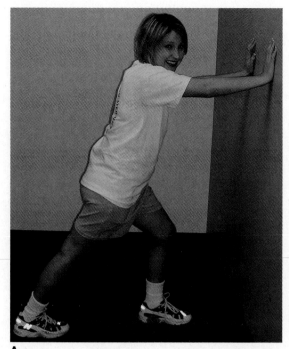 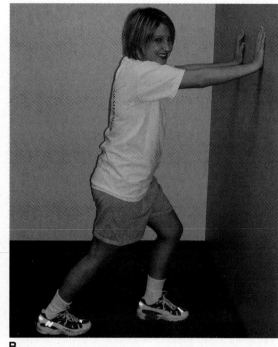

A   **B**

FIGURE 21-14. (A) The gastrocnemius muscle can be stretched by leaning against a wall. Be sure to instruct the patient to keep the foot in the sagittal plane. Any turn-out of the foot will contribute to pronatory forces. (B) The soleus muscle can be stretched with the knee slightly flexed. Again, instruct the patient to keep the foot in the sagittal plane.

Lower extremity biomechanics must be considered when progressing dorsiflexion ROM exercises to a weight-bearing position. If the subtalar joint is pronated in stance, talocrural joint or gastrocnemius stretching will increase the pronation forces. Stretching should be completed with the subtalar joint in a neutral to slightly supinated position. The gastrocnemius can be passively stretched with the patient standing arm's length plus approximately 6 in away from the wall. The involved foot is positioned with its lateral border perpendicular or slightly toe-in to the wall. It is important to be in this position, because gastrocnemius stretching in a toe-out position causes weight-bearing forces to cross the medial longitudinal arch and promote increased subtalar joint pronation (Fig. 21-14). The use of a small hand towel folded under the medial longitudinal arch may help support the subtalar joint and midtarsal joint during stretching.

Active exercises should be incorporated into a patient's functional activities throughout the day. For example, small knee bends from a standing position may reinforce functional mobility of talocrural dorsiflexion instead of subtalar pronation. Progressing small knee bends to a walk stance position reinforces gastrocnemius lengthening as the knee is in extension. As previously stated, the patient must maintain a subtalar neutral position and avoid a toe-out position (see Patient-Related Instruction 21-3: Ankle Mobility and Walking Patterns). Therapeutic exercise progression must incorporate functional retraining of newly gained mobility during swing phase and during late midstance of gait, when maximal dorsiflexion is required. During the late midstance phase, the clinician must ensure the patient maintains a subtalar neutral position and the foot progresses without toeing-out. These compensations prevent talocrural dorsiflexion and produce subtalar pronation and midtarsal abduction.

Step-down training can facilitate controlled eccentric lengthening of the calf muscle group and of the knee and hip extensors. A patient stands on a 2- or 4-in box and is instructed

---

Patient-Related Instruction 21-3

Ankle Mobility and Walking Patterns

To restore the most ideal walking pattern, you must have adequate ankle mobility. You will be asked to perform a specific exercise or series of exercises frequently throughout the day to improve your ankle mobility. The pictures show what your walking pattern should look like. Halfway through the step, you need the most ankle mobility. Be sure that your foot remains pointed forward and does not toe-out (Fig. A). Be sure that you do not allow your arch to flatten (Fig. B).

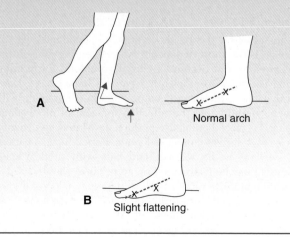

A

Normal arch

B Slight flattening

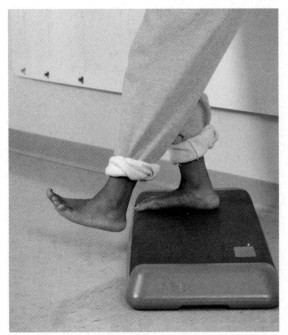

FIGURE 21-15. A step-down exercise is used to improve functional dorsiflexion. The patient must be able to control the pronation component of this motion.

to maintain heel contact of the involved side while lowering the uninvolved heel to the floor (Fig. 21-15). This exercise may be progressed by increasing the step height, speed, and/or direction of movement of the uninvolved limb.

Subtalar Joint

Subtalar joint supination mobility can be addressed with the patient sitting with the involved distal leg placed on the opposite knee. Full active supination is performed, followed by the patient using his hands to progressively pull the calcaneus and foot into greater supination (Fig. 21-16A). If combined with dorsiflexion, this exercise also stretches the peroneal musculature. Subtalar joint pronation mobility can be completed in a similar position by the patient actively pronating and applying graded overpressure (Fig. 21-16B). If combined with dorsiflexion, this exercise also stretches the tibialis posterior muscle. Therapeutic exercise progressions involve functional retraining of the new pronation and supination mobility during the appropriate phase of the gait cycle.

Swelling

Swelling is often the result of impaired joint integrity. As the ankle is the most dependent weight-bearing joint in the body, swelling can become a chronic problem. Early intervention is critical to efficiently treat this impairment. Low-level dynamic exercise and compression in conjunction with frequent elevation can be effective for control of swelling. Emphasis is placed on high-repetition, low-intensity dynamic exercise for adjacent noninjured joints. For example, a patient with swelling at the rearfoot and pain with subtalar joint supination may be instructed how to perform elevated active toe flexion and extension as well as midrange talocrural joint plantar flexion and dorsiflexion (see Self-Management 21-4: Toe and Ankle Active Range of Motion). High-repetition exercise can be prescribed as multiple repetitions at one

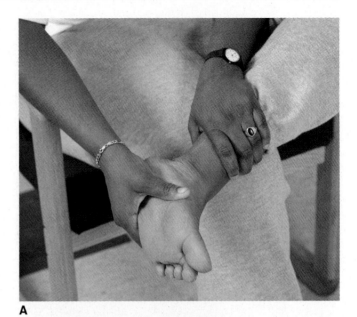

A

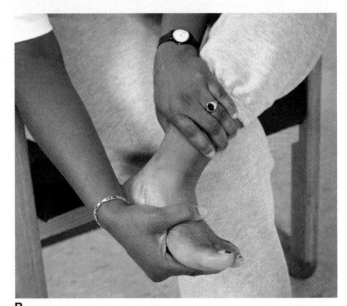

B

FIGURE 21-16. Passive stretching for triplane motion of the foot. (A) Subtalar joint supination. (B) Subtalar joint pronation.

sitting, but it is probably more effective if prescribed as moderate repetitions completed frequently throughout the day (e.g., every 2 hours).

THERAPEUTIC EXERCISE INTERVENTION FOR COMMON ANKLE AND FOOT DIAGNOSES

Although therapeutic exercise prescription should be based on the impairments, activity limitations and participation restrictions of each patient, some generalizations can be made regarding common medical diagnoses. Certain impairments are commonly associated with specific diagnoses; though this section is not exhaustive, it addresses the most common conditions encountered. The problems

SELF-MANAGEMENT 21-4 *Toe and Ankle Active Range of Motion*

Purpose: Increased mobility in the foot and ankle after an injury

Position: Lying on your back with your foot elevated above chest level

Movement Technique: Repeatedly flex and extend your toes. Move your ankle up and down or write the alphabet with your ankle

Dosage
Repetitions: _____
Frequency: _____

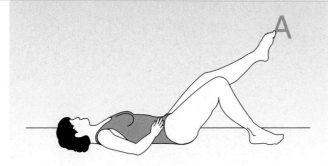

fall into the broad categories of connective tissue disorders (ligament sprains and ankle instability), fractures, functional nerve disorders, localized inflammation (e.g., heel pain/plantar fasciitis, posterior tibialis tendinitis/tendinopathy, medial tibial stress syndrome (MTSS), and Achilles tendinosis), and post surgical rehabilitation (Achilles tendon repair and total ankle arthroplasty [TAA]).

Ligament Sprains

Ligament sprains are the most common sports-related injuries to the foot and ankle.[16–19] Between 70% and 80% of the sprains involve the anterior talofibular ligament (ATFL), calcaneal fibular ligament (CFL), or posterior talofibular ligament (PTFL).[10,20–22] Ligaments of the midfoot, including the dorsal calcaneal cuboid and the bifurcate ligament, may also be involved. The mechanism of injury is usually an inversion and plantar flexion twist. Isolated injuries of the ATFL constitute 65% of ankle sprains, and a combination injury involving the ATFL and CFL comprise 20% of the cases. Isolated injury of the CFL or PTFL is rare.

Ligament sprains are generally classified as one of three grades:

• Grade I represents minor tearing with no functional loss of ankle stability.
• Grade II represents partial tearing of the ligament with moderate instability.
• Grade III describes a complete rupture with significant functional instability.

Grade III sprains are further classified by degrees of injury. First-degree sprains suggest complete rupture of the ATFL.

A second-degree sprain is a complete rupture of the ATFL and CFL. A third-degree sprain suggests a dislocation in which the ATFL, CFL, and PTFL are ruptured.[23]

The patient can usually recall the mechanism of injury, and there is usually a specific site of pain and tenderness. Local edema is often observable. Ecchymosis may occur, indicating injury to blood vessels in the area. Specific stability testing of the affected ligaments may produce guarding and pain.

Syndesmosis sprains, often occurring in conjunction with other injuries, involve a disruption of the distal tibiofemoral ligaments. This results in a diastasis, or widening, of the mortise at the talocrural joint. The mechanism of injury is external rotation on a fixed foot or extreme dorsiflexion. These mechanisms force the talus into the mortise formed by the tibia and fibula, widening this space and disrupting the distal tibiofibular ligaments. If missed on initial evaluation, the patient may subsequently complain of posterior ankle pain, particularly when trying to push-off of the involved ankle. Failure to recognize and treat a significant syndesmosis sprain can produce further widening of the mortise and severe degenerative joint disease. Weight-bearing radiographs are necessary to assess the integrity of the tibiofibular joint with a suspected syndesmosis sprain.

Healing of a ligament sprain, as with most soft-tissue injuries, follows a process of inflammation, repair, and remodeling. These events are sequential but each phase overlaps another. Optimal healing occurs with the introduction of phase-appropriate exercise and functional activity. Controlled stress promotes healing and results in a stronger repair, but excessive loading can interrupt healing and prolong the inflammatory process. The time needed for healing depends on the grade of injury, and clinical decisions should be based on signs, symptoms, and functional assessments.[23]

The initial treatment goals should focus on controlling inflammation and associated pain and swelling. Treatment of grade I and II ankle sprains during the first 1 to 4 days includes protection, rest, ice, compression, and elevation (PRICE). Gradual, early weight bearing[24] is allowed and encouraged, but the injury must be externally protected via a semi-rigid ankle support.[25] Severe grade I and grade II sprains may require the use of axillary crutches for additional protection during ambulation. Patients are instructed to elevate the foot higher than the heart in conjunction with ice applications. Compression with an elastic wrap is beneficial, especially when the foot is in a dependent position, and may be combined with ice application. Elevated edema massage and vasopneumatic compression are also helpful in controlling pain and swelling. Midrange active dorsiflexion and plantar flexion ROM exercises are initiated early, with care not to elongate the injured ligament. Achilles tendon stretching should commence within 48 to 72 hours of injury regardless of weight-bearing capacity, given its tendency to contract after trauma.[12]

Early passive mobilization at the beginning of the talocrural joint's physiologic range is an effective additional treatment for improving pain-free ROM and gait variables such as step length symmetry and stride speed.[26] These gains may occur though the physiological modulation of pain and mechanical alteration of tissues.

Progress exercise as pain and swelling are controlled and weight-bearing tolerance increases. Open chain inversion ROM is progressed as tolerated, but dorsiflexion ROM and calf flexibility can be performed more aggressively. Weight-shifting drills performed with full or partial weight bearing

SELF-MANAGEMENT 21-5 *Dynamic Weight Shifting*

Purpose: Promotes return to weight bearing and proper heel-toe weight transfer during walking

Position: Standing in a stride position

Movement Technique:
1. Step forward with ____ (uninvolved) leg, keeping ____ (involved) leg stable on the ground
2. Step back again with ____ (uninvolved) leg, keeping (involved) stable on the ground

Dosage
Repetitions: _____
Frequency: _____

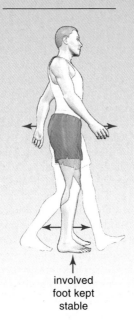

involved
foot kept
stable

and with an external support help to maintain muscle tone and promote balance reactions (see Self-Managements 21-5: Dynamic Weight Shifting and 21-6: Medial/Lateral Weight Shifting). Proprioception boards are helpful, but exercise must be controlled to prevent interruption of tissue repair. Toe raises-off of a step to help maintain strength and flexibility of the calf. Trunk, hip, and knee exercises are helpful in preventing the obvious effects of inactivity as well as promoting proximal control. The hip musculature is vital in maintaining ankle control, influencing foot placement and equilibrium during dynamic activities.[27] The gluteus medius in particular is active through the loading response and midstance phases of gait and can control excessive ankle inversion force moments. A recent study found that individuals with an ankle inversion injury had significantly weaker hip abductors of the involved limb. Early strengthening of the hip abductor musculature, especially the gluteus medius, may promote improved exercise performance and help prevent recurrent ankle sprains (see Building Block 21-4).

The collagen remodelling process is underway 3 to 6 weeks after an injury. Restoration of proprioception and muscle

SELF-MANAGEMENT 21-6 *Medial/Lateral Weight Shifting*

Purpose: Improve control and coordination of standing balance, and prepare for dynamic activities

Position: Standing, using a supportive surface or assistive device if necessary

Level 1: Standing on two legs

Level 2: Standing on one leg

Level 3: Remove support/assistive device

Movement Technique: Shift weight in a slow, circular pattern around the perimeter of the foot. Do this in clockwise and counterclockwise directions

Dosage
Repetitions: ___ times ___ seconds
Frequency: _____

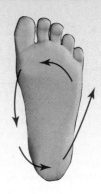

performance are key treatment goals to prevent recurrent hypermobility impairments. Reinjury may occur during this phase because many patients have overconfidence of their ankle's function, so return to a high level of activity should be controlled. Running at slow speeds in straight lines must precede fast speeds and cutting. Slow running in a large figure-eight pattern can be progressed to faster speeds in a smaller figure-eight pattern. Other exercises include double-leg, progressing to single-leg hopping, resisted walking or running using a pulley weight or tubing, and agility exercises. Obstacle courses and agility ladders require minimal resources and can be progressed by speed, direction of movement, and negotiation of the obstacles.[28] Functional strengthening should challenge the entire lower limb to address muscular power as well as promote appropriate body mechanics; exercises may include squats, pushing or pulling weighted objects, stair or ladder climbing.[29] External support should be used during

BUILDING BLOCK 21-4

A patient comes to physical therapy with a grade II ankle sprain. Initially he has non–weight-bearing orders, progressing over 4 weeks to full weight bearing. How might you progress this patient?

high-level activity for 6 to 8 weeks after injury; both taping and bracing are effective in stabilizing the foot and ankle during higher level activity.[30-34]

Immediate treatment of grade III sprains is somewhat debated. One school of thought suggests surgical repair followed by immobilization and then rehabilitation. Recent comparisons suggest that, in the short term, surgical treatments do not show any advantage over functional treatment for grade III sprains.[35] Subotnick[21,22] asserts that surgical repair is indicated in individuals with a history of other disabling sprains; otherwise, conservative treatment should be attempted. The rehabilitation approach for grade III sprains, whether treated with surgical repair or immobilization, is similar to that for grade I and II sprains. A clinician should expect greater deficits in ROM, flexibility, and muscle strength throughout the lower extremity. External supports are important until full strength and proprioception have been obtained.

Even with appropriate intervention and rehabilitation, a significant number of individuals may present with mechanical ankle laxity and report instability up to a year after their sprain.[36] An even greater number will sustain multiple sprains. Chronic recurrent sprain or functional loss is usually related to insufficient recovery of proprioception and strength, hypomobility related to abnormal scarring, or hypermobility resulting from insufficient ligamentous healing. A patient with ankle dysfunction related to hypomobility usually demonstrates limitation and pain with inversion and plantar flexion stress testing. Cross-friction massage, joint mobilization, and mobility exercises are usually beneficial. Postural control may also be compromised with an over-reliance on hip balance strategies in individuals with hypermobility.[11,37] While progressive proprioception and functional strength training are indicated in cases of chronic ankle instability, emerging evidence suggests that patients must complete at least 6 weeks of balance and coordination training to prevent reinjury.[38] Recurrent sprains resulting from hypermobility that do not respond to conservative management may require long-term use of external supports or surgical repair.

Syndesmosis sprains are treated conservatively with cast immobilization for 4 to 6 weeks. An unstable and widened mortise is often treated with surgical fixation. Subsequent rehabilitation is similar to that for medial or lateral ankle sprains (Building Block 21-5).

Ankle Fractures

The talocrural region sustains the highest incidence of fractures in the lower extremity. Excessive talar external rotation, abduction, or adduction within the malleoli can result in shearing or avulsion fractures of the malleoli. Ligament sprains are frequently associated with malleolar fractures. Talocrural joint fractures are commonly classified by the position of the foot (pronated or supinated) and by the direction of force exerted on the malleoli by the talus. Symptoms are similar to those of ankle sprains, although more severe in nature. The following is a description of common talocrural fractures using the Lauge-Hansen classification system.[39-41]

Supination Adduction Injury Extreme lateral loading of the foot results in excessive supination and potential avulsion fracture of the distal fibula in addition to lateral collateral ligament strain. If the force continues, the talus adducts within the distal tibiofibular joint, which results in a shearing fracture of the distal medial malleolus at the joint line.

BUILDING BLOCK 21-5

A 30-year-old female comes to physical therapy two months after sustaining a grade II left ankle inversion sprain. Most of her symptoms have resolved without rehabilitation but she reports increased left foot and medial knee pain that increases when she runs more than ½ mi. This patient's goal is to complete a half marathon in 6 months. Past medical history is significant for multiple left ankle sprains. She has not sought physical therapy until today.

In standing, she presents with an increased left rearfoot valgus angle, apparent left pes planus, and increased medial rotation of the left femur. Left dorsiflexion is stiff and limited but nonpainful. She ambulates and runs with her left lower extremity in lateral rotation and with excessive bilateral lateral trunk flexion. Single limb stance is limited to <10 seconds on each limb with eyes open. Her squat is limited to ½ a range and she demonstrates increased L hip medial rotation and adduction with the activity. Ankle ligamentous stress testing is positive for increased nonpainful gapping of her anterior talofibular and calcaneofibular ligaments.

1. What proximal impairments in body structures and function might you expect to see?
2. Given that this patient presents with multiple problems, what interventions might be most pertinent to address first?

Supination External Rotation Injury Forced external rotation of the talus with a supinated foot can result in tearing of the anterior inferior tibiofibular ligament, followed by fracture of the distal fibula. Continued external rotation force may result in a deltoid ligament rupture or avulsion fracture of the distal medial malleolus. Because the deltoid ligament is very strong, the avulsion fracture of the medial malleolus is more common. Michelson et al. found that a lateral (valgus) load pushes the talus laterally against the fibula resulting in this type of injury adding to this classification system.[41]

Pronated Abduction Injury Excessive abduction of the talus in the distal tibiofibular joint while the foot is pronated results in avulsion fracture of the medial malleolus. Continued abduction of the talus can rupture the anterior and posterior tibiofibular ligament. Separation of the distal tibiofibular joint is referred to as joint diastasis. The final stage of this fracture pattern is shearing off of the lateral malleolus at the level of the joint line.

Pronated External Rotation Injury Forced external rotation of the talus on a pronated foot can result in an avulsion fracture of the medial malleolus, followed by tearing of the anterior tibiofibular ligament and fracture of the fibula. The fibular fracture is usually in the fibular shaft above the talocrural joint. Tibiofibular diastasis may also occur.

Treatment

The key element in the acute treatment of talocrural joint fractures is the restoration of tibiotalar anatomic alignment. Fractures can be treated with closed reduction or with open reduction and internal fixation (ORIF). Fibular fractures without loss of tibiotalar alignment are usually treated with closed reduction. Fractures of both malleoli or one malleolus with a ligament rupture usually result in malalignment and therefore require ORIF. Patients are usually immobilized in a plaster cast for 6 to 10 weeks after ORIF. The clinician should note that muscle profoundly atrophies during even short periods of immobilization with no known method of prevention.[42] Considering the severity of the injury and duration of immobilization is key when designing appropriate interventions.

The initial phase of rehabilitation should include instruction in elevation and active exercise of the noninjured joints. Edema massage, surgical scar mobilization, and modalities for edema reduction are beneficial. Talocrural accessory joint motion must be assessed and joint mobilization techniques initiated as indicated. Active ROM begins in midrange with low intensity and high repetition activity. Controlled, partial–weight-bearing ambulation with an assistive device (i.e., walker or axillary crutches) is often the preferred mode of mobility. Conversely, unprotected ambulation may increase pain and swelling at the foot and ankle and result in undue strain at the lumbopelvic region and opposite lower extremity. Early stationary biking provides a gentle exercise for both lower extremities. Patients should be instructed to pedal with the heel and progress to pedaling with the forefoot.

As the cardinal signs of inflammation resolve, treatment emphasis should focus on aggressive ROM, strengthening, and functional exercise. Involved knee and hip biomechanics should be assessed and treated. The key structural deficit seen in ankle fractures is usually lack of talocrural joint dorsiflexion. Common gait compensations for limited dorsiflexion include the following:

- Abduction and external rotation of the lower extremity
- Genu recurvatum
- Excessive subtalar joint pronation

Early use of heel lifts can help eliminate these compensations (see "Heel and Full Sole Lifts" section). As function normalizes, ROM exercise is generally more tolerable, and progress is usually accelerated. The goal is to remove the heel lifts as soon as ROM is improved. If trauma was extreme and the structural impairment is deemed permanent, heel lifts can be fabricated externally on the shoe for long-term use.

Excessive subtalar joint pronation as a compensation for limited talocrural joint dorsiflexion can create midfoot hypermobility and dysfunction. Foot orthotics may be indicated for the current condition and future foot health. Heel lifts in conjunction with foot orthotics are an adjunct to functional strengthening and proprioceptive training. These supportive devices should be considered early in the rehabilitation process and may be needed for long-term function.

As the median age of the population increases, so has the incidence of ankle fractures among elderly adults.[43] The mechanism of injury is usually low-energy, such as a fall or stumble. It is very important for these individuals to recover function as fast as possible, since bone mineral density, proprioception, and muscle strength are already reduced because of the higher age and decreased activity.

Functional Nerve Disorders

Assessment of impairments associated with nerve dysfunction affecting muscles of the lower leg, ankle, and foot should always begin with screening of proximal entrapment sites. Paresis or paralysis of muscles innervated by the posterior tibial or common peroneal nerves can be the result of lumbar spine impairment. After the spine has been excluded as the source of the nerve disorder, other entrapment sites in the hip (e.g., piriformis syndrome) should be ruled out.

Many nerve disorders are considered to be functional, which means that the nerve is compressed during functional activity. Nerves can be compressed by bony impingements, compartment syndromes, or as a result of joint hypermobility or instability. Occasionally, a nerve can be compressed in multiple locations. It is important to understand the anatomy and innervation patterns to diagnose and treat nerve disorders appropriately (see Review of Neurology in the online supplement to this text). Nerve compression or entrapment may resolve with shoe changes, orthotics, or alteration of impairments in alignment, mobility, and movement patterns through the application of therapeutic exercise. The following sections describe selected sites for injury, compression, or entrapment of the posterior tibial and common peroneal nerves and branches.

Tibial Nerve

The tibial nerve is injured less frequently than the common peroneal nerve because of its deep and protected position within the popliteal fossa. If a lesion or entrapment occurs in the popliteal fossa, all of the calf muscles and plantar muscles of the foot are affected. A complete lesion in the popliteal fossa results in a shuffling gait and difficulty raising the heel during propulsion because of ankle plantar flexion loss. The unopposed action of the muscles innervated by the common peroneal nerve can lead to an increased concavity of the longitudinal arch of the foot (i.e., pes cavus) and clawing of the toes. Sensory loss occurs on the sole of the foot and the plantar surfaces of the toes. Painful disorders, such as causalgia (a form of complex regional pain syndrome), are common with incomplete or irritative lesions.

If entrapment is suspected, the muscles surrounding the popliteal fossa must be assessed for length. If the popliteus, plantaris, and gastrocnemius are short, the tibial nerve may be compressed. Appropriate stretching and changes in alignment and movement patterns that perpetuate muscle shortening may alleviate the pressure and reduce nerve compression.

A more common disorder affecting the tibial nerve is tarsal tunnel syndrome. The tarsal tunnel is a fibro-osseous tunnel formed by the flexor retinaculum, the medial wall of the calcaneus, the posterior portion of the talus, the distal tibia, and the medial malleolus. The tibial nerve travels through this tunnel and may be compressed behind the medial malleolus, under the retinacular ligament. Compression leads to an insidious onset of sensory impairment of the medial and lateral side of the sole of the foot and toes, progressing to muscle atrophy and weakness and of toe flexion, abduction, and adduction.[44,45] Other signs and symptoms include burning, tingling, numbness, pain in the medial portion of the ankle and or the plantar aspect of the foot, local tenderness posterior to the medial malleolus, and a positive Tinel sign. End range ankle dorsiflexion and eversion may reproduce symptoms.[46] These signs and symptoms should be present but often the complete constellation is not found.[47,48]

A hypermobile subtalar joint will stretch the posterior tibial nerve by a prominence of the posteromedial talus. Intervention for compression or entrapment in this region should include treating the impairments associated with subtalar pronation. This may involve stretching a short gastrocnemius, strengthening a weak posterior tibialis, educating the patient regarding altered postural habits, and instruction in proper foot biomechanics during gait and other functional activities. In conjunction with exercise, the use of appropriate footwear alone or with orthotics to control excessive pronation may be necessary for complete resolution of symptoms related to nerve compression. Patients who do not respond to physical therapy interventions may undergo surgical decompression of the tarsal tunnel with mobility activities initiated within the first two weeks postoperatively.[46]

Peroneal Nerve

The common peroneal is the most commonly injured nerve in the lower limb, primarily because of its exposed position as it winds around the neck of the fibula. Injury causes paresis or paralysis of all the muscles supplied by the deep and superficial peroneal nerves. The result is a loss of dorsiflexion and eversion of the foot and extension of the toes, producing footdrop and a steppage gait. An accompanying loss of sensation occurs in the front of the lower leg, dorsum of the foot, and adjacent sides of all toes. Recurrent ankle sprains may also result from peroneal weakness. A thorough knowledge of anatomy, innervation patterns, and function of the affected muscles during gait is necessary to develop an appropriate exercise program during the stages of nerve recovery. Care must be taken to prevent fatigue of a muscle recovering from a nerve injury. An external support (i.e., dorsiflexion assist splint) is usually necessary during the early phases of recovery, when the muscles are weakest.

The deep peroneal nerve may become entrapped distally under the extensor retinaculum, a condition known as anterior tarsal tunnel syndrome. Trauma often plays a role. Recurrent ankle sprains continually place the deep peroneal nerve on maximal stretch as the foot plantar flexes and supinates. Tight-fitting shoes or ski boots have also been implicated. Compression of the deep peroneal nerve usually results in pain radiating into the first web space. The extensor digitorum brevis may be weak or atrophied.[49] One clinical provocative test for tarsal tunnel is maximal foot eversion and dorsiflexion while all of the metatarsophalangeal joints are maximally dorsiflexed. This clinical test is helpful in increasing the sensitivity of the physical examination.[47]

When treating patients with anterior tarsal tunnel syndrome, ensure that nerve compression is not caused by poorly fitting footwear. If the ankle is hypermobile or unstable, associated impairments should be treated with appropriate therapeutic exercise, footwear, bracing, taping, or orthotics to reduce excessive stretch of the deep peroneal nerve. Exercise may include peroneal strengthening combined with drills to train ankle proprioceptors and help prevent recurrent ankle sprains.

Plantar Fasciitis

The plantar fascia provides stability to the foot by supporting the longitudinal arch during the propulsion phase of gait by means of the windlass mechanism.[1,50–53] Injury to the plantar fascia is a result of either intrinsic or extrinsic factors. Intrinsic factors include reduced plantar flexion and intrinsic foot strength, torsional malalignment of the lower extremity,

obesity or sudden weight gain, and foot structure. Recent studies indicate the risk of plantar fasciitis increases as the range of talocrural dorsiflexion decreases.[54] Extrinsic factors include training errors and surfaces, improper or excessively worn footwear.[55,56]

Plantar fasciitis is considered an overuse injury with excessive pronation as the most common cause. Excessive subtalar pronation, pes cavus, and medially shifted weight-bearing forces fatigue the plantar fascia where it arises from the medial calcaneal tuberosity on the anteromedial aspect of the heel. A common symptom is sharp pain at the medial aspect of the heel. However, because of the proximity of the medial calcaneal tuberosity and the origin of the plantar fascia, it is not possible to clinically differentiate a fascial from a bony source of pain by location alone. Patients with plantar fasciitis may report increased heel pain with the first few steps in the morning or after prolonged rest periods, which improves with further ambulation.[57] The clinician may differentiate this pain from a stress fracture or nerve entrapment, as the latter conditions will continue to provoke pain with increased walking.[54]

Dorsiflexion of the toes almost always exacerbates the patient's symptoms because of the windlass mechanism promotes stretching of the fascial fibers.

Other structures may be painful besides the plantar fascia and should be considered for differential diagnosis, including abductor hallucis, flexor digitorum brevis, or abductor digiti minimi muscles, the long plantar ligament, the nearby bursae, and the possibility of compression or diabetic neuropathy.[55,57]

Treatment

Management of plantar fasciitis is classified into three broad categories: decreasing pain and inflammation, reducing tissue stress, and restoring muscle strength and flexibility to involved tissues.[55,56]

The cornerstone of conservative treatment for plantar fasciitis is modification of activity. For the running athlete, mileage reduction, alternate activities, footwear evaluation, work reduction, and shortened workouts should be considered. Low-resistance cycling and swimming pool running are effective alternatives to running on land.

The primary goal of treatment of plantar fasciitis in the acute stage is pain and inflammation control. Therapeutic interventions include the use of nonsteroidal anti-inflammatory medications,[58] steroid injection, iontophoresis,[59,60] phonophoresis, ultrasound, deep tissue massage, cryotherapy, and hydrotherapy.

Taping, foot orthoses, night splints, and modification of footwear are all methods of reducing stress on the plantar fascia. Circumferential or low-dye taping of the foot is usually beneficial as an initial intervention to unload the plantar fascia and reduce inflammation (see Displays 21-2 and 21-3 for longitudinal arch strapping technique).

Abnormal intrinsic rearfoot and forefoot alignment must be assessed for potential orthotic therapy. Proper orthotic prescription with appropriate forefoot and rearfoot posting can support the plantar fascia without direct pressure on the soft tissue underneath the longitudinal arch. Recent literature supports the use of economic prefabricated or over-the-counter orthoses over expensive custom orthotics.[61] Care must be taken to assess the need for orthotics as a long-term solution to the problem.

DISPLAY 21-2
Preparing the Foot for Adhesive Strapping

1. The foot must be clean and dry. Soap and water or alcohol wipes are used to remove perspiration and skin oils, which decrease the tape adherence to the skin.
2. Hair should be shaved to avoid irritation to hair follicles and the pain associated with pulling hair out during tape removal.
3. Skin should be sprayed with a skin preparation or "toughener" that improves tape adherence.
4. Thin foam prewrap used before taping helps protect the skin, but when maximal support is necessary, the tape should be applied directly to the skin. Prewrap has been used successfully when patients are limited to a medium or low activity level.

Low loads applied over a long duration is one of the best methods to stretch tissue. As such, night splints can be another helpful tool when managing plantar fasciitis by preventing plantar flexion during sleep. Using a night splint decreases recovery time when compared to standing gastrocnemius-soleus complex stretching.[62] Individuals with chronic (>6 months duration) plantar fascia pain may derive greater benefit from custom-fabricated versus prefabricated night splints.[57]

 DISPLAY 21-3
Longitudinal Arch Strapping Technique

Tape: 1-in athletic tape.
Taping position: Patient is supine on the treatment table, with his or her foot over the edge.
Taping technique: Place two anchor strips circumferentially just proximal to the metatarsal heads (apply lightly). Begin the first diagonal strip of tape on the medial side of the foot, just proximal to the head of the first metatarsal. Tape posteriorly and around the heel. Angle the tape under the foot, crossing the plantar surface, and return medially near the origin of this strip (A). Place the second diagonal strip of tape on the lateral side of the foot, just proximal to the head of the fifth metatarsal. Tape under the foot, around the heel, and up the lateral side toward the origin of this strip (B). Continue alternating strips in the same pattern until the "fan" is filled in (C). Tie down the entire procedure by placing plantar strips over the previous strips by starting on the dorsolateral aspect of the foot; continue under the arch, and finish on the dorsomedial aspect of the foot. Leave a gap on the top of the foot; bridge this by placing short strips of tape across the gap (D) and (E). Each strip of tape should overlap the previous strip by approximately 1/4 in.

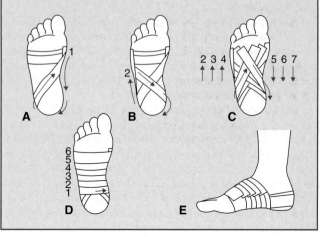

 SELF-MANAGEMENT 21-7 *Plantar Fascia Step Stretch*

Purpose: Increased flexibility of the plantar fascia
Position: Standing with the toes extended against the vertical part of a step and the heel on the floor

Movement Technique: Slowly bend the knee above the toes you are stretching back. Keep your arch from rolling in.

Dosage
Duration: _____
Repetitions: _____
Frequency: _____

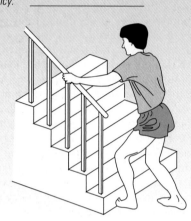

Shoe modification, such as a medial heel wedge to limit pronation, is yet another management technique, as is changing shoes to provide a firm heel counter to control rearfoot motion, or lacing shoes to provide control of midfoot.[56]

In the subacute phase, progressive cross-friction massage and stretching of the plantar fascia helps prevent abnormal scar formation and can improve plantar fascia extensibility (see Self-Management 21-7: Plantar Fascia Step Stretch).

If this stretch increases heel pain, the exercise may be modified to passive toe dorsiflexion in non–weight-bearing position up to the painful range.[57]

Long-term resolution of symptoms of plantar fasciitis can only be achieved by addressing the physiologic and/or anatomical impairments directly affecting the biomechanics of the plantar fascia. If pronation is stressing the plantar fascia, and a stiff talocrural joint and/or short gastrocnemius-soleus complex are contributing to the pronation, mobilization to the talocrural joint or stretching of the gastrocnemius-soleus complex is indicated. The clincian should note, however, that simply stretching the gastronemius has not been demonstrated to significantly decrease plantar pain.[63] In conjunction with mobilization and stretching, strengthening the tibialis anterior and extensor digitorum is critical to maintain and utilize dorsiflexion range during functional activities. If intrinsic muscle weakness is contributing to loss of longitudinal and transverse arch support, strengthening can be initiated to promote dynamic stability against excessive pronation. In addition, lower extremity alignment, muscle flexibility, muscle performance, and movement patterns must be assessed for extrinsic pronatory factors. Functional exercise and proprioceptive training should be initiated to reduce pronatory forces and improve talocrural dorsiflexion.

Posterior Tibial Tendon Dysfunction

The tibialis posterior tendon is the primary dynamic stabilizer of the medial longitudinal arch.[64] During open chain mechanics, the tibialis posterior inverts and plantar flexes the foot, whereas during closed chain mechanics, it decelerates subtalar joint pronation in the loading response phase and supinates the subtalar joint in the midstance and terminal stance phases.[65] Its contraction serves to elevate the medial longitudinal arch, which "locks" (supinates) the midfoot and assists the foot converting to a rigid lever for propulsion. This action allows the gastrocnemius muscle to act with much greater efficiency during gait.[64]

The mechanism of posterior tibial tendon dysfunction is usually excessive subtalar joint pronation and results in acquired flatfoot deformity. However, the tendon can be strained because of poor physical condition or by excessive physical activity. This dysfunction is most common in females who are obese, in their fifth and sixth decade of life, and lead sedentary lifestyles.[66] The least common mechanism of injury is an eversion ankle sprain. Symptoms are commonly located at the distal one third of the medial tibia or inferior and posterior to the medial malleolus resulting from a zone of hypovascularity that correlates to the region of tendon pathology.[66] Typical symptoms include tenderness to palpation along the tendon, pain and/or weakness with resisted inversion and plantar flexion, and pain with closed chain pronation. Walking can become painful if accompanied by excessive pronation. Running, cutting, or jumping may also be impaired because of the posterior tibialis' role during the deceleration phase of these activities. The patient may note feeling increasingly unstable at the ankle, indicating altered proprioception, strength, and coordination.[66]

Treatment

As in plantar fasciitis, a primary goal of treatment in the acute phase is to control inflammation with appropriate medications and therapeutic modalities. Arch or navicular strapping is beneficial to control end-range pronation, thereby decreasing the strain on the tibialis posterior. Low-intensity, high-repetition, open chain plantar flexion and inversion exercises in a pain-free range should be initiated early in the rehabilitation process to control pain and inflammation. Open and closed chain strengthening exercises are commenced as tolerated in the subacute phase. Given the tibialis posterior's role during gait, eccentric and concentric strengthening may yield positive results, though this has yet to be substantiated in the literature.[67] Assess intrinsic and extrinsic pronatory factors and use orthotic therapy and functional exercise as indicated for long-term resolution of symptoms.[68]

Short leg casting with non–weight bearing for 4 to 6 weeks may be necessary for patients with evidence of a partial tear, signified by delayed heel varus with toe raises and weakness.[66] Posterior tibial tendon dysfunction is resistant to conservative treatment and often involves surgery because of the progressive nature of the disorder.[66]

Medial Tibial Stress Syndrome

Although MTSS is one of the most common lower leg injuries sustained in sports, its mechanism remains unknown.[69] It involves a stress reaction by the crural fascia or bone along the posteromedial portion of the tibia most commonly associated with the insertion of the soleus.[70] Some authors have suggested that MTSS is a consequence of repetitive stress that fatigues the soleus and overloads the bone-remodeling capabilities of the tibia.[69] Proposed risk factors include increased pronation, forefoot varus, a positive navicular drop test, high body mass index, hard or inclined running surfaces, inappropriate footwear, and training errors.

Patients may report a dull ache along the middle or distal posteromedial tibia which occurs with exercise.[5,70,71] Initially, the pain may occur at the beginning and end of activity; with continued training, the pain increases in severity and duration.[5,71] Positive physical findings include tenderness to palpation of the middle to distal tibia and pain with heel raises, resisted dorsiflexion, plantarflexion, and/or inversion.[71]

Prevention of MTSS is difficult as the causal factors remain unknown. Methods which show promise in the literature include use of shock-absorbant and pronation-control insoles and graduated running programs. However, stretching of the lower leg has consistently shown to have no effect.[69] Therapeutic exercise considerations should focus on improving the strength and endurance of the soleus in combination with footwear or training alterations. Individuals who exercise daily should commit to at least 1 day per week to a form of cross-training that unloads the tibia and allows bone remodeling to occur, such as a pool workout.

Achilles Tendinosis

Despite its large cross-sectional area, the Achilles tendon is particularly susceptible to injury approximately 2 to 6 cm above its insertion into the calcaneus due to a poor blood supply.[72] The blood supply decreases with age, predisposing this area of the tendon to chronic inflammation and possible rupture.[73]

Overuse pathology of the Achilles tendon is one of the more common tendon injuries of the lower extremity.[74–80] It is especially prevalent among persons participating in running and jumping sports, as the tendon functions eccentrically to lower the heel to the ground upon landing. The tendon is also stressed during the late midstance phase of gait, when it elongates to slow the advancing tibia. This stress is particularly high when walking or running uphill, when the tendon must slow the tibia eccentrically while propelling the body uphill concentrically. Intrinsic factors contributing to injury include rearfoot valgus, gastrocnemius-soleus and hamstring stiffness or shortening,[71] and forefoot varus.[81] Extrinsic factors include running mechanics, type and fit of footwear, and running surface.

Pain is elicited with direct palpation to the tendon and crepitus may occur with active ankle motion.[71] Symptoms may increase with passive talocrural dorsiflexion as a result of Achilles tendon stretch; dorsiflexion ROM may also be diminished. There may be visible edema along the length of the Achilles, as well as tendon thickening secondary to increased collagen deposition.

Recent research into chronic Achilles tendinosis has revealed the findings of high concentrations of an excitatory neurotransmitter, glutamate, in the tendon and absence of inflammatory cells. This may explain the limited success with treatment strategies aimed solely at reducing inflammation and why this condition is so painful.[72,82]

Treatment of Achilles tendinosis should follow the guidelines in Chapter 11. Stretching of the gastrocnemius-soleus complex is essential to increase the length over which the tendon loads can be dispersed. Stretching is recommended only after talocrural mobility is restored; otherwise, excessive tension will be placed on the Achilles if talocrural motion is absent. Stretching should be performed with the knee straight to isolate the gastrocnemius, and with the knee bent to isolate the soleus, while maintaining a neutral foot position (see Fig. 21-14).

Strengthening exercises are an important intervention but should only be introduced following resolution of acute inflammation to avoid exacerbating the patient's condition. If a patient is unable to tolerate weight-bearing activities, an aquatic-based intervention may be appropriate until symptoms decrease; this allows the patient to maintain cardiovascular health while exercising the Achilles in a safe environment.[83] See chapter 16 for further details. The strengthening program is progressed to eccentric activities such as controlled lowering from a plantar-flexed to dorsiflexed position. Use of a decline board may assist these exercises.[81] Eccentric calf strengthening in patients with painful chronic Achilles tendinosis results in significantly better results when compared to concentric strengthening.[75,84] Eccentric exercises may also decrease tendon thickening, possibly indicating a resolution of abnormal collagen deposition described earlier.[85] The speed and load should also be gradually increased to appropraitely and progressively challenge this muscle group (see Self-Management 21-8: Hop-Down Drills), as forces of 2.5 times the body weight act on the tendon during normal gait.[81]

Postoperative Management

Achilles Tendon Rupture

The Achilles tendon is also susceptible to rupture. The typical patient sustaining a rupture is a middle-aged, competitive person involved in intermittent athletic activities. Chronic degeneration is observed in most ruptured tendons, although the majority of ruptures occur without any preexisting complaints.[86] At the time of rupture, the patient complains of feeling as if he or she had been kicked in the back of the leg, despite the fact that most ruptures are the result of noncontact injuries. A defect may be palpated and the Thompson test result is positive.

Achilles tendon ruptures may be treated conservatively with immobilization in a cast or cast boot for up to 12 weeks. The effects of immobilization and the extent of the damage to the Achilles tendon must be considered when planning interventions; prolonged immobilization will have deleterious effects on gastrocnemius-soleus length, strength, and size. ROM activities to restore the length of the gastrocnemius-soleus complex and the mobility of the talocrural joint are necessary. Early rehabilitation activities should commence with non–weight-bearing plantar flexion and slowly progress to closed chain and eccentric activities as outlined for Achilles tendinosis.

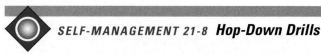

SELF-MANAGEMENT 21-8 *Hop-Down Drills*

Purpose:	Increased balance and coordination during dynamic movement, impact loading, and controlled lengthening of the Achilles
Position:	Standing on a small step of about 4 in.

Movement Technique:

Level 1:	Hop down onto both feet, controlling the landing.
Level 2:	Hop down, landing on a single leg.

Dosage
    Repetitions: _____
    Frequency: _____

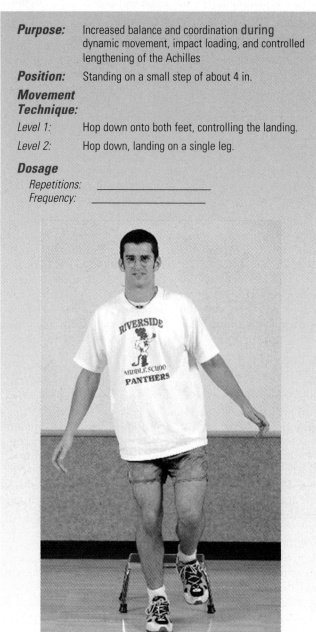

Although Achilles tendon rupture is a relatively common injury, discussion continues regarding whether surgical or nonsurgical treatment is the best management.[87] Recent studies have suggested improved outcomes and superior strength in operatively treated patients, with a decreased rate of rerupture compared to a nonoperatively managed cohort.

Total Ankle Arthroplasty

TAA is a relatively new procedure which still requires significant evidence regarding the best surgical technique, prosthesis, and rehabilitation strategy. The surgery was initially developed to provide an alternative to ankle fusion with the inherent advantage of preserving joint motion. However, early efforts failed to appropriately reproduce the triplanar motion of the talocrural joint and lead to excessive complications.[88] Newer generation prostheses have improved outcomes, though the median survival rate of the component parts is only 5 to 10 years—much lower than for total hip or knee arthroplasty.[89, 90] Surgical complications include prosthesis loosening, infection, boney nonunion or fracture, and persistent pain and stiffness.[89]

Despite these limitations, the popularity of TAA continues to grow. Individuals indicated for the procedure include those with a history of painful rheumatoid or osteoarthritis that limits ROM and functional mobility. In general, most patients who undergo TAA have a good outcome, with the main post-surgical difficulty of limited dorsiflexion.[89]

As with other forms of joint replacement, treatment in the initial post-operative phase should focus on reducing inflammation with manual therapy, cryotherapy, compression, and patient use of an assistive device. Return to full weight bearing is primarily dependent on the surgeon's recommendations and patient tolerance. Stretching of the gastronemius-soleus complex is recommended, but talocrural dorsiflexion may primarily be limited by the replaced talocrural joint. A heel wedge may be appropriate to enable functional mobility and appropriate gait mechanics until full dorsiflexion is achieved, but the patient should be aware that they may not fully gain this motion under current technological limitations. Rehabilitation should progress to improving strength of the proximal, as well as extrinsic and intrinsic foot and ankle, musculature. Balance and equilibrium reactions should be retrained as outlined previously in this chapter.

ADJUNCTIVE INTERVENTIONS

A therapeutic exercise program for the ankle and foot can be enhanced with the use of supportive devices. Adhesive strapping, wedges and pads, biomechanical foot orthotics, and sole or heel lifts can help control excessive compensation and promote early return to functional activity. The supportive devices are an adjunct to a thorough exercise program and, if used independently, may be less successful. In many situations, the converse is also true.

Adhesive Strapping

The use of adhesive strapping is beneficial in controlling the end range of joint motion. Longitudinal arch strapping is valuable when excessive pronation is deemed a primary stressor. Caution must be taken in supportive strapping if the foot is swollen. Strapping should improve the patient's symptoms, and if symptoms increase, the strapping should be removed immediately. The patient must be instructed to remove the strapping slowly by pulling the tape backward on itself. Quick jerking movements and excessive skin distraction with tape removal could pull superficial skin layers off. The foot must be properly prepared before adhesive strapping is applied to enhance support and decrease the risk of skin irritation. Display 21-2 provides guidelines for preparing the foot for adhesive strapping.

The longitudinal arch strapping technique presented in Display 21-3 is designed to decrease soft-tissue strain caused by excessive subtalar joint pronation. Many additions and variations of supportive foot strapping can be explored, such as the navicular strap detailed in Display 21-4.

DISPLAY 21-4
Navicular Strap Technique

Tape: 1 ½" athletic or Leukotape, depending on desired rigidity and patient's functional goals
Taping position: Patient is supine on the treatment table in long or short sitting.
Taping technique: If using Leukotape, begin with Cover Roll and finish with Leukotape. Apply athletic tape directly to skin. The foot should be in a neutral or slightly relaxed position. Apply tape over lateral plantar surface of foot or over the most lateral aspect of dorsal surface of foot and draw the tape medially (A). Gently pull the tape over the medial longitudinal arch, directly crossing the navicular tuberosity. Continue to wind the tape over the dorsal surface of the foot, crossing approximately over the anterior talocrural joint (B), and finishing over the posterolateral distal leg. This process may be repeated twice per foot/ankle to improve midfoot support.

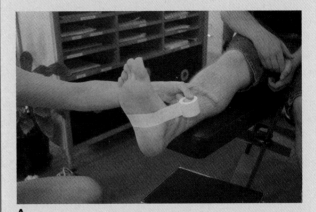
A

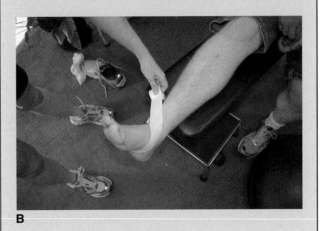
B

Wedges and Pads

Medial heel wedges, longitudinal arch pads, and metatarsal pads can be placed in a shoe or on a flat insole to decrease soft-tissue strain. Medial heel or varus wedges are thick medially and taper laterally. They are made of firm rubber and used with the philosophy of controlling calcaneal eversion and thereby decreasing the degree of subtalar joint pronation. Metatarsal and longitudinal arch pads are made of felt or foam rubber. The metatarsal pad is placed directly proximal to the symptomatic metatarsal head. Medial wedges, longitudinal arch pads, and metatarsal pads are most successful when used in conjunction with adhesive strapping. Longitudinal arch and metatarsal pads can be taped on top of an arch strapping for precise positioning. The medial wedge can be secured in a shoe with the use of double-faced tape. If symptoms are relieved and performance is improved through adhesive strapping and supportive pads, a biomechanical orthotic may be indicated.

Biomechanical Foot Orthotics

It is beyond the scope of this text to provide a detailed description of orthotic evaluation and prescription. This section describes the purpose of orthotic devices, the general fabrication method, the concept of posting, and therapeutic exercise prescription to augment orthotic prescription.

A biomechanical foot orthotic is a device that attempts to control dysfunction by controlling the subtalar joint near its neutral position. Display 21-5 describes the general purposes of a foot orthosis.[91]

A foot orthotic is composed of a shell, which conforms to the contours of the foot, and posting material, which tilts the shell according to the angulation and degree of control desired.

The shell is fabricated from an impression of the foot taken while the subtalar joint is maintained in a neutral position. The shell encompasses the heel, fits closely to the arch, and ends immediately proximal to the metatarsal heads. The shell can be made of a variety of materials, ranging from a flexible foam to a semirigid thermoplastic. Generally, the more rigid shells are indicated for the hypermobile foot requiring motion control. Flexible accommodative shells are used for arthritic conditions, diabetes, and the hypomobile foot. Body weight is also a deciding factor when choosing a shell's rigidity. A heavy individual may require a more rigid shell for more adequate motion control.

Orthotic posting is prescribed from the findings of a biomechanical evaluation of the entire lower extremity. Posting material is added to the shell's undersurface to conform to the foot and ankle angles. A foot orthotic with posting thereby decreases the compensation caused by the individual's structural abnormality. Rear-foot posting is placed under the heel of the shell, and forefoot posting runs under the metatarsal area to the end of the shell. Medial or varus rearfoot posting is indicated for a subtalar varus or a genu varus abnormality. Varus forefoot posting is indicated for a forefoot varus abnormality. Lateral or valgus forefoot posting is indicated for a forefoot valgus abnormality.

Foot and ankle exercises such as calf stretching, arch lifts, toe claws, and single-leg standing balance drills can help prepare the foot before orthotic therapy. Foot orthotic therapy requires a break-in period of 1 to 6 weeks. During the break-in period, the orthotics are worn intermittently, perhaps as little as 1 to 2 hours per day, with a 1-hour progression each day. The break-in period can be accelerated based on orthotic tolerance and nature of the injury. Open chain exercises established before orthotic wear should continue. Closed chain exercise in the orthotics should be progressed slowly. Initially, patients can be instructed to actively supinate off of the orthotic and slowly lower onto it. Static weight-shifting drills can be progressed to exercise involving higher ground reaction forces. Athletic activity should not begin until light activity is well tolerated.

Foot orthotics must be reassessed for wear and breakdown, as periodic refurbishment or upgrading may be necessary. During the orthotic reassessment, the patient's foot and function should also be reexamined. Alignment resulting from anatomic impairments does not change, but the patient's ability to control his or her compensation may improve. Alignment resulting from physiologic impairments may change. Day-to-day orthotic wear and wear for various activities may be adjusted. The reassessment schedule varies with each individual, ranging from 1 week to 1 year after the break-in period.

Heel and Full Sole Lifts

Heel lifts are commonly used for correction of leg length discrepancies. Heel lifts should be isolated for use in equinus contractures and not used for correction of leg length discrepancies. Full sole lifts are more appropriate for the treatment of leg length discrepancies, because the heel is in contact with the ground for only a short period in the gait cycle. After the loading response phase is completed and the foot enters the midstance phase, the forefoot is in contact with the ground. If the lift is only in the heel, the foot functions as if it is descending a small step after the forefoot contacts the ground. The full sole lift eliminates this problem. However, the disadvantage of the full sole lift is that it can occupy excessive room within the shoe. Typically, if a lift beyond 1/8 in is recommended, it should be added to the outside of the shoe. The prescription of a sole lift should be considered carefully, because an apparent leg length discrepancy often is functional and not structural.

Please refer to Chapter 19 for a detailed description of functional versus structural leg length discrepancy. A functional leg length discrepancy often can be treated with therapeutic exercise intervention, focusing on alignment and movement impairments throughout the kinetic chain. The use of a lift for a functional leg length discrepancy can capture and reinforce the alignment impairment rather than resolve the impairment.

Heel lifts can be helpful in the treatment of foot and ankle dysfunctions related to limited motion of the talocrural joint. A lack of 10 degrees of talocrural joint dorsiflexion can result in compensatory subtalar joint pronation during midstance and propulsion. A heel lift places the talocrural joint in a few degrees of plantar flexion at midstance (Fig. 21-17). This increases the available range of dorsiflexion and decreases the abnormal compensation.

Heel lifts can be used in the acute phase to decrease strain on the Achilles tendon, talocrural joint, and subtalar joint. Early ambulation with less pain increases independent

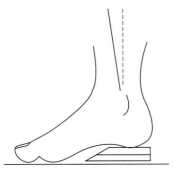

FIGURE 21-17. A heel lift is used to increase the range of dorsiflexion at midstance.

function and enhances the effects of an exercise program. The goal is to normalize the impairment and remove the heel lifts.

If a heel lift is necessary, the following information can guide the proper amount of lift to prescribe. A patient with 0 degrees dorsiflexion may require a 3/4- to 1-in heel lift. Less severe limitations can be treated with smaller lifts. A 1/4- to 3/8-in lift can be placed inside the shoe. The lift depends on shoe style and fit. All or some portion of the lift can be added to the sole of the shoe by a shoe repair service. A lift of the same height should be added to the uninvolved extremity to avoid creating a leg length discrepancy.

 SELECTED INTERVENTION 21-1
For the Lower Quadrant

See Case Study No. 1.

Although this patient requires comprehensive intervention as described in previous chapters, only one exercise prescribed in the final stage of recovery is described.

ACTIVITY: Lunging ball drill

PURPOSE: Improve balance, proprioception, and agility

RISK FACTORS: 10 weeks after second-degree sprain of the right calcaneofibular ligament

ELEMENT OF THE MOVEMENT SYSTEM: Modulator

STAGE OF MOTOR CONTROL: Skill

POSTURE: Standing in "ready" position with knees flexed

MOVEMENT: Step forward and lunge as ball is tossed toward you

SPECIAL CONSIDERATIONS: Be sure foot lands in a good position and that it is in good alignment with respect to the knee, hip, pelvis, and spine.

DOSAGE
   Special Considerations
Anatomic: Calcaneofibular ligament

Physiologic: Late-stage recovery from grade II sprain

Learning Capability: Good body awareness and coordination, should be no trouble

Repetitions/sets: To form fatigue, pain, or 20 to 30 repetitions, up to three sets

Frequency: Every other day

Sequence: Following warm-up of light activity and stretching

Speed: Functional speed

Environment: Home with a partner

Feedback: Initially in clinic with mirror and verbal feedback, tapered to no mirror in home environment

FUNCTIONAL MOVEMENT PATTERN TO REINFORCE GOAL OF SPECIFIC EXERCISE: Play basketball with same form

EXPLANATION OF CHOICE OF EXERCISE: Chosen as skill-level activity to prepare patient for return to basketball. Patient will require excellent balance, proprioception, and agility to return to basketball without recurrent ankle sprain. High repetitions of this exercise for 2 to 3 weeks should prepare patient for basketball without recurrent injury.

▼ **LAB ACTIVITIES**

1. Perform resisted ankle dorsiflexion, plantar flexion, inversion, and eversion using a variety of resistive bands. Perform exercises in long-sitting and short-sitting positions and while standing on one leg. What are the most likely substitutions in each position?
2. Instruct a laboratory partner in correct lower extremity standing posture.
3. Perform the following exercises, maintaining subtalar neutral position and exaggerating pronation. Observe the differences in alignment throughout the lower extremity:

   a. Wall slide
   b. Single-leg wall slide
   c. Step down
   d. Standing on a minitramp
   e. Stair stepper, forward and backward

4. Consider the patient in Case Study No. 1 in Unit 7. Design a rehabilitation program for this athlete in the early, intermediate, and late phases. Instruct your patient in the exercise program, and have your patient perform all exercises.

KEY POINTS

- The three main joints of the ankle and foot are the talocrural, subtalar, and midtarsal, which is further subdivided into the calcaneocuboid and talonavicular.
- The medial collateral ligament controls medial joint stability and controls the extremes of plantar flexion and dorsiflexion in the ankle and foot. The lateral collateral ligament controls lateral joint stability and checks extremes of ROM along with the medial collateral ligament.
- The extrinsic muscles consist of the anterior, lateral, and posterior groups. The anterior group allows dorsiflexion, the lateral group functions as evertors, and the posterior group functions as plantar flexors. The intrinsic muscle group is composed of four layers.
- The functions of the foot during gait are shock absorption, load transmission, surface adaptation, and propulsion.
- The foot and ankle examination must include a subjective history and evaluation of the weight-bearing and non–weight-bearing foot. Relationships of the lower extremity joints must be evaluated.
- Common lower extremity anatomic impairments include subtalar varus, forefoot varus, and forefoot valgus.
- The common physiologic impairments at the foot are mobility loss, loss of force or torque production, impaired posture and movement, pain, and impaired balance and coordination.
- The therapeutic exercise program must consider the kinetics and kinematics of the foot during gait.
- Adjunctive agents may be necessary to treat the structural impairment or to prevent secondary problems associated with physiologic impairments.

CRITICAL THINKING QUESTIONS

1. Consider Case Study No. 1 in Unit 7. How would the treatment program differ if the patient was
   a. A competitive runner
   b. A landscaper walking on uneven surfaces
   c. An elderly individual who is a community walker
   d. A recreational golfer
2. Consider again Case Study No. 1 in Unit 7. The patient has progressed well with your interventions and demonstrates full ankle ROM and extrinsic muscle strength. However, her balance remains faulty. How would you modify your treatment to both address her balance and help her return to basketball? How would you progress the balance program as she improves?
3. Consider Case Study No. 9 in Unit 7. Theorize about potential relationships between this patient's plantar fasciitis, her thigh pain, and other symptoms. Describe a comprehensive treatment program for this individual.
4. Consider again Case Study No. 9 in Unit 7. The patient's thigh pain has improved moderately but has plateaued. Assuming her posture and hip muscle strength is improving and she is regularly performing her home program, what other factors might you consider addressing to drive further symptoms resolution?

REFERENCES

1. Rush SM, Christensen JC, Johnson CH. Biomechanics of the first ray. Part 2: metatarsus primus varus as a cause of hypermobility. A three-dimensional kinematic analysis in a cadaver model. J foot Ankle Surg 2000;39:68–77.
2. Glasoe WM, Yack HJ, Saltzman CL. Anatomy and biomechanics of the first ray. Phys Ther 1999;79:854–859.
3. Kessler RM, Hertling D. Management of Common Musculoskeletal Disorders. New York, NY: Harper & Row, 1983.
4. Donatelli RA, ed. The Biomechanics of the Foot and Ankle. Philadelphia, PA: FA Davis, 1990.
5. Dutton M. Orthopaedic Examinatoin, Evaluation, & Intervention. New York, NY: McGraw-Hill, 2004.
6. Lorimer D, French G, O'Donnell M, et al. Neale's Disorders of the Foot: Diagnosis and Management. 7th Ed. Oxford: Churchill Livingstone, 2006.
7. Hawke F, Burns J. Understanding the nature and mechanism of foot pain. J Foot Ankle Res [serial online]. January 14, 2009.
8. Magee DJ. Orthopedic Physical Assessment. 3rd Ed. Philadelphia, PA: WB Saunders, 1997.
9. Hoppenfeld S. Physical Examination of the Spine and Extremities. New York, NY: Appleton-Century-Crofts, 1976.
10. Gould JA, Davies GJ. Orthopedic and Sports Physical Therapy. St. Louis, MO: CV Mosby, 1985.
11. McKeon PO, Hertel J. Spatiotemporal postural control defiicts are present in those with chronic ankle instability. BMC Musculoskelet Disord 2008;9: 76–81.
12. Mattacola CH, Dwyer MK. Rehabilitation of the ankle after acute sprain or chronic instability. J Athl Train 2002;37:413–429.
13. Coughlan G, Caulfield B. A 4-week neuromuscular training program and gait patterns at the ankle joint. J Athl Train 2007;42:51–59.
14. Bampton S. A Guide to the Visual Examination of Pathological Gait. Philadelphia: Temple University Rehabilitation and Training Center No. 8, 1979.
15. Barton CJ, Bonanno D, Menz HB. Development and evaluation of a tool for the assessment of footwear characteristics. J Foot Ankle Res [serial online]. April 23, 2009.
16. Gerber P, Williams GN, Scoville CR, et al. Persistent disability associated with ankle sprains: a prospective examination of an athletic population. Foot Ankle Int 1998;19:653–660.
17. Adirim TA, Cheng TL. Overview of injuries in the young athlete. Sports Med 2003;33:75–81.
18. Safran MR, Benedetti RS, Bartolozzi AR, et al. Lateral ankle sprains a comprehensive review. Part 1: etiology, pathoanatomy, histopathogenesis, and diagnosis. Med Sci Sports Exerc 1999;31:S429–S437.
19. Liu SH, Jason WJ. Lateral ankle sprains and instability problems. Clin Sports Med 1994;13:793–808.
20. Roy S, Irivn R. Sports Medicine: Prevention, Education, Management and Rehabilitation, Englewood Cliffs, NJ: Prentice-Hall, 1983.
21. Subotnick SI, ed. Sports Medicine of the Lower Extremity. New York, NY: Churchill Livingstone, 1989.
22. Subotnick SI. Podiatric Sports Medicine. Mount Kisco, NY: Futura Publishing, 1975.
23. Safran MR, Zachazewski JE, Benedettie RS, et al. Lateral ankle sprains. Part 2: treatment and rehabilitation with an emphasis on the athlete. Med Sci Sports Exerc 1999;31:S438–S447.
24. Kern-Steiner R, Washecheck HS, Kelsey DD. Strategy of exercise prescription using an unloading technique for functional rehabilitation of an athlete with an inversion ankle sprain. J Orthop Sports Phys Ther 1999;29: 282–287.
25. Kerkhoffs GM, Struijs PA, Marti RK, et al. Different functional treatment strategies for acute lateral ankle ligament injuries in adults. Cochrane Database Syst Rev 2002;3:CDOO2938.
26. Green T, Refshauge K, Crosbie J, et al. A randomized controlled trial of a passive accessory joint mobilization on acute ankle inversion sprains. Phys Ther 2001;81:984–994.
27. Friel K, McLean N, Myers C, et al. Ipsilateral hip abductor weakness after inversion ankle sprain. J Athl Train 2006;41:74–78.
28. Sekir U, Yikdiz Y, Hazneci B, et al. Reliability of a functional test battery evaluating functionality, proprioception, and strength in recreational athletes with functional ankle instability. Eur J Phys Rehabil Med 2008;44:407–415.
29. Kisner C, Colby LA. Therapeutic Exercise: Foundations and Techniques. 4th Ed. Philadelphia, PA: FA Davis Company, 2002.
30. Sacco ICM, Takahasi HY, Suda EY, et al. Ground reaction force in basketball cutting maneuvers with and without ankle bracing and taping. Sao Paulo Med J 2006;124:245–252.
31. Nishikawa T, Grabiner MD. Peroneal motoneuron excitability increases immediately following application of a semirigid ankle brace. J Orthop Sports Phys Ther 1999;29:168–176.
32. Nishikawa T, Ozaki T, Mizuno K, et al. Increased reflex activation of the peroneus longus following application of an ankle brace declines over time. J Orthop Res 2002;20:1323–1326.
33. Refshauge KM, Kilbreath SL, Raymond J. Deficits in detection of inversion and eversion movements among subjects with recurrent ankle sprains. J Orthop Sports Phys Ther 2003;33:166–167.

34. Cordova ML, Ingersoll CD. Peroneus longus stretch reflex amplitude increases after ankle brace application. Br J Sports Med 2003;37:258–262.

35. Specchiulli F, Cofano RE. A comparison of surgical and conservative treatment in ankle ligament tears. Orthopedics 2001;27:686–688.

36. Hubbard TJ, Hicks-Little CA. Ankle ligament healing after an acute ankle sprain: an evidence-based approach. J Athl Train 2008;43:523–529.

37. Riemann BL. Is there a link between chronic ankle instability and postural instability? J Athl Train 2002;37:386–393.

38. McKeon PO, Hertel J. Systematic review of postural control and lateral ankle instability, part II: is balance training clinically effective? J Athl Train 2008;43:305–315.

39. Inman VT, Ralston HJ, Todd P. Human Walking. Baltimore, MD: Williams & Wilkins, 1981.

40. Lauge-Hansen N. Fractures of the ankle: genetic roentgenologic diagnosis of fracture of the ankle. Am J Roentgenol Radium Ther Nucl Med 1954;71:456.

41. Michelson J, Solocoff D, Waldman B, et al. Ankle fractures. Clin Orthop Rel Res 1997;345:198–205.

42. Shaffer MA, Okereke E, Esterhai JL, et al. Effects of immobilization on plantar-flexion torque, fatigue resistance, and functional ability following an ankle fracture. Phys Ther 2000;80:769–780.

43. Nilsson G, Jonsson K, Ekdahl C, et al. Outcome and quality of life after surgically treated ankle fractures in patients 65 years or older. BMC Musculoskelet Disord 2007;8:127–135.

44. Mondelli M, Giannini F, Reale F. Clinical and electrophysiological findings and follow-up in tarsal tunnel syndrome. Electroencephalogr Clin Neurophysiol 1998;109:418–425.

45. Galardi G, Amadio S, Maderna L, et al. Electrophysiologic studies in tarsal tunnel syndrome. Am J Phys Med Rehabil 1994;73:193–198.

46. Antoniadis G, Scheglmann K. Posterior tarsal tunnel syndrome: diagnosis and treatment. Dtsch Arztebl Int 2008;105:776–781.

47. Kinoshits M, Okuda R, Morikawa J, et al. The dorsiflexion-eversion test for diagnosis of tarsal tunnel syndrome. J Bone Joint Surg 2001;83:1835–1839.

48. Reade BM, Longo DC, Keller MC. Tarsal tunnel syndrome. Clin Podiatr Med Surg 2001;18:395–408.

49. Akyuz G, Us O, Turan B, et al. Anterior tarsal tunnel syndrome. Electromyogr Clin Nuerophysiol 2000;40:123–128.

50. Simoneau GG. Kinesiology of walking. In: Neumann DA. Kinesiology of the Musculoskeletal System: Foundations for Physical Rehabilitation. St. Louis, MO: Mosby, 2002.

51. Kappel-Bargas A, Woolf RD, Cornwall MW, et al. The windlass mechanism during normal walking and passive first metatarsalphalangeal joint extension. Clin Biomech 1998;13:190–194.

52. Thordarson DB, Kumar PJ, Hedman TP, et al. Effect of partial versus complete plantar fasciotomy on the windlass mechanism. Foot Ankle Int 1997;18:16–20.

53. Fuller EA. The windlass mechanism of the foot. J Am Podiatr Med Assoc 2000;90:35–36.

54. Roxas M. Plantar fasciitis: diagnosis and therapeutic considerations. Altern Med Rev 2005;10:83–93.

55. Cornwall MW, McPoil TG. Plantar fasciitis: etiology and treatment. J Orthop Sports Phys Ther 1999;29:756–760.

56. Crosby W, Humble RN. Rehabilitation of the plantar fascitis. Clin Podiatr Med Surg 2001;18:225–231.

57. Cole C, Seto C, Gazewood J. Plantar fasciitis: evidence-based review of diagnosis and therapy. Am Fam Physician 2005;72:2237–2242.

58. Barrett SL, O'Malley R. Plantar fasciitis and other causes of heel pain. Am Family Physician 1999;59:2200–2206.

59. Osborne HR, Allison GT. Treatment of plantar fasciitis by LowDye taping and iontophoresis: short term results of a double blinded, randomised, placebo controlled clinical trial of dexamethasone and acetic acid. Br J Sports Med 2006;40:545–549.

60. Costa IA, Dyson A. The integration of acetic acid iontophoresis, orthotic therapy and physical rehabilitation for chronic plantar fasciitis: a case study. J Can Chiropr Assoc 2007;51:166–174.

61. Pfeffer G, Bacchetti P, Deland J, et al. Comparison of custom and prefabricated orthoses in the initial treatment of proximal plantar fasciitis. Foot Ankle Int 1999;20:214–221.

62. Barry LD, Barry AN, Chen Y. A retrospective study of standing gastrocnemius-soleus stretching versus night splinting in the treatment of plantar fasciitis. J Foot Ankle Surg 2002;41:221–227.

63. Radford JA, Landorf KB, Buchbinder R, et al. Effectiveness of calf muscle stretching for the short-term treatment of plantar heel pain: a randomised trial. BMC Musculoskelet Disord 2007;8:36–43.

64. Kohls-Gatzoulis J, Angel JC, Singh D, et al. Tibialis posterior dysfunction: a common and treatable cause of adult acquired flatfoot. BMJ 2004;329:328–1333.

65. Geideman WM, Johnson JE. Posterior tibial tendon dysfunction. J Orthop Sports Phys Ther 2000;30:68–77.

66. Mendicino SS. Posterior tibial tendon dysfunction. Clin Podiatr Med Surg 2000;17:33–55.

67. Kulig K, Pomrantz AB, Burnfield JM, et al. Non-operative management of posterior tibialis tendon dysfunction: design of a randomized clinical trial. BMC Musculoskelet Disord 2006;7:49–54.

68. Chao W, Wapner KL, Lee TH, et al. Nonoperative management of posterior tibial tendon dysfunction. Foot Ankle Int 1996;17:736–741.

69. Craig DI. Medial tibial stress syndrome: evidence-based prevention. J Athl Train 2008;43:316–318.

70. Raissi GRD, Cherati ADS, Mansoori KD, et al. The relationship between lower extremity alignment and medila tibial stress syndrome among non-professional athletes. Sports Med Arthrosc Rehabil Ther Technol 2009;1:11–18.

71. Starkey C, Ryan J. Evaluation of Orthopedic and Athletic Injuries. 2nd Ed. Philadelphia, PA: FA Davis Company, 2002.

72. Alfredson H, Thorsen K, Lorentzon R. In situ microdialysis in tendon tissue: high levels of glutamate, but not prostaglandin E2 (make small) in chronic Achilles tendon pain. Knee Surg Sports Traumatol Arthrosc 1999;7: 378–381.

73. Mazzone MF, McCue T. Common conditions of the Achilles tendon. Am Fam Physician 2002;65:1805–1836.

74. Eriksson E. Tendinosis of the patellar and achilles tendon. Knee Surg Sports Traumatol Arthrosc 2002;10:1.

75. Cook JL, Khan KM, Purdam C. Achilles tendinopathy. Man Ther 2002;7: 121–130.

76. Maffulli N, Khan KM, Pudda G. Overuse tendon conditions: time to change a confusing terminology. Arthroscopy 1998;14:840–843.

77. Humble RN, Nugent LL. Achilles tendonitis: an overview and reconditioning model. Clin Podiatr Med Surg 2001;18:233–254.

78. Schepsis AA, Jones H, Haas AL. Achilles tendon disorders in athletes. Am J Sports Med 2002;30:287–305.

79. Kvist, M. Achilles tendon injuries in athletes. Sports Med 1994;18:173–201.

80. McCrory JL, Martin DF, Lowery RB, et al. Etiologic factors associated with Achilles tendinitis in runners. Med Sci Sports Exerc 1999;31:1374–1381.

81. Rees JD, Wilson AM, Wolman RL. Current concepts in the management of tendon disorders. Rheumatology 2006;45:508–521.

82. Gibbon WW, Cooper JR, Radcliffe GS. Distribution of sonographically detected tendon abnormalities in patients with a clinical diagnosis of chronic Achilles tendinosis. J Clin Ultrasound 2000;28:61–66.

83. Beneka AG, Malliou PC, Benekas G. Water and land based rehabilitation for Achilles tendinopathy in an elite female runner. Br J Sports Med 2003;37:535–537.

84. Mafi N, Lorentzon R, Alfredson H. Superior short-term results with eccentric calf muscle training compared to concentric training in a randomized prospective multicenter study on patients with chronic Achilles tendinosis. Knee Surg Sports Traumatol Arthrosc 2001;9:42–47.

85. Ohberg L, Lorentzon R, Alfredson H. Eccentric training in patients with chronic Achilles tendinosis: normalised tendon structure and decreased thickness at follow up. Br J Sports Med 2004;38:8–11.

86. Kannus P, Jozsa L. Histopathological changes preceding spontaneous rupture of a tendon. J Bone Joint Surg 1991;73:1507–1525.

87. Twaddle BC, Poon P. Early motion for Achilles tendon ruptures: is surgery important? Am J Sports Med 2007;35:2033–2038.

88. Rydholm U. Editorial: is total replacement of the ankle an option? Acta Orthopaedica 2007;78:567–568.

89. Wood PLR, Deakin S. Total ankle replacement: the results in 200 ankles. J Bone Joint Surg [Br] 2003;85-B:334–341.

90. Henricson A, Skoog A, Carlsson A. The Swedish ankle arthroplasty register: an analysis of 531 arthroplasties between 1993 and 2005. Acta Orthopaedica 2007;78:569–574.

91. Cornwall MW. Foot and Ankle Orthoses. La Crosse, WI: APTA Inc., 2000.

RECOMMENDED READING

D'Ambrosia R, Drez D. Prevention and Treatment of Running Injuries. Thorofare, NJ: Slack, 1989.

Kendall FP, McCreary EK, Provance PG. Muscles Testing and Function. Baltimore, MD: Williams & Wilkins, 1993.

Langer S, Wernick J. A Practical Manual for a Basic Approach to Biomechanics. Wheeling, IL: Langer Biomechanics Group, 1989.

McPoil TG, Cornwall MW. The relationship between static measurements of the lower extremity and the pattern of rearfoot motion during walking [abstract]. Phys Ther 1994;74:S141.

McPoil TG, Knecht HG, Schuit D. A survey of foot types between the ages of 18 to 30 years. J Orthop Sports Phys Ther 1988;9:406–409.

Root ML, Orien WP, Weed JH. Neutral Position Casting Techniques. Los Angeles, CA: Clinical Biomechanics Corporation, 1971.

Functional Approach to Therapeutic Exercise for the Upper Extremities

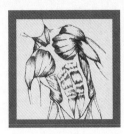

chapter 22

The Temporomandibular Joint

DARLENE HERTLING

WITH CONTRIBUTIONS BY LISA DUSSAULT

The temporomandibular joint (TMJ) cannot be viewed in isolation. Its relationships with the cranium, jaw, and cervical spine are important in function and dysfunction and should be acknowledged in assessment and management strategies. TMJ dysfunction can be the result of a problem anywhere along this kinetic chain. The TMJ is unique because its function is directly related to dentition and the contacting tooth surfaces. Problems with the TMJ can directly influence occlusion and vice versa. A comprehensive approach to the treatment of the TMJ addresses the person as a whole by taking into account these relationships, the performance of functional activities, and the influence of physical and emotional stress on this system.

This chapter provides a brief review of TMJ anatomy and kinesiology and supplies guidelines for the basic examination and evaluation. It covers treatment interventions for common physiologic impairments and common diagnoses affecting the TMJ.

REVIEW OF ANATOMY AND KINESIOLOGY

In referring to the TMJs, the masticatory system, its component structures, and all the tissues related to it, the term *stomatognathic system* is used. This system has several components:

- Bones of the skull, mandible, maxilla, hyoid, clavicle, sternum, shoulder girdle, and cervical vertebrae
- TMJ and dentoalveolar joints (i.e., joints of the teeth)
- Teeth
- Cervical spine
- Regional vascular, lymphatic, and nervous systems
- Muscles and soft tissues of the head and neck and muscles of the cheeks, lips, and tongue

Kinematically, the joints and muscles of this system interact to influence the alignment and function of the mandible in the TMJ. Functional activities such as talking and eating are affected by the kinematics of this system.

Bones

The mandible, the largest and strongest bone of the face, articulates with the two temporal bones and accommodates the lower teeth. It is composed of a horizontal portion, called the body, and two perpendicular portions, called the rami, which unite with the end of the body nearly at right angles. Each ramus has two processes: the coronoid process and the condylar process. The coronoid process serves as an insertion for the temporalis and masseter muscles. The condylar process consists of the neck and the condyle. The condyle, which is convex, articulates with the disk (Fig. 22-1). The two condyles form the floor of the TMJ.

The roof of the TMJ consists entirely of the squamous part of the temporal bone, and it is divided into four descriptive parts:

1. Articular tubercle
2. Articular eminence
3. Mandibular fossa
4. Posterior glenoid spine

The hyoid bone is a horseshoe-shaped bone at the level of C3 and acts as an attachment for the suprahyoid and infrahyoid muscles (Fig. 22-2). The greater wings of the sphenoid bone join into the pterygoid plates that serve as an attachment for the medial and lateral pterygoid muscles (Fig. 22-3).

Osteokinematically, three basic movements exist within the mandible: depression, protrusion, and lateral excursion. These three basic movements can be combined to produce an infinite variety of mandibular motions.

Joints

There are two TMJs, one on either side of the jaw. Both joints must be considered together with the teeth (i.e., the trijoint complex) in an examination.[1] The TMJ is a synovial, condyloid joint found between the mandibular fossa of the temporal bone and the condylar process of the mandibular bone (see Fig. 22-1). The two bony surfaces are covered with collagen fibrocartilage rather than the hyaline cartilage found in most synovial joints of the body. The presence of fibrocartilage is significant because of its ability to repair and to remodel.[2]

The articular disk, or meniscus, also consists of pliable collagen fibrocartilage, but it lacks the ability to repair or remodel. This biconcave disk divides each joint into two cavities (an upper and a lower joint cavities) and compensates functionally for the incongruity of the two opposing joint surfaces (see Fig. 22-1). During opening and closing, the convex surface of the condylar head must move across the convex surface of the articular eminence.

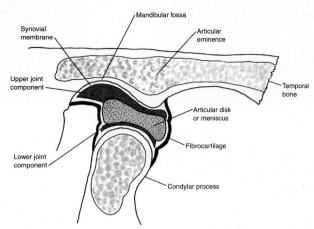

FIGURE 22-1. Articular structures of the TMJ in the closed position.

Kinematically, the mandible may be considered a free body that can rotate in angular directions. It has three degrees of freedom. The basic accessory movements required for functional motion are rotation, translation, distraction, compression, and lateral glide.[3] Accessory movements most often restricted because of periarticular tissue tightness and disk displacement are lateral glide, translation, and distraction. According to Kraus,[4] of these accessory movements, translation causes the most limitation of osteokinematic movement of the mandible and is more difficult to restore. Gliding movements occur in the upper cavity of the joint, whereas rotation or hinge movements occur in the lower cavity. Gliding and rotation are essential for opening and closing the mouth.

The capsule of the TMJ is thin and loose. The capsule and the disk are attached to one another anteriorly and posteriorly but are not attached medially or laterally. Because there are no medial and lateral attachments of the disk and capsule, translation (anteriorly) of the disk can occur within the capsule. The posterior ligament attaches the disk to the posterior aspect of the neck of the mandible, in the bilaminar zone, and the posterior portion of the TMJ.[1–6]

The strongest ligamentous attachments are on the medial side, such as the mediodisco ligament (i.e., Tanaka ligament).[5,6] The TMJ has no capsule on the medial half of the anterior

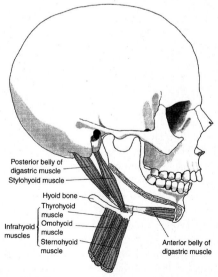

FIGURE 22-2. Hyoid bone and the digastric, stylohyoid, and infrahyoid muscles.

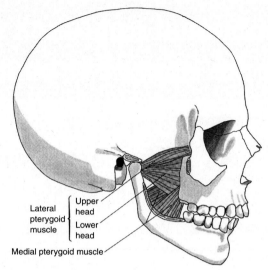

FIGURE 22-3. Medial and lateral pterygoid muscles.

aspect, which allows excessive translation of the condyle, leading to joint pathology.[7] The TMJ can actively displace anteriorly and slightly displace laterally.[2]

The rest position, or loose-packed position, for the TMJ is with the mouth slightly open so the teeth are not in contact. The rest position of the tongue, often referred to as the postural position, is with the first half of the tongue against the hard palate of the mouth.[8,9] Tongue up, teeth apart, and lips closed (TUTALC) is the functional rest position that should be taught to the patient.

There are two closed-packed positions: maximal anterior position of the condyle with maximal opening and maximal retrusion in which the ligaments are taut and the condyle cannot go farther back. The mouth is closed, and the teeth are clenched. In bilateral restriction, the capsular pattern of restriction produces significant loss of lateral movements and limits opening of the mouth and protrusion. In unilateral capsular patterns of restriction, contralateral excursions are most limited. During mouth opening, the mandible deviates toward the restricted side.

The normal range of mandibular opening is 40 to 50 mm. The range of motion (ROM) is considered functional for most jaw activities if 40 mm of opening is possible. This motion should be composed of 25 mm of rotation and 15 mm of translation.[10] To achieve the initial 25-mm opening, rotation occurs between the mandibular condyle and the inferior surface of the disk. The last 15 to 25 mm is the result of anterior translation between the superior surface of the disk and the temporal bone.

Muscles

The functions of all the muscles of the upper quadrant need to be understood because of their impact on TMJ function and dysfunction. The movements of the mandible are the result of the action of the cervical and jaw muscles:

- Elevation
- Depression
- Protraction
- Retraction
- Lateral gliding

All of these movements are used to some extent when chewing. Because the TMJ is bilateral, the muscles of mastication must activate and relax in a regular pattern and in perfect synchronization with the muscles on the contralateral side. Muscles often need to be reeducated after trauma; surgical procedures; and long-standing parafunctional activity, including habitual excessive use of biting force, such as clenching, nail biting, and forced mandibular opening on an unstable occlusion. Muscles can be reeducated by the use of exercise, biofeedback, and functional electrical stimulation.

Main Muscles of Temporomandibular Joint Motion

Five main muscles contribute to TMJ motion:

1. Temporalis
2. Masseter
3. Medial pterygoid
4. Lateral pterygoid
5. Digastric

These muscles also connect the cranium to the mandible along with the buccinator and superior pharyngeal constrictor.[11]

The three major elevator muscles of the mandible are the temporalis, the masseter, and the medial pterygoid. All of the fibers of the temporalis (Fig. 22-4 and Table 22-1)

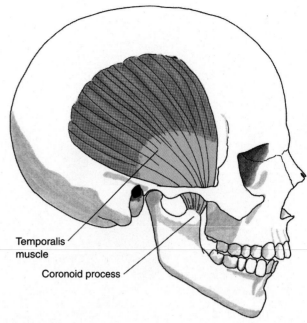

Temporalis muscle

Coronoid process

FIGURE 22-4. Temporalis muscle.

TABLE 22-1 Muscles and Nerves of the Mandible

MUSCLE AND NERVE (N)	ORIGIN	INSERTION	FUNCTION
Digastric N: trigeminal and facial	Anterior belly: depression on the inner side of the inferior border of the mandible. Posterior belly: mastoid notch of the temporal bone	Common tendon to the hyoid bone	Mandibular depression and elevation of the hyoid (in swallowing)
Temporalis N: mandibular division of the trigeminal nerve	Temporal fossa and deep surface of the temporal fascia	Medial and anterior coronoid processus and anterior ramus of the mandible	Elevates mandible to close the mouth and approximates teeth (biting motion); retracts the mandible and participates in lateral grinding motions
Masseter N: mandibular division of the trigeminal nerve	Superficial: zygomatic arch and maxillary process. Deep portion: zygomatic arch	Angle and lower half of the lateral ramus. Lateral coronoid and superior ramus	Elevates the mandible; active in up and down biting motions and occlusion of the teeth in mastication
Medial pterygoid N: mandibular division of the trigeminal nerve	Greater wing of the sphenoid and the pyramidal processus of the palatine bone	Medial ramus and angle of the mandibular foramen	Elevates the mandible to close the mouth; protrudes the mandible (with lateral pterygoid). Unilaterally, the medial and lateral pterygoids rotate the mandible forward and to the opposite side
Lateral pterygoid N: mandibular division of the trigeminal nerve	Superior: inferior crest of the greater wing of sphenoid bones. Inferior: lateral surface of the pterygoid plate	Articular disk, capsule, and condyle. Neck of the mandible and the medial condyle	Protracts mandibular condyle and disk of the TMJ forward, while the mandibular head rotates on the disk; aids in opening the mouth. Joint action of the medial and lateral pterygoids rotates the mandible forward and to the opposite side
Mylohyoid N: mylohyoid branch of the trigeminal nerve	Medial surface of the mandible, entire length	Body of the hyoid bone (floor of the mouth)	Elevates the hyoid bone and tongue for swallowing; depresses the mandible when fixed
Geniohyoid N: ventral ramus of C1 through the hypoglossal nerve	Mental spine of the mandible	Body of the hyoid bone	Assists in depression of the mandible; elevates and protracts the hyoid bone; moves the tongue forward
Stylohyoid N: facial	Styloid process of the temporal bone	Body of the hyoid bone	Draws the hyoid bone upward and backward in swallowing; assists in opening the mouth and participates in mastication

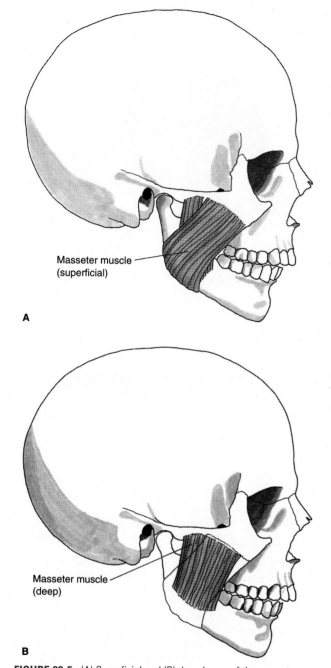

FIGURE 22-5. (A) Superficial and (B) deep layers of the masseter muscle.

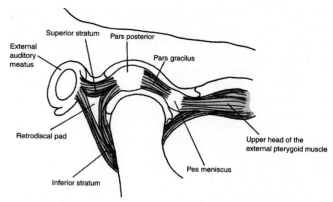

FIGURE 22-6. Sagittal section of the TMJ. The lateral pterygoid inserts into the mandibular condyle and the disk. The disk has three parts: (1) a thick anterior band (pes meniscus), (2) a thicker posterior band (pars posterior), and (3) a thin intermediate zone (pars gracilis) between the two bands.

suprahyoids are active during forced opening of the mandible, when the hyoid bone is fixed by the infrahyoid muscle group.

The lateral pterygoid inserts into the mandibular condyle and articular disk and plays a large role in stabilization of the TMJ (Fig. 22-6). The inferior fibers are active in conjunction with mandibular depressors during mandibular opening and protraction. The superior fibers (upper head) of the lateral pterygoid (see Fig. 22-3 and Table 22-1) act in concert with the elevator muscles during closing. Their role is to decelerate and prevent invagination of the joint capsule with the closure of the mandible.[5] Because the attachment of the superior and inferior fibers is mostly medial, they pull the condyle and disk in a medial direction.

Suprahyoid and Infrahyoid Muscles

The lingual surface of the mandible, anterior to the muscles of mastication, is composed of the suprahyoid muscles. These muscles influence jaw position and play an important role in tongue mobility, speech, mandibular depression, manipulating boluses of food, and swallowing.[11] The suprahyoids consist of the mylohyoid, geniohyoid (Fig. 22-7 and see Table 22-1), and the paired digastric and stylohyoid muscles (see Fig. 22-2).

The infrahyoid muscles (i.e., sternohyoid, thyrohyoid, sternothyroid, and omohyoid) act together to stabilize the hyoid bone. This provides the suprahyoids with a stable base from which to contract and move the mandible (see Fig. 22-2).

Tongue

The tongue is composed of various intrinsic and extrinsic muscles. The genioglossus is the main muscle responsible for positioning of the tongue in the oral cavity.[4] It is primarily responsible for establishing and maintaining the rest position of the tongue and is active in protracting and elevating the tongue. The resting position of the tongue provides the foundation for the resting muscle tone of the mandibular elevators (i.e., temporalis, masseter, and medial pterygoid)

contribute to elevation for closure, particularly for positioning of the condyle at the end of closure.[5] The masseter (Fig. 22-5 and see Table 22-1) is composed of the deep and superficial bellies. The superficial fibers protract the jaw to some degree, and the deep portion acts as a retractor. The medial pterygoid's function (see Fig. 22-3 and Table 22-1) is similar to the masseter's function, although it is less powerful than the masseter.

The primary muscle responsible for mandibular depression is the digastric (see Fig. 22-2 and Table 22-1).[2,12] The lower portion of the lateral pterygoid and the other

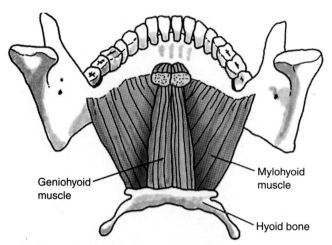

Geniohyoid muscle

Mylohyoid muscle

Hyoid bone

FIGURE 22-7. Mylohyoid and geniohyoid muscles viewed from above and behind the floor of the mouth.

and establishes resting activity of the tongue musculature itself (i.e., jaw-tongue reflex).[4,13–17]

Tongue thrust and other parafunctional habits are often accompanied by an abnormal tongue position against the lingual surface of the mandibular incisors rather than the normal palatal tongue posture.[14–16] Excessive masticatory muscle activity is thought to occur in patients who acquire an altered sequence of swallowing in which tongue thrust occurs.[4] The most frequently cited signs of tongue thrust activity during swallowing include protraction of the tongue against or between the anterior teeth and excessive muscle activity.[15] As a result, the masseter muscles contract incompletely, and there is a concomitant variable state of tension of the orbicularis oris and buccinator muscles.[15] Although tongue thrust is more common in children, it also occurs in adults and is referred to as an acquired adult tongue thrust.[4] It is theorized that tongue movement and positioning in the oral cavity are influenced by the dysfunctional mobility and positioning of the cervical spine[18] (see Building Block 22-1).

Nerves and Blood Vessels

The region is supplied by cranial and cervical nerves. Overlapping of the branches from both types of nerves complicates the neurologic analysis of this region and may account for the extensive range of symptoms in head, TMJ, and cervical dysfunctions.

The innervated tissues of the TMJ are supplied by three nerves that are part of the mandibular division of cranial nerve V. The posterior deep temporal and masseteric nerves supply the medial and anterior regions of the joint, and the

auriculotemporal nerve supplies the posterior and lateral regions of the joint. The auriculotemporal nerve is the major nerve innervating the capsular blood vessels, the retrodiskal pad, the posterolateral capsule, and the TMJ ligament of the TMJ. These tissues have an abundant supply of type IV receptors (i.e., articular pain receptors). Because branches of the auriculotemporal nerve supply the tragus, external acoustic meatus, and tympanic membrane, temporal mandibular dysfunction is often associated with hearing problems, tinnitus, and vertigo.

The external carotid arterial system provides the main vascular supply to the TMJ, masticatory muscles, and associated soft tissues. This vessel divides at the level of the neck of the condyle into the superficial temporal and internal maxillary arteries. The internal maxillary artery and its branches supply the maxilla and mandible, the teeth, and the muscles of mastication. The arterial supply and venous and lymphatic drainage can be clinically significant in patients with head and neck pain. These circulatory systems can be compromised by trauma, disease, changes of the head and neck positions, and muscle spasm.

Kinetics

An overview of the management of the cervical spine muscle imbalances and the relationship of head posture and the rest position of the mandible are included because of the frequently associated muscle hyperactivity and accompanying symptoms observed in the mandibular and cervical spine areas. Functionally, the TMJ, the cervical spine, and the articulations between the teeth are intimately related (Fig. 22-8).

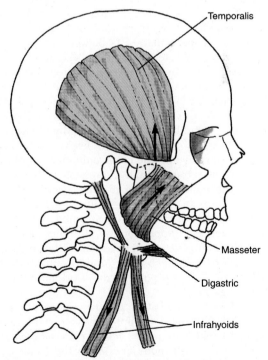

Temporalis

Masseter

Digastric

Infrahyoids

FIGURE 22-8. A lateral view of the head, neck, and mandible showing the muscular forces that flex the head. The infrahyoid muscles pull downward on the hyoid bone. The suprahyoids pull down on the mandible, and the muscles of mastication stabilize the jaw.

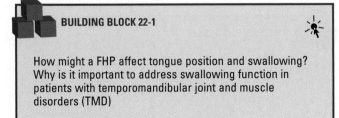

BUILDING BLOCK 22-1

How might a FHP affect tongue position and swallowing? Why is it important to address swallowing function in patients with temporomandibular joint and muscle disorders (TMD)

Muscles attach the mandible to the cranium, the hyoid bone, and the clavicle. The cervical spine is, in essence, interposed between the proximal and the distal attachments of some of the muscles controlling the TMJ.[2] The balance between the flexors and the extensors of the head and neck is affected by the muscles of mastication and the suprahyoid and infrahyoid muscles.[19] Dysfunction in the muscles of mastication or the cervical musculature can easily disturb this balance. The neuromusculature of the cervical and masticatory regions actively influences the function of mandibular movement and cervical positioning.[20-22]

Cervical posture change affects the mandibular path of closure, the mandibular rest position, masticatory muscle activity,[20,21,23] and the occlusal contact patterns. A forward head posture (FHP) is a common postural defect that increases the gravitational forces on the head and often leads to hyperextension of the head (i.e., posterior cranial rotation [PCR] on the neck) (Fig. 22-9A). When the head is held anteriorly, the line of vision extends downward if the normal angle at which the head and neck meet is maintained. To correct for visual needs, the head tilts backward, the neck flexes over the thorax, and the mandible migrates posteriorly.[24] The posterior cervical muscles are shortened and forced to contract excessively to maintain the head in this position, while the anterior submandibular muscles are stretched, resulting in a retraction force on the mandible and an altered occlusal contact pattern. The contracted posterior cervical muscles may entrap the greater occipital nerve and refer pain to the head.[25] Excessive mandibular shuttling (i.e., excursions) between opening and closing, which are necessary for functional activities such as chewing and eating, may lead to hypermobility of the TMJ from overstretching of the capsule.[26]

In the presence of an FHP with no significant PCR (Fig. 22-9B), the suprahyoids shorten, and the infrahyoids lengthen, consequently decreasing or eliminating the freeway space, a space that exists between the upper and the lower arch of the teeth when the mandible is in the rest position.[27,28] The hyoid bone is repositioned superiorly, and the degree of elevation is proportional to the decrease in the cervical lordosis or the increase in the FHP.[27,28] Hyperactivity of the suprahyoids produces a depressive force on the mandible. According to Mannheimer and Rosenthal,[28] when combined with hyoid anchoring by means of the infrahyoids, the net mandibular repositioning effect is one of retraction and depression with increased contact in the molar region. The tonic neck reflex plays a primary role in an individual's ability to achieve correct head-neck posture. FHP is often assumed if tonic neck reflexes or cervical proprioceptive afferents are injured (e.g., whiplash, direct trauma) or are overused (e.g., sports activities, daily postures). The proprioceptive afferents may lose their ability to position the head and neck[7] (see Building Block 22-2).

The FHP is exacerbated by many occupations and activities of daily living (i.e., improper home, work, or driving postures) that require the upper extremities and the head to be positioned more anterior to the trunk than is normal or comfortable.[13,27-29] Another contributing factor is the effect of mouth breathing. The dysfunctional patterns of the mouth-breathing syndrome constitute a chain reaction of body adaptation to abnormal breathing patterns.

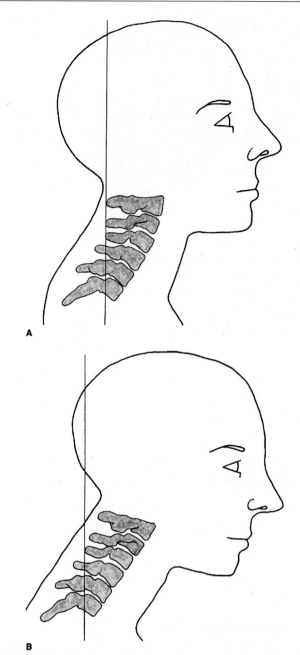

FIGURE 22-9. Types of forward head: (A) increased cervical lordosis with PCR and (B) total flattening out of the cervical lordosis without PCR.

Various investigations have shown that postural relationships change to meet respiratory needs.[16,29] Breathing through the mouth facilitates FHP, a low and forward tongue position (as a result of this pattern, abnormal swallowing ensues),

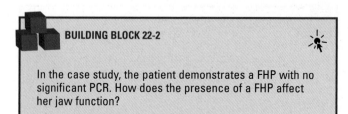

BUILDING BLOCK 22-2

In the case study, the patient demonstrates a FHP with no significant PCR. How does the presence of a FHP affect her jaw function?

CASE STUDY 22-1

The patient is a 21-year-old college student with complaints of 6-week history of limited opening and right-sided jaw pain. Present symptoms include limited opening, right jaw pain, and difficulty with speaking, chewing, and brushing teeth due to pain. History includes 3-year history of right TMJ clicking with occasional pain. The patient reports that she has pain and described it as a dull ache, which worsens with chewing, yawning, and talking. Pain is reported on the visual analogue scale (VAS) at 2/10 at rest, and it will increase to 5/10 with function. Aggravating factors include talking, chewing, yawning, brushing teeth, sleeping position, and clenching. Ease factors include heat, rest, and ibuprofen (600 mg) for pain. 24-hour report: the patient reports increased pain upon waking in the morning and following meals. The patient reports difficulty finding a comfortable sleeping position due to pain, reporting mild sleep disturbance of 1- to 2-hours

sleeplessness. The patient's medical and dental history is noncontributory, and she takes oral contraceptives in addition to the ibuprofen. Management to date included an evaluation by student health services, who recommended scheduled ibuprofen (600 mg three times a day (TID)), soft diet, warm compresses, and referral to therapy.

On opening, the patient demonstrates 25 mm of opening, with pain at end range. No clicking or crepitation is noted. Lateral excursion is 10 mm to the right and 4 mm to the left with pain at end range. Deflection to the right is noted on opening. She reported tenderness with palpation of the right TMJ at the joint line and with palpation of the masseter on the right. Joint play assessment demonstrates decreased mobility of the right TMJ in all planes. The patient demonstrates a FHP; swallowing and breathing functions are normal.

and increased activity of the accessory muscles of respiration (i.e., sternocleidomastoids, scaleni, and pectorals).[7,16,30] This pattern is perpetuated by decreased activity of the diaphragm and hypotonicity of the abdominal musculature.[16] Consequently, many abnormal force vectors are created by abnormal swallow.

EXAMINATION AND EVALUATION

A thorough evaluation of the TMJ includes all components of the stomatognathic system. This assessment assists the therapist in determining the cause of the dysfunction and the influence of other factors and in designing an effective treatment plan.

Subjective Data

A comprehensive history is essential and helps to direct the objective evaluation. The client should provide detailed information about the onset of symptoms, incidence of joint locking, presence of joint noise, history of surgery and trauma, and medical history. Pain should be described in terms of location, intensity, frequency, time of day, and activities that reproduce it. Activity limitations should be addressed along with parafunctional habits. Clients should be asked about their level of psychosocial, environmental, and postural stress, noticing if they sense an increase in clenching or other parafunctional habits when under stress. The type of job a patient has can provide information about posture. Use of a functional outcome questionnaire is helpful in evaluating these patients.

Mobility Impairment Examination

Structures, which must be examined as a possible cause of symptoms, include the TMJ, upper cervical spine, cervical spine, thoracic spine, soft tissues, muscles, and neural tissue. Mobility testing should look at the quality and symmetry of the motions performed to determine the type of dysfunction:

- Active and passive physiologic joint movements of the cervical and thoracic spine
- TMJ: vertical opening, lateral excursion, protrusion (active and passive joint movements)
- Joint function including TMJ rotation and translation
- Joint play
- Muscle tests including muscle length, strength, and control
- Mobility of the nervous system (if indicated)

Pain Examination

Subjective complaints of pain should be evaluated. The client should be asked to point to the site of greatest pain while the therapist notices whether the pain is in the joint or muscular region. Tenderness, warmth, and inflammation should be assessed during palpation and especially when examining several areas:

- Mandible, hyoid bone, and TMJ (note position and prominence)
- Relevant joints of the upper quadrant cervical and upper thoracic spine
- Muscle (masseter, temporalis, medial and lateral pterygoids, splenius capitis, suboccipital, trapezius, sternocleidomastoid, digastric), tendon, tendon sheath, bone, ligament, and nerve
- Relevant trigger points and tender points of fibromyalgia

Special Tests and Other Assessments

Several tests address the functional component of the TMJ complex:

- Segmental stability tests for the atlantoaxial joint
- Oral function
- Occlusion pattern
- Swallowing pattern
- Breathing pattern

The therapist also should evaluate the patient's posture and screen for systemic hypermobility.

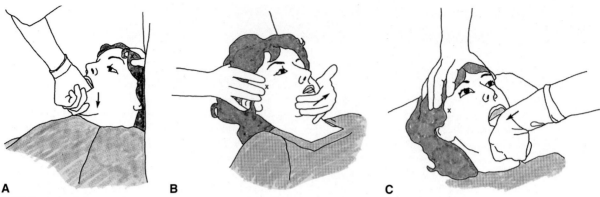

FIGURE 22-10. (A) Interoral distraction. The clinician's thumb is positioned to apply a distraction force. (B) Lateral glide. The clinician's thumb is positioned to apply a lateral glide force. (C) Intraoral translation (ventral glide). The clinician's index and third fingers are positioned to apply translation.

THERAPEUTIC EXERCISE INTERVENTIONS FOR COMMON PHYSIOLOGIC IMPAIRMENT

A treatment plan is implemented after a thorough examination and determination of the diagnosis, activity limitations, and prognosis. Therapeutic exercise interventions should address specific impairments and seek to increase functioning of the TMJ.

Mobility Impairment

Hypomobility

Etiology Mandibular hypomobility (i.e., limitation of functional movements) may result from disorders of the mandible or cranial bone, which include aplasia, dysplasia, hypoplasia, hyperplasia, fractures, and neoplasms.[31] Temporomandibular dysfunctions that can contribute to mandibular hypomobility are ankylosis (fibrous or bony); arthritides, especially polyarthritides involving the periarticular tissue (capsule) and structural bony changes; disk displacement (i.e., acute disk displacement that does not reduce); and inflammation or joint effusion. Also contributing to hypomobility are masticatory muscle disorders such as myofascial pain, muscle splinting, myositis, spasm, contracture, and neoplasia.[31]

Hypomobility may lead to capsular fibrosis (a result of the intermolecular cross-linking adhesions of collagen fibers). It most commonly accompanies one or some combination of three situations:

1. Resolution of an acute articular inflammatory process
2. A chronic, low-grade articular inflammatory response
3. Immobilization in which the capsule may be partially or totally involved

This condition may or may not be painful. If painful, the pain is felt over the side of involvement, with possible reference into areas innervated by cranial nerve V. Pain increases during functional and parafunctional movements of the mandible. If complete capsular shortening exists, the mandibular opening is less than functional, and the patient presents with a capsular pattern of restriction. Lateral movements of the mandible to the opposite side are decreased. With bilateral restriction, lateral movements are most restricted; opening of the mouth and protrusion are limited, but closing is free.

Treatment Therapeutic modalities such as ice or heat can help to decrease pain and muscle guarding. Ultrasound in conjunction with active motion or prolonged static stretch is used to increase extensibility of the capsular tissues.[32] Joint mobilization techniques are used to further enhance capsular extensibility. Joint mobilization procedures for the TMJ include distraction, medial glide, and translation (Fig. 22-10).[4,19,24,33] In each case, the manual hold is performed over the mandible or over the inner aspect of the lower molars. Direct joint mobilizations may also be used, with contact of the therapist's thumbs over the lateral or posterior surface of the condyle of the mandible.[32] Mobilization of the involved soft tissues can facilitate stretching techniques and joint mobilization procedures, making them more tolerable and effective.

Most patients with hypomobility impairment require a home program of active ROM exercises, self-mobilization, and a passive stretching program with tongue depressors or the Thera Bite (Therabite Inc., Bryn Mawr, PA) to maintain and facilitate capsular extensibility along with instructions on proper posture and avoidance of aggravating factors.[34] As part of their home program, they are educated about maintaining the normal rest position of the tongue and mandible (i.e., TUTALC).

Limited mandibular movement can be corrected by a number of self-treatment techniques. Frequent active stretch (i.e., active opening and closing of the mandible) during the day should be encouraged. The therapeutic value of this exercise is to develop mandibular movement in a controlled manner. The tongue-up exercise can control translation. Active protrusion and lateral excursions (with or without tongue blades positioned between the teeth) can be used to actively mobilize the mandible (Fig. 22-11).

Passive stretch (i.e., prolonged static stretch) may be used by placing a number of stacked tongue blades horizontally between the upper and the lower incisors to increase the mandibular opening. The stretch position is maintained for 5 to 10 minutes or until the muscles relax. As the ROM increases, the patient can gradually increase the number of tongue depressors until he or she can open far enough to insert the knuckle of his or her index and middle fingers between the anterior teeth. Normal translation begins after 11 mm or about six tongue blades.[13]

The simplest method of self-stretch is to use the thumb crossed over the index finger. The index finger is placed on

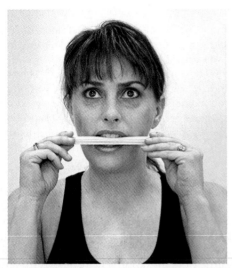

FIGURE 22-11. Active exercise to increase mandibular lateral excursions and protrusion. The patient is given enough tongue blades to place between the teeth to allow for approximately 10 to 11 mm of opening. The patient is then asked to protrude the mandible at this opening to improve translation. The patient may also be instructed to protrude and glide the mandible to one side to improve translation of one side.

the lower teeth, as far posteriorly as possible, and the thumb is placed on the upper teeth. The patient actively opens the jaw and applies gentle pressure in opening until a stretch is felt (Fig. 22-12). This technique should be performed bilaterally to avoid compression of one joint while trying to stretch the other side.

Techniques used for mandibular opening may be helpful in joint restrictions caused by anterior disk displacement with and without reduction. In the case of a nonreducing disk, it is important to limit intracisal opening to approximately 30 mm to protect the retrodiskal tissue from being overstretched.[13]

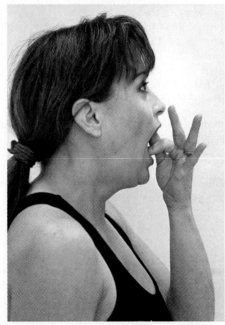

FIGURE 22-12. Active-passive mandibular exercise. The patient is instructed to actively open the mouth. Then, finger pressure is applied to the maxillary and mandibular dentitions with one or both hands.

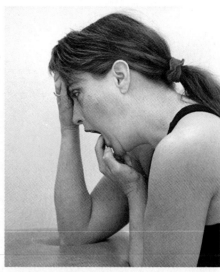

FIGURE 22-13. Postisometric relaxation self-exercise for mandibular opening (temporal, masseters, and medial pterygoid muscles). The patient sits at a table with one elbow on the table and the hand propping his or her forehead; the fingers of the other hand are on the maxillary teeth. After taking up the slack of mouth opening, the patient breathes out. During inhalation, he or she opens the mouth as wide as possible. The hand on the forehead should prevent flexion, which would interfere with maximum opening.

Postisometric relaxation techniques (PIRs) use active muscle contractions at various intensities from a precisely controlled position in a specific direction against a counterforce to facilitate motion.[35] For one PIR technique for mandibular opening, the patient sits at a table, with one elbow on the table and with the hand propping his or her forehead; the fingers of the other hand are on the mandibular dentition.[35] After opening his or her mouth to take up the slack, the patient breathes out; during inhalation, he or she opens his or her mouth as wide as possible, as if yawning (Fig. 22-13). This is followed by closing the mouth against isometric resistance with minimal force; the exercise is then repeated. Deviation of the mandible to the side during the relaxation phase may be introduced as a separate exercise.

For PIR self-treatment for relief of tension of the lateral pterygoid, the patient assumes a supine position. Using his or her thumbs on the mandible, the patient presses his or her chin forward against the isometric resistance of the thumbs with minimal force while breathing. The patient next holds his or her breath and then breathes out while relaxing and letting the chin drop back (Fig. 22-14).[35] The exercise should be done with minimal effort; the relaxation phase is most important.

Tension of the digastric is best diagnosed by trying to shift the hyoid from side to side. When tightness or tension is marked on one side, deviation of the thyroid cartilage to the ipsilateral side may be evident. For self-treatment using PIR, the thumb of one hand lies lateral to the hyoid on the restricted or tense side. During the resistance phase, the patient slightly opens his or her mouth and breathes in, holds his or her breath, and then relaxes while breathing out. The patient closes the mouth while his or her thumb moves the hyoid very gently to the opposite side (Fig. 22-15).[35]

The goal of functional kinetic exercises developed by Klein-Vogelbach[36,37] is for the patient to learn to move the

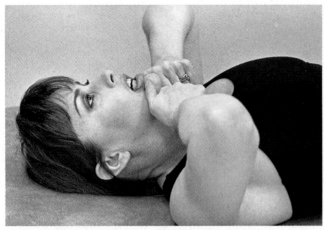

FIGURE 22-14. Postisometric relaxation self-exercise of the lateral pterygoid. The patient is supine, with the mouth slightly open. He or she places both thumbs on the mandible and is instructed to press the chin forward against his or her thumbs while breathing in. The patient holds his or her breath and then breathes out, letting the chin drop back.

TMJs freely and with precision in all directions. In normal TMJ activity, it is the mandible that moves while the head remains stationary. If movement at the TMJ is restricted, it is often helpful to reverse these roles. Normally, jaw elevation, depression, protraction, retraction, and lateral gliding are initiated at the mandible (i.e., distal lever). To facilitate increased motion and to functionally circumvent and break faulty habit patterns, the levers are reversed; the head (i.e., proximal lever) initiates the motion. The head moves but not the mandible. These movements are transmitted to the upper cervical spine joints (i.e., atlanto-occipital and atlantoaxial joints).

While the patient sits with good vertical alignment, the therapist or the patient provides fixation of the mandible; the fingers of both hands should grasp the mandible. Exercises include opening and closing of the mouth, lateral deviations,

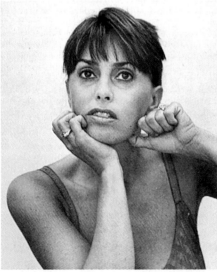

FIGURE 22-15. Postisometric relaxation self-exercise for the digastric muscle. While sitting, one hand is placed under the chin, and the other hand contacts the lateral aspect of the hyoid bone (tense side) with the thumb. After the resistance phase, the thumb gently moves the hyoid medially.

and protrusion and retrusion (Fig. 22-16). These precise and unfamiliar movements of the TMJ must be performed at low intensity and slowly, because the body is learning movements that it does not need in normal motor behavior but that can be used effectively to reduce restriction.[37] These exercises are followed up with normal mandibular motions to assess progress and maintain function. A sensory awareness exercise tape, using these same principles of initiating motion of the jaw with the head and other neuromuscular learning techniques based on the Feldenkrais Method, has been developed by Wildman[38] for home use.

A variation of Klein-Vogelbach kinetic exercises for opening and closing the jaw freely and with precision is an exercise with the head in the inverted position (for patients who can assume the position) (Fig. 22-17). Opening of the mouth in this position must be performed against gravity, providing eccentric isotonic work of the masseter muscle in opening and concentric work in closing. The reverse is true of the jaw-opening muscles, the suprahyoids.

Hypermobility

Etiology　The cause of TMJ hypermobility is unknown. Potential predisposing factors range from joint laxity to psychiatric disorders to skeletal disorders.[39] Investigations suggest that systemic hypermobility (i.e., ligament laxity) may be closely related to TMJ hypermobility, and other investigations suggest disk displacement and osteoarthrosis.[39-41] Parafunctional habits that contribute to hypermobility of the TMJ include prolonged bottle feeding, thumb sucking, and pacifier use in children.[16] Many adult patients present with a history of habitually opening their mouths excessively wide when yawning or eating. Both joints usually are involved, but unilateral hypermobility can occur as a compensatory reaction to hypomobility of the contralateral side.

Believed to be the most common mechanical disorder of the TMJ, hypermobility of the TMJ is characterized by early or excessive anterior translation or by early and excessive anterior translation of the mandible.[42] In cases of hypermobility, translation occurs within the first 11 mm of opening rather than the last 15 to 25 mm. Excessive anterior translation results in laxity of the surrounding capsule and ligaments. The breakdown of these structures allows disk derangement in one or both TMJs. Ultimately, impairments such as functional loss and arthritic changes may occur.

Intervention　Therapeutic modalities such as heat and ice are beneficial if the condition is painful. An important step is to educate the patient regarding the functioning of his or her joints, the reason for the symptoms, and how to modulate these symptoms. The following sections describe treatment options for hypermobility impairment.

Muscle Performance: Temporomandibular Joint Rotation and Translation Control.　For the therapist to teach control of the jaw muscles, the patient must first recognize the resting position of the mandible: lips closed, teeth slightly apart, and the tongue on the hard palate. The patient should breathe in and out through the nose and use diaphragmatic breathing.

The initial exercise limits TMJ mechanics to condylar rotation through an active assistive technique using the index finger and thumb to assist the movement. While maintaining the tongue on the roof of the mouth, one index finger is placed on the involved TMJ, and the other index finger is placed

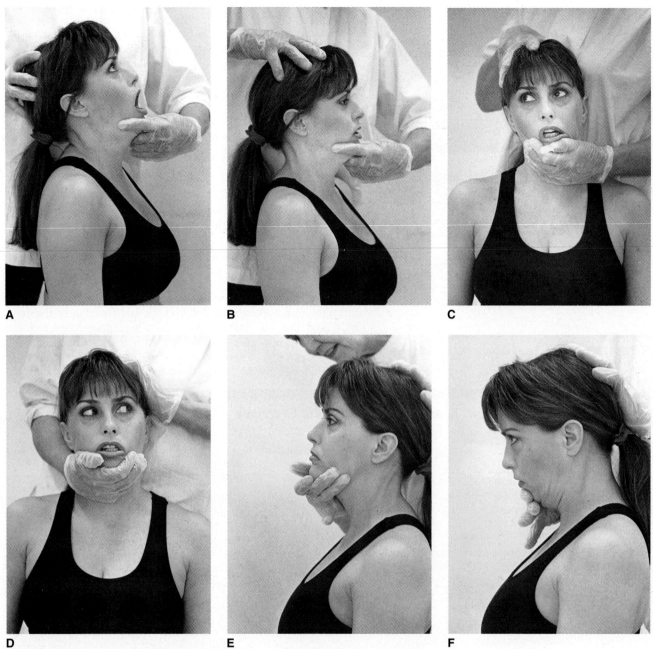

FIGURE 22-16. Functional kinetic exercises using the proximal lever for (A) opening. With the mandible stabilized, the patient extends the head (the tip of the nose moves cranially and dorsally). As the mouth opens, the joints of the upper cervical spine extend, and the TMJs open. (B) Closing. The patient flexes the head (the tip of the nose moves caudally and ventrally) as the mouth closes; the joints of the upper cervical spine flex and the TMJs close. (C) Functional kinetic exercises using the proximal lever for lateral movements to the right. With the mandible stabilized, the right upper teeth slide laterally to the right of the stabilized mandible and (D) to the left (the opposite applies for movement to the left). The movement is one of rotation of the atlanto-occipital and atlantoaxial joints of the cervical spine and lateral translation in the TMJ. (E) Functional kinetic exercises using the proximal lever for protrusion. With the mandible stabilized, the upper teeth slide dorsally in relation to the lower teeth. (F) Retrusion. With the upper teeth moving ventrally to the lower. Functional kinetic protrusion and retrusion include dorsal or ventral glide of the cervical spine and dorsal or ventral translation the TMJs respectively.

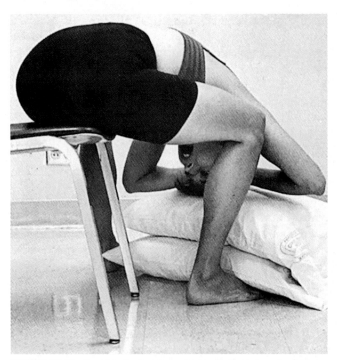

FIGURE 22-17. Opening the mouth exercise with the long axis of the body inverted.

on the chin. The lower jaw is allowed to drop down and back with the guidance of the index finger and thumb (Self-Management 22-1: Concentric and Eccentric Exercises). The use of a mirror to monitor motion is helpful in achieving normal tracking and in ensuring that the tongue stays up and the jaw does not deviate.

The exercise is progressed by placing both index fingers on the TMJs (Fig. 22-18). The lower jaw is allowed to drop down and back, bringing the chin to the throat, as in the first exercise but without the guidance of the index finger on the mandible. As the patient learns to control movement by proprioceptive feedback, he or she may then attempt rotation on opening without the tongue on the palate (without condylar translation), first with the guidance of the index finger and thumb on the mandible, as shown in Self-Management 22-1, and then with both index fingers on the TMJs (see Fig. 22-18).

Muscle Performance: Strengthening and Stabilization Exercises. After or concurrently with an exercise program to develop TMJ rotation and translation control, a mandibular stabilization program should be started to strengthen the jaw muscles and balance the strength and function of the right and the left TMJs. These strengthening exercises are also used to control excessive translation and establish a normal jaw position at rest and in the open-mouth position. Isotonic exercises may be used in the management of painless clicking,

 SELF-MANAGEMENT 22-1 *Concentric and Eccentric Exercises*

Purpose:	To restore proper "tracking" to the TMJ, to limit TMJ mechanics to rotation through an active assisted technique (the patient's thumb and finger of one hand are needed to assist the movement), and to decrease or eliminate clicking, cracking, popping, or excessive movement occurring in the TMJ.		Place the opposite thumb and index finger lightly on the tip of the chin.
Precaution:	Carefully monitor the axis of rotation of the TMJ joint, eliminating any subsequent translatory motion.		Allow the lower jaw to drop down and back with guidance from the thumb and index on the chin.
	Monitor this trial jaw opening in a mirror to ensure a straight opening (i.e., tongue stays on the roof of the mouth).		After learning to control movement by proprioceptive feedback, rotation-controlled movement without the tongue on the roof of the mouth may be attempted.
	Exercise must be done slowly and rhythmically within the pain limits	***Dosage:***	Repeat this exercise five times, five times per day. The patient is instructed to use this pattern of movement frequently during the day or whenever observing himself or herself in a mirror.
Position:	The patient sits on a firm chair, close to the front edge, with feet on the floor about 12 in apart.		
	Instruct the patient to maintain neutral pelvis, lumbar thoracic, and cervical spine alignment.		
	Instruct the patient to think of the head leading up and the torso lengthening and widening to achieve full spinal length. The cervical spine should remain in neutral (eyes focused to horizontal).		
	Assistive positioning devices may be used.		
	The patient can sit with the back and cervical spine supported against a wall (towels behind the head to maintain neutral cervical spine if FHP is stiff or rigid).		
Movement Technique:	*Instruct the patient to*		
	Keep the tongue on the roof of the mouth.		
	Place one index finger on the TMJ.		

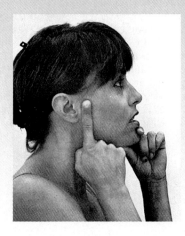

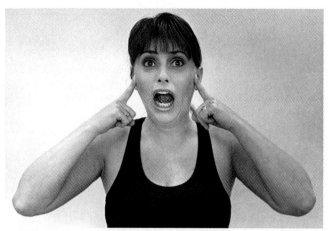

FIGURE 22-18. Neuromuscular reeducation for rotation and translation control. The patient starts with the tongue on the roof of the mouth and index fingers on both TMJs. The mandible is allowed to drop down and back; the tongue is dropped from the roof of the mouth and opening is completed. A mirror is used to monitor complete opening and to ensure a straight opening.

after a painful episode is resolved, and when the click is not caused by a displaced articular disk.[43] Strengthening exercises are also indicated after TMJ operations and for a variety of other TMJ dysfunctions and disorders.

Muscle   Performance: Isometric   or   Static Exercises. Proprioceptive neuromuscular facilitation (PNF) techniques, such as the contract-relax exercise and rhythmic stabilization technique, are used. Light pressures are applied to the jaw with the index finer and thumb on either side of the mandible. The patient is asked to place the tip of the tongue up against the palate, with the teeth slightly apart. Gentle pressures are applied for a short time. Pressure is applied as the patient attempts to open and close the mandible, glide it to the left or right, and glide it ventrally and dorsally or in a diagonal direction back toward or away from either ear (see Patient-Related Instruction 22-1: Mandibular Stabilization Instructions). Motion in each direction is repeated several times to exercise various muscles and stimulate neuromuscular awareness. These exercises may then be performed with the jaw in a position with the teeth one knuckle apart and then two knuckles apart (Fig. 22-19).

PNF techniques of resisted isometric opening contractions of the lateral pterygoids and suprahyoids promote relaxation of the primary closing muscles of the mandible (i.e., temporalis and masseter) through reciprocal inhibition. This technique can also facilitate maximum interincisal distance.[44,45]

Muscle Performance: Isotonic or Dynamic Exercises. Isotonic exercises are performed against the manual resistance of the patient's or therapist's hand on the mandible. The amount of chin resistance allows controlled jaw movements over a restricted ROM, allowing full activity of all the muscles operating about the joint. Exercises include resisted opening and closing and lateral movements (Fig. 22-20). Open-close movements are limited to about 15 mm of opening (i.e., width of one knuckle). The patient should be reminded not to push the jaw forward during the opening movement and to allow the jaw to open in an arc toward the chest. Resistance to closing should be done slowly. Lateral movements are limited to about 5 mm. These exercises

---

◆ Patient-Related Instruction 22-1

Mandibular Stabilization Instructions

The objectives are to strengthen the jaw muscles and to establish a normal jaw position at rest and in the open-mouth position. The following exercises require the application of light pressure to the jaw with your index fingers. The intensity of pressure should be 2 on a scale of 1 to 10 (10 = highest force). The jaw should not move during the application of pressure. Monitor this exercise in front of a mirror.
Maintain the following mouth and jaw position:

1. Keep your teeth apart. Let your jaw and mouth drop open slightly and remain in that position.
2. The tip of the tongue remains on the roof of the mouth, just behind the upper two front teeth.

Maintain good head, neck, and back posture. It is helpful to imagine two strings. One string pulls straight up from the top and back of the head to the ceiling; the second string pulls up from the breast bone.

1. Place the index fingers and thumbs of your hands on either side of your jaw.

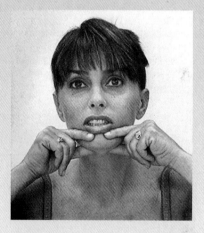

2. Apply gentle pressure (2 on a scale of 1 to 10) in the following directions
   a. To the left side of the jaw
   b. To the right side of the jaw
   c. Up to the ceiling
   d. In toward the neck
   e. Diagonally back toward the left ear
   f. Diagonally back toward the right ear
3. Hold each pressure for 2 seconds.
4. Repeat each direction ___ times, ___ times per day

---

should never be performed so that pain or clicking sounds occur. ROM should stop before the onset of pain or clicking (see Building Block 22-3).

Posture and Movement Impairments

Signs and Symptoms

FHP with resultant rounding of the shoulders can produce dysfunction of the craniocervical and temporomandibular systems. Symptoms associated with FHP can be extremely variable. Patients complain of stiffness, tiredness, tingling,

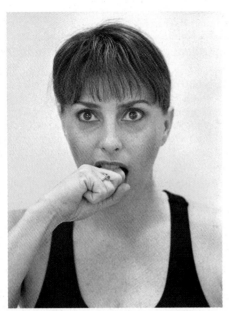

FIGURE 22-19. Isometric stabilization exercises (one- and two-knuckle-width opening). First one and then two knuckles are placed between the upper and the lower teeth. The knuckle or knuckles are removed, keeping the teeth apart. Apply gentle pressure to the lower jaw as in Patient-Related Instruction 22-1. These exercises build on the exercise shown in the Patient-Related Instruction. The earlier stabilization exercise is continued as these exercises are added. Not all patients are progressed automatically to the two-knuckle-width opening exercise.

aching, numbness, and vertigo. A patient may also complain of limitation of neck motion and various pain referrals to the head, arms, and upper thoracic spine.

To restore balance to the system, patients must address excess tension, head and shoulder girdle alignment, jaw

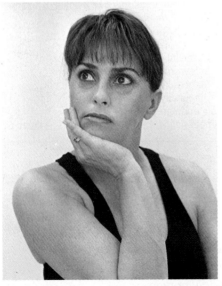

FIGURE 22-20. Isotonic strengthening exercise. Resistive exercise strengthens the left lateral pterygoids against the right lateral force provided by the patient's right hand. Resistance is provided by placing the palm against the chin with the arm stabilized (i.e., the elbow resting against a firm surface or with the arm held firmly against the chest).

> **BUILDING BLOCK 22-3**
>
> A patient demonstrates 55 mm of vertical opening with early and excessive translation noted on opening. What is the movement fault for this patient? What exercises would you teach to help correct this fault?

and tongue position, and breathing. Postural reeducation exercises; manual therapy techniques applied to tight muscles, soft tissue, and joints; and neuromuscular relaxation training may be needed. In general, treatment should begin by developing a home program of relaxation training and postural correction programs monitored jointly by the patient and therapist. Ergonomic advice and spinal supports should be provided as needed. Ultimately, management should become the patient's responsibility. The therapist assists with reinforcement and periodic follow-up visits for adapting programs based on the patient's changes and progress.

Intervention

Therapeutic Exercise: Neuromuscular Relaxation Training Effective self-regulatory and neuromuscular relaxation training involves development of more flexible habits of attention, which must be fully transferred by the trainee to everyday activities. Various relaxation procedures that employ physical and mental exercises and exercises called therapeutic awareness have been devised.[46–48] Relaxation therapies may be integrated into biofeedback-assisted attention training.

Progressive relaxation involves a structured isometric approach that asks the patient to contract the muscles and then relax.[49,50] Another form of progressive relaxation uses a reverse approach in which the muscles are passively stretched and then relaxed.[51,52]

Autogenic training employs adaptive mental imagery.[53,54] The verbal content of the standard exercises is focused on the neuromuscular system (e.g., heaviness of the limbs), the vasomotor system (e.g., warmth of the limbs, coolness of the forehead), and slowing of the cardiovascular system and respiratory mechanisms.

Yoga, meditational mantra, and diaphragmatic breathing techniques are adapted from Eastern disciplines.[55–58] Particularly valuable approaches, which focus on integrated functions of the tongue, jaw, and breathing, include the use of sensory awareness techniques[56,59–62] and sensory-motor learning exercises.[38,63–67]

Therapeutic Exercise: Head, Neck, and Shoulder Postural Exercises A significant aspect of the therapy for the head, neck, and shoulder is a postural exercise program. The principles proposed by Kendall et al.[68] and Sahrmann[69,70] are most beneficial for these patients (see Chapters 9, 17, 23–25). Therapists may also use a variety of movement reeducation approaches to attain balanced posture, alignment, structure, and function. Therapeutic approaches include a variety of methods, such as Aston Patterning,[71,72] the Alexander Technique,[59,60,73] the Feldenkrais Method,[63–67] tai chi,[74–76]

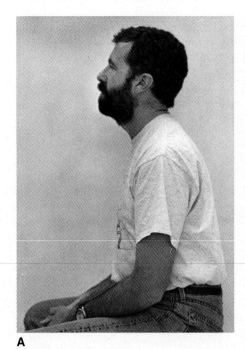
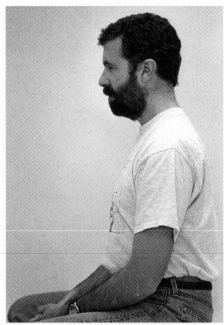

A   **B**

FIGURE 22-21. Head and neck release.
(A) Incorrect: head pulled back and down.
(B) Correct: head releasing forward and up.

and Trager Psychophysical Integration,[72] which use sensory, kinesthetic, and proprioceptive feedbacks to the body-mind system.

A useful method of achieving good postural alignment in sitting and standing is to imagine two "strings" attached to the body: one to the sternum and the other to the top of the head posteriorly. As these strings are pulled up to the ceiling, the head posture is made more axial, with increased opening of the suboccipital space. As the sternum becomes elevated, the shoulder girdle becomes more retracted and depressed. However, flattening of the cervical curve should be avoided. According to Rocabado,[24] cranial flexion should not exceed 150 degrees.

The sternum must be lifted without hyperextension of the thoracic or lumbar spine. The concept of allowing the neck to release so the head can balance "forward and up" should be used to encourage length in the spine.[59] The forward instruction does not mean that the head moves forward of the rest of the body; it is implemented only to undo the backward pull or PCR on the neck. In a patient with PCR, the distance between the occiput and the atlas is decreased, narrowing the suboccipital region. This pulls the occiput posteriorly and inferiorly, resulting in upward and backward displacement of the mandible in the fossa. The Alexander use of the word *up* means away from the top of the spine, with the purpose of eliminating any muscle tension that pulls the head down into the neck. The head *forward and up* movement is allowed to happen by releasing tension in the posterior neck muscles (Fig. 22-21).[59]

Therapeutic Exercise: Mandibular and Tongue Postural Exercises   Proper resting position of the tongue, in addition to helping maintain normal posturing of the mandible and axial spine, enhances normal swallowing patterns and makes daytime clenching more difficult.[77] The correct resting position of the tongue (i.e., comfortably resting against the hard palate) should be discussed with the patient and

demonstrated.[8] The most anterosuperior tip of the tongue should lie in an area against the palate just posterior to the back side of the upper central incisors. Instructing the patient to maintain TUTALC helps to achieve the resting position of the jaw and tongue and overcome parafunctional and functional muscle hyperactivity.[16]

Tongue push-ups may be used as an initial exercise to strengthen the tip of the tongue and familiarize the patient with the correct placement of the tongue.[15] The tongue tip is pointed and pressed against the hard palate (just above the upper teeth) and then released, and the exercise is repeated.

One exercise involves instructing the patient to "cluck" the tip of the tongue against the hard palate and leave it there.[24] Another requires the patient to practice certain sounds, such as those made by the letters T, D, L, and N, that raise the tip of the tongue to the incisal papilla. Words such as Ted, dad, love, and nut can be practiced with added force to activate the tongue muscles.[15]

Neuromuscular control can be achieved by practicing tongue-up exercises along with opening and closing of the mouth with speed.[4] This exercise involves having the patient open and close the mouth wide with the tongue in its resting position. The patient should be instructed to stop short of a "click" with no deviations of the mandible or excessive anterior translation. After controlled opening is achieved, the patient increases the speed of movement. Kraus[4] found this a useful technique in reducing symptoms associated with inflammatory disorders such as synovitis and capsulitis and when inflammation coexists with hypermobility, hypomobility, or excessive parafunctional activities (see Building Block 22-4).

Therapeutic Exercise: Exercises to Correct Dysfunctional Swallow Sequence and Breathing Patterns   A commonly overlooked problem in patients presenting with TMJ and craniocervical disorders is an altered swallowing sequence, which is most often associated with tongue thrust swallow or

BUILDING BLOCK 22-4

Why is it important to teach the normal resting position of the tongue to patients with TMD? How would you teach this to a patient?

abnormal breathing. In abnormal breathing, such as mouth breathing, the tongue is usually depressed, and the upper and the lower parts of the teeth are apart during swallowing. Persons who swallow abnormally usually bring their tongues forward to meet the glass or cup when taking a drink, and excessive lip activity may be evident. Because of the FHP, the hyoid bone may elevate on swallowing, and abnormal contraction of the suboccipital musculature may occur.[13] One of the methods, according to Funt and colleagues,[15] of changing this pattern when drinking from a cup or glass is to instruct the patient to bite the back teeth together, put the tongue to "the spot" on the anterior palate directly behind the upper incisors, siphon the water in between the teeth, and swallow (Fig. 22-22).[15] As water is siphoned during the initial phase of swallowing, the tip of the tongue should return to its resting position without putting pressure on the posterior teeth. When this is accomplished, many sips of water are taken and swallowed without any movement of the facial muscles. Because a tongue thrust habit is usually well rooted, this exercise should be practiced several times daily. After the patient can use the new swallowing pattern for all eating and drinking activities and has learned proper posturing, he or she must apply (at a subconscious level) what he or she has learned to all swallowing activities and become aware of the rest position of the tongue throughout the day.

Proper diaphragmatic breathing is also important to normal TMJ function.[55,59,61,78–80] Mouth breathers, patients with allergies, or patients with nasal obstruction often breathe with increased activity of the accessory muscles of respiration (i.e., scaleni, sternocleidomastoids, and pectoralis minor), leading to FHP with PCR.[81] The patient should be instructed in nasodiaphragmatic breathing (see Patient-Related Instruction 22-2: Diaphragmatic Breathing). Diaphragmatic

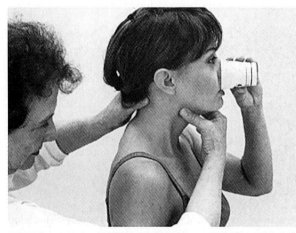

FIGURE 22-22. Swallowing exercise. As water is siphoned during the initial phase of swallowing, the tip of the tongue should return to its resting position. When this is accomplished, many sips of water are taken and swallowed without any movement of the facial muscles.

Patient-Related Instruction 22-2
Diaphragmatic Breathing

- Initially, assume a comfortable position on the floor with your hands on your stomach.
- Relax your belly as much as possible.
- During the first third of inhalation, the belly should expand slightly (on its own) in an outward direction as the diaphragm pushes down on the contents of the abdomen.

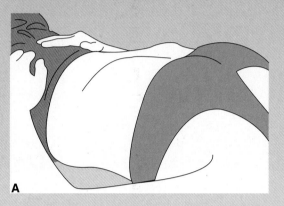

A

- Next, the air should move into the middle portion of the lungs, causing the area of the lower and middle ribs to expand. Complete inhalation means filling the lungs forward, sideways, and backward.

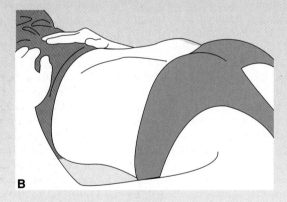

B

- The dimension of breathing often neglected is sideways intercostal breathing.
- Exhalation is largely a passive occurrence. The chest muscles and diaphragm relax, the ribs drop back close together, and the lungs recoil as air is quickly expelled.

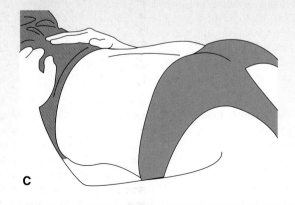

C

breathing occurs more easily by breathing through the nose and with correct positioning of the tongue. A correct rest position of the tongue forces nasodiaphragmatic breathing. Diaphragmatic breathing is best learned in supine, followed by practice during sitting, standing, and activity. Diaphragmatic breathing controls stress, promotes general relaxation of the body, strengthens the diaphragm, improves oxygenation with increased depth of respiration, and decreases the use of the accessory muscle of respiration. This is an important technique taught to patients with dysfunctional involvement of other regions, such as the pelvic floor, lumbar spine, thorax, and cervical spine.

Attempts to alter breathing patterns are often difficult. However, a more normal breathing pattern can be facilitated by altering the head and neck posture. This may be facilitated by an exercise proposed by Fielding.[82] A soft ball (e.g., old tennis ball) or equivalent is placed behind the patient's back at the level of the scapula as he or she sits in a straight-back chair (Fig. 22-23). The mechanism for improvement is not clear, but observation of the patient reveals a slower rate of breathing, improved spinal alignment, mouth closure, and relaxation of the shoulder girdle. The patient should be encouraged to make a conscientious effort to keep the tongue on the roof of the mouth and to practice diaphragmatic breathing.

To fully transfer these ideas to other activities on a subconscious level, it is often helpful for the trainee to practice awareness exercises directed at restoration of the neutral resting position of the head, neck, jaw, and shoulder girdle throughout the day. The RTTPB system (relaxation, teeth apart, tongue on the palate, posture, and breathing) proposed by Ellis and Makofsy[77] is one way to help the trainee remember and practice frequently. This helpful acronym addresses the common imbalance seen in the upper quadrant (see Building Block 22-5).

THERAPEUTIC EXERCISE INTERVENTIONS FOR COMMON DIAGNOSES

In an average clinical setting, the most common disorder of the TMJ is dysfunction involving the capsule and intra-articular structures. TMJ dysfunction can occur as a separate entity or can be a complication of disease, trauma, or developmental abnormalities. Some of the more common diagnoses of the TMJ are reviewed in the following sections.

Capsulitis and Retrodiskitis

Signs and Symptoms
Overloading of the joint from bruxism, excessively hard chewing, trauma, strain, or infection may cause an inflammatory response in the fibrous capsule, synovial membrane, and retrodiskal tissues. The condition is called capsulitis. Habits such as bruxing, tongue thrusting, gum chewing, and pencil chewing can offset the normal pattern of masticatory behavior and lead to asymmetric muscle activity and mandibular malalignment. Overload problems are often related to emotional stress causing excessive muscular activity.

Retrodiskitis occurs with encroachment of the condyle on the articular disk. This causes inflammation or exacerbation

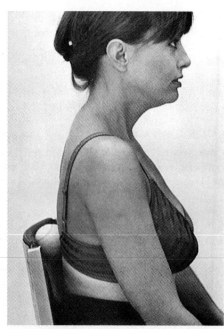

FIGURE 22-23. Posterior co-contraction using a ball behind the back at the level of the scapula to facilitate a more normal breathing pattern.

of an existing inflammatory condition. It can occur gradually, as a result of chronic repetitive microtrauma when the condyles are displaced posteriorly because of anterior disk displacement, or by acute external trauma to the chin, forcing the condyles posteriorly into the tissues.

Persistent, subtle changes in joint kinematics may cause muscular imbalance between the elevators and the depressors and produce abnormal stresses sufficient to result in improper loading of the articular cartilage. This pattern can lead to potential fatigue failure and possible arthritic changes in the articular cartilage. Repeated overload leads to microtrauma and an inflammatory reaction in the capsule, the peripheral parts of the disk, and the lateral pterygoid insertion. The overfatigued lateral pterygoid's ability to move the disk harmoniously during jaw movements can be upset and result in disk displacement and damage.[7]

Signs and symptoms of capsulitis include pain at rest (intensified during functional maximum intercuspation of the teeth) and parafunctional (bruxism) movements of the mandible. Pain occurs on the side of involvement in the area of the TMJ, with possible reference of pain into areas innervated by cranial nerve V. Impairment resulting from capsulitis ranges from minor joint restriction to total immobilization.

Signs and symptoms of retrodiskitis include constant pain and palpable tenderness posterior and lateral to the joint. Pain

BUILDING BLOCK 22-5

Your patient has a history of asthma and allergies. How may this affect his or her jaw symptoms?

is usually increased by clenching or by moving the mandible to the affected side, which permits the condyle to press against the inflamed tissue. With swelling, the condyle may be forced anteriorly, resulting in acute malocclusion. Because chewing on the contralateral side can increase pressure in the inflamed joint, causing more pain, the patient should be advised to chew on the side of the involved joint.[12,83]

Intervention

Treatment depends in large part on the cause. If caused by a single traumatic event, a program of limited mandibular function, mild analgesics, ice, and moist heat or ultrasound may be effective. To decrease pain and muscle guarding, use of phonophoresis, ionophoresis, or laser therapy may be indicated.[13,16,84] The most commonly used therapeutic modality after trauma or surgical intervention is cryotherapy.[13] Cold is used to reduce inflammation, muscle spasm, and edema. Cold packs, ice massage, or vapocoolant sprays are used. Massage, biofeedback, relaxation techniques, and electrical stimulation of the mandibular elevators can help promote muscle relaxation. If minor tenderness persists unduly, judicious use of ultrasound with exercises to extend translatory movement may be needed. Because hemarthrosis may occur in an acutely traumatized joint, measures should be taken to prevent ankylosis. As soon as the occlusion remains stabilized, cautious movement of the joint should be encouraged until resolution is complete.

When the inflammation is related to chronic microtrauma or disk displacement, more definitive therapy may be indicated. Placement of a joint-stabilization splint may reduce bruxism and decrease pressure on the joint.[85] Surface electromyography is often beneficial in the treatment of diurnal parafunction.[86,87] When retrodiskitis is caused by disk displacement, anterior repositioning therapy is indicated to reestablish the normal disk-condyle relationship. Maintaining the mandibular rest position by adapting to the normal rest position of the tongue against the palate with normal lip closure also reduces joint pressure.

After inflammation, pain, and muscle guarding are under control, a program of stretching and muscular reeducation should be instituted. The stretching and PIR techniques discussed in the "Hypomobility" section help to increase capsular extensibility and restore muscle length. Functional kinetic exercises and strengthening and stabilizing exercises can assist in muscular reeducation and relaxation.

Degenerative Joint Disease

Signs and Symptoms

Osteoarthritis, often referred to as degenerative joint disease, of the TMJ is considered primarily a disease of middle or older age. Osteoarthritis alters the force-bearing surfaces of the TMJ, often leading to secondary inflammation of the capsular tissue. The joint space narrows with spur formation and marginal lipping of the joint. There is often erosion of the condylar head, articular eminence, and fossa.[7] Advanced joint disease may lead to atrophy of associated muscles. Some causes of this degenerative process include internal derangement of the disk, an anteriorly placed disk, and repetitive overloading.

The clinical features of osteoarthritis are similar to those of other forms of joint dysfunction. Typically, pain and crepitation occur during mandibular motions. Usually, crepitation remains after the other symptoms disappear. Most persons experience restriction of the mandible.

Intervention

The primary therapy is directed at symptoms and may involve surgery, drug therapy, and physical therapy. Active ROM exercises, mobilization techniques, and stretching, as discussed in the "Hypomobility" section, may be used during the chronic phase. Graded exercises involving a few simple movements performed frequently during the day are often prescribed as a home treatment. Joint protection techniques, such as avoidance of excessive opening and parafunctional habits, and proper resting position of the tongue and mandible should be taught. Advanced bony changes within the joint may necessitate arthroplasty and joint debridement.

Derangement of the Disk

Two general classifications of this disorder are recognized: the anteriorly displaced disk that reduces during joint translation and the anteriorly displaced disk that does not reduce during joint translation.[88] These two conditions may exist indefinitely or may be one of the stages in the continuum of a disease process that leads to degenerative joint disease.[89]

Malocclusion (i.e., overclosure of the mouth with backward displacement of the condyle) or trauma may cause derangement of the disk. Trauma to the disk may cause a partial tearing of the disk from its capsular attachment. Among the various theories regarding the cause of disk derangement are excessive pressure on the joint from clenching or trauma; incoordinate contraction of the two bodies of the lateral pterygoid so that the disk snaps over the condyle rather than following the movement smoothly and coordinately when the mouth is open; deterioration of the disk and cartilaginous surfaces; and stretching of the joint ligaments by frequent subluxation.[85,90,91]

Joint sounds such as clicking are considered one of the hallmarks of disk derangement. The frequency and quality of clicking or other sounds and their association with specific functional movements and pain often help to provide important clues regarding the condition of bony and soft tissues within the joint. Clicking may occur as one or more clicks in one or both joints, and it may or may not be associated with pain. Various types of clicking noises have been observed during sagittal opening, including an opening click, an intermediate click during the opening phase, and an end-range click at full opening.

An opening click is believed to be caused by an anterior displacement of the disk, with the condyle displaced posteriorly and superiorly. As the mandible opens, the condyle must pass over the posterior band of the disk and fall into its normal position in the concave articular surface beneath the disk (Fig. 22-24).[91] Clicking during various parts of opening is probably caused by ruptures or rents of the disk or by anteroposterior displacement.[92] A click occurring early in jaw opening indicates a small degree of anterior disk displacement; a click occurring near maximal opening suggests farther anterior displacement.

On closing, a soft, closing click may also be detected as the condyle slips behind the posterior edge of the band of the

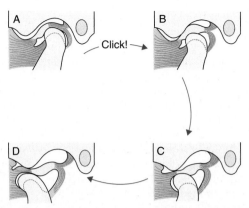

FIGURE 22-24. Mandibular depression with disk displacement. (A) TMJ with the mouth closed. (B) Early in the translatory cycle, the condyle is unable to pass under the posterior aspect of the disk. It overrides the posterior disk material and clicks. (C, D) Normal joint motion allows complete opening.

disk, leaving the disk displaced anteriorly and medially. The opening click occurs as the disk snaps back into its normal position, and the closing click results in disk displacement. Clicking can worsen with time as the posterior ligamentous attachments become further stretched and damaged. In addition to clicks produced during mandibular opening, clicks may be produced by eccentric movements. These clicks may result from structural changes in the disk or incoordinate function of the parts of the joint.

Associated Impairments

The classic sign of the type of anterior disk dislocation with reduction is a distinguished, somewhat loud click or pop on opening accompanied by a coincident palpable jarring of the joint. This signifies that the disk has relocated itself with respect to the condyle. The opening click is followed by a subtler click, usually occurring during closing and signifying that the disk has displaced anterior to the mandibular condyle. Mandibular ROM is usually normal in disk displacement with reduction, and the amount of vertical opening may be greater than normal.[85]

The sign of an anterior disk dislocation that does not reduce is the absence of joint noises with a series of reproducible restrictions during mandibular movements. These restrictions are caused by the disk blocking translatory glide. This results in limited condylar translation in the affected joint, and the disorder is often referred to as a closed lock.[93–95] A restricted maximum opening of 20 to 25 mm is the most obvious sign of an acute anterior disk displacement without reduction. The mandible is sharply deflected to the affected side at the end of opening. Lateral excursion to the contralateral side is limited. Over time, a more normal range is achieved because of elongation of the posterior attachment and continued stretching and tearing of the diskal attachments.[84,90,96]

Pain may be felt in the region of the TMJ on the side of involvement, with possible reference of pain into areas innervated by the trigeminal nerve. Pain increases or is altered during functional and parafunctional movements of the mandible. Most patients with chronic anterior disk displacement without reduction report a history of clicking and occasional locking. The most common sound is crepitus, which represents degenerative changes in the articular

surfaces. Moffett et al.[97] demonstrated that perforation of the disk is usually followed by osteoarthritic changes on the condylar surface, which is followed by similar bony alterations on the opposing surface of the fossa.

Intervention

Anteriorly Dislocated Disk with Reduction A common treatment for an anteriorly dislocated disk with reduction is to use an anterior repositioning appliance or a nonrepositioning appliance applied by a dentist specializing in the treatment of TMJ. Physical therapy modalities such as heat and ice help to decrease pain and muscle guarding, enhancing the effectiveness of the appliance. Instituting a home program to decrease the incidence of parafunctional activity is a first step in management. After parafunctional activities such as gum chewing, nail biting, clenching, excessive opening, and overuse are identified, the client is instructed to avoid these habits. With clenching, the client should be instructed in self-cuing techniques to decrease frequency. The client should check the position of the tongue and mandible frequently throughout the day. A visual cue, such as a clock, in the patient's environment should be used as a reminder. When he or she notices clenching, a deep breath is taken, and the tongue and mandible are restored to their normal resting positions. Education and exercises in facilitating relaxation of muscle tone of the jaw and cervical muscles are often beneficial; these exercises were discussed in previous sections.

Temporomandibular Joint Clicking In the absence of obvious malocclusion, simple exercises designed to allow controlled joint movement under load with simultaneous activity of the extensor and flexor muscles operating about the joint have been found to alleviate the annoying problem of TMJ clicking. Gerschmann[98] found that simple exercises, such as lower jaw thrust exercises in a forward, backward, or anterior direction with the teeth disengaged with a pencil and performing chewing exercises with the pencil, could decrease clicking in about 2 weeks (Fig. 22-25).

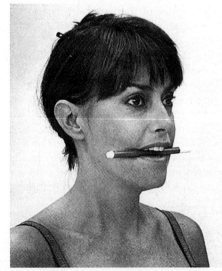

FIGURE 22-25. Chewing the pencil exercise. A soft cylindrical rod (1.5 to 2 mm) is placed horizontally at the back of the mouth so that the object thrusts forward with the mandible. The patient is instructed to bite on the rod with a grinding movement.

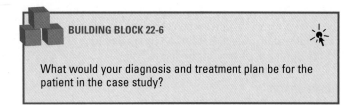

BUILDING BLOCK 22-6

What would your diagnosis and treatment plan be for the patient in the case study?

Au and Klineberg,[43] in a study of young adults, found that clicking was a reversible condition that could be treated successfully with noninvasive isometric exercises (i.e., jaw opening as a hinge movement and lateral deviations) (see Patient-Related Instruction 22-1), which suggests that there is a neuromuscular cause for many TMJ clicking problems.

Anteriorly Dislocated Disk Without Reduction Joint mobilization techniques of distraction (i.e., caudal glide) and translation (i.e., protrusion) to the involved side may be beneficial when hindrance in function warrants treatment (see Fig. 22-10). Therapeutic modalities and soft tissue mobilization techniques, such as myofascial release and massage, can be used to decrease pain and increase tissue extensibility. If articulation techniques in relocating the disk are successful, proceed immediately with the treatment discussed for an anterior disk dislocation that reduces.

Management in disk derangements may best be accomplished by normalization of muscle tone and function. When pain or hindrance of function is significant and therapeutic intervention and appliances are unsuccessful, consultation with an oral surgeon is indicated (see Building Block 22-6).

Surgical Procedures

Postoperative rehabilitation can take 6 months to 1 year. A preoperative physical therapy evaluation should include obtaining a complete medical history and conducting a craniomandibular evaluation, which includes assessment of posture, tongue position, and swallowing sequence. Patient education and patient compliance are critical to successful postoperative treatment. At the preoperative visit, patients should be made aware of the surgical procedure and what to expect postoperatively. Patients should be instructed in techniques of pain control and the reduction of swelling (e.g., cryotherapy, transcutaneous electrical nerve stimulation, diaphragmatic breathing) to be used immediately after surgery. Active and passive exercises that may be indicated after surgery should be explained before surgery. Physical therapy procedures after surgery consist of modalities to decrease inflammation, edema, reflex muscle guarding, and pain. The patient's diet is often limited to soft foods for up to 3 months, depending on the extent of surgery and possible scar growth. It is important to emphasize that the home program is the most significant part of the patient's rehabilitation program.

Postoperative Arthroscopic Surgery

Arthroscopic surgery is indicated for diagnosis and treatment of intracapsular derangement and joint adhesions.[99] Before the advent of TMJ arthroscopy, physical therapy referrals were made usually no earlier than 2 weeks and as late as 6 weeks postoperatively.[100] Arthroscopy has changed this course dramatically. Patients are seen in physical therapy 24 to 48 hours after surgery.

The patient should be reevaluated postoperatively. Changes in pain patterns, sensation, occlusion, and active motions should be recorded along with evidence of intracapsular or extracapsular swelling. In most postoperative procedures, an immediate goal is to maintain the interincisal opening achieved under anesthesia by the surgeon.[13] Postoperative adhesions between the articular surfaces and the disk may occur if mobility is not maintained. Intraoral joint mobilization techniques include distraction and lateral glides (see Fig. 22-10). These techniques are designed to inhibit reformation of adhesions, decompress the TMJ, enhance synovial lubrication, promote muscle relaxation, and restore functional ROM.[4,101] Joint mobilization techniques must be performed gently and slowly within the pain-free range and usually to both TMJs to prevent hypomobility from long-standing dysfunction on the nonsurgical side.

One of the most important exercises postoperatively is teaching the patient to open the mouth with the tip of the tongue on the hard palate to inhibit early translation (see Self-Management 22-1). Studies by Osborne[102,103] and Salter[104] have shown that constant mobility after joint trauma or surgery usually lyses blood clots, forestalling organization into connective tissue. Active isometric and isotonic exercises are performed as previously described (see Patient-Related Instruction 22-1 and Figs. 22-19 and 22-20). Time and effort should be spent on achieving normal tracking and balancing lateral movements. Self-distraction (Fig. 22-26) and gentle active-passive mandibular opening exercises (see Figs. 22-12 and 22-18 and Self-Management 22-1) and lateral deviation of the mandible (see Fig. 22-11) should be performed without causing pain.

If hypomobility develops as healing progresses and the problem is attributed to capsular constriction, ultrasound treatment (under the constant force of tongue blades or a Therabite unit) and more vigorous joint mobilization techniques may be considered. Emphasis should be placed on lateral and medial gliding and on protrusive movements. If hypomobility is attributed to fascial restriction or muscle dysfunction, myofascial release techniques, PNF techniques (i.e., contract-relax exercises and rhythmic stabilization), PIR techniques (see

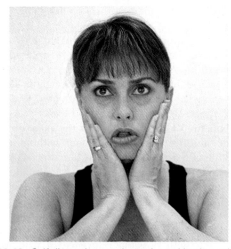

FIGURE 22-26. Self-distraction may be performed by the patient by gently squeezing the face and pulling forward and downward on the mandible. The elbows should rest on a firm surface, or the patient should hold the forearms firmly against the chest. To enhance the mobilization techniques, active participation by the patient is encouraged. The patient actively opens or closes the mouth using minimal muscle contraction, and after relaxing, additional distraction can be applied.

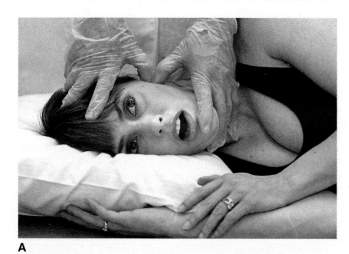 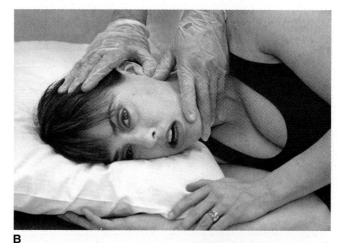

A   **B**

FIGURE 22-27. Extraoral articulation techniques are performed with the patient sidelying on the noninvolved side with the head supported on a pillow. (A) Extraoral medial glide. Gentle oscillatory mobilizations are performed over the lateral pole of the condyle in a medial direction with the thumbs. (B) Extraoral protrusion. Gentle oscillatory mobilizations are performed over the posterior aspect of the condyle in an anterior direction.

Figs. 22-12–22-15), and isotonic exercises may be used to increase mandibular motion and promote relaxation.

At all times, the therapist must consider the cervical spine and any abnormal forces that the exercise may place on the TMJs. The therapist must consider the suprahyoid-infrahyoid length-tension relationship and its influence on tongue physiology and the resting position of the jaw.[17,105] Treatment of the cervical spine, based on the evaluation findings, may be directed at postural corrective exercises for the head and neck, releasing myofascial restrictions, restoring joint mobility, or providing segmental stabilization exercises for hypermobile segments.[106] The typical postarthroscopic surgical patient is followed up for 5 to 7 weeks.[13]

Postarthrotomy Surgery

The most common indication for postarthrotomy surgery is a derangement of the disk that has not responded to nonsurgical management. Arthrotomy (i.e., open joint) procedures vary, depending on the existing pathology and the technique of the maxillofacial or oral surgeon. Surgical options include disk plication and partial or total diskectomy with grafts or without replacement. The degree of disk deformation and the health of the intercapsular disk attachments dictate the feasibility of the plication.

The patient should be seen within the first 3 to 4 days postoperatively to administer appropriate anti-inflammatory modalities and to begin active or passive ROM.[107] Most surgeons request that only active motion without resistance be used during the first 3 postoperative days.[13] They believe passive mobilization can disrupt healing and cause surgical failure.

Physical therapy after a disk plication procedure is based on an understanding of revascularization and healing of the involved tissues. The greatest change in vascularity and healing occurs in the second and third week after surgery, and complete healing occurs in 6 weeks.[108] If a disk has been reconstructed or retrodiskal tissue repair performed, motion may be quite limited, initially allowing only condylar rotation. Splint therapy is usually an integral part of the patient's overall treatment.

After the fifth or sixth week postoperatively, condylar rotation is allowed. Careful early mobilization prevents the potential loss of mandibular movement associated with immobilization. The method of choice is extraoral medial glides, protrusion (Fig. 22-27), and distraction, which can also be done by the patient (see Fig. 22-26).[13] The patient should be instructed in active and passive mandibular exercises (see Fig. 22-12; Self-Management 22-1; and Patient-Related Instruction 22-2). Reeducation of the masticatory muscles is usually started in the third or fourth week. Resisted opening (Fig. 22-28) and active lateral glide with tongue blades (see Fig. 22-11) or surgical tubing is first initiated on the contralateral side (Fig. 22-29). Lateral glide exercises may then be performed with submaximal isometrics. Lateral deviations are usually limited to 5 mm on the side opposite the surgery.

Massage of the temporalis and inferior to the masseter in particular permits a better stretch.[103] Soft tissue mobilization techniques may include deep pressure-point massage,[109] friction massage,[110] acupressure,[111] strain-counterstrain,[112] craniosacral therapy,[113–115] and myofascial release or manipulations.[13,116,117]

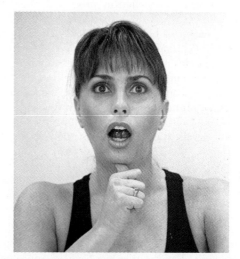

FIGURE 22-28. Resisted concentric opening at the midline is performed by the closing force provided by the therapist's or the patient's hand. Emphasis is placed on straight, midline mandibular depression and protrusion with the tongue on the hard palate. To avoid provoking pain or clicking, opening should be restricted to <20-mm interincisor separation.

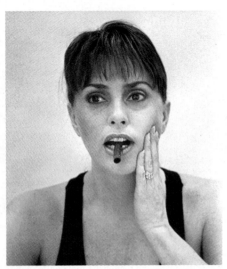

FIGURE 22-29. Lateral deviation of the mandible. Tubing is maintained with the frontal incisors at an end-to-end position. Active exercises are performed by rolling it side to side. A mirror should be used for visual feedback to ensure that no retrusion occurs.

ADJUNCTIVE THERAPY

Surface electromyography (EMG) of the muscles of mastication is used routinely by some dentists and therapists as part of the diagnosis and treatment of TMJ disorders. Muscle hyperactivity, spasms, and imbalance have been suggested in the literature for many years to be major features of TMJ disorders, but evidence to support such concepts is lacking.[118–120] The use of surface EMG is based on the assumption that various dysfunctional or pathologic conditions can be discerned from records of EMG activity of the masticatory muscles, including muscle imbalances,[85,121–123] functional hyperactivity and hypoactivity,[124–128] postural hyperactivity,[85,126,129–131] muscle spasm,[125,126,132,133] fatigue,[134,135] and abnormal occlusal positions.[123,136–140]

Records of EMG activity before and after therapeutic intervention have been used to document changes in muscle function and have been cited as proof that the treatment was successful.[121,122,133] Most researchers agree that surface EMG can measure a behavioral event such as bruxism or clenching.[138,141] With portable EMG devices, relaxation of the masticatory muscles may be attained by the patient through biofeedback at home or work. Nocturnal biofeedback exercise can produce a significant decrease in the frequency and duration of nighttime bruxism.[142–146] However, the benefits of this treatment did not last long, and a return to pretreatment EMG levels was observed as soon as biofeedback

stopped.[143,144] A few controlled studies have shown significant reduction of diurnal masseter muscle activity by using diurnal biofeedback.[65,86]

KEY POINTS

- The relationships of the stomatognathic system, in terms of structure and function, require a thorough evaluation and integrated treatment approach.
- FHP affects the position of the mandible, tongue, and hyoid, altering mandibular rest position, swallowing function, breathing pattern, and muscle balance.
- Proper positioning of the tongue on the roof of the mouth helps to maintain normal resting position of the mandible and promotes normal swallowing function.
- Hypomobility of the TMJ may result from various conditions involving the bones, muscles, joint capsule, retrodiskal tissue, or disk. Treatment seeks to decrease inflammation and pain and increase motion and function.
- In the case of a nonreducing disk, it is important to limit interincisal opening to approximately 30 mm to protect the retrodiskal tissue from being overstretched.
- Hypermobility of the TMJ is characterized by early and excessive translation of the mandible. Treatment seeks to increase joint proprioception and retrain motion, limiting translation through controlled motions and stabilization exercises.
- Hypermobility is usually bilateral; however, it occurs unilaterally when the contralateral joint is hypomobile.
- Postoperative rehabilitation can take 6 months to 1 year. Therapeutic intervention should begin as soon as possible to administer appropriate anti-inflammatory modalities and to begin active or passive ROM. One of the most important exercises postoperatively is teaching the patient to open the mouth with the tip of the tongue on the hard palate to inhibit early translation.
- It is important to involve patients actively in their treatment plan and to emphasize that the home program is the most significant part of their rehabilitation program.

CRITICAL THINKING QUESTIONS

1. Describe the following:
   a. The rest position of the tongue
   b. The motions available to the TMJ
   c. The relationship of the cervical spine and the TMJ
   d. The muscular control necessary for normal TMJ motion

LAB ACTIVITIES

1. Outline a conceptual model of musculoskeletal TMJ dysfunction and its sequelae.
2. List nine generic treatment goals appropriate for treatment of a patient with musculoskeletal pain and dysfunction of the TMJ.

3. Provide a sequential treatment plan using the goals identified in question no. 2 for the following:
   a. A soft tissue lesion without a mechanical deficit
   b. A soft tissue restriction without an articular deficit
   c. An articular deficit with soft tissue lesions or length and flexibility deficit

2. Differentiate

  a. Between the motions available in the upper and lower joint components of the TMJ

  b. Between the classic sign of anterior disk location with reduction and anterior disk location that does not reduce

3. What are the major elements of the exercise prescription after

  a. Postoperative arthroscopic surgery

  b. Postarthrotomy surgery

REFERENCES

1. Magee DJ. Temporomandibular joints. In: Magee DJ, ed. Orthopedic Physical Assessment. 2nd Ed. Philadelphia: WB Saunders, 1992.
2. Norkin CC, Levangie PK. The temporomandibular joint. In: Norkin CC, Levangie PK, eds. Joint Structure and Function: A Comprehensive Analysis. 2nd Ed. Philadelphia: FA Davis, 1992.
3. Moss M. The functional matrix concept and its relationship to temporomandibular joint dysfunction and treatment. Dent Clin North Am 1983;27:445–455.
4. Kraus S. Physical therapy management of TMD. In: Kraus S, ed. Temporomandibular Disorders. 2nd Ed. New York, NY: Churchill Livingstone, 1994.
5. Eggleton TM, Langton DP. Clinical anatomy of the TMJ complex. In: Kraus SL, ed. Temporomandibular Disorders. 2nd Ed. New York, NY: Churchill Livingstone, 1994.
6. Tanaka TT. Advanced Dissection of the Temporomandibular Joint. Chula Vista, CA: Instructional Video, Clinical Research Foundation, 1988.
7. Hartley A. Temporomandibular assessment. In: Hartley A, ed. Practical Joint Assessment: Upper Quadrant. 2nd Ed. St. Louis, MO: Mosby, 1995.
8. Fish F. The functional anatomy of the rest position of the mandible. Dent Pract 1961;11:178.
9. Sauerland EK, Mitchell SP. Electromyographic activity of intrinsic and extrinsic muscles of the human tongue. Tex Rep Biol Med 1975;33:445–455.
10. Pertes RA, Attanasio R, Cinotti WR, et al. The temporomandibular joint in function and dysfunction. Clin Prev Dent 1988;10:23–29.
11. Assael LA. Functional anatomy. In: Kaplan AS, Assel LA, eds. Temporomandibular Disorders: Diagnosis and Treatment. Philadelphia, PA: WB Saunders, 1991.
12. Bell WE. Temporomandibular Disorders: Classification, Diagnosis, Management. 3rd Ed. Chicago, IL: Year Book Medical Publishers, 1990.
13. Dunn J. Physical therapy. In: Kaplan AS, Assael LA, eds. Temporomandibular Disorders. Philadelphia, PA: WB Saunders, 1991.
14. Fricton JR, Kroening RJ, Hathaway KM. TMJ and Craniofacial Pain: Diagnosis and Management. St. Louis, MO: Ishiyzku EuroAmerica, 1988.
15. Funt LA, Stack B, Gelb S. Myofunctional therapy in the treatment of the craniomandibular syndrome. In: Gelb H, ed. Clinical Management of Head, Neck, and TMJ Pain and Dysfunction: A Multi-Disciplinary Approach to Diagnosis and Treatment. 2nd Ed. Philadelphia, PA: WB Saunders, 1985.
16. Racabado M, Iglarsh ZA. Musculoskeletal Approach to Maxillofacial Pain. Philadelphia, PA: JB Lippincott, 1991.
17. Moumoto T, Kawamura Y. Properties of tongue and jaw movements elicited by stimulation of the orbital gyrus of cat. Arch Oral Biol 1973;18:361–372.
18. Kraus SL. Influences of the cervical spine on the stomatognathic system. In: Donatelli R, Wooden M, eds. Orthopaedic Physical Therapy. 2nd Ed. New York, NY: Churchill Livingstone, 1993.
19. Racabado M. Advanced Upper Quarter Manual. Tacoma, WA: Rocabado Institute, 1981.
20. Halbert R. Electromyographic study of head position. J Can Dent Assoc 1958;23:11–23.
21. Perry C. Neuromuscular control of mandibular movements. J Prosthet Dent 1973;30:714–720.
22. Wyke BD. Neuromuscular mechanisms influencing mandibular posture: a neurologist's review of current concepts. J Dent 1972;2:111–120.
23. Prieskel HW. Some observations on the postural position of the mandible. J Prosthet Dent 1965;15:625–633.
24. Rocabado M. Diagnosis and treatment of abnormal craniomandibular mechanics. In: Solberg W, Clark G, eds. Abnormal Jaw Mechanics: Diagnosis and Treatment. Chicago, IL: Quintessence Publishing, 1984.
25. Cailliet R. Neck and Arm Pain. 3rd Ed. Philadelphia: FA Davis, 1991.
26. Friedman MH, Weisberg J. Temporomandibular Joint Disorders: Diagnosis and Treatment. Chicago, IL: Quintessence Publishing, 1985.
27. Mannheimer JS, Dunn J. Cervical spine. In: Kaplan AS, Assael LA, eds. Temporomandibular Disorders. Philadelphia, NY: WB Saunders, 1991.
28. Mannheimer JS, Rosenthal RM. Acute and chronic postural abnormalities as related to craniofacial pain and temporomandibular disorders. Dent Clin North Am 1991;35:185–208.
29. Darnell M. A proposed chronology for events for forward head posture. J Craniomandib Pract 1983;1:50–54.
30. Proffit W. Equilibrium theory revisited: factors influencing position of the teeth. Angle Orthod 1978;48:175–186.
31. McNeill C, ed. Temporomandibular Disorders: Guidelines for Their Classification and Management. Chicago, IL: Quintessence Publishing, 1993.
32. Maitland GDP. Peripheral Manipulations. 3rd Ed. Boston, MA: Butterworth, 1991.
33. Hertling DM. The temporomandibular joint. In: Hertling DM, Kessler R, eds. Management of Common Musculoskeletal Disorders. 3rd Ed. Philadelphia, PA: JB Lippincott, 1995.
34. Mannheimer J. Physical therapy modalities and procedures. In: Pertes RA, Gross SG, eds. Clinical Management of Temporomandibular Disorders and Orofacial Pain. Chicago, IL: Quintessence Publishing, 1995.
35. Lewit K. Therapeutic techniques. In: Lewit K, ed. Manipulative Therapy in Rehabilitation of the Locomotor System. 2nd Ed. Oxford: Butterworth-Heinemann, 1991.
36. Klein-Vogelbach S. Functional Kinetics: Observing, Analyzing, and Teaching Human Movement. Berlin: Springer-Verlag, 1990.
37. Klein-Vogelbach S. Therapeutic Exercises in Functional Kinetics: Analysis and Instruction of Individually Adaptive Exercises. Berlin: Springer-Verlag, 1991.
38. Wildman F. The TMJ Tape for Jaw, Head and Neck Pain. The Intelligent Body Tape Series. Berkeley, CA: Institute of Movement Studies, 1993.
39. Keith DA. Surgery of the Temporomandibular Joint. 2nd Ed. Boston, MA: Blackwell Scientific Publications, 1992.
40. Buckingham RB, Braun T, Harinstein DA, et al. Temporomandibular joint dysfunction: a close association with systemic joint laxity (the hypermobile joint syndrome). Oral Surg Oral Med Oral Pathol 1991;72:514–519.
41. Westling L, Mattiasson A. General joint hypermobility and temporomandibular joint derangement in adolescents. Ann Rheum Dis 1992;51:87–90.
42. Morrone L, Makofsky H. TMJ home exercise program. Clin Manag 1991;11:20–23.
43. Au AR, Klineberg JJ. Isokinetic exercise management of temporomandibular joint clicking in young adults. J Prosthet Dent 1993;70:33–38.
44. Carstensen B. Indications and contraindications of manual therapy for TMJ. In: Grieve G, ed. Therapy of the Vertebral Column. New York, NY: Churchill Livingstone, 1986.
45. Plante D. Postoperative physical therapy. In: Keith DA, ed. Surgery of the Temporomandibular Joint. Chicago, IL: Blackwell Scientific Publishers, 1988.
46. Benson H, Stuart EM. The Wellness Book: The Comprehensive Guide to Maintaining Health and Treating Stress-Related Illness. New York, NY: Simon & Schuster, 1992.
47. Cannistraci AJ, Fritz G. Biofeedback—the treatment of stress-induced muscle activity. In: Gelb H, ed. Clinical Management of Head, Neck and TMJ Pain and Dysfunction: A Multi-Disciplinary Approach to Diagnosis and Treatment. 2nd Ed. Philadelphia, PA: WB Saunders, 1985.
48. Davis M, Robbins Eshelmann E, McKay M. The Relaxation and Stress Reduction Workbook. 3rd Ed. Oakland, CA: New Harbinger Publishers, 1988.
49. Jacobson E. Progressive Relaxation. 4th Ed. Chicago, IL: University of Chicago Press, 1962.
50. Jacobson E. Anxiety and Tension Control. Philadelphia, PA: JB Lippincott, 1964.
51. Carlson CR, Collin FL, Nitz AJ, et al. Muscle stretching as an alternative relaxation training procedure. J Behav Ther Exp Psychiatry 1990;21:29–83.
52. Carlson CR, VenTrella MA, Sturgia ET. Relaxation training through muscle stretching procedures: a pilot case. J Behav Ther Exp Psychiatry 1987:18:121–123.
53. Luthe W, ed. Autogenic Therapy. Vol 1–6. New York, NY: Grune & Stratton, 1969–1972.
54. Schultz JH, Luthe W. Autogenic Training: A Psychophysiological Approach in Psychotherapy. New York, NY: Grune & Stratton, 1959.
55. Jenks B. Your Body: Biofeedback at Its Best. Chicago, IL: Nelson, Hall, 1977.
56. Iyengar BKS. Light on Yoga. New York, NY: Schocken, 1979.
57. Proctor J. Breathing and Meditative Techniques, tape 12. New York, NY: Bio-Monitoring Applications, 1975.
58. Schatz MP. Back Care Basics: A Doctor's Gentle Yoga Program for Back and Neck Pain Relief. Berkeley, CA: Rodmell Press, 1992.
59. Caplan D. Back Trouble. Gainesville, FL: Triad Publishing, 1987.
60. Alexander FM. The Use of Self. London: Re-education Publications, 1910.
61. Barlow W. The Alexander Technique. New York, NY: Alfred A Knopf, 1973.
62. Masters R, Houston J. Listening to the Body: the Psychophysical Way to Health and Awareness. New York, NY: Delta, 1978.
63. Feldenkrais M. Body and Mature Behavior. New York, NY: International University Press, 1949.
64. Feldenkrais M. Awareness Through Movement. New York, NY: Harper & Row, 1972.
65. Feldenkrais M. The Master Moves. Cupertino, CA: Meta Publishers, 1984.
66. Feldenkrais M. The Potent Self. Cambridge: Harper & Row, 1985.
67. Feldenkrais M. Bodily expressions. Somatics 1988;4:52–59.
68. Kendall FP, McCreary, EK, Provance PG. Muscle Testing and Function. 4th Ed. Baltimore, MD: Williams & Wilkins, 1993.
69. Sahrmann S. A program for correction of muscular imbalances and mechanical imbalances. Clin Manag 1983;3:23–28.
70. Sahrmann S. Adult posturing. In: Kraus S, ed. TMJ Disorders: Management of the Craniomandibular Complex. New York, NY: Churchill Livingstone, 1988.
71. Low J. The modern body therapies. Part four: Aston patterning. Massage 1988;16:48–52.

72. Miller B. Alternative somatic therapy. In: Anderson R, ed. Conservative Care of Low Back Pain. Baltimore, MD: Williams & Wilkins, 1991.
73. Jones F. Body Awareness. New York, NY: Schocken Books, 1979.
74. Crompton P. The Elements of Tai Chi. Shaftesbury, Dorset: Element, 1990.
75. Crompton P. The Art of Tai Chi. Shaftesbury, Dorset: Element, 1993.
76. Kotsias J. The Essential Movements of Tai Chi. Brookline, MA: Paradigm Publishers, 1989.
77. Ellis JJ, Makofsky HW. Balancing the upper quarter through awareness of RTTPB. Clin Manag 1987;7:20–23.
78. Frownfelter DL. Chest Physical Therapy and Pulmonary Rehabilitation. 2nd Ed. Chicago, IL: Year Book Medical Publishers, 1987.
79. Kisner C, Colby LA. Chest therapy. In: Kisner C, Colby LA, eds. Therapeutic Exercise: Foundation and Techniques. Philadelphia, PA: FA Davis, 1990.
80. Allen RJ, Leischow SJ. The effect of diaphragmatic and thoracic breathing on cardiovascular arousal. In: Proceedings of the VIIth International Respiratory Psychophysiology Symposium. The Nobel Institute for Neurophysiology, Stockholm Sweden, 1987.
81. Tallgren A, Solow B. Hyoid bone position, facial morphology and head posture in adults. Eur J Orthod 1987;9:1–8.
82. Fielding M. Physical therapy in chronic airway limitation. In: Peat M, ed. Current Physical Therapy. Toronto: BC Decker, 1988.
83. Okeson JP. Management of Temporomandibular Disorders and Occlusion. 3rd Ed. St. Louis, MO: Mosby, 1993.
84. Mannheimer JS. Physical therapy concepts in evaluation and treatment of the upper quarter. In: Kraus SL, ed. Disorders: Management of the Craniomandibular Complex. New York, NY: Churchill Livingstone, 1988.
85. Pertes RA, Gross SG. Disorders of the temporomandibular joint. In: Pertes RA, Gross, eds. Clinical Management of Temporomandibular and Orofacial Pain. Chicago, IL: Quintessence Publishing, 1995.
86. Dohrmann RJ, Laskin DM. An evaluation of electromyographic biofeedback in the treatment of myofascial pain and dysfunction. J Am Dent Assoc 1978;96:656–662.
87. Gale EN. Biofeedback treatment for TMJ pain. In: Igersoll BD, McCutcheon WR, eds. Clinical Research in Behavioral Dentistry: Proceedings of the Second National Conference on Behavioral Dentistry, 1979; University School of Dentistry; Morgantown, WV.
88. Farrar W, McCarty W Jr. Outline of Temporomandibular Joint Diagnosis and Treatment. 6th Ed. Montgomery, AL: Normandy Study Group, 1980.
89. Lawrence ES, Razook SJ. Nonsurgical management of mandibular disorders. In: Kraus S. ed. Temporomandibular Disorders. 2nd Ed. New York, NY: Churchill Livingstone, 1994.
90. Ross JB. Diagnostic criteria and nomenclature for TMJ arthrography in sagittal section. Part 1: Derangement. J Craniomand Disord Facial Oral Pain 1987;1:185–201.
91. Shore MA. Temporomandibular Joint Dysfunction and Occlusal Equilibration. Philadelphia, PA: JB Lippincott, 1976.
92. Whinery JG. Examination of patients with facial pain. In: Alling C, Mahan P, eds. Facial Pain. Philadelphia: Lea & Febiger, 1977.
93. Farrar WB, McCarty WL, Normandie Study Group For TMJ Dysfunction. A Clinical Outline of Temporomandibular Join Diagnosis and Treatment. 7th Ed. Montgomery, AL: Normandie Publications, 1982.
94. Schwartz HC, Kendrick RW. Internal derangement of the temporomandibular joint: description of clinical syndromes. Oral Surg Oral Pathol 1984;58:24–29.
95. Westesson PL. Clinical and arthrographic findings in patients with TMJ disorder. In: Moffett BC, ed. Diagnosis of Internal Derangement of the Temporomandibular Joint. Vol. 1. Seattle: University of Washington, 1984.
96. Eriksson L, Westesson PL. Clinical and radiological study of patients with anterior disc displacement of the temporomandibular joint. Swed Dent J 1983;7:55–61.
97. Moffett BC, Johnson LC, McCabe JB, et al. Articular remodeling in the adult human temporomandibular joint. Am J Anat 1964;115:10–130.
98. Gerschmann JA. Temporomandibular dysfunction. Aust Fam Physician 1988;17:274.
99. Vriell P, Bertolucci L, Swaffer C. Physical therapy in the postoperative management of temporomandibular joint arthroscopic surgery. J Craniomandib Pract 1989;7:27–32.
100. Mannheimer JS. Postoperative physical therapy. In: Kraus SL, ed. Temporomandibular Disorders. New York, NY: Churchill Livingstone, 1994.
101. Racabado M. Physical therapy management for the post surgical patient. J Craniomandib Disord Facial Oral Pain 1989;3:75–82.
102. Osborne JJ. A physical therapy protocol for orthognathic surgery. J Craniomandib Pract 1989;7:132–136.
103. Osborne JJ. Postorthognathic surgery. In: Kraus SL. ed. Temporomandibular Disorders. 2nd Ed. New York, NY: Churchill Livingstone, 1994.
104. Salter RD. Regeneration of articular cartilage through continuous passive motion: past, present and future. In: Stab R, Wilson PH, eds. Clinical Trends in Orthopedics. New York, NY: Thieme Stratton, 1982.
105. Daly P, Preston CD, Evans WG. Postural response of the head to bite opening in adult males. Am J Orthod 1982;82:157–160.
106. Blakney M, Hertling D. The cervical spine. In: Hertling D, Kessler R, eds. Management of Common Musculoskeletal Disorders. Philadelphia, PA: JB Lippincott, 1995.
107. Keith T. Postarthrotomy surgery. In: Kraus SL, ed. Temporomandibular Disorders. 2nd Ed. New York, NY: Churchill Livingstone, 1994.

108. Satko C, Blaustein D. Revascularization of rabbit temporomandibular joint after surgical intervention: histological and micro-angiographic study. J Oral Maxillofac Surg 1986;44:871–876.
109. Travell JG, Simons DG. Myofascial Pain and Dysfunction: the Trigger Point Manual. Baltimore, MD: Williams & Wilkins, 1983.
110. Cyriax J. Text of Orthopedic Medicine: Diagnosis of Soft Tissue Lesions. Vol. 1. 8th Ed. London: Bailliere Tindall, 1982.
111. Bradley JA. Acupuncture, acupressure, and trigger point therapy. In: Peat M, ed. Current Physical Therapy. Toronto: BC Decker, 1998.
112. Jones LH. Strain and Counterstrain. Colorado Springs, CO: The American Academy of Osteopathy, 1981.
113. Lay EM. The osteopathic management of temporomandibular joint dysfunction. In: Gelb H, ed. Clinical Management of Head, Neck and TMJ Pain and Dysfunction: a Multi-Disciplinary Approach to Diagnosis and Treatment. Philadelphia, PA: WB Saunders, 1985.
114. Upledger JE. Temporomandibular joint. In: Upledger JE, ed. Craniosacral Therapy II: Beyond the Dura. Seattle: Eastland Press, 1987.
115. Upledger JE. The Workbook of Craniosacral Therapy. Palm Beach Gardens, FL: The Upledger Institute, 1983.
116. Manheim CJ, Lavett DK. The Myofascial Release Manual. Thorofare, NJ: Slack, 1989.
117. Cantu RL, Grodin AJ. Myofascial Manipulations: Theory and Clinical Application. Gaithersburg, MD: Aspen Publications, 1992.
118. Lund JP, Widmer CG. An evaluation of the use of surface electromyography in the diagnosis, documentation, and treatment of dental patients. J Craniomand Disord 1989;3:125–137.
119. Mohl ND, Lund JP, Widmer CG, et al. Devises for the diagnosis and treatment of temporomandibular disorders. Part II: electromyography and sonography. J Prosthet Dent 1990;63:332–335.
120. Widmer CG. Evaluation of diagnostic tests for TMD. In: Kraus SL, ed. Temporomandibular Disorders. 2nd Ed. New York: Churchill Livingstone, 1994.
121. Festa F. Joint distraction and condyle advancement with a modified functional distraction appliance. J Craniomand Pract 1985;3:344–350.
122. Jankelson B, Pulley ML. Electromyography in Clinical Dentistry. Seattle: MyoTronic Research, 1984.
123. Moyers RE. Some physiologic considerations of centric and other jaw relations. J Prosthet Dent 1956;6:183–194.
124. Moller E. Muscle hyperactivity leads to pain and dysfunction: position paper. In: Klineberg I, Sessle BJ, eds. Oro-facial Pain and Neuromuscular Dysfunction. Oxford, UK: Pergamon, 1985.
125. Moller E, Sheikoleslam A, Louis I. Response of elevator activity during mastication to treatment of functional disorders. Scand J Dent Med 1984;92:64–83.
126. Sheikoleslam A, Moller E, Lous I. Postural and maximal activity in elevators of mandible before and after treatment of functional disorders. Scand J Dent Res 1982;90:37–46.
127. Stohler C, Yamada Y, Ash MM. Antagonistic muscle stiffness and associated reflex behavior in the pain–dysfunction state. Helv Odont Acta 1985;29:13–20.
128. Yemm R. A neurophysiological approach to the pathology and aetiology of temporomandibular dysfunction. J Oral Rehabil 1985;12:343–353.
129. Cooper BC, Rabuzzi DD. Myofascial pain dysfunction syndrome: a clinical study of asymptomatic subjects. Laryngoscope 1984;94:68–75.
130. Dolan EA, Keefe FJ. Muscle activity in myofascial pain-dysfunction patients: a structural clinical evaluation. J Craniomand Disord 1988;2:101–105.
131. Lous I, Sheikoleslam A, Moller E. Postural activity in subjects with functional disorders of the chewing apatus. Scand J Dent Res 1970;78:404–410.
132. Gordon TE. The influence of the herpes simplex virus on jaw muscle function. J Craniomand Pract 1983;2:31–38.
133. Ramfjord SP. Bruxism, a clinical and electromyographic study. J Am Dent Assoc 1961;62:21–44.
134. Naeije M, Hansson TL. Electromyographic screening of myogenous and arthrogenous TMJ dysfunction patients. J Oral Rehabil 1986;13:433–441.
135. Van Boxtel A, Goudswaard P, Janssen K. Absolute and proportional resting EMG levels in muscle contraction and migraine headache patient. Headache 1983;23:223–228.
136. Frank AST. Masticatory muscle hyperactivity and temporomandibular joint dysfunction. J Prosthet Dent 1965;15:1122–1121.
137. Funakoshi M, Fujita N, Takehana S. Relations between occlusal interference and jaw muscle activities in response to changes in head position. J Dent Res 1976;55:684–689.
138. Michler L, Moller E, Bakke M, et al. On-line analysis of natural activity in muscles of mastication. J Craniomand Disord 1988;2:65–82.
139. Mongini F. The Stomatognathic System. Chicago, IL: Quintessence Publishing, 1984.
140. Gelb M. Diagnostic tests. In: Kaplan AS, Assael LA, eds. Temporomandibular Disorders: Diagnosis and Treatment. Philadelphia, PA: WB Saunders, 1991.
141. Rivera-Morales WC, McCall WD. Reliability of a portable electromyographic unit to measure bruxism. J Prosthet Dent 1995;73:184–189.
142. Kardachi BJ, Clarke NG. The use of biofeedback to control bruxism. J Periodontol 1977;48:639–642.
143. Pierce CJ, Gale EN. A comparison of different treatments for nocturnal bruxism. J Dent Res 1988;67:597–601.
144. Rugh JD, Johnston RW. Temporal analysis of nocturnal bruxism during EMG feedback. J Periodontol 1981;52:233–235.

145. Rugh JD, Solberg WK. Electromyographic studies of bruxist behavior before and during treatment. J Calif Dent Assoc 1975;3:56–59.

146. Solberg WK, Rugh JD. The use of biofeedback to control bruxism. J South Calif Dent Assoc 1972;40:852–853.

RECOMMENDED READINGS

Bell WE. Temporomandibular Disorders, Classification, Diagnosis, Management. 3rd Ed. Chicago, IL: Year Book Medical Publishers, 1990.

Bush FM, Dolwick MF. The Temporomandibular Joint and Related Orofacial Disorders. Philadelphia: JB Lippincott, 1994.

Cohen S. A cephalometric study of rest position in edentulous persons: influence of variations in head position. J Prosthet Dent 1957;7:467–472.

Dutton M. The temporomandibular joint. In: Dutton M. Manual Therapy of the Spine, an Integrated Approach. New York, NY: McGraw-Hill, 2002.

Kaplan AS, Assel LA. Temporomandibular Disorders: Diagnosis and Treatment. Philadelphia, PA: WB Saunders, 1991.

Kraus SL ed. Temporomandibular Disorders. New York, NY: Churchill Livingstone, 1994.

Okeson JP. Bell's Orofacial Pains. 5th Ed. Chicago, IL: Quintessence Publishing, 1995.

Rocabado M, Iglarsh ZA. Musculoskeletal Approach to Maxillofacial Pain. Philadelphia, PA: JB Lippincott, 1991.

Skaggs CD. Diagnosis and treatment of temporomandibular disorders. In: Murphy DR, ed. Cervical Spine Syndromes. New York, NY: McGraw-Hill, 2000.

Vitti M, Basmajian JV. Integrated actions of masticatory muscles: simultaneous intramuscular electrodes. Anat Rec 1977;187:173–189.

chapter 23
The Cervical Spine

CAROL N. KENNEDY

Therapeutic exercise interventions are crucial in the rehabilitation of any cervical spine disorder, particularly those of a recurrent or chronic nature. However, exercise programs designed for the treatment of the cervical spine cannot function in isolation. Because of the close relationship between the neck, thoracic spine, shoulder girdle, and temporomandibular joint (TMJ), a complete and successful exercise program must also deal with impairments found in these regions. This chapter briefly reviews cervical spine anatomy and kinesiology and provides guidelines for examination and evaluation. Therapeutic exercise interventions are described for common impairments of body structure and functions and common diagnoses affecting the cervical spine.

REVIEW OF ANATOMY AND KINESIOLOGY

A detailed description of the anatomy and biomechanics of the cervical spine is beyond the scope of this chapter, and the reader is directed to other texts for this information.[1-3]

The cervical spine is composed of two functional units: the craniovertebral (CV) complex and the middle to lower cervical spine. The two units are different in structure and biomechanics, but act together to enable the large range of motion (ROM) available in the cervical spine, while supporting and protecting the vital structures found in this region. One important function of the cervical spine is to place the head in space for the vital functions of sight, hearing, and feeding.

The CV complex includes the atlanto-occipital (AO) and atlantoaxial (AA) joints. The biomechanics of the CV complex are governed by the articular surfaces, the complex ligamentous system, and, to a large degree, the intricate specialized muscular system.

Laxity of the CV ligamentous system results in increased motion of the complex. Signs and symptoms are those related to pressure on the cervical cord, vertebral artery insufficiency, or overreactivity of the articular structures themselves.

The midcervical spine consists of the region from the C2–3 intervertebral segment to the C7–T1 segment. Each mobile segment of the midcervical spine consists of several joints, including the paired zygapophyseal and uncovertebral (UV) joints and the interbody (disk) joint.

Panjabi[4] divided the full ROM of an intervertebral segment into two parts (Fig. 23-1A).

Neutral zone: portion of the ROM that produces little resistance from the articular structures.

Elastic zone: portion of the ROM from the end of the neutral zone up to the physiologic limit of motion.

The entire cervical spine, particularly the CV region, has a large neutral zone of motion. Because of the lack of tension in the capsular or ligamentous system in this middle part of the range, there is less passive control and the muscular system must be recruited to actively control the motion in the neutral zone. If there is damage to the ligamentous system, resulting in an increased neutral zone, muscular control becomes even more important (Fig. 23-1B).

An important aspect of cervical spine anatomy is the vertebral artery. It provides vital blood supply and is close to various structures of the cervical spine that could impede its flow.

The vertebral artery supplies the cervical spinal cord, the cervical spinal column, and the posterior cranial fossa. Intrinsic factors affecting arterial flow are atherosclerosis and thrombus formation. Flow in the artery can also be compromised by various anomalies of the artery itself or the muscles through which it passes. Swelling, degenerative thickening, and osteophytic formation of the UV and zygapophyseal joints can encroach on the artery. These processes should be considered in the patient with a history of degenerative disk disease, cervical osteoarthritis, or trauma. Excessive ROM at the CV joints, as in cases of hypermobility, can kink the artery during rotation. Decreased arterial flow may occur during rotation of the neck, and the addition of extension and traction may further reduce flow. Some of the signs and symptoms of vertebral artery insufficiency include dizziness, drop attacks, diplopia, dysarthria, dysphasia, and nystagmus. Screening for vertebrobasilar insufficiency should be performed for each patient before using these motions during treatment, including exercise.

The cervical nerve roots exit from the intervertebral foramen above the vertebra. The C1 nerve root exits through the osseoligamentous tunnel formed by the posterior AO membrane, which puts it at risk for impingement. As the cervical nerve roots exit the intervertebral foramen, they are surrounded by several structures:

- Zygapophyseal joint
- UV joint
- Cervical disk
- Bony pedicle

Degenerative changes affecting any of these structures may diminish the foramen size and alter nerve function. Cervical roots 4 through 6 have strong attachments to the transverse processes. The dural sleeve at each level forms a plug that protects the nerve and cord from traction forces. Tension in the neuromeningeal structures may produce a pull on the cervical vertebrae.

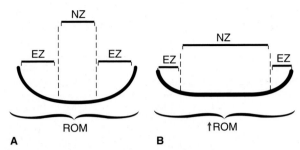

FIGURE 23-1. Neutral zone. (A) Normal. (B) Hypermobile. EZ, elastic zone; NZ, neutral zone; ROM, range of motion.

Muscles

The musculature of the cervical spine is complex, and anatomy texts[3] should be consulted for descriptions of origins and insertions and their actions.

Table 23-1 lists the muscles of the CV complex and their actions (Fig 23-2). These muscles enable the specific, fine movements of the head on the neck that are required for sight, hearing, and balance. They are richly supplied with mechanoreceptors, which are integral to the muscles' strong proprioceptive function and implicated in the production of dizziness in patients with dysfunctions of this region. The upper cervical flexors are crucial in obtaining and maintaining optimal postural balance of the head on the neck. Several long muscles, such as the sternocleidomastoid, link the head directly to the trunk.

The muscles of the midcervical spine, arranged as elsewhere in the spine, consist of slips traversing a various number of segments. Table 23-2 lists these muscle groups and their actions. In individuals with forward head posture (FHP), the deep anterior cervical musculature lengthens and becomes functionally weak, and conversely the posterior group tends to shorten.

As in other regions of the spine, the muscle system can be grouped into three components: deep, intermediate, and superficial. The deep groups tend to be single segmental muscles that function as local stabilizers of the spine rather than prime movers. These muscles tend to become weak or inhibited in pathological states. The intermediate groups are multisegmental but still tend to attach into each segment. They also stabilize the spine, particularly during movement. They often become facilitated or overactive but also at times test weak. The superficial muscle groups tend to have little if any segmental insertions and function to move the head on the trunk. They generally become overactive and tighten, and have a tendency toward protective spasm which inhibits the

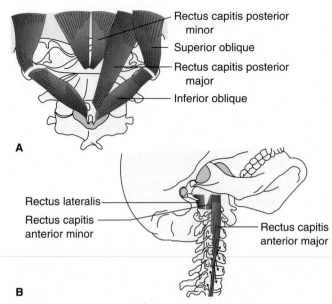

FIGURE 23-2. CV muscles. (A) Posterial suboccipitals muscles. (B) Short upper cervical flexor muscles.

deeper muscle groups. Despite this overactivity, they may still also test weak.

Deep Cervical Flexors

The deep cervical flexors include rectus capitis anterior minor, longus capitis, and longus colli. These muscles function as the deep segmental stabilizers of the cervical spine. Contraction of these muscles decreases the cervical lordosis. Longus colli has been shown to be active bilaterally as a stabilizer during talking, coughing, swallowing, and rotation/side flexion motion of the head and neck. The deep anterior segmental muscles have been shown to weaken and lose their endurance capacity in various types of cervical spine dysfunction, thus producing loss of dynamic stability.

Suprahyoid and Infrahyoid Muscle Groups

The suprahyoid and infrahyoid muscle groups are primarily involved with the functions of swallowing, speech, mastication, and the TMJ. These muscle groups are discussed in Chapter 22. This muscle group can be used to flex the cervical spine, but are inefficient and produce excessive shear forces at the TMJ. Dysfunction of these muscle groups can have a significant effect on cervical posture, and they should be assessed in persons with chronic neck conditions.

Scalene Muscle Group

Of particular clinical interest is the scalene muscle group (Fig. 23-3). These muscles have a tendency to become dominant neck flexors, especially the anterior scalene, and are also often overused during a poor pattern of apical respiration. Because of the angle of pull, increased muscle activity creates compressive and lateral forces on the intervertebral segment. Because of its insertion onto the first and second ribs, the increased activity elevates these ribs. This elevation decreases the space available in the thoracic outlet, which can eventually lead to the symptoms of thoracic outlet syndrome.

TABLE 23-1	CV Region Musculature
MUSCLE	**ACTION**
Rectus capitis posterior minor	AO joint extension
Rectus capitis posterior major	CV complex extension and ipsilateral rotation
Superior oblique	AO joint ipsilateral side flexion and extension
Inferior oblique	AA joint ipsilateral rotation
Rectus capitis lateralis	AO joint ipsilateral side flexion
Rectus capitis anterior	AO joint flexion

TABLE 23-2 Midcervical Musculature

MUSCLE	ACTION			
	FLEXION	EXTENSION	ROTATION	IPSILATERAL SIDE FLEXION
Longus colli	X	NA	MC—bilateral	MC—bilateral
Longus capitis	X	NA	Ipsilateral—MC	NA
Scalenes (elevates first or second rib)				
Anterior	X	NA	Contralateral—MC	X
Medius	MC	NA	NA	X
Posterior	NA	MC	Ipsilateral—MC	X
Sternocleidomastoid	X	X	Contralateral	X
Trapezius upper fibers	NA	X	Contralateral	X
Levator scapula	NA	X	Ipsilateral	X
Splenius, capitis, and cervicis	NA	X	Ipsilateral	X
Spinalis, capitis, and cervicis (inconsistent—blends with semispinalis)	NA	X	NA	NA
Semispinalis, capitis, and cervicis	NA	X	Ipsilateral	NA
Longissimus, capitis, and cervicis	NA	X	Ipsilateral	X
Iliocostalis cervicis	NA	X	NA	X
Interspinalis (most distinct in cervical spine)	NA	X	NA	NA
Multifidus	NA	X	Ipsilateral—MC	MC
Rotatores (inconsistent)	NA	X	Ipsilateral	MC
Intertransversarii (most distinct in cervical spine)	NA	NA	NA	MC

MC, minimal contribution; NA, no action; X, active.

Adaptive shortening of this group also can impinge on the cervical nerve roots as they travel between the scalenes.

Sternocleidomastoid Muscle

With FHP, the sternocleidomastoid muscle (SCM) tends to shorten, increasing the compression load on the cervical spine. It is a prime mover of CV extension and head on trunk flexion, but the movement pattern it produces causes substantial amounts of anterior translation and a poking chin. When flexing the head forward on the trunk, it may increase cervical lordosis. A study by deSousa[3] demonstrated sternocleidomastoid activation in both cervical extension and flexion.

Cervical Extensors

The deep segmental stabilizers in the posterior aspect of the spine are the posterior suboccipitals, multifidus, and interspinalis. The middle layer of the erector spinae, specifically semispinalis cervicis and longissimus cervicis, also have segmental insertions and likely act primarily as stabilizers, as suggested by Conley et al.[5] The cervical extensors also play a role in producing and controlling rotation. These muscles have been shown to both shorten and weaken in the presence of cervical dysfunction, possibly secondary to shortening with a FHP, or reflex inhibition from underlying joint pathology. The more superficial erector spinae muscles tend to extend the head on the trunk. As mentioned previously, SCM is also an upper cervical extensor and increases the cervical lordosis.

Levator Scapula and Upper Fibers of Trapezius

Several muscles can be classified as cervical or shoulder girdle muscles. The levator scapula and the upper fibers of the trapezius have broad insertions into the cervical spine that originate at the scapula. Alterations in the shoulder girdle resting position change the length of these muscles, affecting the cervical spine as well. For example, a depressed scapular resting position lengthens the upper fibers of the trapezius muscle and produces a lateral translation and compression force on the cervical spine. Continuous translational forces on the cervical spine can lead to hypermobility in certain planes and restriction of motion in others.

EXAMINATION AND EVALUATION

Examination of the cervical spine should include evaluation of the entire spine, particularly the thoracic region, the TMJ, and shoulder girdle complex. These regions directly influence the posture and mobility of the cervical spine. The clinician must have the knowledge and skills necessary to perform all the appropriate tests to diagnose impairments and functional losses of the cervical spine.

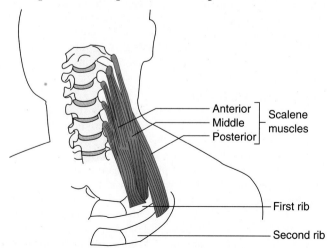

Anterior ⎤
Middle — Scalene muscles
Posterior ⎦

First rib

Second rib

FIGURE 23-3. Scalene muscles.

History and Clearing Tests

In addition to the questions included in any musculoskeletal subjective examination, some questions specifically address the cervical region. These questions are detailed in Grieve's *Common Vertebral Joint Problems*.[6] Functional questionnaires provide an excellent baseline determination and can be used to monitor the progress of treatment over time. For example, the "Neck Disability Index" was developed by Vernon and Mior[7] to provide a reliable and valid measure of cervical spine disability.

Shoulder girdle tests should be performed on the patient if indicated by the subjective history and outcomes of alignment tests.

Posture and Movement Examination

Standing alignment should be assessed in all three planes. The examination includes the spinal curves (i.e., CV region, midcervical region, and cervicothoracic [CT] junction), pelvic alignment, and the scapular resting position.

Sitting alignment should be evaluated in all three planes. The examiner should look for changes that occur from standing to sitting. Supine alignment also is evaluated. The examiner should assess the resting position of each vertebral segment through palpation.

Various motion tests are used to assess the patient's flexibility and ability to move in certain ways:

Movement assessments
Active ROM
Combined movements
Assessment of cervical spine passive mobility
Passive intervertebral movements
Passive accessory vertebral movements
Assessment of myofascial extensibility
Muscle lengths
Assessment of neuromeningeal extensibility
Upper limb neurodynamic test
Median nerve bias
Radial nerve bias
Ulnar nerve bias

Muscle Performance, Neurologic, and Special Tests

Assess the patient's cervical musculature by performing manual muscle tests for recruitment, strength, and endurance. Neurologic tests of sensation, motor activity (i.e., key muscle strength), and reflexes are performed to detect any nerve root conduction signs in the cervical region.

Stability tests, vertebral artery tests, and the foraminal compression test are performed to exclude pathology of the cervical spine.

THERAPEUTIC EXERCISE INTERVENTIONS FOR COMMON IMPAIRMENTS OF BODY FUNCTIONS

Any comprehensive therapeutic exercise program for the cervical spine must address various impairments of body structures and functions. This section describes exercise interventions for impairments of muscle performance (including endurance), mobility (i.e., hypomobility and hypermobility), and posture. Appropriate modifications may be necessary for some patients, depending on their signs and symptoms.

Impaired Muscle Performance

Etiology

Janda has suggested that certain muscles in the cervical spine tend to weaken; the most common of these are the deep, anterior cervical flexors. Studies of patients with cervicogenic headache (CHA) symptoms have found decreased maximal isometric strength and endurance of the short upper cervical flexor muscles compared with those of normal subjects.[8] A group of patients with mechanical neck pain also showed significant weakness of the neck flexor muscles compared with controls.[9] A study of patients with osteoarthritis showed more pronounced fatigue curves for anterior and posterior neck muscles than for the muscles of normal subjects.[10] Patients with whiplash associated disorder (WAD), show inability to isolate and tonically hold the deep cervical flexors,[11] without recruitment of the more superficial muscles as compared to controls. There is decreased EMG output of the deep neck flexor (DNF) muscles during a craniocervical flexion test.[12] Similar impairment of the extensors has also been found, although the effect seems to be greater on the flexors.[13] On real-time ultrasound and MR imaging, atrophy of both multifidus and semispinalis capitis, the deep and intermediate groups, have been found in subjects with neck pain.[14-16] The atrophy was more profound on the side of the pain. Transition of muscle fiber type has been demonstrated in subjects with cervical pain, causing a loss of tonic function,[17] as well as fatty infiltration of the posterior suboccipital muscles.[18,19] Fatiguability is increased in both the flexors and extensors, although at low loads the flexors are more affected.[10,20] This finding is also asymmetrical, worse on the side of pain.[21]

Along with loss of strength and endurance, motor patterning is disturbed in patients with neck pain. In a study of WAD subjects, Jull et al.[22] found early and excessive activation of both the anterior scalene and SCM muscles even at low loads during craniocervical flexion. There was also increased superficial neck muscle activity during arm movements. Falla et al.[23] found a timing delay for all cervical flexors, particularly the DNF group during arm movements, suggesting a lack of control of the neck with arm activities in neck pain patients. During simulated keyboarding tasks, there is increased activation of UFT, SCM, and the anterior scalenes, but less activation of the cervical extensors.[24-27] This was more profound in WAD subjects as compared to mechanical neck pain subjects, with both being increased over controls. Following repetitive arm movements, relaxation times for the excessive activity of UFT, SCM, and anterior scalenes are prolonged in subjects with neck pain, again more noticeably in the WAD than mechanical neck pain subgroups. The superficial neck muscles also demonstrated increased relaxation times following a head lift.[28]

Changes in motor function have been shown to occur quickly after the onset of neck pain.[29] Despite complete resolution of symptoms, these motor impairments have been shown to remain and may contribute to the high recurrence rates for neck pain.

In summary, regardless of the cause of neck pain, there is a reduction in strength and endurance in both the deep neck flexors and extensors, an inability to isolate and tonically hold these muscles, as well as weakness of the more superficial groups. Motor patterning is impaired with delay in deep segmental muscle activation, excessive activity in the superficial muscles, and an inability to relax them following activity.

Many articles in the literature describe cervical strengthening protocols, mainly for the prevention of athletic injuries.[30–33] A program that may be safe for training the healthy neck of an athlete may have little application to the injured neck and particularly to the hypermobile cervical spine. In a study of 90 patients with cervical pain, subjects participated in an 8-week strengthening program that involved concentric-eccentric and variable resistance cervical extension exercises. As a group, the patients gained strength and range and experienced a reduction in pain.[34] Patients receiving supervised and individually tailored exercise programs have been shown to achieve greater improvement than those instructed in a home exercise program.[35,36] Jull et al.[37] found a significant improvement in pain intensity, duration, and frequency in patients with chronic CHA receiving physiotherapy consisting of manual therapy and/or specific low load therapeutic exercise. Results were maintained at 12-month follow-up. In mild, chronic neck pain, a higher load, nod-lift type exercise was as effective as the low load craniocervical flexion exercise in improving pain and disability measures, and was more effective in increasing strength and endurance.[38] This exercise was pain free in this subject population, but may not be suitable for patients with a more irritable or intense level of neck pain. Rosenfeld et al.[39–41] found that an active exercise group had less pain, less sick time, and better ROM at 3 years than standard treatment group consisting of advice to exercise with head and shoulder movements after 2 to 3 weeks. A systematic review of 16 random controlled trials found strong evidence supporting the efficacy of proprioceptive and dynamic neck and shoulder exercises in the treatment of chronic neck pain, and moderate evidence for early active mobilization exercises in early WAD.[42]

Exercise dosage should be determined on an individual basis, depending on the variables of strength, endurance, and irritability. A better response seems to occur when loads are initially very low (less than the weight of the head) and progressed slowly. An exercise is considered too difficult or is stopped when it produces pain, muscle tremors occur because of fatigue, or the exercise cannot be executed correctly. The endurance function of many of these cervical postural muscles should be emphasized by encouraging longer, sustained contractions.

Therapeutic Exercise Intervention

Deep Cervical Flexors The most common muscles to become weak with neck dysfunction are the deep, single segment cervical flexors. It is important to teach the patient to isolate these dynamic stabilizers without substituting with the more superficial muscle groups. The primary exercise to recruit these muscles is the head nod exercise of CV flexion, continuing segmentally into midcervical flexion. During this exercise it is important to control the tendency to substitute with the overactive superficial flexors that would excessively translate anteriorly (see Patient-Related Instruction 23-1: How to Activate your Cervical Core Muscles). If done initially in the upright position at the wall, the exercise is gravity assisted, but the head must stay back in contact with

the wall at all times to prevent any forward movement that would change the exercise into an eccentric contraction of the cervical extensors (see Fig. 23-4). The retracted position also discourages the use of the SCM muscle. The DNFs are recruited to nod the CV unit, decrease the cervical lordosis, and then overcome the resistance of the extensors. The patient is taught to palpate at the front of the neck for any unwanted contraction of the SCM or scalene muscles and to rest the tongue on the roof of the mouth to inhibit hyoid muscle activity. The patient slowly nods the chin down, while sliding the back of the head up the wall. The nod is stopped at the furthest point in range that can be achieved without superficial activity, held for 10 seconds to encourage the endurance function, and is repeated 10 times. The assistance of gravity can be decreased by performing the exercise supine on an incline board, with difficulty increased by progressively tilting the board backward toward horizontal.

When this same nod exercise is performed with the patient in supine, the DNFs work against the resistance of gravity, theoretically making the exercise slightly more difficult. However,

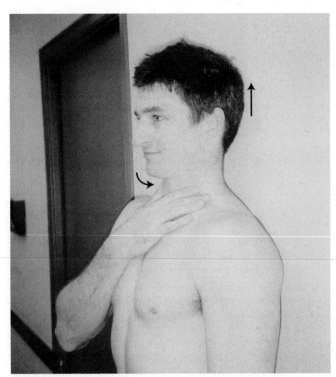

FIGURE 23-4. Wall slide DNF muscle recruitment, palpating for unwanted superficial muscle activity.

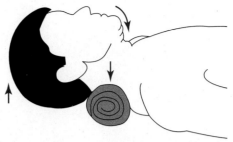

FIGURE 23-5. Short flexor muscle strengthening over a towel roll with slight head liftoff. The patient no longer palpates, because the superficial muscles must now be active to lift the weight of the head against gravity. The neck should not lose contact with the towel, or the chin poke forward, because this is a sign of excessive anterior translation caused by relative dominance of sternocleidomastoid and scalenes substituting for the weaker DNFs.

this position is both well supported and non–weight-bearing so for some patients, and this might be more easily executed than at the wall, despite the gravity assist in that position. The head is positioned in neutral, either resting on a pillow, or with a small folded towel placed under the occiput as needed to achieve a neutral posture. A small rolled towel can be placed under the hollow of the midcervical spine to support the normal cervical lordosis. As a low load recruitment exercise, the head nod is performed with no lifting of the head off the surface, with the patient again palpating anteriorly to ensure no superficial muscle activity. The patient is also instructed to avoid using a neck retraction strategy as compensation during this exercise. If the patient is unable to obtain much excursion of motion because of tight extensors or an extremely ingrained pattern of superficial recruitment, the exercise can be started in more outer range of some extension, nodding toward neutral. Using eye motion to look down as the movement is initiated can also assist in correct muscle activation.

The CV nod exercise can also be performed in a prone position over an exercise ball or in the four-point kneeling (FPK) position. In this position, gravity draws the head forward into a position of upper cervical extension, which is countered by the head-nod motion into upper cervical flexion. This exercise recruits the upper cervical flexors only; gravity is assisting the lower cervical flexors in this position. If the patient maintains the retracted neutral posture of the spine while nodding, it is very difficult to substitute with SCM because this muscle protrudes the neck, and so this is a useful option for patients with very dominant SCM muscles.

Eventually, the patient should be progressed to higher load exercises to increase strength, rather than just recruitment. In supine, the head nod is continued using the towel roll as a fulcrum, and the back of the head is lifted off the surface during

the motion. The patient no longer palpates, because the superficial muscles must now be active to lift the weight of the head against gravity (see Fig. 23-5). The neck should not lose contact with the towel; in other words, the chin should remain tucked, as a chin poke would be a sign of excessive anterior translation caused by relative dominance of sternocleidomastoid and scalenes over the weaker DNFs. The ROM allowed depends on the muscle balance and the ability to continue the head nod without excessive anterior translation. A head nod into a flexion quadrant (e.g., flexion, side flexion, rotation to the same side) emphasizes contraction of the flexors more unilaterally and may be appropriate in cases of asymmetric weakness.

As an alternate progression, a nod liftoff motion can be performed supported on a high incline (Fig. 23-6). The patient is instructed to nod to the point of cervical spine

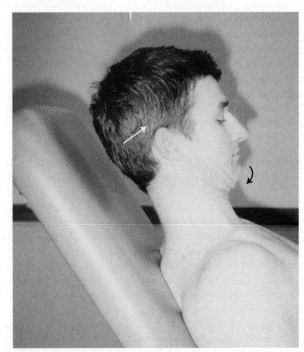

FIGURE 23-6. A nod liftoff motion can also be performed supported on a high incline. The patient is instructed to nod to the point of cervical spine neutral and then just lift the head off the supporting surface to take the weight of the head as resistance. The neutral posture of the neck must be maintained, not allowing dominant superficial muscles to cause a chin poke of anterior translation.

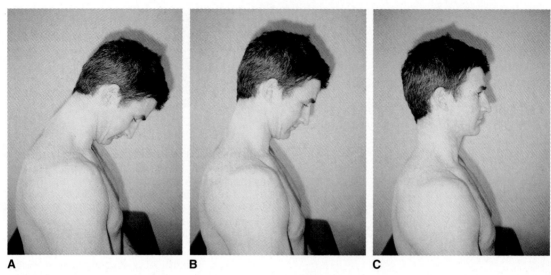

A   **B**   **C**

FIGURE 23-7. RTN in sitting to recruit the segmental extensors. (A) Start in the forward flexed position. (B) Keeping the head dropped forward and the chin tucked, initiate segmental extension starting at the upper thoracic spine. (C) Continue the extension starting at the lower segments, up the cervical spine to the neutral position.

neutral and then just lift the head off the supporting surface to take the weight of the head as resistance. The neutral posture of the neck must be maintained using a balance of both deep and superficial muscles, not allowing dominant superficial muscles to cause a chin poke and anterior translation. The patient will progress to holding this sustained neutral position for 10 seconds, repeating 10 times. The exercise can be further progressed by gradually bringing the incline down toward the horizontal, as long as the patient can control the neutral posture of the neck.

In the upright or sitting positions, autoresistance can be applied to the head-nod motion to increase the load on the muscle. Resistance must be applied at such an angle to appropriately resist the head-nod motion and not encourage a head forward translation movement. Resistance under the chin rather than at the forehead can encourage the proper movement. This might be considered an easier progression than the other two exercises, as the autoresistence can be graded to be substantially less than the weight of the head.

Cervical Extensor Muscles   Both the deep and middle layers of the cervical extensors atrophy and decrease in strength and endurance in response to neck pain. The use of electrical muscle stimulation is effective in the initial stages of retraining, especially when the patient has a high level of pain that precludes resisted exercise. With the patient lying supine with the head supported, small electrodes are placed over the extensor muscles bilaterally at the vertebral level with poor segmental recruitment. Contraction should be a sustained tonic hold, and the patient can simultaneously perform a nod to obtain co-contraction of both the flexors and extensors.

It is more difficult to isolate the deep segmental extensors than the flexors. A study by Mayoux-Benhamou et al.[43] suggested that the motions of return to neutral (RTN) from the flexed posture, and retrusion, are less likely to recruit the superficial extensors. If this motion is performed segment by segment, it is likely that the segmental extensors will need to be recruited. The patient starts in the forward flexed position and initiates the extension in the thoracic spine first, starting at the lower

segments, and sequentially extending until the trunk is in upright neutral position. As the motion moves into the cervical spine, the chin tuck position is maintained as the patient continues to extend segmentally, incorporating a component of slight posterior motion (Fig. 23-7). The patient should be cautioned to not over retract the neck as this is not the cervical neutral posture. Maintaining the CV region in flexion until the end of the motion will tend to inhibit the superficial capitis group of the erector spinae muscles. Tactile cues can be given at each level to encourage the segmental nature of the motion. The exercise can also be progressed by performing the motion in the FPK position. The addition of pure rotation to the exercise in FPK further activates the suboccipital muscles.

The patient can be taught to apply autoresistance to the contraction of a specific muscle determined to be weak on assessment. For example, a weak superior oblique muscle can be retrained by applying autoresistance to AO joint side flexion into extension on the same side (Fig. 23-8). Contraction of the multifidus at the C4–5 level can be obtained by pressure applied to the C4 lamina, as the patient attempts side flexion to the same side into extension.

Multisegmental extension exercises for more generalized weakness can be performed in a supine position with pillow support. The cervical lordosis should be further supported

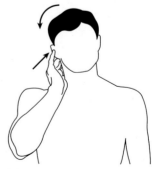

FIGURE 23-8. Retraining a weak right superior oblique muscle by applying autoresistance to AO joint side flexion into extension on the same side.

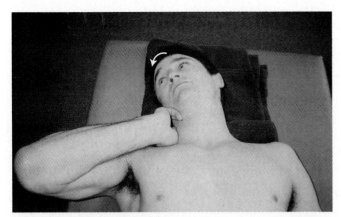

FIGURE 23-9. Concentric muscle contraction into the right extension quadrant over a foam roll or rolled towel. Palpation will encourage more local recruitment.

with a foam roll or rolled towel. While the patient squeezes the roll by the extension movement, the therapist must ensure that the motion remains angular and no shearing occurs. This exercise can be made more specific in cases of asymmetric weakness by working into the extension quadrant (i.e., combined extension, side flexion, and rotation to the same side). The roll is then squeezed between the head and the shoulder on the affected side (Fig. 23-9).

In the prone position over an exercise ball, midcervical extension exercises can be performed against gravity. The position tends to encourage the poking-chin posture of CV extension. The patient should be taught to control the upper cervical flexion while working the middle and lower cervical spine into extension. The exercise can be done into the quadrant position to target the muscles unilaterally. The same exercise can be performed in the FPK position at home. Adding arm motion further challenges the maintenance of the cervical neutral posture and with multiple repetitions, would also reinforce the endurance requirements of these muscles.

With any exercise into cervical extension or an extension quadrant, it is important to consider the following effects:

- Effects on the vertebral artery
- Compression load on the zygapophyseal joints
- Foraminal compression and its effect on the neurologic structures
- Risk of encouraging the cervical lordosis of the FHP

Rotation and Side Flexion Component By exercising into a quadrant position, the muscles that are primarily side flexors and rotators are also recruited. In supine with the head offset on a foam wedge, the slope can be used to apply resistance to combined flexion, side flexion, and rotation of the cervical spine (see Self-Management 23-1: Side Flexor and Rotator Activation).

In the sidelying position with the head supported on a pillow and a towel roll under the neck, these muscles can also be trained more specifically and intensely at higher load. The muscles opposite to the side the patient is lying on can be contracted against gravity as the head is lifted off the pillow. The roll is used as the fulcrum, and the deeper muscles can be emphasized by ensuring that the neck remains in contact with the roll, decreasing the amount of translation taking place (Fig. 23-10).

 SELF-MANAGEMENT 23-1 *Side Flexor and Rotator Activation*

Purpose: To activate and strengthen the neck side flexors and rotators on each side

Starting Position: Lie on your back with your head supported on the foam wedge. Knees are bent. Move the wedge so your head is resting off to one side on the slope of the wedge (A). You will immediately feel that you have to use your neck muscles on the side closest to the peak to hold your head in place.

Movement Technique:
- Perform a slight nod to activate the deep neck muscles. Hold this nod throughout the exercise.
- Slowly, in a controlled fashion, lower your head down the slope to the end of range. Stop before there is any pain. Pause at the end of range, then slowly bring the head back up the slope, maintaining the slight nod throughout (B). Go past your center position, continuing up the slope of the wedge to the end of range. Again pause at this point. In a controlled fashion, bring your head back to mid line. Relax from the nod position. This is one repetition.
- Repeat for the designated number of repetitions, beginning with the preset nod for each.
- Move the wedge over to have the head resting on the other side of the peak. Repeat the same sequence as above for the designated number of repetitions.

Dosage:
Set/repetitions _____
Right _____
Left _____
Frequency _____

A   B

For both of these exercises, the patient is taught to perform a preset nod to activate the deep stabilizing muscles prior to any motion of the head. This would also encourage retraining of the appropriate timing of the motor pattern that is impaired with neck pain.

Strengthening Functional Movement Patterns Several strengthening exercises use combined movements. Because many of the movement patterns required for functional activity are multiplanar, it is beneficial to train the muscle group using these movements. The movement patterns chosen for a particular patient depend on the assessment findings (i.e., specific weakness or reproduction of pain) and on the requirements of work and leisure activities.

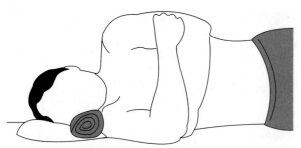

FIGURE 23-10. Recruiting the side flexors and rotators more specifically. The patient is in the sidelying position, with the head supported on a pillow with a towel roll under the neck. The roll is used as the fulcrum, and the deeper muscles can be emphasized by ensuring that the neck remains in contact with the roll, decreasing the amount of translation taking place.

The patient can be taught the correct movement pattern by using a modified muscle energy technique for muscle recruitment rather than mobilization. With the patient sitting, the therapist palpates at the affected level as the patient performs the motion against the resistance of the therapist (Fig. 23-11). The recruitment of the muscles at that segment and any excessive translation can be monitored. Concentric or eccentric muscle contractions can be used.

After the patient can perform these movements correctly (without excessive translation), autoresistance throughout the range can be applied by the patient. Heavy resistance should be avoided, because it tends to encourage faulty movement patterns, as do static maximal isometric contractions. Concentric contractions can be used first through short-arc movements, progressing to full-arc motion and then to eccentric contractions (Fig. 23-12).

Pulley systems or theraband can be used to apply graded resistance. Head pieces can apply resistance to the weak cervical muscles as determined at assessment. It is important to provide the correct angle of pull to encourage an optimal movement pattern of the neck. The weight must be kept low enough to allow the patient to perform the motion smoothly and without substitution of unwanted muscle groups. Supervision is important, because there is a tendency to use a translation motion against

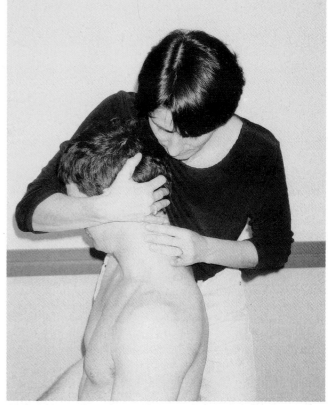

FIGURE 23-11. Strengthening in functional movement patterns. With the patient sitting, the therapist palpates at the affected level as the patient performs the motion against the resistance of the therapist.

the resistance, which often exacerbates the problem, especially in cases of hypermobility. Additional resistance beyond the weight of the head is often not necessary, as not many activities involve lifting more than the weight of the head.

Mobility Impairment

Impairment of mobility can be classified as hypomobility (i.e., reduced motion) or hypermobility (i.e., increased motion).

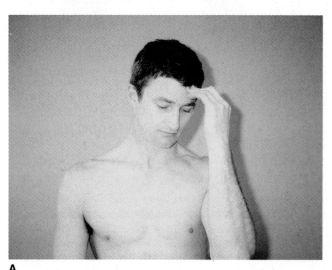

A

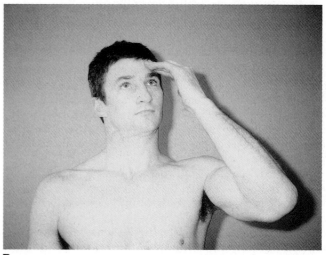

B

FIGURE 23-12. Strengthening in functional movement patterns using autoresistance. (A) Concentric contractions into the left flexion quadrant. (B) Eccentric contractions back into the right extension quadrant (early in range).

In the case of hypomobility, exercises are given to regain and maintain motion. For hypermobility, a stabilization exercise program is used to regain control of the excessive motion.

Hypomobility

Etiology   ROM is often reduced in patients with neck pain regardless of cause. There is a decrease in ROM in all WAD II subjects at 1 month post accident, but this has recovered by 3 months in the subgroups that are classified as either mild or recovered.[44–46] In both the moderate and severe subgroups of WAD II, the reduced ROM persists at 3 months. Decrease in ROM is present in subjects with CHA, but not in migraine or tension type headache and so may be used as a diagnostic feature. Reduction in motion as determined by the flexion-rotation test has been found to correlate highly with CHA related to AA joint rotation restriction.[47] Rosenfeld et al.[39–41] demonstrated that subjects that performed early active repeated rotation movements 10 times hourly, had less pain at both 6 months and 3 years, as well as better mobility and less sick time at 3 years.

Cervical mobility can be reduced for several reasons:

- Segmental articular mobility restriction
- Capsular thickening and contracture
- Degenerative bony changes
- Segmental muscle spasm
- Myofascial extensibility
- Adverse neuromeningeal tension

Cervical mobility also can be affected by syndromes involving the shoulder girdle, and treatment may need to include interventions for impairments in that region.

Therapeutic Exercise Interventions   Even in the early stages of treatment for an acute neck problem, ROM exercises can be taught for each of the restricted planes of motion. Care must be taken in teaching these exercises to ensure that the normal movement pattern is performed and that this pattern is reinforced with repetition. With the patient lying supine with the head supported on a pillow, the weight of the head is eliminated, decreasing the compression load. This position can be helpful for patients with painful neck motion. The use of rhythmic respiration during the exercise can aid in relaxation of the scalene muscles and create a pumping action to help reduce swelling. This activity can be progressed to rotation exercises with the head positioned on the peak of a foam wedge (Fig. 23-13). The amplitude of motion obtained is increased and there is some extension incorporated with the movement on rotation and flexion on return to midline. ROM exercises can also be performed in the upright position.

If a mobility exercise into extension or the extension quadrant is being contemplated, the effects on articular, vascular, and neurological tissues should be considered. Keep in mind that a considerable weight-bearing force is sustained by the articular facet and the intervertebral foramen is being compressed in these positions.

Segmental Articular Restrictions   Segmental articular restrictions generally respond well to manual therapy mobilization techniques unless there is excessive degeneration of the bony structures (see Chapter 7). Self-mobilization

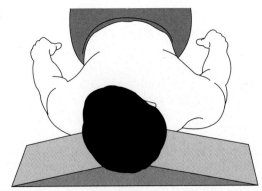

FIGURE 23-13. ROM exercises on a foam wedge. Allows non–weight-bearing motion, combining rotation and side flexion with flexion-extension.

exercises are a useful adjunct to this treatment. The patient is taught to localize to the involved segment with his or her fingers or a towel support and perform a specific, sometimes multiplanar motion to mobilize the joint restriction as determined by mobility testing (see Self-Management 23-2: Self-Mobilization for the Cervical Spine). A specific AA rotation technique as proposed by Mulligan has been shown to be effective in increasing upper cervical motion and decreasing headaches.[48]

Muscle Extensibility   Assessment of muscle lengths is necessary because of muscle imbalances and postural asymmetries that are unique to each individual. Janda[49] states that certain muscle groups in the cervical spine have a greater tendency to shorten. This may be related to the effect of the limbic system on these muscles, the large percentage of afferent fibers supplying these muscles, and the more tonic rather than phasic properties of many of these muscles. According to Janda, the following muscles tend to shorten:

- Posterior suboccipital muscles
- Cervical superficial erector spinae muscles
- Scalenes (anterior, medius, posterior)
- Sternocleidomastoid
- Levator scapula
- Trapezius, upper fibers

A study of cervical musculoskeletal function in postconcussional headache[50] and CHA[51] showed a higher incidence of moderate muscle tightness compared to those with migraines or controls. This finding of tightness was not isolated to any one of the muscles tested (e.g., upper fibers of the trapezius, levator scapula, scalenes, upper cervical extensors), but it was most frequently identified in the upper cervical extensors. In subjects with CHA, many of these muscles were found to be of normal length. A study by Edgar et al.[52] showed a relationship between decreased neuromeningeal extensibility and decreased length of upper fibers of the trapezius, possibly as a protective mechanism. Patients with WAD showed greater electromyelography activity of both their ipsilateral and contralateral upper fibers of the trapezius during repetitive upper extremity activity and were less able to relax that muscle following activity as compared with controls.[24] This may suggest that feelings of tightness in patients with cervical

SELF-MANAGEMENT 23-2 *Self-mobilization for the Cervical Spine*

Purpose: To maintain the range gained during treatment at a particular joint.

AO Joint

Starting Position: Sit tall in a chair with back support. Clasp your hands behind your neck with your little fingers just under the base of your skull. Stabilize the neck, but be careful not to drag the neck forward by pulling forward with your hands.

Movement Technique: Flexion on the right (A)

- Nod your head on your neck. The head must tip away (left) from the stiff side, and chin must deviate toward (right) the stiff side. In other words, tuck your chin toward your armpit on the side of the stiff joint.

Extension on the right (B)

- Tip your head back on your neck over your fingers. Tip the head slightly toward (right) the stiff side and poke the chin away from (left) the stiff side. In other words, poke your chin toward the opposite elbow.

Dosage:
Hold_____count
Repetitions   _____
Frequency   _____

AA Joint

Starting Position: Wrap your hands behind your neck with your little fingers resting at the level of the large bump at the top of the neck below the skull. Stabilize the neck, but be careful not to drag the neck forward by pulling forward with your hands.

Movement Technique:
- Keep eyes level as you rotate the head in the stiff direction, being sure not to let the rest of the neck move with the head.
- If instructed, bias the movement to the joint on one side or the other by
  - tucking the chin into a bit of flexion as you turn, and slightly pull the supporting hand forward on the side you are turning to (C).
  - tipping the chin slightly up as you turn, and hold back with the supporting hand on the side opposite to the direction you are turning to (D).
- Do not let the neck collapse as you turn the head; stay tall.

Dosage:
Hold_____count
Repetitions   _____
Frequency   _____

Midcervical joints

Starting position: Find the stiff joint as instructed. It often will feel tender, or thick under your finger. Hold the bottom bone stable by pushing in gently with your fingers. Alternatively, place the salvage edge of a towel along the effected joint to stabilize it.

Movement Technique: Flexion
- Nod your chin forward until you feel a pull at the stiff joint. Tip the head away from the stiff side and rotate the head away (E). The movement to stretch the joint maximally will be off on the opposite diagonal.
- The fixing fingers should hold the bottom bone down toward the floor.
- You should feel a strong stretch on the side of the neck at the stiff joint.

Extension
- Tip your head back over the stabilizing fingers or towel. The head should also tip and rotate to that same side on a diagonal (F).
- You can push in and up slightly with the fixating fingers.
- Focus the movement to the level that is stiff. Do not arch your whole neck back over the fingers.

Dosage:
Hold_____count
Repetitions   _____
Frequency   _____

A

B

C

D

E

F

spine dysfunction may be more related to overactivity than to true shortening.

Alterations in resting posture may cause a muscle that is of normal length to be placed on tension because of the increased distance between the origin and insertion caused by the posture. For example, a depressed scapular resting position puts tension on the levator scapula, potentially reducing opposite-side flexion and rotation of the cervical spine. The neck motion can be regained immediately on elevating the scapula, confirming that the tension on the levator scapula, resulting from the depressed position of the scapula, was contributing to the loss of neck ROM. Other muscles may adaptively shorten because of long-standing changes in posture. The sternocleidomastoid, for example, tends to adaptively shorten in response to FHP. When the head is brought back into a more normal position, the muscle may appear to be a tight band, inhibiting attempts to retrain optimal posture. Treatment of both cases consists of postural correction exercises. Chapter 26 illustrates taping techniques to correct scapula position and normalize length-tension properties of the cervical muscles that attach to the scapula (i.e., levator scapula and upper trapezius).

The posterior suboccipital muscle group can be lengthened by using the CV flexion head-nod exercise (Fig. 23-14). The stretch can be localized by supporting the rest of the neck with clasped hands and further localized by side flexion away and rotation toward the tighter side.

Further neck flexion must be incorporated to obtain a stretch into the middle to low cervical erector spinae. CV flexion must be maintained throughout the exercise to maintain the stretch on the long superficial extensors. If any anterior translation is allowed, cervical lordosis is produced, which results in a shortening of these muscles. Performing this stretch with the trunk against the wall helps fixate the

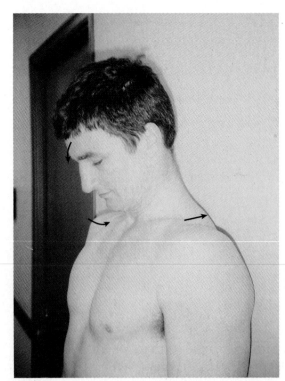

FIGURE 23-15. Stretching into the middle to low cervical erector spinae at the wall.

CT junction (Fig. 23-15). Adding side flexion and rotation to the opposite side biases the stretch to the right or left side.

The scalene muscle group also tends to shorten and become overactive, often reinforced by improper breathing patterns. Teaching proper diaphragmatic breathing while palpating the scalenes can decrease recruitment of this group as a secondary muscle of inspiration (see Chapter 22). Exercises designed to stretch this muscle must allow for adequate fixation of the first and second ribs, which can be achieved through manual or belt fixation. The scalene group is lengthened by side flexion away (Fig. 23-16). Slight rotation toward the affected side will focus the stretch to the anterior group, and rotation away from the effected side will bias the posterior scalene. Performing pure side flexion at the wall prevents the neck from collapsing into an FHP and will allow a more effective stretch. The patient must be instructed to stop at the point of tension, because the muscle pull can produce an unwanted lateral translation force on the cervical spine.

An effective method of regaining normal SCM length is to correct the FHP. Retraining the use of the deep cervical flexors for the habitual movement pattern of neck flexion also decreases overuse tightness of the sternocleidomastoid. If the muscle has become shortened by posttraumatic adhesions, it may be necessary to stretch the muscle. This can be achieved by extension, side flexion away from, and rotation toward the side being treated, while keeping the chin tucked. Lordosis must be controlled, because that position shortens the muscle. This effect can be achieved by bringing the CV flexed head on a straight neck back behind the line of the trunk (Fig. 23-17).

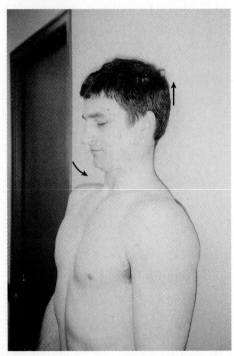

FIGURE 23-14. Stretching the posterior suboccipital muscles using the CV flexion head-nod exercise.

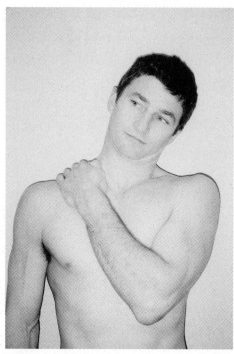

FIGURE 23-16. Stretching the scalene muscles—first rib fixed, side flexion away, and slight rotation toward the affected side at the wall.

When attempting to lengthen the levator scapula muscle, it is important to fix the scapula into depression, upward rotation, or both. Upward rotation of the scapula can be achieved by arm elevation, but this position may be difficult for patients with pain on arm elevation. In the sitting position, depression can be maintained by holding the underside of a chair. The muscle is then stretched by cervical side flexion and rotation to the opposite side and cervical flexion (Fig. 23-18).

To stretch the upper fibers of the trapezius, the scapula must be fixed into depression, downward rotation, or both. Scapular depression and downward rotation can be achieved by reaching the arm down and behind the back. The stretch is then performed into neck flexion, with side flexion away from and rotation toward the affected side (Fig. 23-19).

The concern about the latter two stretches is the resultant forces on irritable zygapophyseal joints from the end-range combined movements. These two muscles and the scalene muscles, because of their angle of pull, may also produce

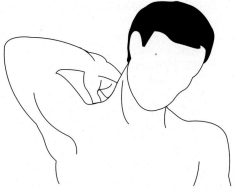

FIGURE 23-18. Stretching the levator scapula—arm overhead (scapular upward rotation), scapular depression, side flexion away, rotation away from affected side, and flexion.

an excessive lateral translation force on the vertebrae when stretched. An alternative exercise is to have the patient face the wall, with the ulnar border of the hands and forearm in contact overhead, and perform a wall slide. The arms are slid downward and slightly inward, creating scapular depression. The cervical spine can then be moved into flexion. From this position, contralateral rotation lengthens the levator scapula muscle, and ipsilateral rotation lengthens the upper fibers of the trapezius muscle (Fig. 23-20).

Adverse Neuromeningeal Tension   Adverse tension in the neuromeningeal structures of the cervical spine can affect the mobility of the neck, thoracic spine, shoulder girdle, and upper extremity.[53] Signs of decreased extensibility of these structures are found on the Upper Limb Neurodynamic Tests, with a median, radial, or ulnar nerve bias. When prescribing

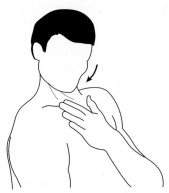

FIGURE 23-17. Sternocleidomastoid stretch-extension, side flexion away from and rotation toward the side being treated.

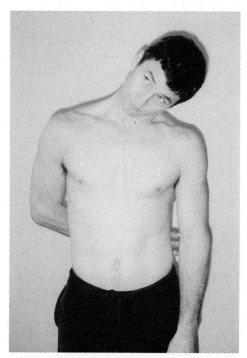

FIGURE 23-19. Stretching the upper fibers of the trapezius—scapular depression and downward rotation, neck flexion, side flexion away, and rotation toward the affected side.

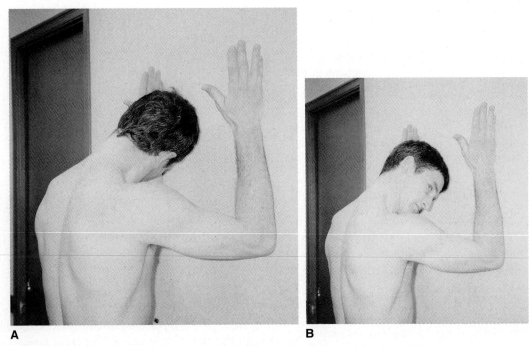

FIGURE 23-20. Alternative wall slide exercise. (A) Contralateral rotation lengthens the right levator scapula muscle. (B) Ipsilateral rotation lengthens the upper fibers of the right trapezius muscle.

an exercise designed to improve neuromeningeal extensibility, the effect on the cervical spine should be considered. Because of direct attachment of dural structures into the cervical vertebrae, tightness in the neuromeningeal system may cause lateral translation of the vertebrae with each attempt to stretch the structures, which can lead to hypermobility of the segment. The affected segment should be manually fixated by the opposite hand supporting under the neck so that the fingers wrap around to the affected side and prevent the lateral translation (Fig. 23-21). The DNF can also be used to stabilize the spine through an active nod, setting the spine in neutral.

The stretch can be performed by the patient in supine lying, with a belt wrapped over the shoulder and around the knee to maintain the scapular depression. Median, radial, and ulnar nerves are biased via various arm, elbow, forearm, and wrist positions as shown in Figure 23-22. It may be more effective initially to emphasize mobility of the system, by using

"slider" exercises that add tension in one component of the movement, while removing tension in another component. For example, tipping the head toward the arm as the elbow is extended.

For median nerve bias, the arm, flexed at the elbow, is abducted to the tension point and externally rotated, with the forearm supinated and the wrist and fingers extended. The elbow is then slowly extended to produce the stretch (Fig. 23-22A).

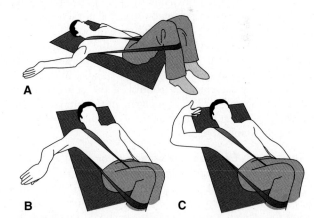

FIGURE 23-22. Dural stretch in supine lying with a belt wrapped over the shoulder and around the knee to maintain scapular depression. (A) For median nerve bias, the arm, flexed at the elbow, is abducted to the tension point and externally rotated, with the forearm supinated and the wrist and fingers extended. The elbow is then slowly extended to produce the stretch. (B) For radial nerve bias, the arm, flexed at the elbow, is abducted and internally rotated, the forearm is pronated, with the wrist flexed. The stretch is produced by slowly extending the elbow. (C) For ulnar nerve bias, the arm, flexed to a right angle at the elbow, is abducted and externally rotated, the forearm is pronated, with the wrist extended. The stretch is produced through further flexion of the elbow.

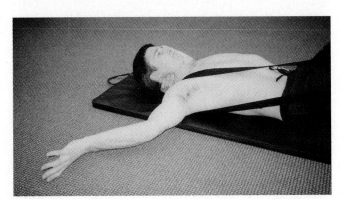

FIGURE 23-21. Dural stretch with manual stabilization and fixation of lateral shear.

Similar stretches can be performed by the patient in standing. The opposite hand is required to maintain depression of the scapula. With each of these exercises, a more intense stretch can be obtained by the addition of contralateral side flexion or rotation of the neck. For more detailed descriptions of these types of exercises, the reader is directed to other sources.[54]

Hypermobility

Etiology   Hypermobility is excessive motion of the intervertebral segment. As hypothesized by Panjabi,[4] spinal stability is obtained through three subsystems:

- Passive musculoskeletal subsystem: inert osseoligamentous column, including the vertebra, disk, capsule, and ligament
- Active musculoskeletal subsystem: the muscle and tendon units
- Control subsystem: the neural and feedback mechanisms

The role of the spinal stability system is to provide sufficient stability through all three subsystems to match the demands made on the spine. Deficiencies in one subsystem can be compensated for, within certain limits. Gross instability, as documented by functional radiographs, may require surgical fixation. Otherwise, hypermobilities are best addressed by conservative measures, including a progressive stabilization exercise program. Exercise programs can be used to enhance both the active and control subsystems.

Specific passive stability testing is performed to determine the degree and planes of laxity. Special attention is given to the amount of translation and the end feel. This assessment determines the structural integrity of the passive subsystem of the spine. To determine the dynamic stability of the cervical spine, the passive tests can be repeated during an active preset DNF nod to neutral. If recruitment of the deep segmental stabilizers decreases the amount of translation on passive testing, there is a degree of dynamic stability present. The neck can also be observed or palpated during bilateral or unilateral elevation of the arm in the relaxed upright posture and then repeated with the cervical spine under the dynamic control of a preset nod (Fig. 23-23). Because of the large neutral zone in the cervical spine, much of the stability in this region is imparted by the dynamic control of the active muscular system. In the case of loss of integrity of the inert stabilizing structures, training of neuromuscular control may result in a functionally stable spine.

Therapeutic Exercise Intervention   For the hypermobile cervical spine, care must be taken in prescribing ROM or stretching exercises that may exaggerate the excessive translation. The neck must be passively fixed at the affected segment during the stretch, or another exercise should be chosen that does not incorporate the unwanted motion. For example, a patient may have a tight right levator scapula muscle but also be hypermobile into right lateral translation at the C3–4 intervertebral segment. Attempts to stretch the levator scapula muscle by left side flexion encourage right lateral translation at C3–4. The patient can control the right lateral translation with the left hand cupping behind the neck, offering a counteracting left translation at the C4 vertebra (Fig. 23-24). It may be more appropriate in this case to choose the wall slide exercise described in the "Hypomobility" section, using contralateral rotation rather than side flexion.

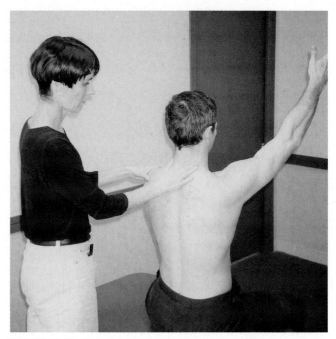

FIGURE 23-23. To determine the stability of the cervical spine during dynamic upper extremity movements, the neck can be observed or palpated during bilateral or unilateral arm elevation in the relaxed upright posture, and then repeated with the cervical spine under the dynamic control of a preset nod. If recruitment of the deep segmental stabilizers decreases the amount of translation, there is a degree of dynamic stability present.

For the patient with lateral translation hypermobility, attempts to incorporate dural stretch exercises cause repetitive lateral translation at the affected joint. A stretch can be performed effectively by first stabilizing that segment for lateral translation (see Fig. 23-21).

Postural correction exercises are an integral component in unloading the hypermobile segment in the cervical spine. Any deviation from the optimal posture of the cervical spine increases the translational forces that the spine is subjected to. The resting posture of the shoulder girdle also plays a role in imparting translational forces to the cervical spine. For example, weakness or poor recruitment of the upper fibers of trapezius leads to a depressed and downwardly rotated scapula, which places the muscle in a lengthened position. Constant pull on the insertion into the cervical spine may eventually lead to hypermobility into lateral translation. In cases of preexisting lateral hypermobility, the continuous lateral force exacerbates symptoms arising from that segment. Exercise should focus on correcting the impairments found on assessment of the

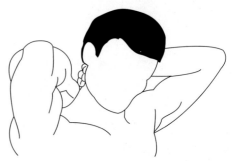

FIGURE 23-24. Levator scapula stretch: fixing C4 to prevent right lateral translation.

shoulder girdle. Taping to reposition the scapula into elevation and upward rotation can reduce this force, allow a more normal movement pattern of the cervical spine, and relieve the increased dural tension caused by the abnormal resting position (see Chapter 25).

Cervical hypermobility can also be addressed through training to facilitate neuromuscular control of the cervical spine with graduated exercise. A series of cervical strengthening exercises can be implemented as determined by specific muscle testing. These exercises, as described in the "Impaired Muscle Performance" section, enhance the active subsystem of the spinal stability system. Alternatively, a cervical stabilization program can be developed to focus on both the active and control subsystem. A stabilization program can be divided into three stages:

- Stage 1: Isolated contraction of the deep segmental flexors and extensors and co-contraction in the cervical neutral position
- Stage 2: Cervical stability during various upper extremity movement patterns
- Stage 3: Cervical stability during functional neck movements

Display 23-1 provides examples of exercise that can be prescribed in each stage.

Throughout the stabilization program, motion at the hypermobile segment must be controlled, particularly for the excessive translation component. In many cases, the patient can be taught to palpate the translation motion of the vertebra and stop moving when it begins. The patient can also be taught to stabilize the affected level manually or through active muscle co-contraction by performimg a preset nod as an exercise is performed. Progressing in the presence of translation of the affected level does not succeed in developing stability, and through increased stresses on the capsule and ligaments, it may result in painful exacerbation to the point that the program has to be discontinued.

Because of the importance of the role of muscles in dynamic stability of the spine, it can be deduced that, despite the presence of hypermobility, functional stability can be regained through neuromuscular retraining. The key is gradually challenging the cervical musculature over several months while preventing excessive motion at the involved segment.

Posture Impairment

Etiology

Although posture is affected by the whole of the axial skeleton, the cervical spine plays an important role in the control of posture. The rich supply of mechanoreceptors in the articular capsules and muscles of the cervical spine provides proprioceptive input and feed into the vestibular system.[55] Any attempt to alter cervical spine posture must include an evaluation of the thoracic spine, shoulder girdle, and pelvis. Many of the involved muscles are multijoint muscles, spanning the first three of these related regions. Changes in the lengths of muscles such as the levator scapula, trapezius, pectoralis major and minor, or rhomboids have profound effects on the shoulder complex and the cervical spine. Changes in the strength of these scapular stabilizers also alter the resting posture of the neck. Alterations of the pelvic base in any plane have effects throughout the spinal column, including the cervical spine.

Patient-Related Instruction 23-2
Optimal Posture of the Neck

It is important to practice proper posture of the head and neck. Good posture decreases the stresses on muscles, joints, and ligaments of the cervical spine, which can reduce pain and prevent wear and tear on these structures. Your therapist will instruct you in additional exercises to enable you to achieve and maintain this posture.

The upper back should be straightened, the shoulder blades pulled back together, and the chin brought back so that the head is centered over the trunk. A useful guideline is that the ear should be over the midline of the shoulder. Do not overcorrect, because a slight curve in the neck is normal. Proper posture must be practiced frequently throughout the day so that this position becomes habitual. This posture must also be adopted during exercise for the neck and upper extremity.

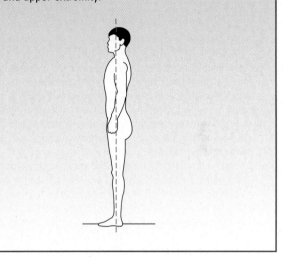

The optimal posture for the cervical spine is the position of cervical neutral or axial extension (Fig. 23-25A and Patient-Related Instruction 23-2: Optimal Posture of the Neck). In cervical neutral, minimal muscle work is required to maintain the position, the spine is in an elongated state, and compressive and translatory forces on the spinal structures are reduced compared with those in the FHP. The most common postural impairment of the cervical spine is the FHP.

A patient with FHP can present with several variations. In some individuals, the lower cervical spine flexion juts the whole cervical spine forward above that level, and extension mainly occurs at the CV region with little increase in the midcervical lordosis (Fig. 23-25B). In others, the lower cervical spine flexion is compensated for by an exaggerated cervical lordosis that may start abruptly, sometimes as low as the C6–7 segment. In these cases, the midcervical lordosis tends to be accompanied by an excessive anterior translation that is an unphysiologic coupling of motion, because extension (i.e., lordosis) should couple with posterior translation (Fig. 23-25C). Each individual should be assessed to determine the exact components of his or her abnormal posture, the levels at which changes in the spinal curves are taking place, and what the emphasis of the postural correction should be. Table 23-3 summarizes alignment findings at various levels of the cervical spine in the optimal position and FHP.

DISPLAY 23-1
Cervical Spine Stabilization Program

STAGE I
The first goal of the stabilization program is to isolate the deep neck flexors and extensors. The next goal is to perform co-contraction patterns in the cervical neutral position. The following exercises can be used to achieve these goals. The exercises are described in more detail in the "Impaired Muscle Performance" section.

Isolation of the deep cervical flexors:
- Cervical core activation in variety of positions (Patient-Related Instruction 23-1 and Fig. 23-4)
- Autoresistance to the deep flexors

Isolation of the deep cervical extensors:
- Electrical muscle stimulation to the cervical extensors in supine
- RTN from flexion (Fig. 23-7)
- Autoresistance to specific multifidus or suboccipital muscles (Fig. 23-8)
- Concentric extension over a foam roll (Fig. 23-9)

Rotation and side flexion components:
- Supine head roll on a foam wedge, offset (Self-Management 23-1)

Co-contraction of the deep cervical flexors and extensors:
- Early co-contraction training can be accomplished in supine lying with the cervical lordosis supported over a towel roll. The extensors are recruited using the electrical muscle stimulator while the patient prevents the extension motion by simultaneously performing the head-nod exercise such that the cervical spine remains in neutral.
- Co-contraction can also be practiced with the patient positioned prone over an exercise ball or in FPK. These positions encourage CV extension. The patient should be taught to control the upper cervical flexion while working the middle and lower cervical spine into extension. The head-nod motion is performed concurrently with lower cervical extension. If done properly, the cervical lordosis should straighten to a neutral position.

STAGE II
After the patient is able to achieve co-contraction of the anterior and posterior muscles of the cervical spine in resting positions, the next goal is to be able to maintain cervical stabilization during arm motion. The exercises consist of initial co-contraction of the cervical musculature (a preset nod to obtain neutral), which is maintained while the patient performs repetitive motions of the upper extremity in various positions (i.e., supine, FPK, sitting, standing). The pattern of the arm motion, amplitude, and position of the exercise is based on what combination challenges the patient optimally while maintaining neutral position of the affected segmental level(s). The goal is to accomplish segmental cervical stability in a variety of positions with an assortment of arm movements and a range of amplitudes.

- Because the most stable position is supine, it is used as the initial starting position.
- Various movements of the upper extremity (e.g., flexion, abduction, diagonals) are performed while palpating the affected segment for unwanted translation. Only those motions in which the segment remains neutral can be performed.
- Bilateral arm motions below 90 degrees often are the least challenging. Unilateral, overhead movements place higher demands on the stabilization system. (However, these effects depend on factors such as the plane or direction of the hypermobility, dural tension, and shoulder or thoracic mobility.)

- Progression includes adding hand weights, which increases the resistance, or lying on a half roll, which reduces the stability of the base (Fig. A).
- These same exercises can be progressed by having the patient perform them in a sitting or standing position (Fig. 23-23), because these positions are more challenging to spinal stability. To make the transition to upright less challenging, the patient can be instructed to sit with the back to the wall to provide feedback of where the head is in space (Fig. B). Upper extremity motion can be altered in direction, amplitude, and pattern.
- The therapy ball can be used as another surface to promote cervical spine stability with upper extremity movements. Ball sitting and the use of pulley systems are beneficial at this stage (Fig. C). In prone on the ball, the patient can be taught to maintain a controlled cervical spine position while performing simple rocking motions. Increased demands can be made on the cervical spine by adding unilateral or bilateral arm motions, with or without weights. This can be progressed to more complicated arm and leg patterns (Fig. D). Similar exercises performed in supine on the ball are of a much higher load to the cervical spine and should be added later in the retraining process, only once a higher level of motor control has been developed.
- The use of proprioceptive neuromuscular facilitation patterns or sport- and work-specific movements introduce a more functional approach (Fig. E).
- Various wobble board systems can be used; the unstable base can further challenge the control of posture as the patient performs various upper or lower extremity movements.

At this stage, heavier loads can also be added to resist cervical musculative to truly achieve strength gains. Control of the unstable segment must be carefully monitored.
- Head nod with liftoff on high incline (Fig. 23-6) and in supine (Fig. 23-5)
- Sidelying head lift (Fig. 23-10)

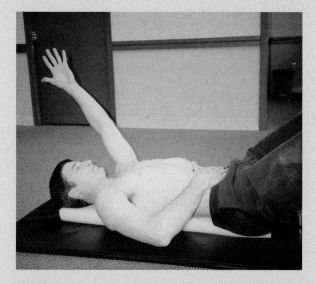

FIGURE A. Maintaining axial extension on a half roll with unilateral overhead motion.

(continued)

DISPLAY 23-1
Cervical Spine Stabilization Program *(Continued)*

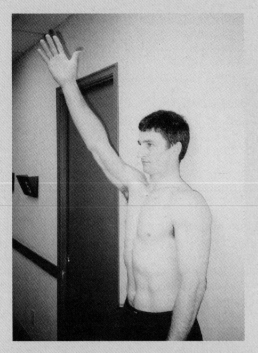

FIGURE B. Wall posture with preset nod and unilateral arm elevation.

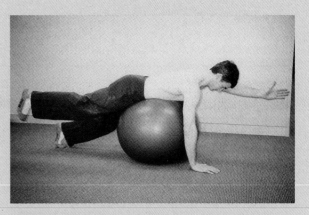

FIGURE D. Maintaining axial extension prone over a ball—opposite arm and leg pattern.

STAGE III
This stage challenges the patient to maintain segmental control during various neck motions. A preset nod activates the deep segmental flexor muscles as stabilizers, permitting the more superficial muscles to perform the movement pattern without excessive segmental translation patterns. Position is based on the ability to control segmental stability during neck motion with gravity-assisted versus gravity-resisted. The amplitude of motion is graded based on the range in which the patient can control segmental stability.

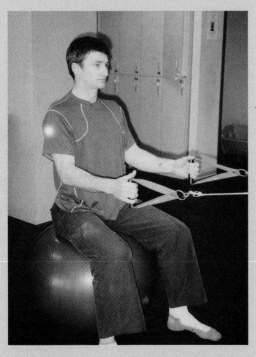

FIGURE C. Maintaining sitting axial extension on a ball—arm motion with pulley resistance.

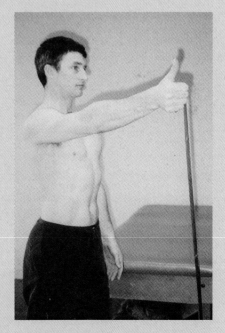

FIGURE E. Maintaining axial extension with proprioceptive neuromuscular facilitation pattern against tubing resistance.

(continued)

DISPLAY 23-1
Cervical Spine Stabilization Program *(Continued)*

- Controlled, non–weight-bearing side flexion and rotation can be initiated in supine using a foam wedge, starting at the peak (Fig. 23-13), progressing to the offset position (Self-Management 23-1).
- Pure rotation and side flexion motions can be practiced at the wall in front of a mirror to give feedback and prevent the tendency to collapse into the hypermobile plane of movement.
- Cervical segmental flexion and RTN from the flexed position are movement patterns that require segmental stabilization during a dynamic movement pattern (Fig. 23-7).
  - Pure rotation in FPK challenges the extensor group of muscles, particularly activation of the suboccipital muscles, as well as proprioceptive control.

- A faulty extension movement pattern using excessive anterior translation can be corrected and practiced in either a sitting or FPK position.
- Manual resistance to a movement pattern can be provided by the therapist (Fig. 23-11).
- Autoresistance in functional patterns (Fig. 23-12).
- Sidelying head lift (Fig. 23-10).
- Nod liftoff (Figs. 23-5 and 23-6).

Note: Although Stage I activities must be practiced prior to moving onto the other two stages, some of the first exercises in both Stages II and III are relatively easy to control and may be added to the program early on.

Reversal of the normal cervical lordosis is a less common postural impairment. In this situation, the patient presents with a very straight cervical spine or even a kyphosis. Treatment focuses on regaining extension in the cervical spine to encourage the normal cervical lordosis.

Postural abnormalities may be observed in the frontal plane with the head and neck tilted to one side. This posture can be caused by factors such as muscle imbalance, articular hypomobilities, habitual work or leisure positions, and hearing or sight deficits necessitating altered head position. Treatment should be directed at the cause of the asymmetry.

Therapeutic Exercise Interventions

Treatment for FHP should address muscle imbalance, neuromeningeal extensibility, articular hypomobility, and proprioception.

Muscle Imbalance The following short muscles should be lengthened:

- Posterior cervical extensors
- Scalene muscles
- Upper fibers of the trapezius
- Levator scapula
- Pectoralis major and minor

It also is important to strengthen the following weak muscles:

- Deep, short cervical flexors (upper and midcervical)
- Scapular stabilizers (middle and lower fibers of the trapezius, rhomboids, and serratus anterior)
- Upper thoracic erector spinae

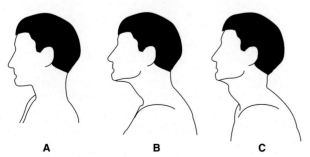

FIGURE 23-25. (A) Axial extension. (B) Forward head position: minimal midcervical lordosis. (C) Forward head position: excessive midcervical lordosis.

Neuromeningeal Extensibility Abnormal cervical postures may be caused by an attempt to decrease stretch on shortened or mechanosensitive neuromeningeal structures. Ipsilateral side flexion of the cervical spine and elevation of the scapula decrease tension in these structures. Exercises designed to alter these postures without first addressing the adverse neural tension can exacerbate the pain and possibly amplify the neurologic symptoms.

Articular Hypomobility Manual therapy techniques may be indicated in conjunction with mobility exercises to regain the restricted motions of

- Upper cervical flexion
- CT junction extension
- Upper thoracic extension

Postural Correction To correct the FHP, the head must be brought back over the trunk. This can often be achieved by directing the patient to "lift the sternum upward," thus decreasing the upper to midthoracic kyphosis. In many patients in whom the thoracic posture is the main component of their faulty posture, this sternal lift is sufficient to automatically draw the head back in line with the trunk. It is important to not allow overcorrection, with patients adopting a flat or even lordotic mid to upper thoracic curve, as they overbrace with their superficial thoracic extensors.

Another primary exercise for achieving many of the goals of postural correction is the head-nod exercise. It corrects the upper cervical extension, and because it also tightens ligamentum nuchae, it simultaneously reduces cervical lordosis. In patients with excessive lordosis of the midcervical spine, continuing the head nod into further cervical flexion stretches the posterior structures that have become shortened by the lordotic position. The head-nod exercise can be modified to include posterior displacement (retraction) of the head and neck complex to encourage extension at the lower cervical spine and CT junction.

One study on the effect of repeated neck retractions in normal subjects found that there was a significant change in resting posture toward a more retracted position after two sets of repeated retractions.[56] It is important to control the amount of flexion and retraction motion to prevent overcompensation into a kyphotic cervical spine position. Supine is a good position for the patient learning this exercise, because there is more proprioceptive feedback from the contact of

TABLE 23-3 Summary of Optimal and Faulty Regional Cervical Spine Positions		
OPTIMAL CERVICAL SPINE POSTURE (SEE FIG. 23-25A)	**FORWARD HEAD POSITION—MINIMAL MIDCERVICAL LORDOSIS (SEE FIG. 23-25B)**	**FORWARD HEAD POSITION—EXCESSIVE MIDCERVICAL LORDOSIS (SEE FIG. 23-25C)**
CV flexion	CV extension	CV extension
Midcervical spine neutral (slight cervical lordosis)	Midcervical lordosis	Excessive midcervical lordosis, can extend as low as C6–7. Accompanied by abnormal anterior vertebral translation.
CT extension	Low cervical and upper thoracic flexion	Upper thoracic flexion
Upper thoracic neutral (slight kyphosis)	Excessive thoracic kyphosis	Excessive thoracic kyphosis

the head. Lying lengthwise along an epifoam roll, with the roll directly under the spine, also encourages the thoracic extension component of postural correction (Fig. 23-26). In this position, the patient controls the lumbar curve with a sustained contraction of transversus abdominis and then performs the head-nod exercise. Sitting and standing against wall support are natural progressions of the exercise (see Fig. 23-4). The patient must maintain a neutral lumbar spine position, and a towel may have to be used behind the head initially to support the forward head or later to maintain a neutral neck position.

Exercises must be included to help regain thoracic extension. Chapter 24 provides descriptions of these exercises.

Maintaining this cervical neutral posture while incorporating upper extremity motion is the next progression; the exercise is done first with wall support and then in free-standing. Resisted upper extremity exercises can be added through the use of free weights, elastic tubing, or pulley systems. Exercises can be chosen to address strength impairments found on assessment or to simulate work or leisure movement patterns. Various wobble board systems can be used; the unstable base can further challenge the control of posture as the patient performs various upper or lower extremity movements. Because many daily activities require a bent-forward position, maintaining proper axial extension while in FPK or prone over the exercise ball can simulate this position, and upper extremity movements can be incorporated as described previously.

Kinesthetic Awareness. Several studies[11,57–61] have shown that subjects with neck pain, particularly those with WAD who complain of dizziness are less accurate in their ability to perceive a neutral resting posture, and return to a cervical neutral posture after motion in either the horizontal or vertical plane. Standing balance is also impaired in these subject groups.[62,63] Patients were able to improve their kinesthetic awareness following manual therapy, vestibular exercises, or by practicing RTN movements using a target.[64,65]

THERAPEUTIC EXERCISE INTERVENTIONS FOR COMMON DIAGNOSES

Some of the more common diagnoses of cervical spine disorders are discussed in the following sections. The impairments that occur with each diagnosis are identified, and examples of exercises for treatment of that condition are given.

Disk Dysfunction

Etiology

Although disk herniation is less common in the cervical spine than in the lumbar spine, various dysfunctions of cervical disks do occur. The term *disk dysfunction* could be used whenever changes in the disk alter its biomechanical properties and prevent normal function. Included in this grouping are degenerative disk disease, excessive disk clefting, and rim lesions (i.e., separation of the disk from the end plate).[66,67] In the acute stages, disk dysfunction can manifest as an irritable condition, with painful limitation of active ROM in all planes, particularly flexion; pain on cough or sneeze; painful cervical muscle contraction from guarding; and difficulty in maintaining upright postures because of the compression load of the head on the neck. There may or may not be associated neurologic signs, depending on the degree of foraminal encroachment by the disk and the condition of other structures surrounding the foramen, such as the zygapophyseal joint capsule, ligaments, and bone. Radiculopathy is discussed in a subsequent section.

Treatment

Treatment initially is aimed at resting the neck, which is achieved through education about proper resting positions to unload the compressive and translatory forces on the cervical spine. Therapeutic modalities may be useful to help alleviate the inflammatory response, decrease the associated muscle spasm, and manage the pain. Manual therapy techniques can be used to mobilize the involved segment if segmental hypomobility is found during mobility testing. Muscle energy techniques can also be used to mobilize and alter muscle activity at that segment.

Manual traction techniques help to decompress the disk and increase intervertebral foramen size. If the condition

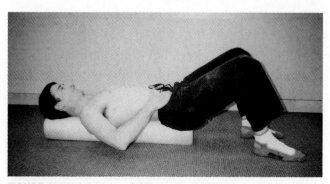

FIGURE 23-26. Lying on an Epifoam roll to encourage thoracic extension.

is very irritable, excessive traction may increase symptoms because of the stretch on the nerve and dura. Breathing pattern reeducation is an appropriate exercise during the acute stages, because excessive use of the secondary muscles of inspiration, such as the scalene muscles, can add a compression load to the cervical spine and should be avoided. Instruction in diaphragmatic breathing while monitoring scalene muscle activity through palpation encourages an optimal breathing pattern and unloads the cervical spine. Using postural correction exercises reduces translational forces. Supine exercises, such as gentle head nod (i.e., CV flexion) may be tolerated at this stage and will help improve posture as well as begin to recruit the cervical stabilizers. Any exercise that causes peripheralization of symptoms must be avoided.

As the condition improves, impairments can be identified and addressed. After a period of protected function, the patient will usually exhibit signs of hypomobility impairment. Degenerative changes at that vertebral segment may also decrease its mobility. Care must be taken in selecting and teaching ROM exercises to minimize compressive or translatory forces, or to close down the intervertebral foramen if there is nerve root involvement.

Because muscle extensibility may be decreased as a result of muscle guarding during the acute phase, stretching exercises should be implemented. Neuromeningeal extensibility should also be assessed at later stages, particularly in cases of neurologic involvement. Exercises to increase the mobility of these structures should not be started when there are still signs of decreased nerve conduction, because the movements can easily exacerbate the condition.

The disk is an important structure in the control of motion of the intervertebral segment, and hypermobility impairment may occur as a result of disk dysfunction. Stability testing at the affected segment may detect increased motion because of the loss of the disk's ability to control translational forces in the spine. This impairment must be addressed with a progression of stabilization exercises. The "Hypermobility" section describes these exercises. It is important to progress slowly, as higher load exercises will also load the healing disk.

To prevent further disk degeneration and reduce the incidence of recurrence of an acute episode, it is important to correct all postural impairments of the cervical spine, thoracic spine, and shoulder girdle. Postural asymmetry of the pelvic girdle also influences the cervical spine, and impairments should be addressed as previously discussed.

Cervical Sprain and Strain

Etiology

Any traumatic incident can produce a sprain or strain of the cervical spine. The most common incident is the WAD that occurs after a motor vehicle accident.

The complex injuries sustained by the neck can affect many different tissues. The soft-tissue structures involved may include muscle, ligament, capsule, articular cartilage, and the disk (including rim lesions). Concurrent bony injuries can include fractures of the articular subchondral bone, transverse and spinous processes, lateral masses of the atlas, and the vertebral body.[66] Suspicion of these injuries requires referral to the physician for management. Patients exhibiting signs of instability from traumatic injury should also be referred to the physician for further diagnostic tests and appropriate medical intervention. The severity of these injuries varies widely, and

the irritability of the condition must be assessed individually. As discussed earlier in this chapter (see "Impaired Muscle Performance" section), patients with WAD have been shown to have decreased recruitment, strength and endurance of their deep cervical flexors, early and excessive recruitment of the more superficial flexors even at low loads, and decreased strength along with atrophy of the deep cervical extensors. Motor patterning is altered during upper extremity tasks, and there are prolonged relaxation times for some of the superficial muscles. In WAD subjects with dizziness, joint position sense, balance, and gaze stability are also impaired when compared with controls.[57–63]

Treatment

During the acute inflammatory stage, treatment is aimed at reducing pain and inflammation and promoting optimal healing. Education about proper resting positions, limitations of activity, and the use of ice can assist in reaching these goals. If segmental hypermobility is suspected, bracing should be considered to reduce stresses on the healing structures. Exercise at this time involves the use of breathing exercises and ROM exercises within the pain-free range. The supine position is often best tolerated at this stage, because it unloads the weight of the head, and the wedge pillow can be used to assist the mobility exercise. Rhythmic neck rotation movements performed in a supine position in conjunction with relaxed breathing can increase mobility and assist vascular flow. Rosenfeld et al.[39–41] showed that regular rotation ROM exercises performed 10 times hourly, resulted in significantly less pain, better mobility, and less time loss from work.

Therapeutic modalities such as ice, interferential current, pulsed ultrasound, or transcutaneous electrical nerve stimulation may also be indicated at this stage to reduce inflammation, decrease muscle spasm, and assist in pain control.

In the subacute stage, it is important to continue to protect the injured structures and to introduce stresses that encourage optimal healing. Grade I and II manual therapy mobilization techniques are effective in pain relief, and grade III and IV mobilizations can help restore motion of the involved segments (see Chapter 7). Impairment of mobility may continue to be the primary dysfunction. Mobility exercises may be progressed into larger arc movements, more specific to the multiplanar articular restrictions found on manual mobility testing. Specific muscle length tests may also indicate that certain muscles are short. However, the effect on the whole spine (e.g., dural stretch, disk compression) must be taken into consideration when choosing mobility exercises. Depending on the degree of ligamentous or disk injury, there may be a mobility impairment of hypermobility. As studies have shown that decreased dynamic stability occurs early in this patient population, stabilization exercises should be included as soon as possible. The Stage I exercises put very little stress on the cervical spine and can be implemented early in rehab. Development of a stabilization program must take into consideration the direction, severity, and irritability of the hypermobility (see the "Hypermobility" section). It is also prudent to begin postural reeducation, progressing through the exercises as tolerated. Overhead arm motions are often too stressful on the cervical spine at this stage because of increased translation and compression forces.

During the remodeling phase or as the condition becomes more chronic, other impairments can be addressed. The muscles strained at the time of injury and the segmental muscles related to levels of articular dysfunction often show impairment of force production. A specific strengthening program can be designed to improve muscle function. Higher load Stage II and III stabilization exercises (see Display 23-1) should be taught and progressed as tolerated. It has been shown that the lower load nod type exercises do not regain strength to the same extent as higher load head lift type exercises,[38,68] so these should be included when the healing structures of the neck are able to tolerate the larger forces. In some chronic cases, the overactivity of the superficial muscles is the predominant feature, and so continuing to use low load exercises to focus on the downtraining of these superficial muscles may be more appropriate than a focus on strengthening with no consideration given to the motor pattern. Postural impairments continue to be a concern, and treatment interventions should include dynamic exercises that encourage movement patterns that incorporate optimal posture.

Neural Entrapment

Etiology

The cervical nerve roots can become entrapped at their exit at the intervertebral foramen. The foramen is bounded by the zygapophyseal joint, the UV joint, the disk, and the pedicle. Any pathologic condition increasing the size of these surrounding structures can lead to narrowing or stenosis of the foramen, potentially entrapping the nerve root. Foramen size is also reduced by the movements of extension and ipsilateral side flexion and rotation. Any muscle imbalance producing this resting position of the cervical spine would further aggravate the problem. The FHP can place the upper and midcervical spine into a posture of increased cervical lordosis, decreasing the intervertebral foramen size. Any scapular resting position that encourages this cervical position (e.g., elevated scapula) or stretches the nerve root (e.g., depressed or protracted scapula) would also aggravate the condition. Changes in neural conduction depend on the degree of pressure or traction on the nerve root.

The term *double crush syndrome* or *multiple crush syndrome* has been used to describe the syndrome in which the nerve is affected at multiple sites along its course from the cervical spine to the hand. Common sites of entrapment are the cervical intervertebral foramen, the thoracic outlet, the elbow, and the carpus. Pressure at any one of these sites in isolation may be insufficient to produce symptoms, but there can be a summation effect as subsequent sites add their "crush" to the nerve.

A common example of crush syndrome is carpal tunnel syndrome. There may be decreased space in the carpal tunnel locally, but it may not be as marked as the symptoms suggest. There may be additional proximal symptoms that are unexplained by pressure at the carpal tunnel alone. In the cervical spine, there may be some mild degenerative changes involving the zygapophyseal joint and uncinate process that decrease the intervertebral foraminal dimensions. A superimposed FHP places the upper and midcervical spine into a resting position of extension, further compromising intervertebral foramen size. A short scalene muscle on the same side, because of a faulty respiratory pattern or the habitual crooking of a phone between head and shoulder, causes a side-flexed posture of the cervical spine and further decreases the intervertebral foramen space. At the thoracic outlet, a short-ened scalene muscle can also elevate the first rib, decreasing the size of the thoracic outlet and creating another potential site of neural entrapment. A depressed scapular resting position places a traction force on the brachial plexus, which can also decrease neural conduction, and increases tension in the neuromeningeal system in the upper quadrant, which can aggravate the condition.

Treatment

Thorough assessment at each of the sites of entrapment can identify the impairments contributing to the condition. Treatment interventions address the impairments found at the cervical spine, thoracic spine, shoulder girdle, and wrist. If wrist dysfunction is treated in isolation, the symptoms tend to recur or change, often working their way proximally. Exercise treatment interventions for the impairment of posture are particularly useful, as is addressing the findings of neuromeningeal hypomobility.

Cervicogenic Headache

Etiology

CHA can be caused by two mechanisms. First, the posterior aspect of the skull, as far forward as the vertex, is supplied by the greater occipital nerve (a branch of the C2 and C3 posterior rami). Any structure supplied by the second or third cervical nerve can refer pain into that distribution. Second, the spinal nucleus of the trigeminal nerve descends into the spinal cord to at least the level of C3. Branches of the trigeminal nerve supply the mandibular, maxillary, and frontal areas of the face. Afferents from the first three or four cervical nerves converge with afferents of the trigeminal nerve. Any structure supplied by these neurologic segments can refer pain into the head and face, causing headache of cervical origin.[55]

There has been conflicting results in studies that have looked for the presence of FHP in subjects with CHA as compared to other headache types.[8,50,51,69] Hypomobility is a feature of cervicogenic headache particularly symptomatic segmental stiffness in the upper cervical spine[15,51,69,70]. As with other subjects with neck pain, those with cervicogenic headache demonstrate weakness and lack of endurance of the deep cervical flexors and extensors along with excessive activity of the superficial groups.[15,51,70] Zito et al.[51] found a higher incidence of muscle tightness in these subjects as compared to other headache types, but this tightness was not confined to a specific muscle. Jaeger[71] found a significant number of myofascial trigger points on the symptomatic side compared with the asymptomatic side in patients presenting with cervicogenic headache.

Treatment

Treatment interventions should mainly target impairments of posture, mobility, and muscle performance. Mobility exercises may be performed as generalized ROM exercises or designed as specific articular mobilization exercises to address the segmental mobility restrictions found on manual mobility testing, most often of the upper cervical intervertebral levels (see the "Hypomobility" section). Specific muscle stretches can address the myofascial tightness and trigger points that may be contributing to the headache. Progressive exercises to increase muscle performance and endurance of the deep cervical flexor and extensor muscles should be included in the exercise program. Jull et al.[37] showed that a combination

BUILDING BLOCK 23-1
Constructing New Knowledge

1. Consider a 45-year-old male patient with long-standing mild neck pain. On testing the cervical flexors, there is weakness of both the DNF and the superficial muscles as well. Describe a progression of exercises to first address the deeper muscle weakness and then the more generalized flexor weakness. Be sure to include dosage.
2. Consider a 22 -old-female patient who has resolved from a recent episode of acute wry neck. This is her third episode in the past year. Your examination reveals some hypermobility on testing at the C4–5 segment. Outline the progression of exercises you would prescribe to develop dynamic stabilization of her cervical spine.
3. A 35-year-old female patient sustained a WAD II injury in a motor vehicle accident 2 weeks ago. She is reluctant to move her neck, and you note excessive bracing of the superficial musculature on many of your tests. Describe three exercises that you could prescribe on this first visit to assist in improving her mobility and relaxation of her superficial muscles. Be sure to provide information about the education component to assist this patient in confidently performing the appropriate dosage for this group of exercises.
4. Your patient is a 65-year-old male with poor static resting posture. He has a FHP along with an increased thoracic kyphosis. A number of his neck muscles have shortened because of this constant position, and his SCM muscle is overdominant. List those muscles which are likely to have shortened in this situation. Create an exercise program to address both the muscle length and balance impairments and to gain control over the forward head posture.
5. Consider a patient with a restriction of left side flexion, with the tightness felt on the right side of the neck. List three different types of structures which could be contributing to this restriction of motion. Describe one mobility exercise you could teach to address each one. Give a progression wherever possible.
6. Describe the situations in which you would use a higher load neck flexor strengthening exercise as compared to a low load DNF recruitment exercise.
7. Your patient presents with an asymmetric loss of strength of rotation/side flexion to the right. Which exercises could you use to specifically target this asymmetric pattern?
8. Your patient is a painter with neck pain, aggravated by overhead work, particularly when painting ceilings. You notice that his neck collapses forward into anterior translation in the mid cervical spine on active neck extension. You have already helped him to retrain and strengthen the DNFs, but you notice that his extension pattern has not really changed. Describe a progression of exercises you could use to retrain an optimal extension pattern, leading to control of the anterior translation tendency while painting ceilings.
9. Your patient presents with a diagnosis of thoracic outlet syndrome. On examination you determine that one of the more important contributing factors is overactivity of her anterior scalene muscles. Describe three exercises you could prescribe to assist in downtraining the excessive activity of this muscle.

of manual therapy and specific therapeutic exercise gave significant improvement in intensity, frequency, and duration of headaches in a population with chronic cervicogenic headache as compared to controls. This improvement was maintained at 12 months.

KEY POINTS

- The cervical spine examination and evaluation consists of a patient report (subjective history) and the physical (objective) examination. The patient report should include information about the client's job, sitting position, and type of exercise performed. The physical examination includes visual observation; active and passive movement tests, including myofacial and neuromeningeal extensibility tests; manual muscle testing; neurologic tests; various special tests; and clearing tests of the thorax, shoulder girdle, and TMJ.
- Common impairments of body structures and functions affecting the cervical spine include muscle performance impairment, posture impairment, and mobility impairment (i.e., hypomobility and hypermobility).
- A therapeutic exercise program is developed to address each impairment and improve overall function of the individual.
- The following are common diagnoses of the cervical spine:

- Disk dysfunction: Impairments that are often associated with this diagnosis include mobility (i.e., hypomobility and hypermobility) and posture.
  - Sprain or strain: Impairments associated with this diagnosis include mobility, posture, and muscle performance.
  - Neural entrapment: Impairments associated with this diagnosis include mobility and posture.
  - CHA: Associated impairments include mobility, posture, and muscle performance production, particularly endurance.
- For any patient presenting with a particular diagnosis, the associated impairments are identified. They must then be prioritized according to their relative importance as those requiring immediate attention and those most likely to be tolerated by the patient.

REFERENCES

1. White A, Panjabi M. Clinical Biomechanics of the Spine. Philadelphia: JB Lippincott, 1990.
2. Twomey L, Taylor J. Functional and applied anatomy of the cervical spine. In: Grant R, ed. Physical Therapy for the Cervical and Thoracic Spine. Melbourne: Churchill Livingstone, 1994.
3. De Sousa OM, Furlani J, Vitti M. Etude Electromyographique du m. stemo-cleidomastoideus. Electromyogr clin Neurophysiol 1973;13:93–106.
4. Panjabi M. The stabilizing system of the spine. Part 1: Function, adaptation, and enhancement. Part 2: neutral zone and instability hypothesis. J Spinal Disord 1992;5:383–397.
5. Conley MS, Meyer RA, Bloomberg JJ, et al. Noninvasive analysis of human neck muscle function. Spine 1995;20:2505–2512.

6. Grieve G. Common Vertebral Joint Problems. Edinburgh: Churchill Livingstone, 1981.
7. Vernon H, Mior S. The neck disability index: a study of reliability and validity. J Manipulative Physiol Ther 1991;14:409–415.
8. Watson D, Trott P. Cervical headache: an investigation of natural head posture and upper cervical flexor muscle performance. Cephalgia 1993;13: 272–282.
9. Silverman J, Rodriquez AA, Agre JC. Quantitative cervical flexor strength in healthy subjects and in subjects with mechanical neck pain. Arch Phys Med Rehabil 1991;72:679–681.
10. Gogia P, Sabbahi M. Electromyographic analysis of neck muscle fatigue in patients with osteoarthritis of the cervical spine. Spine 1994;19:502–506.
11. Jull G. Deep neck flexor dysfunction in whiplash. J Musculoskeletal Pain 2000;8:143–154.
12. Falla DL, Jull GA, Hodges PW. Patients with neck pain demonstrate reduced electromyographic activity of the deep cervical flexor muscles during performance of the craniocervical flexion test. Spine 2004;29:2108–2114.
13. Vernon HT, Aker P, Aramenko M, et al. Evaluation of neck muscle strength with a modified sphygmomanometer dynamometer: reliability and validity. J Manipul Physiol Ther 1992;15:343–349.
14. Kristjansson E. Reliability of ultrasonography for the cervical multifidus muscle in asymptomatic and symptomatic subjects. Man Ther 2004;9:83–88.
15. Amiri M, Jull G, Bullock-Saxton J, et al. Cervical musculoskeletal impairment in frequent intermittent headache. Part 1: subjects with single headaches. Cephalgia 2007;27:793–802.
16. Elliott J, Jull G, Noteboom JT, et al. MRI study of the cross sectional area for the cervical extensor musculature in patients with persistent whiplash associated disorders (WAD). Man Ther 2007;13:258–265.
17. Uhlig Y, Weber BR, Grob D, et al. Fibre composition and fibre transformation in neck muscles of patients with dysfunction of the cervical spine. J Orthop Res 1995;13:240–249.
18. Hallgren RC, Greenman PE, Rechtien JJ. Atrophy of suboccipital muscles inpatients with chronic pain: a pilot study. JAOA 1994;94:1032–1038.
19. Elliott J, Jull G, Noteboom JT, et al. Fatty Infiltration in the cervical extensor muscles in persistent whiplash-associated disorders: a magnetic resonance imaging analysis. Spine 2006;31:847–855.
20. Falla D, Rainoldi A, Merletti R, et al. Myoelectric manifestations of sternocleidomastoid and anterior scalene muscle fatigue in chronic neck pain patients. Clin Neurophysiol 2003;114:488–495.
21. Falla D, Jull G, Rainoldi A, et al. Neck flexor muscle fatigue is side specific in patients with unilateral neck pain. Eur J Pain 2004;8:71–77.
22. Jull G, Kristjansson E, Dall'Alba P, et al. Impairment in the cervical flexors: a comparison of whiplash and insidious onset neck pain patients. Man Ther 2004;9:89–94.
23. Falla D, Jull G, Hodges PW, et al. Feedforward activity of the cervical flexor muscles during voluntary arm movements is delayed in chronic neck pain. Exp Brain Res 2004;157:43–48.
24. Nederhand MJ, Ijzerman MJ, Hermens HJ, et al. Cervical muscle dysfunction in the chronic whiplash associated disorder grade II (WAD-II). Spine 2000;25:1938–1943.
25. Nederhand MJ, IJzerman MJ, Hermens HJ, et al. Cervical muscle dysfunction in chronic whiplash associated disorder grade II. Spine 2002;27:1056–1061.
26. Szeto GP, Straker LM, O'Sullivan PB, et al. A comparison of symptomatic and asymptomatic office workers performing monotonous keyboard work. Man Ther 2005;10:270–291.
27. Falla D, Bilenkij G, Jull G, et al. Patients with chronic neck pain demonstrate altered patterns of muscle activity during performance of an upper limb task. Spine 2004;13:1436–1440.
28. Barton PM, Hayes KC. Neck flexor muscle strength, efficiency, and relaxation times in normal subjects and subjects with unilateral neck pain and headache. Arch Phys Med Rehabil 1996;77:680–687.
29. Sterling M, Kenardy J, Jull G, et al. Development of motor dysfunction following whiplash injury. Pain 2003;103:65–73.
30. Stump J, Rash G, Semon J, et al. A comparison of two modes of cervical exercise in adolescent male athletes. J Manipulative Physiol Ther 1993;16:155–160.
31. Deange J. Strengthening the neck for football. Athlet J 1984;Sept:46–48.
32. Leggett S, Graves JE, Pollock ML, et al. Quantitative assessment and training of isometric cervical extension strength. Am J Sport Med 1991;19:653–659.
33. Pollock ML, Graves JE, Bammon MM, et al. Frequency and volume of resistance training: effect on cervical extension strength. Arch Phys Med Rehabil 1993;74:1080–1086.
34. Highland T, Dreisinger TE, Vie LL, et al. Changes in isometric strength and range of motion of the isolated cervical spine after eight weeks of clinical rehabilitation. Spine 1992;17(Suppl 6):S77–S82.
35. Taimela S, Takala EP, Asklof T, et al. Active treatment of chronic neck pain: a prospective randomized intervention. Spine 2000;25:1021–1027.
36. Bunketorp L, Lindh M, Carlsson J, et al. The effectiveness of supervised physical training model tailored to the individual needs of patients with whiplash-associated disorder – a randomized controlled trial. Clin Rehabil 2006;20:201–217.
37. Jull G, Trott P, Potter H, et al. A randomized controlled trial of exercise and manipulative therapy for Cervicogenic headache. Spine 2002;27:1835–1843.
38. O'Leary S, Jull G, Kim M, et al. Specificity in retraining craniocervical flexor muscle performance. J Orthop Sports Phys Ther 2007;37:3–9.
39. Rosenfeld M, Gunnarsson R, Borenstein P, et al. Early intervention in whiplash-associated disorders. Spine 2000 25:1782–1787.
40. Rosenfeld M, Seferiadis A, Carlsson J, et al. Active intervention in patients with whiplash-associated disorders improves long term prognosis. Spine 2003;28:2491–2498.
41. Rosenfeld M, Seferiadis A, Gunnarsson R, et al. Active involvement and intervention in patients exposed to whiplash trauma in automobile crashes reduces costs. Spine 2006;31:1799–1804.
42. Sarig-Bahat H. Evidence for exercise therapy in mechanical neck disorders. Man Ther 2003;8:10–20.
43. Mayoux-Benhamou MA, Revel M, Vallee C. Selective electromyography of dorsal neck muscles in humans. Exp Brain Res 1997;113:353–360.
44. Dall'Alba PT, Sterling MM, Treleaven JM, et al. cervical range of motion discriminates between asymptomatic persons and those with whiplash. Spine 2001;26:2090–2094.
45. Kasch H, Stengaard-Pedersen K, Arendt-Nielsen L, et al. Headache, neck pain and neck mobility after acute whiplash injury. Spine 2001;26:1246–1251.
46. Sterling M, Jull G, Vicenzino B, et al. Characterization of acute whiplash associated disorders. Spine 2004;29:182–188.
47. Ogince M, Hall T, Robinson K, et al. The diagnostic validity of the cervical flexion-rotation test in C1/2-related cervicogenic headache. Man Ther 2007;12:256–262.
48. Hall T, Chan HT, Christensen L, et al. Efficacy of a C1–2 self sustained natural apophyseal glide (Snag) in the management of cervicogenic headache. J Orthop Sports Phys Ther 2007;37:100–107.
49. Janda V. Muscles and motor control in cervicogenic disorders: assessment and management. In: Grant R, ed. Physical Therapy for the Cervical and Thoracic Spine. Melbourne: Churchill Livingstone, 1994.
50. Treleaven J, Jull G, Atkinson L. Cervical musculoskeletal dysfunction in post-concussional headache. Cephalgia 1994;14:273–279.
51. Zito G, Jull G, Story I, et al. Clinical tests of musculoskeletal dysfunction in the diagnosis of Cervicogenic headache. Man Ther 2006;11:118–129.
52. Edgar D, Jull G, Sutton S. The relationship between upper trapezius muscle length and upper quadrant neural tissue extensibility. Aust Physiother J 1994; 40:99–103.
53. Butler DS. Mobilization of the Nervous System. Melbourne: Churchill Livingstone, 1991.
54. Butler D. The Neurodynamic Technique. Adelaide: Noigroup Publications, 2005.
55. Bogduk N. Cervical causes of headache and dizziness. In: Grieves G, ed. Modern Manual Therapy of the Vertebral Column. Edinburgh: Churchill Livingstone, 1986.
56. Pearson ND, Walmsley RP. Trial into the effects of repeated neck retractions in normal subjects. Spine 1995;20:1245–1250; discussion 1251.
57. Revel M, Andre-Deshays C, Minguet M. Cervicocephalic kinesthetic sensibility in patients with cervical pain. Arch Phys Med 1991;72:288–291.
58. Heikkila H, Astrom PG. Cervicocephalic kinesthetic sensibility in patients with whiplash injury. Scand J Rehabil Med 1996;28:133–138.
59. Loudon JK, Ruhl M, Field E. Ability to reproduce head position after whiplash injury. Spine 1997;22:865–868.
60. Treleavan J, Jull G, Sterling M. Dizziness and unsteadiness following whiplash injury: characteristic features and relationship with cervical joint position error. J Rehabil Med 2003;35:36–43.
61. Treleavan J, Jull G, Low Choy N. The relationship of cervical joint position error to balance and eye movement disorders in persistent whiplash. Man Ther 2006;11:99–106.
62. Michaelson P, Michaelson M, Jaric S, et al. Vertical posture and head stability in patients with chronic neck. J Rehabil Med 2003;35:229–235.
63. Treleavan J, Jull G, Low Choy N. Standing balance in persistent whiplash: a comparison between subjects with dizziness and without dizziness. J Rehabil Med 2005;37:224–229.
64. Karlberg M, Magnusson M, Malmström E, et al. Postural and symptomatic improvement after physiotherapy in patients with dizziness of suspected cervical origin. Arch Phys Med Rehabil 1996;77:874–882.
65. Revel M, Minguet M, Gregoy P, et al. Changes in cervicocephalic kinesthesia after a proprioceptive rehabilitation program in patients with neck pain. Arch Phys Med Rehabil 1994;75:895–899.
66. Taylor JR, Kakulas BA, Margolius K. Road accidents and neck injuries. Proc Australas Soc Hum Biol 1992;5:211–231.
67. Taylor JR, Kakulas BA, Margolius K. Acute injuries to the cervical joints. Spine 1993;18:1115–1122.
68. O'Leary S, Falla D, Jull G, et al. Muscle specificity in tests of cervical flexor muscle performance. J Electromyogr Kinesiol 2007;17:35–40.
69. Dumas JP, Arsenault AB, Boudreau G, et al. Physical Impairments in Cervicogenic headache: traumatic vs. nontraumatic onset. Cephalgia 2001;21:884–893.
70. Jull G, Amiri M, Bullock-Saxton J, et al. Cervical musculoskeletal impairment in frequent intermittent headache. Part 2: subjects with multiple headaches. Cephalgia 2007;27:891–898.
71. Jaeger B. Are "cervicogenic" headaches due to myofascial pain and cervical spine dysfunction? Cephalgia 1989;9:157–163.

chapter 24

The Thoracic Spine

ROB LANDEL AND CARRIE M. HALL

The thoracic spine is unique in its structure and function from the remainder of the spine because of its articulations with the sternum and ribs and its critical role in ventilation. The thoracic spine's location between the cervical and lumbar spine allow it to be vulnerable to impairments in these related regions. Conversely, impairments in the thoracic region affect function of the surrounding spinal regions. As a critical link in the kinematic chain, functions of other regions of the body (e.g., shoulder girdle, hip, foot, ankle) affect function of the thoracic spine and vice versa.

Unlike the lumbar and the cervical spine, there is a paucity of literature regarding the management of thoracic spine impairments, particularly with regard to interventions for impaired muscle performance. Much of the approach to exercise for the region must be extrapolated from the lumbar and cervical regions, with allowance made for differences due to the thoracic cage. This chapter presents principles and examples of therapeutic exercise prescription for common pathologies and impairments affecting the thoracic region and contributing to a person's activity limitations.

As you progress through this chapter, it may be helpful to keep patient scenarios in mind. For each scenario in Display 24-1, ask yourself how you would address the patient's impairments, activity limitations, and participation restrictions through an appropriate exercise program. What exercises would you choose? How would you dose the exercises (number of repetitions, sets, speed of movement, amount of rest, progression from initial session to discharge, and so on).

EXAMINATION AND EVALUATION

A comprehensive examination, including the history, systems review, and tests and measures, enables the physical therapist to determine the diagnosis (based whenever possible on impairments, activity limitations, and participation restrictions), prognosis, and interventions.[1-3] The physical therapist must follow an organized, sequential approach in order to avoid omitting crucial information that may prevent an accurate interpretation of the findings. In addition, a detailed history must be taken to determine the nature and extent of the dysfunction. Throughout this process, good listening skills and skill in asking questions to promote open communication in an effective, efficient manner is necessary. Beyond the general data generated from a patient/client history as defined in Chapter 2, the following information is important to obtain from a patient with impairment, activity limitations, or participation restrictions involving the thoracic spine.

History

Because the thoracic region is a site of many visceral causes and sources of pain (e.g., chest pain due to acute myocardial infarction, pain located at the costovertebral angle of the lower thoracic segments that actually originates in the kidneys), questions must be asked which will help determine whether or not physical therapy is the appropriate management option for the patient. The findings from a thorough history can indicate possible nonmechanical sources of symptoms (see Appendix 1). If the therapist suspects that the pain is derived from nonmechanical or visceral sources, the patient should be referred to the appropriate medical practitioner.

Systems Review

A systems review provides a quick screen of the pertinent systems. If problems are observed during this review, more detailed tests should be done as the next phase of the examination process. Information about disorders of other systems (e.g., cardiopulmonary, genitourinary, gastrointestinal) that may mimic thoracic musculoskeletal disorders should be obtained during the medical history portion of the examination, and used to guide the subsequent systems review. For example, a systems review of the cardiopulmonary system includes screens of the lungs (e.g., respiratory rate, breath sounds), heart (e.g., heart rate, heart sounds), and blood pressure.

A systems review of the skeletal system is also called a scan examination. The scan examination is a quick procedure that includes tests and measures listed in Display 24-2. Because the thoracic spine spans the upper and lower quadrants, screens of both regions are advisable, particularly as they relate to the transitional zones (i.e., C7–T1 and T12–L1). Chapter 23 provides a more detailed explanation of the upper quadrant scan examination, and Chapter 17 explains the lower quadrant scan examination.

Kyphotic individuals, especially elder women with a history of osteoporosis, should be screened for vertebral body fractures. Individuals with excessive spinal stiffness should be examined radiographically for ankylosing spondylitis. To be considered significant, radiographic findings must be correlated with the clinical examination findings.

Additional medical screening is highly indicated in individuals whose symptoms do not appear to be mechanical in nature, who have a history of cancer, risk factors for vascular disease, a history of exposure to tuberculosis, or bilateral lower extremity neurologic complaints with or without reports of incontinence (see Appendix 1). It is important to understand the origin of the problem, because the decision to refer on an emergency basis rather than on a routine follow-up visit with

DISPLAY 24-1
Patient Cases

Pain

Orson Buggy is a 60-year-old horse-drawn carriage driver who complains of mid-back pain that limits his work tolerance. He describes an ache that increases the longer he sits, which he must do to drive tourists. He also reports a sharper pain of short duration that occurs when the carriage hits a bump or hole, relatively often in the area he must drive. You observe that he sits in a flexed posture. His pain is aggravated by flexion with overpressure, and vertical compression of his trunk while in his resting sitting position. His pain is less with extension. Compression of his trunk when sitting upright is painfree.

Osteoporosis/Insufficiency Fracture

Viola Fuss is a 64-year-old meditation and stress relief counselor with moderate osteoporosis who complains of mid-back pain. Radiographs reveal a stable compression fracture of the T6 vertebral body; both her orthopedist and radiologist feel it is stable and she is cleared for exercise. Her primary activity limitation is decreased walking endurance due to fatigue and shortness of breath.

Hyperkyphosis/Parkinson Disease

Denton Fender is a 56-year-old auto body mechanic who was diagnosed with Parkinson disease 3 years ago, and is still in the early stages. Individuals with this disorder typically acquire a flexed posture as they age and the disease progresses. In addition, their voice volume is often low, reflecting a decrease in chest and diaphragm excursion due to the resulting hyperkyphosis.

Dustin Dubree is a 72-year-old construction company owner with Parkinson disease who's "on" periods last about 3 hours. He remains active running his company, including overseeing work at job sites. His major complaint at this time is having to take three or more attempts at rising from a chair, and taking up to a minute some times to straighten into an upright posture upon standing. You note on physical exam that he has limited hip flexion and lumbar extension.

Thoracic Outlet

Laura Biden is a 22-year-old policewoman with diffuse neck, shoulder, arm and hand pain and numbness in the fifth digit. These problems make it difficult to write traffic tickets. You note that she sits and stands with an exaggerated kyphosis and forward, drooping shoulders. Passively or actively holding her shoulders back and straightening her back improves her UE symptoms after several minutes. She notes she is unable to maintain this position for long, however.

DISPLAY 24-2
Outline of a Scan Examination

Observation

Range of motion

During trunk flexion observe for rib hump (scoliosis)
- Motor assessment
- Sensory assessment
- Vascular status
- Reflexes
- Palpation
- Clearing tests

Upper quadrant (see Chapters 23 and 25)
- Foraminal encroachment
- Compression or distraction
- Upper limb tension test (ulnar bias may indicate upper thoracic pathology)
- TOS tests

Lower quadrant (see Chapters 17 and 19)
- Prone knee bend (may indicate low thoracic pathology)
- Straight-leg raising
- Slump test
- hip flexion, abduction, external rotation (FABER)
- Scour test

problem. Proceeding in this manner eliminates unnecessary procedures and streamlines the examination.

Tests for regions other than the thoracic spine, for example, the lumbopelvic, hip, or cervical areas, may be chosen should the provisional diagnosis list require them. Display 24-3 lists impairments that may require examination in patients with thoracic complaints. For a detailed explanation of each test and measure the reader is referred to Magee's text on orthopedic physical assessment.[8]

DISPLAY 24-3
Component Impairments Related to Thoracic Kyphosis During Gait

Stance Limb
- **Initial Contact:** Hip extensor strength is necessary to prevent backward lean by means of lumbar lordosis. Lumbar lordosis can lead to thoracic kyphosis.
- **Terminal Stance:** Hip flexor length and hip joint extension mobility are necessary to prevent lumbar lordosis and secondary thoracic kyphosis.

Swing Limb
- Hip extensor length, hip joint flexion mobility, and hip flexor strength are necessary to perform proper hip flexion during swing and prevent backward lean by means of lumbar lordosis to advance the limb. Lumbar lordosis can lead to thoracic kyphosis.

Trunk
- Balance between length and performance of oblique abdominal or spinal extensor muscles is necessary to prevent thoracic kyphosis.
- Counterrotation between the pelvis and trunk is necessary to promote optimal trunk function during gait to prevent compensatory thoracic flexion.

the physician will depend upon the system involved, the nature and severity of the complaint, and the clinical findings.

Tests and Measures

The next step in the examination process is the selection of one or more tests and measures to ascertain the impairments, activity limitations, and participation restrictions of the patient. This determination leads to the development of the final diagnosis and the prognosis, which should guide the physical therapist's choice of management options. The selection of tests and measures, like the choice of questions asked, should be driven by the provisional diagnosis list. The choice of performing any tests and measure therefore depends on the results of the history and systems review. Each test or measure should contribute to the process of either confirming or disconfirming a potential cause of the

THERAPEUTIC EXERCISE INTERVENTIONS FOR COMMON IMPAIRMENTS OF BODY STRUCTURES AND FUNCTIONS

The basic steps in designing the plan of care for a patient or client are to (1) identify the impairments that relate to the observed posture or movement pattern, activity limitation and participation restriction, and (2) address each causative impairment as necessary. Therapeutic exercise interventions for the thoracic region include activities and techniques that address impairments that directly and indirectly affect thoracic spine function. Comprehensive treatment of thoracic activity limitations and impairments requires treatment of related areas, including the cervical spine, the shoulder girdle, and the lumbopelvic region.

The ultimate goal of all therapeutic exercise interventions should be to regain maximum pain-free function. This requires addressing impairments contributing to the faulty movement that are related to the activity limitation and participation restriction. Analysis of complex movements (e.g., gait, forward bending, reaching, rising from sitting, ascending or descending stairs) requires division of the movement into component parts to analyze the contribution from each segment or region involved in the movement. The examination and evaluation should reveal specific regional physiologic impairments such as hypomobility in the hips or impaired muscle performance of the shoulder girdle. Combining the information obtained from movement analysis and specific examination of selected regions can determine which impairments need to be addressed to improve the strategy of movement for the given task. For example, a goal of maintaining a neutral spine while walking for an individual with pain related to thoracic kyphosis may require improving any one or all the impairments listed in Display 24-4.

DISPLAY 24-4
Required Tests and Measures for Thoracic Spine Examination

Aerobic Capacity: Assessment of vital signs may be necessary, particularly when working with patients with a cardiopulmonary disorder or patients at risk for falls.

Ergonomics and Body Mechanics: The ergonomics of the patient's work station(s) can provide vital information regarding the pathomechanics of the condition. Observation of the activities of daily living and the patient's occupational and recreational movement patterns can reveal impairments in movement in the thoracic and related regions. For example, when reaching across the body one might observe excessive thoracic flexion and lateral flexion that may occur as compensatory movements for insufficient hip and thoracic rotation.

Gait, Locomotion, and Balance: Assessment of these skills can determine risk for falls.

Joint Mobility and Integrity: Arthrokinematic testing of the zygapophyseal, costotransverse, sternocostal, and sternochondral joints. Motion findings in these tests should correlate with osteokinematic findings. Specific testing of osteokinematic function of the ribs can be assessed during inhalation and exhalation.[4]

Motor Function: Altering impaired movement patterns and observing for an associated change in symptoms will assist in determining the pathomechanics of the symptoms. For example, in the case of compensatory thoracic flexion and lateral flexion because of reduced hip and thoracic rotation, having the patient rotate the hip and thoracic spine to the limit of mobility while thoracic flexion and lateral flexion are restricted should alter the movement. This can be achieved manually by the therapist or actively if the patient is able to make the change from verbal instruction alone. If the symptoms are reduced with the new movement pattern, the flexion or lateral flexion movement patterns are assumed to be contributing to the symptoms.

Muscle Performance: Include muscle performance tests to determine presence of nerve root dysfunction in the cervicothoracic and thoracolumbar regions. Manual muscle testing can identify imbalances in muscle performance between synergists and agonist–antagonist muscle pairs in the trunk and shoulder girdles (see Chapters 17 and 25).

Pain Tests and Disability Measures: The Functional Rating Index[5] (measures the magnitude of clinical change in spinal conditions), Oswestry,[6] and Roland-Morris Disability

Questionnaires[7] (disability scales developed for the cervical and lumbar spines which, although not specific to the thoracic spine, can be used to gain insight into the condition's effect on the patient's life; see Chapters 17 and 23).

Posture: Particularly as it relates to the head and neck and lumbar-pelvic-hip complex in standing, sitting, and recumbent positions, signs of asymmetry and scoliosis.

Range of Motion and Muscle Length: Assess the quality and quantity of motion in general as well as intersegmental mobility during active and passive osteokinematic thoracic and upper extremity movements; observe for localized areas of hypermobility with associated areas of hypomobility. Assessment of unilateral upper extremity elevation can assist in the assessment of mobility of the upper thoracic region. For example, upper thoracic extension and rotation to the ipsilateral side should accompany upper extremity arm elevation.[2]

If articular function in a specific joint is found to be normal, and yet overall mobility is limited, lack of myofascial extensibility can be suspected as a primary cause. For example, a stiff or short right external and left internal oblique can limit right thoracic rotation. If this were the case, accessory joint play assessment would reveal normal joint mobility.

Sensory Integrity: Function of the intercostal nerves; special tests, such as those for TOS and neural tension.

Ventilation, Respiration, and Circulation: Observation of breathing patterns can be very useful in fully understanding underlying contributing factors to numerous diagnosis such as kyphosis related diagnoses and TOS. Assess the quality (e.g., proper pump and bucket handle motions of the rib cage, looking for movement in all three directions) and quantity (rate, inspirometry) of respiration. (Lee DG. Manual Therapy for the Thorax—A Biomechanical Approach. Delta, British Columbia, Canada: DOPC, 1994.)

Other: Radiographs (diagnosis and curve angle in scoliosis, Scheuermann disease, and kyphosis related to osteoporosis, signs of ankylosing spondylitis); MRI (soft tissue pathology such as herniated nucleus pulposis); additional medical screening for visceral sources of thoracic pain (see Appendix 1).

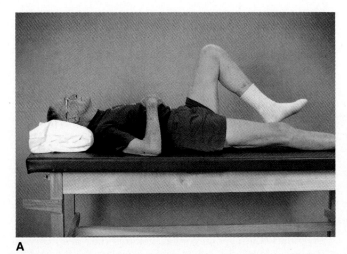

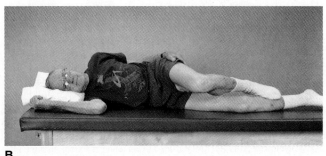

A   B

FIGURE 24-1. This exercise promotes simultaneous hip flexion and trunk counterrotation to prepare for the complex movement of the swing phase of gait on the left. (A) The start position is supine with hip and knee flexion. (B) The end position is sidelying with hip and knee flexion and left trunk rotation.

In an appropriate treatment progression, component impairments are first addressed, followed by integrated movements with relatively simple activities or techniques, progressed to more challenging activities or techniques, and then progressed to complex, integrated functional movement patterns. Figure 24-1 demonstrates an integrated movement in sidelying, which is gravity-lessened for the hip flexors and gravity-assisted for the oblique abdominal muscles and spinal extensors. This movement pattern can be progressed to the upright position of the swing phase of step-up (Fig. 24-2) and eventually into the swing phase of gait (after the stance phase of gait components have adequately improved through another set of exercises).

Because the thoracic spine lies between the shoulder girdle and lumbar-pelvic-hip complex, correction of movement impairments of these regions may be necessary to improve the movement pattern of the thoracic spine. Movement impairments at the foot and ankle also can contribute to impairments in the thoracic spine. The link between the foot and the thoracic spine is reviewed in a subsequent section on scoliosis. Chapter 21 details the exercise prescriptions for impairments in the foot and ankle.

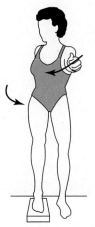

FIGURE 24-2. During the swing phase of the step-up, trunk counterrotation can be emphasized to facilitate the complex movement during the swing phase of gait.

Impaired Muscle Performance

Patients with impairments, activity limitations, or performance restrictions related to impaired muscle performance require resistive exercise with dosage parameters targeted toward a goal of increased force or torque production, power, or endurance (see Chapter 5). The cause of the altered muscle performance must be determined to ascertain the appropriate intervention to treat the impairment. The intervention plan developed is specific to the source or cause. There are several possible sources of reduced force or torque production:

- Neurologic impairment or pathology (e.g., peripheral nerve injury, nerve root injury, CNS disorder)
- Muscle injury or strain
- Disuse resulting in atrophy and general deconditioning
- Length-associated changes resulting in altered length-tension properties

Neurologic Impairment or Pathology Intervention

When muscle performance is impaired because of neurologic injury or pathology, the neural input must be restored in order for muscle performance to improve. If the nerve injury or pathology is permanent and paresis or paralysis is the outcome, the clinician must consider the effect of the resulting muscle weakness and subsequent adaptive shortening or contracture in the opposing muscles. In the case of paresis, the clinician must consider the effect of stretch on the weak muscle due to antagonist action superimposed on the initial weakness caused by the nerve damage. If reinnervation is latent, these same considerations must be heeded during the recovery process. Weak muscles must be protected from overstretch with proper support and stimulated with appropriate-dosage resistive exercise in the short range. The strong muscles must be stretched to maintain proper extensibility and prevent contracture and deformity.

One example of impaired muscle performance related to neurologic injury or pathology is reduced muscle force production in the diaphragm resulting in faulty breathing mechanics. Diaphragmatic breathing exercises cannot be effective until the source of the weakness is appropriately addressed. Because the diaphragm is innervated by the

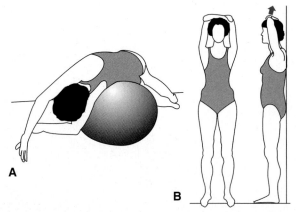

FIGURE 24-3. (A) Lateral trunk flexion stretch is assisted by gravity over a gymnastic ball. (B) Lateral trunk flexion while standing against a wall with arms overhead. The wall guides movement in the frontal plane. The arms-overhead position facilitates stretch to the intercostals. Diaphragmatic breathing into the stiff region can augment the stretch.

phrenic nerve (C3–5), treatment of any cervical dysfunction at these levels may be necessary to improve diaphragmatic function. Subsequently, appropriate diaphragmatic breathing must be taught along with stretch of the lateral trunk and intercostal muscles (Fig. 24-3). The lateral trunk and intercostal muscles may become stiff because of the unilateral rib approximation that may result from inadequate rib expansion, causing weakness in the diaphragm.

In the case of paraplegia with thoracic spine involvement, impaired respiration may result. Full excursion of chest expansion should be encouraged via deep breathing exercises utilizing the diaphragm. Resistance can be applied to the chest walls, diaphragm, and sternum via manual contacts using principles of proprioceptive neuromuscular facilitation (see Chapter 15) or using equipment. For example, inspiration can be facilitated using elastic bands wrapped around the chest. Resistance can be given to the diaphragm by placing weight on the abdomen while in supine (Fig. 24-4). The patient should be instructed to take full, deep breaths.

Muscle Strain or Injury

Causes   Trauma, such as a blow to the chest or a sudden rotational injury sustained in a motor vehicle accident, can lead to muscle injury. An insidious-onset strain can also occur in muscles surrounding the thoracic region. Possible mechanisms of gradual insidious-onset muscle strain include overuse or overstretch.

One example of overuse in the thoracic region is provided by the scalene muscle group, particularly the anterior scalene. The actions of the anterior scalene include cervical flexion, ipsilateral cervical lateral flexion, contralateral cervical rotation, and elevation of the first rib (i.e., acting as an accessory muscle of respiration). Overuse of the anterior scalene can result from underuse or weakness of the deep cervical flexors (i.e., longus colli and capitis and rectus capitis anterior), other contralateral cervical rotators (i.e., deep cervical rotators, semispinalis cervicis, sternocleidomastoid, or upper trapezius), or primary muscles of inspiration (i.e., diaphragm, levator costarum, and intercostals). Chronic overuse can lead to stiffness or adaptive shortening of the anterior scalene, which can contribute to elevation of the first rib. Elevation of the first rib can disrupt cervicothoracic joint mechanics and contribute to thoracic outlet syndrome (TOS; see the section "Thoracic Outlet Syndrome").

Another example is middle and lower trapezius strain, which refers to the painful upper back condition resulting from gradual and continuous tension on the middle and lower trapezius muscles[9] (Kendall). The strain in these muscles is caused by overstretch from a habitual position of forward shoulders (see Chapter 25), kyphosis, or a combination of these two faults. Treatment of the thoracic region must include treatment of the impairments related to the postural fault and/or the kyphosis to reduce the habitual stretch on the tissues (see the sections "Posture and Movement Impairment" and "Kyphosis").

Intervention   Treatment of overuse of a particular muscle group must improve muscle performance of underused synergists and address the posture and movement patterns contributing to excessive use. In the anterior scalene example described above, instructing the patient in proper

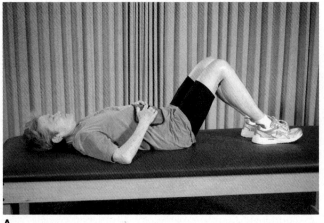

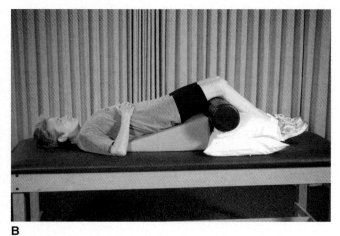

FIGURE 24-4. Resisted diaphragmatic breathing. (A) A weight can be placed on the patients abdomen while in supine to provide resistance to diaphragm excursion. (B) Alternatively, by positioning the patient supine with the head inclined downward the diaphragm must work against the weight of the abdominal contents during inhalation.

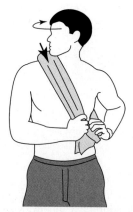

FIGURE 24-5. It is important to stabilize the first rib while stretching the anterior scalene. After the rib is stabilized, *gentle* active range of motion into ipsilateral rotation stretches to the same side anterior scalene without undue cervical shear or first rib elevation.

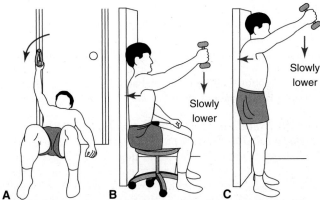

FIGURE 24-7. Activity promoting strength of the thoracic spine extensors in the short range in various start positions. In each position, the patient is instructed to maintain neutral cervical, thoracic, and lumbar spine positions using core activation strategies (see Chapters 18 and 24 for details on core activation strategies for the lumbar and cervical regions, respectively). Supine (A), resisted upper extremity extension from a flexed position using elastic tubing. The thoracic extensors stabilize against the flexion moment. Sitting (B) and standing (C) upper extremity eccentric lowering from a flexed position stimulates thoracic extensor activity to stabilize against a flexion moment.

diaphragmatic breathing (see Patient-Related Instruction 22-2: Diaphragmatic Breathing) rather than using accessory muscle strategies may be an important intervention to reduce the stress placed on the anterior scalene. The deep neck flexors are often weak, particularly after a neck injury (such as whiplash), and need to be strengthened in isolation of the overused muscle(s). Chapter 23 provides exercises in the "Impaired Muscle Performance" section to address weak cervical flexors. Stretch of the anterior scalene should be performed with caution. Stabilization of the first rib is essential so that gentle active ROM of the cervical spine in ipsilateral rotation can stretch the scalene without rib elevation or cervical anterior shearing (Fig. 24-5). The patient should be instructed to avoid chronic postures of neck ipsilateral side bending and contralateral rotation to avoid overuse of the muscle in the short range (e.g., talking on the phone for prolonged periods without use of a headset (Fig. 24-6).

Disuse Resulting in Atrophy and General Deconditioning

Disuse and deconditioning can be caused by illness, immobilization, sedentary lifestyle, or subtle shifts in muscle balance from repetitive faulty movement patterns. Progressive resistive exercises for the upper body can address general disuse and deconditioning. Initially, the weight of the limb alone can provide enough stimulus for strength gains in the severely deconditioned individual. Progression in small increments is recommended because the upper body muscles are

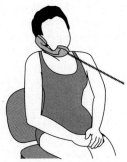

FIGURE 24-6. Resting a telephone on an elevated shoulder with the neck in lateral flexion and opposite rotation can cause shortening and overuse of the anterior scalene muscle.

small compared with those of the lower body, and excessive resistance added prematurely may promote muscle imbalance by strengthening the dominant synergists or antagonists (see Chapter 25). Abdominal and back extensor strengthening (see Fig. 24-7) may be indicated to improve the alignment, movement, and stabilizing function of the thoracic region. Chapter 17 describes proper exercise prescription for the abdominal muscles.

Muscle function in response to injury has not been as well studied in the thoracic spine as it has in the lumbar spine. However, one can extrapolate lumbar findings to the thoracic spine in an attempt to make educated decisions regarding thoracic spine management. Many authors have highlighted the importance of the lumbar multifidus muscle in providing dynamic control,[10-13] and there is cumulative evidence that the cross sectional area of the paraspinal muscles is smaller in patients with chronic[14-17] and postoperative low back pain.[18,19] Furthermore, it has been shown that recovery of multifidi muscle function in the lumbar spine is not automatic following resolution of the pain.[20] This atrophy may permit spinal hypermobility and instability and therefore be an important factor to consider in treatment of persons with spine-related pain.[21]

There is general consensus in the literature supporting the need for active reconditioning exercise in the treatment of spine pain.[22] Add to these findings the natural tendency toward kyphosis (due to the effects of gravity, aging, and habitual usage patterns) and it seems clear that thoracic extension strength should be an emphasis in any plan of care for the region. In addition to strength, since the thoracic extensors are primarily postural muscles, any exercise plan should be dosed so as to improve muscular endurance. Unfortunately, there is little agreement on which exercise regimens are most effective. The use of static stabilization training has been advocated[23] as an ideal means of improving the recruitment of back muscles capable of enhancing spinal stability, particularly the multifidus. This text describes a series of specific exercises to promote spine stability in Chapter 17 (see Patient-Related

Instruction 17-1 and Self-Managements 17-1 and 17-2). The exercises presented in Chapter 17 can be extrapolated to the thoracic spine by adding the focus on thoracic spine alignment and thoracic multifidus activation. Progression of these exercises to use of thoracic multifidus activation during ADLs and occupational and recreational activities are necessary for the best functional outcome.

Length-associated Changes Resulting in Altered Length-Tension Properties

Causes Subtle imbalances in muscle length can lead to length-associated strength changes and positional weakness of one synergist compared with its counterpart or its antagonist muscle group. For example, in the thoracic spine, the erector spinae and upper rectus abdominis are susceptible to length-associated strength changes from chronic kyphotic posture. The thoracic erector spinae are vulnerable to overstretch, and the upper rectus abdominis is susceptible to adaptive shortening. Overstretching and shortening can lead to conditions within the thoracic region such as joint impairments and respiratory dysfunction. The muscle imbalance can contribute to conditions in the adjacent cervical and lumbopelvic areas, and soft tissue dysfunction from the kyphosis-lordosis or swayback posture (see the section "Kyphosis").

Intervention Treatment of muscle length imbalance requires a twofold approach of strengthening the weak and overstretched muscle group (e.g., the thoracic erector spinae) in the shortened range (see Figs. 24-7 and 24-8), and stretching adaptively shortened muscle groups (e.g., the

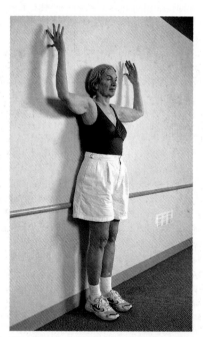

FIGURE 24-8. This exercise stretches superior fibers of the external oblique muscle at the rib angle and the shoulder adductors, and it provides resistance to the spine extensors and scapular upward rotators in the short range. Standing with the back to the wall in a neutral spine position, the patient raises her arms raised in horizontal abduction. The elbows are forward of the wall to maintain the arms in scapular plane. Deep diaphragmatic breathing is performed in this position. The arms can slide up the wall as the length of the pectoralis major allows. The lower abdominals contract to maintain the lumbar spine and pelvis in neutral alignment.

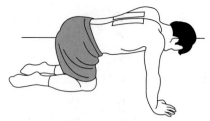

FIGURE 24-9. Longitudinal tape spanning the kyphosis, applied in four-point kneeling to capture neutral spine alignment, can prevent excessive thoracic flexion.

upper rectus abdominis). Supportive taping (see Fig. 24-9) can be used as an adjunctive measure to facilitate positive length-associated changes. Patient-related instruction aimed at correcting posture and movement patterns that perpetuate these length-associated changes is required to prevent recurrence of conditions caused by this muscle performance impairment.

Impaired Range of Motion, Muscle Length, and Joint Mobility/Integrity

Optimal function of the thoracic region requires full and symmetrical cardinal plane motion as well as combined motions. In addition, full thoracic spine and rib motion during breathing should be a goal. The examination should delineate joint versus soft tissue movement impairments, and the plan of care be designed appropriately. Lack of motion (hypomobility) can be the result of either joint or soft tissue impairments, and manual intervention will differ in each case (joint mobilization versus soft tissue mobilization, for example). The exercise intervention, on the other hand, will typically address both causes simultaneously. The general plan for excessive motion (hypermobility) is to stabilize with muscle function while addressing biomechanical factors, such as adjacent hypomobile areas, that transmit increased forces to and produce excess motion in the problem area. Finally, optimal function requires trunk stability during extremity movements. Therefore, appropriate thoracic exercise management will progress from active extremity movement to resisted extremity exercise, while demanding concurrent trunk stability.

Hypermobility

Causes The rational therapeutic exercise intervention plan for hypermobility of the thoracic spine must consider the mechanism or cause of the hypermobility. Spinal mobility must be examined both globally (e.g., the thoracic spine as a whole) and locally (e.g., segmentally). Optimal global spinal movement incorporates motion contributions from each spinal level. Lack of motion in one segment will transfer the mechanical stress to adjacent movement segments. The segments experiencing greater stress over time will become hypermobile. Tissue responses to the increased load may render the region symptomatic. In this case, intervention must address the local impairments. If the underlying cause is an impairment in habitual posture or repetitive movement, the clinician must consider the integrated relationship between the foot and ankle, pelvic girdle, trunk, and upper extremity in developing a plan of care. If there is a history of macrotrauma but the expected healing time has been surpassed, the clinician must consider issues contributing to delayed or interrupted healing.

Interventions Regardless of the mechanism or cause of the hypermobility, central to the success of a program to improve stability of the thoracic spine is the concept that the trunk muscles must hold the vertebral column stable for independent upper and lower extremity movement to occur. This role must be executed regardless of the speed of movement and any additional load the individual may be carrying. Spinal stability must be maintained without sacrificing adequate chest mobility necessary for respiration. Loads must be transferred from the ground upward in an efficient manner, and this can be done without cumulative microtrauma only if the forces are attenuated through an efficient kinematic chain from the foot and ankle upward through to the thoracic spine.

Improved Motor Control. Intervention for hypermobility begins at the stability stage of motor control. The patient is instructed to hold the spine in ideal alignment during movements of the upper and lower extremity. The activity or technique chosen depends largely on the level of intensity the patient can sustain while maintaining ideal alignment with proper recruitment patterns. The prescribed direction of force imposed on the spine depends on the direction of the hypermobility. For example, a patient may present with difficulty in stabilizing against flexion forces such that, when the arm is lowered from a flexed position, the thoracic spine flexes instead of remaining in neutral alignment. A flexion force such as resisted (in some cases, using only the weight of the arm) or rapid upper extremity extension (from an overhead start position) can be used to challenge the spinal extensors. The exercises can begin in sitting with the back against the wall or in supine (see Fig. 24-7), and then progressed to standing. The former positions require stabilization of fewer regions than standing (i.e., sitting eliminates the need to stabilize the foot, ankle, knee, and hips), and the wall or floor provides proprioceptive feedback to enhance stabilization. Similar principles can be used in creating exercises to stabilize against rotational or lateral flexion forces.

Applying an axial load to the thorax and gauging the response can allow the estimation of ideal or optimal alignment in sitting or standing. In the optimal position axial loading forces are distributed equally throughout the vertebral body and intervertebral disk. In symptomatic patients the ideal alignment or "neutral spine" position will often allow asymptomatic axial loading. Additionally, in patients and clients alike, the therapist can feel the increased stability of the spine as the load is applied, as the spine does not give way into either flexion or extension. Specific motion segments that demonstrate hypermobility can be identified and exercises promoting stability can be prescribed. Exercises should target the single segment muscles, such as the multifidi, since multi-segment muscles like the semispinalis or iliocostalis promote multi-segmental motion. Since the primary action of the multifidus is rotation, resisted isometric rotation isolated to the hypermobile segment is a rational starting point. This can be initiated in side-lying with manual resistance. Home exercises can be performed using a straight-backed chair for stability and elastic band or tubing for resistance.

As control of the hypermobile segment(s) improves, several variables can be adjusted to progress the difficulty of the exercises and make them more specific to the activity limitations and participation restrictions of the patient. Utilizing the intervention model described in Chapter 2 can be helpful in this process. For example, once stability control has been achieved

for a given load, adding resistance to the extremities can increase the intensity of the demand. As another example, the speed of extremity movement can be altered based on the functional demands of the patient's work or lifestyle. Slow, controlled movements promote stability and endurance while faster movements such as catching a medicine ball promote fast recruitment.

Motor control and motor learning theory, based on findings in normal individuals[24] suggests that altering the practice conditions and the amount, type and scheduling of feedback is essential to optimal acquisition of motor skills. Accordingly, exercises and activities should be sequenced in a random fashion, rather than repeating the same activity over and over. Feedback should be provided on an intermittent, rather than continuous, basis. Attention to these details will enhance skill acquisition.

Gymnastic balls, foam rolls, and balance boards can modify stabilization activities to provide a greater challenge by destabilizing the base of support (Fig. 24-10). The theory behind

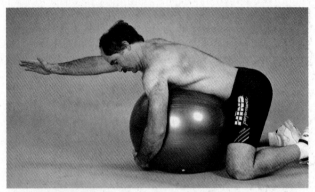

A1

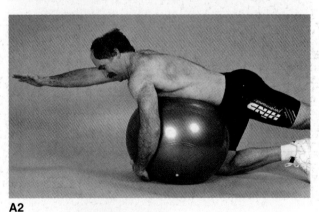

A2

B

FIGURE 24-10. (A) These exercises use the labile surface of the gymnastic ball to stimulate balance and equilibrium reactions. The patient is instructed to maintain axial extension and neutral thoracic and lumbar spine alignment. Teach the patient cervical and lumbopelvic core activation prior to adding any arm or leg movements (see Chapters 18 and 24 for details on lumbar and cervical core activation strategies respectively). (B) The foam rolls further destabilize the base of support.

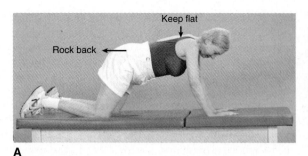
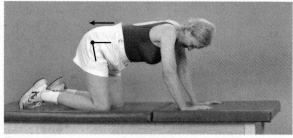

FIGURE 24-11. In four-point kneeling, the patient is instructed to maintain neutral spine position while rocking back toward the heels (A, B). At the point of hip flexion stiffness, the tendency is to flex in the lumbar and/or thoracic spine. The patient is instructed to stop at the onset of spine flexion.

the use of these pieces of equipment is that the labile base of support stimulates balance and equilibrium reactions. Continuous postural adjustments are required, facilitating smooth coordination of posture and movement. Care must be taken to ensure that the patient employs proper trunk stabilization strategies when using equipment that destabilizes the base of support.

Adjacent Areas of Hypomobility. Difficulty stabilizing against flexion forces is a common problem for the thoracic spine. The therapist must consider that excessive thoracic flexion may occur because of lack of mobility in related regions. For example, in sitting a decrease in hip flexion mobility may be compensated for by thoracic flexion with forward-reaching or forward-bending movements. Four-point kneeling with a sit-back movement (Fig. 24-11) can promote hip flexion mobility and thoracic spine stability. This movement pattern must eventually be transferred to controlled mobility and skill level activities in sitting and standing positions, such as reaching forward with hip flexion while maintaining neutral spine position (Fig. 24-12).

Another common cause of excessive thoracic spine motion is lack of thoracic and hip rotation combined with excessive shoulder girdle protraction. For example, in cross-body reaching tasks, the elbow extends and the shoulder flexes and horizontally adducts until the full length of the arm has been reached. If further reach is required, the thoracic spine should rotate, followed by lumbar spine and hip joint flexion and rotation. If standing, a step toward the object can increase the reach span. The arm can effectively reach across the body if the scapula provides a stable base for arm movement and the thorax provides a stable base for the shoulder girdle. This movement requires appropriate recruitment and length-tension properties of the scapulothoracic, glenohumeral, spinal extensor, and oblique abdominal muscles. There must be ample mobility in the glenohumeral joint for upper extremity horizontal adduction and in the thoracic spine and hip joints for rotation. A prevalent faulty movement pattern is to reach instead with scapular abduction and thoracic flexion (Fig. 24-13). Impairments in the shoulder girdle, thorax, and hips may need to be addressed separately

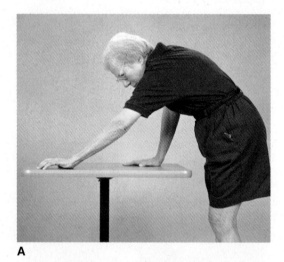

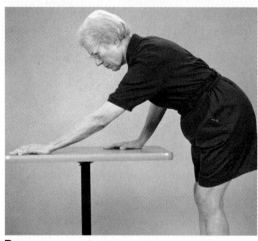

FIGURE 24-12. (A) The standing subject reaches forward with excessive thoracic flexion. (B) The movement pattern is altered such that flexion takes place at the hips, knees, and shoulder, and the thoracic spine remains in neutral.

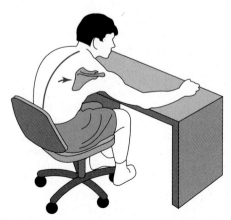

FIGURE 24-13. A prevalent movement pattern is to reach with scapular abduction and thoracic flexion.

to improve the movement pattern of cross-body reaching and thereby reduce the tendency toward excessive thoracic flexion. One useful activity to retrain independent motion among the upper extremity, thoracic spine, and hip joints is shown in Self-Management 24-1: Cross-body Reaching. The prerequisites for correct performance of this exercise are proper movement patterns at the scapulothoracic, glenohumeral, and hip joints (see Chapters 19 and 25).

External Support. Treatment of hypermobility in the thoracic spine may also include supportive devices such as a posture brace (to prevent thoracic flexion; Fig. 24-14)

and taping. Taping can be used to facilitate and remind against excessive flexion and rotation (Fig. 24-9). As strength, endurance, and control improve the patient can be weaned-off the supportive devices.

Hypomobility

Impaired mobility of the thoracic spine and ribs may manifest as dysfunctions in other regions. For example, patients with cervical pain can have decreased pain and increased ROM after manipulation of the thoracic spine. The last degrees of end-range shoulder flexion require thoracic extension

---

 SELF-MANAGEMENT 24-1 *Cross-body Reaching*

Purpose:	To promote independent motion of the shoulder joint from the shoulder blade, torso, and hip. You should not progress to the next level without mastering the previous level. Use the movement pattern acquired in Level 4 when reaching across the body for an object farther away than the span of the arm. Avoid reaching by moving your shoulder blade or flexing in your thoracic spine excessively.
Starting Position:	Stand with feet about 2 in away from the wall and the pelvis and spine in neutral. If your hip flexors are short or stiff, you may need to flex your hips and knees to achieve a neutral spine and pelvis position.

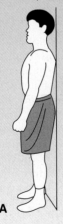

A

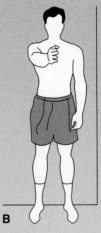

B

Level 2: After you can reach your arm to the midline of your body, rotate your torso as far as you can without moving at the hips, knees, ankles, or feet. Do not move your shoulder blade from its starting position. Do not let your thoracic spine flex; *rotate* it.

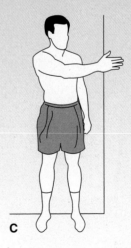

C

Movement Technique:

Level I: Move your arm across your body to the midline without letting your shoulder blade move from its starting position. This may require a submaximal contraction of your interscapular muscles.

(continued)

SELF-MANAGEMENT 24-1 *Cross-body Reaching* (Continued)

Level 3: After you have mastered independent rotation of your torso, add hip rotation to the movement. Do not move your feet from the starting position (i.e., do not take a step forward, but allow your ankles and feet to rotate naturally with hip rotation). Do not move your shoulder blades from the original position or allow your thoracic spine to flex forward.

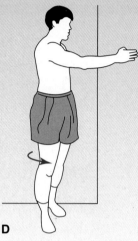

D

Level 4: After you have performed rotation sequentially at the torso and hips, take a step diagonally forward across midline of your body. Do not

let your shoulder blade move from its starting position, but achieve a greater reach by stepping across your body.

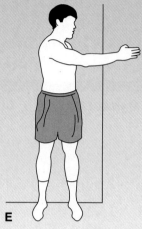

E

Dosage:
Repeat: _____ times
Sets: _____
Frequency: _____
Variations: _____After a wall is no longer required for feedback, a pulley or elastic can be used to resist the movement pattern.
_____Increase the speed of the movement.
_____Add a weight in your hand.

and rotation. Lumbar spine pain may result from excessive lumbar mobility that is related to relative thoracic hypomobility. In addition, poor thoracic spine and costovertebral

mobility can remain asymptomatic while anteriorly pain can develop at the costosternal joints, resulting in costochondritis. Poor thoracic spine and rib mobility will result in decreased chest expansion and therefore decreased lung capacity. This can result from disease processes such as ankylosing spondylitis, from structural deformities such as scoliosis, or from habitual postures such as seen in the patient with Parkinson's who spends most of his time sitting in flexion. Because of gravity, the tendency is to sit in a flexed posture; therefore, restrictions and extension mobility and a relatively fixed kyphosis are typical findings on examination. See Building Block 24-1.

Causes Hypomobility can result from pain or altered tone, restrictions in neural or dural mobility, trauma-inducing osteokinematic restriction, degenerative joint changes,

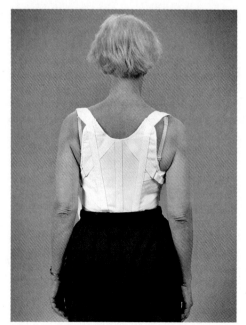

FIGURE 24-14. A posture brace can be used to control excessive thoracic flexion.

BUILDING BLOCK 24-1

Consider the patient with Parkinson disease in Case No. 3, Display 24-1. You are finding it difficult to hear the patient because of low vocal volume. Describe one postural change and two exercises that would likely improve the patient's vocalization.

disease processes, or generalized stiffness in the joints or myofascial tissues from self-induced or externally induced immobility. Self-induced immobilization can result from pain or repetitive altered movement patterns. Repetitive altered movement patterns can produce sites and directions of relative mobility and concurrent sites and directions of hypomobility. For example, the movement strategy of scapular abduction and thoracic flexion to reach across the body can lead to hypomobility in thoracic rotation. One must consider the effect that postoperatively induced immobility, such as open heart surgery or mastectomy, has on the mobility of the thoracic cage.

Hypomobility can be caused by limitations in myofascial length or mobility. In the case of myofascial restriction in the absence of articular hypomobility, correlating articular glides are normal, but osteokinematic motion is limited in rotation. For example, restriction in right rotation can indicate short or stiff right external and left internal oblique muscles. Hypomobility of the thoracic spine can also be found in relation to breathing, with reduced movement in pump or bucket handle breathing mechanics.

Intervention Patients with long-standing joint mobility restrictions are likely to develop myofascial restrictions, requiring concurrent intervention to both. Treatment of joint restrictions usually requires joint mobilization techniques, and treatment of myofascial tissue requires passive stretching, active ROM exercises, or both. Therefore, to maintain mobility gained with joint mobilization techniques, it is important to teach the patient a self-management exercise program that includes a passive stretch, active ROM exercise, or both. Functional movement patterns should be learned that reinforce the mobility gained through mobilization and specific exercise.

A clinical example may best illustrate this point. A patient presents with left rotation and left lateral flexion restrictions in the thoracic spine at the T7 segmental level. The examination determines that this restriction is articular. The appropriate joint mobilization technique is performed to restore the arthrokinematic glide.[2,3] To maintain the mobility gained, the patient is instructed to perform specific mid-thoracic lateral flexion, blocking motion at the relatively hypermobile segments below T7, to facilitate motion at the stiff segmental level (Fig. 24-15). Repeated thoracic left rotation can also be instructed (Fig. 24-16). The patient should be instructed to use left rotation of the thoracic spine frequently throughout

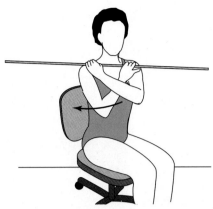

FIGURE 24-16. Holding onto a light dowel rod can encourage thoracic rotation by keeping the dowel rod level while rotating the torso. The patient is instructed to rotate the sternum. Lower segments can be stabilized by keeping the lower back flat against the back of the chair.

the day to further facilitate maintenance of articular mobility. All exercises should be done with high repetitions (up to 20 times) and frequently throughout the day (up to 10 times), and in the pain-free range to prevent aggravation of symptoms.

Proper diaphragmatic breathing is essential to the treatment of many impairments in the thoracic spine and related regions (see Chapters 17 and 22). The Patient-Related Instruction 22-2: Diaphragmatic Breathing in Chapter 22 describes proper diaphragmatic breathing, with emphasis on pump and bucket handle breathing. After mastering diaphragmatic breathing in a supine position, the patient should progress to sitting and standing while applying the same breathing techniques.

In older adults, aerobic conditioning may provide significant improvements in spinal mobility, physical function, and overall health.[25] The effects of a 3-month supervised program of spinal flexibility and aerobic exercises was compared to one with aerobic exercise alone on axial rotation, maximal oxygen uptake (VO_2max); functional reach, timed-bed-mobility; and the Physical Function Scale (PhysFunction) of the Medical Outcomes Study SF-36. Both groups improved in all measures although there was no difference between the groups, suggesting that for this population either type of exercise would be beneficial.

Muscle/Myofascial Length

Specific myofascial tissue length impairments that promote poor thoracic mobility can be gleaned from analyzing the movements created by each muscle. Commonly impaired muscles include the pectoralis major and minor, rectus abdominis, and oblique abdominals (extension); the paraspinals and the more lateral iliocostalis (flexion); and the intercostals, which can limit motion in all directions. Specific soft tissue mobilization and longitudinal stretching techniques are often necessary to restore full mobility but must always be followed by exercises aimed at maintaining the new mobility if not gaining more range of motion.

Restrictions in oblique abdominal muscle length can limit thoracic rotation. In the case of myofascial restriction in the absence of articular hypomobility, correlating articular glides are normal, but osteokinematic motion is limited in rotation. Restriction in right rotation can indicate short

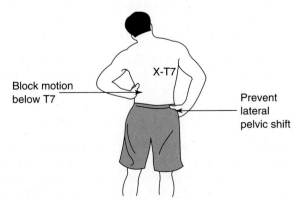

FIGURE 24-15. Left thoracic spine lateral flexion can be encouraged at T7 by blocking excessive lateral flexion below T7.

Block motion below T7

X-T7

Prevent lateral pelvic shift

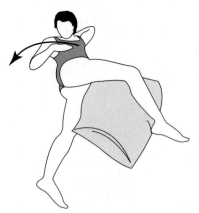

FIGURE 24-17. Rotation stretch for short or stiff right external and left internal oblique muscles.

or stiff right external and left internal oblique muscles. A passive stretch (Fig. 24-17) can be used in conjunction with diaphragmatic breathing (see Patient-Related Instruction 22-2: Diaphragmatic Breathing) into the right thoracic rib cage. Lying on a foam roller can increase the stretching force. Postural habits and repetitive movement patterns must be analyzed for potential causes of myofascial restrictions. Comprehensive treatment may include changing the ergonomics of the workstation to reduce factors contributing to myofascial restrictions (e.g., rearranging the workstation to reduce sustained and repeated left rotation and promote occasional right rotation). The patient's movement patterns and activities may need to be altered to limit repeated left rotation and promote more activities requiring symmetric rotation. For example, the patient should reduce the time spent playing tennis (an asymmetric activity) and begin walking, jogging, biking, or swimming (symmetric activities). See Building Block 24-2.

Patients who have undergone surgery such as a coronary artery bypass graft (CABG) or mastectomy will develop thoracic spine and rib hypomobility if not exercised properly. Early exercises should focus on maintaining deep inspiration ROM as tolerated by the patient. Diaphragmatic breathing will also assist in lymphatic drainage post-mastectomy. Gentle stretching of the chest musculature should be undertaken, within the confines of post-operative precautions. In general, such precautions would include avoiding undue stress to the involved tissues in the early stages of healing. Resisted exercises that stress the involved musculature and their associated joints should be avoided until such time as allowed by post-operative protocols. For example, pectoralis major

BUILDING BLOCK 24-2

Consider the buggy-driving patient in Case No. 1, Display 24-1. This patient, like many large equipment operators, spends much of his day rotating to one side due to the nature of the traffic flow. He is having pain when rotating to the left, the direction he must turn to most frequently at work. Provide some recommendations for his work and leisure activities as well as exercise intervention choices.

strengthening after a CABG should not take place until the sternum has healed. As the surgical incisions heal shoulder ROM exercises should be introduced, gradually progressing to full arcs of motion and adding resistance (Fig. 24-8).

Pain

Pain in the thoracic region has many possible causes or mechanisms. The onset of pain may be the result of joint dysfunction (i.e., thoracic vertebrae or rib articulations), soft tissue injury or strain, or of non-visceral (e.g., osteoporosis, ankylosing spondylitis, Scheuermann disease) or visceral diseases (see Appendix 1).

Treatment must focus on the cause or mechanism of the pain, not just the source. This chapter should provide you with theoretical strategies and clinical examples of exercises used to alleviate impairments that could be contributing to the causes and mechanisms of musculoskeletal origin pain.

Impaired Posture and Motor Function

Optimal postural alignment is discussed in detail in Chapter 9. As noted previously, it is important to distinguish between postural faults that are due to permanent changes in the structure of the spine and those that are amenable to change. The impairments of body structures common to the thoracic spine were discussed earlier. This section will deal with non-structural impairments of posture.

Head posture is contingent upon thoracic posture which in turn is dependent on the lumbar spine, pelvis and lower extremities. In addition, as noted earlier, full upper extremity motion requires thoracic mobility. Therefore, all aspects of the kinetic chain must be examined and evaluated.

Kyphosis

Causes   Postural kyphosis is caused by habitual trunk flexion, for which there are several reasons. An individual with poor postural habits, for example a student who spends most of her time sitting in class in a flexed posture, is likely to develop a kyphosis. Weak trunk extensors can exacerbate already poor posture. A dominant daily activity that encourages thoracic flexion, for example working daily sitting at a computer writing a book chapter on thoracic spine exercise while using a chair with poor trunk and pelvic support, will likely encourage a kyphotic spine. Finally, there are diseases that tend to manifest with thoracic kyphosis as a secondary complication. Parkinson disease is an example of one such disorder, in which there is a lack of movement into extension, and is discussed later in this chapter.

Intervention   Any plan of care for kyphosis must consider the structural impairment and pathology in addition to the related impairments in body function. Display 24-5 lists potential impairments of body functions associated with kyphosis, and Table 24-1 lists general exercise recommendations to address these impairments.

Although diseases such as osteoporosis and Scheuermann's cause structural changes in the vertebrae that create the kyphosis, postural habits and movement patterns can exaggerate the posture impairment. Although exercise cannot correct the structural changes that have occurred in the vertebrae, it can positively influence physiologic factors that exaggerate the

DISPLAY 24-5

Impairments of Body Fuctions Associated With Kyphosis

Alignment
Forward head
Cervical lordosis
Abducted scapulae

Kyphosis-lordosis: Lumbar lordosis, anterior pelvic tilt, hip joint flexion, knee joint hyperextension, ankle plantar flexion

Swayback: Lumbar flexion, posterior pelvic tilt, hip joint hyperextension, knee joint hyperextension, neutral ankle

Kyphosis-Lordosis	Swayback
Short and Strong*	
Neck extensors	Hamstrings
Hip flexors	Upper fibers of internal oblique
Lumbar spinal extensors	
Shoulder adductors	Shoulder adductors
Pectoralis minor	Pectoralis minor
Intercostals	Intercostals
Elongated and Weak	
Neck flexors	Neck flexors
Upper back spinal extensors	Upper back spinal extensors
External oblique	External oblique
Hamstrings	One-joint hip flexors
Middle and lower trapezius	Middle and lower trapezius

Findings associated with short muscles must be tested by muscle length and manual muscle tests, because not all muscles held in short positions develop shortness.

kyphosis. Only through a comprehensive program of exercise and patient-related instruction can these contributing factors be properly addressed.

In patients without a structural kyphosis in whom lack of extension ROM is the primary impairment, manual joint and soft tissue mobilization is a key part of successful management. Joint mobilization techniques are described and discussed in Chapter 7. Often a kyphotic posture is associated with shortened soft tissues on the anterior aspect of the thorax. Soft tissue mobilization and manual stretching of the pectoralis major and minor is often required, followed by a home stretching program (Fig. 24-8).

Patient-related instruction is indicated to improve posture alignment and avoid positions that contribute to the kyphosis. Support to the lower back may be indicated to help

relax the musculature holding the spine in lordosis in the lordosis-kyphosis posture, and a shoulder support may be indicated for the kyphosis to help stretch the pectoralis minor and relieve strain on the middle and lower trapezius, and thoracic paraspinal muscle group (see Fig. 24-14).

As illustrated by Table 24-1, exercise prescription for the treatment of kyphosis may need to go well beyond strengthening the thoracic erector spinae. The thoracic spine must function as part of a kinematic chain, and treatment of body function impairments in each region influencing the kyphosis is indicated. Ultimately, improved physiologic capabilities in each region can provide a good foundation for enhanced function and quality of life. Specific exercises must progress to functional movements meaningful to that patient. For example, a patient with Scheuermann disease with a desk job needs to maintain his best neutral spine when working. He would benefit from learning to lean forward and backward from the hip joints while maintaining a neutral spine. Thinking about the distance between the symphysis pubis and the base of the sternum and keeping this distance constant during forward and backward movements at the hip joints can be useful in changing movement patterns that promote thoracic flexion.

Home exercises that promote extension throughout the thoracic spine often end up exacerbating segments that are already hypermobile, because the hypomobile segments resist being moved and only transfer the motion to the segments that move easily. It is therefore important to utilize self-management exercises that target the stiff segments while protecting the mobile ones. Figure 24-18 illustrates an effective self-mobilization technique.

Another relatively specific extension exercise involves the use of a foam roll. Lying on the foam roll with it positioned horizontally encourages extension of the thoracic spine but also serves to mobilize the ribs. If positioned in the hook-lying position, rolling the knees to one side encourages trunk rotation. With the roll positioned at 45 degrees, mobilization into extension and rotation is possible. Throughout all these mobility exercises, deep breathing should be emphasized, to incorporate chest mobility. As with the use of tennis balls, the key element in this exercise's potential for success is maintaining the mobilization for a sufficient amount of time (1 minute per segment to start), being consistent (every day without fail), and staying with the program (2 to 4 months). Considering that gravity is forcing the thoracic spine into flexion every

TABLE 24-1	**Therapeutic Exercise Management for Kyphosis**
STRETCH	**STRENGTHEN**
Kyphosis	
Cervical spine extensors (See Figs. 23-14 and 23-15)	Cervical spine flexors (See Display 23-1)
Intercostals (See Figs. 24-3, 24-8)	Thoracic spine extensors (See Fig. 24-7)
Lumbar spine extensors (See Fig. 24-11)	
Pectoralis minor, shoulder adductors (See Fig. 24-8)	Middle and lower trapezius (See Self-Management 25-2)
Lordosis	
Lumbar spine extensors (See Fig. 24-11)	External oblique (See Self-Management 17-1)
Hip flexors (See Self-Management 19-9)	Hip extensors (See Self-Management 20-1)
Swayback	
Intercostals (See Figs. 24-3, 24-8)	External oblique (See Self-Management 17-1)
Hamstrings (See Fig. 19-20A and Self-Management 19-7)	Hip flexors (See Self-Management 19-5)

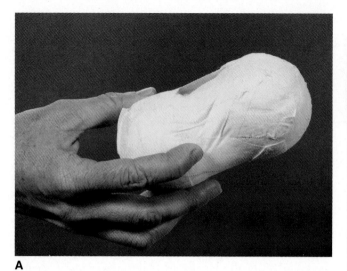

A

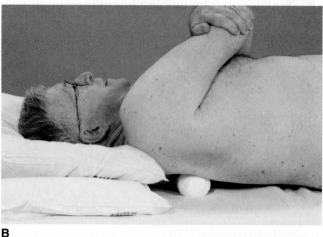

B

C

FIGURE 24-18. A self management exercise can be used to mobilize stiff segments in the thoracic spine. One way to accomplish this is to have the patient lie supine on two tennis balls that have been taped together into a peanut shape. (A) The balls themselves contact the transverse processes while the spinous processes are spared direct contact by the indentation between the balls. The patient positions the tennis balls first at the thoracolumbar junction (B), and lies on top of them for 1 minute. The patient repositions the tennis balls at 1-minute intervals, progressing superiorly one segment at a time to address each spinal level. The primary forces at work are gravity and time. The balls act as a fulcrum selectively forcing each movement segment into extension. Adding active shoulder abduction, flexion or protraction (C) can increase the amount of force. Since the forces are relatively small, a relatively long time is required. The exercise must be done daily at least, and results typically occur over weeks or months.

second of every day that the patient is upright, encouraging extension 10 minutes per day seems a paltry amount of time in comparison. Asking for more time than this, however, risks losing the patient's compliance.

Taping the thoracic spine for proprioceptive feedback and as a reminder to avoid flexion postures is a powerful way to teach patients new habits. The patient is asked to assume a quadruped position with the thoracic spine held flat, not in flexion. The tape is applied along the paraspinal region on each side and spans several segments above and below the hypermobile segment or "hinge point" (Fig. 24-9). Each time the patient flexes from this area the tape will provide proprioceptive feedback in the form of a pull on the skin, reminding the patient to stay in more extension. This type of feedback is very successful when used during symptomatic activities, alerting the patient to how often and how unaware they are that potentially harmful movements occur. Leaving the tape on for several hours at a time helps to counteract the constant force of gravity compressing the spine into flexion. The use of tape is gradually decreased as the patient develops improved awareness and the endurance necessary to actively maintain their positioning.

Finally, exercises to address kyphosis need to be prescribed that address muscle performance impairments in the thoracic extensors. This was described previously in the section on "Muscle Performance Impairment."

Intervention in Patients with Scheuermann Disease

Intervention is usually limited to patients with a painful deformity, documented progression, and at least 2 years of growth remaining. Younger children with a mild deformity can be initially treated with a program of exercise to strengthen spinal extensor muscles (see Fig. 24-7) and stretch the hamstring (see Fig. 19-22), pectoralis major (see Fig. 25-19), and superior fibers of the rectus abdominis muscles and anterior longitudinal ligament (see Self-Management 17-7: Prone Press-up Progression, level II, in Chapter 17) Though there is a paucity of research on the effect of spinal exercise on spinal parameters in Scheuermann disease, one study did demonstrate the beneficial effect of regular exercise.[26] In adolescents, Scheuermann disease is effectively managed with bracing until skeletal maturity has been reached (see the section "Scoliosis"). Contraindications to brace treatment include curves >70 degrees, severe apical wedging, and a rigid curve. Surgery (spinal fusion) is considered as an option for patients with severe deformity and disabling pain and as necessary in cases of neurologic compromise. At any stage in life, management of the resulting kyphosis can be effective in preventing increased postural kyphosis overlaid over the anatomic kyphosis (see the section "Kyphosis").

Scoliosis

Causes Non-structural scoliosis may result from highly repetitive, asymmetric activities related to hand dominance.

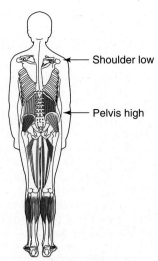

FIGURE 24-19. In a typical dominant right-hand pattern, the right iliac crest is high and the shoulder low. The darkly shaded muscles can develop adaptive shortening, while the lightly shaded muscles can develop adaptive lengthening. (From Kendall FP, McCreary EK, Provance PG. Muscles: Testing and Function. 4th Ed. Baltimore, MD: Williams & Wilkins, 1993:89.)

A common pattern of muscle imbalance and alignment changes for right-handed individuals is pictured in Figure 24-19. The therapist should be aware of the postural habits of a child in the various positions of the body, such as sitting, standing, and lying, because habits developed in childhood can persist into adulthood. A right-handed child may sit at his desk to write with the upper body laterally flexed to the right. If this posture is also assumed in sidelying to perform homework (Fig. 24-20), sitting (Fig. 24-21), and to carry his homework in a backpack slung over the right shoulder, he is prone to develop muscle imbalance problems that can lead to acquired scoliotic deviations of the spine that persist into adulthood.

The pronation of one foot, standing on one leg, or standing with the same knee always bent (these habits often occur together) can contribute to the development of acquired scoliosis. The imbalances in hip musculature or faulty foot alignment or knee position that result in lateral pelvic tilt are more closely related to primary lumbar or thoracolumbar curves than to primary thoracic curves.

Intervention To develop a comprehensive approach to treatment, a comprehensive musculoskeletal evaluation must be performed. The evaluation should include the tests and measures described in Display 24-6. Exercises should be carefully selected on the basis of the examination findings. The general principles of exercise prescription for patients with scoliosis

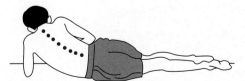

FIGURE 24-20. Children sometimes assume a sidelying position on the floor or bed to do their homework. A right-handed person lies on the left side so that the right hand is free to write or turn the pages in a book. Such a posture places the spine in a left convex curve.

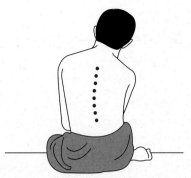

FIGURE 24-21. Sitting on one foot (the left in this illustration) causes the pelvis to tilt downward on the left and upward on the right. This places the spine in a left convex curve.

are listed in Display 24-7. Exercises to be avoided by individuals with scoliosis include those listed in Display 24-8. An alternative exercise is shown in Self-Management 24-2: Postural Exercise With Back to Wall. Exercises for muscle imbalances associated with acquired scoliosis were described previously.

Patients with mild scoliotic curves often do not require treatment, as long as the curve does not progress. Periodic observation is required to make sure the degree of curvature is not increasing. After skeletal maturity has been reached, a curvature (by the Cobb method) of <25 degrees[27] to 30 degrees[28] typically does not progress. In the patient with an immature spine, if the curve is between 25 and 40 degrees there is a high risk of further progression. These patients need to be treated using a brace, which in 70% to 80% of the cases will prevent further progression.[27] In one study, a brace worn 16 or more hours each day was shown to

---

DISPLAY 24-6
Tests and Measures Included in a Scoliosis Evaluation

Posture Alignment
- Plumbline and segmental, in back, front, and side views

Muscle Length Tests
- Hip flexor (differentiating psoas from tensor fascia lata and rectus femoris)
- Hamstrings
- Forward bend for length of posterior muscles
- Tensor fascia lata–iliotibial band
- Teres major and latissimus dorsi

Muscle Strength Tests
- Back extensors
- Abdominal muscles (differentiating trunk curl from pelvic stabilization roles)
- Lateral trunk
- Oblique abdominals
- Hip flexors
- Hip extensors
- Hip abductors (differentiating posterior gluteus medius)
- Middle and lower trapezius

Movement
- Forward bending to determine a structural curve and the location of the curve

DISPLAY 24-7
Principles of Exercise Prescription for Scoliosis

- Symmetric exercises should not be attempted.
- If one group or one muscle within a group is too strong for its antagonist or synergist, that muscle or group should be stretched, and the weaker, longer antagonist or synergist should be strengthened and supported to provide balance to the region.
- The lateral and anterior abdominal muscles, pelvic girdle, and leg muscles usually have asymmetric strength, causing the body to deviate about all three planes of motion but primarily in the transverse and frontal planes. Because the posterior spinal muscles are relatively less affected, the program should emphasize promoting strength of the relatively weak muscle or groups of muscles in the anterior thoracolumbar region and the pelvic-hip complex.

DISPLAY 24-8
Exercises to Avoid in Treating Scoliosis

- Exercises that promote flexibility of the spine should be avoided without counterbalancing exercises or support promoting opposing shortening and strength to maintain corrections.
- A subject who is also developing kyphoscoliosis should avoid back extension exercises performed in prone because it promotes further lumbar extension (Self-Management 24-2: Postural Exercise with Back to Wall).
- Trunk curl exercises or sit-ups should be avoided even if the rectus abdominis and internal oblique muscles are weak, because thoracic flexion promotes the kyphosis (see **Chapter 17** for alternative methods of abdominal strengthening).

SELF-MANAGEMENT 24-2 *Postural Exercise With Back to Wall*

Purpose: To reduce the tendency for excessive mid-back forward flexion and forward shoulder posture. After this exercise is mastered in sitting, it can be progressed to standing.

Starting Position: Sit on a stool with the lower back nearly flat against the wall. You should be able to fit your hand behind your lower back if your spine is in optimal position. If you have an exaggerated upper and mid-back curve, you may have a larger space between the wall and your back. Try to reduce this space as much as possible by contracting your lower abdominal muscles. *Caution:* Do not let your upper and middle back forward flex more in an attempt to reduce the curve of your lower back.

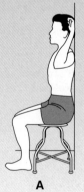

A

Press your head back with your chin tucked down. If you have an exaggerated curve of your upper or middle back, you may not be able to get your head to the wall. Place one or two towel rolls behind your head with your head as close to the wall as possible and with your eyes and nose positioned horizontally. *Caution:* Do

not let your chin rise upward in an attempt to get your head closer to the wall.

Place your thumbs on the wall with your elbows pointing slightly forward. If you have an exaggerated curve of your upper or middle back, you may not be able to get your thumbs to the wall (A).

Movement Technique: Keep your thumbs in contact with the wall, keep your head and low back in the starting position, and slide your arms to a diagonal position overhead. When your head or low back deviates from the start position or your shoulders shrug excessively, stop the movement (B).

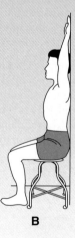

B

Dosage:
Repeat: _____ times
Sets:
Frequency:

be effective in preventing 90% or more of the curves from getting worse, particularly mild curves (25 to 35 degrees).[29] Most authorities recommend wearing the brace for 23 hours each day, because using it part time can create compliance problems about when to take it off and put it on. When it becomes part of a daily routine, it becomes a standard function. However, the brace cannot correct a curve. At best, it can prevent it from worsening. In adults, the curve may progress slowly over the years, and bracing may not be a practical solution.

Early detection and intervention is the key to the treatment of scoliosis. A few carefully selected exercises that help to maintain muscle balance and a kinesthetic sense of good alignment are recommended over a vigorous, complex program. This means providing good patient-related education about how to avoid habitual positions and activities that can increase the curvature. It also means providing incentives that help keep the child, adolescent, or adult interested and cooperative in an ongoing program.

The use of exercise in the management of scoliosis is controversial. Muscle imbalance that exists as a result of postural or other non-structural scoliosis theoretically can be treated through the use of exercise to prevent further exaggeration of the scoliosis beyond that which the disease has caused. The message that exercise is of little or no value prevails in the literature, leaving individuals with scoliosis the treatment options of doing nothing, bracing, or surgery. In the American Academy of Orthopedic Surgeons 1985 lecture series, this statement appears:

"Physical therapy cannot prevent a progressive deformity, and there are those who believe specific spinal exercise programs work in a counterproductive fashion by making the spine more flexible than it ordinarily would be and, by so doing, making it more susceptible to progression."[30] Kendall et al.[9] warns that overemphasis on flexibility is the exercise approach that leads to the view that exercise is of little value or even counterproductive in the treatment of scoliosis. She states that adequate musculoskeletal evaluation has been lacking, and as a result, there has been little scientific basis on which to justify the selection of therapeutic exercises. Kendall's premise for using therapeutic exercise is that scoliosis is a problem of symmetry and that restoring symmetry requires the use of asymmetric exercises along with appropriate support. Stretching of stiff or short muscles is desirable only if it is performed with simultaneous exercise and appropriate support to shorten and strengthen what is too long and relatively weak.

The correction of asymmetrical postural habits may be helpful in preventing the development of scoliosis during childhood. Exercises should be carefully selected on the basis of thorough examination findings, and adequate instruction is needed to ensure that the exercises will be performed correctly and with precision. The object is to use asymmetric exercises to promote symmetry. To illustrate this point, consider the following case.

The patient is a gymnast with a right thoracic, left lumbar curve (Fig. 24-22). Along with other findings, right iliopsoas and right external oblique weaknesses are diagnosed. An example of an asymmetric exercise is resisted exercise to the right iliopsoas (Fig. 24-23). Because the iliopsoas muscle attaches to the lumbar vertebrae, transverse processes, and the intervertebral disks, this muscle

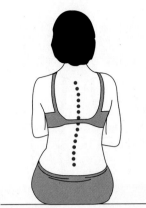

FIGURE 24-22. This person has a right thoracic and left lumbar curve.

can pull directly on the spine. Figure 24-24A demonstrates the adverse effect of resisting the left iliopsoas, and Figure 24-24B illustrates the positive effect of resisting the right iliopsoas. A left upper extremity diagonal reaching movement pattern can facilitate right thoracic lateral flexion. Simultaneous right hip flexion and left upper extremity diagonal reaching should promote lateral deviation, correcting both curves (Fig. 24-25). If performed as a home program, this movement should be monitored (by an observer or using a mirror) to ensure that the appropriate spine correction occurs.

Kendall et al.[9] describes an exercise in supine to address the weakness of the right external oblique. In the supine position, the subject places the right hand on the right lateral chest wall and the left hand on the left side of the pelvis. Keeping the hands in position, the object of the exercise is to bring the two hands closer by contraction of the abdominal muscles without flexing the trunk. It is as if the upper part of the body shifts toward the left, and the pelvis shifts toward the right. By not allowing trunk flexion and contracting the posterior lateral fibers of the external oblique, there will be a tendency toward some counterclockwise rotation of the thorax in the direction

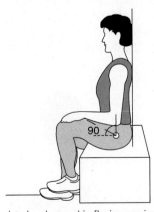

FIGURE 24-23. Resisted end-range hip flexion can isolate the iliopsoas from the other hip flexors that do not attach directly to the spine. The patient is instructed to passively lift the thigh to end range and hold the position against gravity while maintaining a neutral spine position. The patient is instructed to activate the lumbopelvic core prior to letting go of the leg (see Chapter 18 for core activation strategies). Resistance is applied only after the patient is able to hold the limb against gravity without resistance.

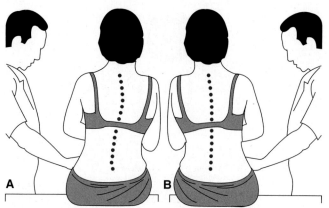

FIGURE 24-24. (A) The dotted line shows the adverse effect of resisting the left iliopsoas in a left lumbar curve. (B) The dotted line shows the positive effect of resisting the right iliopsoas in a left lumbar curve.

of correcting the thoracic rotation that accompanies a right thoracic curve.

There is some evidence in small groups that exercise using trunk rotation may inhibit the progression of adolescent scoliosis.[31] However, there was no control group in this trial and there were only 20 subjects. One study has looked at the effect of axial unloading in changing the spinal curvature and found some improvement but without lasting results.[32] Again, the group was small (six subjects) and there was no control group for comparison. A review of the literature found that physical exercise prevents or reduces disabilities, and facilitates the neutralization of postural deficits to produce a stationary or regressive curve.[33]

Often adolescents with scoliosis will have impairments in their overall fitness level. This has to do as much with poor self-image and reluctance to participate in activities while wearing the brace as it has to do with impairments in respiratory function. These children must be encouraged to remain as physically active as possible, and the parent must take an active role in this process. If the curve is severe enough, aerobic capacity may become impaired and appropriate endurance exercises should be prescribed. Thirty minutes of bike ergometry four times a week over 2 months produced a significant improvement in aerobic capacity in young girls

with scoliosis compared to a control group of girls with scoliosis who did not exercise.[34]

Consider a case of asymmetry and muscle imbalance found in acquired and structural scoliosis associated with unilateral pronation. For example, the combination of left pronation, shortness of the left tensor fascia lata, left gluteus medius and right hip adductors, and weakness of the right gluteus medius, left hip adductors, and left lateral abdominals can be seen in a person with a right thoracic curve and left lumbar curve. In cases such as these, along with specific exercises to improve the length of the left tensor fascia lata and strength of the right gluteus medius, left hip adductors, and lateral abdominal muscles (see Chapters 17 and 19), the use of an orthotic to support the left foot may be indicated (see Chapter 21). Correction of lateral pelvic tilt associated with a lumbar curve can be helped by proper lift on the side of the low iliac crest. However, no lift can help if the patient continues to stand in an asymmetric posture, such as with weight predominantly on the leg with the higher iliac crest and with the knee flexed on the side of the lift.

Lordosis

Causes   Thoracic lordosis is a loss of the normal posterior curve of the thoracic spine, and it can be associated with abnormal posture correction strategies. For example, in an attempt to correct forward shoulders, the individual extends the thoracic spine, rather than adduct the shoulder girdle on the stable thorax. If this is done habitually, the thoracic spine becomes a site of relative flexibility.

Intervention   Attempts to improve impairments of the shoulder girdle with lower trapezius resistive exercises (Fig. 24-26A) cause thoracic extension instead of scapular adduction. Use of a support under the sternum (Fig. 24-26B) can somewhat block the undesired thoracic extension to allow resistive exercises to transmit forces to the scapula instead of the thoracic spine. Applying tape anteriorly as a proprioceptive feedback mechanism to prevent excessive thoracic extension will facilitate movement in the lumbar spine and pelvis. Patient-related instruction is necessary to alter the strategy of posture correction performed by the patient. Self mobilization into thoracic flexion can be performed, using the back of a firm chair to stabilize caudal segments while the cranial vertebrae are actively flexed (Fig. 24-27).

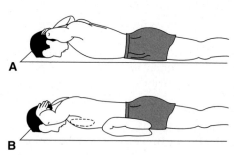

FIGURE 24-26. (A) In a person with thoracic lordosis, attempts at performing resisted lower and middle trapezius exercises promote thoracic extension instead of scapular adduction. (B) Use of a firmly rolled towel placed under the sternum can stabilize the thoracic spine in flexion, allowing the force of the middle and lower trapezius to adduct the scapula instead of extending the thoracic spine.

FIGURE 24-25. The dotted line shows the effect of reducing the right thoracic and left lumbar curve by simultaneously reaching diagonally upward with the left arm and resisting right hip flexion.

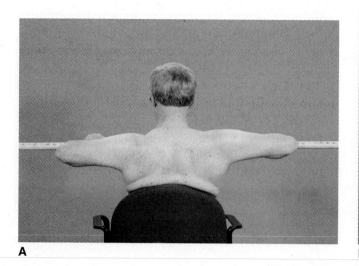

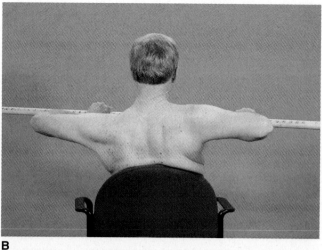

FIGURE 24-27. Blocking motion of the caudal segments by stabilizing against the back of a chair, while mobilizing the segments above. (A) Starting position. (B) End position, rotation. Be sure to instruct the patient to rotate the spine versus adduct the scapula. (C) End position, extension. Be sure to instruct the patient to stabilize the thoracolumbar and lumbar regions to prevent extension.

THERAPEUTIC EXERCISE INTERVENTION FOR COMMON DIAGNOSES

This section contains selected medical diagnoses that have a bearing on the muscular, skeletal, and nervous systems as they relate to the thoracic region. Although there are numerous musculoskeletal diagnoses associated with the thoracic region, only a few are discussed to provide examples of therapeutic exercise prescriptions for the related activity limitations, participation restrictions, and related impairments.

Prevention and Intervention in Patients with Osteoporosis

When treating patients with vertebral compression fractures secondary to osteoporosis, the therapist must know whether the fracture is stable or unstable. Physiologic forces or movement will not displace a stable fracture. Fortunately, compression fractures are normally stable secondary to their impacted nature. Traditional treatment is nonoperative and conservative. Patients are treated with a short period (no more than a few days) of bedrest. Prolonged inactivity should be avoided, especially

in elderly patients. Pain control can be in the form of oral or parenteral analgesics, muscle relaxants, external back-braces, and physical therapy modalities.[34,35] See Building Block 24-3.

Patients who do not respond to conservative treatment or who continue to have severe pain may be candidates for surgical intervention. However, most patients can make a full recovery or at least significant improvements in 6 to 12 weeks

BUILDING BLOCK 24-3

Why is extended bed rest and prolonged inactivity to be avoided?

A 77-year-old male spent the last 2 weeks in bed recovering from pneumonia. His cough is nearly gone and his breathing is no longer impaired. He is otherwise healthy. What impairments and activity limitations might be found in this patient? Design an exercise program that will effectively treat his impairments and improve his function, using two in-clinic visits and a home program.[37,38]

and can return to a normal exercise program after the fracture has fully healed. A well-balanced diet, regular exercise, calcium and vitamin D supplements,[36,39] smoking cessation, and medications to treat osteoporosis may help prevent additional compression fractures. Age should never preclude treatment.

There is now good evidence that diagnosing and treating osteoporosis does indeed reduce the incidence of compression fractures of the spine.[40–42] Regular activity and muscle strengthening exercises have been shown to decrease vertebral fractures and back pain.[43] Inactivity leads to bone loss, but weight-bearing exercise can reduce bone loss and increase bone mass. The optimal type and amount of physical activity that can prevent osteoporosis has not been established, but moderate weight-bearing exercise such as walking is recommended. Resisted upper extremity exercise is also recommended to induce weight-bearing stress on the spine and wrist. Exercise to reduce the stress of kyphosis are discussed in a later section of this chapter (see the section "Kyphosis"). See Building Block 24-4.

Measures to prevent falls must be initiated by patients and their caregivers, because a fall in this population can lead to morbidity or death from the secondary effects of immobilization and reduced activity. Specific exercise techniques addressing impairments related to balance are addressed in Chapters 8 and 19. Table 24-2 lists items that should be assessed when determining what preventive measures should be followed.[44]

Exercise Management of Parkinson Disease

Parkinson disease is a progressive neurologic disorder that results in the loss of L-dopa in the substantia nigra. The clinical findings of the disease include rigidity, facial masking, resting tremor, dyskinesia, bradykinesia, difficulty initiating movement, and a flexed posture.

TABLE 24-2 Items to Assess in Determining Risk for Falls in the Elderly	
AVOIDANCE OF RESTRAINTS	**MUSCLE STRENGTH**
Balance assessment	Neurologic function; cortical, extrapyramidal, and cerebellar functions; lower extremity peripheral nerves; proprioception; reflexes
Cardiac function, cardiac rhythm, heart rate, orthostatic pulse, and blood pressure	Vision
Gait	

Intervention

Appropriate treatment for Parkinson disease includes a combination of drug therapy, usually a form of L-dopa replacement, and exercise. A consideration in designing exercise programs in Parkinson disease is the typical waxing and waning of the drug effectiveness, often termed the "on" and "off" periods. The patient may swing from a fully functional and mobile individual while "on" to one who is immobilized and "frozen," all in a matter of minutes. As the disease progresses, the "on" periods may become very short despite appropriate medication doses. See Building Block 24-5. The patient in this situation may not wish to spend this valuable "on" time exercising, opting instead for performing highly valued or necessary tasks. In these cases, the exercise program must be economical in effect given the time needed to perform it. That is, only the few, most effective and broadly useful exercises should be chosen. The patient must be made aware of the importance of the exercises in order to consider them worth the time investment. This can be accomplished in a powerful way if the patient can experience the benefit of performing the exercise. For example, a simple exercise practicing a forward weight shift in sitting using an exercise ball or a stick (Fig. 24-28) often will result in dramatic improvement in sit to stand ability (from unable to independent). Experiencing this improvement will make it more likely that the patient will attach importance to it and will therefore increase compliance.

Even so, it may be that the "on" periods are so short as to make it unreasonable to ask the patient to spend it doing exercises. In these cases the help of a family member or caregiver is crucial, in the form of a program of primarily ROM exercises. Utilizing inexpensive equipment such as exercise balls and wands or canes, and teaching positioning techniques that promote spinal extension, can allow even a frail spouse to assist in the exercises (see Fig. 24-28).

There is growing evidence that exercise can play an important role in the management of Parkinson disease. For example, the effectiveness of an exercise intervention for people in early and midstage Parkinson disease (stages 2 and 3 of Hoehn and Yahr) in improving spinal flexibility and physical performance in a sample of community-dwelling older people was described by Schenkman et al.[45] They compared people with Parkinson disease who received 10 weeks (30 sessions) of exercise instruction with a group of patients who received no exercise instruction found improved functional axial rotation, functional reach, and timed supine to stand. See Building Block 24-6.

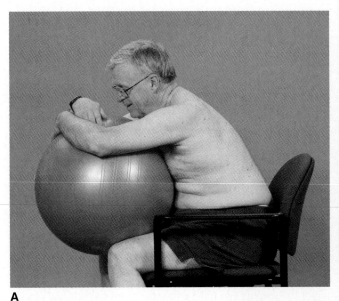

A

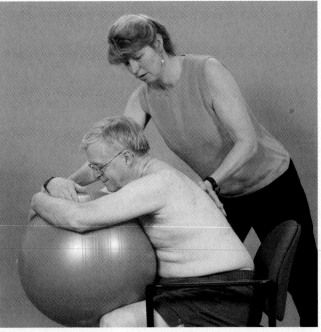

B

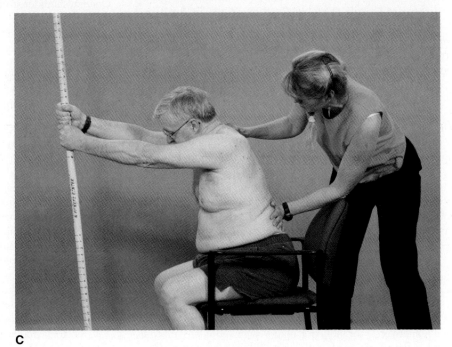

C

FIGURE 24-28. Encouraging thoracic extension coupled with shoulder elevation, using a forward weight shift. (A) With the exercise ball resting in the patient's lap and his arms resting on top of the ball, the patient shifts his weight forward, causing shoulder elevation and thoracic extension. (B) Assistance with the movement can be provided by a family member or friend. (C) A stick, dowel or broomstick can be substituted for the ball. These exercises can be especially effective in encouraging spinal extension with simultaneous hip flexion as a pre-transfer activity in patients with Parkinson disease. Be sure to instruct the patient to stabilize against lumbar flexion during this motion by activating lumbar erector spinae. The hips must have enough mobility to move into flexion without associated lumbar flexion.

BUILDING BLOCK 24-6

Consider the patient in Case No. 3, Display 24-1. The patient is a 56-year-old auto body mechanic who was diagnosed with Parkinson disease 3 years ago, and is still in the early stages. Develop a preventative home exercise program that would address impairments of decreased extensor strength, endurance, and extension mobility.

Thoracic Outlet Syndrome

TOS was first described by Peet et al.[46] as a syndrome caused by compression or stretching of the brachial plexus and/or the subclavian artery and vein as they transverse the thoracic outlet. All the symptoms attributed to TOS imply compression or stretching of the brachial plexus, subclavian artery and vein, or both areas. See Building Block 24-7.

Traditionally, the etiology of TOS has been thought to be due to mechanical, nontraumatic brachial plexus compression caused by bony, ligamentous, or muscular obstacles anywhere between the cervical spine and lower border of the axilla.

BUILDING BLOCK 24-7

Consider the patient in Case No. 5, Display 24-1. The patient is a 22-year-old policewoman with diffuse neck, shoulder, arm and hand pain and numbness in the fifth digit. These problems make it difficult to write traffic tickets. She is referred to PT with a diagnosis of Type 3 TOS. List the findings you would expect on her history and physical examination.

BUILDING BLOCK 24-8

Let us return to Laura Biden, the 22-year-old policewoman with diffuse neck, shoulder, arm, and hand pain and numbness in the fifth digit. Recall that these problems make it difficult for her to write traffic tickets. You note that she sits and stands with an exaggerated kyphosis and forward, drooping shoulders. Passively or actively holding her shoulders back and straightening her back improves her UE symptoms after several minutes. She notes she is unable to maintain this position for long, however. Given the impairments you expected to find in Laura, design an exercise program that addresses these impairments, and progress the dosage parameters from initial visit to discharge from physical therapy.

Common sites of compression include the anterior scalene, between the clavicle and first rib, and under the pectoralis minor. Several types of impairments of body structures, such as a cervical rib, a J-curve structural variation of the first rib, and a long transverse process of C7, may predispose the neurovascular bundle to compression. Fibrous bands between the cervical vertebrae and first rib may also be a source of compression. Less commonly, a tumor in the thoracic outlet may compress the neurovascular bundle.

Recently, Ide et al.[47] identified three subsets of patients with TOS; those with compression only (Type 1), those with combined compression and stretching or traction (Type 2), and those with only stretching/traction (Type 3). Swift and Nichols[48] reported that some patients with TOS had *droopy shoulder syndrome* suggesting that their symptoms resulted from stretching of the brachial plexus. Nakatsuchi et al.[49] proposed that the symptoms of TOS might be related to increased tension of the brachial plexus and surrounding vasculature due to muscular imbalance and the resultant downward traction.

Diagnosis

A careful evaluation is necessary to diagnose the subsets of TOS and to differentiate it from a spinal tumor, multiple sclerosis, cervical disk pathology, carpal tunnel syndrome, angina, tendinitis, and other brachial plexus injuries. Patients with TOS present with the following signs and symptoms: (a) persistent diffuse pain and/or paresthesia involving the neck, shoulder, arm, forearm, or wrist and hand, (b) sensory and motor loss most commonly involves the C8–T1 segmental level (because of the C8–T1 sensory and motor changes, fine coordination may be affected, and patients may complain of symptoms when holding a newspaper, combing hair, or buttoning clothes), (c) a positive Tinel sign over the brachial plexus, (d) elicitation of reproducible pain and/or paresthesia by at least one provocation maneuver[50–53] or induction and/or aggravation of symptoms upon pulling downward on the arm and their improvement or elimination upon supporting the arms upward, and (e) exclusion of diseases of the cervical spine and a peripheral neuropathy.

Treatment

Once the patient is diagnosed into the appropriate subset, treatment can be specified toward relieving compression, stretching, or both. Ultimately, the patient must be instructed in self-management techniques that treat the site and cause(s) of TOS and prevent recurrences.[54]

Treatment of Type 3 TOS

Characteristically, patients with Type 3 TOS are young, slender women with drooping shoulders and poor posture.[47] The distance between the first thoracic spinous process and coracoid process indicates the stretch placed on the neurovascular bundle.

Presumably, the greater the distance, the greater the magnitude of stretch.[47] Therefore, treatment aimed at improving the muscle performance and reducing the elongation of the upper trapezius and middle trapezius would be highly beneficial. Supportive taping of the scapula can relieve the stretch on the brachial plexus. General shoulder strengthening exercises with taping to prevent traction on the brachial plexus and posture education is recommended. Conservative treatment is often successful with this type of TOS. Thoracic outlet decompression surgery may not be effective in patients whose major symptoms are due to stretching of the brachial plexus.[55,56] See Building Block 24-8.

General Treatment Concepts for Type 1 and Type 2 TOS

- Correct posture and movement impairments relevant to neurovascular compression and/or stretching, such as correcting a depressed and anterior tilted scapula
- Taping the scapula into elevation (see Fig. 25-24) often reduces compression and alleviates symptoms until the related impairments are remedied.
- Alter sleep habits such as sleeping on the stomach with the neck extended and rotated, or arms overhead.
- Improve diaphragmatic breathing patterns. Accessory breathing patterns using scalenes and pectoralis minor may elevate the first rib and pull the scapula, and therefore the clavicle, closer to the first rib, causing compression of the fibers of the anterior scalene, within the costoclavicular space, or under the pectoralis minor.
- Correct impairments of body functions linked to posture and movement impairments, such as improving the length of the scalenes and pectoralis minor to increase the space of the thoracic outlet and mobility of the first rib; force-generating capacity or length–tension properties of underused synergists or antagonists such as the upper trapezius to alleviate a depressed scapula or lower trapezius to offset a short pectoralis minor.
- Alter movement patterns during instrumental ADLs. Examples include changing work station ergonomics, body mechanics, or sport-specific movements.
- Appropriately refer for treatment of any patients with cognitive-affective elements or exacerbating health habits that may be causing tension in the relevant musculature. For example, anxiety may cause cervical or brachial tension, or smoking may cause poor breathing habits.

LAB ACTIVITIES

1. Your patient has trouble stabilizing against rotational forces in the upper thoracic region. Develop and teach your partner three sequentially more difficult exercises to improve stabilization skills against rotational forces.
2. Refer to the Patient-Related Instruction 22-2: Diaphragmatic Breathing. Assess your partner's breathing in the supine position. Does your partner have integrated pump and bucket handle rib motions? Are they symmetric? Teach your partner proper breathing mechanics.
3. Play the role of a person with Scheuermann disease with a desk job at a visual display terminal. Teach your partner proper ergonomics at the workstation. Teach your partner to reach across the desk and into a file cabinet. Avoid exaggerating the kyphosis.
4. Design an exercise program for a patient with right thoracic and left lumbar scoliosis. Teach each activity to your partner. Can you see or feel the effect of asymmetric exercise on the spine?
5. Referring to Critical Thinking Question 4, what alternative exercise would you prescribe to your patient with osteoporosis if she had weak abdominal muscles? Teach your partner this activity. Which abdominal muscle would you expect to dominate in the exercise you instruct for someone with kyphosis?
6. Referring to Critical Thinking Question 5, what alternative exercise would you prescribe to your patient with osteoporosis if she had weak thoracic erector spinae? Teach your partner this activity. Be sure to role-play someone with moderate to marked kyphosis.

KEY POINTS

- A comprehensive examination of all patients, including the history, systems review, and tests and measures, must be performed to enable the therapist to determine the diagnosis (based on impairments, activity limitations, and participation restrictions), prognosis, and interventions.
- When considering therapeutic exercise interventions for common impairments of body functions of the thoracic region, the therapist must consider the role of the thoracic spine in the kinematic chain and how other segmental levels can affect the physiologic function of the thoracic spine.
- Although few exercises solely address the thoracic region, those that address respiration, mobility, and performance of the trunk, shoulder girdle, and cervical muscles are important for optimal thoracic function.
- Thoracic spine function can be enhanced by treating the cervical and lumbar spine, shoulder girdle, pelvic-hip complex, and foot and ankle complex.
- Therapeutic exercise intervention is thought to affect the course of non-structural scoliosis if the disorder is treated through asymmetric exercises, patient-related instruction, and movement retraining.
- There are many causes of kyphosis. If the cause is a disease such as Scheuermann's or osteoporosis, exercise intervention cannot reverse the pathology, but it may be able to retard or prevent further exaggeration of the kyphosis.
- Exercises may play an important role in the management of Parkinson disease. Exercises should be chosen carefully to maximize their effect without stealing precious "on" time from the patient.
- Diagnosis and treatment of TOS requires extensive knowledge of the anatomy and kinesiology of the cervical, thoracic, and shoulder girdle regions.

CRITICAL THINKING QUESTIONS

1. Describe how function of the foot and ankle, hip, and shoulder girdle could affect function of the thoracic spine. Provide one example for each region.
2. You have been referred an 18-year-old boy with Scheuermann disease.
   a. What two posture types would this patient probably exhibit?
   b. List the possible shortened and lengthened muscles around the trunk and pelvis for each posture type.
3. You have been referred a 16-year-old female with right thoracic and left lumbar scoliosis.
   a. What are the possible shortened and lengthened muscles in the anterior and posterior trunk and pelvic girdle?
   b. What foot and ankle alignment faults could contribute to this scoliosis?
4. Why would trunk curl exercises be contraindicated for someone with Scheuermann disease or osteoporosis?
5. Why would prone hyperextension exercises be contraindicated for someone with Scheuermann disease or osteoporosis?
6. What five exercises would you choose to teach to a patient with Parkinson disease who complains of an increasingly flexed posture, if he has only 3 hours each day when he is "on?"
7. List common postural impairments found in someone with TOS.
8. Given the list you created in No. 7, what muscles would you want to stretch versus strengthen?

REFERENCES

1. Guide to physical therapist practice. 2nd Ed. American Physical Therapy Association, 2001.
2. Lee DG. Manual Therapy for the Thorax—A Biomechanical Approach. Delta, British Columbia, Canada: DOPC, 1994.
3. Flynn TW. The Thoracic Spine and Rib Cage: Musculoskeletal Evaluation and Treatment. Boston, MA: Butterworth-Heinemann, 1996.
4. Lee DG. Biomechanics of the thorax: a clinical model of in vivo function. J Manual Manipulative Ther 1993;1:13.
5. Feise RJ, Menke JM. Functional rating index–A new valid and reliable instrument to measure the magnitude of clinical change in spinal conditions. Spine 2001;26:85–86.
6. Fairbank JC, Couper J, Davies JB, O'Brien JP. The Oswestry low back pain disability questionnaire. Physiotherapy 1988;66:271–273.
7. Roland M, Morris R. A study of the natural history of back pain. Part I: Development of a reliable and sensitive measure of disability in low back pain. Spine 1983;8:141–144.

8. Magee DJ, ed. Orthopedic Physical Assessment. Philadelphia, PA: W.B. Saunders Co., 2002.

9. Kendall FP, McCreary EK, Provance PG. Muscles Testing and Function. Baltimore, MD: Williams & Wilkins, 1993.

10. Panjabi M. The stabilizing system of the spine. Part I Function, dysfunction, adaptation, and enhancement. J Spinal Disord 1992;5:383–389.

11. Daneels LA, Vanderstraeten GG, Cambier DC, et al. A functional subdivision of hip, abdominal and back muscles during asymmetric lifting. Spine 2001;26:E114–E121.

12. Goel V, Kong W, Han J, et al. A combined finite element and optimization investigation of lumbar spine mechanics with and without muscles. Spine 1993;18:1531–1541.

13. Wilke H, Wolf S, Claes L, et al. Stability increase of the lumbar spine with different muscle groups. A biomechanical in vitro study. Spine 1995;20:192–198.

14. Daneels L, Vanderstracten G, Cambier D, et al. SSE Clinical Science Award 2000: computed tomography imaging of trunk muscles in chronic low back pain patients and healthy control subjects. Eur Spine J 2000;9:266–272.

15. Gibbons L, Videman T, Battié M. Isokinetic and psychophysical lifting strength, static back muscle endurance, and magnetic resonance imaging of the paraspinal muscles as predictors of low back pain in men. Scand J Rehabil Med 1997;29:187–191.

16. Kader D, Wardlaw D, Smith F. Correlation between the MRI changes in the lumbar mustifidus muscles and leg pain. Clin Radiol 2000;55:145–149.

17. Hides JA, Stokes MJ, Saide M, et al. Evidence of lumbar multifidus muscle wasting ipsilateral to symptoms in patients with acute/subacute low back pain. Spine 1994;19:165–172.

18. Kawaguchi Y, Matsui H, Tsui H. Back muscle injury after posterior lumbar surgery. Spine 1994;19:2598–2602.

19. Sihvonen T, Herno A, Paljarvi L, Airaksinen O, Partanen J, Tapaninahos A. Local denervation of paraspinal muscles in postoperative failed back syndrome. Spine 1993;18:575–581.

20. Hides J, Richardson C, Jull G. Multifidus recovery is not automatic following resolution of acute first episode of low back pain. Spine 1996;21:2763–2769.

21. Daneels LA, Vanderstraeten GG, Cambier DC, et al. Effects of three different training modalities on the cross sectional area of the lumbar multifidus muscle in patients with chronic low back pain. Br J Sports Med 2001;35:186–191.

22. Carpenter D, Nelson B. Low back strengthening for the prevention and treatment of low back pain. Med Sci Sports Exerc 1999;31:18–24.

23. Jull G, Richardson C. Rehabilitation of active stabilization of the lumbar spine. In: Twomey LT, Taylor JR, eds. Physical therapy of the low back. 2nd Ed. New York, NY: Churchill-Livingstone, 1994:251–273.

24. Winstein C. Knowledge of results and motor learning–Implications for physical therapy. Phys Ther 1991;71:140–149.

25. Schenkman M, Morey M, Kuchibhatla M. Spinal-flexibility-plus-aerobic versus aerobic-only training: effect of a randomized clinical trial on function in at-risk older adults. J Gerontol A Biol Sci Med Sci 1999;54:M335–M342.

26. Somhegyi A, Ratko I, Gomor B. Effect of spinal exercises on spinal parameters in Scheuermann disease. Orv Hetil 1993;20:401–403.

27. Roach. Adolescent idiopathic scoliosis. Orthop Clin North Am 1999;30:353–365, vii–viii.

28. Soucacos PN, Zacharis K, Soultanis K, et al. Risk factors for idiopathic scoliosis: review of a 6-year prospective study. Orthopedics 2000;23:833–838.

29. Blackman R, O'Neal K, Picetti G, Estep M. Scoliosis treatment. Oakland, CA: Children's Hospital, Kaiser Permanente Hospital, 1998.

30. American Academy of Orthopedic Surgeons Staff. Instructional Course Lectures. St. Louis, Missouri: CV Mosby, 1985;34:103–104.

31. Mooney, Brigham. The role of measured resistance exercises in adolescent scoliosis. Orthopedics 2003;26:167–171; discussion 171.

32. Hales, et al., Treatment of adult lumbar scoliosis with axial spinal unloading using the LTX3000 Lumbar Rehabilitation System. Spine 2002;27:E71–E79.

33. Negrini A, Versini N, Parzini S, et al. Role of physical exercise in the treatment of mild idiopathic adolescent scoliosis: review of the literature. Europa Medicophysica 2001;37: 181–190.

34. Athanasopoulos S, Paxinos T, Tsafantakis E, et al. The effect of aerobic training in girls with idiopathic scoliosis. Scand J Med Sci Sports 1999;9:36–40.

35. Ernst E. Exercise for female osteoporosis. A systematic review of randomized clinical trials. Sports Med 1998;25:359–368.

36. Old JL, Calvert M. Vertebral compression fractures in the elderly. Am Fam Phys 2004;69:111–116.

37. Gill TM, Allore H, Guo Z. The Deleterious Effects of Bed Rest Among Community-Living Older Persons. J Gerontol A Biol Sci Med Sci 2004;59(7):M755–M761.

38. Convertino VA, Bloomfield SA, Greenleaf JE. An overview of the issues: physiological effects of bed rest and restricted physical activity. [Miscellaneous Article]. Med Sci Sports Exerc 1997;29(2):187–190.

39. Reid IR. The role of calcium and vitamin D in the prevention of osteoporosis. Endocrin Metab Clin North Am 1998;27:389–398.

40. Ullom-Minnich P. Prevention of osteoporosis and fractures. Am Fam Physician 1999;60:194–202.

41. Maricic M, Adachi JD, Sarkar S, et al. Early effects of raloxifene on clinical vertebral fractures at 12 months in postmenopausal wimen with osteoporosis. Arch Intern Med 2002;162:1140–1143.

42. Black DM, Thompson DE, Bauer DC, et al. Fracture risk reduction with alendronate in women with osteoposoris: the Fracture Intervention Trial. FIT Research Group. J Clin Endocrinol Metab 2000;85:4118–4124.

43. Sinaki M, Itoi E, Wahner HW, et al. Stronger back muscles reduce the incidence of vertebral fractures: a prospective 10 year follow-up of postmenopausal women. Bone 2002;30:836–841.

44. American Geriatrics Society, British Geriatrics Society, and American Academy of Orthopedic Surgeons Panel on Falls Prevention. Guideline for the prevention of falls in older persons. J Am Geriatr Soc 2001;49:664–672.

45. Schenkman M, Cutson TM, Kuchibhatla M, et al. Exercise to improve spinal flexibility and function for people with Parkinson's disease: a randomized, controlled trial. J Am Geriatr Soc 1998;46:1207–1216.

46. Peet RM, Henriksen JD, Anderson TP, et al. Thoracic outlet syndrome: evaluation of a therapeutic exercise program. Mayo Clin Proc 1956;31:281–287.

47. Ide J, Katoka Y, Yamaga M, et al. Compression and stretching of the brachial plexus in thoracic outlet syndrome: correlation between neuroadiographic findings and symptoms and signs produced by provocation manoeuvres. J hand Surg 2003;3:218–223.

48. Swift TR, Nichols FT. The droopy shoulder syndrome. Neurology 1984;34: 212–215.

49. Nakatsuchi Y, Saitoh S, Hosaka M, et al. Conservative treatment of thoracic outlet syndrome using an orthosis. J Hand Surg 1995;20B:34–39.

50. Adson AW. Surgical treatment for symptoms produced by cervical ribs and the scalenus anticus muscle. Surgery. Gynecol Obstet 1947;85:687–700.

51. Eden KC. The vascular complications of cervical ribs and first thoracic rib abnormalities. Br J Surg 1939;27:111–139.

52. Roos DB. New concepts of thoracic outlet syndrome that explain etiology, symptoms, diagnosis, and treatment. Vascular Surg 1979;13:313–320.

53. Wright IS. The neurovascular syndrome produced by hyperabduction of the arms. Am Heart J 1945;29:1–19.

54. Edgelow PI. Neurovascular consequences of cummulative trauma disorders affecting thoracic outlet: a patient centered approach. In: Donatelli RA, ed. Physical Therapy of the Shoulder. 3rd ed. New York: Churchill Livingstone; 1997.

55. Ide J, Ide M, Yamaga M. Longterm results of thoracic outlet decompression. Neuro-orthopedics 1994;16:59–68.

56. Tagaki K, Yamaga M, Morisawa K, et al. Management of thoracic outlet syndrome. Arch Orthop Trauma Surg 1987;106:78–81.

RECOMMENDED READINGS

Ascani E, Bartolozzi P. Natural history of untreated idiopathic scoliosis after skeletal maturity. Spine 1986;11:784–789.

Brown C, Deffer P. The natural history of thoracic disc herniation. Spine 1992;17(Suppl 6):S97–S102.

Cantu R, Grodin A. Myofascial Manipulation Theory and Clinical Application. Gaithersburg, MD: Aspen Publishers, 1992.

Donatelli R, Wooden M. Orthopaedic Physical Therapy. New York, NY: Churchill Livingstone, 1989.

Gould J, Davies G. Orthopedic and Sports Physical Therapy. St. Louis, MO: CV Mosby, 1985.

Gross J, Fetto J, Rosen E. Musculoskeletal Examination. Cambridge, MA: Blackwell Science, 1996.

Irwin S, Tecklin J. Cardiopulmonary Physical Therapy. 3rd Ed. St. Louis, MO: Mosby, 1995.

Malone T, McPoil T, Nitz A. Orthopedic and Sports Physical Therapy. 3rd Ed. St. Louis: Mosby–Year Book, 1997.

Mitchell FL, Moran PS, Pruzzo NA. An Evaluation and Treatment Manual of Osteopathic Muscle Energy Procedures. Valley Park, MO: Mitchell, Moran, and Pruzzo, 1979.

Pratt N. Clinical Musculoskeletal Anatomy. Philadelphia, PA: JB Lippincott, 1991.

Richardson J, Iglarsh ZA. Clinical Orthopaedic Physical Therapy. Philadelphia, PA: WB Saunders, 1994.

Winkel D. Diagnosis and Treatment of the Spine. Gaithersburg, MD: Aspen Publishers, 1996.

chapter 25

The Shoulder Girdle

CARRIE M. HALL

The shoulder girdle functions with the arm, forearm, wrist, and hand in a kinetic chain with the trunk and lower extremity. Therefore, dysfunction of the shoulder girdle can affect function of related regions, and conversely dysfunction of related regions can affect function of the shoulder girdle. For example, faulty movement patterns and associated impairments of the shoulder girdle can affect function of the cervical spine because of shared musculature (i.e., levator scapula and upper trapezius). In addition, faulty movement patterns and associated impairments of the spine and pelvis can affect function of the shoulder girdle. For example, asymmetric spine and pelvis alignment can contribute to faults in shoulder girdle alignment and subsequent movement patterns.

This chapter will first present information related to anatomy, kinesiology, and evaluation of the shoulder girdle. This information will set the stage for the sections on therapeutic exercise intervention for common impairments of body structures and functions. As with all other chapters in this book, the goal is not to provide a list of exercises for shoulder girdle impairments and conditions, but rather to provide the necessary information to become a critical thinker and perceptive problem solver such that you will be prepared with the knowledge necessary to develop an efficient and effective exercise prescription for any case involving the shoulder girdle.

REVIEW OF ANATOMY AND KINESIOLOGY

The anatomy and kinesiology of the shoulder girdle is one of the most complex regions of the body. The combined coordinated movements of the three distinct articulations and the involved muscles and periarticular structures allow the arm and hand to be positioned in space for a variety of functions. The result is a range of motion (ROM) that exceeds that of any other joint complex in the body.

The shoulder girdle is composed of the sternoclavicular (SC), acromioclavicular (AC), and glenohumeral (GH) joints. Scapulothoracic (ST) motion occurs through combined SC and AC joint motions.[1]

Each of these joints function interdependently and in synchrony to provide movement of the upper extremity.
The importance of understanding the complexity of the anatomy and kinesiology of the shoulder girdle as it pertains to therapeutic exercise prescription cannot be underestimated. For that reason, a thorough review can be found on the Web site.

EXAMINATION AND EVALUATION

More than 50 physical diagnostic tests have been described for the shoulder girdle.[1-5] Diagnosis of dysfunction in the shoulder girdle is challenging because of the complex anatomy and kinesiology and interrelationships of the AC, SC, and GH joints and the cervicothoracic spine. Furthermore, functions of the elbow, forearm, wrist, and hand are related to the function of the shoulder girdle as part of the upper quarter kinetic chain. Dysfunction in one segment of the chain affects the function of other segments.

A clinical example of the close relationship between joints in the upper quarter is an individual presenting with reduced forearm pronation ROM. The compensation for this restriction during the activities of daily living (ADLs) requiring forearm pronation may be medial rotation and abduction of the GH joint to orient the palm of the hand downward. If this pattern is performed repetitively, particularly in elevated arm positions biased toward the frontal plane, impingement of the subacromial structures of the shoulder may develop.

The descriptive examination and evaluation information discussed in this section is not intended to be comprehensive or reflect any specific philosophical approach. It is presented in alphabetical order and should simply serve as a review of pertinent tests performed in shoulder girdle examinations.

Patient/Client History

In addition to the general data collected from a patient/client history as defined in Chapter 2, Display 25-1 illustrates a sampler of information that is important to obtain from a patient with impairment, activity limitation or participation restriction involving the shoulder girdle complex.

Clearing Examinations

Routine cervicothoracic spine screening should be included during the examination of any patient with shoulder girdle signs and symptoms. Dysfunction of the cervicothoracic region may contribute to shoulder dysfunction.[6-8] Additionally, the elbow-wrist-hand complex should be excluded as a source of pain, although it rarely refers pain proximally to the shoulder.

Visceral referral of symptoms should be considered in cases refractory to physical therapy intervention. Appendix 1 lists specific visceral pain referral patterns into the shoulder girdle. A thorough health history can assist in identifying signs that may designate visceral sources of symptoms.

DISPLAY 25-1
Functional Index Questionnaire

FUNCTIONAL INDEX

Part 1:

Answer all five sections in Part 1. Choose the one answer in each section that best describes your condition.

Walking
- ❑ Pain does not prevent me walking any distance.
- ❑ Pain prevents me walking more than 1 mi.
- ❑ Pain prevents me walking more than 1/2 mi.
- ❑ Pain prevents me walking more than 1/4 mi.
- ❑ I can only walk using a stick or crutches.
- ❑ I am in bed most of the time and have to crawl to the toilet.

Work
(Applies to work in home and outside)
- ❑ I can do as much work as I want to.
- ❑ I can only do my usual work, but no more.
- ❑ I can do most of my usual work, but no more.
- ❑ I cannot do my usual work.
- ❑ I can hardly do any work at all (only light duty).
- ❑ I cannot do any work at all.

Personal Care
(Washing, dressing, etc.)
- ❑ I can manage all personal care without symptoms.
- ❑ I can manage all personal care with some increased symptoms.
- ❑ Personal care requires slow, concise movements due to increased symptoms.
- ❑ I need help to manage some personal care.
- ❑ I need help to manage all personal care.
- ❑ I cannot manage any personal care.

Sleeping
- ❑ I have no trouble sleeping.
- ❑ My sleep is mildly disturbed (<1 hour sleepless).
- ❑ My sleep is mildly disturbed (1 to 2 hours sleepless).
- ❑ My sleep is moderately disturbed (2 to 3 hours sleepless).
- ❑ My sleep is greatly disturbed (3 to 5 hours sleepless).
- ❑ My sleep is completely disturbed (5 to 7 hours sleepless).

Recreation/Sports
(Indicate sport if appropriate_____)
- ❑ I am able to engage in all my recreational/sports activities without increased symptoms.
- ❑ I am able to engage in all my recreational/sports activities with some increased symptoms.
- ❑ I am able to engage in most, but not all of my usual recreational/sports activities because of increased symptoms.
- ❑ I am able to engage in a few of my usual recreational/sports activities because of my increased symptoms.

- ❑ I can hardly do any recreational/sports activities because of increased symptoms.
- ❑ I cannot do any recreational/sports activities at all.

Acuity
(Answer on initial visit.)
- ❑ How many days ago did onset/injury occur? _____days

Part II:
Choose the one answer that best describes your condition in the sections designated by your therapist.

UPPER EXTREMITY

Carrying
- ❑ I can carry heavy loads without increased symptoms.
- ❑ I can carry heavy loads with some increased symptoms.
- ❑ I cannot carry heavy loads overhead, but I can manage if they are positioned close to my trunk.
- ❑ I cannot carry heavy loads, but I can manage light to medium loads if they are positioned close to my trunk.
- ❑ I can carry very light weights with some increased symptoms.
- ❑ I cannot lift or carry anything at all.

Dressing
- ❑ I can put on a shirt or blouse without symptoms.
- ❑ I can put on a shirt or blouse with some increased symptoms.
- ❑ It is painful to put on a shirt or blouse and I am slow and careful.
- ❑ I need some help but I manage most of my shirt or blouse dressing.
- ❑ I need help in most aspects of putting on my shirt or blouse.
- ❑ I cannot put on a shirt or blouse at all.

Reaching
- ❑ I can reach to a high shelf to place an empty cup without increased symptoms.
- ❑ I can reach to a high shelf to place an empty cup with some increased symptoms.
- ❑ I can reach to a high shelf to place an empty cup with a moderate increase in symptoms.
- ❑ I cannot reach to a high shelf to place an empty cup, but I can reach up to a lower shelf without increased symptoms.
- ❑ I cannot reach up to a lower shelf without increased symptoms, but I can reach counter height to place an empty cup.
- ❑ I cannot reach my hand above waist level without increased symptoms.

Adapted from Therapeutic Associates Outcomes System, Therapeutic Associates, Inc., Sherman Oaks, CA, with permission.

Motor Function (Motor Control and Motor Learning)

Visual observation and palpation of the 3D motions of the scapula on the thorax and GH joints can be augmented by surface electromyography (EMG). The use of surface EMG can assist in determining patterns and timing of recruitment of the trapezius, serratus, deltoid, and infraspinatus muscles. The infraspinatus is the only rotator cuff muscle that can be examined with palpation or surface EMG. Surface EMG can be useful in determining faulty motor control patterns responsible for many shoulder diagnoses. This type of qualitative testing is important, because active ROM may be within normal limits (WNLs) but have abnormal associated kinematics contributing to shoulder dysfunction.

Muscle Performance

Impaired muscle performance can result from numerous causes/sources (refer to Chapter 5). Various tests can determine the

DISPLAY 25-2
Shoulder Girdle Muscles to Include in Manual Muscle Testing*

- Upper, middle, and posterior deltoid
- Glenohumeral lateral rotators
- Glenohumeral medial rotators (with isolation of subscapularis)
- All portions of the trapezius
- Serratus anterior
- Rhomboids and levator scapula
- Pectoralis major
- Latissimus dorsi

The reader is referred to the appropriate reference for specific MMT techniques.

TABLE 25-1 **Diagnosis Based on Resistive Tests**

FINDING OF RESISTIVE TEST	LESION
Strong and painless	Normal
Strong and painful	Minor muscle lesion
	Minor tendon lesion
Weak and painful	Gross macrotraumatic lesion such as fracture
	Partial rupture of muscle or tendon
Weak and painless	Muscle or tendon rupture
	Neurologic dysfunction

presence and potential cause or source of impaired muscle performance.

Specific manual muscle testing (MMT) provides information regarding the amount of force or torque that a musculotendinous unit can generate. Display 25-2 provides a list of muscles that should be included in MMT of the shoulder girdle. MMT is traditionally done, but testing of muscle performance can be performed with a dynamometer, and both types of testing can be performed in conjunction with surface EMG when appropriate. Texts on manual testing for specific protocols should be consulted.[9,10]

Positional strength testing is a specialized form of MMT that tests the muscle at a specific length to obtain information regarding the length-tension properties of the muscle (see Chapter 5). Positional strength testing is particularly useful in determining whether a muscle is weak because of altered length-tension properties. If a muscle is lengthened, it tests weak in the short range but strong in a slightly more lengthened range. If a muscle is weak because of other causes, it tests weak throughout the range. Sahrmann has provided more information on positional strength testing of muscles in the shoulder girdle.[11]

Selective tissue tension tests combine active and passive ROM with resisted tests of muscles about the shoulder girdle.[12] The sum total of the results of each test assists the practitioner in determining which tissue is the probable source of the shoulder condition.[13,14] Many clinicians use Cyriax's selective tissue tension model for the diagnosis of soft-tissue lesions of the shoulder.[15] The Cyriax model has been shown to be a reliable scheme for assessing patients with shoulder pain.[16] If selective tissue tension test results are positive for a contractile lesion, the resisted test can further diagnose the severity of the lesion. Table 25-1 highlights diagnostic findings of resisted tests.

Pain

Evaluation of pain is done throughout the examination process. Palpation of suspected tissues is used to evaluate tissue tension, temperature, swelling, and provocation of pain.[17] Cyriax[12] and Maitland[18] advocate use of the sequence of pain and resistance during passive movement testing to establish the irritability level of a tissue. This information can guide the aggressiveness with which stretching and mobilization techniques are performed.

Because a subjective report of the pain associated with specific activities can help in the assessment, the clinician should question the patient about which activities are associated with pain. Pain often is latent (i.e., experienced after the activity), which makes it difficult to relate a cause or source. The range of pain, from the least pain to the worst pain experienced, should be examined through some accepted method of pain assessment (e.g., visual analog scale).[19]

The clinician must attempt to determine a mechanical cause of the pain during the course of the examination. This is often quite challenging but necessary to ensure full recovery and prevention of recurrences. For example, although the supraspinatus tendon can be diagnosed as the source of pain through selective tissue tension testing and palpation, the cause of the pain may be insufficient scapular posterior tilt.[20] Insufficient posterior tilt can lead to pain because of mechanical impingement of the supraspinatus under the acromion process. Local treatment of the supraspinatus may decrease the pain in the short term. However, treatment of the faulty postures and movement impairment in addition to related intrinsic and extrinsic physiological impairments is essential to manage the condition long term.

Peripheral Nerve Integrity

Results of thoracic outlet,[21] neural tissue provocation testing,[22] peripheral nerve integrity tests, and resisted tests diagnose a pattern of muscle weakness due to peripheral nerve injury. Tests of shoulder girdle musculature, combined with elbow, forearm, wrist, and hand musculature, can indicate whether a nerve deficit is at the level of the cervical spine (i.e., nerve root) or is a peripheral nerve lesion. The pattern of weakness indicates peripheral or nerve root involvement or possibly forms of myopathy (i.e., fascioscapulohumeral muscular dystrophy).

Posture

Atypical positions of the scapula on the thorax, GH joint, and cervicothoracic spine have been noted in patients with shoulder girdle dysfunction.[6,7,8,23,24] Although there is inconsistent clinical reliability and validity with tests to measure scapula and humerus resting position,[25] there is research supporting the relationship between the incidence of pain in the shoulder girdle and aberrant scapula and humerus posture.[6,7]

Therefore, the clinician should observe and document the following:

- Total body alignment—particularly related to symmetry in limb lengths
- Head position, cervical, thoracic, and lumbar spine alignment
- Pelvic position about all three planes
- Analysis of alignment of the scapula, clavicle, and humerus about all three planes of motion

Range of Motion, Muscle Length, Joint Mobility, and Joint Integrity

Elements to include in testing ROM, muscle length, joint mobility, and joint integrity of the shoulder girdle are listed in Display 25-3.

Work (Job/School/Play), Community, and Leisure Integration or Reintegration (Including Instrumental ADLs)

Functional testing, whether in the form of performance testing or subjective grading, should be included in the examination. One form of subjective grading that can be time efficient is a health-related quality of life scale. The Shoulder Pain and Disability Index (SPADI)[37,38] is a self-administered questionnaire that consists of two dimensions, one for pain and the other for functional activities, and requires 5 to 10 minutes for a patient to complete. Display 25-5 lists the SPADI items. Roach et al.[37] and Williams et al.[38] have explained the administration of this test.

THERAPEUTIC EXERCISE INTERVENTIONS FOR COMMON IMPAIRMENTS OF BODY STRUCTURES AND FUNCTIONS

After a thorough examination and evaluation of the shoulder girdle, the clinician should have a good understanding of the

---

DISPLAY 25-4
Shoulder Girdle Muscles Prone to Adaptive Length Changes

Adaptive Shortening	Adaptive Lengthening
Rhomboid major and minor	Middle trapezius
Levator scapula	Lower trapezius
Upper trapezius	Upper trapezius
Subscapularis	Subscapularis
Teres major	Serratus anterior
Latissimus dorsi	
Pectoralis major and minor	
Long head of biceps	
GH lateral rotators	

---

activity limitations and participation restrictions affecting the patient as well as the related body function and structure impairments. A diagnosis and prognosis are formulated, and an intervention is planned. After it is determined which body function impairments should be treated to restore activity and participation level, a plan of care must be developed to treat the appropriate impairments and limitations/restrictions. Therapeutic exercise intervention is vital in the restoration of shoulder girdle function in order to restore the precise coordinated muscular force couples acting on the three integrated joints in the shoulder girdle complex. The following sections provide information about therapeutic exercise interventions for common impairments of body structures and functions. Pain is presented as the first impairment because of the importance of understanding the underlying impairments contributing to and/or causing pain.

Pain

Differential diagnosis of pain in the upper quarter is difficult in part because of the interdependence in the anatomy of the shoulder, elbow, wrist, hand, and cervicothoracic spine. Pain stemming from tissues in the shoulder girdle may be experienced locally or referred distally down the arm as far as the wrist and hand.[39] Confounding the diagnosis of the source of

---

DISPLAY 25-3
Elements to Include in Testing ROM, Muscle Length, Joint Mobility, and Joint Integrity of the Shoulder Girdle

- Active and passive osteokinetic ROM of the ST, GH, and cervicothoracic spine joints
- Passive arthrokinematic mobility tests of the SC, AC, GH, ST joints, and cervicothoracic spine
- Capsuloligamentous integrity[26–30]
- Glenoid labrum integrity tests[31–34]
- Rotator cuff integrity[33,34]
- Subacromial impingement tests[35,36]
- Muscle length testing for scapulohumeral, axioscapular, and axiohumeral muscle groups. Examples of muscles that fall into each category are summarized in Display 25-4. Sahrmann[11] and Kendall et al.[9] have described the appropriate muscle length testing procedures.
- Functional movements should be examined, including reaching behind the back, touching the back of the head and neck, and reaching across to the opposite shoulder.

DISPLAY 25-5
Shoulder Pain and Disability Index

Pain dimension: How severe is your pain?

1. At its worst?
2. When lying on the involved side?
3. Reaching for something on a high shelf?
4. Touching the back of your neck?
5. Pushing with the involved arm?

Disability dimension: How much difficulty do you have?

1. Washing your hair?
2. Washing your back?
3. Putting on an undershirt or pullover sweater?
4. Putting on a shirt that buttons down the front?
5. Putting on your pants?
6. Placing an object on a high shelf?
7. Carrying a heavy object (e.g., 10 lb)?
8. Removing something from your back pocket?

shoulder pain is the fact that the shoulder girdle is a common region for referral from sites extrinsic to the shoulder girdle such as the cervicothoracic spine[40,41] and nonmusculoskeletal sources, such as the heart and diaphragm (see Appendix 1).[42]

If the *source* of the pain is determined to be located in the shoulder girdle, treatment may involve a combination of interventions, including manual therapy, physical agents or electrotherapeutic modalities, and therapeutic exercise aimed at the shoulder girdle region. A clinical example can illustrate the use and interaction of physical therapy interventions. Display 25-6 outlines hypothetical examination and evaluation findings of a person diagnosed with rotator cuff tendinopathy. Treatment of the source of the pain may include the following interventions:

- Transverse friction massage to the affected rotator cuff tenoperiosteal or musculotendinous junctions to assist in the formation of a strong and mobile scar[12]
- Active exercise, electrical stimulation in mid range, or both to broaden the muscle (serving a similar purpose to that of transverse friction massage)[12]
- Physical agents (e.g., cryotherapy) or electrotherapeutic modalities (e.g., phonophoresis, ultrasound) used to treat the inflammatory process[43]

Treatment isolated to the *source* of the pain can assist in the healing process and provide relief of discomforting the short term, but will not be able to manage the condition long term, particularly if the cause of the pain is repetitive microtrauma from faulty postures or movement patterns. The clinician must address the underlying *cause* of the pain for long-term resolution of the condition.

It has been shown that there is an association between faulty scapulohumeral kinematics and rotator cuff disease.[11,48,49] Treating the *cause* of the rotator cuff impingement requires eliminating or modifying the sustained postures and repetitive movement patterns believed to contribute to or perpetuate the faulty kinematics. This training is far more specific than the basic activity modification described under treatment of the *source* of the pain. Altering sustained postures and repetitive movement patterns usually requires prior therapeutic exercise intervention focused on muscle performance, joint mobility, and sift tissue extensibility. Improved physiologic capabilities provide a better foundation for precise posture and movement control. For example, lower trapezius and serratus anterior muscles with an MMT grade of 3–/5 cannot fully participate in a muscular force couple to upwardly rotate, posterior tilt, and laterally rotate the scapula during arm elevation against gravity. Therapeutic exercise aimed at improving muscle performance of the upward rotators until they achieve a minimal MMT grade of 3 to 3+/5 is a prerequisite for retraining the coordinated muscular force couples required for functional movement patterns against gravity. Posture and movement education must be initiated as soon as possible, but premature introduction of functional activities can perpetuate the faulty postures and movement patterns causing the pain and inflammation.

In the case presented in Display 25-6, the following impairments must be addressed to promote optimal posture and movement patterns:

- Muscle performance of the rotator cuff (see Self-Management 25-1: Facelying Shoulder Rotation, scapular

upward rotators (see Self-Management 25-2: Facelying Arm Lifts, and Self-Management 25-3: Serratus Anterior Progression)
- Muscle extensibility of the pectoralis minor (Fig. 25-1), rhomboids and levator scapula (Fig. 25-2), and GH lateral rotators (see Self-Management 25-4: Lateral Rotator and Posterior Capsule Stretch)
- Joint mobility of the AC, SC, GH joints, and the cervicothoracic junction, first rib articulations at T1 and the manubrium, and all thoracic vertebrae.

Often, altered length-tension properties of the scapular upward rotators exist due to prolonged posture habits (i.e., thoracic kyphosis leading to scapular tilt and lengthening of the serratus anterior and lower trapezius), the exercises prescribed must be initiated at relatively low levels of intensity. For example, the patient should begin with level I of the lower trapezius (see Self-Management 25-2) and serratus anterior progressions (see Self-Management 25-3). Even so, improving the muscle performance of the lower trapezius, serratus anterior, and rotator cuff may not translate directly into improved function. Transitional exercises should be prescribed to train the muscle to function with the appropriate magnitude and timing during ADLs or instrumental ADLs. Examples of transitional exercises are shown in Figure 25-3 (see Building Block 25-1).

Ineffective treatment of pain may result from failing to determine that the source of symptoms is not within the shoulder girdle. Even if the source is determined to come from an associated musculoskeletal region, ineffective treatment may nonetheless result from failing to recognize that the shoulder girdle may be contributing to the cycle of pain and dysfunction. For example, a patient may be diagnosed with radicular pain originating from an inflamed C5–6 nerve root caused by a protruding nucleus pulposus at that level. However, it may be determined that faulty postures and movements of the shoulder girdle are contributing to faulty postures and movements of the cervical spine because of the shared musculature and joint articulations.[50] An example is a person with a depressed scapula at rest (Fig. 25-4) and insufficient elevation of the scapula during movement, particularly during the first half of the movement. This person may experience excessive tension on the cervical spine because of overstretching of the upper trapezius at rest and levator scapula during upward scapula rotation.[51] This excessive tension may compromise normal movement of the cervical spine and restrict cervical rotation with the arms at the side or simultaneously with movement of the shoulder girdle (e.g., driving a car and needing to look behind the shoulder). In this case, treating the cervical spine in isolation may not result in full functional recovery.[52] However, in this case, adding treatment of the posture and movement patterns of the shoulder girdle and the related shoulder impairments to the plan of care would be critical to treating symptoms originating in the cervical spine (see Building Block 25-2).

Range of Motion and Joint Mobility Impairments

This category of impairments covers the scope of osteokinematic and arthrokinematic mobility from excessive ROM or joint hypermobility to reduced ROM or joint hypomobility.

DISPLAY 25-6
Clinical Case of Rotator Cuff Impingement (Primary Rotator Cuff Disorder)

Examination and Evaluation

History
A 35-year-old, right-handed man complains of right shoulder pain. His occupation requires him to sit at a visual display terminal (VDT) 8 to 10 hours each day, 5 days each week. He also engages in cross-country skiing, climbing, and kayaking. A primary activity limitation includes inability to sleep on his right shoulder due to pain at night that awakens him briefly two to three times each week. His participation restrictions include inability to participate in any recreational activity using his right arm overhead. Work is not disrupted at this time, although he does experience a fatiguing discomfort between his shoulder blades while working at the computer about two-thirds into his workday.

Postural Alignment
Moderate forward head, moderate abducted, anterior tilted, and downwardly rotated scapulae, with the right scapula slightly depressed, bilateral humerus in moderate abduction (R > L), and moderate thoracic kyphosis

Cervical Clearing Examination
Slight stiffness in cervical rotation to the right, otherwise negative for shoulder girdle signs or symptoms

Passive ROM
Elevation in the plane of the scapula (see Fig. 25-8 Web site)—150 degrees
Lateral rotation at 90 degrees of abduction—90 degrees
Medial rotation at 90 degrees of abduction—40 degrees
Elbow, forearm, wrist, hand—WNL

Active ROM
Active arm elevation in flexion and abduction—WNL
Total scapular upward rotation is 45 degrees.
GH lateral rotation with the arm adducted to the side is 60 degrees, but it improves to 80 degrees when the scapula is positioned in neutral instead of the patient's abducted rest position.

Scapulohumeral Rhythm
Faulty scapulohumeral rhythm is present. The scapula is slow to elevate from the initial depressed position and is still depressed relative to the left at 90-degree flexion, but excessively elevates in the last half of flexion. In addition, the scapula fails to fully upwardly rotate and is only rotated upward to 10 degrees at 90 degrees of flexion. The patient experiences pain from 90 degrees to end range. Pain is reduced with assisted elevation and upward rotation of the scapula.

Muscle Length
Moderate shortness in the GH lateral rotators and rhomboids and lengthened right upper trapezius and middle trapezius.

Joint Mobility
Hypomobile GH posterior and inferior glide, ST upward rotation, and AC joint anteroposterior glide

Muscle Performance (tests performed on right only)
GH lateral rotators: 3+/5 (pain)
GH abductors: 4−/5 (pain)
Supraspinatus (full can test)[44]: 3+/5 (pain)
Subscapularis (lift-off position)[13] 3+/5
Upper trapezius: 3+/5
Middle trapezius: 3+/5
Lower trapezius: 3+/5
Serratus anterior: 3+/5

Rhomboids/levator scapula: 5/5
Biceps: 4−/5
Triceps: 5/5

Resisted Tests
General abduction, outer-range lateral rotation, and supraspinatus are weak and painful.

Motor Control
Surface EMG analysis demonstrates latent upper trapezius and serratus anterior activity, when compared to the uninjured side, during scaption.

Palpation
Tenderness was elicited over the tenoperiosteal and musculotendinous junction of the supraspinatus and AC joint.

Special Tests
Neer impingement sign[45] and Hawkins impingement tests[44] are positive
Jobe apprehension test[46] is negative
Negative dropping and hornblower's signs[34]
Sulcus sign[47] is negative

Assessment
This patient appears to have primary rotator cuff disorder. His body function impairments include:

- Altered mobility in periarticular soft tissues limiting posterior and inferior glide of the GH joint
- Reduced muscular extensibility in GH lateral rotators, further contributing to limited GH posterior glide
- Reduced muscular extensibility in scapular downward rotators, limiting scapular upward rotation
- Lengthened scapular elevator and upward rotator group, affecting length-tension properties of muscles participating in the upward rotator force couple
- Decreased muscle performance of the elevator or upward rotator, affecting the muscle's participation in the active force couples
- Altered motor control patterns in scapular rotators
- Positive signs of injury to subacromial tissue, particularly supraspinatus (i.e., positive impingement sign, weak and painful resisted tests, palpation).

Summary of Pathomechanics
This patient is vulnerable to developing impairments that contribute to impingement syndrome. The prolonged faulty posture he sustains during an 8- to 10-hour workday can lead to altered base, modulator, and biomechanical elements of the movement system. The faulty joint alignment (biomechanical), can contribute to GH impingement because of the altered relationship between the ST and GH joints. Prolonged faulty postures can lead to altered muscle length-tension properties (base), which can contribute to altered movement and recruitment patterns (biomechanical and modulator). For example, if the scapula is chronically abducted, downwardly rotated, depressed, and anteriorly tilted at rest, the axioscapular upward rotators could adaptively lengthen and the axioscapular downward rotators and scapulohumeral muscles could adaptively shorten. When he raises the arm overhead, as is required for rock climbing and kayaking, the patient's scapula may not sufficiently upwardly rotate and the humeral head may translate excessively superior in the glenoid fossa. This movement pattern results in impingement of subacromial structures against the AC ligament and possibly the acromion process.

SELF-MANAGEMENT 25-1 **Facelying Shoulder Rotation**

Purpose: To strengthen the shoulder rotators and train independent motion between the shoulder blade and the arm

Starting Position: Kneel next to a weight bench; if at home, lie on your stomach adjacent to the edge of your bed. Place two or more rolled towels under your shoulder joint. Position your arm out to the side with the elbow bent to 90 degrees. Keep as much of your shoulder supported on the bench or bed as possible. Your arm should hang from your elbow down, not from your shoulder. Properly positioned, your elbow should be slightly lower than your shoulder and the "ball" of the "ball-and-socket" joint should be well supported with towel rolls.

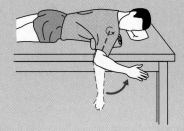

Lateral Rotation

Medial rotation (target muscle: subscapularis)

Movement Technique:

Lateral rotation (target muscles: infraspinatus, teres minor)

- You may perform this exercise just by rotating your arm or with weight. If you are to perform this with weight, see the amount of weight you have been prescribed under dosage.
- Slowly rotate your shoulder so that your forearm moves up toward your head. Stop just short of horizontal.
- Concentrate on letting your arm move independent from your scapula. Your shoulder should "spin" in the socket. There should be no movement of your scapula.
- An alternate activity is to place your forearm on the table in the start position, slowly move your wrist off the supporting surface and hold your wrist and forearm isometrically for 5 to 10 seconds. Return your hand back to the supporting surface. Repeat for the designated number of repetitions.

- You may perform this exercise by rotating your arm with or without added weight. If you perform this with weight, see the amount of weight you have been prescribed under dosage.
- Slowly rotate your shoulder in the opposite direction so that your forearm moves backward.
- Do not let your shoulder displace into the towel roll. Think of keeping your shoulder "pulled away" from the towel roll, or the "ball" in the "socket."
- Your range of motion is more limited in medial rotation than lateral rotation (possibly only 10 to 20 degrees). Remember, it is quality not quantity that is important.

Dosage
Weight _____
Sets/repetitions _____
Frequency _____

Dosage
Weight _____
Sets/repetitions _____
Frequency _____

Medial Rotation

SELF-MANAGEMENT 25-2 *Facelying Arm Lifts*

Purpose: To strengthen the middle and lower trapezius

Starting Position: Lie on your stomach with at least one pillow under your abdomen. Place your hands on the back of your head. Use this position for levels I through III.

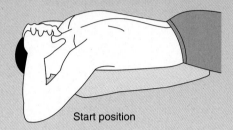

Start position

Movement Technique:

Level I: Stomach-lying elbow lifts(target muscles: middle and lower trapezius)

Barely lift your elbows. Keep your neck muscles (upper trapezius) relaxed, and contract the region between your shoulder blades (lower trapezius). Keep the contraction just enough to lift the elbows so as not to use rhomboids to adduct the shoulder blades.
- Hold the contraction for 5 seconds.
- Lower the elbows and repeat.
- Stop when your neck muscles become more tense; this is an indication that the middle and lower trapezius are fatiguing and that you should stop and rest.

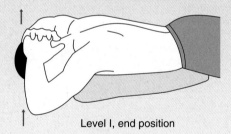

Level I, end position

Dosage
Sets/repetitions _____
Frequency _____

Level II: Stomach-lying elbow lift with arms extended (target muscles: middle and lower trapezius)

Barely lift your elbows. Keep your neck muscles (upper trapezius) relaxed, and contract the region between your shoulder blades (lower trapezius). Keep the contraction just enough to lift the elbows so as not to use rhomboids to adduct the shoulder blades.
- Slowly extend your elbows so that your arms are straight. Bend your elbows so that the hands return to the position behind your head.

- Relax your elbows to the table.
- Stop when your neck muscles become more tense; this is an indication that the middle and lower trapezius are fatiguing and you should stop and rest.

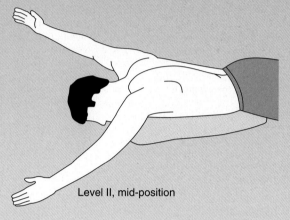

Level II, mid-position

Dosage
Sets/repetitions _____
Frequency _____

Level III: Stomach-lying elbow lift with arm extension overhead (target muscles: middle and lower trapezius)

Barely lift your elbows. Keep your neck muscles (upper trapezius) relaxed, and contract the region between your shoulder blades (lower trapezius). Keep the contraction just enough to lift the elbows so as not to use rhomboids to adduct the shoulder blades.
- As you extend your elbows while raising your arms overhead, be sure not to tense your neck muscles (upper trapezius) during this level of exercise. If you are unable to keep your neck muscles relatively relaxed, you may not be ready for this level of exercise.
- Return your hands to your head, lower your elbows, and relax.

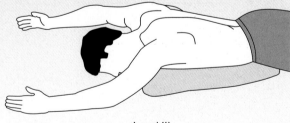

Level III

Dosage
Sets/repetitions _____
Frequency _____

(continued)

SELF-MANAGEMENT 25-2 *Facelying Arm Lifts* (Continued)

Starting Position: Lie on your stomach on a weight bench, piano bench, or low bed. Your chest should be suspended off the edge of the bench. Bend your knees if they extend too far off the bench. Pull your abdomen up and in. Your head should be in line with your spine with your chin tucked. Hold dumbbells with palms facing forward and thumbs up. Arms should be relaxed at chest level and resting on the floor or against the bench if the bench is tall. Keep elbows slightly bent.

Movement Technique:

Level IVA: Stomach lying reverse horizontal fly (target muscle: middle trapezius)

- Raise the dumbbells in a semicircular motion to just below chest height. Do not lift beyond chest level.
- Lower to the starting position using the same path.
- Exhale up; inhale down.

Level IVB: Stomach-lying diagonal reverse fly (target muscle: lower trapezius)

- Raise your elbows in a semicircular motion, diagonally upward toward the head to just below the level of the head. Do not lift the elbows above the level of the head.
- Lower to the starting position using the same path.
- Exhale up; inhale down.
- Repeat in sets of 10 repetitions. Begin using a light weight when you can complete two sets of 10 repetitions maximum with proper technique.

Dosage
Weight _____
Sets/repetitions _____
Frequency _____

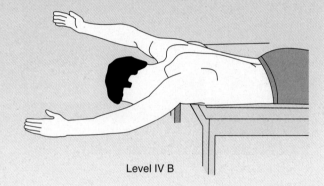

Level IV B

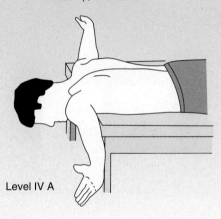

Level IV A

Dosage
Weights _____
Sets/Repetitions _____
Frequency _____

SELF-MANAGEMENT 25-3 *Serratus Anterior Progression*

Purpose: To progressively strengthen your serratus anterior

Level I: Backlying Isometric with Arm Overhead

Starting Position: Lie on your back with one to two pillows positioned above (not under) your head.

Movement Technique:
- Raise your arm overhead, close to your ear, until it reaches the pillow.
- Gently but consistently push your arm backward into the pillow and hold for 10 seconds.

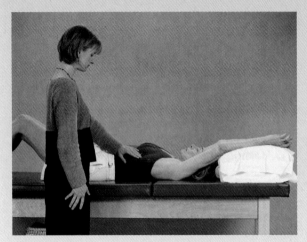

Level I

Dosage
Sets/repetitions _____
Frequency _____

Level II: Sidelying with Dynamic Arm Slide

Starting Position:
Lie on your side with two to three pillows in front of your head and shoulders. Bend your hips and knees. Rest your arm on the pillows with your elbow bent. Grasp the prescribed color of elastic band in your hand and attach the other end to your top foot.

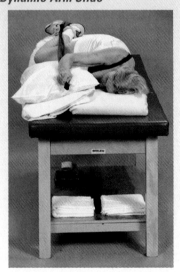

Level II, start position

Movement Technique
- Slide your arm upward toward your head, keeping it in contact with the pillows.
- Slowly lower the arm back down to the starting position. Do not pull the arm back down, but slowly lower it against the resistance of the elastic.

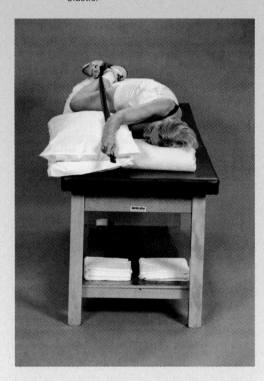

Level II, end position

Dosage
Color of elastic _____
Sets/repetitions _____
Frequency _____

Level III: Standing back to the wall and arm lift

Starting Position: Stand with your feet about 2 to 3 in from the wall. Your head should be against the wall. If you cannot bring your head against the wall, place one or two small, rolled hand towels behind your head. Pull in your stomach to rotate your pelvis backward and reduce the arch in your back. You should be able to place one hand between your lower back and the wall. If there is more space between your back and the wall, bend your hips and knees slightly to reduce the pull from your hip flexors. You should be able to reduce the arch of your back more easily.

(continued)

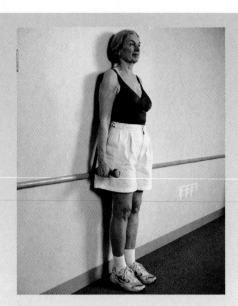

Level III, start position

Movement Technique:
- Lift your arms in front of your body with your elbows straight.
- Try to bring the arms all the way back to the wall, but stop if you feel your back arching or your shoulders shrugging.
- Slowly lower your arms to your side, ensuring your shoulders stay back against the wall and do not roll forward.

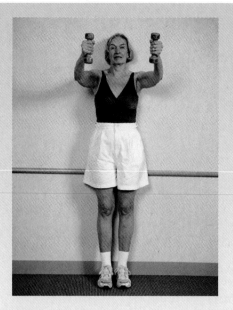

Level III, mid position

Dosage
Weight _____
Sets/repetitions _____
Frequency _____

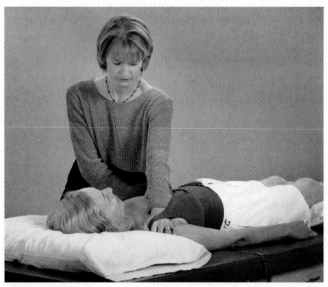

FIGURE 25-1. Manual stretch of the pectoralis minor. The hand applying the stretch force is placed over the coracoid process. A stabilizing hand can be placed over the rib cage. The force applied by the practitioner is in a posterior, superior, and lateral direction.

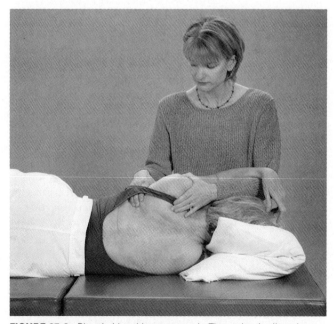

FIGURE 25-2. Rhomboid and levator stretch. The patient's elbow is resting on the practitioner's abdomen. The practitioner cups her hands around the scapula. By shifting the body weight from the caudal to the cranial positioned foot, a rotational force is transmitted to the scapula. The hands rotate the scapula upward like the scapular force couple.

SELF-MANAGEMENT 25-4 *Lateral Rotator and Posterior Capsule Stretch*

Purpose: To stretch the shoulder rotators and train independent movement between the shoulder blade and the arm

Starting Position: Slide your arm out to the side, and bend your elbow to 90 degrees. Position your forearm so that the fingers point to the ceiling. Hold your shoulder down with the opposite hand.

Movement Technique:
- Relax and let your shoulder joint rotate, allowing your forearm to move toward the floor.
- Do not let your shoulder come off the floor and move into your hand as your forearm gets closer to the floor.
- You may hold up to a 2-lb weight in your hand to assist in the stretch.

Dosage
Hold the stretch for _____ seconds
Sets/repetitions _____
Frequency _____

Alternate Position: Lie on the side of your affected arm. Be sure to lie directly over your shoulder joint with your arm positioned at perpendicular to your body and your elbow bent to 90 degrees.

Movement:
- Using your free hand, place it on the dorsum of the hand of the shoulder you are stretching. Gently perform an isometric contraction into your free hand. Hold for 6 seconds. Relax.
- On relaxing, move your forearm downward in the direction of your feet until you feel a mild stretch. Repeat the isometric contraction. Move your hand to the next barrier. Repeat three to four times.

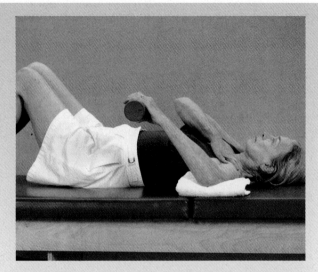

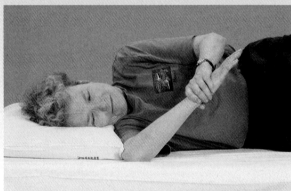

An example of extreme loss of mobility is adhesive capsulitis or frozen shoulder, and an example of extreme excessive mobility is GH dislocation. Mobility is a hallmark characteristic of the shoulder girdle. Even a minor alteration in mobility at any of the three joints of the shoulder girdle, cervicothoracic junction, or thoracic spine can disrupt the normal mechanics of the shoulder girdle.

For the purposes of simplifying terminology in this section, we have chosen to use the terms *hypomobility* when referring to either loss of ROM, reduced extensibility in soft tissues, or reduced joint mobility; and *hypermobility* when referring to excessive ROM, excessive muscle length, or excessive joint mobility.

Hypomobility and hypermobility impairments are intimately related. The "chicken and egg" dilemma exists when assigning causative factors, however, hypomobility is usually associated with a compensatory increase in motion at another joint in the kinetic chain (i.e., scapular elevation as compensation for lack of independent GH motion)[53] or a compensatory increase in a specific direction of motion at the impaired segmental level (i.e., a stiff posterior GH capsule causing excessive anterior GH translation and anterior hypermobility).[54]

Hypomobility

Hypomobility cannot be treated as an isolated impairment. Numerous examples exist in the shoulder girdle complex depicting the intimate relationship between hypomobility and hypermobility. For example, if the scapula does not fully upwardly rotate during arm elevation, the arm and hand can reach the same endpoint by moving into excessive scapula elevation; or the humerus may compensate by translating excessively inferiorly.[24] When restoring balanced and coordinated motion to the shoulder girdle, mobility must be restored in the specific direction of the relatively less mobile joint. Simultaneously, the relatively more mobile segments must be protected from motion in the offending direction (i.e., external support such as bracing or taping and retraining movement patterns).

The method by which mobility is restored must be highly prescriptive and based on individual examination findings. To choose the appropriate intervention, it must be determined which structures are responsible for the loss of mobility (i.e., muscle, periarticular tissue, boney alterations), the direction of the loss of motion, and the severity of restriction. Any one or a combination of the three joints (SC, AC, GH) may be restricted in one or numerous directions because of articular or periarticular soft tissue or

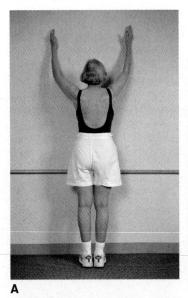
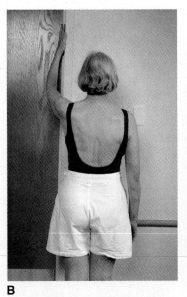
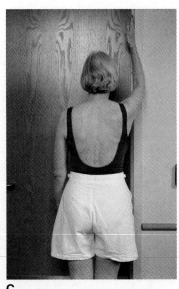

A **B** **C**

FIGURE 25-3. Transitional rotator cuff exercises. (A) The patient places the ulnar aspects of the hands on the wall and slides the hands up the wall in the sagittal or scapular plane, depending on whether the focus is on the serratus anterior or lower trapezius, respectively. (B) Medial rotation bias. The patient places the palm of the hand against the door frame and slides the hand upward and downward while maintaining a mild pressure into medial rotation against the door frame. The patient must not push so hard that she recruits the pectoralis major, latissimus dorsi, and teres major. The goal is to use the subscapularis to encourage an increased rotator cuff force vector during arm elevation by facilitating subscapularis. (C) Lateral rotation bias. The patient places the dorsum of the hand against the door frame and slides the hand upward and downward while maintaining a mild pressure into lateral rotation against the door frame.

bony restrictions or loss of extensibility or adaptive shortening of myofascial tissue. If the restrictions are mild and the compensatory movements can be easily minimized, self-stretching, self-mobilization, and active exercise may suffice. However, if the restrictions are significant (higher levels of stiffness or involving more than one segment) or affect a specific arthrokinematic motion, manual joint mobilization, soft-tissue mobilization, and/or manual stretching may be indicated (see Chapter 7).

Stretching   Stretching short or stiff myofascial tissue with a self management program can be challenging in the shoulder girdle because of the complexity of the joint system and the ease of moving in compensatory patterns. For example, it is difficult to self-stretch a short rhomboid muscle that is limiting scapular upward rotation, because the compensatory motion may be to elevate the scapula, which does not result in a stretch to the rhomboids. Manual stretching (see Fig. 25-2) may be necessary to restore normal tissue extensibility to the rhomboids. Concurrent strengthening exercises for the scapular upward rotators (see Self-Managements 25-2 and

25-3) are encouraged until normal scapular upward rotation mobility is restored during active motion.

The same challenge can occur in attempting to stretch a short pectoralis minor that is limiting scapular posterior tilt of the scapula during arm elevation. The traditional corner stretch (Fig. 25-5) can be ineffective because the head of the humerus

BUILDING BLOCK 25-1

Describe three more examples of faulty posture habits that alter scapula or humerus positions that can lead to altered length tension properties. Name the faulty posture, the affected muscles, and which are prone to lengthening versus shortening.

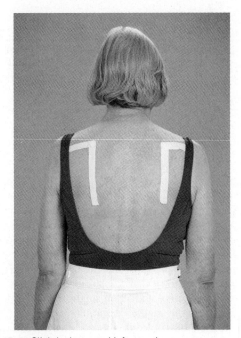

FIGURE 25-4. Slightly depressed left scapula.

BUILDING BLOCK 25-2

Intervention for pain originating from the cervical spine with an associated depressed scapula:
- Scapular taping into elevation and upward rotation (see "Adjunctive Interventions: Taping" later in this chapter)
- Upper trapezius and levator scapula strengthening
- Education regarding posture habits (e.g., do not allow the shoulder to assume a depressed position, keep arms supported at work station and during sustained periods of sitting such as during a movie)
- Movement retraining (i.e., initiating with upper trapezius initially to move the scapula to normal level of elevation, then retraining normal movement and recruitment patterns from an improved start position)

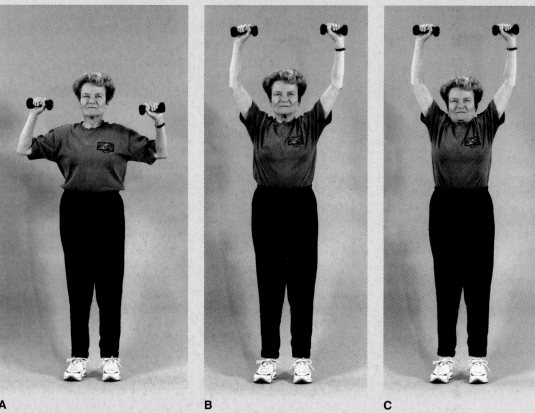

A   **B**   **C**

Upper trapezius strengthening into the short range. For patients with 3/5 muscle strength: the patient faces the wall and slides the ulnar aspect of the hand up the wall (see Fig. 25-11A). At the end range, scapula elevation is performed through available ROM (not pictured). For patients with 3+/5 to 5/5 muscle strength: patient performs an overhead press technique. (A) At end range, scapula elevation is performed through full available ROM (B, C).

can compensate by moving anteriorly into the relatively more flexible anterior capsule instead of stretching a short pectoral muscle. This action reflects a fundamental physical law: objects tend to move through the path of least resistance. The relatively flexible anterior capsule is the path of least resistance, and it stretches more readily than a short pectoralis minor. Even in the absence of compensatory anterior humeral head translation, research has shown that a posterior shift of the coracoid process with horizontal abduction might not be sufficient to stretch the pectoralis minor.[55] A simultaneous posterior and superior shift of the coracoid is more effective in stretching the pectoralis minor. Manual stretching (see Fig. 25-2) may be

necessary until normal extensibility of the pectoralis minor is achieved. Stretching should be combined with strengthening of the lower trapezius (see Self-Management 25-2) and serratus anterior (see Self-Management 25-3) until posterior tilt is restored during active motion.

In these examples, stretching the short muscle was combined with strengthening an antagonist muscle. This principle is important to restore muscle balance. In this case, stretching the pectoralis minor, rhomboid, or both muscles can be complemented with active exercise of the middle and lower trapezius and serratus anterior muscles in the shortened range.

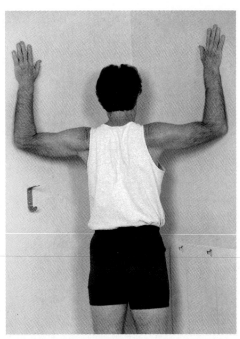

FIGURE 25-5. Traditional pectoralis major and minor stretch.

SELF-MANAGEMENT 25-5 *Latissimus and Scapulohumeral Muscle Stretch*

Purpose: To stretch the trunk muscles that attach to your arm and the muscles that originate on the shoulder blade and attach to your arm.

Starting Position:
- Lie on your back with your hips and knees bent and feet flat on the floor.

To stretch your scapulohumeral muscles, you need to prevent your shoulder blade from sliding out to the side. To do this, you need to hold the outside edge of your shoulder blade with the opposite hand.

Movement Technique:
- Raise your arm over your head, keeping the arm close to your ear. When you feel your back arch or your shoulder blade slide out to the side, stop the movement.
- Rest your arm on the appropriate number of pillows so that your arm may relax in the position previously determined.
- Hold the stretch for the prescribed amount of time, and lower your arm back to your side. Keep your shoulder back as you lower your arm, and do not let it roll forward.

Dosage
Hold the stretch for _____ seconds
Sets/repetitions _____
Frequency _____

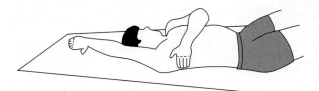

Other common muscles in the shoulder girdle that require stretching include the GH lateral rotators and the medial rotator-adductor group. Although these often can be successfully self-stretched, special self-stabilization techniques should be employed to ensure compensatory motions do not occur. These exercises are illustrated in Self-Management 25-4; Self-Management 25-5: Latissimus and Scapulohumeral Muscle Stretch; and Figure 25-6, respectively.

Stretching is ineffective if the improved flexibility does not translate into an improved functional outcome. Posture education is another important aspect to consider when treating mobility impairments. The patient must be educated to avoid postures that adaptively shorten the target soft tissues and lengthen the opposing ones. In the case of a short pectoralis minor, sitting or standing in kyphosis and forward head posture must be gradually reduced. Scapular taping can assist in improving postural habits (see "Adjunctive Interventions: Scapular Taping" and Building Block 25-3).

Active exercise through a functional range must be instructed and performed precisely to stretch the short soft tissues and recruit the lengthened and weak muscles with the optimal length-tension relationships. Though originally depicted as an exercise to promote function of the rotator cuff, Figure 25-3 can also be used to orient the scapula into upward rotation, placing the rhomboid in an elongated position. The kinematics of the scapula must be closely observed, and biofeedback provided to the patient regarding any deviation from the optimal scapular motion to ensure a lengthening stimulus is applied to the rhomboid muscle.

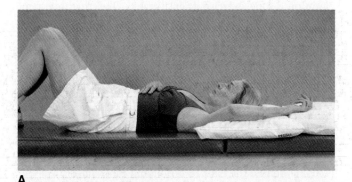

A

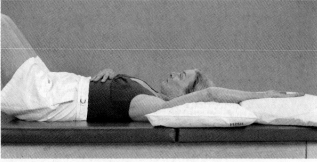

B

FIGURE 25-6. Active pectoralis major stretch. (A) The patient rests her abducted and laterally rotated arms on pillows in the scapular plane. The pillows should be of sufficient height to prevent glenohumeral anterior translation. (B) The patient slides her arms upward until she feels a stretch across the pectoralis region. A static stretch can be maintained at the end position.

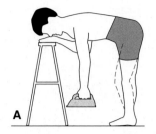

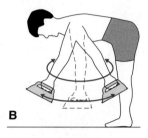

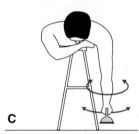

FIGURE 25-7. Pendulum exercise. (A) The patient should bend forward at the hips approximately 90 degrees, and his knees should be slightly bent to allow greater hip flexion and minimize stress to the low back. The patient should place the hand not being used in the exercise on a firm surface (e.g., stool) and place his head on the hand. This permits relaxed movement and concentration on the indicated movement of the involved shoulder. The involved arm should dangle freely, and a weight can be held in the hand. Use of an iron as a weight is suggested for home exercise. A weight adds traction to the glenohumeral joint and widens the pendulum arc. The patient should maintain the thoracic spine in neutral to prevent excessive scapula abduction, so as to transmit the forces from the weight to the GH joint rather than the ST joint. (B, C) Pendulum exercises are done passively; no muscular action of the glenohumeral joint is required. Instead, muscular effort of the trunk and hips allow the body to sway and the arm to swing in sagittal, frontal, and transverse planes of motion. The exercise can be progressed to active exercise by actively swinging the arm in the same planes and arcs of motion. (Adapted from Cailliet R. Shoulder Pain. Philadelphia, PA: FA Davis, 1966.)

Effects of Immobilization Loss of ROM and muscle extensibility and joint hypomobility can occur as a result of imposed immobilization following an injury or self-immobilization resulting from pain, fear, or a deconditioned state. Immobilization should never be prolonged because of the tendency to develop myofascial shortening, loss of capsular extensibility, muscular atrophy, and disturbed motor control. Immobilization resulting in hypomobility can cause activity limitation and profound disability.

To prevent immobilization during painful periods or during the "rest" phase of healing, carefully prescribed ROM exercises can be initiated. Pain, lack of strength, and poor motor control can lead to further pain and injury during elevation against gravity. In the early phases of healing, a traditional gravity-lessened exercise in which GH motion is achieved is the Codman exercise, also called the pendulum exercise (Fig. 25-7). This exercise adds traction to the GH joint, stretches the capsule, avoids active abduction, and minimizes the common faulty movement pattern of scapular elevation during exercise against gravity. The rhythmic pendulum movements are believed to modulate pain.

Hypermobility

To effectively treat hypermobility or instability in the absence of a traumatic onset, the hypomobile segments must be identified. Hypermobility does not improve despite aggressive exercise protocols if it is occurring in response to a less mobile segment. For example, the GH joint may become hypermobile in the anterior direction in response to a hypomobile scapula in the direction of SC retraction. Another scenario is reaching behind the back (see Building Block 25-4).

If the scapula fails to move three dimensionally into a more adducted and downward rotated position, it becomes a barrier to the head of the humerus. If the goal is to reach behind the back, the humerus may compensate by translating into the anterior capsule. Lack of scapular adduction is the result of reduced SC retraction and/or AC lateral rotation; lack of scapular downward rotation is result of reduced SC depression and/or anterior/inferior rotation and/or AC downward rotation. Attention to restrictions in these joints in the related directions is pivotal to treatment of the hypermobile GH joint in the direction of anterior glide that is perpetuated by faulty kinematics during common functional movements such as reaching behind the back.

This is just one functional example of how the humerus may compensate with excessive anterior translation, but if this compensation is repeated throughout daily activities, hypermobility results in the GH joint in the anterior direction. Treatment must focus on the *cause* of the hypermobility by improving mobility of the relatively less mobile

segments and concurrently reducing mobility at the relatively more mobile segments. Improving the muscle performance, length-tension properties, and motor control of the dynamic stabilizers in the relatively more mobile direction is the recommended approach to decrease excessive or abnormal mobility. Specific exercise to remedy impairments associated with faulty movement patterns must be included in the plan of care. Ultimately, the functional movement patterns causing the hypermobility must be addressed (e.g., retraining scapular adduction and downward rotation at the appropriate time in the coordinated hand behind back movement pattern).

An impairment commonly associated with a faulty movement pattern that contributes to an anterior GH hypermobility is impaired muscle performance and altered length-tension properties of the GH medial rotators. Among the dynamic stabilizers, the subscapularis provides the greatest degree of stabilization in external rotation (i.e., cocking phase of pitching).[56] To isolate subscapularis function from the other medial rotators (i.e., pectoralis major, latissimus dorsi, and teres major), its unique function must be promoted by carefully prescribing the posture and movement parameters of the activity chosen.

An exercise to improve the muscle performance and length-tension properties of a lengthened subscapularis is prone medial rotation (see Self-Management 25-6: Subscapularis Isometric Exercise). If the subscapularis can produce enough force to rotate the arm against gravity, prone is the desired position for the patient to perform medial rotation.[24] Prone

medial rotation poses a greater challenge to the subscapularis to prevent the humerus from translating anteriorly than a supine position, in which gravity assists the humerus posteriorly. Theoretically, if the other medial rotators dominate the subscapularis during this exercise, anterior translation during medial rotation will occur. Decker et al.[57] demonstrated that IR at 90-degree abduction produced less pectoralis major activity compared to 0-degree abduction. Pectoralis major and latissimus dorsi activity increase when performing IR exercises in an adducted position or while moving into an adducted position during the exercise.[58] Thus, IR at 90-degree abduction may be performed if attempting to strengthen the subscapularis while minimizing larger muscle group activity.

The goal in this case is to strengthen the subscapularis to prevent abnormal or excessive anterior translation of the head of the humerus during GH medial rotation and during other functional movement patterns. Resolution of this impairment does not necessarily translate into a functional outcome unless the muscle is specifically trained during functional activities. The subscapularis muscle is kinesthetically limited, and it cannot be palpated or recorded with surface EMG. The clinician's best indication that it is working is to observe or palpate movement of the head of the humerus during functional activities. Because movement occurs rapidly and the movement is difficult to observe, videotaping the movement can be useful for carefully analyzing movement.

If the humeral head appears to be translating excessively anteriorly, particularly if symptoms of hypermobility or pain are present, the clinician must determine whether the problem is caused by a base, modulator, or biomechanical element defect. A base element problem may be caused by insufficient subscapularis force capability and/or length-tension properties and indicates that the introduction of functional retraining is premature.

A modulator element problem may be caused by poor motor control of the subscapularis. Methods to improve motor control include verbal, visual (e.g., patient views videotape to gain understanding of the movement pattern), or tactile feedback to provide knowledge of results. Verbal cueing might include "think of sucking the ball into the socket," or "imagine the ball is on a skewer and you are sliding it into the socket." These verbal cues might augment the concavity compression role of the subscapularis and improve GH stability.

A biomechanical element problem may be caused by an increased thoracic flexion preventing adequate scapular adduction during horizontal arm abduction, or limited thoracic rotation in a more global movement (such as with cocking phase of pitching), and thereby leading to excessive GH anterior translation. This condition requires attention to the posture and associated movement of the thoracic spine to ultimately improve the GH movement pattern.

Impaired Muscle Performance

As discussed in the examination/evaluation section, impaired muscle performance can result from numerous causes. This section discusses therapeutic exercise intervention for each major cause of impaired muscle performance.

Neurologic Pathology

Neurologic pathology can lead to sensory or motor changes and occur at the level of the nerve root or in

---

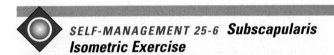

SELF-MANAGEMENT 25-6 *Subscapularis Isometric Exercise*

Purpose: To strengthen the subscapularis in the short range

Starting Position: Kneel next to a weight bench; if at home, lie on your stomach adjacent to the edge of your bed. Place one or two towels rolled under your shoulder. Position your arm out to the side with elbow bent to 90 degrees. Keep as much of your shoulder supported on the bench or bed. Your arm should hang from your elbow down, not from your shoulder. Rotate your arm backward as far as you can before you feel the "ball" drop out of the socket. Position a garbage can or another object sufficient to support your arm.

Movement Technique:
- Raise your hand ½ in off the garbage can, and hold it for 10 seconds.
- Be sure the "ball" does not drop out of the socket.
- Lower your hand back to the garbage can.

Dosage
Sets/repetitions _____
Frequency _____

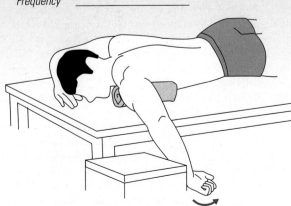

the periphery. Thorough examination and evaluation can determine the anatomic site of the neurologic deficit. A thorough discussion of thoracic outlet syndrome can be found in Chapter 24.

Alterations in neurologic function at the nerve root level from cervical involvement can be a source of impaired muscle performance in the shoulder girdle musculature. For example, mechanical dysfunction of the C4 or C5 levels may result in weak abduction, flexion, medial, or lateral rotation.[59] Strength-related activities will not improve muscle performance in the shoulder until the cause of the mechanical dysfunction of the cervical spine is addressed (see Chapter 23, Cervical Spine, for concepts related to therapeutic exercise intervention of the cervical spine). If the underlying cause of impaired muscle performance is cervical mechanical dysfunction, the position of the cervical spine with respect to the trunk and the shoulders is extremely important when performing shoulder exercises.

Another common neurologic deficit involving the shoulder girdle is injury of a peripheral nerve resulting from traction, compression, trauma, or surgery. Nerves that are vulnerable to injury are the supraspinatus nerve in the suprascapular notch,[60,61] the axillary nerve between teres major and teres minor, the long thoracic nerve along the middle axillary line,[62] spinal accessory in the jugular foramen or posterior triangle[63,64] and the brachial plexus in the thoracic outlet.[65] Nerve injury often results in weakness of the innervated muscles. Injury to the long thoracic nerve is discussed to demonstrate the resulting muscle performance impairments and the related therapeutic exercise intervention.

The pathophysiology of long thoracic nerve palsy is determined by three factors: direct pressure on the nerve, stretching of the nerve, and ischemia. Each factor separately can cause a nerve lesion. The long thoracic nerve is particularly susceptible to stretch from postures or movements of depression of the scapula (e.g., carrying a heavy bag with the strap over the shoulder). The stretching capacity of a peripheral nerve is estimated at 8% to 15%.[66] In research on human cadavers, in which the head was turned to the opposite shoulder while elevating the ipsilateral arm, the long thoracic nerve could be stretched twice its length.[67] The injury manifests as weakness of the serratus anterior, a critical muscle for normal scapular mechanics. A hallmark sign for long thoracic nerve injury is scapular winging at rest that is exaggerated during arm elevation, arm lowering, or pushing. The pathomechanics that contributed to the injury must first be resolved before strength-related activities can be effective. In the case of a traction injury to the long thoracic nerve, the postures and body mechanics that cause depression of the scapula must be addressed. Strength exercises for the scapular elevators (e.g., upper trapezius, levator scapula) are often necessary. Taping the scapula into elevation may also be required to relieve the tension on the nerve (see Adjunctive Interventions: Scapular Taping).

To develop a working prognosis, one must consider the anatomy of the long thoracic nerve. From its origin, the root of C5–7, and the brachial plexus, the long thoracic nerve runs between the first rib and the clavicle to the serratus anterior muscle over a distance of approximately 35 cm. Recovery of the nerve is a very slow process: about 1 cm per week. Recovery may occur between a few months and 2 years.[68] Initially, neuromuscular electrical stimulation (NMES) can be used to prevent muscle atrophy.[69] NMES can be used with biphasic pulses in burst mode applied via

DISPLAY 25-7
Commonly prescribed Serratus Anterior Exercises

- D1 and D2 diagonal PNF pattern flexion (see Chapter 15)
- D2 diagonal PNF pattern extension (see Chapter 15)
- supine scapular protraction
- supine upward scapular punch
- military press
- push-up plus
- GH IR and ER at 90-degree abduction
- shoulder flexion, abduction, and scaption with ER above 120 degrees.

electrodes over the motor points of the affected serratus anterior.[70] Self-Management 25-3 can be used in conjunction with NMES for prevention of atrophy initially and later to reeducate the serratus anterior as motor function returns.

Passive ROM exercises can be prescribed and manual joint mobilization techniques can be applied to the GH and ST joints to prevent loss of mobility in the early stages. As reinnervation of the muscle occurs, a progressive strengthening exercise program must be introduced. Several exercises elicit high serratus anterior activity.[71–75] Display 25-7 lists commonly prescribed exercises.

A general rule of thumb to consider in functionally strengthening the serratus anterior is that its activity tends to increase in a somewhat linear fashion with arm elevation.[72,74,75–78] Though one would not initially consider performing shoulder IR and ER at 90 degrees of abduction (see Self-Management 25-1) to generate serratus anterior activity, these are excellent choices because the role of the serrautus is to stabilize the scapula against the forces exerted by the rotator cuff.[72] For example, the force exerted by the supraspinatus at the supraspinous fossa has the ability to downwardly rotate or internally rotate the scapula if this force is not counterbalanced by the ST musculature. Following the principle of specificity of training, when possible, the exercise should duplicate the function of the serratus anterior.

Decker et al.[71] compared several common exercises designed to recruit the serratus anterior. The authors identified that the three exercises that produced the greatest serratus anterior EMG signal were the push-up with a plus, dynamic hug (see Fig. 25-8) and punch exercises (similar to a jabbing protraction motion; see Fig. 25-9).

Despite the high activiation levels of the serratus anterior during protraction patterns, this author recommends caution in promoting the protraction function of the serratus anterior. Normal UQ kinematics involve a combination of scapula upward rotation, posterior tilt, and external rotation.[78] The clavicle retracts during normal UQ elevation, which is coupled with scapula external rotation (an important function of the serratus as well as an important kinematic to prevent subacromial impingement).[78–81] Training scapular protraction movement patterns could be detrimental to restoring ideal shoulder girdle kinematics.

An alternative exercise that has been shown to be an effective method to strengthen the serratus anterior is the wall slide (see Fig. 25-3).[77] The wall slide begins by slightly leaning against the wall with the ulnar border of the forearms in contact with the wall, elbows flexed 90 degrees, and shoulders abducted 90 degrees in the scapular plane. From this position

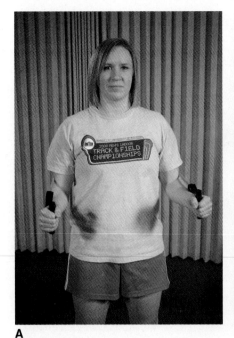 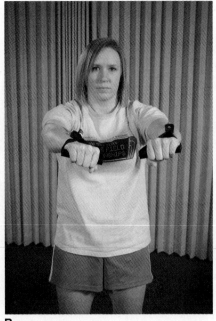 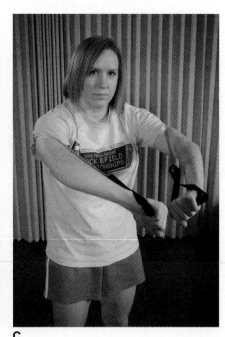

A   B   C

FIGURE 25-8. Dynamic hug for the serratus anterior begins with elbows flexed 90 degrees and arms at side (A). The next motion is elbow extension with humeral internal rotation (B). The ending position is with the humerus in full internal rotation, elbows flexed slightly and humerus moving into horizontal adduction similar to a "hugging" motion until full acromioclavicular protraction is reached (C).

the arms slide up the wall in the scapular plane, while leaning into the wall. Interestingly, the wall slide produces similar serratus anterior activity compared to scapular abduction above 120-degree abduction with no resistance.[77] One advantage of the wall slide compared to scapular abduction is that, anecdotally, patients report that the wall slide is less painful to perform. This may be because during the wall slide the upper

extremities are supported against the wall, making it easier to perform while also assisting with compression of the humeral head within the glenoid. Thus, this may be an effective exercise to perform during the earlier protective phases of some rehabilitation programs.

The hand-knee position is an alternative position to provide resistance to the serratus anterior. Figure 25-10 illustrates an

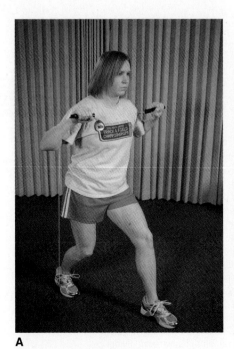 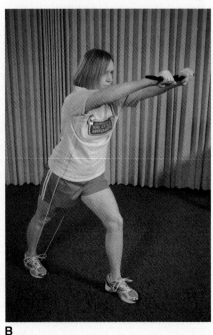

A   B

FIGURE 25-9. Bilateral serratus anterior punch to 120-degree abduction begins with hands by the side (A) before extending elbows and elevating shoulders up to 120 degrees of elevation and full protraction (B).

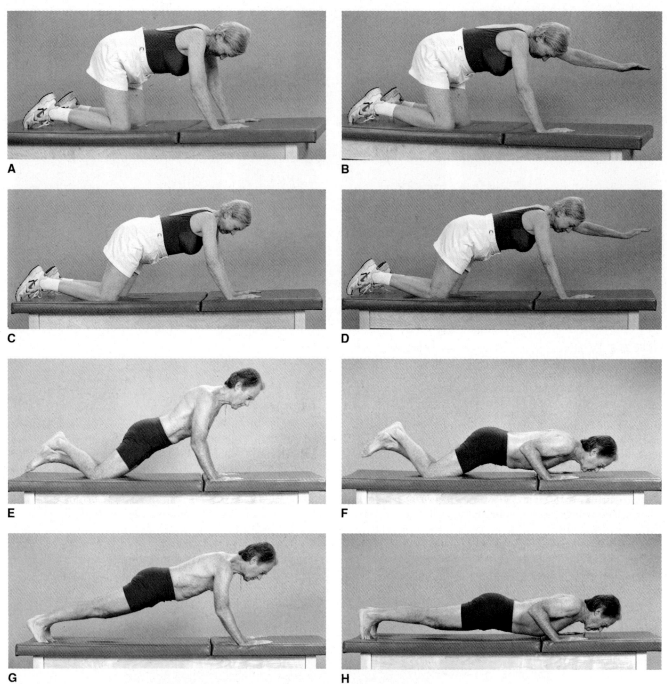

FIGURE 25-10. Progressive serratus strengthening exercises. (A) The patient assumes a quadruped position, with the hips directly over the knees and the shoulders directly over the hands. The scapula should be flat against the rib cage in neutral position. (B) The patient then lifts the opposite hand slightly off the ground. The supporting shoulder girdle should not demonstrate any alteration in scapular position. (C) The patient assumes a quadruped position, with the hips slightly in front of the knees and shoulders directly over the hands. The scapula should be flat against the rib cage in neutral position. (D) The patient then lifts the opposite hand slightly off the ground. The supporting shoulder girdle should not demonstrate any alteration in scapular position. (E) "Serratus push-up." The patient assumes the position shown. The hips should be in neutral with respect to the sagittal plane. This subject is in more hip flexion than is desirable. The scapula should be resting against the rib cage in a neutral position. The elbows should be in the sagittal plane with the olecranon process facing posteriorly and the antecubital fossa facing anteriorly. The fingers should be directed forward with the wrist in extension; a small towel roll may be placed under the palm of the hand to reduce the amount of wrist extension if full wrist extension is uncomfortable. (F) The patient slowly lowers his body toward the floor while maintaining neutral pelvis and spine alignment. The elbows should flex in the sagittal plane (sometimes called a triceps push-up). The scapula should abduct and adduct during the movement. Evidence of winging or lack of abduction indicates the load is too great or the muscle has fatigued. (G) The patient is positioned as in (E) and (F), but the legs are straight. (H) The exercise proceeds as in (E) and (F).

initial progression on hands and knees. The goal with this exercise is to support the body weight through the affected upper extremity without scapular adduction or winging. Stepping the knees behind the hips increases the weight the arms must support, thus increasing the strength demand on the serratus anterior (see Fig. 25-10C and D). This exercise can be progressed to a push-up position. The desired position for a "serratus push-up" is modified from the traditional "pectoral push-up" by positioning the olecranon and antecubital fossa in the sagittal plane. This modified position is also called a "triceps push-up." To progress the level of difficulty, the exercise can be performed first in the bent-knee position (see Fig. 25-10E and F) and then progressed to a straight-body position (see Fig. 25-10G and H) if higher levels of performance using the serratus anterior are required. Though the "plus" movement of the scapula during a push-up does generate high serratus activation levels,[71-75,82] caution is recommended in promoting this additional movement due to aforementioned reasons.

The clinician must consider the most critical function(s) to restore and consider the posture, mode, movement, and dosage parameters based upon the examination findings. A clinical example detailed in Display 25-8 can provide a platform for prescribing a therapeutic exercise intervention (see Building Block 25-5).

Muscle Strain

Muscle strain results from an injurious tension. Muscle strain can result from a sudden and excessive tension or from a gradual and continuous tension imposed on a muscle. Both types of muscle strain commonly occur in the shoulder girdle.

An example of a muscle strain caused by sudden and excessive tension imposed on a muscle is a sudden fall onto the shoulder or outstretched arm, resulting in a rotator cuff strain or complete tear. The examination may reveal weakness in some or all portions of the rotator cuff. Selective tissue tension tests may also reveal pain with resistive testing and stretch, depending on the severity of the strain.

Treatment should follow the guidelines for tissue healing outlined in Chapter 11. Low-load muscle contraction can be introduced in the repair-regeneration phase to impose a load on the healing tissue along lines of stress. Initially, submaximal isometric contractions at various positions within the pain-free range can be prescribed. Alternatively or in addition, concentric-eccentric dynamic exercise can be prescribed. Dosage parameters related to the load, starting and ending positions, and ROM depend on the severity of the strain.

More aggressive strength regimens can be gradually introduced in the later stages of the repair-regeneration phase to prepare the muscle for the final phase of healing (Fig. 25-11). The type of contraction and specific movement pattern required of the muscle should be trained as early as possible. For example, prevention of excessive humeral head superior translation is a specific and necessary function for the rotator cuff during arm elevation (concentric) and the return from arm elevation (eccentric; see Fig. 25-13). The final phase of healing should include activity-specific exercises related to the patient's functional goals. Complex functional movement patterns can be trained, and a gradual return to sport-specific activities, such as returning to a pitching program (Display 25-9),[83,84] can be accomplished. Quality of movement during exercise and functional activities must be emphasized and used as a guide for progression at any stage.

Another form of strain common in the shoulder girdle is the type resulting from gradual and continuous tension. For

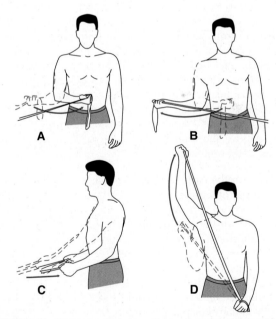

FIGURE 25-11. Higher-level rotator cuff exercise using elastic tubing. The therapist must ensure precise motion at the GH joint and provide biofeedback to the patient regarding the PICR of the ST joint during these movements. (A) Medial rotation. Caution must be taken to prevent scapula abduction and medial rotation during GH medial rotation. (B) Lateral rotation. Caution must be taken to prevent scapula adduction during GH lateral rotation. (C) Extension. Caution must be taken to move the elbow only slightly posterior to the midaxillary line to prevent excessive anterior displacement of the humeral head. (D) Flexion. Caution must be taken to ensure optimal PICR of the ST joint during arm elevation and control over superior translation of the humeral head.

DISPLAY 25-9
Nine-Level Rehabilitation Throwing Program*

Level	Throws/Feet	Throws/Feet	Throws/Feet
1	25/25	25/60	
2	25/25	50/60	
3	25/25	75/60	
4	25/25	50/60	25/90
5	25/25	50/60	25/120
6	25/25	50/60	25/150
7	25/25	50/60	25/180
8	25/25	50/60	25/210
9	25/25	50/60	25/240

*This program is designed for athletes to work at their own pace to develop the necessary arm strength to begin throwing from a mound. The athlete is to throw 2 days in a row and then rest for 1 day. It is not important to progress to the next throwing level with each outing. It is preferred that a number of outings at the same level be completed before progressing. It is important to throw with comfort, which may necessitate moving back a level on occasion.

DiGiovine NM, Jobe FW, Pink M, et al. An electromyographic analysis of the upper extremity in pitching. J Shoulder Elbow Surg 1992;1:15–25.

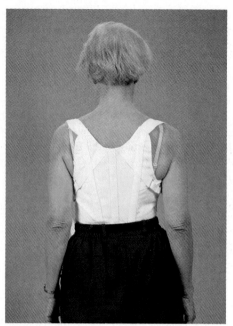

FIGURE 25-12. Posture brace.

example, strain to the middle and lower trapezius often results from a habitual position of abducted and downwardly rotated scapulae found in thoracic kyphosis. Subjective and objective characteristics of middle/lower trapezius strain include24:

- Symptoms of "burning" pain along the course of the middle or lower trapezius may be experienced. If the strain is not accompanied by adaptive shortening of the anterior muscles, pain is not constant and can be relieved in the recumbent position. However, change of position does not affect the symptoms of a person with associated adaptive anterior shortness. This is due to the fact that the anterior shortness (i.e., pectoralis major and minor) maintains the protracted position of the scapula even in the recumbant position.
- Heavy breasts that are not adequately supported
- Positional weakness in the middle and lower trapezius
- Adaptive shortening of the pectoralis major and minor and other internal rotators

Treatment in the early healing phase should include support in the form of taping (see the "Adjunctive Interventions: Taping" section), bracing (Fig. 25-12), or supportive brassiere to relieve the tension on the middle and lower trapezius. If shortness affects the shoulder medial rotator and adductor group, gradual stretching (see Fig. 25-16 and Self-Management 24-2: Postural Exercise with Back to Wall) is indicated before strengthening the middle and lower trapezius. Stretching allows the middle and lower trapezius to be strengthened at the appropriate length.

Exercises to strengthen the middle and lower trapezius muscles should not only consider the function of these muscle fiber directions, but also the length at which the muscles are being strengthened. The lengthened range must be avoided to prevent further strain to the muscle. Lengthened muscles produce less force or torque in the short range; therefore, initial exercises may need to be performed in gravity-lessened positions. The gravity-lessened position decreases the load on the lengthened muscle so it can produce sufficient force or torque in the short range. Figure 25-13 depicts a

strengthening exercise for the lower trapezius in a gravity-lessened position. Prone horizontal abduction between 90 and 135 degrees of abduction in ER has been shown to demonstrate high levels of middle and lower trapezius activation.[72] The progressive exercises shown in Self-Management 25-2 demonstrates a progression of load using these positions to activate the middle and lower trapezius fibers. Exercise prescription can proceed to this progression once when force capability can be produced in the short range against the higher loads imposed by longer lever arms and the introduction of gravity. Figure 25-3 can be used, this time with the emphasis on optimal length-tension properties of the lower trapezius, timing of activation with respect to the upper trapezius and serratus anterior (see Fig. 25-6 on Web site), optimal ST kinematics, and concentric/eccentric control.

One of the ultimate goals is to alter length-tension properties of both lengthened and shortened muscles. New length-tension properties of the affected musculature should be achieved if the following conditions are met:

- Strengthening in the shortened range is combined with proper support for the middle and lower trapezius.
- Stretch is applied to the anterior musculature (i.e., pectoralis minor, pectoralis major, short head of biceps).
- Education is provided regarding improved postures, movement patterns, workstation ergonomics, and body mechanics.

Use of these concepts and principles will result in alleviating the precipitating pathomechanics to allow the strain to heal.

Disuse, Deconditioning, and Reduced Conditioning

In some cases, muscles become weak because of disuse or deconditioning or may not be able to produce enough force or torque to enable an individual to achieve higher levels of performance (i.e., reduced conditioning). Impaired muscle performance due to disuse or lack of conditioning can

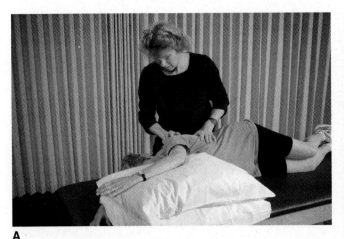 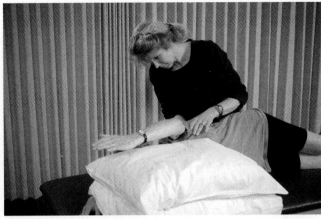

A **B**

FIGURE 25-13. Gravity-lessened position to strengthen lower trapezius. (A) Position the patient in sidelying with as many pillows as necessary to support the arm in the sagittal or scapular plane. The arm rests on the pillow at 90 degrees of elevation with the elbow bent. (B) Slide the arm upward toward full elevation. The ST and glenohumeral joint PICR should be monitored for any deviations. Once full available upward rotation is achieved, the patient lifts the arm 1 to 2 in off the pillow. An isometric contraction of the lower trapezius is held for the specified duration. Care must be taken to lift the entire arm, and not just the elbow. Frame (C) depicts incorrect lifting of the elbow leading to GH MR versus the desired minimal abduction movement necessary to stimulate lower trapezius recruitment.

manifest as alterations in performance of ADLs, instrumental ADLs, recreation, leisure activity, or sports. Muscle performance impairments can be caused by many forms of disuse or deconditioning:

- Gradual development of subtle alterations in agonist–antagonist relationships caused by habitual postures or repetitive movement patterns, which can create problems related to muscle balance (e.g., insidious onset of shoulder impingement without evidence of anatomic impairments as a precipitating factor)[24]
- Generalized weakness from prolonged bed rest or reduction in activity because of illness, preventing performance of ADLs and instrumental ADLs (e.g., dressing, meal preparation, housework)
- Decreased power output preventing maximal performance of a high strength-demand sport, such as swimming, tennis, or throwing.

The shoulder girdle poses a challenge for the clinician prescribing a general strength-conditioning program because of the potential for creating muscle imbalances. A conditioning program should include exercises for all major muscle groups. The posture and movement of the technique are critical to a successful program. For example, if a biceps curl is done with poor technique (i.e., anterior scapular tilt is increased during the elbow flexion motion) rather than optimal technique (i.e., scapula remains neutral with respect to tilt during the elbow flexion motion with proper stabilization from the axioscapular muscles), the patient risks development of impaired muscle length-tension properties of the scapular stabilizers, which could cause secondary impairments or pathology (e.g., subacromial impingement from a scapula functioning in excessive anterior tilt). This risk increases if the same faulty posture is used during a variety of other exercises. Display 25-10 summarizes exercises that are recommended for inclusion in a general shoulder girdle conditioning program.

In the case of a high-level athlete or strenuous industrial worker, general conditioning exercises may not be enough to improve performance of the desired activity. The choice of what type of exercise (e.g., dynamic, isokinetic, isometric) is used in training depends on the performance level and the specific activities to which the individual wishes to return. The prescription of high-level strength conditioning exercises must be specific for mode, contraction type, and velocity whenever possible. For example, when strength training the medial rotators in the pitching athlete, the type of contraction should duplicate the eccentric contraction used in the cocking phase to decelerate motion and a concentric contraction used in the acceleration phase to create pitching velocity.[84] Examples of techniques or activities that can provide concentric and eccentric contraction training include manual resistance by the physical therapist in the clinic, plyometric equipment, and a home program using elastics (Fig. 25-14).

Prevention of injury is a major concern for the athlete or industrial worker. In designing a training program for these persons, the clinician should prescribe exercises to improve the muscle performance of the muscles required for the sport or occupation and prescribe exercises to strengthen opposing muscles to prevent muscle imbalances. For example, sports such as baseball may require training for the shoulder medial rotators. If strengthening for the opposing lateral rotators and scapular adductor and upward rotators (i.e., middle and lower trapezius) is not performed, muscle imbalances may develop and lead to impairments of body structures and functions and pathology.[24] In addition, the clinician should ensure that all the medial rotators are stimulated in a conditioning program and that the larger pectoralis major and latissimus dorsi do not predominate and create an imbalance within the medial rotator group. Specific exercise for the subscapularis as shown in Self-Management 25-6 can be prescribed along with more general medial rotation exercises to maintain muscle balance.

DISPLAY 25-10
Shoulder Girdle Conditioning Program

- Bench press (flat, incline, decline)

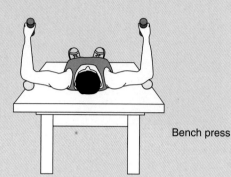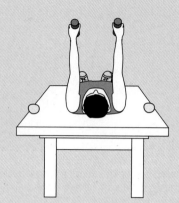

Bench press

- Prone middle and lower trapezius

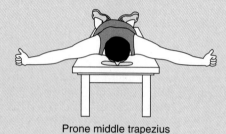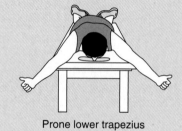

Prone middle trapezius   Prone lower trapezius

- Latissimus pulldown

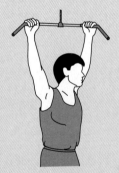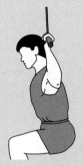

- Lateral deltoid raise—in frontal plane or scaption (through full ROM) or

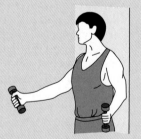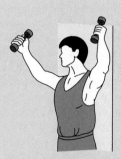

Wall arm lift scapular plane   Lift through full range to wall

(continued)

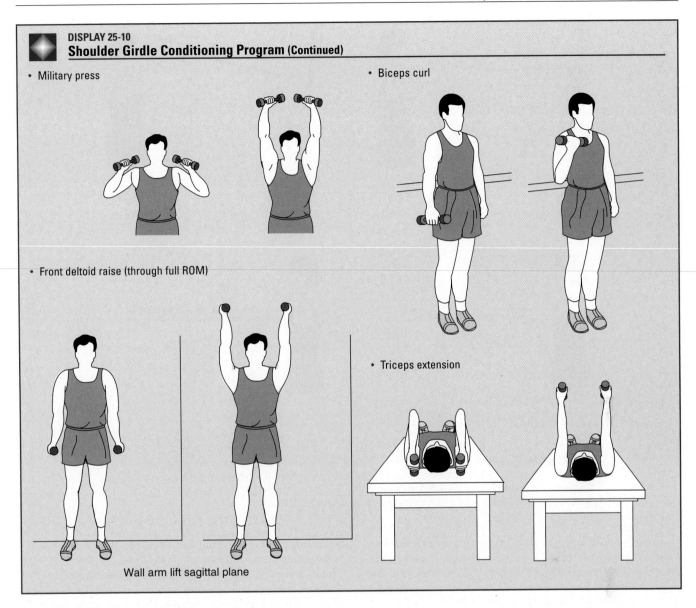

- Military press
- Biceps curl
- Front deltoid raise (through full ROM)
- Triceps extension

Wall arm lift sagittal plane

A component of muscle performance includes muscle endurance. Postural faults in the upper quadrant often are often attributed to lack of muscle endurance. However, little or no muscle activity has been found in upper quadrant muscles during relaxed standing posture.[85] Postural faults are commonly caused by alterations in muscle length whereby some muscles become adaptively lengthened and others adaptively shortened. The altered lengths of muscles do not provide the optimal support to the shoulder girdle structure.

Impairments in muscle endurance have also been implicated in shoulder and neck symptoms. However, despite the methodologic problems associated with quantifying muscle fatigue,[86] most authorities agree that muscle fatigue is not solely responsible for occupational neck and shoulder complaints.[87,88] Indeed, it has been shown that the trapezius, for example, is under constant muscle tension in myalgic

subjects,[89] but that a combined program aimed at restoring ideal muscle length-tension properties, muscle force, endurance, and coordination is more applicable than focusing on muscle endurance alone.[90]

Generally, research indicates that prevention and treatment of neck and shoulder symptoms require a multidimensional approach to reduce the workload on muscle.[91–94] Suggested interventions include ergonomic changes in the workstation and appropriate pacing of activity with rest,[95] combined with measures to reduce stress and anxiety in the work place.[95,96]

In the case of recovery from injury, starting a new job with greater workload demands, or trying to improve performance levels in an upper extremity for a sport, endurance may need to be developed in the upper extremity musculature. Local muscle fatigue has been shown to affect the kinematics of the joints in the shoulder girdle complex.[97] When the ADLs or

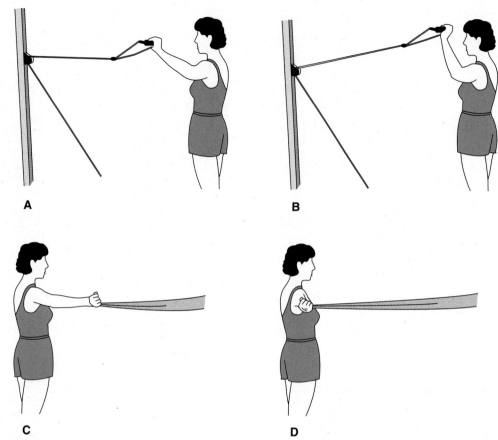

FIGURE 25-14. Plyometric exercise for rotator cuff. (A, B) Starting and ending positions for dynamic plyometric shoulder external rotation (using Impulse Inertial Exercise System). (C, D) Starting and ending positions for dynamic plyometric horizontal abduction using elastic tubing. Monitor the patient to prevent excessive anterior translation of the head of the humerus during horizontal abduction.

instrumental ADLs require more endurance than the muscles possess, endurance must be considered while making decisions about exercise dosage. Chapter 5 provides specific dosage recommendations, but generally, resistance is modified to allow for higher repetitions of a given exercise.

Posture and Movement Impairment

Restoring optimal posture and movement patterns (motor control) to the shoulder girdle complex and the entire upper quadrant (and in many cases, the lower quadrant) should be an integral component of any exercise prescription for the shoulder girdle. Attention to posture and movement patterns is a required component of exercise to remedy-related impairments. The etiology of an overuse injury may be a result of poor structure or function in any of the joints included in the shoulder complex. Additionally, function of the cervical and thoracic spine is important to the maintenance of shoulder girdle complex function. Examination of the structure and function of each of these related regions joints will lead the clinician to the pathomechanics underlying the overuse injury.

Posture

Optimal resting alignment of the shoulder girdle is described in Chapter 9. This alignment facilitates ideal joint positions and resting lengths of the axioscapular, scapulohumeral, and axiohumeral muscles. The resting length of a muscle can be a factor in its participation in active force couples.[24,98] Head, spine, and pelvis alignment additionally affect alignment of the shoulder girdle. For example, forward head, kyphosis, lordosis, and anterior pelvic tilt encourage protracted clavicular position and anterior tilt, and downwardly rotated scapulae.[24] Habitual faulty alignment such as this places the middle and lower trapezius on stretch. Adaptive lengthening can ensue, in turn affecting the length-tension properties of these muscles and thereby affecting their performance in scapular force couples.[49,99]

Optimal alignment of the shoulder girdle complex requires education of habitual cervical, thoracic, and even lumbar and pelvic postures during standing, sitting, and sleeping. Equally important is the education of preferred postural patterns beginning and ending frequently repeated movements. Optimal ergonomics at the workstation (e.g., factory assembly line, desk and chair, kitchen counter, car, baby changing table) are critical to successful postural changes. Support through bracing, taping, and supportive brassieres may be necessary to facilitate the reeducation process and reduce strain on lengthened muscles.

Movement

Restoration of the optimal kinematics during active motion requires knowledge about the kinesiology of the shoulder girdle complex. If the ideal is known, the clinician can devise a program of exercises to remedy the impairments and retrain movements to approach the ideal standard. The goal is to achieve movement as close to the ideal kinematics as possible to enhance the health and longevity of the biomechanical system. The references and reading list at the end of the chapter provide sources for more information about electromyographic or cinematographic analysis of the shoulder girdle during common movement patterns, sport activities, and therapeutic exercises.

THERAPEUTIC EXERCISE INTERVENTIONS FOR COMMON DIAGNOSES

Although comprehensive descriptions and intervention plans for all diagnoses affecting the shoulder girdle are beyond the scope of this book, a few diagnoses are discussed. An overview of the pathogenesis or pathomechanics, examination findings, and proposed treatment plan, with an emphasis on exercise, is provided for each selected diagnosis.

Rotator Cuff Disorders

For the purposes of this text, the broad category of rotator cuff disorders include such medical diagnoses as subacromial impingement syndrome, rotator cuff/glenoid labral tears, posterior shoulder pain, and GH hypermobility/instability. Although each of these classifications merits a separate detailed review of etiology, diagnosis, and treatment concepts, it is beyond the scope of this text to do so. Comprehensive understanding of rotator cuff disorders can be established by means of reviewing the literature sited in this section.

Rotator cuff disorders can be broadly classified as acute or chronic in origin, though acute, avulsive tears of healthy rotator cuff tendons are considered to be rare.[100–102] Most authors believe that rotator cuff tears that appear to be of sudden onset after trauma are extensions of underlying chronic tears or tears of previously degenerated tendons.[100–102]

Two common types of chronic rotator cuff disorders have been described in the literature. One type includes those that can be attributed to mechanical compression of the subacromial structures. Medical diagnoses that are included in this category are primary or external impingement syndrome and bursal surface rotator cuff tears.[103]

The second type includes those disorders that can be attributed to tensile overload of the rotator cuff. Tensile disease is a result of repetitive, intrinsic tension overload. The pathologic changes referred to as "angiofibroblastic hyperplasia" by Nirschl[104] occur in the early stages of tendon injury and can progress to rotator cuff tears from the continued tensile overload.[105] Throwing or racket sport athletes are at high risk for this type of rotator cuff injury because of the high, repetitive eccentric forces incurred by the posterior rotator cuff musculature during the deceleration and follow-through phases of overhead sport activities. Medical diagnoses that are included in this category are internal impingement syndrome and undersurface rotator cuff tears.[106] Tears can be classified as partial or incomplete, complete, or massive.[45] Incomplete tears do not extend through the complete thickness of the tendon. Complete tears extend through the complete thickness of the tendon or muscle. A massive tear indicates more than one rotator cuff tendon or muscle is torn.

Another term, secondary impingement, has been used in the literature to describe a third mechanism of rotator cuff disease. Secondary Impingement by definition implies that there is a problem with keeping the humeral head centered in the glenoid fossa during movement of the arm.[107] Generally is caused by weakness in the rotator cuff (RTC) muscles (functional instability) combined with a GH joint capsule and ligaments that are to loose (micro-instability). The impingement generally occurs at the coracoacromial space secondary to anterior translation of the humeral head as opposed to the subacromial space that is seen in primary impingement. Tearing of the RTC is again extra-articular however intra-articular tearing is also seen in these patients. Patients are typically younger and the pain is located in the anterior or anterolateral aspect of the shoulder. The symptoms are usually activity specific and involve overhand activities. It is important to treat the underlying "micro-instability" in patients with secondary impingement.

Numerous classification systems have emerged in an attempt to logically categorize staging and mechanistic factors of rotator cuff disorders.[46,103,108–110] There is much overlap with these systems, and their terminology is not synonymous; therefore, these systems cannot be used interchangeably to discuss classification of rotator cuff disorders. The literature presents three general categories of rotator cuff disorders: pure impingement in the absence of instability, impingement with instability, and pure instability in the absence of impingement. Table 25-2 presents a modified classification of rotator cuff disorders.

Primary rotator cuff disorders can be further classified into three progressive stages of pathology[111]:

1. Stage I: edema and hemorrhage
2. Stage II: fibrosis and tendinitis
3. Stage III: tendon degeneration and tendon rupture

Because primary rotator cuff disorders have three pathologic stages and may involve the supraspinatus, biceps tendon, subacromial bursa, and AC joint, the presenting activity limitations and impairments can vary greatly. Table 25-3 describes the pathology, presenting and diagnostic signs, impairments, subjective complaints, and activity limitations based on the stage of the disorder.

Stage I can progress to stage II and ultimately to stage III disease if the condition is not appropriately treated. If the condition progresses to stage III, a minor injury to the shoulder (e.g., overuse of the shoulder in raking leaves, loss of balance requiring a sudden upper extremity movement) may advance a degenerative or partial-thickness tear to a full-thickness tear. If this occurs, the individual experiences sudden weakness with diminished ability to raise the arm. For stage III, roentgenograms and arthrograms most often have positive findings of subacromial spurring, calcific deposits, and bursal surface rotator cuff tears.

Posterior shoulder pain, often excluded from most classification systems, is found under secondary impingement with minor instability/hypermobility. The rationale for

TABLE 25-2 A Modified Classification of Rotator Cuff Disorders

	LEVEL OF INSTABILITY	CLINICAL FINDINGS	MEDICAL DIAGNOSIS
Primary impingement	No instability	Older patients (>35 year) Painful arc + Impingement sign – Apprehension sign ± Pain at rest Pain during overhead activity	Primary impingement syndrome Rotator cuff tendinitis Subacromial bursitis Bursal surface rotator cuff tears
Secondary impingement	Minor instability/ hypermobility	Stiffness and slow warm-up Pain during overhead activity + Impingement + Apprehension ± Relocation test	Stable shoulder Early undersurface rotator cuff changes Early labrum changes GH hypermobility Functional instability
	Unidirectional instability (anterior/posterior)	Pain during overhead activity Inability to perform ± Sensation of instability + Apprehension sign + Relocation	Labral lesion undersurface rotator cuff tear Primary instability with secondary impingement
	Multidirectional instability (always inferior)	+ Sulcus	Multidirectional instability Undersurface rotator cuff tear Attenuated but intact labrum
Instability	Posttraumatic instability	+ Impingement sign + Apprehension sign	Glenoid labral damage (Bancart lesion) Humeral head defect (Hill Sacks lesion)

this placement is that researchers suggested,[46,112] and later confirmed both arthroscopically[113–116] and with magnetic resonance imaging,[117] that some of the rotator cuff injuries result from impingement of the inner fibers of the rotator cuff and the fibers of the posterior superior labrum between the greater tuberosity and the posterior superior glenoid. This condition

has been termed "inside (internal) impingement."[46] This mechanism of impingement is not easily identified because the shoulder looks relatively stable and therefore can be easily mistaken for early primary impingement. However, treatment must take into consideration the faults in the kinematics of the ST and GH joints to adequately treat this condition.

TABLE 25-3 Diagnosis of Primary Impingement

STAGE	PATHOLOGY	IMPAIRMENTS	ACTIVITY LIMITATIONS
I	Edema, hemorrhage	1. Pain with impingement test 2. Minimal to no weakness in biceps or supraspinatus 3. Minimal to no decrease in mobility 4. Altered PICR at GH and ST joints	Minimal pain with activity
II	Fibrosis, tendinitis	1. Pain with impingement test 2. Supraspinatus or biceps weak and painful 3. Moderate decrease in mobility at GH joint and probable compensatory motion at ST joint 4. AC joint tenderness	1. Toothache-like pain that disturbs sleep 2. Inability to participate in overhead activity without pain
III	Tendon degeneration or tendon rupture	1. Weakness (depends on pain level and integrity of rotator cuff and biceps) 2. Significant decrease in mobility at GH joint with obvious compensation at ST joint 3. Significant AC joint tenderness	1. Prolonged history of shoulder 2. Minimal pain (complete rotator cuff tear) or severe pain (partial rotator cuff tear) 3. Significant restriction in use of affected upper extremity

AC, acromioclavicular; GH, glenohumeral; PICR, path of instant center of rotation; ST, sternothoracic.
Adapted from Neer CS, Walsh, RP. The shoulder in sports. Orthop Clin North Am 1977;8:583–591.

TABLE 25-4 Etiologic Factors in Rotator Cuff Disorders	
INTRINSIC FACTORS	**EXTRINSIC FACTORS**
Acromial type[92]	GH muscle dysfunction
Degenerative changes in the acromioclavicular[81] joint	Scapulohumeral muscle dysfunction
Vascularity of the rotator cuff	Postural faults
	Capsular stiffness
	Activity type
	Overtraining

Etiologic Factors of Rotator Cuff Disorders

Etiologic factors of rotator cuff disorders are of two basic types: intrinsic or extrinsic. Intrinsic factors are physical characteristics within the subacromial space that predispose an individual to rotator cuff disorders (Table 25-4). Extrinsic factors are conditions or the environment in which an activity takes place that predispose an individual to rotator cuff disorders (Table 25-4).

Because the scapula plays a critical role in controlling the position of the glenoid, relatively small changes in the action of the AS muscles can affect the alignment and forces involved in movement around the GH joint.[24] Athletes with shoulder pathology consistently demonstrate abnormalities in scapular rotator activity, suggesting that motor control is an important factor to consider in extrinsic etiology of rotator cuff disorders.[82,114,118–121] Muscle function has been investigated in healthy shoulders[74,76,82] and in shoulders with GH instability[119,120] or impingement.[82,121] Most authors suggest that alterations exist in muscle activity of the scapular rotators in persons with rotator cuff disorders.

The findings of the study by Wadsworth and Bullock-Saxton[118] indicate that a relationship exists between shoulder injury and the temporal recruitment patterns of the scapular rotators, such that injury reduces the consistency of muscle recruitment. They further suggest that injured subjects have muscle function deficits on their unaffected side, indicative of the possibility that muscle function deficits may predispose athletes to injury. Hence, promotion of motor control of scapular rotators may be an important factor in prevention of rotator cuff disorders.

Muscle dysfunction has also been investigated in the integrated deltoid–rotator cuff mechanism in persons with subacromial impingement.[122] The middle deltoid and rotator cuff muscles were evaluated during isotonic scaption from 30 to 120 degrees. Overall, the impingement group demonstrated decreased mean muscle activity in comparison with the group of normal subjects, particularly in the infraspinatus and subscapularis during the first portion of arm elevation. The inferior force vector is provided by the infraspinatus and subscapularis, thus humeral head depression during the critical first portion of elevation may be insufficient in persons with subacromial impingement.

This body of research suggests that dysfunction in scapular rotator or deltoid-rotator cuff muscle function is present in persons to rotator cuff disorder. Yet, it must be considered that many rotator cuff disorders involve more than one etiologic factor. Consequently, it is critical for the physical therapist to identify *all* intrinsic and extrinsic factors to effectively manage rotator cuff disorders.

Therapeutic Exercise Intervention of Rotator Cuff Disorders

Treatment principles for nonoperative rotator cuff disorders are based on the underlying pathology, presenting impairments, and activity limitations. Treatment for secondary rotator cuff disorders should consider impairments related to hypermobility and instability problems in addition to impingement. A clinical example of rotator cuff disorder is provided in Display 25-5 with general treatment guidelines presented in Display 25-11.

Given that normal muscle activity of the scapula rotators is essential for normal movement of the shoulder girdle,[123–127] the ability to effectively strengthen the serratus anterior and all portions of the trapezius is vital for effective management of rotator cuff disorders (see Display 25-12). EMG analysis of the trapezius and serratus anterior muscles has been performed during therapeutic exercises.[71–73,127–130] Conclusions drawn about activation levels of scapular rotator muscles during specific exercises should be made with caution because of inherent limitations in study design. The EMG data presented in Display 25-13 were derived from studies minimizing common limitations in EMG research. The data presented may assist physical therapists in developing exercise programs that will optimally activate the trapezius and serratus anterior muscles. Because the results of the studies presented were obtained by studying subjects without pathology of the shoulder girdle rather than patients with rotator cuff disorders, caution is warranted in extrapolating these findings to a patient population. Exercises may need to be modified to accommodate a painful shoulder. Display 25-14 summarizes additional exercises for activation of the scapular rotators that are illustrated in this chapter.

Etiologic Factors Contributing to Hypermobility/ Instability of the Glenohumeral Joint

It is not within the scope of this text to discuss diagnoses and treatments of the entire spectrum of GH joint hypermobility/instability, therefore, this section focuses on anterior GH hypermobility leading to GH subluxation (i.e., partial dislocation). Hypermobility and subluxation are difficult to diagnose and terminology can best be understood if joint stability is considered in terms of a continuum of stability (Fig. 25-15).[126] Jobe et al.[46] first described the etiology of secondary rotator cuff disease, or hypermobility, as a continuum (see Display 25-15).

In the absence of trauma, the etiology of GH hypermobility is a circular cause and consequence scenario. Whether the cause or consequence, one should consider that habitual impairments in posture and repetitive movement patterns can result in microtrauma to static and dynamic stabilizers and dysfunction in the relationship between the GH, AC, and SC joints. Attenuation of the static and dynamic stabilizers contributes to mild hypermobility, increasing the demand on the stabilizing function of the rotator cuff. This may lead to a vicious cycle of excessive

DISPLAY 25-11
Treatment for Primary Rotator Cuff Disorder

First Aid

During the early stages, easy self-management measures can assist in decreasing inflammation and pain and promoting early healing.

- Medications: Nonsteroidal antiinflammatory medications may be prescribed by the physician to assist in reducing inflammation to the acromial and subacromial tissues.
- Rest: The patient avoids postures or movements that trigger pain and inflammation. This may require absolute restriction of overhead activity, reduced activity, or modification of the technique used during overhead activity.
- Resting position: This position provides the greatest amount of volume in the shoulder joint, assisting in blood flow and decreasing pain. The patient should use pillows to support the arm in slight elevation, abduction, and neutral rotation while sitting, driving, or sleeping. The patient should avoid sleeping on the involved side. If sleeping on the uninvolved side, pillows should be used to support the shoulder as described.
- Ice: Ice can reduce inflammation and relieve pain. Choices include cold packs, bags of chipped ice, or ice massage. Ice should be applied directly to the affected tissues. This may require special positioning to expose the affected tissues.[15]

Supervised Treatment

After a thorough examination and evaluation, a plan of care is developed based on the presenting activity limitations and related impairments.

- Pain and inflammation: In addition to instructing the patient in first aid self-management, the physical therapist can use physical agents such as ultrasound, phonophoresis, or interferential stimulation.
- ROM, muscle length, joint mobility: Exercise and joint mobilization can be prescribed to increase mobility in periarticular tissues and improve muscle extensibility. Education and exercise can be prescribed to normalize length-tension properties of adaptively shortened and lengthened muscles.
- Muscle performance: Exercise can be prescribed to improve force or torque capability, length-tension properties, and endurance of the rotator cuff and scapular upward rotators. Dosage parameters should be adjusted according to the goal of the exercise as outlined in Chapter 2.
- Posture and movement: For the tissue to heal and to prevent recurrence, the mechanical causes of the impingement must be eliminated. During the early phases of intervention, posture and movement must be addressed to the greatest possible extent given the presenting impairments in force or torque, endurance, and mobility. After the physiologic capabilities have improved, long-term management requires specific training in posture and movement habits, and underlying motor control of the integrated function of the scapular rotators and deltoid–rotator cuff mechanism, to eliminate the mechanical cause of impingement during function. This should including ergonomic modifications, specific movement retraining during ADLs and instrumental ADLs, and alterations in athletic training techniques.

Surgery

If supervised treatment fails, surgery to remove subacromial spurring and increase space for the subacromial tissues may be necessary. Surgery should be considered only when symptoms have persisted despite conservative treatment for more than 1 year. Anterior acromioplasty is the recommended choice for decompression of the rotator cuff in primary impingement.[109] The posterior half of the acromion is not involved in the impingement process and, therefore, lateral or complete acromionectomy is thought to weaken the deltoid unnecessarily. In many cases, repair of the rotator cuff is necessary.

Prevention

Prevention lies in early recognition and prompt and comprehensive treatment of the presenting activity limitations and related intrinsic and extrinsic impairments, particularly those related to motor control of the scapula rotators and deltoid–rotator cuff mechanism.

DISPLAY 25-12
Specific Therapeutic Exercise Intervention for Rotator Cuff Disorder

Pain and inflammation

Short-term resolution as described under "First Aid" in Display 25-11. Long-term resolution requires addressing the remaining impairments.

Muscle length

- Passive manual stretch to rhomboids (see Fig. 25-2)
- Self-stretch to GH lateral rotators (see Self-Management 25-4)

Muscle Performance

- Strengthen middle and lower trapezius in a short range (see Self-Management 25-2)
- Strengthen serratus anterior in the short range (see Self-Management 25-3)
- Strengthen rotator cuff (see Self-Management 25-1)

Posture and movement

- Ergonomic modifications at visual display terminal (VDT) workstation
- Transitional exercises to improve kinematics of GH and ST joints in elevation (see Fig. 25-3)
- Surface EMG training during simple elevation movements to restore temporal relationships in scapular rotators
- Functional retraining for ADLs with focus on motor control and integrated scapula and deltoid–rotator cuff function
- Functional retraining for instrumental ADLs (sports and recreation) with focus on motor control and integrated scapula– and deltoid–rotator cuff function
- Alter sport-specific training as needed to promote optimal motor control and biomechanics

DISPLAY 25-13
Activation Exercises for Trapezius and Serratus Anterior Based on EMG Analysis

Exercises for Upper Trapezius

- Shoulder shrug (Fig. 1)[72,73]

Exercises for Middle Trapezius

- Prone arm lift with arm overhead (Self-Management 25-2: Facelying Arm Lifts, Level IV B)[72,74]
- Prone horizontal extension with lateral rotation (Self-Management 25-2: Facelying Arm Lifts, Level IV A)

Exercises for Lower Trapezius

- Prone arm lift with arm overhead (Self-Management 25-2: Facelying Arm Lifts, Level IV B)[72]
- Prone shoulder lateral rotation at 90-degree abduction (Self-Management 25-1: Facelying Shoulder Rotation)[72,130]
- Prone horizontal extension with lateral rotation (Self-Management 25-2: Facelying Arm Lifts, Level IV A)[72,73]

Exercises for Serratus Anterior

- NOTE: In general, exercises that create upward rotation of the scapula were found to produce much more EMG activity in the serratus anterior than straight scapular protraction exercises.[71-73]
- Shoulder abduction in the plane of the scapula (Fig. 25-8 on Web site) above 120 degrees (Display 25-9)[72,74]

- Diagonal exercise with a combination of flexion, horizontal flexion, and external rotation (Table 15-1)[72]

Exercises for simultaneous activation of the trapezius and serratus anterior

- Prone arm lift with arm overhead (Self-Management 25-2: Facelying Arm Lifts, Level IV B)[72]
- Shoulder abduction in the plane of the scapula (Fig. 25-8 on Web site)[72]

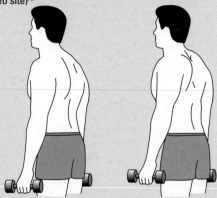

FIGURE 1. Shoulder shrug.

DISPLAY 25-14
Additional Exercises Designed for Isolation of Scapular Rotator Muscles

Exercises for Upper Trapezius
- Upper trapezius strengthening (Fig. 25-5)

Exercises for Middle and Lower Trapezius Activation
- Facelying arm lifts (Self-Management 25-2)
- Wall slides (Fig. 25-3)

- Back-to-wall arm slides in abduction (Fig. 1)
- Isometric scapula upward rotation (Fig. 2)

Exercises for Serratus Anterior
- Serratus anterior progression (Self-Management 25-3)
- Progressive serratus strengthening exercises (Fig. 25-8, 25-9, 25-10)

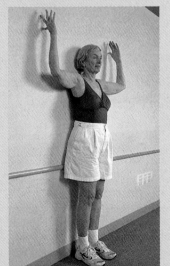

FIGURE 1. Back to wall, arm slides in abduction. With the back to the wall, the elbows and humerus should be in the scapular plane. Thumbs can touch the wall to ensure that the humerus remains in the scapular plane. The patient slides the arms up the wall, and stops when the scapula deviates from the PICR (i.e., excessive elevation). The goal is to achieve full scapular plane elevation with the ideal PICR at the glenohumeral and ST joints.

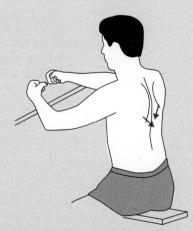

FIGURE 2. Alternative isometric scapular upward rotation. The arms can be positioned in as much elevation as is available. The cue should be to "gently squeeze your shoulder blades together." Caution should be taken to prevent excessive rhomboid or latissimus dorsi contribution.

Stable ——————————————————————————————→ Unstable

| **Normal** | **Lax/Hypermobile** | **Subluxed** | **Dislocated** |
| Normal congruity and loading | Congruity maintained, but joint is unloaded | Partial contact of articular surfaces—congruity lost. | No contact of articular surfaces—congruity lost. |

FIGURE 25-15. Continuum of shoulder stability. (Adapted from Strauss MB, Wrobel LJ, Neff RS, Cady GW. The shrugged-off shoulder: a comparison of patients with recurrent shoulder subluxations and dislocations. Physician Sports Med 1983;11:96.)

translation of the humeral head, mechanical impingement, and attenuation of the subacromial structures.[92,93,101,131] Left unchecked, mild hypermobility can progress to subluxation and dislocation.

GH stability is achieved through a number of different mechanisms, involving the articular geometry, the static capsuloligamentous complex (CLC), the dynamic (muscular) stabilizers, and neuromuscular control.[110] The specific contributions of the shoulder musculature to joint stability are listed in Display 25-16.[123,132–136]

Diagnosis of Hypermobility/Instability
Early diagnosis and treatment of GH hypermobility can prevent serious pathology resulting from dislocation or impingement. However, mild GH hypermobility is difficult to diagnose, because the "microinstability" of the humeral head occurs during active movement without the signs or symptoms associated with subluxation or instability (i.e., positive apprehension or relocation signs). Excessive passive joint mobility in specific directions combined with displaced kinematics of the GH joint during active arm elevation or GH rotation confirm the diagnosis of hypermobility. The most common abnormal GH motions are excessive superior translation during arm elevation, excessive anterior translation during lateral rotation and arm horizontal abduction (also called hyperangulation),[141] and abnormal anterior translation during medial rotation. Excessive translation can be confirmed by palpating the humeral head during active motions and comparing the motion to that on the unaffected side.

The diagnosis of unidirectional instability or multidirectional instability is based on complaints of pain and activity limitation combined with positive apprehension, relocation, and or sulcus signs.[142,143]

Treatment for Glenohumeral Hypermobility/Instability
Treatment of hypermobility and any hypomobility should occur simultaneously. For example, a common examination finding for the anterior hypermobile or subluxating shoulder is posterior capsular stiffness (indicated by restricted GH MR ROM and restricted posterior glide of the humeral head in the glenoid fossa) and possibly a coexisting anteriorly displaced humerus at rest. The stiffness of the posterior capsule can restrict posterior translation of the humeral head, occurring primarily during the osteokinematic motions of medial rotation and flexion and causing an abnormal anterior translation during these osteokinematic motions. The posterior capsular stiffness can also contribute to an anteriorly displaced rest position of the humeral head. With the head of the humerus in an anteriorly displaced position at rest,

---

DISPLAY 25-15
Jobe's Instability Continuum[46]

1. RTC weakness generally occurs first.
2. Functional instability follows prolonged RTC weakness.
3. Capsular laxity, which develops (acquired) or becomes prominent (preexisting congenital laxity).
4. Subluxation (inability of the humeral head to center in the glenoid during motion).
5. RTC/Labral tearing (late stage disease of secondary impingement).

DISPLAY 25-16
Contribution of the Shoulder Musculature to Joint Stability

- Passive muscle tension from the bulk effect of the rotator cuff muscle
- Rotator cuff contraction causing compression of the articular surfaces
- Joint motion that secondarily tightens the passive ligamentous constraints
- Barrier or restrain effect of the contracted rotator cuff muscle
- Redirection of the joint force to the center of the glenoid surface by coordination of muscle forces from both GH and ST joints
- ST muscle balance
  - Efficient compressive forces on the rotator cuff are partially dependent upon the stability of their origins on the scapula[137]
  - Scapular position affects length-tension properties of the rotator cuff
  - Scapula upward rotation, posterior tilt, and lateral rotation is necessary to maximize subacromial space[138–140]

it is more vulnerable to moving into an excessive anterior translation during lateral rotation and abduction. Specific joint mobilization of the posterior capsule combined with passive self-stretching of the GH lateral rotators is the best treatment for the hypomobility (see Self-Management 26-4: Glenohumeral Hypermobility).

As passive mobility is restored, the restoration of precise active mobility must closely follow. The GH joint needs to be trained to move in a precise kinematic pattern without abnormal or excessive anterior translations. This often must occur in conjunction with restoring the normal kinematics of the ST joint (explained later in this section). The subluxating shoulder may require a period of immobilization to allow stiffening of lax structures. Abduction and lateral rotation positions must be avoided to prevent stretching of the anterior capsule. The immobilization period should last no longer than 3 weeks, and pain-free isometric exercises for the scapulohumeral and axioscapular muscles should begin as soon as tolerated to avoid the disuse or deconditioning effects of prolonged immobilization.

Active ROM exercises can be initiated against gravity as the patient regains strength and motor control. Abnormal movement patterns, such as excessive scapular elevation, should be discouraged.

Gradually, resistive exercises can be initiated targeting the pectoralis major, latissimus dorsi, teres major, and subscapularis to provide dynamic restraint to anterior translation into the anterior capsule. However, the main target muscle should be the subscapularis because of its insertion anterior to the GH joint and its proximity to the axis of rotation of the GH joint. Careful observation of the humeral head path of instant center of rotation (PICR) during medial rotation is a good indicator of the participation of the subscapularis in the medial rotation force couple. Anterior translation of the humerus should not take place during medial rotation because it is a sign of insufficient subscapularis participation. In addition, proper scapular stabilization by the serratus anterior and lower trapezius shoulde be encourage to prevent anteiror scapular tilt. Exercises should be prescribed to isolate subscapularis function as much as possible (see Self-Management 25-6).

Infraspinatus and teres minor strengthening can also be targeted to prevent excessive anterior translation of the head of the humerus.[144] For the infraspinatus and teres minor to provide a stabilizing force on the GH joint, stability of the ST joint is a prerequisite. If the scapula is not stabilized by the axioscapular muscles, when the infraspinatus and teres minor contract, instead of providing a posterior force to the GH joint, contraction of the infraspinatus and teres minor can contribute to further anterior displacement. This occurs by reverse action on the scapula; instead of compressing the GH joint into the glenoid fossa, the resultant force pulls the scapula toward the humerus (scapula internal rotation) and forces the head of the humerus anteriorly. During any lateral rotation exercise, care must be taken to ensure that internal rotation at the AC joint is prevented by encouraging serratus anterior, middle, lower trapezius and rhomboid activity and that lateral rotation occurs at the GH joint without excessive anterior translation.

Isokinetic or plyometric upper extremity exercises (see Fig. 25-14) can be incorporated into the resistive training program of individuals returning to a high level of function. Again, it is recommended that the clinician closely monitors

proper stabilization of the scapula during resisted movements of at the GH joint.

If the kinematics are closely monitored, movements into full lateral rotation and abduction should not be contraindicated. If excessive anterior translation occurs because of lack of force-generating capability from the axioscapular or rotator cuff muscles and poor motor control, extremes of ROM should be avoided.

Sport-specific exercises can be gradually incorporated into the treatment program to prepare the patient for transition to functional activity (Fig. 25-16). Attention to the kinematics of the GH joint is the guide to progression. Control over the translatory motions of the GH joint should be emphasized over general strength gains.

The literature supports the notion that motor control is critical in restoring function to the unstable shoulder.[145-148] Research indicates that peak torque gains occur in persons trained with EMG biofeedback in purely functional patterns with no emphasis on "strength exercising." Functional gains and abolition of pain was greater and occurred earlier in the group trained functionally with EMG biofeedback than the group trained in more traditional strength regimens.[145]

Treatment Principles for Postoperative Rotator Cuff Disorders

Tears of the rotator cuff can be managed with non-steroidal anti-inflammatory drugs, intra-articular or subacromial glucocorticosteroid injection, oral glucocorticosteroid treatment, physical therapy, and open or arthroscopic surgery. To date, there is little evidence to support or refute the efficacy of common interventions for tears of rotator cuff in adults.[149] Rowe[150] stated, "the majority of rotator cuff lesions should respond satisfactorily to conservative measures," noting two exceptions: the young adult with a documented full-thickness tear and an elderly patient with a full-thickness

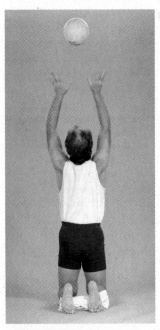

FIGURE 25-16. Sport-specific exercise for someone with glenohumeral hypermobility: ball tossing upward to simulate a set in volleyball.

tear with disabling pain unresponsive to conservative treatment. Additional investigators have stressed the importance of initial nonoperative management of rotator cuff tears.[111,151–154] According to Mantone et al.,[155] there are several instances in which nonoperative treatment would not be indicated. The first is the 20- to 30-year-old active patient with an acute tear and severe functional deficit from a specific event. The second is the 30- to 50-year-old patient with an acute rotator cuff tear secondary to a specific event. These patients are best treated with early operative intervention. The third instance is the highly competitive athlete, particularly one who is involved in overhead or throwing sports. These patients need to be treated operatively because rotator cuff repair is necessary for restoration of the normal strength required to return these athletes to the same competitive preoperative level of function. Patients who do not respond to conservative treatment may require operative intervention. Based upon the review of 14 trials in a Cochrane Database of Systematic Reviews for surgical repair for rotator cuff tears, no firm conclusions about the effectiveness or safety of surgery for rotator cuff disease could be made.[156] There is "Silver" level evidence from six trials that there are no significant differences in outcome between arthroscopic and open subacromial decompression, although four trials reported earlier recovery with arthroscopic decompression.[156]

If surgery is performed, the postoperative exercise regimen after anterior acromioplasty and repair of the rotator cuff is determined by the strength of the rotator cuff. Methodical planning and cooperation by the patient, surgeon, and physical therapist are necessary to plan a program with a successful outcome. The patient will have greater confidence if clear objectives are developed. Preoperatively, the surgeon and physical therapist should explain to the patient that it will take up to 12 months for mature healing of the tendons. However, during this time, activities will be progressively advanced, and strict adherence to the physical therapist's instructions will ensure the most successful outcome. The physical therapist must understand the specific anatomic considerations and limitations to plan a safe and effective postoperative rehabilitation program. Only the surgeon knows the strength and stability of the repair and therefore should work closely with the physical therapist in developing the aftercare program of each patient.

The algorithm shown in Display 25-17 provides guidance for rehabilitation after a standard rotator cuff repair.[45] Because of the unique anatomic arrangement and function of the rotator cuff, rehabilitation after surgery is considered to be more difficult than that of any other joint. In most patients, the muscles involved in the precisely integrated force couples used in upper extremity movements have suffered from months of atrophy and disuse. Early in the rehabilitation process, careful exercises may be prescribed to prevent significant atrophy of key scapular muscles that perform upward rotation, posterior tilt, and/or external rotation functions (Fig. 2 in Display 25-14). Toward the latter stages of rehabilitation, precise integration and coordination of motor control must be restored to all the muscles involved in the functional movements used by the individual. Postoperative care after repair for a massive rotator cuff tear is far more conservative, requiring longer periods of immobilization and slower return to function.

Often repair of a torn rotator cuff effectively improves comfort, active motion, and strength in most patients. According to Romeo et al.,[157] female patients 66 years of age and older are more likely to have an unsatisfactory result. In addition, an associated biceps tear in female patients is a poor prognostic factor.[157] Overall, better results are seen in patients with less that 5 cm^2 tear, and in patients with an intact biceps tendon.[157] At an average of 54 months after open rotator cuff repair and acromioplasty, 94% of patients were satisfied and stated they were better because of the surgery to repair their torn rotator cuff.[157]

Adhesive Capsulitis

Adhesive capsulitis, or frozen shoulder describes a condition characterized by painful and limited passive and active ROM. Factors associated with adhesive capsulitis include female gender,[158] older than 40 years,[158] trauma,[159] diabetes,[160] prolonged immobilization,[161] thyroid disease,[162] stroke or myocardial infarction,[163,164] and the presence of autoimmune diseases.[165] The prevalence of adhesive capsulitis in the general population is slightly >2%,[166] increasing to 10% to 38% in patients with diabetes and thyroid disease.[167,168] Seventy percent of patients with adhesive capsulitis are women, and 20% to 30% of those affected subsequently develop adhesive capsulitis in the opposite shoulder.[169]

Lundberg[170] first described a classification system identifying primary adhesive capsulitis as idiopathic and secondary adhesive capsulitis as posttraumatic. Zuckerman[171] went on to further classify secondary adhesive capsulitis into three subcategories: systemic, extrinsic, and intrinsic (Fig. 25-17)

In primary adhesive capsulitis, an insidious onset of pain causes the individual to gradually limit the use of the arm. Inflammation and pain can cause reflex inhibition of the shoulder muscles, similar to inhibition of the quadriceps after injury to the knee. There is disagreement in the literature as to whether the underlying pathologic process is an inflammatory condition[172–174] or a fibrosing condition.[175] Significant evidence exists[174,176–178] in support of the hypothesis that the underlying pathologic changes in adhesive capsulitis are synovial inflammation with subsequent reactive capsular fibrosis.

Diagnosis

Adhesive capsulitis has been staged based upon arthroscopic findings as described in Table 26-5).[179,180] These stages represent a continuum of the disease rather than discrete well-defined stages. The course associated with adhesive capsulitis typically lasts from 1 to 3 years.[161,181] There is a relationship of the length of each stage to the length of the remaining stages in that the shorter the initial inflammatory component, the shorter the second and third stages and overall course of the condition. Thus, early intervention can reduce the overall duration of the condition. The role of the physical therapist is to hasten the progression through the stages and limit the severity of the earlier stages so that the patient can move to the final stages as quickly as possible with the least amount of impairment, activity limitation, and participation restrictions.

Treatment

Neviaser and Neviaser[179,180] stress the importance of an individualized treatment plan based upon the stage of the disease. Patient-related instruction is a critical component in educating the patient as to the stage and progression of the

DISPLAY 25-17
Rehabilitation After Rotator Cuff Repair

This protocol is a guideline only; actual progression will be based on clinical presentation

Protective Phase (1 to 4 weeks)

- Sling protection is used for 2 to 3 days and up to 6 weeks at night.
- Pendulum exercises (see Fig. 25-7) are initiated within the first 48 hours and should be performed three times a day.
- Self-assisted ROM exercises are initiated at the end of the first week (A, B, and C).

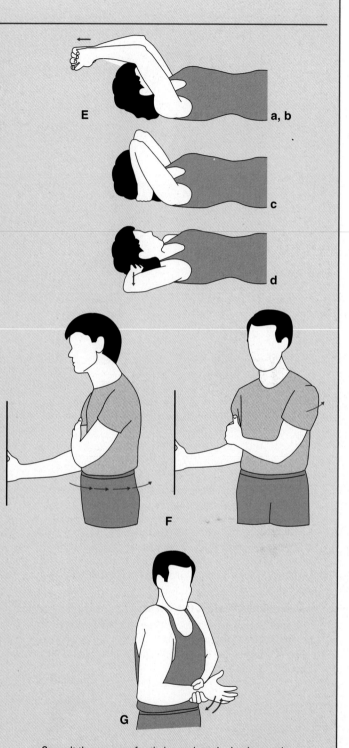

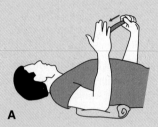

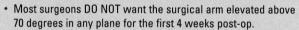

- Most surgeons DO NOT want the surgical arm elevated above 70 degrees in any plane for the first 4 weeks post-op.
- Gentle isometric exercise may be introduced as early as 1 week post op, but is highly dependent on the extent of the surgery (G–J).

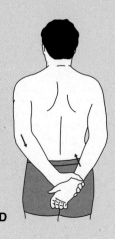

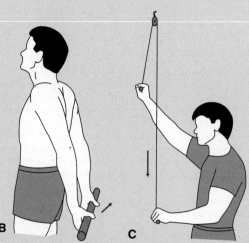

- Consult the surgeon for timing on introducing isometrics.
- Scapular pinches every hour with good upright posture.
- Maintain good upright shoulder girdle posture at all times—especially during sling use.

Early Intermediate Phase (4 to 8 weeks)

- Additional self-assisted ROM exercises are prescribed 6 weeks after surgery (D, E, F).

(continued)

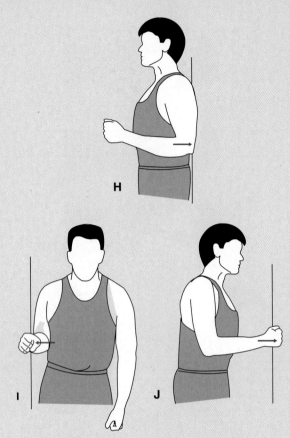

- If motion is restricted at this time, gentle passive stretching by the physical therapist is indicated.
- Mobilization of GH, SC, AC joints as needed to restore joint mobility (this may be started earlier if needed).
- ROM goals should be up to 90 degrees of flexion and abduction without excessive clavicular elevation.
- Isometric exericse is progressed to active ROM as patients symptoms permit (K and L)

Late Intermediate Phase (8 to 12 weeks)

- ROM goals should be full ROM in all planes, flexion, abduction, external rotation, internal rotation.
- Continued mobilization of GH, SC, AC joints as needed to fully restore joint mobility

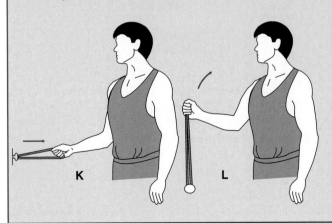

- Light resistance with resistive tubing is added to dynamic exercise for flexion, extension, ER, IR
- More aggressive exercise for serratus anterior and trapezius (Display 25-13) are introduced.

Advanced Rehabilitation Phase (12 weeks and beyond)

- A more aggressive rotator cuff strengthening program is introduced (Self-Management 25-1)
- Add weights to all exercises as tolerated.
- Continue to seek full ROM in all planes with attention to motor control and scapulohumeral rhythm.
- Swimming is allowed at 5 months after surgery.
- Submaximal sport-specific training is progressed to maximal training by the end of 1 year after surgery.

General Precautions and Contraindications

- Flexion should precede abduction when restoring active motion.
- The patient should avoid leaning on the arm or carrying more than 5 lb of weight in the early and intermediate phases of rehabilitation.
- Patients with complete tears of the supraspinatus should avoid lifting more than 15 lb in the first year postoperatively.
- Skiing, skating, roller-blading, and other such activities are forbidden in the first year after surgery to avoid reinjury from a fall.

(A) Assisted lateral rotation in supine. A towel is placed under the elbow to keep the humerus in neutral and prevent excessive anterior displacement. The patient pushes the involved arm into lateral rotation, using the uninvolved arm to supply the power. (B) Assisted extension. The patient pushes backward into extension, using the uninvolved arm to supply the power. Caution should be used to prevent excessive GH extension and anterior displacement of the GH joint. (C) Pulley-assisted elevation in both flexion and scaption planes. The uninvolved arm supplies the power to raise the involved arm. Caution should be used to prevent excessive scapular elevation as compensation for lack of GH mobility. The motion should be stopped as soon as a deviation in the path of instant center of rotation of the GH or ST joint is noted. This exercise can be progressed to active assisted elevation when directed by the physician. (D) Assisted medial rotation. The patient is instructed to medially rotate the arm by pushing the arm backward, followed by pulling the hand upward toward the scapula. Caution should be used to prevent excessive scapular anterior tilt and GH anterior displacement. (E) Assisted abduction. The patient is instructed to (a) lie on the back, (b) lock the fingers together and stretch the arms overhead (the uninvolved arm powers the involved arm), (c) bring the hands behind the neck, and (d) flatten the elbows (reverse by sliding the hands overhead and down). Caution should be taken while abducting to ensure the scapulae are in a neutral position and the clavicle retracts as the arm abducts. (F) Assisted lateral rotation in a doorway. The patient is instructed to stand in a doorway facing the door frame. The elbow is flexed to 90 degrees. The palm is on wall. The elbow is held in adduction. The body turns gradually until the patient faces into the room. Caution should be taken to ensure proper scapular alignment during the lateral rotation process. (G) Isometric medial and lateral rotation. (H) Isometric extension. (I) Isometric abduction. (J) Isometric flexion. (K) Resistive exercise for shoulder extensors. Caution should be taken to prevent thoracic flexion or scapular anterior tilt. The range should be limited to extension to the midaxillary line to prevent contractions of the rhomboid in the short range. (L) Resistive exercise for shoulder flexion. The motion is upward into flexion as if throwing an "upper cut" punch. Caution should be taken to monitor the ST kinematics.

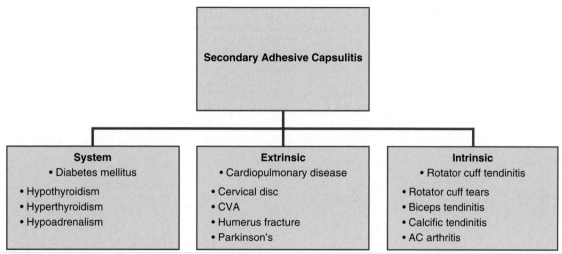

FIGURE 25-17. Secondary adhesive capsulitis categories.

condition and the necessary commitment to self management for the best outcome. The use of therapeutic exercise has been shown to be a common and effective component of intervention used for adhesive capsulitis.[163,182–186] The determination of the type and intensity of exercise depends on the patient's specific strength, ROM, joint mobility, motor control needs, and level of irritability. Kelley et al.[187] propose an irritability classification to assist the practitioner in clinical decisions regarding intervention.

Nonoperative Interventions   The best approach to adhesive capsulitis is prevention. Although this syndrome is considered a self-limited process, complete recovery with no residual limitation and disability is neither ensured nor common. Fibrosis, secondary arthritis, myofascial contracture, disuse atrophy, and altered motor control patterns may be permanent. Only active

use of the arm and full maintenance of GH and ST active mobility with precise shoulder kinematics at all three shoulder girdle articulations can reverse these changes.

Table 25-6 outlines basic interventions for each stage of adhesive capsulitis.

Stage 1.   Patient-related instruction about the natural history of frozen shoulder is important to allay the patient's fears of more serious disease. Discussing how the painful synovitis progresses to fibroplasia and motion restriction prepares the patient for an extended recovery Instruction in compliance with a self management program is vital to positive long term outcomes.

Patients who present with painful limitation of motion are recommended to be given oral nonsteroidal anti-inflammatory medications that are supplemented with other analgesics as necessary.[188–190] An intra-articular injection of steroid and

TABLE 25-5	Adhesive Capsulitis Stages Based on Arthroscopic Findings
STAGE	**FINDINGS**
Stage 1	• Duration of symptoms is 0–3 months • Pain with active and passive ROM • Examination under anesthesia: normal or minimal loss of ROM • Arthroscopy: diffuse GH synovitis, most pronounced in anterosuperior capsule • Pathologic changes: hypertrophic, hypervascular synovitis, rare inflammatory cell infiltrates, normal underlying capsule
Stage 2: Freezing stage	• Duration of symptoms: 3–9 months • Patient presents with continued pain • Severe loss of ROM in all planes • Examination under anesthesia: ROM same as without anesthesia • Arthroscopy: dense, proliferative, hypervascular synovitis. • Pathologic changes: hypertrophic, hypervascular synovitis with perivascular and subsynovial scar, fibroplasias and scar formation in the underlying capsule • Duration of symptoms 5–9 months
Stage 3: Frozen stage	• Continued severe loss of ROM with minimal pain • Examination under anesthesia: same as Stage 2 • Arthroscopy: No hypervascularity seen, remnants of fibrotic synovium can be seen. The capsule feels thick in insertion of the arthroscope and there is diminished capsule volume • Pathologic changes: "burned out" synovitis without significant hypertrophy or hypervascularity. Underlying capsule shows dense scar formation • Duration of symptoms: 15–24 months
Stage 4: Thawing stage	• Minimal pain • Progressive improvement in ROM

TABLE 25-6 Physical Therapy Intervention During Stages 1 to 4 Adhesive Capsulitis

STAGE/GOAL	PRI	MODALITIES	STRENGTHENING	STRETCHING AND ROM	JOINT MOBILIZATION
Stage 1 Goal: interrupt pain and inflammation promote relaxation	Educate (pathogenesis, posture, activity modification)	As needed to control pain, inflammation, and promote relaxation	Early closed chain exercises (i.e., wall slides)	AAROM in pain-free ROM, aquatic exercise gentle PROM, pendulum exercise	Grade I and II mobilizations
Stage 2 Goal: minimize pain, inflammation, capsular adhesions, and restriction of ROM	Posture, necessity for HEP	As needed to decrease pain and inflammation and improve tissue extensibility	More advanced scapular training, specific rotator cuff strengthening	AROM, PROM	Grade II and III mobilizations
Stages 3 and 4 Goal: Increase ROM	Posture, necessity for HEP	To promote relaxation, tissue extensibility and reduce treatment discomfo rt	More specific scapular training to reestablish force couples, continued rotator cuff strengthening	More specific AROM to reestablish scapular and GH mechanics; more aggressive stretching (PNF, STM, low load prolonged stretch)	Grades III and IV

AAROM, active assisted range of motion; AROM, active range of motion; PROM, passive range of motion; HEP, home exercise program; PNF, proprioceptive neuromuscular facilitation; STM, soft-tissue mobilization.

local analgesic can be extremely useful both in the diagnosis and treatment of adhesive capsulitis.[191–195] After injection, passive GH ROM is reevaluated. If the patient has significant decrease in pain and increased ROM, the diagnosis of stage 1 is confirmed. If, however, pain is improved, but ROM has not changed significantly, the diagnosis of stage 2 is confirmed.

Patients should also be started on a supervised physical program to restore function by decreasing the pain and inflammatory response, increasing ROM, improving muscle performance, and reestablishing normal shoulder mechanics. The primary goal of treatment of patients with stage 1 adhesive capsulitis is to interrupt the cycle of pain and inflammation.

Though little data exists to support the use of therapeutic modalities, modalities are suggested to influence pain (high-voltage galvanic stimulation, transcutaneous electrical stimulation,[190] iontophoresis, cryotherapy), reduce inflammation (iontophoresis, phonophoresis, cryotherapy), and to promote relaxation (moist heat, ultrasound).[196] Hydrotherapy can also be effectively used to break the cycle of pain (see Chapter 16).[197]

Applying the correct tensile stress to the tissues is based upon the patient's irritability (see Table 25-7). In patients with high irritability, such as the case in Stage 1, low intensity and short duration joint mobilizations are performed to alter the joint receptors' input, reduce pain, decrease muscle guarding, and increase motion.[198] Grade I and II joint mobilizations and physiologic movements (active assisted ROM) within a pain-free ROM can be used at this stage (see Chapter 7).[199]

Closed chain exercises can be performed to promote the rotator cuff function of GH stabilization (i.e., wall slides),[200] and improve extensibility of the affected muscles, capsule, and ligaments. Stretching should be done in painfree range and may be held from 1 to 5 seconds, two to three times a day. Scapular stabilization exercises can be modified to allow the patient to activate the scapular muscles in pain-free positions (see Fig. 25-20; Self-Management 25-3, level 1, can be modified with more pillows to allow the patient to work in less extreme range of upper extremity elevation). This type of exercise should be initiated as early as possible to promote

TABLE 25-7 Irritability Classification

HIGH IRRITABILITY	MODERATE IRRITABILITY	LOW IRRITABILITY
High pain (≥7/10)	Moderate pain (4–6/10)	Low pain (≤3/10)
Consistent night or resting pain	Intermittent night or resting pain	No resting or night pain
Pain prior to end ROM	Pain at end ROM	Minimal pain at end ROM with overpressure
AROM less than PROM secondary to pain	AROM similar to PROM	AROM same as PROM

Modified from: Kelley MJ, McClure PW, Leggin BG. Frozen shoulder: evidence and a proposed model guiding rehabilitation. J Orthop Sports Phys Ther 2009;39:135–148.

GH stability and optimal ST force couple recruitment. Scapula taping (see "Adjunctive Interventions: Taping") can be used to help promote scapula stability and GH mobility. The home exercise program should include passive ROM exercises in *pain-free* ROM and pendulum exercises to promote capsular stretch (Fig. 25-7).

Postural training is incorporated to discourage forward head and thoracic kyphosis, which places the scapula in anterior tilt, internal rotation, and clavicular protraction.

Stage 2. The continuum of symptoms presenting in this stage may include pain in the paracervical and periscapular region as a result of compensatory scapula elevation. At this stage, the individual may learn to use ST, elbow, or trunk motions to substitute for lost GH motions.[57] "Hiking" of the shoulder girdle is evident during elevation of the arm as a result of capsular stiffness and rotator cuff weakness disallowing normal GH mechanics.[57] Anterior translation of the humeral head may result from a decrease in capsular volume.[201] The limitation of ROM is in a capsular pattern with lateral rotation the most limited, followed by abduction, then medial rotation.[202]

The goal of the second phase of rehabilitation is to continue to decrease inflammation and pain, and to minimize capsular restriction and secondary weakness of the rotator cuff and scapular upward rotator force couple. Passive joint mobilizations are used to stretch the CLC to allow normal GH mechanics. Contracture of the rotator cuff interval (RCI) has been shown in patients with adhesive capsulitis.[203-205] The RCI forms the triangular-shaped tissue between the anterior supraspinatous tendon edge and the upper subscapularis border, and includes the superior GH ligament and the coracohumeral ligament. Stretching, soft tissue and joint mobilization should target the RCI and the CLC. It has been proposed that an inferior glide with the arm at the side, while in external rotation, stretches the RCI.[206]

Johnson et al.[207] found significant improvement in external rotation ROM in patients with adhesive capsulitis after performing posterior glide mobilizations for 1 minute at end range of abduction and external rotation. High-grade mobilizations (Grade III and IV) are used to promote elongation of shortened fibrotic soft tissues. High-grade mobilizations should be performed with the joint positioned at or near its physiologic end range. It should be noted that immediate gains with mobilization represent transient tissue preconditioning and must be followed up with a self management program.[208,215] Stretching passively or with hold-relax techniques to the posterior capsule can be addressed with a home exercise as shown in Self-Management 25-4.

Once passive motion is improved, it must be followed with active exercises to maintain the ROM. If strength is fair or above, active exercises against gravity can be introduced in sagittal, frontal, and the plane of the scapula. The therapist must pay careful attention to ensure restoring motor control patterns to promote 3-D scapular kinematics (versus elevation or excessive upward rotation) and control over GH superior glide.[57] Careful isolated strengthening of the rotator cuff, serratus anterior, middle and lower trapezius is indicated (see Self-Managements 25-1, 25-2, and 25-3).

Taping the ST joint can significantly help to limit scapular substitution patterns and force greater mobility at the GH joint during functional activity (see "Adjunctive Interventions: Taping" section).[209] Taping the ST joint may transfer

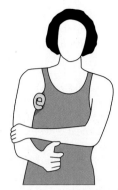

FIGURE 25-18. Self-mobilization of the glenohumeral joint into lateral distraction.

improvements made in mobility and force or torque production with specific exercise to ADLs and instrumental ADLs, including specific movement patterns necessary for sport.

Stages 3 and 4. At these stages, pain may resolve spontaneously.[210] Physical examination will reveal a stiff shoulder with faulty SH kinematics.[211] The goal of physical therapy is to improve GH mobility and restore SH rhythm. In this phase, irritability level reduces and more aggressive stretching and joint mobilization are tolerated and should be a focus of treatment. Figure 25-18, provides an example of a self-mobilization technique. Full active ROM is the goal, because any residual limitation may reinitiate the cycle. Low load, prolonged stretch produces plastic elongation of tissues as opposed to high tensile resistance seen in high load, brief stretch.[212,213] Heat may be used for relaxation, ultrasound may be used to promote tissue extensibility in the axillary fold, and cryotherapy may be used to reduce treatment discomfort. It is important to note that biologic remodeling occurs over long periods (months) as opposed to mechanically induced change which occurs within minutes.[214] Brand calls this tissue growth, not stretch.[215] This growth process is consistent with the recovery process in end stage primary adhesive capsulitis. Strengthening of the rotator cuff and SH muscles continues in this phase to reestablish coordinated force couples (see Self-Managements 25-1, 25-2, and 25-3), although positions may still require modification because of ROM limitations in the GH joint.

Operative Treatment. Conservative treatment will often be successful in patients with stage 2 adhesive capsulitis; however, some patients in late stage 2 and stage 3 may have a refractory motion loss. In patients who continue to have a refractory motion loss that creates disability, operative treatment may be necessary. Operative treatment is demanding, and proper patient selection, anesthesia, and postoperative analgesia are critical to its success. Operative treatment of patients with adhesive capsulitis includes closed manipulation and arthroscopic release. Closed manipulation is contraindicated in patients with significant osteopenia, recent surgical repair of soft tissues about the shoulder, or in the presence of fractures, neurologic injury and instability.

Historically, arthroscopy has been of little diagnostic and therapeutic value in patients with adhesive capsulitis of the shoulder.[159] However, it has been suggested that the arthroscope may be helpful for delineation of disorders, documentation of the result of closed manipulation, and treatment of concomitant intra-articular and subacromial disease.[174,201,216,217] The goal of physical therapy treatment after surgery is to maintain ROM achieved under anesthesia and to decrease pain and inflammation. In the recovery room, the arm is placed in the quadrant position while the patient is still under scalene block anesthesia. A second scalene block is administered during an overnight hospital stay so the patient can tolerate exercise through the ROM.[218,219] Continuous passive motion is recommended throughout the night.[220] After discharge, the patient should receive outpatient physical therapy 5 days per week for the next 2 weeks, then three times per week until treatment is completed. Treatment includes high frequency of interventions directed toward ROM, modalities for pain and inflammation, and hydrotherapy. Strengthening exercises are gradually incorporated into the program, as outlined previously.

ADJUNCTIVE INTERVENTIONS: TAPING

Complex muscular relationships exist among the scapula, humerus, cervical, thoracic spine, lumbar spine, and pelvis. Faulty scapular alignment contributes to a variety of syndromes affecting the upper quadrant. Scapular taping can improve the resting alignment of the scapula on the thorax, thereby improving joint alignment of the related joints and length-tension properties of the shared musculature between the scapula and other regions of the upper quadrant. Scapular taping can be a useful adjunctive intervention when used with therapeutic exercise for the treatment of many upper quadrant diagnoses.[21,221]

Patients can perform exercises and ADLs or instrumental ADLs while taped with the added benefit of improved joint alignment and length-tension properties of the scapular musculature. The benefit of scapular taping over an off-the-shelf brace is that taping allows the specific three-dimensional correction of each patient's unique alignment faults. Short-term taping (2 to 3 weeks) may assist in improved neuromuscular control of faulty movement patterns, whereas long-term taping (8 to 12 weeks) may affect muscle length-tension properties. Taping the ST joint has several goals:

- To improve initial alignment, which promotes improved movement patterns
- To alter length-tension properties by stretching tissues that are too short and reducing tension placed on tissues that are too long
- To provide support and reduce stress to myofascial tissues under chronic tension
- To provide kinesthetic awareness of scapular position during rest and movement
- To guide the kinematics during movement

Each piece of tape provides a specific corrective force on the scapula. Any one piece can be used in conjunction with other directional pieces to provide a multidimensional correction of the alignment of the scapula. The goal is to tape the scapula into improved alignment. If, however, the patient has significant kyphosis, forward-head, or forward-shoulder posture, 100% correction should not be attempted. It is instead recommended to moderately correct the faulty alignment, because too much change in such a short period may not be well tolerated by an individual with a chronic postural problem.

The tape product is specialized for taping the body for alignment and movement. It has the best combination of adhesive, extensible, yet stiff properties. The undertape is called Cover-Roll stretch, a hypoallergenic tape applied to protect the patient's skin from the overtape, called Leukotape (Beirsdorf Inc., Norwalk, CT). On the shoulder girdle, the Cover-Roll stretch often is adequate alone, particularly on a small-framed person with minimal to moderate postural faults.

The description of taping that follows details one method of taping, but other methods of taping can be used on the scapula and the humerus.[222] The goals of improved alignment and function are common to various techniques. Improved alignment and function during ADLs and instrumental ADLs and exercise can be achieved with proper taping techniques, and therefore taping can be a useful adjunctive intervention to therapeutic exercise and functional retraining.

Scapular Corrections

The following illustrations depict corrections of scapula position.

- Correcting Scapular Depression and Improving Scapular Elevation (Fig. 25-19)
- Correcting Scapular Downward Rotation and Improving Scapular Upward Rotation (Fig. 25-20)
- Correcting Scapular Abduction and Improving Scapular Adduction (Figs. 25-21 and 25-22)
- Correcting Scapular Winging
  - Tape as for correction of scapular downward rotation (see Fig. 25-20) and abduction (see Fig. 25-21).
- Correction of Scapular Anterior Tilt (Fig. 25-23)
- Correcting Scapular Elevation (see Fig. 25-24)

Prevention of Allergic Reaction

A common side effect of taping is an allergic reaction to the tape adhesive or skin breakdown. The following are troubleshooting tips to help prevent adverse reactions to taping:

- Use only Cover-Roll stretch, which is hypoallergenic. The allergic reaction is usually to the adhesive in the Leukotape.
- Use a skin preparation solution before application of the tape. A recommended skin preparation solution is Milk of Magnesia. A thin coat applied to the skin should completely dry before the tape is applied to allow easier tape removal.
- Ensure that all tape residue is removed before the next tape application.
- Warn patients of potential skin irritation. Instruct patients to remove the tape immediately if any itching or burning sensations develop.

Prevention of Skin Breakdown

Skin breakdown often occurs because of excessive friction between the skin and the tape. Follow these guidelines to minimize skin breakdown:

- Do not cross the midline of the spine with the tape.
- Do not cross more than one joint at a time.
- Tape the scapulae bilaterally, particularly in elevation.
- Use a skin preparation solution before taping.

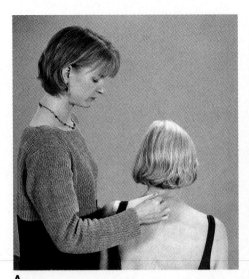
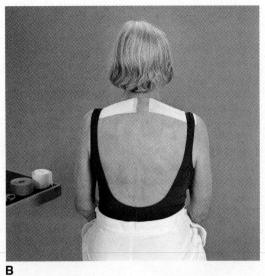

A   **B**

FIGURE 25-19. Correction of scapula depression. (A) Anchor the tape to the lateral edge of the acromion process. Passively elevate the scapula, ensuring the acromial end rotates upward. Pull the tape medially toward the cervical spine along the suprascapular space, following the fiber direction of the upper trapezius. Do not cross the cervical spine. Apply a piece in a similar direction on the opposite side to prevent lateral shearing across the cervical spine. (B) Repeat the application until the correction is made. Often, if tape is applied to correct additional alignment faults, this piece needs to be repeated to ensure that other tape applications have not pulled the scapula into depression.

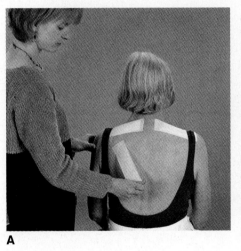
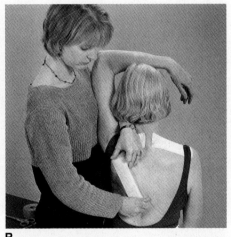

A   **B**

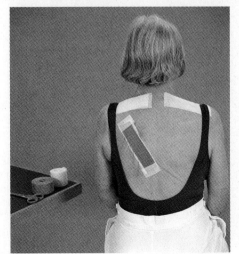

FIGURE 25-20. Taping the scapula into upward rotation. (A) Anchor the tape slightly medial to the root of the scapula. Passively elevate the arm into full flexion. (B) With the scapula in upward rotation, pull the tape medially and caudally toward the lower thoracic spine. (C) This piece provides a center of rotation for scapular upward rotation.

C

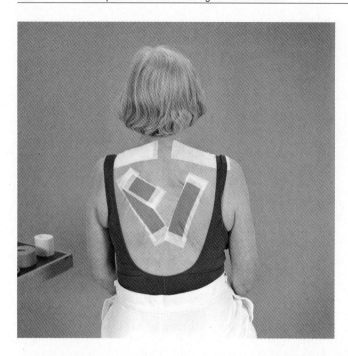

FIGURE 25-21. Taping the scapula into adduction. Tape as in Figure 26-20, but add a piece following the fiber direction of the middle trapezius as shown on the left scapula of this subject.

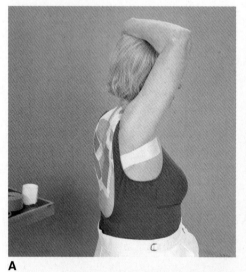

A

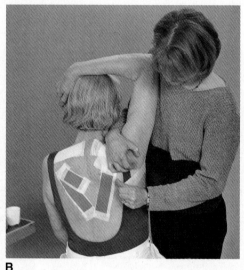

B

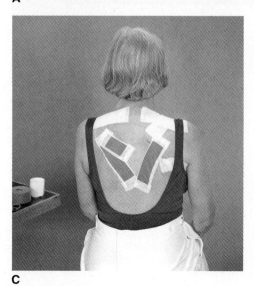

C

FIGURE 25-22. This is an alternative or adjunctive technique for taping the scapula into adduction. A second piece of tape can be used to prevent excessive abduction. (A) Anchor the tape proximally in the axilla and just anterior to the lateral border of the scapula. (B) Pull the tape posteriorly and caudally while adducting and upwardly rotating the scapula. (C) Attach the tape to the medial border of the inferior scapula. As the patient elevates the arm, a pull is felt in the axilla if the scapula begins to abduct.

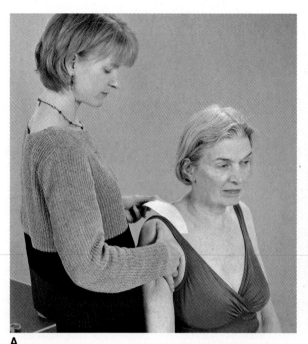
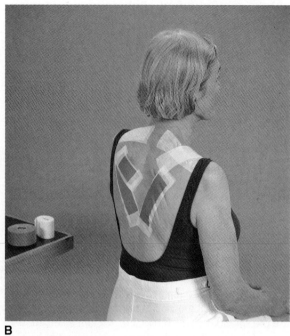

A **B**

FIGURE 25-23. Taping the scapula into a posterior tilt. (A) Anchor the tape to the coracoid process. (B) While tilting the scapula posteriorly, pull the tape posteriorly, caudally, and medially (opposite to the direction of pull of the pectoralis minor). Anchor the tape to the spine of the scapula. Place another tape as for correction of downward rotation (see Fig. 26-20) and scapular abduction (see Fig. 26-21), being sure to cover the inferior pole of the scapula to control tilt.

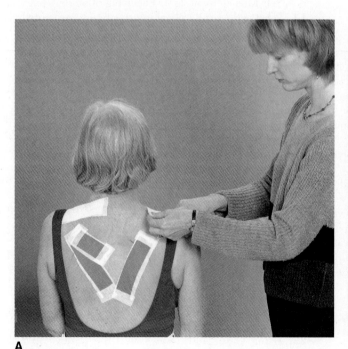
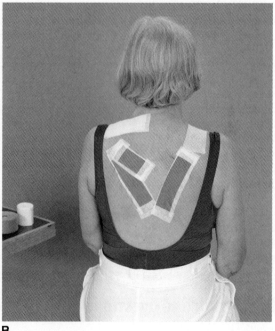

A **B**

FIGURE 25-24. Taping the scapula into depression. Use this technique to correct scapular elevation. (A) Anchor the tape to the anterior border of the upper trapezius. (B) Pull the tape posteriorly and anchor it to the spine of the scapula.

- Remove all tape residue before the next taping. Use Leukotape to dab off most of the residue, and follow up with adhesive tape remover.
- If skin breakdown occurs, allow the skin to heal fully before reapplying the tape. This may take 1 week or longer.

If taped properly, patients can often tolerate taping for 3 to 5 days. Showering with the tape is allowed, but soaking the tape is not recommended. For a person engaged in aggressive activities, the tape is more likely to loosen and not be as effective for as many days as it is for a less active individual.

KEY POINTS

- Critical to the management of the shoulder girdle complex is a thorough understanding of the anatomy and kinesiology of each of the four articulations comprising the complex.
- Precise kinematics at each of the four articulations and the integration of all four articulations with respect to joint function, force couples, and precise motor control to coordinate motion are required for optimal function of the shoulder complex.
- Because the shoulder girdle is one link in a kinetic chain, the function of the shoulder girdle affects and is affected by the function of other regions of the upper and lower quadrants.
- Treatment of impairments, although often necessary for improved function, should be complemented by functional retraining modified to the level of ability at a given time in the rehabilitation process.
- Ideal total body posture is a prerequisite for optimal movement in the shoulder girdle complex.
- A thorough understanding of the integrated approach to therapeutic exercise in the shoulder girdle is key to successful outcomes of shoulder girdle conditions.
- Rotator cuff disorders include such medical diagnoses as impingement syndrome, rotator cuff/glenoid labral tears, posterior shoulder pain, and GH hypermobility and instability.
- Most rotator cuff tears are extensions of underlying chronic tears or tears of already degenerated tendons.
- Adhesive capsulitis has been staged based upon arthroscopic findings as described in Table 25-5.
- Treatment of adhesive capsulitis should be individually based on the stage of the disease.
- Early intervention is key to successful outcome of adhesive capsulitis. Complete recovery with no residual limitation or disability is neither ensured nor common.
- Scapular taping can improve resting posture and proprioception, and thereby affect movement of the shoulder girdle complex.

CRITICAL THINKING QUESTIONS

1. What are the 3D kinematics of the scapula during arm elevation?
2. What are the 3D kinematics at the AC joint?
3. What are the coupled motions of the scapula during:
   a. Clavicle elevation
   b. Clavicle posterior rotation
   c. Clavicle retraction
4. What conjunct GH motion is a prerequisite to restoring full upper extremity elevation?
5. Why is the rotator cuff–deltoid function contingent on the scapular upward rotation force couple?
6. Which muscles can limit scapular upward rotation mobility?
7. Which muscles must have normal force or torque and length-tension relationships to achieve full upward scapular rotation ROM?
8. What is the timing of onset of the scapular muscles during scapular upward rotation to produce the ideal kinematics for scapular rotation?
9. What musculature is shared by the shoulder girdle and cervical spine? What joints are linked by the shared musculature?
10. If the upper trapezius is overstretched, as in a depressed scapula, in what direction is cervical spine rotation limited? What treatment do you propose to correct this problem?
11. If the levator scapula is adaptively shortened, as in a downwardly rotated scapula, in what direction is cervical spine rotation limited? What treatment do you propose to correct this problem?
12. How can cervical nerve root involvement affect the function of the shoulder girdle?
13. Using the case described in Display 25-6 determine the dosage parameters for improving muscular force or torque of the rotator cuff (using the exercise described in Self-Management 25-1: Facelying Shoulder Rotation).
14. What is the most critical intervention to promote healing of a strained muscle caused by adaptive lengthening from faulty postures?
15. How can poor technique during a biceps curl contribute to an anterior tilted scapula?
16. Adapt Self-Management 25-1 dosage parameters to focus on endurance.
17. In what alignment does the scapula rest to develop an elongated serratus anterior? How does this elongation contribute to a faulty kinematics of the scapula during scapular upward rotation?
18. What intrinsic and extrinsic factors predispose an individual to impingement syndrome?
19. Why is restoring the scapular kinematics important in the long-term recovery of impingement syndrome?
20. When is active motion overhead introduced for a patient after rotator cuff repair? As a physical therapist, what physiologic capabilities do you consider to be minimal expectations for exercise progression to overhead positions?
21. How can taping the scapula help adhesive capsulitis to recover? What taping techniques would you use?
22. Using Case Study No. 4 in Unit 7, develop a comprehensive exercise program. Describe each exercise according to the therapeutic exercise intervention model described in Chapter 2. You can follow the format used in the Selective Intervention at the end of Chapter 26.

REFERENCES

1. Maitland GD. Peripheral Manipulation. 3rd Ed. London: Butterworths, 1991.
2. Boublik M, Hawkins RJ. Clinical examination of the shoulder complex. J Orthop Sports Phys Ther 1993;18:379–385.
3. Tomberlin JP. The shoulder. In: Tomberlin JP, Saunder HD, eds. Evaluation, Treatment, and Prevention of Musculoskeletal Disorders. Vol 2. Extremities. Minneapolis, MN: The Saunders Group, 1994.
4. Magee DJ. Orthopedic Physical Assessment. Philadelphia, PA: WB Saunders, 1997.
5. Wilk KE, Andrews JR, Arrigo CA. The physical examination of the glenohumeral joint: emphasis on the stabilizing structures. J Orthop Sports Phys Ther 1997;25:380–389.
6. Griegel-Morris P, Larson K, Mueller-Klaus K, et al. Incidence of common postural abnormalities in the cervical, shoulder, and thoracic regions and their association with pain in two age groups of healthy subjects. Phys Ther 1992;72:426–430.
7. Greenfield B, Catlin PA, Coats PW, et al. Posture in patients with shoulder overuse injuries and healthy individuals. J Orthop Sports Phys Ther 1995;21:287–295.
8. Crawford HJ, Jull GA. The influence of thoracic posture and movement on range of arm elevation. Physiother Theory Pract 1993;9:143–148.
9. Kendall FP, McCreary EK, Provance PG. Muscle Testing and Function. 4th Ed. Baltimore, MD: Williams & Wilkins, 1993.
10. Daniels L, Worthingham C. Muscle Testing: Techniques of Manual Examination. 4th Ed. Philadelphia, PA: WB Saunders, 1980.
11. Sahrmann SA. Diagnosis and Treatment of Movement Impairment Syndromes. (Course outline). St. Louis, MO: Washington University, 1998.
12. Cyriax J. Textbook of Orthopedic Medicine. 8th Ed. London: Bailliere Tindall, 1982.
13. Kelly BT, Kadrmas WR, Speer KP. The manual muscle examination for rotator cuff strength: an EMG investigation. Am J Sports Med 1996;24:581–588.
14. Greis PE, Kuhn JE, Schulheis J, et al. Validation of the lift-off test and analysis of subscapularis activity during maximal internal rotation. Am J Sports Med 1996;24:589–593.
15. Cyriax J. Textbook of Orthopaedic Medicine: Diagnosis of Soft-Tissue Lesions. 7th Ed. London: Bailliere Tindall, 1978.
16. Pellicchia GL, Paolino J, Connel J. Intertester reliability of the Cyriax evaluation in assessing patients with shoulder pain. J Orthop Sports Phys Ther 1996;23:34–38.
17. Mattingly GE, Mackarey PJ. Optimal methods for shoulder tendon palpation: a cadaver study. Phys Ther 1996;76:166–174.
18. Maitland GD. Vertebral Manipulation. 5th Ed. London: Butterworths, 1986.
19. Duncan GH, Bushnell MC, Lavigne GJ. Comparison of verbal and visual analogue scales for measuring the intensity and unpleasantness of experimental pain. Pain 1989;37:295–303.
20. Borstad JD, Ludewig PM. Comparison of scapular kinematics between elevation and lowering of the arm in the scapular plane. Clin Biomech (Bristol, Avon). 2002 Nov–Dec;17(9–10):650–659.
21. Jackson P. Thoracic outlet syndrome: evaluation and treatment. Clin Manag 1987;7:6–10.
22. Butler D. Mobilization of the Nervous System. Melbourne: Churchill Livingstone, 1991.
23. Ayub E. Posture and the upper quarter. In: Donatelli R, ed. Physical Therapy of the Shoulder. New York, NY: Churchill-Livingstone, 1991.
24. Sahrmann SA. Diagnosis and Treatment of Movement Impairment Syndromes. St. Louis: Mosby, 2002.
25. Peterson DE, Blankenship KR, Robb JB, et al. Investigation of the validity and reliability of four objective techniques for measuring forward shoulder posture. J Orthop Sports Phys Ther 1997;25:34–42.
26. Ellenbecker TS, Mattalino AJ, Elam E, et al. Quantification of anterior translation of the humeral head in the throwing shoulder. Manual assessment versus stress radiography. Am J Sports Med 2000;28:161–167.
27. Speer KP, Hannafin JA, Altchek DW, et al. An evaluation of the shoulder relocation test. Am J Sports Med 1994;22: 177–183.
28. Oliashirazi A, Mansat P, Cofield RH, et al. Examination under anesthesia for evaluation of anterior shoulder instability. Am J Sports Med 1999;27:464–468.
29. Gross ML, Distefano MC. Anterior release test: a new test for occult shoulder instability. Clin Orthop Relat Res 1997;339:105–108.
30. O'Brian SJ, Pagnani MJ, Fealy S, et al. The active compression test: a new and effective test for diagnosing labral tears and acromioclavicular abnormality. Am J Sports Med 1998;26:610–613.
31. Mimori K, Muneta T, Nakagawa T, et al. A new pain provocation test for superior labral tears of the shoulder. Am J Sports Med 1999;27:137–142.
32. Kim SH, Ha KI, Han KY. Biceps load test: a clinical test for superior labrum anterior and posterior lesions in shoulders with recurrent anterior dislocations. Am J Sports Med 1999;27:300–303.
33. Itoi E, Tadato K. Sano A, et al. Which is more useful, the "full can test" or the "empty can test" in detecting the torn supraspinatous tendon? Am J Sports Med 1999;27:65–68.
34. Walch G, Boulahia A, Calderone A, et al. The "dropping" and "hornblower's" signs in evaluation of rotator cuff tears. J Bone Joint Surg 1998;80B:624–628.
35. Leroux JL, Thomas E, Bonnel F, et al. Diagnostic value of clinical tests for shoulder impingement syndrome. Rev Rheum 1995; 62:423–428.
36. Riand N, Levigne C, Renaud E, et al. Results of derotational humeral osteotomy in posterosuperior glenoid impingement. Am J Sports Med 1998;26:453–459.
37. Roach KE, Budiman-mak E, Songsiridej N, et al. Development of a shoulder pain and disability index. Arthritis Care Res 1991;4:143–149.
38. Williams JW, Holleman DR, Simel DL. Measuring shoulder function with the shoulder pain and disability index. J Rheumatol 1995;22:727–732.
39. Travell JG, Simons DG. Myofascial Pain and Dysfunction. Baltimore, MD: Williams & Wilkins, 1983.
40. Bogduk N. Innervation and pain patterns in the cervical spine. In: Grant R, ed. Physical Therapy of the Cervical and Thoracic Spine. 2nd Ed. New York, NY: Churchill Livingstone, 1994.
41. Grieve GP. Referred pain and other clinical features. In: Boyling D, Palastanga N, eds. Grieve's Modern Manual Therapy: The Vertebral Column. 2nd Ed. New York, NY: Churchill Livingstone, 1994.
42. Boissonnault WG, Janos SC. Screening for medical disease: physical therapy assessment and treatment principles. In: Boissonnault WG, ed. Examination in Physical Therapy Practice: Screening for Medical Disease. New York, NY: Churchill Livingstone, 1995.
43. McDiarmid T, Ziskin MC, Michlovitz SL, ed. Therapeutic Ultrasound. In: Michlovitz SL, ed. Thermal Agents in Rehabilitation. 3rd Ed. Philadelphia, PA: FA Davis, 1996.
44. Beaudreuil J, Nizard R, Thomas T, et al. Contribution of clinical tests to the diagnosis of rotator cuff disease: a systematic literature review. Joint Bone Spine 2009;76:15–9.
45. Neer CS. Shoulder Reconstruction. Philadelphia, PA: WB Saunders, 1990.
46. Jobe FW, Pink M. Classification and treatment of shoulder dysfunction in the overhead athlete. J Orthop Sports Phys Ther 1993;18:427–431.
47. Stillman JF, Hawkins RJ. Classification and physical diagnosis of instability of the shoulder. Clin Orthop 1993;291:7–19.
48. Hawkins RJ, Dunlop R. Nonoperative treatment of rotator cuff tears. Clin Orthop 1995;321:178–188.
49. Schmidt L, Snyder-Mackler L. Role of scapular stabilizers in etiology and treatment of impingement syndrome. J Orthop Sports Phys Ther 1999;29:131–138.
50. White SG, Sahrmann SA. A movement system balance approach to management of musculoskeletal pain. In: Grant R, ed. Physical Therapy of the Cervical and Thoracic Spine. 2nd Ed. New York, NY: Churchill Livingstone, 1982.
51. Van Dillen LR, McDonnell MK, Susco TM, Sahrmann SA. The immediate effect of passive scapular elevation on symptoms with active neck rotation in patients with neck pain. Clin J Pain 2007 Oct;23:641–647.
52. Andrade GT, Azevedo DC, De Assis Lorentz I, et al. Influence of scapular position on cervical rotation range of motion. J Orthop Sports Phys Ther 2008 Nov;38:668–673.
53. Baybar SR. Excessive scapular motion in individuals recovering from painful and stiff shoulders: causes and treatment strategies. Phys Ther 1996;76: 226–247.
54. Schwartz RE, O'Brian SJ, Warren RF. Capsular restraints to anterior-posterior motion of the abducted shoulder: a biomechanical study. Orthop Trans 1988;17:727.
55. Muraki T, Aoki M, Izumi T, et al. Lengthening of the pectoralis minor muscle during passive shoulder motions and stretching techniques: a cadaveric biomechanical study. Phys Ther 2009 Apr;89:333–341.
56. Abboud JA, Soslowsky LJ. Interplay of the static and dynamic restraints in glenohumeral instability. Clin Orthop Relat Res 2002;400:48–57.
57. Decker MJ, Tokish JM, Ellis HB, Torry MR, Hawkins RJ. Subscapularis muscle activity during selected rehabilitation exercises. Am J Sports Med 2003;31:126–134.
58. Reinold MM, Escamilla RF, Wilk KE. Current concepts in the scientific and clinical rationale behind exercises for glenohumeral and scapulothoracic musculature. J Orthop Sports Phys Ther 2009 Feb;39:105–117.
59. Matsen FA, Arntz CT, Lippitt SB. Rotator cuff. In: Rockwood CA, Matsen FA, eds. The Shoulder. 2nd Ed. Philadelphia, NY: WB Saunders, 1998.
60. Karatas GK, Gogus F. Suprascapular nerve entrapment in newsreel cameramen. Am J Phys Med Rehabil 2003;82:192–196.
61. Fabre T, Piton C, Leclouerec G, et al. Entrapment of the suprascapular nerve. J Bone Joint Surg Br 1999;81:414–419.
62. Elders LM, Van der Meché FA, Burdorf A. Serratus anterior paralysis as an occupational injury in scaffolders: two case reports. Am J Ind Med 2001;40:710–713.
63. Laska T, Hannig K. Physical therapy for spinal accessory nerve injury complicated by adhesive capsulitis. Phys Ther 2001;81:936–944.

64. Logigian EL, McInnes JM, Berger AR, et al. Stretch-induced spinal accessory nerve palsy. Muscle Nerve 1988;11:46–50.

65. Howell JW. Evaluation and management of thoracic outlet syndrome. In: Donatelli R, ed. Physical Therapy of the Shoulder. 2nd Ed. New York, NY: Churchill Livingstone, 1991.

66. Mumenthaler M. Neuropathies. In: Vinken PJ, Bruyn GW, Klawans HL, eds. Handbook of Clinical Neurology. Amsterdam: Elsevier Science, 1987.

67. Oware A, Herskovitz S, Berger AR. Long thoracic nerve palsy following cervical chiropractic manipulation. Muscle Nerve 1995;18:1351.

68. Kauppila LI, Vastamaki M. Iatrogenic serratus anterior paralysis. Long term outcome in 26 patients. Chest 1996;109:31–34.

69. Snyder-Mackler L, Robinson AJ. Clinical Electrophysiology. Baltimore, MD: Williams & Wilkins, 1989.

70. Watkins AL. A Manual of Electrotherapy. 3rd Ed. Philadelphia, PA: Lea & Feabiger, 1972.

71. Decker MJ, Hintermeister RA, Faber KJ, Hawkins RJ. Serratus anterior muscle activity during selected rehabilitation exercises. Am J Sports Med 1999;27:784–791.

72. Ekstrom RA, Donatelli RA, Soderberg GL. Surface electromyographic analysis of exercises for the trapezius and serratus anterior muscles. J Orthop Sports Phys Ther 2003;33:247–258.

73. Hintermeister RA, Lange GW, Schultheis JM, Bey MJ, Hawkins RJ. Electromyographic activity and applied load during shoulder rehabilitation exercises using elastic resistance. Am J Sports Med 1998;26:210–220.

74. Moseley JB, Jr, Jobe FW, Pink M, Perry J, et al. EMG analysis of the scapular muscles during a shoulder rehabilitation program. Am J Sports Med 1992;20:128–134.

75. Myers JB, Pasquale MR, Laudner KG, et al. Bradley JP, Lephart SM. On-the-field resistance tubing exercises for throwers: an electromyographic analysis. J Athl Train 2005;40:15–22.

76. Bagg SD, Forrest WJ. A biomechanical analysis of scapular rotation during arm abduction in the scapular plane. Am J Phys Med Rehabil 1988;67:238–245.

77. Hardwick DH, Beebe JA, McDonnell MK, et al. A comparison of serratus anterior muscle activation during a wall slide exercise and other traditional exercises. J Orthop Sports Phys Ther 2006;36:903–910.

78. Ludewig PM, Cook TM, Nawoczenski DA. Three dimensional scapular orientation and muscle activity at selected positions of humeral elevation. J Orthop Sports Phys Ther 1996;24:57–65.

79. Ludewig PM, Reynolds JF. The Association of Scapular Kinematics and Glenohumeral Joint Pathologies. J Orthop Sports Phys Ther 2009;39:90–104.

80. Graichen H, Bonel H, Stammberger T, et al. Three dimensional analysis of the width of the subacromial space in healthy subjects and patients with impingement syndrome. Am J Roentgenol 1999;172:1081–1086.

81. Ludewig PM, Cook TM. Alterations in shoulder kinematics and associated muscle activity in people with symptoms of shoulder impingement. Phys Ther 2000;80:276–291.

82. Ludewig PM, Hoff MS, Osowski EE, et al. Relative balance of serratus anterior and upper trapezius muscle activity during push-up exercises. Am J Sports Med 2004;32:484–493.

83. Donatelli RA. Physical Therapy of the Shoulder. 3rd Ed. New York, NY: Churchill Livingstone, 1997.

84. DiGiovine NM, Jobe FW, Pink M, et al. An electromyographic analysis of the upper extremity in pitching. J Shoulder Elbow Surg 1992;1:15–25.

85. Basmajian JV, DeLuca CJ. Muscles Alive. 5th Ed. Baltimore, MD: Williams & Wilkins, 1985.

86. Westgaard RH. Measurement and evaluation of postural load in occupational work situations. Eur J Appl Physiol 1988;57:291–304.

87. Jensen C, Nilsen K, Hansen K, et al. Trapezius muscle load as a risk indicator for occupational shoulder-neck complaints. Int Arch Occup Environ Health 1993;64:415–423.

88. Veiersted KB, Westgaard RH, Anderson P. Pattern of muscle activity during stereotyped work and its relationship to muscle pain. Int Arch Occup Environ Health 1990;62:31–41.

89. Elert J, Brulin C, Gerdle B, et al. Mechanical performance, level of continuous contraction and muscle pain symptoms in home care personnel. Scand J Rehabil Med 1992;24: 141–150.

90. Kadi F, Ahlgren C, Waling G, et al. The effects of different training programs on the trapezius muscle of women with work-related neck and shoulder myalgia. Acta Neuropathol 2000;100:243–258.

91. Toivanen H, Helin P, Hanninen O. Impact of regular relaxation training and psychosocial working factors on neck-shoulder tension and absenteeism in hospital cleaners. J Occup Med 1993;35:1123–1130.

92. Greico A, Occhipinti E, Colombini D, et al. Muscular effort and musculoskeletal disorders in piano students: electromyographic, clinical and preventive aspects. Ergonomics 1989;32:697–716.

93. Sundelin G, Hagberg M. The effects of different pause types on neck and shoulder EMG activity during VDU work. Ergonomics 1989;32: 527–537.

94. Schuldt K, Ekholm J, Harms Ringdahl K, et al. Effects of arm support or suspension on neck and shoulder muscle activity during sedentary work. Scand J Rehabil Med 1988;19:77–84.

95. McLean L, Tingley M, Scott R, et al. Computer terminal work and the benefit of microbreaks. App Ergonom 2001;32:225–237.

96. Ketola R, Toivonen R, Hakkanen M, et al. Effects of ergonomic intervention in work with video display units. Scand J Work Environ Health 2002;28:18–24.

97. McQuade KJ, Wei SH, Smidt GL. Effects of local muscle fatigue on three-dimensional scapulohumeral rhythm [abstract]. Phys Ther 1993;73:S109.

98. Gossman MR, Sahrmann SA, Rose SJ. Review of length-associated changes in muscle. Experimental evidence and clinical implications. Phys Ther 1982;62:1799–1808.

99. Paletta G, Warner JJP, Warren RF. Shoulder kinematics with two plane x-ray evaluation in patients with anterior instability or rotator cuff tearing. J Shoulder Elbow Surg 1997;6:516–527.

100. Craven WM. Traumatic avulsion tears of the rotator cuff. In: Andrews JR, Wilk KE, eds. The Athlete's Shoulder. New York, NY: Churchill Livingstone, 1994.

101. Ellenbecker TS. Etiology and evaluation of rotator cuff pathology and rehabilitation. In: Donatelli RA, ed. Physical Therapy of the Shoulder. 3rd Ed. New York, NY: Churchill Livingstone, 1994.

102. Cofield RH. Current concepts review of rotator cuff disease of the shoulder. J Bone Joint Surg Am 1985;67:974.

103. Fu FH, Harner CD, Klein AH. Shoulder impingement syndrome. A critical review. Clin Orthop 1991;269:162–173.

104. Nirschl RP. Shoulder tendonitis. In: Pettrone FP, ed. Upper Extremity Injuries in Athletes: American Academy of Orthopedic Surgeons Symposium. St. Louis, MO: Mosby, 1988.

105. Andrews JR, Alexander EJ. Rotator cuff injury in throwing and racket sports. Sports Med Arthrosc Rev 1995;3:30.

106. Baring T, Emery R, Reilly P. Management of rotator cuff disease: specific treatment for specific disorders. Best Pract Res Clin Rheumatol 2007: 279–294.

107. Kvitne RS, Jobe FW. The diagnosis and treatment of anterior instability in the throwing athlete. Clin Orthop Relat Res 1993:107–123.

108. Neer CS. Impingement lesions. Clin Orthop 1983;173:70–77.

109. Bigliani LU, Levine WN. Subacromial impingement syndrome. J Bone Joint Surg Am 1997;79:1854–1868.

110. Belling Sorensen AK, Jorgensen U. Secondary impingement in the shoulder. An improved terminology in impingement. Scand J Med Sci Sports 2000;10:266–278.

111. Neer CS. Anterior acromioplasty for the chronic impingement syndrome in the shoulder. J Bone Joint Surg Am 1972;54:41–50.

112. Walch G, Boileau P, Noel E, et al. Impingement of the deep surface of the supraspinatous tendon on the posterosuperior glenoid rim: an arthroscopic study. J Shoulder Elbow Surg 1992;1:238–245.

113. Hurley JA, Anderson TE. Shoulder arthroscopy: its role in evaluating shoulder disorders in the athlete. Am J Sports Med 1990;18:480–483.

114. Liu SH, Boynton E. Posterior superior impingement of the rotator cuff on the glenoid rim as a cause of shoulder pain in the overhead athlete. Arthroscopy 1993;9:697–699.

115. Gartsman GM, Milne JC. Articular surface partial-thickness rotator cuff tears. J Shoulder Elbow Surg 1995;4:409–415.

116. Jobe CM. Posterior superior glenoid impingement: expanded spectrum. Arthroscopy 1995;11:530–536.

117. Tirman PF, Bost FW, Garvin GJ, et al. Posterosuperior glenoid impingement of the shoulder: findings at MR imaging and MR arthrography with arthroscopic correlation. Radiology 1994;193:431–436.

118. Wadsworth DJ, Bullock-Saxton JE. Recruitment patterns of the scapular rotator muscles in freestyle swimmers with subacromial impingement. Int J Sports Med 1997;18:618–624.

119. Glousman R, Jobe F, Tibone J, et al. Dynamic electromyographic analysis of the throwing shoulder with glenohumeral instability. J Bone Jt Surg 1988;70A:220–226.

120. McMahon PJ, Jobe FW, Pink MM, et al. Comparative electromyographic analysis of shoulder muscles during planar motions: anterior glenohumeral instability versus normal. J Bone Jt Surg 1996;5:118–123.

121. Ruwe PA, Pink M, Jobe FW, et al. The normal and the painful shoulders during the breaststroke. Electromyographic and cinematographic analysis of twelve muscles. Am J Sports Med 1994;22:789–796.

122. Reddy AS, Mohr KJ, Pink MM, et al. Electromyographic analysis of the deltoid and rotator cuff muscles in persons with subacromial impingement. J Shoulder Elbow Surg 2000;9:519–523.

123. Blasier RB, Guldberg RE, Rothman ED. Anterior shoulder stability: contributions of rotator cuff forces and the capsular ligaments in a cadaver model. J Shoulder Elbow Surg 1992;2:27–35.

124. Howell SM, Kraft TA. The role of the supraspinatus and infraspinatus muscles in glenohumeral kinematics of anterior shoulder instability. Clin Orthop 1991;263:128–134.

125. de Groot JH. The variability of shoulder motions recorded by means of palpation. Clin Biomech 1997;12:461–472.

126. Strauss MB, Wrobel LJ, Neff RS, et al. The shrugged-off shoulder: a comparison of patients with recurrent shoulder subluxations and dislocations. Physician Sports Med 1983;11:85–97.

127. Chandler TJ, Kibler B, Stracener EC, et al. Shoulder strength, power, and endurance in college tennis players. Am J Sports Med 1992;20:455–458.

128. Lear LJ, Gross MT. An electromyographical analysis of the scapular stabilizing synergists during a push-up progression. J Orthop Sports Phys Ther 1998;28:146–157.

129. McCann PD, Wooten ME, Kadaba MP, et al. A kinematic and electromyographic study of shoulder rehabilitation exercises. Clin Orthop 1993;288:179–188.

130. Ballantyne BT, O'Hare SJ, Paschall JL, et al. Electromyographic activity of selected shoulder muscles in commonly used therapeutic exercises. Phys Ther 1993;73:668–677.

131. Smith RL, Brunolli J. Shoulder kinesthesia after anterior glenohumeral joint dislocation. Phys Ther 1980;69:106–112.

132. Lippitt SB, Vanderhooft E, Harris SL, et al. Glenohumeral stability from concavity-compression: a quantitative analysis. J Shouder Elbow Surg 1993;2:27–35.

133. Bach BR, Warren RF, Fornek J. Disruption of the lateral capsule of the shoulder: a cause of recurrent dislocation. J Bone Joint Surg 1988;70B:274–276.

134. Bigliani LU, Kelkar R, Flatow EL, et al. Glenohumeral stability: biomechanical properties of passive and active stabilizers. Clin Orthop 1996;330:13–30.

135. Bigliani LU, Pollock RG, Soslowsky LJ, et al. Tensile properties of the inferior glenohumeral ligament. J Orthop Res 1992;10:187–197.

136. Kumar VP, Balasubramaniam P. The role of atmospheric pressure in stabilizing the shoulder: an experimental study. J Bone Joint Surg 1985;67A:19–21.

137. Kibler WB. Role of the scapula in the overhead throwing motion. Contemp Orthop 1991;22:525–532.

138. Ludewig PM, Cook TM. Translations of the humerus in persons with shoulder impingement symptoms. J Orthop Sports Phys Ther 1996;80:276–291.

139. Flatow EL, Soslowsky LJ, Ticker JB, et al. Excursion of the rotator cuff under the acromion. Patterns of subacromial contact. Am J Sports Med 1994;22:779–778.

140. Brossman J, Preidler KW, Pedowitz RA, et al. Shoulder impingement syndrome: influence of shoulder position on rotator cuff impingement—an anatomic study. AJR Am J Roentgenol 1996;167:1511–1515.

141. Davidson PA, Elattrache NS, Jobe CM, et al. Rotator cuff and posterior-superior glenoid labrum injury associated with increased glenohumeral motion: a new site of impingement. J Shoulder Elbow Surg 1995;4:384–390.

142. Warren R. Subluxation of the shoulder in athletes. Clin Sports Educ 1983;2:339–354.

143. Matthews LS, Oweida SJ. Glenohumeral instability in athletes: spectrum, diagnosis, and treatment. Adv Orthop Surg 1985;8:236–248.

144. Perry J. Anatomy and biomechanics of the shoulder in throwing, swimming, gymnastics and tennis. Clin Sports Med 1983;2:247–270.

145. Reid DC, Saboe LA, Chepeha JC. Anterior shoulder instability in athletes: comparison of isokinetic resistance exercises and an electromyographic biofeedback re-education program—a pilot program. Physiotherapy Canada 1996;48:251–256.

146. McQuade KJ, Dawson J, Smidt GL. Scapulothoracic muscle fatigue associated with alterations in scapulohumeral rhythm kinematics during maximum resistive shoulder elevation. J Orthop Sports Phys Ther 1998;28:74–80.

147. Pascoal AG, van der Helm FF, Pesarat CP, et al. Effects of different arm external loads on the scapulo-humeral rhythm. Clin Biomech 2000;15:S21–S24.

148. Warner JJ, Micheli LJ, Arslanian LE, et al. Scapulothoracic motion in normal shoulders and shoulders with glenohumeral instability and impingement syndrome. A study using more topographic analysis. Clin Orthop 1992;285:191–199.

149. Ejnisman B, Andreoli CV, Soares B, et al. Interventions for tears of the rotator cuff in adults. Cochrane Database Syst Rev 2009:CD002758.

150. Rowe CR. Ruptures of the rotator cuff: Selection of cases for conservative treatment. Surg Clin North Am 1963;43:1531–1540.

151. Hawkins RJ, Kennedy JC. Impingement syndrome in athletes. Am J Sports Med 1980;8:151–158.

152. Cofield RH, Simonet WT. Symposium on sports medicine: Part 2. The shoulder in sports. Mayo Clin Proc 1984;59:157–164.

153. Jobe FW. Thrower problems. Am J Sports Med 1979;7:139–140.

154. Richardson AB, Jobe FW, Collins HR. The shoulder in competitive swimming. Am J Sports Med 1980;8:159–163.

155. Mantone JK, Burkhead WZ Jr, Noonan J Jr. Nonoperative treatment of rotator cuff tears. Orthop Clin North Am 2000;31:295–311.

156. Coghlan JA, Buchbinder R, Green S, Johnston RV, Bell SN. Surgery for rotator cuff disease. Cochrane Database Syst Rev 2008;1:CD005619.

157. Romeo AA, Hang DW, Bach BR Jr, et al. Repair of full thickness rotator cuff tears. Gender, age, and other factors affecting outcome. Clin Orthop Relat Res 1999 Oct;(367):243–255.

158. Binder A, Bulgen DY, Hazelman BL, et al. Frozen shoulder: a long term prospective study. Ann Rheum Dis 1984;43:361–364.

159. Lloyd-Roberts GG, French PR. Periarthritis of the shoulder: a study of the disease and its treatment. BMJ 1959;1:1569–1574.

160. Bridgeman JF. Periarthritis of the shoulder and diabetes mellitus. Ann Rheum Dis 1972;31:69–71.

161. DePalma AF. Loss of scapulohumeral motion (frozen shoulder). Ann Surg 1952;135:193–204.

162. Bowman CA, Jeffcoate WJ, Patrick M. Bilateral adhesive capsulitis, oligoarthritis and proximal myopathy as presentation of hypothyroidism. Br J Rheumatol 1988;27:62–64.

163. Miller MD, Rockwood CA Jr. Thawing the frozen shoulder: the "patient" patient. Orthopedics 1997;19:849–853.

164. Mintner WT. The shoulder-hand syndrome in coronary disease. J Med Assoc GA 1967;56:45–49.

165. Bulgen DY, Binder A, Hazelman BL. Immunological studies in frozen shoulder. J Rheumatol 1982;9:893–898.

166. Anderson BA, Sojbjerg JO, Johannsen HV, et al. Frozen shoulder: arthroscopy and manipulation under general anesthesia and early passive motion. J Shoulder Elbow Surg 1998;7:218–222.

167. Aydeniz A, Gursoy S, Guney E. Which musculoskeletal complications are most frequently seen in type 2 diabetes mellitus? J Int Med Res 2008;36:505–511.

168. Milgrom C, Novack V, Weil Y, et al. Risk factors for idiopathic frozen shoulder. Isr Med Assoc J 2008;10:361–364.

169. Hannafin JA, Chiaia TA. Adhesive capsulitis. Clin Orthop Related Res 2000;372:95–109.

170. Lundberg J. The frozen shoulder. Clinical and radiographical observations. The effect of manipulation under general anesthesia. Structure and glycosaminoglycan content of the joint capsule. Local bone metabolism. Acta Orthop Scand 1969;119(Suppl):111–159.

171. Zuckerman JD. Definition and classification of frozen shoulder. J Shoulder Elbow Surg 1994;3:S72.

172. Hannafin JA, DiCarlo EF, Wickiewicz TL, et al. Adhesive capsulitis: capsular fibroplasia of the glenohumeral joint [abstract]. J Shoulder Elbow Surg 1994;3(Suppl):5.

173. Rodeo SA, Hannafin JA, Tom J, et al. Immunolocalization of cytokines and their receptors in adhesive capsulitis of the shoulder. J Orthop Res 1997;15:427–436.

174. Wiley AM. Arthroscopic appearance of frozen shoulder. Arthroscopy 1991;7:138–143.

175. Bunker TD, Anthony PP. The pathology of frozen shoulder. A Dupuytren-like disease. J Bone Jt Surg 1995;77B:677–683.

176. Bulgen DY, Binder A, Hazelman BL. J Rheumatol 1982;9:893–898.

177. Grubbs N. Frozen shoulder syndrome: a review of literature. J Orthop Sports Phys Ther 1993;18:479–487.

178. Rizk TE, Pinals RS. Histocompatibility type and racial incidence in frozen shoulder. Arch Phys Med Rehabil 1984;65:33–34.

179. Neviaser RJ. Painful conditions affecting the shoulder. Clin Orthop 1983;173:63–69.

180. Neviaser RJ, Neviaser TJ. The frozen shoulder. Diagnosis and management. Clin Orthop 1987;223:59–64.

181. Placzek JD, Roubal PJ, Freeman DC, et al. Long term effectiveness of translational manipulation for adhesive capsulitis. Clin Orthop 1998;356:181–191.

182. Mao C, Jaw W, Cheng H. Frozen shoulder: correlation between the response to physical therapy and follow-up shoulder arthrography. Arch Phys Med Rehabil 1997;78:857–859.

183. O'Kane JW, Jackins S, Sidles JA, et al. Simple home program for frozen shoulder to improve patients' assessment of shoulder function and health status. J Am Board Fam Pract 1999;12:270–277.

184. Carette S, Moffet H, Tardif J. Intraarticular corticosteroids, supervised physiotherapy, or a combination of the two in the treatment of adhesive capsulitis of the shoulder. Arthritis Rheum 2003;3:829–838.

185. Arslan S, Celiker R. Comparison of the efficacy of local corticosteroid injection and physical therapy for the treatment of adhesive capsulitis. Rheumatol Int 2001;21:20–23.

186. Hay EM, Thomas E, Paterson SM, et al. A pragmatic randomized controlled trial of local corticosteroid injection and physiotherapy for the treatment of new episodes of unilateral shoulder pain in primary care. Ann Rheum Dis 2003;62:394–399.

187. Kelley MJ, McClure PW, Leggin BG. Frozen shoulder: evidence and a proposed model guiding rehabilitation. J Orthop Sports Phys Ther 2009;39:135–148.

188. Binder A, Hazelman BL, Parr G, et al. A controlled study of oral prednisone in frozen shoulder. Br J Rheumatol 1986;25:288–292.

189. Huskisson EC, Bryans R. Diclofenac sodium in treatment of the painful stiff shoulder. Curr Med Res Opin 1983;8:350–353.

190. Rhind V, Downie WW, Bird HA, et al. Naproxen and indomethacin in periarthritis of the shoulder. Rheumatol Rehabil 1982;21:51–53.

191. Bulgen DY, Binder A, Hazelman BL, et al. Frozen shoulder: prospective clinical study with an evaluation of three treatment regimens. Ann Rheum Dis 1984;43:353–360.

192. D'Acre JE, Beeney N, Scott DL. Injections and physiotherapy for the painful stiff shoulder. Ann Rheum Dis 1989;48:322–325.

193. DeJong BA, Dahmen R, Hogeweg JA, et al. Intraarticular triamcinolone acetonide injection in patients with capsulitis of the shoulder: a comparative study of two dose regimes. Clin Rehab 1998;12:211–215.

194. Quigley TB. Indications for manipulation and corticosteroids in the treatment of stiff shoulder. Surg Clin North Am 1975;43:1715–1720.

195. Steinbrocker O, Argyros TG. Frozen shoulder: treatment by local injection of depot corticosteroids. Arch Phys Med Rehabil 1974;55:209–213.

196. Wadsworth CT. Frozen shoulder. Phys Ther 1986;66:1878–1883.

197. Speer KP, Cavanaugh JT, Warren RF, et al. A role for hydrotherapy in shoulder rehabilitation. Am J Sports Med 1993;21:850–853.

198. Wyke B. The neurology of joints. Ann R Coll Surg Engl 1967;41:25–50.

199. Owens-Burkhart H. Management of frozen shoulder. In: Donatelli RA, ed. Physical Therapy of the Shoulder. New York, NY: Churchill Livingstone, 1991.

200. Kibler BW. Shoulder rehabilitation: principles and practice. Med Sci Sports Exerc 1998;30(Suppl):S40–S50.

201. Segmuller HE, Taylor DE, Hogan CS, et al. Arthroscopic treatment of adhesive capsulitis. J Shoulder Elbow Surg 1995;4:403–404.

202. Cyriax J. Examination of the Shoulder. Limited Range Diagnosis of Soft Tissue Lesions. Vol. 1. 8th Ed. London: Balliere Tindall, 1982.

203. Ide J, Takagi K. Early and long-term results of arthroscopic treatment for shoulder stiffness. J Shoulder Elbow Surg 2004;13:174–179.

204. Omari A, Bunker TD. Open surgical release for frozen shoulder: surgical findings and results of the release. J Shoulder Elbow Surg 2001;10:353–357.

205. Uhthoff HK, Boileau P. Primary frozen shoulder: global capsular stiffness versus localized contracture. Clin Orthop Relat Res 2007;456:79–84.

206. Kelley MJ, McClure PW, Leggin BG. Frozen shoulder: evidence and a proposed model guiding rehabilitation. J Orthop Sports Phys Ther 2009;39:135–148.

207. Johnson AJ, Godges JJ, Zimmerman GJ, et al. The effect of anterior versus posterior glide joint mobilization on external rotation range of motion in patients with shoulder adhesive capsulitis. J Orthop Sports Phys Ther 2007;37:88–99.

208. Frank C, Amiel D, Woo SL, et al. Normal ligament properties and ligament healing. Clin Orthop Relat Res 1985;15–25.

209. Bush TA, Mork DO, Sarver KK, et al. The effectiveness of shoulder taping in the inhibition of the upper trapezius as determined by the electromyogram [abstract]. Phys Ther 1996;76:S17.

210. Boyle-Walker KL, Gabard DL, Bietsch E, et al. A profile of patients with adhesive capsulitis. J Hand Ther 1997;10:222–228.

211. Vermeulen HM, Stoddijk M, Eilers P, et al. Measurement of three dimensional shoulder movement patterns with an electromagnetic tracking device in patients with a frozen shoulder. Ann Rheum Dis 2002;61:115–120.

212. Light KE, Nuzik S. Low-load prolonged stretch vs high-load brief stretch in treating knee contractures. Phys Ther 1984:64:330–333.

213. Rizk TE, Christopher RP, Pinals RS, et al. Adhesive capsulitis (frozen shoulder): a new approach to its management and treatment. Arch Phys Med Rehabil 1983;64:29–33.

214. Arem AJ, Madden JW. Effects of stress on healing wounds: I. Intermittent noncyclical tension. J Surg Res 1976;20:93–102.

215. Brand PW. The forces of dynamic splinting: ten questions before applying a dynamic splint to the hand. In: Hunter JM, Mackin EJ, Callahan AD, eds. Rehabilitation of the Hand. St. Louis, MO: C.V. Mosby, 1995:1581–1587.

216. Cobb DS, Cantu R, Donatelli RA. Myofascial treatment. In: Donatelli RA, ed. Physical Therapy of the Shoulder. New York, NY: Churchill Livingstone, 1997.

217. Pollock RG, Duralde XA, Flatow EL, et al. The use of arthroscopy in treatment of resistant frozen shoulder. Clin Orthop 1994;304:30–36.

218. Brown AR, Weiss R, Greenberg C, et al. Interscalene block for shoulder arthroscopy: comparison with general anesthesia. Arthroscopy 1993;9:295–300.

219. Kinnard P, Truchon R, St-Pierre A. Interscalene block for pain relief after shoulder surgery. Clin Orthop 1994;304:22–24.

220. McCarthy MR, O'Donoghue PC. The clinical use of continuous passive motion in physical therapy. J Orthop Sports Phys Ther 1992;15:132–140.

221. Host HH. Scapular taping in the treatment of anterior shoulder impingement. Phys Ther 1995;75:803–812.

222. Kim SH, Ha KI, Han KY. Biceps load test: a clinical test for superior labrum anterior and posterior lesions in shoulders with recurrent anterior dislocations. Am J Sports Med 1999;27:300–303.

223. Johnston TB. The movements of the shoulder joint. A plea for the use of the "plane of the scapula" as the name of reference for movements occurring at the humeroscapular joint. Br J Surg 1937;25:252–260.

224. Saha AK. Mechanism for shoulder movements and a plea for the recognition of "zero position" of glenohumeral joint. Indian J Surg 1950;12:153–165.

225. Hoppenfeld S. Physical Examination of the Spine and Extremities. Norwalk, CT: Appleton-Century-Crofts, 1976.

226. Silliman JF, Hawkins RJ. Classification and physical diagnosis of instability of the shoulder. Clin Orthop 1993;291:7–19.

chapter 26

The Elbow, Forearm, Wrist, and Hand

LORI THEIN BRODY

Therapeutic exercise texts have often minimized or excluded the elbow, wrist, and hand, deferring evaluation of this region to other health care providers. This complex region is a challenging and specialized area of rehabilitation. Although numerous texts describe the anatomy, kinesiology, pathology, and surgical repair of this area, few sources relate pathology, impairments, and activity limitations with physical therapy intervention at the distal upper extremity level.[1] This chapter discusses common impairments and activity limitations of the elbow, wrist, and hand and the related therapeutic interventions. A brief review of anatomy and kinesiology provides the basis for the interventions chosen. Further details on the anatomy and kinesiology of this region can be found on the website.

ANATOMY*

Although the anatomy of a given joint is closely related to anatomy of adjacent joints, the elbow, wrist, and hand are discussed separately in the following sections.

Elbow and Forearm

Osteology

The primary osteologic considerations at the elbow and forearm are the humerus, radius, and ulna bones (Fig. 26-1.) The articulation of the humerus with the ulna and the radius forms the elbow joint.[2] The key aspects of elbow and forearm osteology include:

- The spool-shaped trochlea of the humerus articulates with the trochlear notch of the ulna, and the rounded humeral capitulum articulates with the radial head laterally.
- The medial epicondyle is a subcutaneous, blunt projection, easily palpable during elbow flexion, with a posterior shallow groove accommodating the ulnar nerve.
- The lateral epicondyle is also subcutaneous, with its anterolateral surface serving as the origin of the wrist extensor muscles.
- The radius is the shorter and more lateral of the two forearm bones, with the radial tuberosity serving as the distal insertion of the biceps brachii.
- The ulna is the longer of the two forearm bones and serves as the major distal component of the elbow joint proper, with its hook-shaped anterior surface articulating with the humeral trochlea.

Arthrology

The elbow joint is comprised of several articulations, including the humeroulnar, the humeroradial, and the proximal and

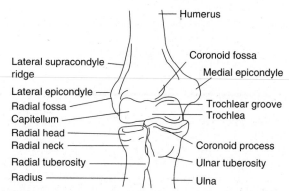

FIGURE 26-1. Elbow osteology with significant bony landmarks. (From Stroyan M, Wilk KE. The functional anatomy of the elbow complex. J Orthop Sports Phys Ther 1993;17:280.)

distal radioulnar. Because of these multiple articulations, it is considered to be a compound synovial joint. The major ligamentous structures are as follows:

- The ulnar collateral ligaments (UCLs), with anterior, posterior, and oblique components.[3] See Figure 26-2.
- The thick, cordlike anterior portion of the UCL is the primary stabilizer against valgus forces throughout most of the range of motion.
- The radial collateral ligament is a triangular, fan-shaped band blending distally with the annular ligament and the origins of the extensor carpi radialis brevis (ECRB) and supinator muscles.[3]
- The interosseus membrane is a broad fascial sheath running distomedially, connecting the radius and ulna and providing attachments for the deep forearm muscles.

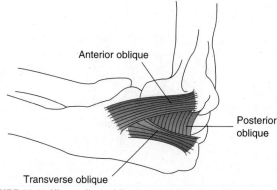

FIGURE 26-2. Ulnar collateral ligaments of the elbow. (From Zarin B, Andrews J, Carson W. Injuries to the Throwing Arm. Philadelphia, PA: WB Saunders, 1985.)

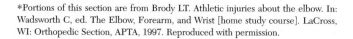

*Portions of this section are from Brody LT. Athletic injuries about the elbow. In: Wadsworth C, ed. The Elbow, Forearm, and Wrist [home study course]. LaCross, WI: Orthopedic Section, APTA, 1997. Reproduced with permission.

TABLE 26-1 Muscles of the Elbow and Forearm

MUSCLE	ORIGIN	INSERTION	ACTION	SPINAL LEVEL	PERIPHERAL NERVE
Pronator teres	Medial epicondyle and coronoid process of ulna	Middle lateral radius	Forearm pronation	C7	Median
Supinator	Lateral epicondyle	Lateral upper 1/3 of radius	Forearm supination	C6	Radial
Biceps brachii	Coracoid process; scapular supraglenoid tubercle	Radial tuberosity	Shoulder flexion; elbow flexion	C5–6	Musculocutaneous
Brachialis	Distal 1/2 of anterior humerus	Coronoid process of ulna	Elbow flexion	C5–6	Musculocutaneous and radial
Brachioradialis	Proximal 2/3 of lateral supra-condylar ridge of humerus	Lateral radial styloid	Elbow flexion	C6	Radial
Triceps	Infraglenoid tubercle of scapula; proximal posterolateral humerus; Distal 2/3 or posteromedial humerus	Olecranon process	Elbow extension	C7–8	Radial

Myology

Despite only a few muscles having a direct action at the humeroulnar joint, numerous muscles attach about the elbow and can be a source of pain and disability. Although many muscles perform multiple actions, they are classified by the articulation of their primary action. Muscles and their innervation can be found in Table 26-1.[4]

Wrist

The bony structures of the carpal bones indicate their roles. The outer bones generally have half of their surfaces covered with articular cartilage (inner surfaces), and their outer surfaces are rough, providing attachment for connective tissues. The inner bones have two thirds of their surfaces covered by articular cartilage, and only the palmar and dorsal surfaces are irregular, providing for ligamentous attachments. A brief overview of anatomy and kinesiology is expanded on the website.

Osteology

The wrist joint is a complex area that includes eight carpal bones, the distal radius and ulna, and the bases of the metacarpal bones (Fig. 26-3). Proximally, the distal radius and radioulnar disk articulate with the scaphoid, lunate, and triquetrum. Laterally, the scaphoid is the largest bone in the proximal carpal row. The distal carpal row consists of the trapezium, trapezoid, capitate (the most central and largest of all carpal bones) and the hamate (Fig. 26-4). Key aspects of wrist osteology include:

- The scaphoid spans the intercarpal joint, linking the proximal and distal rows, making this bone prone to injury.
- The proximal pole of the scaphoid is susceptible to avascular necrosis following a fracture.[5]
- The lunate bone is the most frequently dislocated bone in the wrist and perilunate instability following a wrist injury must be evaluated.[6,7]
- The triquetrum articulates with the lunate laterally, the hamate distally and laterally, and the pisiform medially and the articular disk proximally.
- The pisiform is a small pea-shaped bone that is sesamoid in nature and has several soft tissue attachments.
- Distally, the trapezium articulates with the first and second metacarpals, while lateral and adjacent to it, the trapezoid also articulates with the second metacarpal.

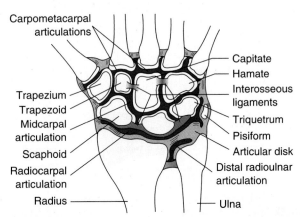

FIGURE 26-3. Wrist osteology. Cross section of the wrist and pertinent bony and soft tissues.

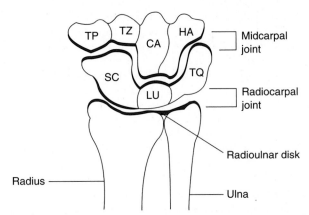

FIGURE 26-4. Wrist complex. The radiocarpal joint is composed of the radius and the articular disk, with the scaphoid (SC), lunate (LU), and triquetrum (TQ) bones. The midcarpal joint is composed of the scaphoid, lunate, and triquetrum with the trapezium (TP), trapezoid (TZ), the capitate (CA), and hamate (HA) bones.

- The capitate is the central and largest of all carpal bones (the "keystone" of the proximal transverse arch), with a central position allowing articulation with seven other bones and serving as a central site for ligamentous attachment.[8]
- The hamate is the most lateral bone of the distal carpal row, articulating with the fourth and fifth metacarpals and containing a palmar hook which protects the ulnar nerve passing beneath.

Arthrology

The wrist is generally divided into radiocarpal, midcarpal, carpometacarpal (CMC), and intercarpal joints. The radiocarpal joint is surrounded by an articular capsule that is lined with a synovial membrane, and this joint is formed by the articulations of the distal radius and the triangular articular disk with the scaphoid, lunate, and triquetrum bones.[2,9] See Figure 26-4. The key aspects of wrist arthrology are as follows:

- The medial portion of the radiocarpal joint includes a network of structures called the triangular fibrocartilage complex (Fig. 26-5).[9]
- The radiocarpal joint is reinforced by several ligaments which are true intracapsular ligaments. The radiocarpal and ulnocarpal joints are considered to be extrinsic because of attachments outside the wrist. (Fig. 26-6).[2]
- The intercarpal joints consist of articulations between individual bones within the proximal carpal row and the distal carpal row.
- The midcarpal joint is the articulation between the proximal and distal rows. The ligaments in this area are considered to be intrinsic and are divided into interosseous and midcarpal ligaments.[10] The specific ligaments are listed in Table 26-2.
- The CMC joints are also enclosed in a loose articular capsule, and are joined by dorsal, palmar, and interosseous ligaments.

Myology: Muscles Acting at the Wrist Joint

Several important muscles that function at the wrist have their origin at the elbow. These are the major wrist flexors and extensors. These muscles can be a source of epicondylitis from overuse activities at the wrist. Interventions should be directed at the muscle function at the wrist. A list of the key muscles can be found in Table 26-3.

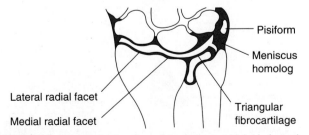

FIGURE 26-5. The proximal surface of the radiocarpal joint is formed by the medial and lateral facets of the distal radius and by the triangular fibrocartilage or articular disk. The articular disk and meniscus homolog are together part of the triangular fibrocartilage complex.

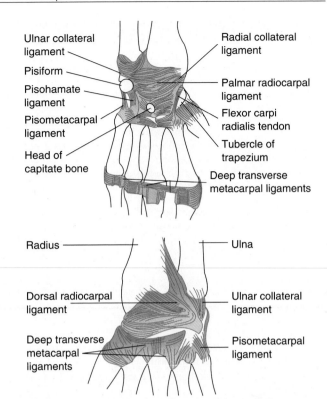

FIGURE 26-6. (A) Palmar aspect of the ligaments of the left wrist and metacarpal area. (B) Dorsal aspect of the ligaments of the left wrist.

Hand
Osteology
The key aspects of the osteology of the hand are as follows:

- Five metacarpals and fourteen phalanges compose the bony structure of the hand.
- Each metacarpal has a distal head, shaft, and base.[2]
- The medial four metacarpals articulate proximally with each other and with the distal row of carpal bones while the first and second metacarpals do not articulate with each other.

TABLE 26-2 Intrinsic Ligaments of the Wrist

CLASSIFICATION OF INTRINSIC LIGAMENTS	LIGAMENT NAMES
Interosseous	
Distal row	Trapezium-trapezoid
	Trapezoid-capitate
	Capitohamate
Proximal row	Scapholunate
	Lunotriquetral
Midcarpal	
Dorsal*	Scaphotriquetral
	Dorsal intercarpal
Palmar*	Scaphotrapeziotrapezoid
	Scaphocapitate
	Triquetrocapitate
	Triquetrohamate

*Midcarpal ligaments span the proximal and distal rows on the palmar or dorsal surfaces. (From Berger RA. The anatomy and basic biomechanics of the wrist joint. J Hand Ther 1996;9:84–93.)

MUSCLE	ORIGIN	INSERTION	ACTION	SPINAL LEVEL	PERIPHERAL NERVE
Extensor carpi radialis longus	Distal 1/3 of lateral supracondylar ridge	Base of second metacarpal	Wrist extension and abduction	C6–7	Radial
Extensor carpi radialis brevis	Common extensor tendon, lateral epicondyle	Base of third metacarpal	Wrist extension and abduction	C6–7	Radial
Extensor carpi ulnaris	Common extensor tendon	Base of fifth metacarpal	Wrist extension and adduction	C7–8	Radial
Flexor carpi radialis	Common flexor tendon of medial epicondyle	Base of second metacarpal	Wrist flexion and abduction	C6–7	Median
Flexor carpi ulnaris	Common flexor tendon; proximal posterior ulna	Pisiform bone, hamate, fifth metacarpal	Wrist flexion and adduction	C8–T1	Ulnar
Pronator quadratus	Medial anterior distal ulna	Lateral anterior distal radius	Forearm pronation	C8–T1	Median

TABLE 26-3 Muscles of the Wrist

Other muscles with primary function at the hand also assist function at the wrist. These will be included in Table 26-4.

- The first metacarpal is saddle shaped proximally to articulate with the trapezium
- There are three phalanges in each finger and two in the thumb.
- Each phalanx has a distal head, shaft, and proximal base.
- The thumb contains two sesamoid bones at the MCP joint.

Arthrology

The MCP and interphalangeal (IP) joints have similar arthrologic structures. Each is composed of an articular capsule and synovial lining. The MCP joints contain volar ligaments, which are thick and fibrocartilaginous, loosely attached to the metacarpal, and firmly attached at the phalangeal bases.[2] Because of the incongruence of the MCP joints, the volar ligament (i.e., volar plate) does more than reinforce joint capsule. Its fibrocartilaginous structure adds surface area to the base of the proximal phalanx to more closely approximate the size of the larger metacarpal head. This plate also checks hyperextension. Its flexible attachments permits motion into flexion without restricting motion or impinging the long flexor tendons.[9] The transverse metacarpal ligament connects the volar ligaments of the second through fifth MCP joints. Collateral ligaments are found on either side of the joint and are strong, rounded cords.[2] The capsular, volar, and collateral ligament arrangement at the MCP joints is the same structure found in the IP joints (Fig. 26-7).

Myology: Muscles Acting at the Hand

The muscular anatomy of the hand can be classified as thumb and finger musculature. Many muscles contribute to the fine motor function of the wrist and hand. Although a mere listing of the muscles along with their anatomy does not address the fine motor skill necessary for hand function, it is a place to begin consideration of hand function. A listing of muscles as well as figures of some key musculature can be found in Tables 26-4 and 26-5 and Figures 26-8 and 26-9.

REGIONAL NEUROLOGY

Several important nerves serve the elbow, wrist, and hand. These nerves may be injured locally by trauma, stretched during activities, or compressed within a confined space. Understanding the area anatomy aids the clinician in determining the source of symptoms.

The median nerve originates from two roots from the lateral (C5–7) and medial (C8–T1) cords. It descends along the brachial artery to enter the distal arm of the cubital fossa. It passes between the brachialis posteriorly and the bicipital aponeurosis anteriorly. At the elbow, the median nerve passes under the ligament of Struthers and the lacertus fibrosus and then enters the forearm between the heads of the pronator teres. This nerve can be injured or entrapped in any of these areas. It continues distally behind and adhered to the flexor digitorum superficialis (FDS) and anterior to the flexor digitorum profundus (FDP). As the median nerve passes the distal margin of the pronator teres muscle, it divides into the median nerve and the anterior interosseous nerve.[2] The anterior interosseous nerve supplies the first and second FDP, flexor pollicis longus (FPL), and pronator quadratus. Just proximal to the flexor retinaculum, the

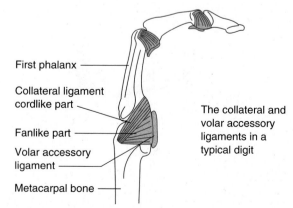

First phalanx

Collateral ligament cordlike part

Fanlike part

Volar accessory ligament

Metacarpal bone

The collateral and volar accessory ligaments in a typical digit

FIGURE 26-7. Ligaments of the fingers.

TABLE 26-4 Muscles Functioning Primarily at the Hand

MUSCLE	ORIGIN	INSERTION	ACTION	SPINAL LEVEL	PERIPHERAL NERVE
Extensor digitorum	Common extensor tendon of lateral epicondyle	Middle and base of distal phalanx of digits 2–5	Extends MCP joints and assists extension of IP joints	C6–8	Radial
Extensor indicis	Posterior ulna	Extensor expansion of index finger	Extends MCP joint and assists IP joint extension	C7–8	Radial
Extensor digiti minimi	Common extensor tendon	Extensor expansion of fifth digit	Extends MCP joint and assists with IP joint extension	C7–8	Radial
Palmaris longus	Common flexor tendon	Flexor retinaculum, palmar aponeurosis	Tenses palmar fascia	C7–8	Median
Flexor digitorum superficialis (FDS)	Common flexor tendon; coronoid process; radius	Middle phalanges of digits 2–5	Flexes proximal IP joints, assists MCP joint and wrist flexion	C7–8	Median
Flexor digitorum profundus (FDP)	Anteromedial ulna	Bases of distal phalanges digits 2–5	Flexes DIP joints; assists flexion of IP and MCP joints		
Flexor digiti minimi	Hook of hamate	Proximal phalanx of fifth digit	MCP flexion of fifth finger	C8	Ulnar
Opponens digiti minimi	Hook of hamate	Length of fifth MC	Opposes CMC of fifth finger	C8–T1	Ulnar
Dorsal interossei	Metacarpal bones	Radial and ulnar sides of fingers	Digit abduction and assists flexion and extension	C8–T1	Ulnar
Palmar interossei	Metacarpal bones	Ulnar and radial sides of fingers	Adduction of fingers	C8–T1	Ulnar

IP, interphalangeal; MCP, metacarpophalangeal.

TABLE 26-5 Muscles Functioning at the Thumb

MUSCLE	ORIGIN	INSERTION	ACTION	SPINAL LEVEL	PERIPHERAL NERVE
Adductor pollicis	Capitate; second and third MC	Proximal phalanx of thumb	Adduction of CMC joint	C8–T1	Ulnar
Abductor pollicis longus (APL)	Posterior ulna and radius	First MC	Abducts and extends CMC joint	C7–8	Radial
Abductor pollicis brevis (APB)	Trapezium and scaphoid	Proximal phalanx of thumb	Abduction of CMC and MCP joints	C6–8	Median
Opponens pollicis	Trapezium	First MC	Opposes CMC of thumb	C6–8	Median
Flexor pollicis longus	Interosseus membranes, medial epicondyle	Distal phalanx of thumb	Flexes IP joint	C8–T1	Median
Flexor pollicis brevis	Trapezius, trapezium, and capitate	Proximal phalanx of thumb	Flexes MCP and CMC joints of thumb	C6–8, T1	Median and ulnar
Extensor pollicis longus	Posterior ulna	Distal phalanx of thumb	Extends IP joint	C7–8	Radial
Extensor pollicis brevis	Posterior radius	Proximal phalanx of thumb	Extends MCP joint	C7–8	Radial

CMC, carpometacarpal; MC, metacarpal; MCP, metacarpophalangeal.

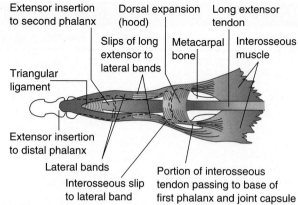

FIGURE 26-8. Dorsal view of extensor mechanism of the fingers.

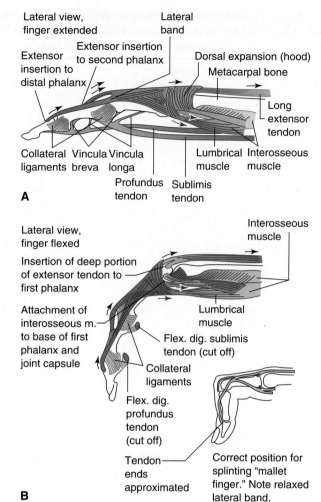

FIGURE 26-9. Intrinsic muscle anatomy. (A) Extended position. (B) Flexed position.

median nerve becomes superficial and then passes deep to the flexor retinaculum into the palm. It then passes through the carpal tunnel, where it may become compressed. After passing through the tunnel, the median nerve divides into five or six branches, providing motor and sensory innervation to the hand.

The ulnar nerve arises from the medial cord (C8–T1) of the brachial plexus, but it may receive fibers from the ventral ramus of C7. Because of its location and anatomic relationships, the ulnar nerve is susceptible to compression, traction, and friction. The ulnar nerve courses distally through the axilla along with the axillary artery and vein and the brachial artery. At the middle of the humerus, it moves medially, descending anterior to the medial head of the triceps. The ulnar nerve can become entrapped here by the arcade of Struthers, approximately 8 cm proximal to the medial epicondyle.[2] At the elbow, the ulnar nerve passes superficially through a groove on the dorsum of the medial epicondyle, entering the forearm in the cubital tunnel between the two heads of the flexor carpi ulnaris. The ulnar nerve can become entrapped here as well, because the cubital tunnel narrows 55% during elbow flexion.[11] Traction across an unstable medial elbow joint can also injure the ulnar nerve. Through the forearm, the ulnar nerve descends along the medial side of the FDP. Just proximal to the wrist, it sends off a dorsal branch that continues distally across the flexor retinaculum. The ulnar nerve continues distally with the ulnar artery, beneath the most superficial aspect of the flexor retinaculum, and divides into superficial and deep terminal branches. The ulnar nerve can be compressed as it crosses the distal edge of the pisohamate portion of the retinaculum. The superficial and deep branches provide motor and sensory innervation to the hand.

The radial nerve arises from the posterior cord (C5–8) and is the largest branch of the brachial plexus. It courses distally between the medial and long heads of the triceps and then passes obliquely posterior to the humerus and deep to the lateral head of the triceps to the lateral aspect of the humerus to penetrate the anterior compartment.[2] Its proximity to the humerus makes it susceptible to injury in mid-humeral fractures. As the radial nerve continues distally, it bifurcates to become the posterior interosseous and superficial radial nerves. The superficial radial nerve has only sensory fibers. The posterior interosseous nerve is analogous to its anterior correlate (i.e., anterior interosseous nerve) in that it has only motor fibers. The posterior interosseous nerve passes through the supinator muscle, around the proximal radius, and beneath the extensor muscle mass, and the superficial radial nerve passes beneath the brachioradialis muscle and continues distally to the hand. The superficial radial nerve continues distally along the anterolateral aspect of the forearm. Proximal to the wrist, it passes deep to curve around the radius and divides into four or five dorsal digital nerves. This nerve innervates the skin of the dorsolateral hand. It is susceptible to injury in the distal forearm and hand, where it lies superficially. Compression can by caused by casts, watchbands, and similar items.[12]

KINESIOLOGY

Elbow and Forearm

Normal ROM at the elbow joint is 0 to 135 degrees actively and 0 to 150 degrees passively. Much of this mobility is necessary for the normal activities of daily living (ADLs). For example, putting on a shirt requires a range of 15 to 140 degrees, and drinking from a cup requires range of 72 to 130 degrees.[13] ROM in flexion is limited by anterior muscle bulk, and ROM in extension is limited by the bony articulation of the olecranon in the olecranon fossa. The extended position of the humeroulnar joint is the close-packed position; additional inherent stability occurs in extreme flexion. Motion occurs primarily by gliding of the ulna on the trochlea.

Pronation and supination technically occur through the forearm at the proximal and distal radioulnar joints. The normal range of pronation and supination is 0 to 80 degrees in each direction. Pronation occurs as the radius crosses over the ulna at the proximal radioulnar joint. Although most ADLs occur with the forearm in a middle position, some activities, such as receiving change in the palm of the hand, require full supination.

Resistance to valgus stress in full extension is limited equally by the UCL, bony congruity, and the anterior capsule.[9] As the elbow moves into flexion, most of the resistance to valgus stress is provided by the anterior band of the UCL. Morrey and An[14] found the UCL to contribute approximately 54% of the resistance to valgus stress in flexion. The joint articulation contributed 33% of the resistance to valgus.

Resistance to varus in full extension is provided by the bony congruity and by the radial collateral ligament and capsule.[9] Resistance to distraction is provided by soft-tissue components, and the anterior portion of the joint capsule provides the primarily resistance to anterior displacement.

A cadaveric study of the flexor pronator group relative to the UCL throughout the ROM has significant implications for rehabilitation of individuals with medial elbow injuries. At 30 degrees of elbow flexion, the pronator teres and flexor carpi radialis muscles were entirely anterior to the UCL, and the flexor carpi ulnaris muscle was found over or posterior to the UCL.[15] The FDS muscle was over the UCL in most cases. The findings were similar at 90 degrees, except the flexor carpi ulnaris muscle was completely over the UCL, and the FDS muscle was anterior to the UCL in most cases. At 120 degrees, the pronator teres, flexor carpi radialis, and FDS muscles were all anterior to the UCL, and only the flexor carpi ulnaris muscle was over the UCL. This pattern suggests that the flexor carpi ulnaris muscle is the primary dynamic medial elbow stabilizer throughout the ROM and particularly at 120 degrees of flexion.[15]

Wrist

The normal wrist ROM is from 80 degrees of flexion to 70 degrees of extension. The resting position of the wrist is between 20 and 35 degrees of extension and 10 to 15 degrees of ulnar deviation while in the close-packed position.[16] The wrist functions primarily through a range of 10 degrees of flexion to 35 degrees of extension when performing most ADLs.[17] However, some activities, such as rising from a chair, require significantly more extension.[17] Movement at the radiocarpal joint is predominantly a gliding movement of the concave distal radius and articular disk on the convex proximal carpal row. The proximal carpal row is considered to be an intercalated segment, a relatively unattached middle segment of a three-segment link, because of its position between the radius and distal carpus.[9]

Mechanically, the scaphoid plays a critical role in stabilizing this segment by means of its position bridging the proximal and distal carpal rows (i.e., the midcarpal joint). The radiocarpal and midcarpal joints provide variable proportions of the motion during wrist extension and flexion. When the

proportion contributed by radiocarpal joint exceeds that of the midcarpal joints in one direction, this pattern reverses in the other direction.[9] Wrist extension is initiated at the distal carpal row, with this row gliding on the relatively stable proximal row. As the wrist passes into extension, these rows begin to move together, with the scaphoid intervening as the bridge to this process.[9] Full extension is the close-packed position of the wrist.

In general, the distal carpal row functions as a unit because of the interlocking of articular surfaces and the ligamentous connections between the distal row and the metacarpals distally.[10] The distal row tends to move in unison with the second and third metacarpals, palmar flexing when these metacarpals palmar flex and dorsal flexing when they dorsally flex. The proximal carpal row differs in its movement pattern from the distal row. In general, the bones in the proximal row move together, although greater motion occurs between the bones in the proximal row than in the distal row. This is true of the direction and magnitude of motion between the bones in the proximal row. The proximal row tends to move in the same direction as the distal row and therefore in the same direction as the second and third metacarpals.[10] Between-bone motion also occurs, and, during wrist extension, the scaphoid supinates while the lunate pronates, functionally separating these bones. This motion underlies perilunate instabilities occurring as a result of forceful extension.

Frontal plane motion is normally from 15 degrees of radial deviation to 30 degrees of ulnar deviation. The ulnar styloid is shorter than the radial styloid, accounting for the greater range in ulnar deviation than radial. Greater ulnar and radial deviation is possible when the wrist is in a neutral flexion-extension position. Arthrokinematic motion in radial and ulnar deviation is more complex than in flexion and extension. During radial deviation, the proximal carpal row glides ulnarly and flexes while the distal row pivots radially. During ulnar deviation, the proximal row glides radially and moves into extension while the distal row moves ulnarly.[10]

The mobility of the wrist depends on the position of the fingers because of the length of extrinsic tendons crossing the wrist and hand joints. For example, wrist flexion is decreased when the fingers are simultaneously flexed because of the length of the extrinsic finger extensor muscles. Likewise, the mobility of the fingers depends on the position of the wrist, as evidenced by the inability to fully flex the fingers when the wrist is flexed.

Load transmission across the wrist is significant and varies with wrist position. With the wrist and forearm in neutral, approximately 80% of the force is transmitted across the radiocarpal joint and 20% across the ulnocarpal joint.[18] Further breakdown of the radiocarpal loads shows that approximately 45% of these forces are transmitted across the radioscaphoid joint and 35% across the radiolunate joint.[18] Forearm pronation increases the load transmitted across the ulnocarpal joint to approximately 37%, with a proportional reduction of load at the radiocarpal joint. Radiocarpal forces increase to 87% when the wrist is in radial deviation.[10]

Hand

Carpometacarpal Joints

CMC joints two through five are similar in structure and function, but the first CMC is different. The second through fourth CMC joints permit one degree of freedom in flexion and extension, and the fifth CMC allows some abduction and adduction as well. Motion at the CMC joints is limited primarily by the ligamentous structure. Motion increases at the CMC joints from the radial to the ulnar side of the hand.[9] Almost no motion occurs at the second and third CMC joints, the fourth is slightly more mobile, and the fifth moves through a range of nearly 10 to 20 degrees.[9]

The first CMC joint is saddle shaped and has two degrees of freedom and some axial rotation. This mobility allows for opposition, a key function of the thumb. The thumb is involved in nearly all forms of prehension, or handling activities, and loss of the thumb accounts for the greatest portion of disability in the hand.[19] ROM is approximately from 20 degrees of flexion to 45 degrees of extension and from 0 degrees of adduction to 40 degrees of abduction. Mobility at the CMC is limited by the ligamentous and interposed soft tissues.

A primary role of the CMC joints is to contribute to cupping of the hand, forming palmar arches. This hollowing allows the hand to conform to the shape of the object being held (Fig. 26-10A and B). Two arches are visible: the longitudinal arch that spans the length of the hand and the metacarpal arch that transverses the palm.

Metacarpophalangeal Joint

The four medial metacarpophalangeal (MCP) joints possess two degrees of freedom, flexion and extension, and abduction and adduction. The mobility at these joints increases from the radial to ulnar sides of the hand, with an active ROM from 90 degrees of flexion to 10 degrees of extension. Passively, variable amounts of extension are available. Functional flexion at the MCP joint is approximately 60 degrees.[16] The range in abduction and adduction is approximately 20 degrees in each direction. The range in the frontal plane is limited by articular surface geometry, and the range in flexion is limited by joint geometry and capsule, and the range in extension is limited by the volar plates.

The MCP joint of the thumb also possesses two degrees of freedom. The ROM is more limited here than in fingers two through five. Almost no hyperextension is available in normal hands, and only approximately 50 degrees of flexion can be obtained. Extension at this joint is further limited by the presence of two sesamoid bones, stabilized by collateral and intersesamoid ligaments. The primary function of MCP mobility of the thumb is providing additional range for opposition and prehension activities.

Interphalangeal Joints

The IP joints of the fingers and thumb are similar in function. Each is a hinge joint with one degree of freedom. ROM at the

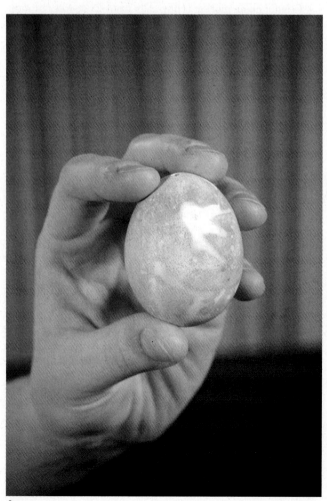
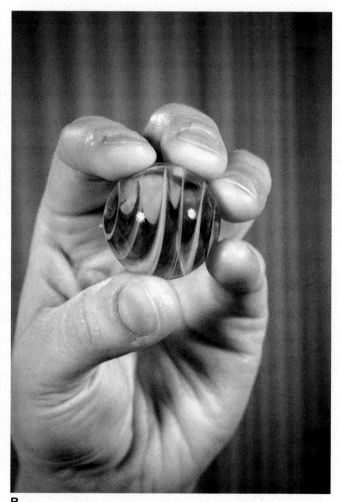

A **B**

FIGURE 26-10. (A, B) Hollowing of the hand allows it to conform to different size and shape objects.

IP joints, as with the other joints in the hand, increases from the radial to the ulnar side of the hand. This is easily observed when making a fist. The ROM at the proximal interphalangeal (PIP) is from 0 degrees of extension to 100 degrees of flexion at the radial side of the hand and nearly 135 degrees of flexion at the ulnar side. Little hyperextension is available because of the volar plates. The distal interphalangeal (DIP) joint demonstrates less ROM, from 10 degrees of extension to 80 degrees of flexion. Functional flexion at the PIP joints is approximately 60 degrees, and functional flexion at the DIP joints is 40 degrees.[16]

Extensor Mechanism

The extensor mechanism of the fingers is composed of the extensor hood (i.e., extensor expansion or dorsal aponeurosis) and the extensor digitorum (ED), palmar interossei, dorsal interossei, and lumbrical muscles. Each finger contains a similar mechanism that is necessary for successful extension of the finger. As the ED courses distally, it flattens into an aponeurotic hood over the metacarpal, and just distal to the MCP joint, the ED is joined by tendon fibers from the interossei muscles. The interossei arise from the lateral borders of the metacarpals (see Fig. 26-9). This aponeurosis formed by the ED and interossei continues distally, where, proximal to the PIP, the hood splits into three branches. All three branches receive fibers from the interossei, and the medial branch also receives fibers from the lumbricals. A central tendon continues distally and crosses the PIP to insert at the base of the middle phalanx. Two lateral bands on either side continue distally, cross the PIP joint, and reunite into a single tendon that terminates at the distal phalanx. Several local ligaments attach to the extensor hood and prevent bowstringing during movement. The oblique retinacular ligaments are important in simultaneous PIP and DIP extension.

A complete description of the mechanics of the extensor hood is beyond the scope of this text, but a few generalizations can be made. At the MCP joint, contraction of the ED produces extension while activation of the lumbricals and interossei produce flexion. The torque produced by the ED exceeds the that of others, and extension results. At the PIP joint, the ED, interossei, and lumbricals together produce extension (Figure 26-11). Isolated contraction of the ED causes the finger to claw or to produce MCP hyperextension with IP flexion[9] because of the passive pull of the long finger flexors at the IP joints. Extension of the PIP joint also produces DIP extension (and vice versa), and when the PIP is held in flexion, the DIP is incapable of isolated extension. This mechanism is finely tuned to produce fine movements and strong grip. Any imbalance in the lateral slips disrupts this mechanism and significantly alters hand function.

Prehension

The hand is well suited for the major task of grasping, gripping, and manipulating objects. Prehension is the global term for the usual tasks of grasping, holding, and manipulating objects. Many terms are commonly used to describe hand functions. Most functions can be grouped into the categories of grip and pinch. These can be further subdivided into categories such as power grip, precision grip, hook grip, key pinch, and precision pinch. The power grip is used for developing firm control, while the precision grip is used when accuracy and precision are needed. The precision grip allows the hand to conform to different size and shape objects. Examples of power grip include hook, spherical, cylinder, and fist grasps. Examples of pinch types include the key, and tip-to-tip and pulp-to-pulp pinches.

Grip activity has been broken down into four stages. In the first step, the hand opens by simultaneous action of the long extensor and hand intrinsic muscles. The fingers then close about the object, requiring activity of the intrinsic and extrinsic flexor and opposition muscles. The third step is an increase in force in these same muscles to a level appropriate for the task. The hand again opens to release the object.[16] While the flexors are grasping the object, the wrist extensor muscles must fire simultaneously to prevent the long flexors from producing wrist flexion.

The innervation of the hand is related to the two types of grip. The ulnar nerve controls the motor and sensory distribution of the medial digits, and these digits are used more for the power grip. The median nerve controls the lateral digits, which are used more for the precision grip. The thumb musculature, used in both types of grip, is innervated by both nerves.[16]

The power grip is used when force generation is the primary objective (Fig. 26-12A). Carrying a suitcase, climbing on a jungle gym, making a fist, and grasping a baseball to throw are all examples of power grip. In this situation, the ulnar digits stabilize the object, holding it against the palm, with or without the assistance of the thumb. The fingers are fully flexed while the wrist is extended and ulnarly deviated.

The precision pinch is used when fine control is necessary. This grip is used when holding a writing implement, putting a key in the door, or holding a piece of paper between two fingers (Fig. 26-12B and C). The precision pinch includes primarily the MCP joints and the radial side of the hand. The index and middle fingers work with the thumb to create a tripod. In contrast with the power grip, the object in a precision pinch may never come in contact with the palm.

EXAMINATION AND EVALUATION

Examination and evaluation of the elbow, wrist, and hand must include a comprehensive assessment of the upper quarter. The upper extremity relationships between the cervical spine and distal joints requires a full examination to ensure identification

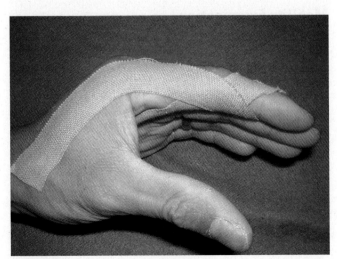

FIGURE 26-11. Patient with a lumbrical strain who improved with kinesiotaping.

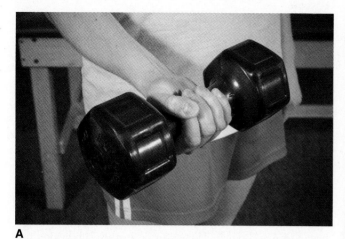

A

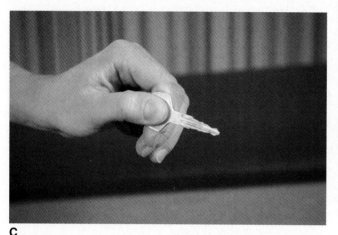

C

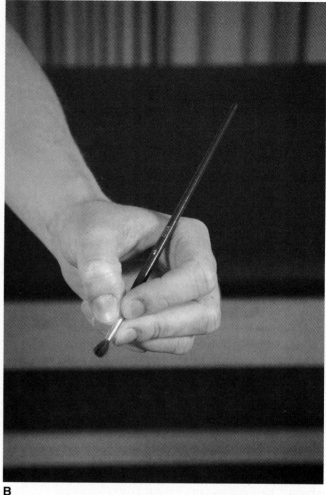

B

FIGURE 26-12. (A) Power grip. (B) Precision grip (C) Key grip.

of the problem source. Many of the examination techniques depend on the situation. The presence of comorbidities such as diabetes or rheumatoid arthritis (RA) necessitates different examination techniques from those used for the patient without such additional issues. The following sections address the key aspects of elbow, wrist, and hand examinations.

History and Observation

The history and subjective information focuses the remainder of the examination. In addition to the medical history and evaluation of the current problem, subjective information about the signs and symptoms after the injury is valuable. Information is gathered about the activity limitations (e.g., inability to manipulate buttons, zippers and other small objects, inability to carry out hygiene activities, difficulty writing or typing, problems opening jars) and participation restrictions (e.g., unable to work because of inability to type, unable to care for child because of pain and weakness in elbow) associated with the current complaint. Information to differentiate primary elbow, wrist, and hand problems from those referred from the cervical spine must be ascertained.

The resting position of the hand also should be observed, including these deformities:

- Swan-neck deformity
- Boutonnière deformity

- Ulnar drift
- Clubbing of DIPs
- Heberden or Bouchard nodes
- Claw fingers
- Dupuytren contracture
- Mallet or trigger finger

Mobility Examination

Mobility examination of the elbow, wrist, and hand includes osteokinematic and arthrokinematic testing and tests of muscle extensibility. It is particularly important to find the sources of mobility loss in the hand, because this impairment is associated with significant activity limitations and disability. Examination procedures should distinguish between contractile and noncontractile tissues and between intrinsic and extrinsic muscle limitations. In most cases, both osteokinematic and arthrokinematic tests of mobility should be performed, as well as tests of muscle flexibility.

Muscle Performance Examination

Muscles functioning at the elbow, wrist, and hand should be tested in a logical order on the basis of the subjective information provided, history, and the results of the examination. Many of the hand muscles are quite small, and therapists must consider their relative strength when applying traditional manual muscle testing criteria. Stabilization, particularly when trying to isolate small intrinsic muscles of the hand, ensures that the muscle of interest is being tested. Kendall[4] has described the testing procedures for the relevant muscles in the region. Grip and pinch (tip pinch and key pinch) force measurements are commonly used and have high reliability. However, large changes (i.e., improvements) in these measures are necessary before they can be reliably detected with standard measuring devices.[20]

Other Tests

Many special tests assess the integrity of tissues throughout the upper quarter. These tests examine ligament stability, soft-tissue mobility, neurologic status, and functional tasks. Magee[16] has provided a complete listing and description of special tests. Some of the more common tests used are listed in Display 26-1.

THERAPEUTIC EXERCISE INTERVENTIONS FOR COMMON IMPAIRMENTS OF BODY FUNCTIONS

Mobility of Joint Functions: Impaired Range of Motion

Impaired mobility in the distal upper extremity can be very disabling. Fine motor skills are necessary for the simplest of daily activities. Mobility activities must restore full ROM throughout the distal segments to maintain independence in many household tasks. Impaired mobility in this region is

treated with a combination of therapeutic modalities, exercise, and splinting.

Hypomobility

Hypomobility in this region can occur for a number of reasons. Injuries that necessitate a period of immobilization can produce profound mobility loss. Surgery, neurologic injuries, burns, and falls can significantly impair mobility. Because of the mobility required for functional use of the upper limb, loss of motion in this region can be quite disabling.

Intervention for mobility loss requires a thorough evaluation to determine the structures responsible for or contributing to the motion loss. The joint capsule, short musculotendinous structures, immobile fascial tissues, or restricted nervous tissues are a few examples of tissues that may be at fault. Evaluation techniques aimed at differentiating contractile from noncontractile tissues, followed by specific tension testing, can pinpoint the source of limitation. Only then can appropriate intervention be initiated.

Mobility impairment at the **elbow** includes loss of flexion and extension. Loss of elbow extension occurs frequently after fractures or dislocations at the elbow. Loss of motion occurs rapidly at the elbow, and therefore immobilization is kept to the minimum acceptable time. Degenerative joint disease has a lower impact on the upper extremity joints than the lower, and loss of motion because of arthritic changes at the elbow therefore is less common than at the knee. Loss of motion at the elbow is often compensated by trunk, shoulder, and wrist motion, all of which may place additional loads on these structures.

Mobility loss at the **forearm** includes loss of pronation and supination. The capsular pattern shows equal loss of pronation and supination. Loss of motion at the forearm is common after immobilization for wrist and hand fractures. Loss of pronation and supination results in difficulties with turning knobs, opening jars, receiving change, and turning a key. These motions are frequently transferred to the shoulder, with the person performing external and internal rotation to compensate. Restoration of motion is important to prevent secondary injury to the shoulder.

Loss of motion at the **wrist** is common after falls or fractures injuring the wrist. Fractures of the distal radius or ulna require immobilization and potentially surgical stabilization. Scaphoid fractures are prone to avascular necrosis due to the local blood supply, and therefore require immobilization. This immobilization leads to loss of mobility at all joints of the forearm, wrist and hand. RA also affects the wrist joint causing deformity, pain and loss of hand function.

Loss of motion in the **hand** is frequently caused by rheumatoid arthritic changes. Loss of motion in the hand may also result from osteoarthritis (OA), and this process tends to affect the PIP and DIP joints but not the MCP joints (see Self-Management 26-1: Proximal and Distal Interphalangeal Joint Flexion). The thumb CMC is significantly affected by OA and RA. Injuries such as fractures, dislocations, and burns produce limitations in mobility after treatment. Dupuytren contraction, or contraction of the palmar fascia, usually affects the fourth or fifth fingers, where the skin is adherent to the underlying fascia. This progressive fibrosis of the palmar fascia has no known cause and affects men older than 40 years of age more than women.[16] These impairments can lead to activity limitations (e.g., inability to grasp a pen) and therefore

SELF-MANAGEMENT 26-1 *Proximal and Distal Interphalangeal Joint Flexion*

Purpose: To increase the mobility in the joints and tendons of your fingers

Starting Position: Start with all the joints of your fingers as straight as possible.

Movement Technique: Keeping your knuckle joints (MCP) straight, bend the middle and fingertip joints (PIP and DIP) as far as possible. Return to the starting position.

Dosage
Repetitions: _____
Frequency: _____

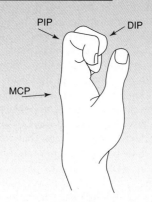

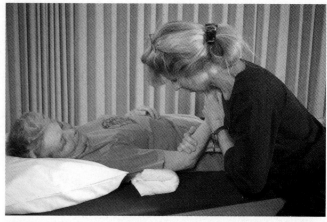

FIGURE 26-13. Elbow joint mobilization. Distal traction at humerounlnar joint to increase elbow flexion and extension range of motion.

participation restrictions (e.g., unable to work because of inability to grasp objects).

Activities to increase mobility begin with an intervention to warm the tissue (i.e., active exercise, superficial or deep heat), followed by stretching the musculotendinous tissue, or mobilizing the joint depending upon the source of the restriction. For example, limited motion because of capsular restriction at the elbow may be treated with humeroulnar distraction techniques and some anterior and posterior glides (see Chapter 7; Fig. 26-13). After mobilization techniques, passive prolonged stretching in the direction of limitation may be performed along with concurrent application of heat or cold. Active mobility in the new range should follow (Fig. 26-14 A and B). For example, active pronation and supination may be followed

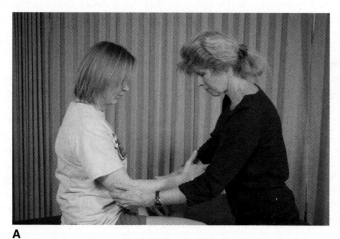

A

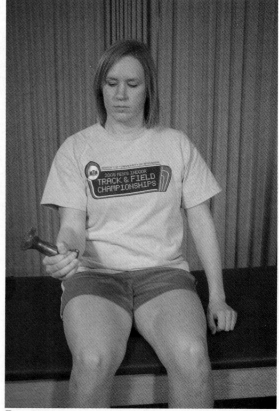

B

FIGURE 26-14. (A) Contract-relax stretching of the forearm into supination, followed by (B) active use of the forearm into elbow flexion with forearm supination.

SELF-MANAGEMENT 26-2 *Metacarpophalangeal and Proximal Interphalangeal Joint Flexion With Distal Interphalangeal Joint Extension*

Purpose:	To increase the mobility of your finger joints and tendons
Position:	Start with all joints of your fingers as straight as possible.
Movement Technique:	Bend your knuckle (MCP) and middle (PIP) joints while keeping the fingertip joints (DIP) straight. Return to the starting position.

Dosage
Repetitions: _____
Frequency: _____

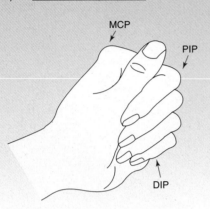

by active hand to mouth exercises or active forward reaching. When immobility is caused by a short or stiff muscle, traditional stretching techniques may be employed. At the same time, postural correction and strengthening of the antagonist (which is often weak because of its lengthened position) must occur. Immobile fascial connective tissues are mobilized by manual techniques such as massage and manual deep pressure application. As with stretching, this intervention should be followed with active use of the limb (see Self-Management 26-2: Metacarpophalangeal and Proximal Interphalangeal Joint Flexion With Distal Interphalangeal Joint Extension). See Building Block 26-1.

Treatment for immobility of the hand of a patient with RA depends on the acuteness of the situation and the degree of deformity. Immobilization may be the treatment of choice in some phases of this disease process (see the "Stiff Hand and Restricted Motion" section). Neural gliding techniques

---

BUILDING BLOCK 26-1

A 56-year-old forklift driver has pain with active pronation and supination following a radial head fracture which is now healed. Outline a typical treatment session for this patient in the early phase.

---

are employed when neural tension test reveals immobility of neural tissue to be the source of the patient's symptoms.

Hypermobility

Hypermobility is an uncommon problem at the elbow and forearm; hypomobility is a much more common complaint. Elbow hyperextension ROM is one criteria for a diagnosis of systemic hypermobility. However, hypermobility at this joint is rarely symptomatic because of the limited weight bearing occurring in the upper extremities. Individuals participating in upper extremity weight-bearing sports such as gymnastics or wrestling may have difficulty associated with elbow hyperextension during sports.

Similarly, hypermobility is uncommon at the wrist and hand. Hypermobility should not be confused with instability. Instabilities occur in the wrist and the hand. Lunate dislocation with perilunate instability and scapholunate dissociation are common, and instability in the fingers is evident in the hand of the patient with RA. However, physiologic hypermobility rarely exists without pathology or injury, and if hypermobility is present, it rarely produces symptoms.

Impaired Muscle Power Functions

Several injuries or pathologies can impair a patient's ability to produce torque in the distal upper extremity. Fractures, dislocations, contusions, sprains, tendon lacerations, burns, nerve entrapments, and crush injuries are some of the conditions that can limit a person's torque-producing ability. The relationship between the force or torque impairment and activity limitations or participation restrictions must be established to justify and guide treatment. Specific muscular strengthening exercises must be progressed to activities that reproduce the function of the upper extremity. This includes self-care activities such as dressing, grooming, and bathing and work activities such as pushing, pulling, grasping, pinching, typing, and other dexterous movements.

Any strengthening exercises for the elbow, wrist, and hand must consider the kinetic chain relationship across these joints. The joints are interconnected and related, and the muscular anatomy often crosses several joints. Strengthening exercises for the elbow often load the wrist and finger muscles as the individual holds a weight or other resistive equipment in the hand. Strengthening exercises requiring a grip differ from those using resistance around the wrist (e.g., a cuff weight). For example, strengthening exercises for lateral epicondylitis focus on strengthening the wrist extensor muscles in their roles as active wrist extensors (concentrically and eccentrically) and as stabilizers against finger flexor activity such as gripping or shaking hands. Any wrist extension exercise that concurrently requires gripping may overload these muscles (Fig. 26-15). This relationship is one reason why prescribing shoulder exercises while holding a 16-oz can in the hand can produce lateral epicondylitis in previously asymptomatic individuals.

Neurologic Causes

Neurologic pathology or injury is a common source of impaired muscle function in the distal upper extremity. Cervical degenerative joint disease, degenerative disk disease, and cervical spine injuries can cause symptoms distally in the respective nerve root distributions. After exiting the cervical spine, the nerves may be entrapped in a number of locations throughout

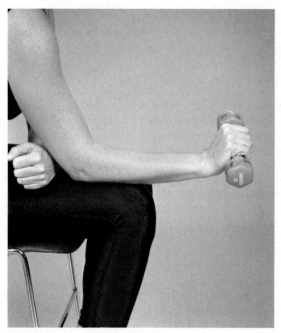

FIGURE 26-15. Resisted wrist extension with free weights.

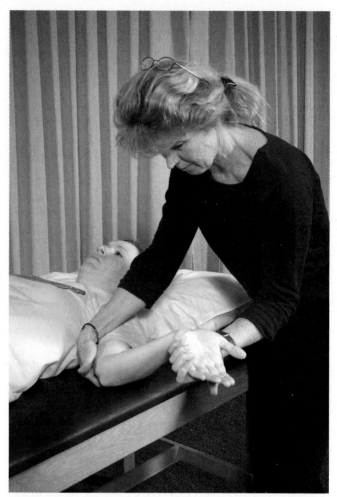

FIGURE 26-16. Neural gliding techniques with an emphasis on median nerve.

the neck and thorax. Entrapment may produce distal neurovascular symptoms such as thoracic outlet syndrome. In this situation, the neurovascular bundle is compressed at one or more sites (e.g., cervical rib, scalene muscles) producing a variety of intermittent to constant symptoms.

More distally, the radial nerve may be compressed in the radial tunnel, the ulnar nerve at the medial elbow or at the pisiform, and the median nerve in the carpal tunnel. The ulnar nerve is also subject to traction injuries at the medial elbow in the thrower. Similarly, the mobility of any nerve within its nerve sheath may become restricted (Fig. 26-16).

Injury, compression, traction, or ischemia of these nerves, proximally or distally, results in various symptoms, including loss of the ability to produce torque in the muscles served by the damaged nerve. Treatment for a limited ability to produce torque depends on the specific situation. For example, the individual with distal weakness caused by cervical spine disk herniation may benefit from traction, postural retraining, and cervical spine exercises, followed by progressive resistive exercises for distal musculature only after the proximal symptoms have resolved. Nerve entrapments at the elbow, wrist, or hand must be treated first by release techniques to mobilize the nerve. In contrast, traction injuries to the ulnar nerve at the elbow should be initially treated with stabilization techniques. Only then can strengthening exercises be initiated. These exercises may be performed in positions or postures that minimize the traction or compressive forces on the nerve. Progression to more provocative and functional patterns should follow. See Building Block 26-2.

Muscular Causes

Muscle injuries in this region range from tendinopathies at the elbow (i.e., medial and lateral epicondylitis) and wrist (i.e., de Quervain tenosynovitis) to tendon lacerations in the hand. Intervention to increase the ability to produce torque

after injury to the muscle depends on the location and severity of injury, the role of that muscle in functional activities, and the stages of healing. The ability of the muscle to tolerate loads, whether stretching loads or isometric, or shortening or lengthening muscle contractions, is the first step in determining an individual's readiness for strengthening exercises. Eccentric contractions are frequently used to treat tendinopathy at the elbow joint (see Chapter 11).

After the appropriate level of load is determined, progressive isometric to dynamic exercises may be initiated for elbow musculature (e.g., extensors, flexors), forearm musculature (e.g., pronators, supinators), and wrist and hand (e.g., flexors, extensors, ulnar and radial deviators). Exercises may be

 BUILDING BLOCK 26-2

A 16-year-old softball pitcher experiences weakness in the muscles innervated by the ulnar nerve due to valgus stress traction injury. She has been taken off pitching until symptoms resolve and needs to rehabilitate key musculature. What are the key muscle groups to consider for rehabilitation? What types of exercises might be recommended?

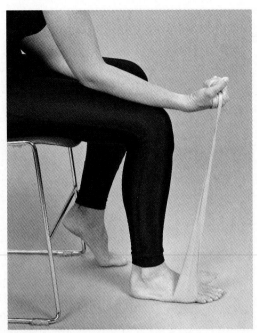

FIGURE 26-17. Resisted wrist flexion combined with grip strengthening using a resistive band.

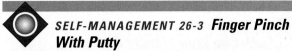

SELF-MANAGEMENT 26-3 *Finger Pinch With Putty*

Purpose:	To increase the strength of the muscles used to pinch
Starting Position:	Form the putty into the shape of a ball. Hold it between your fingertips.
Movement Technique:	Pinch the putty between your fingertips and your thumb until your fingers press through the putty. Reshape the putty and repeat.

Dosage
  Repetitions: _____
  Frequency: _____

performed in an open chain, using light weights, bands, or other functional objects (Fig. 26-17). Closed chain activity such as leaning against a wall or on a countertop to provide resistance is also appropriate. In the hand, manual resistance is often used. After surgery for tendon repairs, PROM in the direction of pull of the lacerated tendon is allowed first, followed by Active Assisted ROM (AAROM) and AROM when sufficient healing allows. Mobilization occurs early to prevent adhesions of the tendon within the sheath. However, resistance is applied only after satisfactory healing at the surgical site (about 8 weeks). At that point, simple gripping exercises using sponges, putty, or other small resistive objects may be initiated (Fig. 26-18). Resistance to extension can be provided manually or by using small resistive bands. In addition to restoring torque producing abilities, the fine motor function of the muscles must be retrained. Several dexterity tasks are available for training these skills (see Self-Management 26-3: Finger Pinch With Putty).

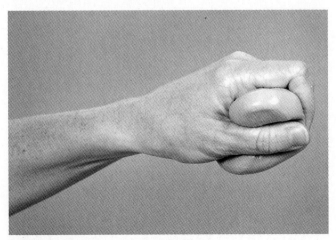

FIGURE 26-18. Grip strengthening using putty.

Disuse and Deconditioning

Proximal muscle deconditioning can lead to distal muscle overuse injuries. This occurs with repetitive work or activity and reinforces the importance of a thorough upper quarter examination. Effective repetitive distal activity requires proximal stabilization, maintaining posture within a neutral range. When the proximal muscles fatigue, posture is compromised, and a greater load is placed on the distal muscles. For example, as the rotator cuff fatigues during a repetitive lifting task, more of the lifting may be performed by the elbow flexors and wrist extensors, predisposing the individual to lateral epicondylitis. As one group of distal muscles fatigues, the load is shifted to alternate muscle groups, overworking these muscles. Appropriate muscle endurance for the required task is necessary throughout the kinetic chain.

Endurance Impairment

Muscular endurance impairment is often seen at the wrist and hand in individuals who perform repetitive work with their hands. Imbalance between the endurance of wrist flexors and extensors, along with a number of other factors (i.e., posture, tool design, volume of activity, etc.), contribute to forearm, wrist, and hand pain. Overwork of the wrist and finger flexors during repetitive gripping or typing can contribute to overuse problems of the forearm, wrist and hand. Forms of epicondylitis at the elbow may be considered forms of endurance impairment as well. Epicondylitis may develop as an acute injury because of a muscular strain, or it may result from fatigue of the overworked musculature. In this situation, impaired muscle endurance is contributing to the situation.

Particular attention should be given to the posture assumed during performance of these exercises. Wrist extensor

SELF-MANAGEMENT 26-4 *Wrist Extension Exercise With Grocery Bag*

Purpose:	To increase the strength of your forearm, wrist, and hand muscles
Starting Position:	Find a bag or purse with a comfortable handle. An object with too large or too small a handle can increase your pain. Place objects such as cans or bags of beans in the bag according to the weight recommendations of your clinician. Hold the handle of the bag over the edge of a table with your palm down.

Movement Technique:

Level 1:	Hold the bag for a count of 10. Rest by setting the bag down or by holding it with your other hand.
Level 2:	Raise and lower the bag through a comfortable range.

Dosage

Repetitions: _____
Frequency: _____

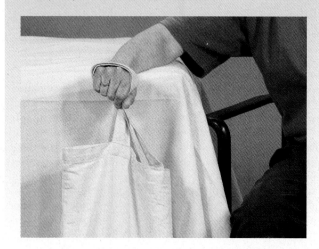

strengthening exercises should focus on the position of interest; if the individual functions at work with the wrist in a specific posture, that posture should be assessed and corrected if necessary. Subsequent exercises should focus on strengthening the muscle at the length it will be during functional activity. In contrast, training the wrist extensor muscles in the case of lateral epicondylitis will likely use a dynamic range of strengthening, given the wide ROM for most activities producing lateral epicondylitis (e.g., tennis, painting, hammering; see Self-Management 26-4: Wrist Extension Exercise With Grocery Bag). See Building Block 26-3.

Pain and Inflammation Impairment

Pain and inflammation occur throughout the distal upper extremity for a variety of reasons. Injury or surgery can result in pain and inflammation. Central or local nerve compression usually produces pain locally and pain radiating from the site

BUILDING BLOCK 26-3

An artist specializing in pottery complains of fatigue in her wrist and finger flexors after a day of working at the pottery wheel. She reports that this is due to putting in long hours preparing for a show. She has no neurological symptoms nor signs of systemic disease. Design an initial therapeutic exercise program for her. Her show is completed, but she would still like to work at her wheel to keep up her inventory. What advice do you have regarding her work at the wheel?

of compression. Inflammatory conditions such as RA or OA produce pain and inflammation in the affected joints, and tendinopathies also are painful.

Inflammation is easily detected in this region because of the superficial nature of the structures. The MCP, PIP, and DIP joints in the hand are easily observed for swelling and redness and palpated for warmth and tenderness. Crepitus in tendons such as the abductor pollicis longus (APL) and extensor pollicis brevis (EPB) tendons in a person with de Quervain syndrome is readily palpable, as is the local tenderness associated with medial and lateral epicondylitis.

Intervention for inflammation is based on the acuteness of the inflammation (see Chapter 11). Gentle active, active assisted, or passive motion to maintain mobility during the acute phase may be indicated. In some situations, immobilization with splints may be necessary, with occasional removal for gentle mobility activities. After the acute phase has passed, more aggressive activities may be initiated.

Gentle grade I oscillations may be used to decrease pain in some situations. This approach along with ice and other adjunctive agents can decrease pain enough to allow resumption of a therapeutic exercise program.

Muscle Endurance Functions: Impaired Posture and Movement

The most common posture and movement impairments in this region are work- and hobby-related cumulative injuries. Lateral and medial epicondylitis at the elbow and carpal tunnel syndrome (CTS) and de Quervain tendinitis at the wrist result from impairments in posture and movement. The posture of the wrist and hand influences symptoms at the elbow. Grasping and pinching always cause a flexion moment at the wrist that must be offset by extensor muscle activity. This places loads on the common extensor tendon at the elbow. Hand grip strength is a function of the object's size and the posture of the wrist. For a given size of object, an optimal wrist position for maximum grip strength exists.[21] In the examination of the individual with a disorder related to work or hobbies, the size of the tool and its impact on elbow, wrist, and posture must be considered. These tools can be hobby related (e.g., golf club, racquet, gardening tools, knitting needles) or work related (e.g., hammers, screwdrivers, shovels, welding tools, sewing tools). When grip is involved, the posture of the upper quarter relative to that tool must be examined. Posture during nongrip activities such as keyboard operating also is important. The guidelines for posture while sitting at a

Patient-Related Instruction 26-1

Computer Workstation Posture

The following information can help you to evaluate your computer workstation. If you have specific medical problems, consult your clinician for any special needs you may have.

Computer

Correct keyboard position

- Elbows bent at 90 degrees
- Wrists straight or slightly bent up
- Keyboard downwardly sloped
- Try placing the keyboard on a commercially available keyboard tray with a wrist rest.

Correct monitor position

- About 16 to 22 in away (about an arm's length)
- Top of the screen even with top of forehead
- Use a stand or adjustable monitor arm to regulate height.

Mouse

Correct mouse position

- Elbows bent at 90 degrees
- Wrist straight or slightly bent up
- Shoulders relaxed and arm at your side
- Elbow supported on armrest if available

Your Work

- Your document and screen should be at similar heights.
- Use a document holder.
- Sit directly in front of the keyboard, monitor, and document holder.

Sitting posture

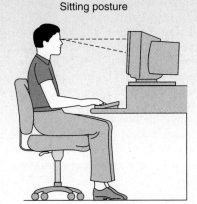

computer work terminal can be found in the Patient-Related Instruction 26-1: Computer Workstation Posture.

Movement factors may contribute to injuries in this region. Fatigue during repetitive activity produces changes in movement patterns and subsequent overuse injuries. As muscles begin to fatigue, the individual has more difficulty controlling force production, and substitution occurs. Substitution may occur with a synergistic muscle or a muscle group more proximal or distal in the kinetic chain. In either case, the primary muscle and the substituting group are vulnerable to overuse injuries. Allowing adequate rest time, using proper tool size, reinforcing good posture, and controlling cycle time, recovery time, and exertion frequency can decrease repetitive loads.

THERAPEUTIC EXERCISE INTERVENTIONS FOR COMMON DIAGNOSES

Osteoarthritis and Rheumatoid Arthritis

OA and RA commonly affect the wrist and hand.[22,23] The hands are the most frequent site of OA in the elderly, and can have a significant impact on function and disability in this population.[22] Radiographic hand OA ranges in prevalence from 29% to 76% with this variation the result of genetic backgrounds and environment.[24] Hand OA can have different presentations depending upon individual factors. Some predictors of hand OA include: older age, genetics, female sex, menopausal, manual labor with pneumatic vibratory tools and metal, high impact physical activity, and repetitive use of the hand.[22] In patients with RA, hand and wrist dysfunction are common, with 75% of patients with a 15- to 20-year history of RA having erosive wrist disease.[25]

Hand OA occurs more frequently in women over the age of 50, and in the elderly population, the prevalence of hand OA is as high as 80%.[22,26] The joints most severely affected in are often the second and third DIP, the first IP and both first CMC joints with the PIP with the lowest OA prevalence. Symmetry of OA between rows of joints was the most common pattern of interrelationship found.[27] Hand OA is associated with pain and loss of function, particularly when both the thumb and fingers are involved.[28,29] Pinch and grip strength and hand function measures are decreased with hand OA, while the high grip strength appears to be a predictor of the development of OA in the proximal hand joints but not the DIP joints.[30]

RA is a chronic, systemic inflammatory disease affecting multiple joints, with its greatest impact on the synovial membranes. The wrists and hands are typically involved, and strength impairments can significantly impact the patient's quality of life.[31] The distal radioulnar joint is affected causing the ulna to dorsally subluxate on the radius at the distal radioulnar joint. The patient with RA often has a wrist deformity of flexion, radial deviation, and volar subluxation of the carpal bones.[19] Ankylosis may eventually ensue, severely restricting mobility at the wrist. This motion loss is particularly disabling for the individual with RA, because adjacent joints are also affected and unable to compensate for wrist immobility.

At the hand, this disease produces MCP joint ulnar deviation and volar subluxation of the proximal phalanges. The synovial changes associated with RA weaken connective tissues surrounding the joints, leading to joint subluxation and/or dislocation. For example, swan-neck deformity, or hyperextension of the PIP and flexion of the DIP, results from flexor and extensor imbalance and PIP joint laxity.[19] A boutonniere ("buttonhole") deformity arises when the extensor mechanism fails over the PIP joint causing hyperextension of the DIP and flexion of the PIP with failure of the extensor mechanism. At the thumb, a "zig-zag" deformity can cause significant functional impairments for people with RA (Fig. 26-19). Additionally, mucous cysts and nodules impact the function of tendons, causing "trigger fingers" in tendons with sheaths.

Intervention for patients with RA affecting the wrist and hands typically consists of therapeutic exercise to maintain joint mobility and musculotendinous strength and integrity, night

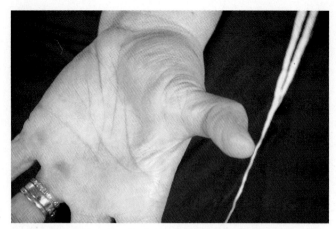

FIGURE 26-19. Early stages of rheumatiod arthritis of the thumb.

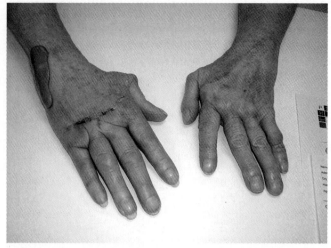

FIGURE 26-20. RA of the hands before and after surgery to correct deformities.

splinting, as well as patient education in joint protection.[32,33] A program that includes education in joint protection has been shown to produce outcomes with less early morning stiffness and better measures of ADLs than those without such education programs.[34] However, advice alone is insufficient to improve outcomes in patients with RA. A therapeutic exercise program consisting of strengthening and mobilization activities has shown superior outcomes to programs consisting of advice or simple stretches alone.[35] Programs consisting of strengthening exercises have shown improvements in strength and hand function at 6 weeks, that was further improved by 12 weeks.[36] The dosage of therapeutic exercise needs to be individualized based upon the stage and severity of the disease. Research has shown that intense exercise is tolerated in some patients with RA. Mobility, hand pain and functional ability improved in patients undergoing an intense rehabilitation program compared with a conservative program.[37] However, for those with significant loss of hand function, surgical intervention can improve the quality of life (Fig. 26-20).

Splints or orthoses used for RA include resting hand splints, wrist supports, and finger splints.[38] A variety of splints are available and can be customized for use during functional activities or at night or other times of rest. Splinting should be accompanied by an appropriate therapeutic exercise program

to ensure optimal mobility, strength, and function of the hand (Fig. 26-21A and B).

Cumulative Trauma Disorders

Most musculoskeletal injuries that occur in the workplace are not caused by accidents or acute injuries that sprain ligaments; they result from wear and tear stresses on the musculoskeletal system. Wear and tear injuries are frequently referred to as cumulative trauma disorders (CTDs). The most common CTS is carpal tunnel syndrome which will be discussed in further detail in a subsequent section. There has been a significant increase in the number of reported cases of CTDs in the workplace (Display 26-2). According to the Bureau of Labor Statistics, 23,800 cases were reported in 1972, a number that steadily increased to 332,000 in 1994. In 1995, the number of cases decreased by 7% to 308,000.[39] Jobs with the highest risk of CTDs include those in the meat- and fish-processing industries, work using chain saws and electronic assembly work.[40]

CTDs are by definition work-related phenomena, although these disorders may also occur with certain hobbies and other

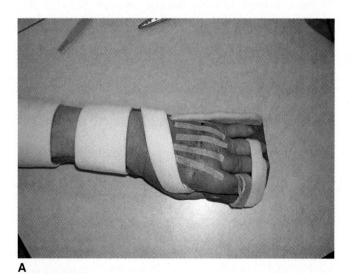

A

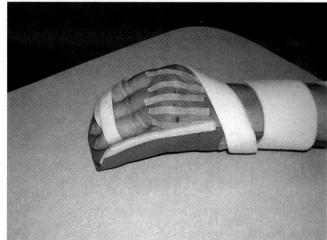

B

FIGURE 26-21. (A, B) A night splint is used to rest and maintain the position of the wrist and hand.

nonwork-related activities. The World Health Organization has defined CTDs as being multifactorial in nature, indicating that a number of risk factors contribute to these disorders, including physical risk factors, environment, work organization, and psychosocial, sociocultural, and individual risk factors. Because of the multifactorial nature of CTDs, there is some controversy about the role these risk factors play in the development of CTDs.

Physical risk factors include repetition, awkward postures, prolonged activities, forceful exertions, and fatigue (Display 26-3).[41] Specific modifiable factors include work tasks with high vibration, working in flexion or extension for prolonged periods of time, tasks demanding heavy resistance, lack of variability in tasks, insufficient break time, and work that is highly repetitive.[40,42] The magnitude, duration, and repetition need to be considered for each of these risk factors. Environmental risk factors, such as vibration and cold, may also be present, further complicating the picture. The worker exposed to these factors and not given adequate recovery time may develop a CTD. The worker is unable to recover from the microinjuries or microtrauma that occurs at the tissue level over time. CTDs typically have a slow onset, with only minimal symptoms noticed initially. Many people ignore the early symptoms and do not seek medical attention until the symptoms prevent them from participating in work or in recreational or home activities.

Work may also aggravate or exacerbate an existing health or musculoskeletal problem. For example, forceful gripping at work may aggravate a previous sport injury at the elbow, such as lateral epicondylitis. The diagnosis of lateral epicondylitis is frequently used to describe a CTD injury at the elbow involving the lateral extensor mechanism.

Acting alone or in combination, awkward postures, excessive forces, and frequent repetitions may cause mechanical and physiologic stress on the soft tissues. When a person is positioned in an awkward posture, the body is unable to function at an optimal level. For example, wrist deviations may stretch the soft tissue, irritating the tendons and tendon sheaths. When in a lengthened position, the wrist muscles may be unable to exert the required force for the task. When the wrist is in a 45-degree flexed position, the grip strength may be reduced by 40%.[43] The individual may be functioning at a greater percentage of their maximum capabilities. Fatigue is more likely to occur when functioning at a higher percentage of the maximum voluntary contraction. Fatigue, coupled with excessive repetitive motions, may exceed the tendon sheath's capacity to lubricate the tendon, causing increased friction and eventual wear and tear of the tendon.

Vibration is a significant stressor contributing to a variety of wrist and hand musculoskeletal disorders. Termed *hand-arm vibration syndrome* this primarily work-related musculoskeletal disorder is comprised of vascular, neurological and musculoskeletal components.[44] People regularly exposed to high frequency vibratory tools (i.e., spinning/rotating tools, saws, grinders).

Workplace design and ergonomics must be carefully evaluated when a patient is diagnosed with a CTD. Ergonomics is the study of fitting the job to the individual. Certain occupational risk factors such as repetitive gripping or forceful pushing with the wrist in an ulnar-deviated position may prevent the person from successfully returning to that job without symptoms recurring. A job analysis or ergonomic analysis should be completed to assess the risk factors present in the individual's work environment. An example is an individual grasping a straight-handled tool such as a knife. This tool and activity places the wrist in an ulnar-deviated position. By angling the tool handle instead of the wrist, the wrist's position is improved. By ensuring appropriate preventive maintenance (e.g., sharpening the knife on a timely basis), the stress on the tool operator is decreased.

Nerve Injuries

A variety of nerve injuries occur throughout the elbow, wrist, and hand because of the anatomic structures in the upper extremity and the functional demands in the region. A thorough knowledge of the local anatomy provides a foundation for understanding the impairments found with these nerve injuries.

Carpal Tunnel Syndrome

CTS at the wrist is the most common peripheral compression neuropathy, affecting a greater proportion of women than men.[19,45,46] The prevalence of CTS in the general population has been estimated between 0.6% and 16% with a 10% lifetime risk of development.[46,47] CTS in the working population is associated with significant costs at many levels (individual, employer, third party payer, etc.).[45]

The carpal tunnel is a small tunnel on the volar aspect of the wrist that is occupied by the median nerve and by nine tendons. The base of the carpal tunnel is formed by the carpal arch, one of three concave arches on the volar aspect of the wrist and hand. The carpal arch is concave on its palmar surface and is spanned by the flexor retinaculum. At this level, the median nerve contains motor fibers innervating the abductor pollicis brevis, the superficial head of the flexor pollicis brevis, the opponens pollicis, and the first and second lumbrical muscles. Sensory fibers provide innervation to the volar thumb and to the index, middle, and one half of the ring fingers.

The average cross-sectional area of the carpal tunnel is 1.7 cm² with the wrist in neutral. Pressure in the carpal tunnel varies with wrist position. Normal tissue fluid pressure with the wrist in neutral is 2.5 mm Hg. Passive flexion and extension of the wrist has been shown to increase carpal tunnel pressure significantly.[48] With the wrist in 40 degrees of flexion, the carpal tunnel pressure increases to 47 mm Hg.[48] The mean wrist position associated with the lowest carpal tunnel pressure is approximately 2 degrees of flexion and 3 degrees of ulnar deviation. Wrist extension increases carpal tunnel pressure more than wrist flexion.[48,49] Digital fingertip pressure also increases carpal tunnel pressure.

CTS is caused by a decrease in the size of the carpal tunnel or an increase in the size of its contents, which compresses the median nerve. A single insult (e.g., Colles fracture), systemic conditions or disease (e.g., pregnancy, diabetes, RA), anomalous anatomy, and cumulative trauma within the carpal tunnel (e.g., flexor tenosynovitis) can compress the median nerve. Physical factors associated with CTS include repetitive motion, force, mechanical stresses, posture, vibration, and temperature.

CTS can manifest with sensory or motor impairments of the median nerve. Diagnosis is based on the presence of one or more common symptoms and on the results of provocative tests. Electrodiagnostic studies can be valuable in confirming the diagnosis and detecting other neuropathies. Associated impairments can include nocturnal pain and numbness, clumsiness when holding small objects, paresthesias in the median nerve distribution, and occasionally pain that radiates proximally. Symptoms of shoulder pain or upper arm pain are not uncommon.[26] Diagnosis is based on the history, a positive Tinel test result, direct compression tests, Phalen sign, manual muscle testing, sensation testing, upper limb tension tests, and extrinsic muscle length tests.

Intervention for CTS is multifaceted and may include a variety of interventions. The most commonly assessed outcomes include: sensory functions, muscle functions, sensations of pain in the median nerve distribution, sleep functions, structure of the median nerve, structures of the area of the skin (ICF Body Structures and Functions impairments); self care, domestic life, hand and arm use, fine hand use (ICF Activities limitations); and, participation in work and employment (ICF Participation restrictions).[50] Review of conservative management has shown limited or no benefit to the use of nonsteroidal antiinflammatory medications (NSAIDs) or vitamin B6. Oral corticosteroids show greater benefit than NSAIDs, but are associated with greater side effects.[46,51,52] Local cortisone injections have shown significant but short term (<6 months) relief. (same) Ultrasound treatments have shown conflicting evidence with no improvement seen with short term treatment, but significant improvements with longer term (7 weeks) treatment.[51] Night (and occasionally day) wrist splints positioned at 0 to 15 degrees of extension have been advocated (Fig. 26-22).[53–55] Full-time splinting may be better than night-time splinting only, but compliance may be difficult.[53] Splinting in neutral may be better than extension

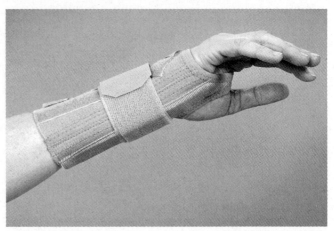

FIGURE 26-22. A wrist splint is used to rest the forearm and wrist musculature.

due to decreased tension on the median nerve in the neutral position.[54]

Exercise intervention for CTS has been shown to have limited effectiveness.[51,52] Therapeutic exercises focuses on maintaining mobility and function without producing an exacerbation. Although not curative, therapeutic exercise may be beneficial for maintaining the integrity of associated soft tissues. Stretches for the extrinsic and intrinsic muscles are prescribed for several times each day (Fig. 26-23). If working, a patient should perform them before work, on breaks, or after work. They should be performed slowly and gently; the patient should feel only a gentle stretching sensation. Differential tendon gliding exercises are performed to lubricate and increase gliding of the FPL, FDS, and FDP tendons. These are best performed with the hand elevated to concurrently control local edema. Carpal bone mobilization techniques may also be helpful in decreasing CTS symptoms.[56] Finally, one study of yoga found improvements in Phalen sign, grip strength and pain, but no change in Tinel sign, sleep disturbance or nerve conduction studies.[57]

Median nerve gliding exercises and the upper limb tension test with median nerve bias can be used as treatment techniques, although research has not found consistent improvement in CTS with the addition of nerve gliding exercises.[45,46,58] The upper limb tension test with median nerve bias requires a position of shoulder girdle depression, shoulder abduction to approximately 110 degrees, forearm supination, wrist and finger extension, and shoulder lateral rotation.[1] After assuming this stretch position while standing, the patient should perform repetitions of elbow flexion and extension or wrist flexion and extension. Strengthening is generally not prescribed for patients with CTS who also have flexor tenosynovitis. If the precipitating factors have been eliminated and weakness creates a functional limitation, resistive exercises are closely monitored. The focus should be on balancing mobility and strength about the wrist.

Patient education is a key intervention in the treatment and prevention of CTS. Patients are instructed to maintain a neutral upper extremity joint position during seated or standing work. This position is accomplished with the wrist in neutral, elbow flexed in the middle range, shoulders relaxed in adduction, scapula slightly depressed and adducted, and the cervical spine positioned with the earlobe in line with the

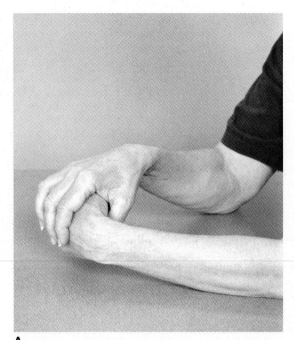

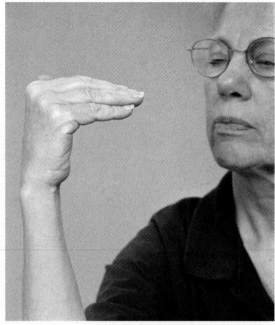

A   **B**

FIGURE 26-23. (A) Stretching exercise for wrist extensor muscles. (B) Flexion at the metacarpal joints with extension at the IP joints can maintain mobility in the ED tendon and the collateral ligaments.

glenohumeral joint. The patient is also instructed to avoid a sustained pinch and grip, especially with the wrist in flexion, and to avoid repetitive overuse of the wrist and fingers. Patients should avoid direct pressure over the carpal tunnel by using a wrist rest or padded table edge or use a downwardly sloped keyboard. This type of keyboard has been shown to decrease the wrist extension angle and decrease muscle activity.[59] (see Patient-Related Instruction 26-1: Computer Workstation Posture).

Ergonomic intervention includes use of ergonomic tools that are padded with appropriately sized grips and handles. Data processing station revision should allow an adjustable chair height and keyboard height and tilt. Antivibration gloves are helpful for preoperative and postoperative carpal tunnel release to pad and protect the carpal tunnel and flexor tendons (Fig. 26-24).[58,60]

Patients treated acutely for CTS related to flexor tenosynovitis often respond well to conservative treatment without recurrence of symptoms if finger and wrist position

and activities are monitored.[58] Conservative treatment is recommended for patients with transient symptoms and negative nerve study results. Patients who fail conservative treatment (usually a 3-month trial) often require carpal tunnel release surgery. Studies have shown that the carpal tunnel increases in size with the release of the volar carpal ligament. Symptoms often improve immediately after surgery in mild to moderate cases. Because of the progressive nature of CTS, surgical outcomes appear to be improved by earlier surgical intervention (within 3 years of diagnosis).[46] Open carpal tunnel release offers good symptom relief for most patients.[61]

Cubital Tunnel Syndrome

Cubital tunnel syndrome is the second most common entrapment neuropathy in the upper extremity.[60] This syndrome is characterized by ulnar nerve pathology at the elbow in the absence of trauma. The cubital tunnel is formed by the medial epicondyle, olecranon, medial collateral ligament of the elbow, and a fibrous band called the arcade of Struthers.[62] Several muscles in the wrist and hand are innervated by the ulnar nerve, and the ulnar nerve provides sensation to the dorsal and volar ulnar side of the hand, the fifth finger, and the ulnar half of the ring finger.

Ulnar nerve entrapment may produce nerve injury through ischemia or mechanical deformation of the nerve. These forces can occur from trauma to the elbow, external compression, repetitive elbow motion, or prolonged elbow flexion. The more superficial positions of the sensory fibers within the ulnar nerve at the elbow make them susceptible to compression. With elbow motion, normal nerve excursion has been reported to be as great as 10 mm. Traction on the nerve may occur with repetitive activities such as throwing. The nerve may also undergo increases in traction forces when its excursion is limited by posttraumatic adhesions.[28] As the elbow moves from extension to flexion, intraneural pressure

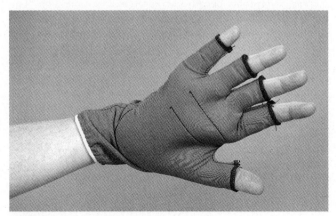

FIGURE 26-24. Antivibration gloves.

in the cubital tunnel increases from 7 to 24 mm Hg. Pressure as high as 209 mm Hg has been recorded in a patient with cubital tunnel syndrome with elbow flexion and flexor carpi ulnaris contraction.[29]

Symptoms of cubital tunnel syndrome can include aching in the medial forearm and ulnar side of the hand. The aching can radiate proximally or distally. Paresthesias or anesthesias in the ulnar nerve distribution often accompany the pain.[29] Prolonged or repeated end-range elbow flexion tends to exacerbate symptoms. Functional activities eliciting symptoms include sleeping with the elbow flexed at night, combing the hair, driving, or holding the telephone. Leaning on the medial elbow can directly compress the ulnar nerve. Early in the syndrome, patients typically control the paresthesias by repositioning the elbow in a more extended position. As the syndrome progresses, activity limitations caused by motor changes cause activity limitations such as difficulty in turning keys, a weak grip and pinch, and dropping objects held in the ulnar side of the hand.

Focused physical examination techniques include Tinel testing over the ulnar nerve, provocative elbow flexion testing (including direct compression over the cubital tunnel), upper limb tension testing with ulnar nerve bias, observation of muscle bulk and clawing in the fourth and fifth digits, muscle testing, Froment sign, and sensory testing. The differential diagnoses include C8–T1 nerve root pathology, thoracic outlet syndrome, and compression of the ulnar nerve at Guyon canal.

Conservative management of cubital tunnel syndrome consists of eliminating all sources of external and dynamic ulnar nerve compression at the elbow, antiinflammatory medication, elbow splinting in 40 to 60 degrees at night, elbow pads, and stretching exercises. Stretching exercises focus on extrinsic flexor and extensor muscles along with ulnar nerve–innervated intrinsic muscle stretches. Nerve gliding techniques may be appropriate for patients with intermittent symptoms. The ulnar nerve's normal longitudinal excursion can be limited by adherence to adjacent structures. Nerve gliding can be achieved by assuming a modified ulnar nerve bias tension test position while standing. This position requires shoulder depression and abduction, wrist extension, and forearm supination, followed by elbow extension.[1] Several repetitions of elbow or wrist flexion and extension can be performed. This intermittent stretch is usually better tolerated than a prolonged stretch (Fig. 26-25).

Key adjunctive interventions are focused on patient education. Posture correction and proximal stretching or strengthening to maintain posture are indicated when the patient has faulty posture. Short pectoralis minor and weak scapular stabilizer muscles are often observed in individuals working at computers or on assembly lines. Although ADLs can be modified to allow rest of the involved arm, it is more challenging to modify work conditions. Use of the uninvolved arm is encouraged to wash and comb hair, eat, or perform any activity requiring prolonged or repeated elbow flexion. Use of a telephone headset is helpful in cases of frequent or prolonged telephone use. A transcutaneous electrical nerve stimulation unit may provide some relief. Four electrodes can be placed along the ulnar nerve, with two proximal to the cubital tunnel and two distal.

If conservative treatment of cubital tunnel syndrome does not reduce or resolve symptoms in 3 months, surgical treatment may be considered. In the absence of clinically identifiable sensory loss or muscle weakness, conservative treatment may be continued indefinitely in the form of a home exercise program. Ulnar nerve transposition surgery involves mobilizing the ulnar nerve at the ulnar groove and anteriorly transposing it subcutaneously, intramuscularly, or submuscularly to the flexor pronator muscle group.

Radial Tunnel Syndrome

Radial nerve entrapment at the elbow, also called radial tunnel syndrome, is entrapment of the posterior interosseous nerve in one of five locations within the radial tunnel:

- The entrance to the tunnel where fibrous bands encircle the nerve
- The leash of Henry, where the radial recurrent vessels supply the brachioradialis and the extensor carpi radialis longus (ECRL) muscles
- The fascia and medial portion of the ECRB tendon
- The arcade of Frohse
- Distally between the tendinous origins of the supinator muscle[11,62]

Radial nerve entrapment occurs much less frequently than median and ulnar nerve compressions. Radial nerve compression may be caused by direct trauma or anatomic structures compressing the nerve. Nerve compression commonly results from repetitive pronation and supination or wrist flexion and extension activities. Occasionally, a single strenuous effort initiates the problem, and subsequent repetitive motion perpetuates it.

The patient with radial tunnel syndrome often has symptoms similar to those produced by lateral epicondylitis. Frequently, these persons have undergone unsuccessful treatment for lateral epicondylitis. Tennis elbow straps may increase symptoms because of additional compression. The most common symptom is that of aching in the extensor-supinator muscle mass that is distal to the lateral epicondyle. Tenderness is approximately 3 in distal to the lateral epicondyle, with occasional pain radiating distally. No overt sensory deficits are found, because the posterior interosseous nerve contains only motor fibers. A brachial plexus or C7 nerve root injury should be excluded in the differential diagnosis. The upper limb tension test with radial nerve bias may provide additional information.

Intervention for radial tunnel syndrome is conservative, including rest, antiinflammatory medication, therapeutic exercise, and wrist cock-up splinting for 3 to 6 months. The goal of stretching is to restore full extrinsic wrist extensor and flexor muscle length and tendon excursion. If extensor stretches are painful, initial stretches can be performed with

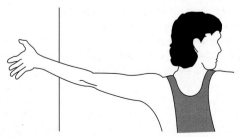

FIGURE 26-25. Nerve gliding stretch with elbow extension, forearm supination, and wrist extension.

the elbow flexed and forearm supinated, followed by fisted wrist flexion. The exercise is progressed until full elbow extension and forearm pronation are achieved with fisted wrist flexion without forcing through pain. Radial nerve gliding techniques may be helpful to encourage adequate nerve gliding from the cervical spine to the wrist and hand level.

Adjunctive treatments include iontophoresis or phonophoresis applied over the supinator muscle or moist heat before stretching. Soft-tissue massage to the forearm flexors and extensors may help to relax involved muscles and improve the extensibility and circulation in the area. Upper extremity activities should be performed with the forearm in neutral to prevent prolonged stretching or overuse of the supinator muscle. This activity modification is particularly important in lifting tasks. Job rotation or diversification can prevent prolonged use of the extensor-supinator muscle group.

Functional outcomes after conservative management of radial tunnel syndrome are difficult to determine because of the challenge in identifying the correct diagnosis, the relative rarity of the syndrome, and the frequent surgical intervention in clearly diagnosed cases. The clinician should be alert to radial tunnel syndrome as a differential diagnosis in cases of recalcitrant lateral epicondylitis. When radial tunnel is properly diagnosed, surgery is often the treatment of choice. Patients commonly are seen postoperatively for scar and pain management, stretching, and strengthening programs.

Musculotendinous Disorders

Lateral Epicondylar Tendinopathy

Tendinopathy of the common wrist extensor musculature is the most frequent problem seen in the lateral elbow. The incidence of this syndrome in recreational and professional tennis players is 39% to 50%.[63] The prevalence of lateral epicondylitis in the general population has been found to be approximately 1.3%.[64] Although "lateral epicondylitis" and "tennis elbow" are common names for this problem, lateral epicondylar tendinopathy is seen as frequently in persons who are not tennis players and inflammatory cells are almost always absent.[65] Any individual using hand tools for work or hobbies are susceptible to developing symptoms. The combination of continuous grip along with repeated wrist and elbow activity precipitates symptoms. Repetitively handling tools weighing >1 kg, repetitive movements, low job control, and low social support have also been shown to increase the risk of lateral epicondylitis.[66] Additionally, smoking has been found to be a risk factor for lateral epicondylitis.[64]

Wrist extension is accomplished by the combined actions of the ECRL, ECRB, and extensor carpi ulnaris. These muscles all originate on the lateral epicondyle and supracondylar ridge of the humerus. The lateral epicondyle is also the origin of the ED and extensor digiti minimi. Of the extensor muscles involved in lateral epicondylar tendionopathy, the ECRB is generally the greatest contributor to symptoms.[67] The ECRB may be involved in 100% of cases, and the ED is involved in 30% of cases.[67] The wrist is stabilized by the extensors working in synergy with the flexors. Biomechanical models have shown that grasping and pinching tasks always produce a flexion moment at the wrist that must be countered by the wrist extensors. Many tasks requiring use of hand tools or writing instruments require wrist extensor activity. Because optimal hand function occurs when the hand is in a complete fist and the wrist is extended 15 to 20 degrees, the grip size of the implement and the resting posture of the wrist can have a great impact on producing and alleviating symptoms. These factors are important aspects of patient education.

Individuals with lateral epicondylar tendinopathy describe pain with any activity that requires gripping and lifting, such as shaking hands, lifting a carton of milk, or turning doorknobs. Use of hand tools, writing, and lifting bags also produce symptoms. Tenderness to palpation over the lateral epicondyle is common, and resisted wrist and finger extension is painful.

The treatment approach for lateral epicondylitis is conservative, consisting of relative rest, occasional bracing, inflammation control, and therapeutic exercise. Exercise includes stretching to restore the normal length of the musculotendinous unit. Stretching the wrist into flexion and pronation should reproduce a sensation of tightness in the forearm. Reproduction of pain at the elbow indicates that stretching is too vigorous.

Strengthening should focus on the role of the wrist extensors in upper extremity function. The wrist extensor function to stabilize the wrist against the wrist and finger flexors as well as functionally extending the wrist. Because the wrist extensors work during wrist extension and gripping, the clinician must approach use of hand-held weights cautiously. The initial strengthening program may include gripping and wrist extension as separate exercises, gradually progressing to concurrent wrist extension and gripping (Fig. 26-26). Depending on the symptoms, the program may begin with isometric muscle contractions and progress to dynamic concentric and eccentric exercises.

There is a growing body of literature supporting the use of eccentric exercise in the treatment of tendinopathy.[68–71] It is theorized that chronic tendinopathy-related pain may be due to neovascularization that occurs in this disorder. The eccentric exercise is suggested to hinder the angiogenesis found with chronic tendinopathy. The eccentric program should be progressive and focus on the parameters of length, load, and speed.[68] The program starts with exercise in a self-selected range of comfort and progresses to full range of motion. The speed is initially slow (~30 degrees per second) and progresses up to a fast speed (~90 degrees per second) while maintaining a set resistance of approximately 30% of a maximum voluntary contraction of the pain-free contralateral side.[68] Once the patient tolerates this intensity at the fastest speed, the intensity is increased and the speed returns to the slower rate and is again gradually increased. When the fastest speed is again reached, the intensity increases, and so on. This type of program has been shown to significantly decrease pain, increase strength, decrease performance restriction and improve the tendon image as measured by ultrasound.[68,69] See Chapter 11 for more information on the principles of treating tendinopathy.

Adjunctive interventions include therapeutic modalities such as ice, cross-friction massage, prolotherapy, patient education and bracing. Bracing may include a counterforce brace such as a tennis elbow strap or a wrist splint (Fig. 26-27). A counterforce brace decreases loads on the extensor origin by creating a new origin of the muscle that bypasses the inflamed portion of the tendon. Counterforce bracing also limits the maximum contraction of the muscles, thereby decreasing forces. A wrist splint can limit wrist extensor activity necessary

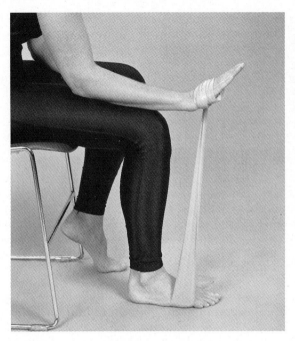
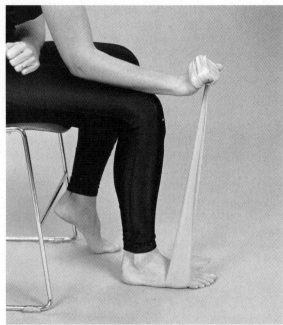

A   **B**

FIGURE 26-26. Wrist extension exercises. (A) Without grip. (B) With grip.

by providing an external stabilization to the wrist. Patient education regarding home and work ergonomics should be provided. Lifting with the forearm supinated decreases wrist extensor muscle activity. Tasks should be modified to limit repetitive elbow and wrist motion when possible. Judicious use of cortisone injections by the physician can decrease inflammation in cases of a true tendinitis rather than a tendinosis.

When conservative management of lateral epicondylitis fails, surgical management may be considered. Nirschl[63] observed that most patients have inadequate and fragmented conservative treatment plans. Good documentation and appropriate follow-up care are necessary to ensure that all conservative measures have been appropriately exhausted before surgery is considered.

Medial Epicondylitis

Medial epicondylitis is encountered less frequently than lateral epicondylitis and accounts for 10% to 20% of all epi-

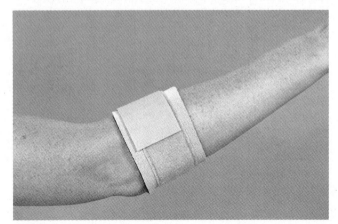

FIGURE 26-27. Tennis elbow strap.

condylitis cases.[29] Its prevalence in the general population has been estimated at 0.4%.[64] The muscles involved are the flexor-pronator group, including the flexor carpi radialis, palmaris longus, pronator teres, and flexor carpi ulnaris. Repetitive wrist flexion in recreational activities such as golf or fly fishing or at work subject the common wrist extensors to overuse. Repetitive movements, high hand grip forces, and working with vibrating tools have been associated with medial epicondylitis.[66] Smoking, obesity, repetitive movements, and forceful activities are also significantly associated with medial epicondylitis.[64] Affected persons usually describe pain at the medial epicondyle with resisted wrist flexion and forearm pronation. Passive stretch into extension and supination also may reproduce symptoms.

Management of medial epicondylitis is conservative, with a focus on controlled activity matched with appropriate rest, stretching and strengthening exercises, and interventions to reduce pain and inflammation. Therapeutic exercises include stretching for the flexor and pronator muscles, as long as stretching does not reproduce elbow symptoms (Fig. 26-28). As symptoms resolve, a progressive strengthening program with an emphasis on the demands specific to the individual patient is implemented. Like lateral epicondylar tendinopathy, similar symptoms at the medial elbow can be successfully treated with eccentric exercise.[72] Therapeutic modalities such as ice, iontophoresis, and phonophoresis and prolotherapy can provide relief from the pain. This intervention creates a better environment in which the therapeutic exercise program can be more effective. When conservative management fails, surgical resection of the diseased portion of the tendon may be undertaken.

De Quervain Syndrome

De Quervain syndrome, also called stenosing tenosynovitis, is an inflammation of the tendons of the first dorsal wrist

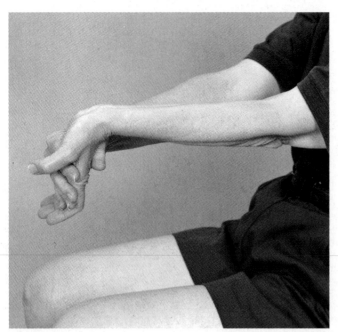

FIGURE 26-28. Wrist flexor stretch.

compartment. The muscles in this compartment are the EPB and APL. The most common cause is overuse of the hand and wrist, particularly in movements requiring radial deviation while the thumb is stabilized in a grip.[73] Women are affected about 3 to 10 times more often than men.

Persons with de Quervain syndrome notice pain on the radial aspect of the wrist in the region of the radial styloid. Flexing the thumb across the palm is quite painful, and resisted extension and abduction may be painful as well. Palpable tenderness and bogginess may be noticed over the tendons of the first compartment. Radial and ulnar deviation may produce clicking or pain. The Finkelstein test is the most commonly used test to diagnose de Quervain syndrome. Measurements may reveal that pinch and grip are weak and painful.

Therapeutic exercise intervention for de Quervain syndrome includes stretching for the EPB and APL and the extrinsic wrist flexor and extensor muscles. Strengthening should be initiated after full pain-free ROM has been achieved. Strengthening includes the thumb and wrist musculature and full gripping exercises. To prevent further overuse to these tendons during the initiation of a rehabilitation program, immobilization using a forearm base thumb spica splint may be necessary. The splint should be worn during symptomatic times or periods of high activity. The splint is removed to perform exercises throughout the day.

Other adjunctive measures include cross-friction massage over the first dorsal compartment and activity modification. Work, hobby, or sport modifications to decrease the frequency and forces involved with wrist and thumb motion may be necessary to allow the rehabilitation program to succeed. Therapeutic modalities to reduce inflammation such as ice and iontophoresis may be helpful. The physician may place the patient on an antiinflammatory medication, inject the area with steroid or analgesic medication, or surgically release of the first dorsal compartment. Patient education to avoid or limit situations contributing to the symptoms is essential to prevent recurrence.

Trigger Finger

Trigger finger, also known as digital tenovaginitis stenosans, is a result of thickening of the flexor tendon sheath. Thickening causes catching of the tendon as the finger actively flexes.[16] The flexor tendons of the fingers have an intricate anatomy that includes a synovial sheath extending from the mid-metacarpal area to the DIP joints. Overlying the sheath is a series of annular and cruciform fibrous bands or pulleys. These pulleys hold the flexor tendons close to the metacarpals and phalangeal bones, thereby improving the efficiency of motion. Thickening of the sheath at the A-1 pulley (i.e., fibrous band that overlays the synovial sheath at the MCP joint level) and enlargement of the flexor tendons are the basis for the symptoms found. This thickening may be caused by repetitive trauma or by direct pressure over the MCP joint in the palm, as when grasping.

Impairments associated with trigger finger include pain and tenderness in the finger from the volar MCP to the PIP level and intermittent triggering or "snapping" of the finger. The triggering usually occurs with flexion, and it may require passive assist to fully extend the finger.

Intervention for trigger finger is usually conservative and involves active IP flexion and tendon gliding exercises on an hourly basis. Ultrasound, massage, and icing can be used to relieve symptoms of pain and swelling. Splinting is common, and the hand-based splint or digital splint holds the MCP joint at full extension while leaving all other joints free. The splint is worn at all times for 1 to 3 weeks. Thereafter, it is worn for periods of high activity. The splint prevents triggering at the A-1 pulley and rest to minimize inflammation. The physician may inject into the synovial sheath at the level of the A-1 pulley to decrease local inflammation.

If conservative management is unsuccessful, surgery may be performed to release the A-1 pulley. Postoperative therapeutic intervention includes the same active exercise program and potential splinting as conservative management. Progressive grip strengthening may be required to return the patient to full functional use of the hand for work and ADLs. Education and work modification to avoid or limit repetitive grasping and releasing activities of the hand also are necessary.

Tendon Laceration

Tendon lacerations and repair require a complex series of treatments that must account for wound healing, tendon healing, and surgical techniques. Tendon repair treatment is complicated by the need for tendon excursion to prevent adhesions while allowing stability and protection to the healing tendon. Controlled motion helps prevent tendon adhesion, which limits motion and therefore limits function. Too much motion may compromise the repair. The clinician must provide a system of controlled motion, based on physician preference, surgical technique, mechanism of injury, and patient adherence.

The extensor tendons are divided into eight zones that determine treatment protocol used. Because of the extensiveness of each protocol, we review only the highlights for each zone (Fig. 26-29A).[74] In zones I and II, laceration causes a mallet finger. A mallet finger splint is fitted to the patient's DIP joint in 0 to 15 degrees of hyperextension from postoperative day 1 through 6 weeks. The PIP joint is left free to allow movement at the PIP level and proximally. The DIP joint should not be allowed to flex during this time. AROM

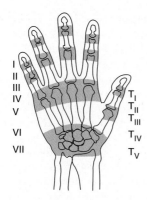
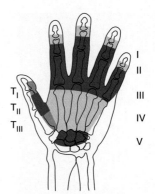

Zones of extensor tendon injury:

I — DIP joint and distal phalanx
II — Middle phalanx
III — PIP joint
IV — Proximal phalanx
V — MP joint
VI — Metacarpal bone
VII — Wrist
T_I — IP joint and distal phalanx of the thumb
T_{II} — Proximal phalanx of the thumb
T_{III} — Thumb MP joint
T_{IV} — Metacarpal bone of the thumb
T_V — Wrist

A

Zones of flexor tendon injury:

I — Distal to the FDS insertion
II — Between the A_1 pulley and the FDS insertion
III — Area between the distal carpal tunnel border and the A_1 pulley
IV — Within the carpal tunnel
V — Proximal to the carpal tunnel
T_I — From the thumb IP joint distally
T_{II} — Between the thumb A_1 pulley and the IP joint
T_{III} — Area of the first metacarpal bone

B

FIGURE 26-29. (A) Extensor tendon zones of the hand. (B) Flexor tendon zones of the hand.

exercises at the PIP joint are initiated at 4 to 6 weeks with flexion to 25 degrees. Strengthening is started at 6 to 8 weeks with monitoring for an extensor lag. If a lag is present, the patient returns to wearing the splint and AROM.

For zones III and IV, a digital gutter splint is fabricated to include the DIP and PIP joints (MCP is left free) at 2 weeks after surgery. If the lateral bands were not repaired, mobilization of the DIP may begin at 10 to 14 days. If the lateral bands were repaired, the DIP should be immobilized for 4 weeks. The PIP joint may be immobilized for up to 6 weeks. At 6 to 8 weeks, AROM is begun, with progressive flexion and extension exercises. Treatment must be modified if an extensor lag develops and will be individualize based upon consultation with the hand surgeon. Gentle strengthening is begun after 8 weeks.

For zone V (distal to tendonae junctionae), a hand-based splint is custom fabricated at 3 days to 1 week. This hand-based splint holds the MCP in 70 to 80 degrees of flexion and the digit in full extension. This position prevents contracture of the lateral bands at the MCP. AROM, PROM, and strengthening are continued as for zones III and IV.

For zones V (proximal to tendonae junctionae), VI, VII, and VIII, a volar forearm splint is fabricated at 3 to 5 days postoperatively. This splint extends from just proximal to the PIP joint, crosses the MCP joint, and continues two thirds of the way up the forearm, with the wrist positioned in 30 degrees of extension. This allows controlled movement of the extensor tendons through PIP and DIP joint movement, which prevents tendon adhesions. AROM, PROM, and strengthening exercises are continued as for the more distal zones.

Flexor tendon repairs also rely on zones to determine the appropriate protocol. There are five flexor tendon zones (see Fig. 26-29B). Current treatment protocols focus on controlled motion to prevent scar adhesions that limit functional movement. They also rely on the use of a dorsal blocking splint to prevent disruption of the surgical repair. This dorsal blocking splint is custom fabricated with the wrist in 20 degrees of flexion, the MCPs in 50 degrees of flexion, and the PIP and DIPs in full extension (Fig. 26-30).[33]

The program for zones I, II, and III consists of passive flexion and extension motion at the PIP and DIP joints and composite passive flexion and extension at the MCP, PIP, and DIP joints within the confines of the splint. This program is started on postoperative day 1 or 2 and continued through week 5.[33] AROM is started at 31/2 weeks, PROM into extension is begun at 6 weeks, and strengthening is started at

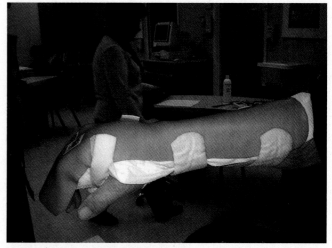

FIGURE 26-30. A dorsal blocking splint.

TABLE 26-6 Flexor tendon repair post-operative protocol with early passive motion

STAGE	PRECAUTIONS	GOALS	INTERVENTION
Early: Weeks 1–3	No active flexion. No wrist motion Active extensión only to DBS. Splint at all times	1. Protect healing structures 2. Decreased edema and pain 3. Minimize tendon adhesion 4. Full protected IP joint extension 5. Decreased PIP joint contracture 6. Maintain ROM of uninvolved joints 7. HEP independence	*Dorsal Blocking Splint:* 1. Wrist flexion 20–30 degrees 2. MP flexion 60–70 degrees 3. IPs 0 degree 4. Dynamic traction of fingers into flexion 5. Palmar pulley at DPC to attain increased IP flexion 6. Night block to hold IPs in extensión *Exercise:* 1. Active extension to DBS with passive flexion 2. Protected PROM 3. Edema control 4. Scar massage 5. Sensory education
Intermediate: Weeks 3 or 4–6	Guarded AROM No composite digit and wrist extension No passive composite extension Protect repaired pulleys	1. Protect healing structures 2. Decrease edema and pain 3. Restore tendon glide 4. Decrease scar adherence 5. Restore PROM of restricted joints 6. Maintain ROM of uninvolved joints 7. Gradually increase active/passive extension to full range	1. Gente AROM 2. Isometric exercise 3. Active assisted flexion 4. Progress to tendon gliding exercise *Blocking exercise:* (if tendon restricted) FDS at 4 weeks. FDP at 6 weeks. *Splinting* with wrist in neutral to increased extension 5. Edema control 6. Scar management 7. Progress to light prehensile activity
Late: Weeks 6–12	Prevent tendon rupture Prevent tenodynovitis of repaired tendons	1. Maximize full tendon glide and musculotendinous length 2. Maximize grip and pinch strength 3. Resume work and avocational activity	*Splinting:* 1. Phase out of protective splint 2. To decrease contractures 3. To increase excursion of long flexors or extensors *Exercise:* 1. Blocking, if needed 2. Isolated FDS glive 3. Muscle tendon unit stretching 4. Sustained gripping 5. Progress to strengthening Gradually resume full ADLs, return to work and avocational activities

DBS, Dorsal Blocking Splint; IP, interphalangeal joint; PIP, proximal interphalangeal joint; DPC, dorsal palmar crease.

8 weeks. Full functional use is allowed at 10 to 12 weeks postoperatively. The program for zones I, II, and III uses the dorsal blocking splint with rubber-band traction. The addition of a palmar pulley allows for greater FDP tendon excursion. The rubber band traction holds the digit into near full composite flexion, and the patient is instructed to extend the finger against the force of the rubber band to the dorsal blocking splint. The patient is instructed to do this 20 to 30 times per hour. This protocol is initiated 2 to 6 days postoperatively. AROM is started 5 weeks postoperatively, with PROM into extension started 7 to 8 weeks postoperatively. Strengthening is performed after 8 weeks.[33] The outcomes for flexor tendon repairs with early active mobilization are good.[75–78] Table 26-6 provides guidelines following flexor tendon repair. However, it has been noted that current clinical practice patterns vary widely and often differ from those reported in the literature.[78] See Table 26-6.

For zones IV and V, both protocols are overall as previously delineated, but they progress faster. AROM is initiated at 3 weeks within the dorsal blocking splint. AROM out of the splint occurs at 4 weeks. PROM into extension and strengthening is initiated at 6 weeks. A four-strand suture technique allows controlled active movement beginning on postoperative day 2. A wrist-hinged dorsal blocking splint is used to allow a tenodesis movement in which the digits are held at the end range by active digit contraction. PROM may be used to achieve full composite flexion. This splint and active motion is continued until week 8, with full active and passive exercise and strengthening started at that time.[33]

Bone and Joint Injuries

Injuries to the bones and joints of the elbow, wrist, and hand can cause significant impairments, activity limitations, and participation restrictions. Fractures of the hand are the most common fractures in the body.[79] Fracture management requires an understanding of the fracture's stability, healing process and potential, and need for surgery to establish stability and healing potential.[80] It is essential that these injuries are properly evaluated and appropriate interventions applied.

Medial Elbow Instability

Medial elbow instability is seen in children and adults and is found most often in individuals involved in throwing. High forces on the medial elbow structures during the cocking and acceleration phases can result in attenuation and rupture of the static ligamentous structures. During the acceleration phase of throwing, the elbow extension speeds can reach 2,300 degrees per second.[81] In the adult, acute rupture of the UCL can occur. More often, continued valgus loading and loss of dynamic muscular support places loads on the UCL, leading to gradual instability. Progressive instability can lead to rupture or tension of the ulnar nerve. In some cases, this progressive instability and load on the ulnar nerve leads to surgical reconstruction of the UCL. Table 26-7 provides guidelines for rehabilitation following UCL reconstruction.

In the child or adolescent, medial elbow instability is commonly known as "little league elbow." The growth plate and associated ligamentous and tendinous structures are at risk until the fusion at the growth plate is complete. In the child, the valgus stress on the medial side of the elbow is countered with a compressive force on the lateral side at the radiocapitellar joint. This can lead to compression and shearing of the radial head on the capitellum. Osteochondrosis of the capitellum can occur with loose body formation.

Treatment of the child or adult with valgus instability depends on the pathologic stage. Controlled rest is essential, along with strengthening exercises for the involved musculature. Dynamic support of the medial elbow to minimize loads on the static structures is a critical component of the treatment program. This approach includes strengthening the trunk, shoulder, elbow, forearm, and wrist muscles (Fig. 26-31). Proximal weakness can transfer loads distally, and a rotator cuff problem can produce instability problems at the elbow. In addition to strengthening, consideration of throwing form and the throwing schedule (e.g., number of throws, games, inning) is important to prevent a recurrence of the problem.

Elbow Dislocations

Elbow dislocations are second in incidence only to dislocations of the shoulder in the adult population. The elbow is the most frequently dislocated joint in children younger than 10 years

---

TABLE 26-7 Rehabilitation Guidelines Following UCL Reconstruction

PHASE	PRECAUTIONS	GOALS	INTERVENTIONS
Early: Weeks 4–6	*Brace:* Week 1: immobilization fixed at 90 degrees. Week 2: hinged brace from 30 to 100 degrees. Week 3: hinged brace from 15 to 100 degrees. Week 4: hinged brace from 10 to 120 degrees	1. Protect healing tissues 2. Decrease pain and inflammation 3. Prevent muscular atrophy 4. Initiate elbow ROM	1. Gentle A/AAROM for elbow and wrist 2. Gentle mobility to achieve ROM goals 3. Submaximal isometric for shoulder IR, abduction, elbow flexion and wrist flexion/extension at week 2 4. Gripping exercise 5. Cervical spine and shoulder ROM
Intermediate: Weeks 6–12	Week 5: hinged brace from 0 to 130 degrees. Week 6: discontinue brace except in risky environments. Avoid all valgus posiitons and minimize valgus stress to elbow during rehab	1. Increased ROM to nearly full ROM by week 10 2. Prevent reinjury 3. Increased total arm strength	1. Gentle A/AAROM for elbow and wrist 2. Light dynamic resistance for shoulder IR, abduction, elbow flexion and wrist flexion/extension 3. Scapular strengthening and stabilization 4. Core, hip and lower extremity strengthening 5. Continued upper quarter mobility
Late: Weeks 12–20	No pain with strengthening exercises. Post-exercise pain should be minimal and resolve within 24 hours	1. Maximize shoulder strength in key muscle groups and functional activities 2. Increased distal muscle function and strength	1. Shoulder and elbow strengthening in functional movements and activities, controlling valgus force at elbow 2. Progressive scapular strengthening 3. Rhythmic stabilization for elbow and shoulder with progressively less protected positions 4. Core, hip, and lower extremity strengthening 5. Address any remaining impairments
Return to activity: Weeks 20–36	No pain with strengthening or functional progression; post-exercise pain should resolve within 24 hours	1. Good dynamic neuromuscular control in functional activities 2. Biomechanically sound functional activities to minimize medial elbow stress 3. Return to pain-free activity	1. Multi-joint, multi-plane strengthening program 2. Shoulder and elbow strength and stabilization drills, specific to work or sport 3. Plyometric program using ball or other tools specific to the work or sport tasks 4. Functional progression, including interval throwing program in thrower, or other sport or work specific activities

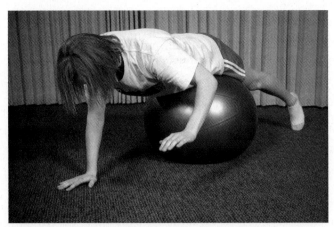

FIGURE 26-31. Therapeutic exercise on a ball, weightbearing on the upper extremity to strengthen in a closed chain.

of age.[82] Elbow dislocations are classified by the direction of movement of the radius and ulna on the humerus, and most are posterior. A fall on an outstretched hand or hyperextension are the most common mechanisms of injury. Dislocation also can injure the UCL, the lateral collateral ligament, the anterior capsule, and common flexor and extensor muscle origins or fracture the medial epicondyle. The ulnar, median,

or radial nerves may be injured. After dislocation, the elbow is reduced (and stabilized if necessary) and immobilized for 1 to 2 weeks.

Impairments after dislocation include loss of motion, pain, inability to produce torque, and occasionally neurovascular problems. Restoration of full motion may be difficult and should be a priority in the treatment program. Many patients retain a residual loss of extension of 10 to 15 degrees, and full recovery of motion and strength takes 3 to 6 months for most patients.[83]

Intervention after dislocation includes AROM and AAROM initiated 2 to 7 days after the dislocation and PROM 2 weeks after the dislocation. Motion should be performed in a variety of shoulder positions. Dynamic splinting may be necessary to restore motion. Prefabricated splints are available to restore flexion or extension. A static night splint can maintain current range if a dynamic splint cannot be tolerated all night. Caution is necessary to avoid overly aggressive PROM, because it may contribute to heterotopic bone formation. Individuals with head injuries or those with a combined fracture-dislocation with prolonged immobilization face the greatest risk of heterotopic bone formation.

Isometric muscle contractions are initiated early and progressed to dynamic contractions as tolerated (Fig. 26-32). Open and closed chain exercises and proprioceptive neuromuscular facilitation techniques are useful for restoration of function.

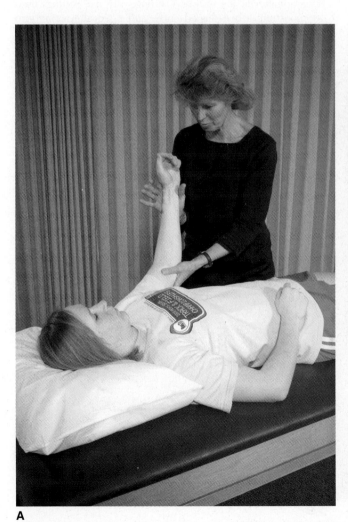
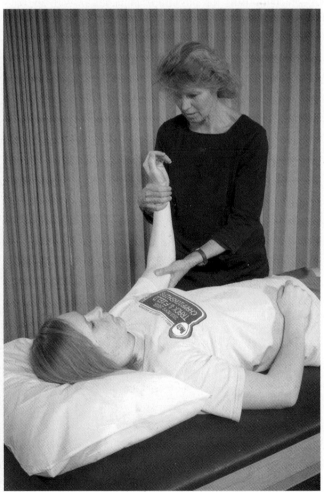

A B

FIGURE 26-32. Rhythmic stabilization for muscles supporting elbow joint.

If instability is present, a hinged elbow support with extension blocks may allow functional use of the elbow within a limited range. Exercises are performed throughout the day, in or out of the brace. If the patient has hypomobility, joint mobilization techniques can help restore full elbow and forearm mobility (see Chapter 7).

Carpal Instability

The bony and ligamentous anatomy of the wrist is intricately balanced to allow flexibility and stability. Williams[2] observed that the carpal bones are spring loaded like a jack-in-the-box and kept under control by ligament restraints. The palmar ligaments are very substantial compared with the dorsal wrist ligaments. An area between the capitate and lunate where no ligamentous support is maintained is an area of potential weakness. A fall on an outstretched hand can result in damage to the scapholunate ligament and produce instability. This instability may result in dislocation of the lunate where its dorsal surface faces dorsally, called *dorsal intercalated segment instability*. Injury resulting in a volarly facing distal lunate is called *volar intercalated segment instability*.

Many types and descriptions of static and dynamic carpal patterns exist. Static instability patterns demonstrate radiographic changes such as abnormal gapping between carpal bones. A static instability generally indicates a significant injury such as a complete ligament tear. Dynamic instability patterns are detected during the physical examination or with special imaging techniques. Dynamic instability patterns generally indicate increased laxity or partial ligament tears. Scapholunate dissociation is the most common form of carpal instability and occurs when ligaments from the proximal pole of the scaphoid are torn. This injury can occur from a fall on an extended, ulnarly deviated wrist; degeneration resulting from RA; a direct blow to the wrist; or in association with a distal radius fracture, carpal fracture, or carpal dislocation. Scapholunate instability is the most frequent cause of carpal instability and accounts for a large proportion of impairments, activity limitations, and time lost from work.[84] The severe form of instability is termed the SLAC (scapholunate advanced collapse) wrist and may be the result of the undetected or untreated injury. Isolated injury to the scapholunate interosseous ligament may be difficult to detect with standard clinical examination or radiographs, and may be the first step in progressive decline to degenerative changes (Fig. 26-33 A and B).[84]

Impairments associated with a scapholunate dissociation include point tenderness over the involved ligament, swelling of the dorsal wrist, pain or limited AROM and PROM of the wrist, a painful click or clunk with radial deviation, grip weakness, and decreased wrist and hand function because of pain. In addition to routine examination procedures such as documentation of pain with rest and functional activities, ROM, and strength of the forearm, wrist, and hand musculature, the clinician should assess grip and pinch strength. Grip strength is performed with a dynamometer at the standard setting, with five settings used to demonstrate a bell-shaped curve and rapid alternating grip strength. Lateral and three-point pinch strength is also assessed.

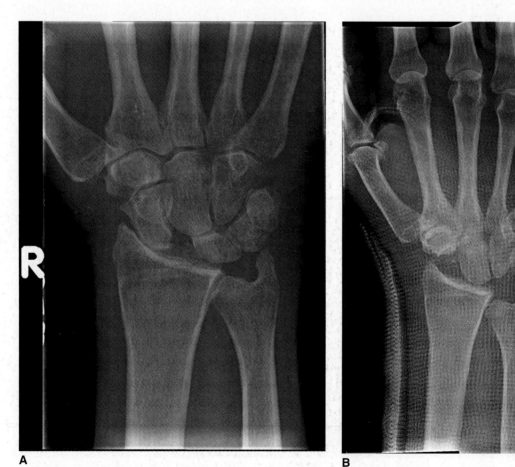

FIGURE 26-33. (A) SLAC wrist before surgery. (B) SLAC wrist after proximal row carpectomy.

Severe instabilities are treated with surgical reduction and ligament reconstruction. Fusions may also be performed for a number of carpal instability patterns. After surgery or for mild cases of instability, the patient is referred for rehabilitative management.[84,85]

Therapeutic exercises for carpal instability include grip and pinch strengthening exercises. Putty exercises and isolated muscle strengthening exercises are incorporated to restore strength and dynamic function throughout the region. With a lunate dislocation and ligament injury, a painful grip may indicate instability leading to lunate destruction. In this situation, grip strengthening should be avoided. Any mobility deficits are treated with active, passive, and AAROM.

Intervention for carpal instability also includes protective splinting of the wrist. The thumb MCP is included in cases of scaphoid involvement, such as scapholunate dissociation. If the ligament disruption is on the ulnar side of the wrist, a wrist cock-up or ulnar gutter splint suffices. Therapeutic modalities may be used for pain and inflammation, and patient education is a critical component of successful management.

Gamekeeper's Thumb

The MCP joint of the thumb functions primarily in flexion and extension because of the condyloid shape of the joint surface. Small degrees of abduction, adduction, and rotation also occur. Tautness in the UCL limits abduction and extension and adds stability to the joint in a functional position. However, this functional position also places the UCL at risk for injury. The most common injuries to the thumb MCP involve the UCL.

Gamekeeper's thumb, or a sprain to the UCL of the MCP joint, is the result of abduction or hyperextension forces. This injury occurs frequently in skiing when a fall catches the thumb in the strap of the ski pole, pulling the thumb into abduction. Complete ruptures lead to instability and significant disability. A thorough examination, with valgus stress performed in extension (collateral ligament and volar plate) and flexion (collateral ligament only), should be done to differentiate partial from complete tears. Impairments associated with gamekeeper's thumb include tenderness along the ulnar aspect of the MCP joint, localized edema, and instability of the joint.

Treatment of partial tears requires immobilization in a thumb spica cast for 3 weeks, followed by a thumb spica splint (Fig. 26-34). The splint is removed throughout the day to allow exercise of the wrist and hand. Acute injuries with gross

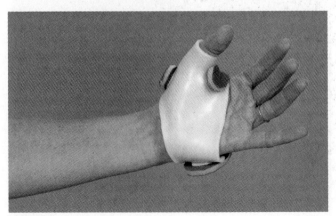

FIGURE 26-34. Thumb spica splint.

Purpose:	To increase the strength of your thumb muscles
Starting Position:	Form the putty into a barrel shape, and place it in the palm of your hand, resting against your thumb.
Movement Technique:	Press your thumb into the putty with as much force as is comfortable until your thumb has pressed through the putty into your hand. Reshape the putty and repeat.

Dosage
Repetitions: _____
Frequency: _____

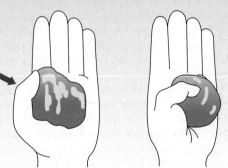

instability require surgical stabilization. Therapeutic exercise after immobilization after surgical and nonsurgical treatment include pain-free thumb MCP flexion and extension and gradually adding pain-free rotation and opposition. After 4 to 6 weeks, grip and pinch strengthening exercises are initiated with putty or gripper equipment (see Self-Management 26-5: Thumb Press). Lateral (key) pinch is initiated, but the patient should be instructed to limit or avoid tip pinch stress until 6 to 8 weeks. Exercises should be progressed to activities pertinent to the patient's lifestyle as quickly as possible within the constraints of healing.

Olecranon Fractures

Olecranon fractures are generally the result of a direct blow or a fall. A fall on an outstretched hand with the elbow in flexion, followed by a strong contraction of the triceps, can cause an olecranon fracture. A nondisplaced fracture is immobilized in 45 to 90 degrees of flexion for a short time. A displaced fracture may be treated with open reduction and internal fixation (ORIF) using tension band wiring or plate and screw fixation. A small comminuted fracture may be excised with reattachment of the triceps tendon. Excision of loose bodies is required during surgery to prevent a loss of mobility from these fragments. The impairments seen after fracture or surgery are pain, limited ROM, and loss of the ability to produce torque. The proximity of the ulnar nerve makes it vulnerable to injury in a olecranon fracture. Close examination is necessary to assess the status of the nerve.

Intervention after fracture begins with AROM in a forearm neutral position. AROM and AAROM may be initiated as early as 2 days after fracture. These individuals usually are immobilized, and the immobilization is removed for ROM activities. The length of immobilization is decreased for the elderly, and ROM exercise is initiated sooner.[49,86] Active ROM is progressed to PROM and stretching.

The biceps muscle often shortens because of the flexed elbow position during immobilization or protection periods. Suggested forms of exercise to restore muscle length include elbow and shoulder extension, walking with a normal arm swing, and contract-relax stretching.

The adaptive shortening may result in weakness, and strength should be addressed concurrently. Suggested strengthening exercises include isometric contractions throughout the available range for all major muscle groups, resistive band exercises for shoulder musculature, resisted elbow flexion in a variety of forearm positions, resisted elbow extension, and resisted wrist and forearm exercises. A stationary bicycle with combined arm movements or a cross trainer allowing repetitive elbow flexion and extension is helpful to restore motion and strength. If forearm rotation strength is limited, a light hammer can be used to train pronation and supination (Fig. 26-35).

Adjunctive interventions include elevation, ice, and active shoulder, wrist, and finger exercises to control edema. Scar massage should be initiated early after surgical stabilization. Generally, the scar is mature enough to tolerate massage 10 to 14 days postoperatively. The triceps may become adherent to the scar and should be treated with cross-friction massage and triceps resistive exercises. Joint mobilization with distraction may be initiated in later stages if loss of motion is a problem. The prognosis after an olecranon fracture is good, but loss of terminal extension is a common residual impairment.

Radial Head Fracture

Radial head fractures occur most often as a result of falls on an outstretched hand with the forearm in supination. These fractures also occur in combination with dislocation. The individual with a radial head fracture has pain over the radial head in the lateral elbow, and forearm rotation is painful. A nondisplaced fracture can be treated with sling immobilization for 1 to 2 days, whereas a displaced fracture may be treated with ORIF. For severe fractures, the radial head may be excised. Any pathology at the distal radioulnar joint can complicate this form of treatment. The patient may be immobilized with the forearm in neutral but allowing elbow ROM (i.e., sugar tong or Muenster splint) for 2 to 3 weeks.

The most common impairment after a radial head fracture is a loss of 10 to 20 degrees of elbow extension. Crepitus or clicking at the radial head may occur with supination and pronation.

Treatment of a nondisplaced radial head fracture includes initiation of elbow and forearm AROM 1 week after injury. Successful treatment demands early ROM. The progression is similar to that for olecranon fractures. After ORIF of displaced fractures, motion may begin immediately postoperatively, barring any secondary injuries. Strengthening and functional use of the limb should be progressed as for other upper extremity injuries.

Colles Fracture

The distal radius is fractured more frequently than any other bone in the body.[19] The Colles fracture is a dorsally angulated fracture of the distal radius with or without concurrent ulnar fracture. This fracture occurs most often from falling on an outstretched hand. The volarly angulated distal radius fracture is known as a Smith fracture. The Colles fracture is initially treated with closed reduction and cast immobilization in an above-elbow cast to prevent pronation and supination or with ORIF. If healing is progressing well, a short forearm cast may be applied after 2 weeks.

The major impairments after cast removal are pain, decreased mobility and strength, and swelling. Control of edema is critical to prevent a stiff hand. Elevation, ice, edema massage, and compression garments can be used to reduce

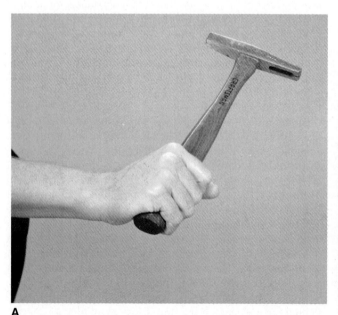
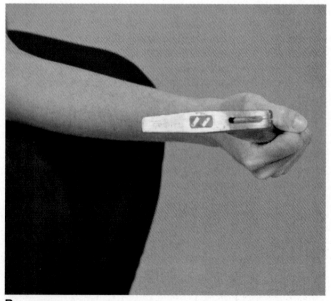

A   **B**

FIGURE 26-35. Range of motion of the forearm using a hammer. (A) Pronation. (B) Supination.

edema. Education about controlling edema must be emphasized to prevent further complications.

Restoration of mobility is essential for full functioning of the hand. The priority in the early phase of mobility exercises should be to regain wrist flexion, extension, and supination, because these are usually the most limited motions and important for a functional outcome (see Self-Management 26-6: Finger and Wrist Flexor Stretching). Exercises should include AROM and self-PROM techniques using the opposite extremity. If mobility remains limited, joint mobilization may facilitate gains in ROM (see Chapter 7). When dealing with complicated Colles fractures, splinting may be necessary to maintain gains in ROM achieved while at rest or at night or to assist in increasing mobility. Static splinting provides support and maintains range between exercise sessions. This intervention may be supplied by prefabricated wrist supports or custom-made splints. Dynamic splinting may also be of value in cases of limited mobility. These splints include a constant or variable tension across the wrist, forearm, or both areas to facilitate increasing motion in the direction desired. Many commercial devices are available, or a custom splint may be fabricated.

Strengthening exercises may be initiated with isometric contractions, grip strengthening, and resisted elbow exercises. Watch for substitution, and utilize proximal stabilization to ensure motion at the joint(s) of interest (Fig. 26-36) As range

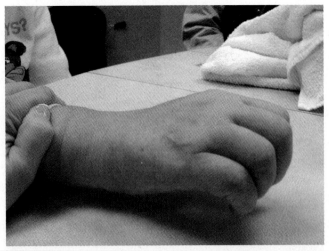

FIGURE 26-36. Wrist extension exercise after Colles fracture. Wrist stabilization is necessary to prevent substitution by finger extensor muscles.

improves, dynamic exercises for the wrist may be employed using free weights or resistive bands (Fig. 26-37). The clinician must consider the patient's preinjury status to establish relevant goals.

Scaphoid Fracture

The scaphoid is often fractured as a result of a fall on an outstretched hand but frequently goes unrecognized. Individuals often pass these fractures off as sprains because of the lack of obvious deformity. The scaphoid is highly susceptible to injury because of its shape and its position. Its narrow midline makes it more vulnerable to stress, and its position crosses the two rows of carpal bones, predisposing it to more frequent injury.

The individual with a scaphoid fracture relates a history of a fall on or other trauma to an extended wrist, with subsequent pain and loss of motion. Pain is particularly apparent with any overpressure in extension, such as in pushing a heavy door open. Athletes are unable to bench press because of the pressure into wrist extension. Palpable tenderness over the anatomic snuffbox and painful extension warrant medical evaluation.

SELF-MANAGEMENT 26-6 *Finger and Wrist Flexor Stretching*

Purpose:	To increase the mobility of the soft tissues in your wrist and hand
Starting Position:	With your palm facing up and wrist at the edge of a table
Movement Technique:	Using your other hand, gently press your wrist and fingers down toward the floor. Hold 15 to 30 seconds, relax, and repeat.

Dosage
Repetitions: _____
Frequency: _____

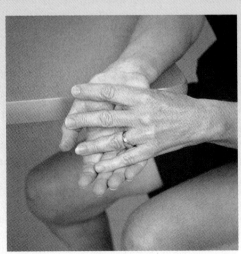

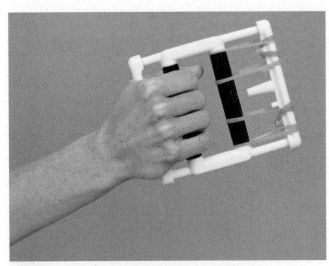

FIGURE 26-37. Grip strengthening exercises. Resistance is easily altered by increasing or decreasing the number of bands.

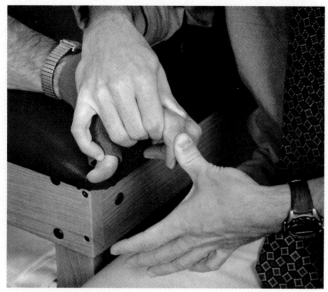

FIGURE 26-38. Resisted finger extension at the PIP joint.

Medical intervention for scaphoid fractures is immobilization for 8 to 12 weeks. Because the poor vascular supply predisposes the scaphoid to nonunion, these fractures are treated conservatively. If the fracture is severe or displaced, ORIF with a Herbert screw may be used. Because of the importance of the scaphoid in providing stability to the wrist, healing of this fracture is important. A bone stimulator may be used to facilitate bone healing. The thumb is immobilized along with the wrist because of its involvement in thumb mobility.

The rehabilitation after immobilization is similar to that for a Colles fracture. Edema control and restoration of mobility, strength, and function relative to the individual's needs are the primary goals. Self-stretching exercises, mobilization, and strengthening exercises are indicated (Fig. 26-38). Specific thumb AROM and PROM exercises should also be included. Specific grip, pinch, and thumb opposition strengthening exercises also are important after a scaphoid fractures. Putty or other household products (e.g., racquetball, Nerf ball, clothespin, rubber bands) may be used. Include the patient in discovering objects at home or work that may be used to accomplish the established goals (Fig. 26-39).

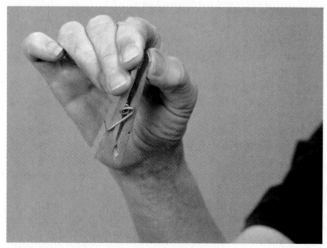

FIGURE 26-39. Resisted pinching using a clothespin.

Metacarpal Fracture

Metacarpal fractures account for 30% to 50% of all hand fractures.[79,87] Metacarpal fractures can occur from a fall onto an outstretched hand with initial ground contact along the metacarpals, from industrial accidents (e.g., punch press machines), or from fist fights. When the fifth metacarpal is the only involved bone, it is commonly referred to as a boxer's fracture. Metacarpal fractures can occur at the base, shaft, neck, or head. Tension in the long finger flexors can cause angulation, shortening, and/or rotation of metacarpal fractures. Importantly, these tendons must be considered during the healing process to avoid adhesions and loss of tendon mobility during the fracture healing process.[80]

Impairments associated with fracture in the acute stage include pain, swelling, loss of motion and strength, and deformity. The MCP joints of fingers two through five are essentially ball and socket joints with a slack joint capsule in extension and taut collateral ligaments in flexion. The dorsal and palmar interossei muscles arise from the metacarpal bones and insert into the extensor mechanism. These muscle groups need special attention during evaluation, because their length and strength may be affected after injury or immobilization for metacarpal fractures.

Medical intervention depends on the severity of the fracture. If the fracture is nondisplaced, it is usually casted for 2 to 3 weeks. A custom static splint that crosses the wrist and includes only the affected MCP joints up the PIP level may be worn for 2 to 3 weeks. Radial or ulnar gutter splints allow immobilization of only the affected metacarpals and permit passive range of motion while in the splint. If the MCP joint is flexed during immobilization, the position can prevent collateral ligament contracture. If the fracture is displaced or unstable surgical fixation with pins, Kirschner wires, or a plate is indicated.

The start of rehabilitation depends on the medical intervention. If the fracture is surgically stabilized, treatment begins as early as 1 to 3 days after surgery. Early intervention avoids associated impairments of dorsal hand edema, extensor tendon adhesions, MCP collateral ligament adhesions, and intrinsic muscle contractures. Exercises in the first phase emphasize gentle AROM of the wrist and all fingers and blocked MCP flexion and extension exercise (see Self-Management 26-7: Metacarpophalangeal Joint Extension With Distal Interphalangeal Joint Flexion). This specific exercise prevents collateral ligament adhesions and encourages extensor tendon gliding with minimal stress placed on the fracture site. Aggressive interosseous and lumbrical stretching along with thumb-index web space stretching also should be initiated in this phase. Intrinsic muscle stretching can only be accomplished by maintaining the MCP in neutral or hyperextension while flexing at both IP joints (Fig. 26-40).

At 2 weeks, scar mobilization may begin, and at 4 to 6 weeks after surgery, passive MCP flexion may be initiated. At 6 to 8 weeks after surgery, intervention may focus on aggressive MCP flexion (i.e., joint mobilizations), wrist strengthening, and grip and pinch strengthening, including the intrinsic muscles (e.g., putty exercises for finger abduction and adduction).

The patient treated with immobilization may begin after cast removal at 2 to 3 weeks after the injury. Gentle AROM of the wrist and MCP joints is initiated at this time. PROM is initiated after 4 to 6 weeks. All other noninvolved joints and

SELF-MANAGEMENT 26-7 *Metacarpophalangeal Joint Extension With Proximal and Distal Interphalangeal Joint Flexion*

Purpose:	To increase the mobility in your finger extensor tendon
Starting Position:	Keep the middle (PIP) and end (DIP) joints flexed
Movement Technique:	Keeping those joints flexed, actively extend at your knuckle joints
Dosage	
Repetitions:	_____
Frequency:	_____

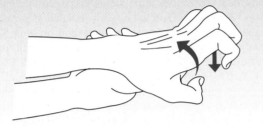

fingers should be completing AROM exercises from the beginning of immobilization to prevent functional loss. The program is progressed similar to that for surgical management.

Adjunctive agents include education, elevation, ice, and compression garments to control edema. Dynamic splinting may be used to promote passive stretching of the MCP joints for 20-minute sessions performed 6 to 8 times per day. Massage is used to manage scar formation in the operative cases.

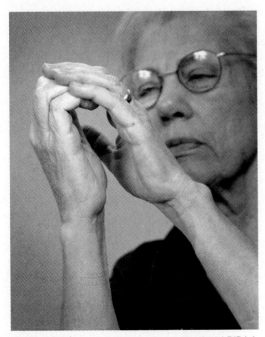

FIGURE 26-40. Stretching exercises at the proximal and DIP joints.

Phalangeal Fracture

Phalangeal fractures usually occur as a result of trauma. Approximately 45% to 50% of all hand fractures involve the distal phalanx, 15% to 20% the proximal phalanx, and 8% to 12% the middle phalanx.[37] Unlike metacarpal fractures, phalangeal fractures are more often unstable due to the lack of soft tissue support and the additional tension in the long finger flexors.[80] Additionally, immobilized phalangeal fractures result in loss of motion at a higher rate than metacarpal fractures, in both the injured and adjacent fingers.[80]

Impairments observed in the acute stage include localized swelling, pain, and tenderness over the fractures; hypomobility at IP joints and possibly MCP joint; and abnormal alignment of the IP joint. Patients may also experience lateral instability. Associated impairments after immobilization usually include restricted PIP joint flexion and extension (from volar plate contracture), DIP flexion and extension, and flexor tendon adhesions.

As with metacarpal fractures, the intervention depends on the severity of the fracture. If nondisplaced, the immobilization is accomplished by a custom splint or foam-covered metal splint. The period of immobilization varies according to the location of the fracture. If located at proximal or distal ends, only 3 to 4 weeks are required because of the good vascularity in cancellous bone. Mid-shaft middle phalangeal fractures require 10 to 14 weeks or longer because of the poor blood supply in the bony cortex. Displaced fractures require internal fixation with Kirschner wires or pinning. Extreme care is taken to avoid rotation, and often a buddy splint or buddy taping technique is used to help minimize this complication.

Intervention after nonsurgical postimmobilization care of phalangeal fractures is usually initiated at 3 to 6 weeks after injury or when immobilization is no longer necessary. Exercises of active and passive motion for all MCP, PIP, and DIP joints should be initiated along with tendon gliding exercises. For PIP joint restrictions of 20 degrees or more, dynamic PIP extension splinting may be required. Several commercial prefabricated splints are available, or custom splints can be fabricated. Static progressive splinting can be used at night. The finger splint is fabricated in full extension, and tension-adjustable straps are used to allow gradual finger extension toward the splint.

After surgical internal fixation, intervention may begin as early as 2 days after surgery. Gentle AROM of the MCP, PIP, and DIP joints, with emphasis on full PIP joint motion, is initiated. Tendon gliding, scar management, and edema control also should be encouraged. At 4 to 8 weeks after surgery, dynamic PIP extension splinting may be initiated, along with buddy taping during exercises or ADLs. Again, these general guidelines will vary depending upon the phalanx fractured, as well as the fixation, healing and associated considerations.

Complex Regional Pain Syndrome

Reflex sympathetic dystrophy (RSD) is a term used to describe a cluster of signs and symptoms, including pain disproportionate to the injury, vasomotor and trophic changes, stiffness, swelling, and decreased function. Other terms for RSD have included sympathetically maintained pain, causalgia, sympathetic dystrophy without pain, shoulder-hand syndrome, and Sudeck atrophy. The uncertain role of the sympathetic nervous system in RSD led the International Association for the Study of Pain and the American Pain Association to recommend use of the term complex regional pain syndrome (CRPS) to replace the term RSD.[88]

Several common features and two classifications of CRPS have been identified. The common features are local tissue damage or nerve damage that initiates a reflex response in the peripheral and central nervous systems. Several disorders with the same abnormal clinical findings share these criteria with CRPS. The two types have been classified by the absence or presence of nerve involvement, the first resembling RSD (without nerve involvement) and the second equivalent to causalgia (with nerve involvement).[88] Several impairments are associated with CRPS and may include pain and inflammation, swelling, stiffness, vasomotor disturbances, trophic changes, bone demineralization, and dystonia.[38] Initial activity limitations are numerous and are based on pain-limited use of the extremity. An ADL checklist is helpful to monitor even small improvements in functional tasks.

Pain disproportionate to the injury severity is the primary clinical feature of CRPS. In the upper extremity, the pain is found throughout a large part of the arm, from the upper arm distally to and fully including the hand. The pain is often described as burning initially and eventually changing to pressure, aching, and binding sensations. Pain is often constant, starting locally at the original injury site and spreading throughout the extremity. The pain often leads to disuse and self-immobilization of the extremity, along with the known consequences of this response. In addition to constant pain, hypersensitivity to touch occurs, with extreme sensitivity to any kind of tactile stimulation. Occasionally, sympathetic and trophic changes occur with minimal complaints of pain or pain related only to motion of stiff joints.

Excessive swelling at the injury site is often the first objective sign noticed in the early phase. Swelling can subsequently spread throughout the distal upper extremity. Initially, it has a fusiform and pitting appearance, but it later takes on a hard and brawny character that contributes to joint stiffness. Periarticular thickening is observed at the IP joints. Edema is difficult to control even with otherwise successful intervention techniques.

Joint restriction with CRPS is often more profound than expected for the associated diagnosis. Unlike the traditional joint stiffness experienced after injury that decreases with ROM and functional use, individuals with CRPS tend to lose motion over time and seem to be refractory to improvement with traditional active and passive exercises and dynamic splinting. Fibrosis of ligaments limits motion about joints, and adhesions in tendon sheaths limit the gliding properties of the tendon, producing inflammation and pain. These changes contribute to the vicious circle of pain and inflammation. Palmar fascitis can be seen, and nodules and thickening of the palmar fascia can be palpated. This stiffness contributes to limited MCP and IP extension.

Discoloration of various degrees occurs with vasomotor instability. Pallor results from with vasoconstriction of the arterial and venous systems. Redness is evident when there is dilation of both sides of the vascular tree. Blueness (cyanosis) is usually present with vasoconstriction of the venous system.[89] Sudomotor changes occurring include hyperhidrosis (excessive sweating) early and dryness in later stages.

Bone demineralization is a reliable sign of CRPS and assists in making the diagnosis. Although some demineralization takes place with immobilization, the bulk of calcium loss results from increased blood flow in the periarticular bone.[89]

Sudeck[90] described the condition as "inflammatory bone atrophy." Untreated cases progress from "spotty" osteoporosis to diffuse osteoporosis.

Trophic changes in the skin are initially caused by swelling and later by nutritional changes in the hand. The skin appears glossy or shiny, and evidence of subcutaneous tissue atrophy is present. Excessive and dark hair growth may be present. The nails become coarse, rigid, and curved.[89]

Intervention for CRPS must be approached practically and cautiously. Traditional exercises for restricted joints are often painful and exacerbate the pain cycle and vasomotor instability. Pain must be controlled before progressing to other treatment techniques. Modalities such as heat and cold may be helpful in reducing pain but must not aggravate the vasomotor tone. Elevation and moist heat before edema massage and exercise can improve tissue extensibility and tolerance to exercise.

Therapeutic exercise interventions include AROM, joint mobilization techniques, and continuous passive motion (CPM) devices. Exercise is best tolerated if initiated at proximal and less painful joints. Supine shoulder flexion or simple posture correction with the patient's back against a wall promotes upper extremity blood flow and improved proximal joint alignment. Active exercise of the wrist and hand should be performed elevated and directed to individual joints and motions. Blocked finger flexion exercises encourage more complete joint motion and specific tendon gliding (see Self-Management 26-8:

SELF-MANAGEMENT 26-8 *Blocked Finger Extension*

Purpose:	To increase the mobility of your finger joints and tendons.
Starting Position:	
Level 1.	Hold the knuckle joint of your finger straight.
Level 2.	Hold the knuckle and middle joints of your finger straight.
Movement Technique:	
Level 1.	Bend your middle joint, keeping your fingertip joint straight.
Level 2.	Bend only your fingertip joint.

Dosage
Repetitions: _____
Frequency: _____

Level I   Level II

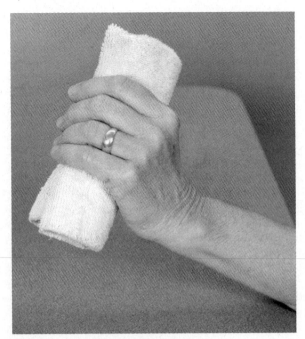

FIGURE 26-41. Grasping exercise using a towel.

Blocked Finger Extension). Holding a towel or soft ball while gripping can improve motor function by the assistance of palmar sensory stimulation (Fig. 26-41). Patients are encouraged to keep the wrist in slight extension during gripping exercises to ensure maximal efficiency of the flexor tendons.

A three-component stress-loading program has been a successful technique for treatment of CRPS. The components include compressive loading of the upper extremity, distraction, and use of other modalities, including splinting.[91] The object is to provide stress to the tissues while minimizing painful joint motion. Loading activities can include rocking on hands and knees or standing with weight applied through the upper extremity by leaning on a table (Fig. 26-42). Therapy putty or a foam ball under the palm can be used to allow feedback on the pressure being applied with the weight-bearing activities. Fingers can be flexed over the edge of the table if composite

finger extension is painful. Resistive band exercises can also be used to provide stress to upper extremity joints without introducing painful joint motion.

Other interventions may be used to decrease pain and edema and to improve mobility. Joint mobilization techniques specific to pain control, such as joint distraction and volar-dorsal glides, are often tolerated well and promote normal joint proprioceptive sensory input (Fig. 26-43). End-range techniques may produce pain early with increased local inflammation and a resulting loss of joint motion. These techniques should be introduced gradually and instructed for home use when tolerated. CPM devices can be used periodically, alternating with active use and exercises. The device can be adjusted and controlled by the patient to allow slow and repetitive joint motion in pain-free ranges. The CPM may also contribute to pain relief (i.e., gate control theory) and improve periarticular and cartilage nutrition.

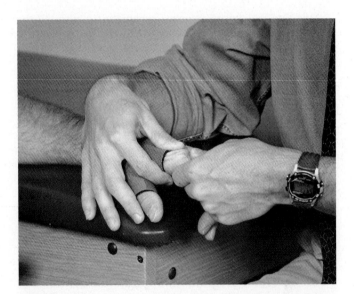

A

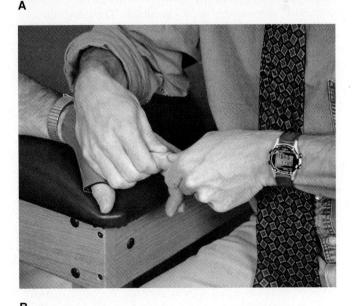

B

FIGURE 26-43. Mobilization at the MCP joint. (A) Dorsal glides. (B) Volar glides.

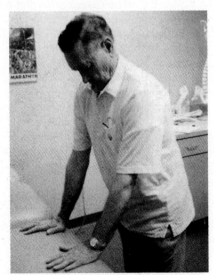

FIGURE 26-42. Leaning on a table can facilitate weight bearing through the wrist.

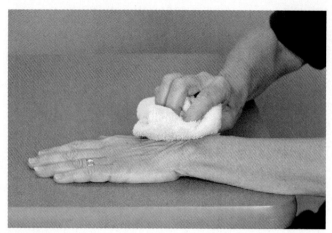

FIGURE 26-44. A variety of textures can be used to desensitize the hand.

Splinting can be an effective technique to maintain or regain joint motion. Tissue responds positively to the appropriate amount of force and negatively to excessive force. Static splinting can be effective in early stages to maintain the joints of the hand in their functional positions at rest. The functional position is described as the wrist in mid-extension, the thumb abducted, the MCP joints flexed 60 to 70 degrees, and the IP joints near full extension. A resting hand splint for an entire hand or a joint-specific PIP extension splint can prevent anticipated development of joint motion restrictions. Dynamic splinting may be tolerated when edema is stabilized to allow a slow and gradual stretch of contracted joint tissues. Dynamic splinting should be done intermittently with gentle tension provided for 20 to 30 minutes. Vascularity should be monitored closely. Increases in edema or pain indicate the need to decrease tension or wearing time.

Hypersensitivity leads to disuse and tactile overprotection, and desensitization programs can be designed on the initial visit. These programs allow the patient a graded and controlled series of activities to improve tactile tolerance and raise the sensory pain threshold. The program can include textures (e.g., denim, terry cloth, corduroy), massage or percussion (e.g., light progressing to firm) with the opposite hand, and tapping a sensitive finger tip on a table (Fig. 26-44). Effort should be made to avoid cyclic stimulation to avoid increased pain. Protective padding or splinting may be helpful for temporary and intermittent use to protect a hypersensitive area from repeated painful environmental stimuli.

Transcutaneous electrical nerve stimulation has been effective for pain modulation, vasodilation, and vasoconstriction. Reports describe improvement in RSD pain as high as 90%.[92-94] Electrode placement and stimulating parameters may vary in effectiveness. Effective sites may include direct placement over the anatomic pain site, over peripheral or superficial cutaneous nerves, or proximal to the area of discomfort. The initial home program should promote pain relief to ensure adherence.

Elevation to decrease arterial hydrostatic pressure and assist in lymphatic and venous damage, elevated massage, and compression are techniques used to decrease edema. Elevated massage from distal to proximal aspects can mobilize edema, assist in pain relief, and improve ROM and

desensitization. Maintaining continuous contact with the skin can decrease the chance for pain exacerbation during massage. Compression can be performed by intermittent sequential compression pumps and continuous compression devices. Acute edema may require only 2 hours of sequential compression pump use daily to be effective in edema reduction. Chronic fibrotic edema may require more prolonged use. Acute edema may require near continuous use of external compression. Compression gloves with exposed fingertips allow use of the hand while controlling edema. A light, self-adhering wrap can be used for individual finger edema reduction.

Physicians often perform stellate ganglion blocks in the treatment of CRPS. These procedures block all efferent sympathetic impulses. After a successful block, the patient may find significant relief and be more successful in exercise attempts. The sympathetic block is therapeutic and helps to confirm the diagnosis.

Treatment of a patient with CRPS must be approached with patience, sympathy, and flexible planning. Improvement is often slow, and the stiffness and pain may worsen before improving. Psychologic help is often necessary to assist with pain management. Individuals with acute symptoms often respond quickly with a decrease in pain and swelling after one treatment. Those in latter stages respond slowly and often unpredictably. Their impairments and activity limitations can be overwhelming. Keeping their program focused on one or two priority activities at a time increases adherence and the ability to assess the effectiveness of each treatment.

Stiff Hand and Restricted Motion

The diagnosis of the "stiff hand" is often used to describe joint limitation from a variety of causes. The primary diagnosis can include lacerations, burns, fractures, soft-tissue crush injuries, and nerve and vascular trauma. The common cause is tissue trauma resulting in an inflammatory response. The resulting edema, fibrosis, and collagen alteration limits tissue gliding (i.e., tendons) and extensibility (i.e., skin, ligament, and joint capsule). Restricted motion is categorized as articular or extraarticular by the tissue causing the limitation. Joint stiffness that follows simple immobilization is attributable to fixation of the joint ligaments to bone in areas normally meant to be free from such fixation, as well as shortening of the ligament by new collagen synthesis.

Knowledge of the normal anatomy and kinesiology of the wrist and hand help to understand, predict, and effectively treat limited mobility. At the MCP joints, the capsule is very elastic dorsally to allow for full MCP joint flexion. The extensor expansion glides over the dorsal capsule. With dorsal hand swelling, the MCP joints often lose joint flexion. This is initially caused by limited extensibility of the dorsal skin and progressively by adhesions of the collateral ligaments in their position of joint extension. The PIP and DIP joints are similar to the MCP joints with two exceptions. First, the collateral ligaments at the IP joints do not become slack in flexion; they remain taut throughout joint range, preventing lateral motion of the IP joints. Second, unlike the MCP joint, the loose-packed position for the IP joints is flexion. The volar plate becomes slack with IP joint flexion and taut in extension, preventing hyperextension, as seen at the MCP

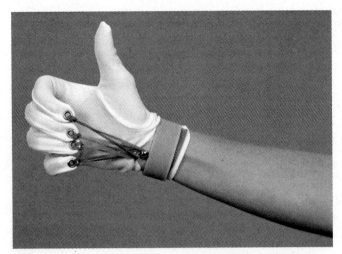

FIGURE 26-45. A flexion glove can improve the range of motion into flexion.

joint. After prolonged local swelling, the IP joints tend to lose joint extension, and the volar plate can become adhered in its slack position, preventing the necessary lengthening for full IP joint extension.

Structures outside the joint such as muscle, tendon, or skin adhesions can also limit joint motion. After prolonged immobilization in wrist and finger flexion, the flexor muscles become shortened. After tendon repair or fractures adjacent to tendons, tendon gliding is often limited by scar tissue or fracture calluses. For complete finger flexion, 7 cm of excursion is needed in the FDP tendons.[3] After a dorsal hand burn, metacarpal fracture, or prolonged dorsal hand edema resulting in decreased skin mobility, adjacent joint motions may be lost. Approximately 4 cm of dorsal skin laxity is needed for full MCP joint flexion and complete fisting.

Patients with articular and extraarticular tissue restriction describe activity limitations such as an inability to hold a fork or grip a steering wheel and difficulty getting their hands into their pockets. Examination must distinguish between articular and extraarticular sources of limited motion. A thorough evaluation, performed with an understanding of the local anatomy and kinesiology, can result in effective intervention.

Interventions for articular limitations include heat before joint mobilization, strengthening, and splinting. Splinting can include dynamic splints (worn for 20 to 30 minutes six to eight times each day or 2 to 3 hours for one or two times each day) or static splints (worn at night). A flexion glove can apply nonspecific tension to the dorsal tissue of the fingers, with an elastic strap used to increase forces at the IP joints (Fig. 26-45).

Extra-articular restriction rely heavily on tendon gliding activities such as differential tendon gliding and blocked IP flexion. As with articular restrictions, static or dynamic splinting plays a role in improving mobility. When intrinsic muscles are shortened or the tendons adhere to surrounding tissues, stretching, gliding, and splinting are the treatments of choice. Along with exercise and splinting, edema can be controlled with compression gloves, compression pumps, elevation, and wraps. Scar massage is important in treating surgical or burn cases.

KEY POINTS

- The ulnar nerve may become entrapped in the cubital tunnel, the median nerve compressed in the carpal tunnel, and the radial nerve entrapped in any of several locations at the lateral elbow.
- The UCL is the primary static stabilizer and the flexor carpi ulnaris muscle the primary dynamic stabilizer of the medial elbow.
- The carpal tunnel is located on the volar aspect of the wrist and contains nine tendons and the median nerve.
- Grip is generally divided in power grip, used when force generation is the primary objective, and prehension grip, used when precision is the main goal.
- Activities to increase mobility include traditional stretching exercises, joint mobilization, and tendon and nerve gliding exercises.
- CTDs are usually the result of a combination of factors such as work pace, decreased rest intervals, and little variability in the task.
- Conservative management of CTS is often successful if hand and wrist postures and hand activities are monitored.
- Radial tunnel syndrome is often misdiagnosed as lateral epicondylitis.
- Cases of lateral and medial epicondylitis often result from repetitive wrist and hand activities at work, at home, or during recreation.
- Medial elbow instability occurs in children and adults who participate in throwing sports. Progressive instability in the child can lead to osteochondrosis of the capitellum and loose body formation.
- Sprain of the thumb's UCL (or gamekeeper's thumb) can result in degenerative joint disease of the CMC joint if instability continues.
- The anatomy of the scaphoid predisposes it to nonunion after a fracture. Any individual with wrist pain and wrist extension loss after a fall on an outstretched hand should be evaluated for fracture of the scaphoid.
- Individuals with CRPS have various degrees of pain, trophic changes, loss of mobility, and a variety of activity limitations and disability.
- Interventions for individuals with a stiff hand include mobility activities, splinting, and strengthening exercises.

CRITICAL THINKING QUESTIONS

1. Consider Case Study No. 8 in Unit 7. Design a workstation for this individual given his physical examination and subjective history. How would your treatment differ if the patient's occupation was
   a. A carpenter
   b. A house painter
   c. A portrait painter
   d. A violinist
   e. A pianist
2. Consider potential reasons why this patient's symptoms did not resolve after his workstation update several months ago.
3. Discuss the relationship between this patient's head and neck examination and his distal complaints.

SELECTED INTERVENTION 26-1
Upper Quadrant

See Case Study No. 8

Although this patient requires comprehensive intervention, one specific exercise addressing motor control is described.

ACTIVITY: Simulated typing with surface electromyography (SEMG).

PURPOSE: Develop motor control strategy to use appropriate levels of wrist extensor activation, wrist flexor relaxation, production of microrests, and complete baseline recovery between timed bouts of data entry.

RISK FACTORS: Watch for cervical posture as part of repetitive strain; injury to extensor group may be secondary to cervical dysfunction.

ELEMENT OF MOVEMENT SYSTEM EMPHASIZED: Modulator

STAGE OF MOTOR CONTROL: Skill

MODE: Isometric wrist extensor and flexors, concentric and eccentric finger flexors and extensors.

POSTURE: Sitting at a simulated workstation in optimal ergonomic posture, with SEMG appropriately placed on right and left forearm flexor and extensor groups.[41]

MOVEMENT: While simulated typing is performed on a keyboard using a palm and wrist rest and optimal ergonomic posture, SEMG monitors forearm flexor and extensor activity bilaterally. The right forearm attempts to follow the template developed by the left forearm. Random stopping is called out to determine the spontaneous speed and level of recovery to baseline. Timed rest breaks are scheduled to determine planned speed and level of recovery to baseline.

SPECIAL CONSIDERATIONS: Closely monitor cervical position and paracervical muscle tension.

DOSAGE

Special Considerations
Anatomic: Lateral epicondyle, musculotendinous and tenoperiosteal junction of wrist and finger extensor group.
Physiologic: Subacute strain.
Learning capability: May be difficult as patient works up to 60 hours a week at visual display terminal. Probably has strong patterns of overuse of wrist and finger extensors.

Repetitions/sets: Five minutes of typing form one repetition. Perform up to five sets.

Rest period: Random 5-second rest breaks are called out during each repetition; 15-second breaks are taken after each 5-minute bout of exercise.

Frequency: If SEMG is rented, practice should be twice daily for 2 to 4 weeks. If only used in clinic, recommend three times a week for 3 to 6 weeks. For cost-effectiveness, unit rental is preferred.

Sequence: Perform after stretching exercises are performed, but not after muscle performance exercises so as not to overly fatigue muscles.

Speed: Functional speed.

Environment: Initially in quiet home environment, then progress to work environment.

Feedback: Initially, continuous audio feedback from the SEMG unit. Threshold is set so as not to exceed left side wrist and finger extensor activity. Visual feedback is used to see the speed and level of recovery to baseline during microrests and rest breaks. The patient is reassessed once each week, and the decision to progressively fade feedback is based on performance. Progressive fading of feedback occurs during exercise sessions to eliminating either audio or visual feedback every third set, to every other set, and so forth. A second party relaying the results between sets provides verbal knowledge of the results.

Functional movement pattern to reinforce goal of exercise: In addition to using an improved motor strategy during data entry, the patient is encouraged to use elbow flexors instead of forearm extensors during lifting tasks (e.g., lift in forearm supination versus pronation) to reduce the strain to the wrist/finger extensors.

Rationale for exercise choice: This exercise was chosen as a skill-level activity to reduce the overuse of the wrist and finger extensors during a highly repetitive functional activity. Through the use of SEMG feedback with a proper faded feedback schedule,[42] the patient can develop an intrinsic reference for muscle activation and error detection to improve motor control strategies to reduce recruitment effort and improve the speed and level of relaxation to baseline.

SELECTED INTERVENTION 26-2
Total Body

See Case Study No. 10

Although this patient requires comprehensive intervention, one specific exercise prescribed in the intermediate stage of recovery is described.

ACTIVITY: Step-ups; swing phase, with counterrotation (see Fig. 24-29 in Chapter 24).

PURPOSE: Incorporate proper total-body movements in a functional context.

RISK FACTORS: None

ELEMENT OF THE MOVEMENT SYSTEM EMPHASIZED: Modulator.

STAGE OF MOTOR CONTROL: Controlled mobility.

POSTURE: Standing in front of a 6-in step in front of a mirror.

MOVEMENT: Lift the right leg onto the step with simultaneous right thoracic rotation and left forward arm swing.

SPECIAL CONSIDERATIONS: Be sure the patient does not hike his right hip during the hip flexion phase and does not drop his right shoulder (right thoracic lateral flexion) or adduct his right scapula instead of right thoracic rotation during the upper body counterswing maneuver.

DOSAGE

Special considerations
Anatomic: Right hamstring and adductor, right subscapularis, right glenohumeral joint.
Physiologic: Chronic moderate strain and tendinitis, questionable instability of right glenohumeral joint.
Learning capability: Very ingrained movement pattern from a long history of high-mileage running; may require high repetitions and significant feedback in early stages of learning.

Repetitions/sets: Initially to form fatigue as evidenced by hip hike, shoulder drop, and scapula adduction; work up to three sets of 20 to 30 repetitions.

Frequency: Six to seven days each week.

Duration: Expect at least 2 weeks before evidence of motor control changes and 6 to 8 weeks before skill level is achieved.

Sequence: Perform after specific exercises for psoas muscle performance, thoracic rotation mobility, and abdominal muscle performance exercises have been performed. Follow with step-up: stance phase.

Speed: Slow progressed to functional speed.

Environment: Home in front of a mirror.

Feedback: Initially in clinic with mirror providing visual feedback and clinician providing verbal feedback. Taper to continued use of mirror, but with knowledge of results of verbal feedback after every 3 to 4 repetitions. Withdraw mirror and verbally provide KR every 3 to 4 repetitions. Progress toward skill.

FUNCTIONAL MOVEMENT PATTERN TO REINFORCE GOAL OF EXERCISE: Ascending stairs, gait.

RATIONALE FOR EXERCISE CHOICE: The total-body movement pattern of right hip hike and right shoulder drop during swing phase of gait may be perpetuating the upper and lower extremity conditions. Without adequate hip flexion, the gluteus maximus is less efficient at assisting the stance phase of gait or step up; the persistent right shoulder drop and scapula adduction and downward rotation can perpetuate posture and movement impairments consistent with glenohumeral impingement and hypermobility. As a result, this pattern of movement must be altered to fully recover from the upper and lower body conditions.

LAB ACTIVITIES

For each of the following case scenarios, evaluate your patient and design and execute an exercise program. Teach your patient a home exercise program.

1. A 56-year-old woman sustained an ulnar shaft fracture when she slipped and fell on the ice 6 weeks ago. She was casted for 3 weeks above the elbow and then recasted with a below-elbow cast. Her cast was removed 3 days ago. Evaluation reveals loss of AROM and PROM for elbow extension, pronation, and supination, wrist flexion and extension, and radial and ulnar deviation. Strength testing was not performed. She had no edema. Joint play assessment was not performed, but atrophy was visible.

2. A 12-year-old boy complains of medial elbow pain. He is active in Little League and pitched 14 innings over the weekend. He complains of pain along the medial collateral ligament, pain with passive elbow extension, flexion, pronation, and supination (with a guarded end feel). A mild effusion is observed, and there is increased laxity with valgus stressing. Radiographic findings are negative.

3. A 44-year-old patient presents with lateral elbow pain after shoveling wet, heavy snow. He complains of pain with activities such as picking up his briefcase, turning the doorknob, and grasping objects. He also has difficulty using the mouse on his computer. Examination reveals a loss of AROM and PROM of wrist flexion (and finger flexion increases symptoms), decreased strength with wrist extension and supination, and pain with palpation at the lateral epicondyle. There is no effusion, but slight warmth is noticed.

4. Three weeks ago, a 22-year-old collegiate gymnast dislocated her elbow (the olecranon displaced posteriorly) from a fall on an outstretched hand when she missed grasping the high bar and fell to the floor. She was in a sling for 2 weeks and has been out of the sling for 1 week, but she is carrying her arm in a guarded position. Examination reveals a loss of elbow extension (actively and passively with a springy end feel), full anteroposterior flexion, and a loss of pronation and supination anteroposteriorly. Joint play assessment reveals decreased humeroulnar joint distraction.

5. A 70-year-old woman fell on the ice and sustained a Colles fracture 8 weeks ago. She underwent a closed reduction and was immobilized in a series of casts. She also has insulin-dependent diabetes mellitus and has decreased sensation over for distal forearm, wrist, and hand. Examination reveals a loss of all active and passive wrist motion, decreased joint play in the inferior radioulnar joint, visible atrophy, and a loss of strength with resisted movements in neutral.

6. A 32-year-old man sustained a scaphoid fracture 10 weeks ago when he fell on an outstretched hand while skiing downhill. He was casted for 8 weeks, and periodic radiographs revealed nonunion of his scaphoid. He underwent surgical stabilization of the fracture using a bone graft from his iliac spine. He has been immobilized for 12 weeks since surgery. He is referred to physical therapy to begin ROM out of the splint four times each day. Examination reveals a loss of all wrist motions, decreased thumb flexion and extension, and decreased opposition.

7. A 40-year-old meat cutter sustained a laceration of his finger extensors (proximal to his MCP joints) while working. He underwent surgical fixation and was allowed to actively contract only the finger flexors. He has been removed from his splint and is allowed to begin active finger extension. Examination reveals decreased active finger extension (at the MCP joints) from weakness but full passive finger extension. Mobility of the MCP joints is decreased.

8. A 50-year-old man sustained a crush injury to his hand when his shirt sleeve got caught in a printing press and pulled his hand in. He sustained multiple metacarpal and carpel fractures, some of which were surgically stabilized through pinning. He has been casted for 8 weeks and presents to physical therapy today. Examination reveals a massive loss of motion of all wrist and fingers joints, atrophy in the thenar and hypothenar eminence, and decreased joint mobility in the carpal and MCP joints and all finger joints.

REFERENCES

1. Butler DS. Mobilization of the Nervous System. New York, NY: Churchill Livingstone, 1991.
2. Williams PL, Warwick R, Dyson M, Bannister LH, eds. Gray's Anatomy. 37th Ed. New York, NY: Churchill Livingstone, 1989.
3. Tubiana R. Architecture and functions of the hand. In: Thomine JM, Mackin EJ, eds. Examination of the Hand and Upper Limb. Philadelphia, PA: WB Saunders, 1984.
4. Kendall FP, McCreary EK, Provance PG. Muscles Testing and Function. 4th Ed. Baltimore, MD: Williams & Wilkins, 1993.
5. Russe O. Fracture of the carpal navicular. J Bone Joint Surg Am 1960;42: 759–768.
6. Ambrose L, Posner MA. Lunate-triquetral and midcarpal joint instability. Hand Clin 1992;8:653–668.
7. Culver JE. Instabilities of the wrist. Clin Sports Med 1986;5:725–740.
8. Chase RA. Anatomy and kinesiology of the hand in rehabilitation of the hand. In: Hunter JM, Mackin EJ, Callahan AD, eds. Rehabilitation of the Hand: Surgery and Therapy. 4th Ed. St. Louis: CV Mosby, 1995.
9. Norkin CC, Levangie PK. Joint Structure and Function: A Comprehensive Analysis. 2nd Ed. Philadelphia, PA: FA Davis, 1992.
10. Berger RA. The anatomy and basic biomechanics of the wrist joint. J Hand Ther 1996;9:84–93.
11. Safran MR. Elbow injuries in athletes: a review. Clin Orthop 1995;310: 257–277.
12. Pratt NE. Clinical Musculoskeletal Anatomy. Philadelphia, PA: JB Lippincott, 1991.
13. Morrey BF, Askew KN, Chao EYS. A biomechanical study of normal functional elbow motion. J Bone Joint Surg Am 1981;63:872–887.
14. Morrey BF, An KN. Articular and ligamentous contributions to the stability of the elbow joint. Am J Sports Med 1983;11:315–319.
15. Davidson PA, Pink M, Perry J, et al. Functional anatomy of the flexor pronator muscle group in relation to the medial collateral ligament of the elbow. Am J Sports Med 1995;23:245–250.
16. Magee D. Orthopedic Physical Assessment. 3rd Ed. Philadelphia, PA: WB Saunders, 1997.
17. Brumfield RH, Champoux JA. A biomechanical study of normal functional wrist motion. Clin Orthop 1984;187:23–25.

18. Viegas SF, Tencer AF, Cantrell J, et al. Load transfer characteristics of the wrist: part I. The normal joint. J Hand Surg 1987;12:971–978.

19. Wadsworth C. The wrist and hand. In: Malone TR, McPoil T, Nitz AJ, eds. Orthopedic and Sports Physical Therapy. 3rd Ed. St. Louis: CV Mosby, 1997.

20. Schreuders TAR, Roebroeck ME, Goumans J, et al. Measurement error in grip and pinch force measurements in patients with hand injuries. Phys Ther 2003;83:806–815.

21. O'Driscoll SW, Horii E, Ness R, et al. The relationship between wrist position, grasp size and grip strength. J Hand Surg Am 1992;17:169–177.

22. Kalichman L, Hernandez-Molina G. Hand osteoarthritis: an epidemiological perspective. Arthritis Rheum 2009.

23. Cavaliere CM. Chung KC. A systematic review of total wrist arthroplasty compared with total wrist arthrodesis for rheumatoid arthritis. Plast Reconstr Surg 2008;122:813–825.

24. Lawrence RC, Felson DT, Helmick CG, et al. Estimates of the prevalence of arthritis and other rheumatic conditions in the United States. Part II. Arthritis Rheum 2008;58:26–35.

25. Belt EA, Kaarela K, Lehto MUK. Destruction and reconstruction of hand joints in rheumatoid arthritis: a 20 year follow-up study. J Rheumatol 1998;25:459–461.

26. Caspi D, Flusser G, Farber I, et al. Clinical, radiologic, demographic, and occupational aspects of hand osteoarthritis in the elderly. Semin Arthritis Rheum 2001;30(5):321–331.

27. Kalichman L, Cohen Z, Kobliansky E, et al. Patterns of joint distribution in hand osteoarthrtitis: contribution of age, sex and handedness. Am J Hum Biol 2004;16(2):125–134.

28. Bagis S, Sahin G, Yapici Y, et al. The effect of hand osteoarthritis on grip and pinch strength and hand function in postmenopausal women. Clin Rheumatol 2003;22(6):420–424.

29. Marshall M, van der Windt D, Nicholls E, et al. Radiographic hand osteoarthritis: patterns and associations with hand pain and function in a community-dwelling sample. Osteoarthritis Cartilage 2009;17(11):1440–1447.

30. Chaisson CE, Zhang Y, Sharma L, et al. Higher grip strength increases the risk of incident radiographic osteoarthritis in proximal hand joints. Osteoarthritis Cartilage 2000;8(Suppl A):S29–S32.

31. Bodur H, Yilmaz O, Keskin D. Hand disability and related variables in patients with rheumatoid arthritis. Rheumatol Int 2006;26(6):541–544.

32. Hammond A, Freeman K. The long-term outcomes from a randomized controlled trial of an educational-behavioural joint protection programme for people with rheumatoid arthritis. Clin Rehabil 2004;18(5):520–528.

33. Silva AC, Jones A, Silva PG, et al. Effectiveness of a night-time hand positioning splint in rheumatoid arthritis: a randomized controlled trial. J Rehabil Med 2008;40(9):749–654.

34. Buljina AI, Taljanovic MS, Avdic DM, et al. Physical and exercise therapy for treatment of the rheumatoid hand. Arthritis Rheum 2001;45(4):392–397.

35. O'Brien AV, Jones P, Mullis R, et al. Conservative hand therapy treatments in rheumatoid arthritis – a randomized controlled trial. Rheumatology 2006;45(4):577–583.

36. Brorsson S, Hilliges M, Sollerman C, et al. A six-week exercise programme improves strength and hand function in patients with rheumatoid arthritis. J Rehabil Med 2009;41(5):338–342.

37. Ronningen A, Kjeken I. Effect of an intensive hand exercise programme in patients with rheumatoid arthritis. Scand J Occup Ther 2008;15(3):173–183.

38. Egan M, Brosseau L, Farmer M, et al. Splints/orthoses in the treatment of rheumatoid arthritis. Cochrane Database Syst Rev 2003;(1):CS004018.

39. National Institute for Occupational Safety and Health. Musculoskeletal Disorders and Workplace Factors: A Critical Review of Epidemiologic Evidence for Work-Related Musculoskeletal Disorders of the Neck, Upper Extremity, and Low Back. NIOSH Publication No. 97–141. Cincinnati, OH: NIOSH, 1997.

40. Van Rijn RM, Huisstede BM, Koes BW, et al. Associations between work-related factors and the carpal tunnel syndrome—a systematic review. Scand J Work Environ Health 2009;35(1):19–36.

41. Putz-Anderson V. Cumulative Trauma Disorders: A Manual for Musculoskeletal Diseases of the Upper Limbs. Bristol, PA: Taylor & Francis, 1992.

42. Roquelaure Y, Mechali S, Dano C, et al. Occupational and personal risk factors for carpal tunnel syndrome in industrial workers. Scand J Work Environ Health 1997;23(5):364–369.

43. Eastman Kodak Company. Ergonomic Design for People at Work, Vol 2. New York, NY: Van Nostrand Reinhold, 1986.

44. Kakosy T, Nemeth L. Musculoskeletal disorders caused by hand-arm vibration. Global Occupational Health Network 2003;4:3–6.

45. Heebner ML, Roddey TS. The effects of neural mobilization in addition to standard care in persons with carpal tunnel syndrome from a community hospital. J Hand Therapy 2008;21(3):229–241.

46. Goodyear-Smith F, Arroll B. What can family physicians offer patients with carpal tunnel syndrome other than surgery? A systematic review of nonsurgical management. Ann Fam Med 2004;2(3):267–273.

47. Papanicolaou GD, McCabe SK, Firrell J. The prevalence and characteristics of nerve compression symptoms in the general population. J Hand Surg (Am) 2001;26:460–466.

48. Rempel D. Musculoskeletal loading and carpal tunnel pressure. In: Gordon SL, Blair SJ, Fine LJ, eds. Repetitive Motion Disorders of the Upper Extremity. Rosemont, IL: American Academy of Orthopaedic Surgeons, 1995.

49. Ditmars DM, Hovin HP. Carpal tunnel syndrome. Hand Clin 1986;2525–2532.

50. Jerosch-Herold C, Leite JCC, Song F. A systematic review of outcomes assessed in randomized controlled trials of surgical interventions for carpal tunnel syndrome using the International Classification of Functioning, Disability and Health (ICF) as a reference tool. BMC Musculoskelet Disord 2006;7:96–106.

51. O'Connor D, Marshall S, Massy-Westropp N. Non-surgical treatment (other than steroid injection) for carpal tunnel syndrome. Cochrane Database Syst Rev 2003;(1):CD003219.

52. Piazzini DB, Aprile I, Ferrara PE, et al. A systematic review of conservative treatment of carpal tunnel syndrome. Clin Rehabil 2007;21(4):299–314.

53. Walker WC, Metzler M, Cifu DX, Swartz Z. Neutral wrist splinting in carpal tunnel syndrome: a comparison of night-only versus full-time wear instructions. Arch Phys Med Rehab 2001;56:1565–1567.

54. Burke DT, Durke MM, Stewart GW, et al. Splinting for carpal tunnel syndrome: in search of the optimal angle. Arch Phys Med Rehab 1994;75: 1241–1244.

55. Michlovitz SL. Conservative interventions for carpal tunnel syndrome. J Orthop Sports Phys Ther 2004;34(10):589–600.

56. Muller M, Tsui D, Schnurr R, Biddulph-Deisroth L, Hard J, MacDermid JC. Effectiveness of hand therapy interventions in primary management of carpal tunnel syndrome: a systematic review. J Hand Ther 2004;17(2):210–228.

57. Garfinkel MS, Singhal A, Katz WA, et al. Yoga-based intervention for carpal tunnel syndrome: a randomized trial. JAMA 1998;280:1601–1603.

58. Medina McKeon JM, Yancosek KE. Neural gliding techniques for the treatment of carpal tunnel syndrome: a systematic review. J Sport Rehabil 2008;17(3):324–341.

59. Simoneau GG, Marklin RW, Berman JE. Effect of computer keyboard slope on wrist position and forearm electromyography of typists without musculoskeletal disorders. Phys Ther 2003;83:816–830.

60. Idler RS. Anatomy and biomechanics of the digital flexor tendons. Hand Clin 1985;1:3–11.

61. Gerritsen AA, Uitdehaap BM, van Geldere D, et al. Systematic review of randomized clinical trials of surgical treatment for carpal tunnel syndrome. Br J Surg 2001;88(10):1285–1295.

62. Plancher KD, Peterson RK, Steichen JB. Compressive neuropathies and tendinopathies in the athletic elbow. Clin Sports Med 1996;15:331–372.

63. Nirschl RP. Soft tissue injuries about the elbow. Clin Sports Med 1986;5:637–652.

64. Shiri R, Viikari-Juntura E, Varonen H, et al. Prevalence and determinants of lateral and medial epicondylitis: a population study. Am J Epidemiol 2006;164(11):1065–1074.

65. Khan KM, Cook JL, Bonar F, et al. Histopathology of common tendinopathies. Sports Med 1999;6:393–408.

66. Van Rijn RM, Huisstede BM, Koes BW, Burdorf A. Associations between work-related factors and specific disorders at the elbow: a systematic literature review. Rheumatology 2009;48(5):528–536.

67. Kibler WB. Pathophysiology of overload injuries around the elbow. Clin Sports Med 1995;15:447–457.

68. Croisier J-L, Foidart-Dessalle M, Tinant F, et al. An isokinetic eccentric programme for the management of chronic lateral epicondylar tendinopathy. Br J Sports Med 2007;41:269–275.

69. Woodley BL, Newsham-West RJ, Baxter GD. Chronic tendinopathy: effectiveness of eccentric exercise. Br J Sports Med 2006;4:188–198.

70. Stasinopoulos D, Stasinopoulou K, Johnson M. An exercise programme for the management of lateral elbow tendinopathy. Br J Sports Med 2005;12:944–947.

71. Martinez-Silvestrini JA, Newcomer KL, Gay RE, et al. Chronic lateral epicondylitis: comparative effectiveness of a home exercise program including stretching alone versus stretching supplemented with eccentric or concentric strengthening. J Hand Ther 2005;4:411–419.

72. Knobloch K, Spies M, Busch KH, et al. Sclerosing therapy and eccentric training in flexor carpi radialis tendinopathy in a tennis player. Br J Sports Med 2007;12:920–921.

73. Kirkpatrick WH. De Quervain's disease. In: Hunter JM, Schneider LH, Mackin EF, Callahan AD, eds. Rehabilitation of the Hand. 3rd Ed. St. Louis: CV Mosby, 1990.

74. Cannon NM, ed. Diagnosis and Treatment Manual for Physicians and Therapists. 3rd Ed. Indianapolis, IN: Hand Rehabilitation Center of Indiana, 1991.

75. Osada D, Fujita S, Tamal K, et al. Flexor tendon repair in zone II with 6-strand techniques and early active mobilization. J Hand Surg Am 2006;31(6): 987–992.

76. Al-Qattan MM, Al-Turaiki TM. Flexor tendon repair in zone II using a six-strand 'figure of eight' suture. J Hand Surg Eur 2009;34(3):322–328.

77. Grewal R, Chan Saw SS, Varitimidus S, et al. Evaluation of passive and active rehabilitation and of tendon repair for partial tendon lacerations after three weeks of healing in canines. Clin Biomech 2006;21(8):804–809.

78. Groth GN. Current practice patterns of flexor tendon rehabilitation. J Hand Ther 2005;18(2):169–174.

79. McNemar TB, Howell JW, Chang E. Management of metacarpal fractures. J Hand Ther 2003;16(2):143–151.

80. Hardy MA. Principles of metacarpal and phalangeal fracture management: a review of rehabilitation concepts. J Orthop Sports Phys Ther 2004;34(12):781–799.

81. Werner SL, Fleisig GS, Dillman CH, et al. Biomechanics of the elbow during baseball pitching. J Orthop Sports Phys Ther 1993;17:274–278.

82. Sobel J, Nirschl RP. Elbow injuries. In: Zachazewski JE, Magee DJ, Quillen WS, eds. Athletic Injuries and Rehabilitation. Philadelphia, PA: WB Saunders. 1996.

83. Josefsson PO, Johnell O, Gentz CF. Long term sequelae of simple dislocation of the elbow. J Bone Joint Surg Am 1984;66:927–930.

84. Kuo CE, Wolfe SW. Scapholunte instability: current concepts in diagnosis and management. J Hand Surg Am 2008;33(6):998–1013.

85. Slade JF III, Milewski MD. Management of carpal instability in athletes. Hand Clin 2009;25(3):395–408.

86. Rowe C. The management of fractures in elderly patients is different. J Bone Joint Surg Am 1965;47:1043–1059.

87. Meyer FN, Wilson RL. Management of nonarticular fractures of the hand. In: Hunter JM, Schneider LH, Mackin EF, Callahan AD, eds. Rehabilitation of the Hand. 4th Ed. St. Louis: CV Mosby, 1995.

88. Stralka SW, Akin K. Reflex sympathetic dystrophy syndrome. In: Orthopaedic Section Home Study Course. LaCrosse, WI: Orthopaedic Section, APTA, December 1997.

89. Lankford LL. Reflex sympathetic dystrophy. In: Hunter JM, Schneider LH, Mackin EF, Callahan AD, eds. Rehabilitation of the Hand. 3rd Ed. St. Louis: CV Mosby, 1990.

90. Sudeck PMH. Ueber die acute entzundliche Knockenatrophie. Arch Klin Chir 1900;62:147–156.

91. Watson HK, Ryu J. Degenerative disorders of the carpus. Orthop Clin North Am 1984;15:337–354.

92. Lee VH, Reynolds CC. Clinical application of transcutaneous electrical nerve stimulator in patients with upper extremity pain. In: Hunter JM, Schneider LH, Mackin EF, Callahan AD, eds. Rehabilitation of the Hand. 3rd Ed. St. Louis: CV Mosby, 1990.

93. Cram JR, Kasmann GS, Holtz J. Introduction to Surface Electromyography. Rockville, MD: Aspen Publishers, 1998.

94. Kasman GS, Cram JR, Wolf SL. Clinical Applications in Surface Electromyography. Rockville, MD: Aspen Publishers, 1998.

Case Studies

DOROTHY BERG, CARRIE M. HALL, AND LORI THEIN BRODY

 CASE STUDY NO. 1

Lisa is a 17-year-old high school student who complains of right (R) ankle pain and swelling. She describes injuring herself yesterday during basketball practice. Coming down after a rebound attempt, she landed on the foot of another player, twisting her ankle and falling to the ground. Immediately after the injury, she was able to move her ankle and walk off the court. Now Lisa reports difficulty bearing full weight on her R foot and is unable to walk or run without a significant limp. Her team is contending for the state championship in 6 weeks, and Lisa hopes to play.

EXAMINATION

Pain: 4/10 at rest, constant in nature in non–weight-bearing: 6/10 with weight-bearing

Gait: R foot flat, "step to" pattern with use of axillary crutches.

Active Range of Motion: Plantar flexion/dorsiflexion 20 to 5 degrees; foot inversion/eversion 3 to 5 degrees with pain end range

Passive Range of Motion: Plantar flexion/dorsiflexion 40 to 15 degrees; foot inversion/eversion 3 to 8 degrees with muscle guarding

Accessory Motion: Subtalar and talocrural distraction hypomobile; subtalar medial/lateral glide hypomobile with muscle guarding; talonavicular, cuboid/navicular and cuneiform/navicular all hypomobile

Palpation: Moderate localized swelling in region distal to R lateral malleolus; marked tenderness and early signs of ecchymosis in same region

Strength Testing: Anterior tibialis 4/5 (pain elicited); posterior tibialis 5/5; gastrocnemius/soleus 5/5; peroneus longus 4–/5 (pain elicited)

Resisted Testing: Dorsiflexors and evertors weak and painful

Balance: Unable to assess because of patient discomfort in weight bearing

EVALUATION: Acute, traumatic ligamentous injury to the R ankle.

Impairment	*Functional Limitation*	*Disability*
• Localized pain, and swelling of lateral R ankle • Decreased active and passive range of motion for R ankle • Midfoot hypomobility • Faulty R foot alignment in stance into calcaneal eversion • Decreased static and dynamic standing balance	• Weakness in ankle evertors and dorsi-flexors • Limited weight bearing and movement tolerance in standing and walking, necessitating the use of crutches	• Unable to run or jump on R foot • Unable to play basketball

DIAGNOSIS: Second degree sprain of the R calcaneofibular ligament

PROGNOSIS

Short-Term Goals (7 to 10 days)
1. Ambulate without an assistive device, step-through pattern, 15 minutes, no ankle pain
2. Tolerate low-intensity running and jumping

Long-Term Goals (3 to 4 weeks)
1. Ambulate unlimited, no ankle pain
2. Return to full-intensity basketball practice

CASE STUDY NO. 2

Sarah is a 69-year-old, retired college professor with a medical diagnosis of osteoarthritis in both knees. She is widowed and living alone in a third-floor apartment with elevator access. Yesterday, Sarah underwent elective surgery for bilateral (B) total-knee arthroplasties. Her medical history includes emphysema, myocardial infarct 2 years ago, moderate obesity, and hypertension. She lives independently but has a maximum walking tolerance of one-half block when using a cane for support.

EXAMINATION

Arousal/Cognition: Alert and oriented; follows complex commands; motivated to get out of bed

Cardiovascular: Pale with complaints of nausea; short of breath with exertion; diaphoretic in sitting; vital signs: pulse 96 supine, 108 sitting; blood pressure 144/66 mm Hg supine, 126/64 mm Hg sitting

Wounds: Dressed with gauze and clear tape, moderately soaked with bloody drainage; periwound regions warm to touch, hypererythemic, and swollen

Pain: 3/10 at rest, 8/10 with movement

Active Range of Motion: R knee extension/flexion 20 to 47 degrees (pain elicited); L knee extension/flexion 15 to 52 degrees (pain elicited)

Endurance: Maximum sitting tolerance 15 minutes; maximum standing tolerance 20 seconds

Strength Testing: Iliopsoas (B) 2+/5; gluteus maximus (B) 4/5; gluteus medius (B) 2+/5; quadriceps (R) 2/5, (L) 3–/5; hamstrings (R) 2+/5, (L) 3–/5

Resisted Testing: Shoulder girdle extension and depression, elbow extension all strong and pain free

Posture: Semiflexed both knees, with L > R valgus knee deformity

Gait: Wide base of support, stiff knees, flexed trunk, maximum upper extremity support on walker

EVALUATION: Acute, postoperative pain, inflammation, muscle weakness, and decreased active motion of both knees

Impairment
- Bilateral decreased knee active range of motion
- Bilateral weak quadriceps and hamstrings
- Postoperative pain and inflammatory response
- Markedly limited activity tolerance

Functional Limitation
- Required moderate assist for bed mobility and basic sit to stand transfer
- Unable to sit >15 minutes
- Unable to stand >20 seconds
- Unable to walk

Disability
- Unable to resume independent basic and instrumental activities of daily living
- Unable to walk household distances
- Unable to resume teaching and writing interests
- Unable to access family, church, and clubs for social interaction

DIAGNOSIS: Postoperative day 1 after bilateral total knee arthroplasties

PROGNOSIS

Short-Term Goals (7 to 10 days)
1. Independent bed mobility and basic transfer with walker
2. Independent ambulation 30 m with walker
3. Active knee range of motion >10 to 70 degrees to enable up/down stairs
4. Out of bed and up in chair >5 hours per day

Long-Term Goals (12 weeks)
1. Ambulation >100 m, rest breaks as needed, allowing for baseline compromised cardiopulmonary status
2. Return to independent driving for community access
3. Return to preoperative vocational routine

CASE STUDY NO. 3

Cathy is a 61-year-old journalist with a number of complaints, including trunk weakness, leg weakness, and generalized fatigue. She has a history of osteoporosis, osteoarthritis, and a recent 2-week bout with diarrhea caused by her medication. Recently, Cathy has had difficulty managing a 40- to 50-hour work week. She has no history of regular exercise nor any home exercise equipment. Her maximum walking tolerance is reportedly one block, limited by shortness of breath, general fatigue, and hip discomfort.

EXAMINATION

Posture/Alignment: Long kyphosis with posterior displacement of the upper trunk and a forward head. Lumbar spine is flattened. Posterior pelvic tilt. B hips extended and internally rotated. B knees in recurvatum; tibial external rotation; scapulae abducted and elevated

Muscle Length: Hamstrings: passive straight-leg raise to 50 degrees (B)

Strength Testing: Trunk curl 3–/5; leg lowering 2–/5; iliopsoas (R) 3/5 degrees, (L) 3–/5; gluteus medius (R) 3/5, (L) 2+/5; gluteus maximus (B) 3+/5; quadriceps (R) 4/5, (L) 4–/5; hamstrings (R) 4–/5, (L) 3+/5

Active and Passive Range of Motion:

Thoracolumbar spine: forward bend thoracic > lumbar flexion with lumbar spine remaining in neutral; back bend with excessive extension at thoracolumbar junction;

Hip: internal rotation (R) 0 to 20 degrees, (L) 0 to 15 degrees, external rotation (R) 0 to 35 degrees, (L) 0 to 33 degrees, flexion (bent knee) 0 to 85 degrees, extension 0 to 25 degrees

Shoulder: flexion in scapular plane 0 to 140 degrees, with early upward rotation of scapulae and lacking thoracic extension component at end range

Endurance: Standardized 12-minute walk test completed with subjective complaints of shortness of breath and lower extremity muscle fatigue; distance, 900 m; standing rest required at 10 minutes, peak heart rate of 132, blood pressure of 153/88 mm Hg

EVALUATION: Generalized deconditioning with gradual onset of faulty alignment because of changes in joint mobility and muscle strength and length, compounded by recent illness

Impairment	Functional Limitation	Disability
• Muscle weakness pelvic girdle • Faulty spinal, pelvic and lower extremity alignment • Muscle shortening of hamstrings and rectus abdominis • Decreased cardiovascular endurance • Decreased lower extremity muscle endurance • Restrictions at thoracolumbar spine intervertebral and thoracic spine costovertebral joints • Faulty shoulder girdle movement patterns • Hip joint restrictions	• Unable to walk >10 minutes without shortness of breath and fatigue • Stairs require rail support • Difficulty getting up from low chairs • Rest breaks required during AM and PM self-care routine	• Unable to tolerate exertion of a full work week • Unable to complete basic and instrumental activities of daily living in a timely manner • Avoidance to social activities because of fatigue

DIAGNOSIS: Generalized deconditioning superimposed on baseline medical diagnoses of osteoporosis and osteoarthritis

PROGNOSIS

Short-Term Goals (2 weeks)

1. Demonstration of energy conservation and pacing techniques to maximize activity tolerance at work and home

Long-Term Goals (4 to 6 months)

1. Increase in musculoskeletal and cardiovascular endurance to allow resumption of full duties at work and home

CASE STUDY NO. 4

Jack is a 58-year-old retired banker who presented with complaints of right (R) shoulder pain that was most noticeable when reaching overhead or behind. His pain occasionally wakes him at night. Jack's medical history is significant for a nonspecific R shoulder injury sustained playing tennis 2 years ago. This went untreated, and the symptoms resolved. Jack has been refurbishing his 35-ft wooden sailboat and noticed the onset of shoulder pain after sanding the deck. He is R-hand dominant.

EXAMINATION

Posture/Alignment: Forward head with upper cervical extension, cervical-thoracic junction flexion, and flattened thoracolumbar spine; scapulae elevated, abducted, and downwardly rotated R > L; R humerus anteriorly displaced in the glenohumeral joint

Active Range of Motion: R shoulder flexion 0 to 90 degrees, extension 0 to 30 degrees, abduction 0 to 100 degrees, external rotation 0 to 25 degrees, internal rotation 0 to 50 degrees; pain elicited end range all directions

Passive Range of Motion: R shoulder flexion 0 to 110 degrees, extension 0 to 33 degrees, abduction 0 to 110 degrees, external rotation 0 to 25 degrees, internal rotation 0 to 55 degrees; end-range pain elicited in all directions

Accessory Motion Testing:

Glenohumeral: diffusely hypomobile, especially posterior and inferior glides

Scapulothoracic: hypomobile medial glide and upward rotation; hypermobile lateral/cephalic glides

Upper thoracic: hypomobile segmental anterior/posterior glides T2–8

Strength Testing: Upper trapezius/levator scapula (R) 5/5, (L) 5/5; middle trapezius (R) 2/5, (L) 3/5; lower trapezius (R) 1/5, (L) 3/5; rhomboids (R) 3/5, (L) 4/5; serratus anterior (R) 4/5, (L) 5/5

Resisted Testing (neutral position): Strong and painless R shoulder flexion, extension, internal rotation, abduction and adduction; weak and painless external rotation

Quality of Movement: Glenohumeral flexion/abduction achieved through 30 degrees of glenohumeral motion, followed by 1:1 scapulohumeral rhythm to roughly 90 degrees; remaining motion achieved through shoulder girdle elevation

EVALUATION: Decreased osteokinematic and arthrokinematic motion of R shoulder girdle and cervical-thoracic spine, resulting in faulty movement patterns and pain with end-range shoulder function

Impairment	Functional Limitation	Disability
• Decreased physiologic and accessory motion	• Unable to reach, lift, or pull overhead	• Difficulty retrieving wallet from back pocket
• Faulty scapulothoracic, glenohumeral, and cervical-thoracic spine alignment	• Disturbed sleep	• Difficulty unlocking car passenger door from driver's seat
• Faulty shoulder girdle movement patterns		• Unable to complete moderate- or heavy-duty boat refurbishing tasks
• Pain with end-range shoulder girdle motion, especially forward flexion		

DIAGNOSIS: Subacute R shoulder adhesive capsulitis

PROGNOSIS

Short-Term Goals (3 weeks)

1. Decrease night pain by 50%
2. Light weight lifting and reaching activities up to shoulder height without pain

Long-Term Goals (3 to 4 months)

1. No night pain
2. Ability to tolerate resisted motion at end range of shoulder motion; thus able to complete heavy-duty jobs on boat

CASE STUDY NO. 5

Irene is an 85-year-old woman who fell at home, resulting in acute low back pain and right more than left (R > L) lower extremity radiculopathy and necessitating bed rest for more than 2 weeks. She is weak, deconditioned, unsteady on her feet, and fearful of falling. She now uses a walker for ambulation. Her back still gives her pain, although she no longer suffers lower extremity symptoms. Irene lives in her own apartment in an assisted-living environment. Before the fall, she independently handled her basic activities of daily living and was socially active with fellow residents.

EXAMINATION

Posture: Kyphotic/lordotic thoracolumbar alignment; anterior pelvic tilt; hips slightly flexed

Strength Testing: Leg lowering 2/5; gluteus maximus (R) 2+/5, (L) 3+/5; gluteus medius (R) 2/5, (L) 3/5; iliopsoas (R) 3/5, (L) 4–/5; quadriceps (R) 4/5, (L) 4+/5; hamstrings (R) 3–/5, (L) 3+/5

Muscle Length: Moderate shortening of quads > iliopsoas, R > L; (B) hamstrings unremarkable

Functional Movement Testing: Pain with standing or walking (4/10). Pain relief with sitting or sidelying. Standing forward bend at 20 degrees; standing backward bend trace with reproduction of symptoms

Gait: Positive Trendelenburg with stance R > L; wide base of support; flexed at hips with forward displaced trunk over pelvis; markedly diminished lumbopelvic rhythm

Balance: Standardized stand reach test of 6 inches; provoked balance response demonstrates delayed step response with hip > ankle strategies

Reflexes: Knee jerk (B) 2+; ankle jerk (R) 1+, (L) 2+

Sensory: Light touch intact, mildly decreased proprioception R > L

EVALUATION: Fixed kyphosis and lordosis malalignment, with corresponding muscle length and tension changes; painful with active or passive extension, affecting static and dynamic standing balance, and standing tolerance

Impairment	Functional Limitation	Disability
• Fixed kyphotic-lordotic alignment of thoracolumbar spine • Muscle weakness, especially trunk and proximal lower extremity • Shortened iliopsoas and quadriceps, R > L • Decreased static and dynamic standing balance • Fear of falling • Pain with lumbar extension	• Assistance required to get out of bed or up from a chair • Inability to stand >2 minutes • Inability to walk >10 m • Mobility avoidance	• Loss of independence performing basic activities of daily living • Loss of independence with ambulation • Unable to walk to dining room • Reluctant to participate in usual social activities (bridge, films, out for dinner with family)

DIAGNOSIS: Lumbar spinal stenosis exacerbated by fall. Now with subacute pain, deconditioning, balance deficits, and increased fear of falling.

PROGNOSIS

Short-Term Goals (2 weeks)
1. Independent ambulation with walker, 25 m
2. Independent transfer out of bed
3. Independent stand for 10 minutes for morning self-care routine

Long-Term Goals (8 weeks)
1. Independent ambulation within building complex; no assistive device
2. Resume all previous social activities with friends and family

CASE STUDY NO. 6

Scott, a 32-year-old man, presented 1 week after right (R) anterior cruciate ligament autograft reconstruction. He is on medical leave of absence from his position as a full-time driver and delivery man for a shipping company. Scott is an outdoor enthusiast and has hopes of returning to rock climbing, kayaking, and skiing after his rehabilitation.

EXAMINATION

Gait: Toe-touch pattern with use of axillary crutches; knee held semiflexed

Active Range of Motion: Knee extension/flexion 15 to 60 degrees with subjective sensation of "tightness" at both extremes

Passive Range of Motion: Knee extension/flexion 12 to 70 degrees with spasm end feel

Palpation: Moderate suprapatellar swelling; posterior capsule distention; girth (3 cm proximal to superior patellar pole) R = 44 cm, L = 38 cm; moderate joint line tenderness

Strength Testing: Resisted testing contraindicated; surface electromyographic testing confirms 35% decreased vastus medialis oblique recruitment relative to nonsurgical leg

Accessory Motion: Hypomobile patellar glides, all directions

EVALUATION: Postoperative R knee joint effusion, pain, decreased range of motion, and altered muscle recruitment patterns

Impairment	Functional Limitation	Disability
• Localized swelling in suprapatellar and posterior capsule regions	• Unable to tolerate foot flat stance on R with a step through pattern	• Unable to lift from floor height or drive; therefore, unable to work
• Acute surgical pain with end-range knee motion	• Crutches required secondary to above gait problems	• Unable to participate in usual outdoor sports
• Impaired vastus medialis recruitment	• Unable to tolerate prolonged static extension	
• Decreased patellofemoral accessory joint mobility		
• Loss of R lower extremity coordination		

DIAGNOSIS: R knee dysfunction from primary structural injury and corrective surgery

PROGNOSIS

Short-Term Goals (2 to 4 weeks)
1. Ambulate without assistive device
2. Return to modified work routine

Long-Term Goals (6 to 12 months)
1. Return to preoperative work routine
2. Resume low-to-moderate intensity sports

CASE STUDY NO. 7

Mary is a 36-year-old wife and mother of two young children. She has a 6-month history of chronic back, hip, neck, and shoulder pain, recently diagnosed as fibromyalgia. She is not working, although she is trained as a research laboratory technician. Mary reports she's having a hard time keeping up with her husband and children and increasing difficulty managing her home. Even minor activities such as lifting or carrying her children can result in profound pain, fatigue, or weakness just a few hours later. She once was very active and now is skeptical but hopeful that she can return to a regular exercise program. Ultimately, she would like to return to part-time work.

EXAMINATION

Posture and Observation: Tall, slim build; stands in ankle plantar flexion, knee recurvatum, anterior pelvic sway relative to thorax, posterior pelvic tilt with lumbar flexion and thoracic kyphosis. Cervical spine in R sidebend. Resting muscle tension apparent in facial, neck, and shoulder muscles. Upper chest breathing pattern; respiratory rate 24 at rest

Active Range of Motion:

Cervical: flexion 0 to 30 degrees; extension 0 to 25 degrees; rotation (R) 0 to 40 degrees, (L) 0 to 28 degrees; sidebending (R) 0 to 30 degrees, (L) 0 to 22 degrees

Thoracolumbar: flexion to floor with lumbar > hip motion, pain elicited at initial and end range; extension, rotation, and sidebending all mildly decreased with guarding

Muscle Length: Shortened hamstrings; shortened gastroc/soleus; shortened two joint hip flexors; shortened pectoralis major and minor; lengthened middle and lower trapezius; shortened latissimus dorsi

Strength Testing: Upper trapezius (B) 5/5; middle trapezius (R) 3–/5, (L) 2/5; lower trapezius (B) 2/5; sternocleidomastoid (R) 2–/5, (L) 2+/5; trunk curl 3–/5; leg lowering 2/5; gluteus maximus (B) 3+/5; gluteus medius (R) 3–/5, (L) 3/5; iliopsoas (B) 3+/5; quads (R) 4/5, (L) 4–/5; hamstrings (R) 4+/5, (L) 4–/5

Surface Electromyography: Elevated resting muscle tension prevalent (temporalis, upper trapezius, sternocleidomastoid, lumbar paraspinals); same groups demonstrate erratic and asymmetric recruitment with static and active range of motion testing

Palpation: Tender to light pressure in suboccipital region, medial upper trapezius, sternocleidomastoid origin and insertion R > L, interscapular region, anterior thigh and posterior iliac crest

EVALUATION: Diffuse soft tissue and muscle pain, weakness, and fatigue

Impairment
- Multifocal soft-tissue pain, aggravated with activity
- Profound muscle fatigue
- Abnormal static and dynamic muscle tension and recruitment patterns, generally elevated
- Mild diffuse loss of active physiologic range of motion, especially spine and hips

Functional Limitation
- Unable to sit >10 minutes
- Unable to stand >15 minutes
- Unable to walk >1/2 mile
- Unable to lift >10 lb from floor height

Disability
- Unable to play on the floor with children
- Unable to tolerate sexual intercourse
- Unable to return to work as laboratory technician

DIAGNOSIS: Chronic pain of fibromyalgia with secondary weakness, fatigue, loss of motion, and abnormal motor recruitment

PROGNOSIS

Short-Term Goals (6 to 8 weeks)
1. Ambulate 15 minutes twice per day without residual symptoms
2. Lift 20 lb from floor height
3. Static lift 20 lb for 3 minutes

Long-Term Goals (1 year)
1. Return to work part time
2. Continuous ambulation for 30 to 40 minutes without residual pain or fatigue

CASE STUDY NO. 8

George is a 35-year-old computer data entry specialist with a 9-month history of multiple complaints, including interscapular pain, head and neck pain with associated headaches, and right (R) lateral forearm pain. No specific traumatic event preceded these symptoms, although they have progressively worsened over the last couple of months such that they now interfere with his ability to work. His employer completed a workstation assessment several months ago and provided state-of-the-art office equipment, but this has provided no significant relief of George's symptoms. Typically, he can spend several uninterrupted hours on the computer without awareness of time passed. A typical work week is 60 hours. George is moderately obese and admits to a sedentary lifestyle.

EXAMINATION

Posture/Alignment: Forward head, elevated shoulders L > R, excessive lumbar lordosis with anterior pelvic tilt. Scapulae excessively abducted and downwardly rotated L > R. Cubital fossa oriented medially bilaterally. Laterally rotated femurs with hyperextended knees in postural knock-knees

Active Range of Motion:

Cervical: flexion 0 to 25 degrees; extension 0 to 60 degrees, pain elicited; rotation (R) 0 to 55 degrees, (L) 0 to 60 degrees; sidebend (R) 0 to 35 degrees, (L) 0 to 45 degrees

Shoulder: forward flexion (R) 0 to 120 degrees, (L) 0 to 140 degrees; extension (R) 0 to 30 degrees, (L) 0 to 45 degrees; external rotation (R) 0 to 35 degrees, (L) 0 to 50 degrees

Hip: hip external rotation (B) 0 to 45 degrees, internal rotation (B) 0 to 10 degrees

Muscle Length: Shortened latissimus dorsi; lengthened rhomboids and mid-lower trapezius; shortened pectoralis major

Strength Testing: Serratus anterior 3/5; rhomboid major 4/5; upper trapezius 5/5; middle and lower trapezius 1 to 2/5; infraspinatus/teres minor 4/5; anterior/middle deltoid 5/5; biceps (R) 4–/5, (L) 5/5; triceps (B) 5/5; flexor carpi radialis/ulnaris (R) 4/5, (L) 5/5; extensor carpi radialis longus brevis (R) 3+/5, pain elicited, (L) 5/5; pronator teres/supinator (R) 4–/5, (L) 5/5; trunk curl 3/5; leg lowering 2/5; iliopsoas (R) 3+/5, (L) 4/5

Accessory Motion Testing: Cervical: L > R hypomobile posterior/anterior and rotation segmental testing at C1/2 and C2/3; shoulder girdle: decreased anterior/inferior glenohumeral glides; decreased scapulothoracic inferior glide and downward rotation; excessive scapulothoracic lateral glide and upward rotation

Palpation: Suboccipital region moderately tender; diffusely tender interscapular L > R; tender R lateral epicondyle

Deep Tendon Reflexes: Biceps (R) 1+, (L) 2+; triceps 2+ and symmetric

Sensation: Diminished light touch R lateral forearm and thumb

EVALUATION: Chronic postural malalignment resulting in multifocal postural and movement dysfunction most evident in overstretched and weakened scapular stabilizers and upper cervical segmental hypomobility; subsequent musculoskeletal pain and headaches; subacute overuse injury to R wrist extensor group

Impairment	*Functional Limitation*	*Disability*
• Upper cervical, asymmetric facet joint motion dysfunction	• Unable to sit >30 minutes	• Unable to complete job requirements
• Painful and shortened deep suboccipital extensors	• Daily headaches, limiting concentration	• Loss of job satisfaction
• Faulty shoulder girdle alignment	• Difficulty keying with right hand because of forearm pain	
• Overstretched and weakened shoulder girdle adductors, upward rotators, and depressors		
• Postural muscle weakness and fatigue		
• Pain and inflammation R extensor carpi radialis longus		

DIAGNOSIS: Chronic grade 1 muscle strain of middle and lower trapezius; upper cervical facet joint movement dysfunction and possible fixed deformity; R extensor carpi radialis longus tendinitis

PROGNOSIS

Short-Term Goals (2 to 4 weeks)
1. Reduce headache frequency and intensity by 50%
2. Increase sitting tolerance to 60 minutes, incorporating postural adjustments and short breaks

Long-Term Goals (6 months)
1. Reduce headache frequency and intensity by 75% to 100%
2. Return to baseline work level

CASE STUDY NO. 9

Janet is a 47-year-old nurse with primary complaints of posterolateral right (R) thigh pain. The pain is worse with weight bearing first thing in the morning, gets better with limited activity, but worsens by the end of the day—especially if she has been on her feet quite a bit during the day. Secondary complaints include intermittent, dull low back pain and occasional bouts of sharp pain in the arch of her R foot.

EXAMINATION

Posture and Alignment: Thoracic kyphosis, lumbar lordosis, posterior pelvic tilt with anterior displacement of pelvis over base of support; elevated iliac crest R > L; medially rotated femurs R > L; laterally rotated tibias R > L; foot pronation R > L

Active Range of Motion: Hip internal rotation 0 to 55 degrees, external rotation 0 to 30 degrees; thoracolumbar flexion full and pain free with reversal of lumbar lordosis

Muscle Length: Shortened tensor fascia lata/iliotibial band (TFL/ITB) with end-range stretch pain; shortened hamstrings (medial > lateral); shortened gastroc/soleus

Strength Testing: Leg lowering 2/5; trunk curl 4/5; gluteus medius (R) 2+/5, (L) 3/5; gluteus maximus (R) 3/5, (L) 3+/5; TFL (R) 3+/5 (pain elicited), (L) 4/5; iliopsoas (R) 2+/5, (L) 3/5; quadriceps (R) 4–/5, (L) 4+/5; hamstrings (R) 4+/5, (L) 4+/5; posterior tibialis (B) 5/5 (R > L muscle fatigue)

Accessory Motion Testing: Hypermobile posterior/anterior glides T10–L2 with relative hypomobility of lower lumbar segments; hypomobile dorsal glide great toe R > L

Movement Testing: Single-leg stance (R) with pain and excessive medial rotation of femur; decreased pain when femur held in lateral rotation

Gait: Positive Trendelenburg (R), medial rotation of femur midstance (R), excessive foot pronation early and late stance R > L

Palpation: Tender along R ITB; slight tenderness to deep palpation of plantar fascia at calcaneus origin

EVALUATION: Acute, easily irritable pain arising from R ITB resulting from compensatory TFL patterns associated with weakness and length-tension imbalance of TFL synergists; intermittent bouts of foot pain arising from plantar fascia, excessive pronation, and great toe hypomobility, currently nonsymptomatic

Impairment	*Functional Limitation*	*Disability*
• Postural alignment fault of posterior pelvic tilt, medially rotated femur, and foot pronation • Muscle weakness of TFL synergists, including gluteus medius, iliopsoas, and quadriceps • Shortened iliotibial band • Lengthened gluteus medius • Faulty movement patterns during gait	• Unable to walk 20 minutes without onset of R leg pain	• Unable to perform all job requirements for full 8-hour shift • Unable to walk for fitness • Difficulty performing household tasks because of leg pain

DIAGNOSIS: ITB fascitis and intermittent plantar fascitis

PROGNOSIS

Short-Term Goals (4 to 6 weeks)
1. Perform light duty work 40 hours per week
2. Walk 1.5 miles per day, paced at 20 minutes per mile, without leg or foot pain
3. Perform housework without leg pain if paced at 30- to 40-minute work intervals

Long-Term Goals (12 to 16 weeks)
1. Resume full duty work at 40 hours per week
2. Walk 3 miles per day, paced at 20 minutes per mile, without leg or foot pain
3. Perform all housework without limitations

CASE STUDY NO. 10

Pete is a 38-year-old man with complaints of right (R) shoulder and hip pain. He fell onto his R shoulder 6 months ago. He complains of clicking and instability, particularly during movements of hand behind back. He also has impingement pain at the middle to end range of arm elevation. He is an avid runner (30 to 40 miles per week) and has posterior, superior, and medial hip pain after about 2 miles of running. The hip pain resolves about 45 to 60 minutes after the run. His occupation requires prolonged sitting at a computer, and he has increased hip pain after 45 to 60 minutes of sitting. His shoulder also begins to ache after approximately the same time period.

EXAMINATION

Alignment: Slight forward head and head tilt to left (L); R head of humerus slightly anterior displaced; R scapula in moderate depression, tilt, downward rotation, adduction; R iliac crest elevated relative to left; R femur adducted and in slight medial rotation relative to L; R tibia slightly laterally rotated; R foot in slight abduction and pronation. Total body posture is a classic swayback. Sitting alignment is with pelvis in posterior tilt and R trunk sidebending with R scapula depressed, downwardly rotated, and tilted

Gait: At loading response, R trunk is in R sidebending with R scapula depressed, downwardly rotated, and adducted; throughout R stance phase, the pelvis demonstrates a compensated Trendelenburg on the right; throughout swing phase on the L, the pelvis moves in excessive R forward rotation (clockwise approximately 12 degrees); foot mechanics appear unremarkable with exception of slight excessive supination at terminal stance

Lumbar and Cervical Scan Examinations: Negative for reproduction of symptoms or neurologic signs

Range of Motion:
Right shoulder: flexion 0 to 150 degrees, scaption 0 to 150 degrees, lateral rotation/medial rotation (with arm abducted 90 degrees) 90 to 40 degrees
Right hip: flexion/extension 95 to 10 degrees, abduction/adduction 30 to 5 degrees, lateral/medial rotation (prone) 50 to 20 degrees
Thoracic rotation: 25% limitation right rotation

Scapulohumeral Rhythm: During arm elevation, scapula is slow to upwardly rotate; most of rotation occurs in last phase of arm elevation; reduced overall scapulothoracic (ST) upward rotation on R relative to L; scapular winging on return from elevation

Muscle Length: Moderate shortness in right medial hamstrings, R tensor fascia lata/iliotibial band (TFL/ITB), excessive length of R iliopsoas, moderate shortness in R rhomboid, significant shortness in (R) infraspinatus/teres minor, excessive length in R trapezius and serratus anterior

Strength Testing (short-range positional strength): Gluteus medius (R) 3+/5, (L) 4+/5; gluteus maximus (R) 4−/5, (L) 4+5; iliopsoas (R) 3/5, (L) 4/5; medial hamstrings (R) 4−/5 (pain elicited), (L) 5/5; adductors (R) 4−/5 (pain elicited), (L) 5/5; hip lateral rotators (R) 3+/5, (L) 4+/5; subscapularis (R) 3+/5, (L) 4+/5; infraspinatus/teres minor (R)/(L) 5/5; upper trapezius (R) 4−/5, (L) 5/5; middle trapezius (R) 3+/5, (L) 4/5; lower trapezius (R) 3+/5, (L) 4/5; serratus anterior (R) 3−/5, (L) 4/5; trunk curl 5/5; leg lowering 3/5

Joint Mobility: Moderate restriction in glenohumeral (GH) posterior and inferior glide (capsular end feel, pain after resistance), moderate excessive mobility in GH anterior glide (capsular end feel); moderate restriction in ST upward rotation (muscular end feel), and acromioclavicular joint anterior glide (capsular end feel); moderate restriction in hip posterior and inferior glide (capsular end feel, pain after resistance)

Resisted Tests: Weak and painful R medial hamstrings, adductors, and subscapularis

Special Tests: Positive apprehension and relocation signs R shoulder, positive impingement sign for R shoulder, positive slump test R lower extremity (pain reproduced in posterior, superior, and medial hip)

Palpation: Tenderness over subscapularis and supraspinatus insertions; tenderness in region of medial ischial tuberosity and inferior pubic ramus

Functional Tests: Pain and apprehension with reaching R hand behind back; painful arc with touching R hand to head; during hand behind back maneuver, R scapula fails to adduct, and humeral head translates excessively anteriorly when compared with L. Step-ups illustrate hip hike with hip flexion phase on R and compensated R Trendelenburg with R stance limb; squats reveal asymmetrical hip flexion with R hip hike at end range

(continued)

CASE STUDY NO. 10 *(Continued)*

EVALUATION: Chronic strain to R hamstring and adductor muscles; chronic strain to R subscapularis; impingement R shoulder; questionable R shoulder instability

Impairment

- Localized pain R anterior and superior shoulder and right hip
- Hypermobility/instability(?) of R shoulder
- Capsular restriction R hip
- Short ST downward rotators, GH lateral rotators, medial hamstrings, TFL/ITB, R adductors
- Long ST upward rotators, subscapularis, iliopsoas
- Thoracic spine, GH, ST, hip joint restrictions
- Weakness in R shoulder upward rotators, subscapularis, gluteus medius, gluteus maximus, iliopsoas, hip lateral rotators

Functional Limitation

- Unable to reach R hand behind back or overhead without discomfort or unstable feeling
- Unable to sit, climb more than five flights of stairs, or run 2 miles without right hip discomfort

Disability

- Unable to sit at computer for more than 45 to 60 minutes at a time at work
- Unable to participate in recreational activity of running at desired level

DIAGNOSIS: R shoulder impingement and hypermobility and instability; R subscapularis strain; R medial hamstrings and adductor magnus strain with secondary sciatic nerve injury or entrapment. Need to rule out R glenoid labrum tear and long thoracic nerve injury, which may have occurred during the fall.

PROGNOSIS

Short-Term Goals (2 to 3 months)

1. Elevate R arm through full range of motion and reach behind back without pain or instability
2. Sit 45 minutes without R hip pain
3. Climb 5 flights of stairs without R hip pain
4. Run 15 miles per week without increased R hip pain

Long-Term Goals (6 to 8 months)

1. Unlimited use of right arm without pain or instability
2. Sit unlimited periods (in good alignment) without R hip pain
3. Climb up to 10 flights of stairs without R hip pain
4. Run 30 miles per week without R hip pain

COMPLETE INTERVENTION

A complete intervention for this case study follows on the next few pages: Complete Intervention: Lower Quadrant and Complete Intervention: Upper Quadrant.

COMPLETE INTERVENTION—LOWER QUADRANT
For Case Study No. 10

Following is a comprehensive exercise program for lower quadrant intervention for Pete. It is prescribed in the first week.

AT WEEK 1

ACTIVITY: Hand-knee rocking (see Self-Management 20-6 in Chapter 20).

PURPOSE: To improve the flexibility of the hips, stretch the posterior hip muscles, and train independent movement between the hips, pelvis, and spine.

RISK FACTORS: Watch for symmetry when rocking backward.

ELEMENT OF MOVEMENT SYSTEM EMPHASIZED: Base.

STAGE OF MOTOR CONTROL: Mobility.

MODE: Passive movement exclusively of the hips.

POSTURE: Hands and knees with hips directly over the knees and shoulders directly over the hands. Hip joints should be at a 90-degree angle. Knees and ankles are hip-width apart with feet pointing straight back. Hands shoulder-width apart with hands pointing straight forward. Keep a slight extension curve in the low back.

MOVEMENT: First set inner core (see Patient-Related Instruction 18-1 in Chapter 18). The patient is instructed to rock backward at the hip joint only, stopping before onset of back movement.

SPECIAL CONSIDERATIONS: Motion at the hips should be independent from the lumbopelvic region.

DOSAGE

> *Special Considerations*
>
> > *Anatomic:* Hip joints, not the lumbopelvic region
> >
> > *Physiologic:* Asymmetric hip stiffness at end range hip flexion
> >
> > *Learning Capability:* Ingrained movement pattern of hip hiking with functional activities; may require high repetitions and significant feedback in early stages of learning
>
> *Repetitions/Sets:* 30 repetitions, 1 set
>
> *Frequency:* 7 days per week
>
> *Sequence:* Begin with this exercise, followed by the open kinetic chain strengthening exercises.
>
> *Speed:* Slowly to monitor accessory lumbopelvic movements
>
> *Environment:* At home on a flat, firm surface, initially, in front of a mirror
>
> *Feedback:* Initially in the clinic with clinician providing tactile and verbal feedback and a mirror providing visual feedback. Begin with knowledge of performance for every repetition then taper every three to four repetitions with knowledge of results.

FUNCTIONAL MOVEMENT PATTERN TO REINFORCE GOAL OF EXERCISE: Ascending stairs, gait, and running without asymmetric pattern.

RATIONALE FOR EXERCISE CHOICE: This exercise was chosen to improve hip flexion mobility resulting from reduced extensibility in the capsule, ligament, muscle, or myofascial stiffness. For Pete to have a symmetric walking, stair-climbing, and running pattern, hip mobility needs to be WNL bilaterally. It is assumed that the stiffness in his right hip contributes to the hip hiking pattern and that this pattern contributes to the upper quarter asymmetry as well. To recover from both lower and upper quarter conditions, hip mobility impairment should be resolved.

ACTIVITY: Iliopsoas strengthening (see Self-Management 20-5, Level I, in Chapter 20).

PURPOSE: Iliopsoas neuromuscular education to promote recruitment in the shortened range with hip flexion.

RISK FACTORS: Ensure use of iliopsoas and not TFL or RF recruitment. Watch for hip hiking on the right.

ELEMENT OF MOVEMENT SYSTEM EMPHASIZED: Base and modulator.

STAGE OF MOTOR CONTROL: Mobility.

MODE: Isometric iliopsoas contraction.

POSTURE: Seated with unilateral hip flexion and slight hip lateral rotation.

MOVEMENT: First set inner core. The patient passively flexes the hip into end range flexion with slight lateral rotation. Avoidance of hip hike or lumbar flexion is critical. The patient simply holds the limb without any resistance provided.

SPECIAL CONSIDERATIONS: Hip medial rotation will recruit the dominant hip flexor muscle, TFL, over the iliopsoas contributing to further shortening of the IT band. Hip hiking will contribute to lateral pelvic tilt versus hip flexion and should be avoided.

DOSAGE

> *Special Considerations*
>
> > *Anatomic:* Right iliopsoas, right hip joint
> >
> > *Physiologic:* Length associated changes in strength; stronger in the lengthened range than the shortened range
> >
> > *Learning Capability:* Very ingrained movement pattern from a long history of high-mileage running; may require high repetitions and significant feedback in early stages of learning
>
> *Repetitions/Sets:* To form fatigue, pain, or 20 to 30 repetitions, up to 3 sets
>
> *Frequency:* 6 to 7 days per week
>
> *Sequence:* After quadruped rocking

Speed: Hold for 10 seconds

Environment: At home on a firm surface

Feedback: Initially in clinic with clinician providing tactile and verbal feedback. Begin with knowledge of performance for every repetition then taper every three to four repetitions with knowledge of results.

FUNCTIONAL MOVEMENT PATTERN TO REINFORCE GOAL OF EXERCISE: Ascending stairs, gait, and running.

RATIONALE FOR EXERCISE CHOICE: This exercise was chosen to improve muscle performance and motor control strategies of hip flexor muscles. Hip flexion without contributing to IT band shortening or hip hiking patterns depends on proper recruitment of the iliopsoas muscle in the shortened range. This method of neuromuscular re-education is necessary before translating to dynamic activity and function.

ACTIVITY: Stomach lying gluteus medius strengthening (see Self-Management 20-4, Level I, in Chapter 20).

PURPOSE: Gluteus medius muscle strengthening in the shortened range.

RISK FACTORS: Medial hamstring and adductor magnus strain.

ELEMENT OF MOVEMENT SYSTEM EMPHASIZED: Base.

STAGE OF MOTOR CONTROL: Mobility.

MODE: Concentric and eccentric gluteus medius contractions.

POSTURE: Stomach lying with a pillow under the pelvis if indicated by the physical therapist. Legs should be in line with hips and slightly rotated outward.

MOVEMENT: First set inner core. Next perform an isometric contraction of the gluteus maximus. Slightly lift the leg into extension and abduction until lateral tilt is seen. Stop just short of lateral tilt of the pelvis. Hold at end range. Ensure the knee remains slightly rotated laterally.

SPECIAL CONSIDERATIONS: Keep the lumbopelvic region stable using the inner core. Hold slight hip lateral rotation throughout the range to avoid TFL muscle recruitment. Recruit the gluteus maximus and relax the hamstring muscles.

DOSAGE

Special Considerations

Anatomic: Right gluteus medius, right hip joint

Physiologic: Length associated changes in strength; stronger in the lengthened range than the shortened range

Learning Capability: May be difficult secondary to capsular restrictions. Ingrained muscle recruitment pattern of the TFL muscle and lateral trunk muscles from a long history of high-mileage running; may require high repetitions and significant feedback in early stages of learning

Repetitions/Sets: To form fatigue, pain, or 20 to 30 repetitions

Frequency: 6 to 7 days per week

Sequence: After quadruped rocking

Speed: Slowly

Environment: At home on a firm surface

Feedback: Initially in clinic with clinician providing tactile and verbal feedback. Begin with knowledge of performance for every repetition then taper every couple repetitions with knowledge of results.

FUNCTIONAL MOVEMENT PATTERN TO REINFORCE GOAL OF EXERCISE: Ascending stairs, gait, and running.

RATIONALE FOR EXERCISE CHOICE: This exercise was chosen to improve motor control strategies and strength of gluteus medius, and gluteus maximus muscles. Lumbopelvic stability and IT band extensibility depends on proper recruitment of the gluteus medius muscle throughout the range. This method of neuromuscular re-education and strengthening is necessary before returning to functional activities.

AT 3 WEEKS

ACTIVITY: Iliopsoas strengthening (see Self-Management 20-5, Level 2, in Chapter 20).

PURPOSE: Iliopsoas strengthening to improve muscle balance of hip flexor muscles.

RISK FACTORS: Watch for TFL substitution or lateral pelvic tilt.

ELEMENT OF MOVEMENT SYSTEM EMPHASIZED: Base.

STAGE OF MOTOR CONTROL: Mobility.

MODE: Resistive isometric iliopsoas contraction.

POSTURE: Sitting with unilateral hip flexion and slight hip lateral rotation.

MOVEMENT: First set inner core. The patient passively flexes the hip as far as possible while maintaining neutral lumbopelvic position. Next, the patient holds the position and provides gentle resistance to the hip in the direction of extension and slight lateral rotation. The contraction should be isometric.

SPECIAL CONSIDERATIONS: Hip medial rotation will recruit the dominant hip flexor muscle, TFL, over the iliopsoas contributing to further shortening of the IT band.

DOSAGE

Special Considerations

Anatomic: Right iliopsoas, right hip joint

Physiologic: Length associated changes in strength; stronger in the lengthened range than the shortened range

Learning Capability: Very ingrained recruitment pattern from a long history of high-mileage running; may require high repetitions and significant feedback in early stages of learning

Repetitions/Sets: To form fatigue, pain, or 15 repetitions, up to 3 sets

Frequency: 3 to 4 days per week

Sequence: After quadruped rocking

Speed: Hold for 10 seconds

Environment: At home on a firm surface

Feedback: Initially in clinic with clinician providing tactile and verbal feedback. Begin with knowledge of performance for every repetition then taper every three to four repetitions with knowledge of results.

FUNCTIONAL MOVEMENT PATTERN TO REINFORCE GOAL OF EXERCISE: Ascending stairs, gait, and running.

RATIONALE FOR EXERCISE CHOICE: This exercise was chosen to improve strength of iliopsoas muscle. This is the progression from isometric hold without resistance. Hip flexion without contributing to IT band shortening depends on proper recruitment of the iliopsoas muscle in the shortened range. Iliopsoas strengthening decreases TFL muscle dominance during dynamic activity and function.

ACTIVITY: Sidelying gluteus medius strengthening (see Self-Management 20-4, Level 4, in Chapter 20).

PURPOSE: Gluteus medius muscle strengthening in the shortened range.

RISK FACTORS: Medial hamstring and adductor magnus strain.

ELEMENT OF MOVEMENT SYSTEM EMPHASIZED: Base.

STAGE OF MOTOR CONTROL: Mobility/stability.

MODE: Concentric and eccentric gluteus medius contractions.

POSTURE: Sidelying against a wall with a small towel roll behind the superior gluteal. The towel roll ensures the hip slides up the wall in slight extension. Superior hip should be slightly laterally rotated.

MOVEMENT: First set inner core. Slide the leg up the wall, keeping the heel in contact with the wall to ensure hip extension, to end range. Stop before lateral pelvic tilt. Hold at end range. Be sure the hip stays laterally rotated.

SPECIAL CONSIDERATIONS: Keep the lumbopelvic region stable using the inner core to prevent lateral pelvic tilt. Hold slight hip lateral rotation and extension throughout the range to avoid TFL muscle recruitment.

DOSAGE

Special Considerations

Anatomic: Right gluteus medius, right hip joint

Physiologic: Length associated changes in strength; stronger in the lengthened range than the shortened range

Learning Capability: May be difficult secondary to capsular restrictions. Ingrained muscle recruitment pattern of the TFL muscle from a long history of high-mileage running; may require high repetitions and significant feedback in early stages of learning

Repetitions/Sets: To form fatigue, pain, or six to eight repetitions

Frequency: 3 to 4 days per week

Sequence: After iliopsoas strengthening

Speed: Slowly

Environment: At home on a firm surface

Feedback: Initially in clinic with clinician providing tactile and verbal feedback. Begin with knowledge of performance for every repetition, then taper every couple repetitions with knowledge of results.

FUNCTIONAL MOVEMENT PATTERN TO REINFORCE GOAL OF EXERCISE: Ascending stairs, gait, and running.

RATIONALE FOR EXERCISE CHOICE: This exercise was chosen to improve strength of the gluteus medius muscle. Lumbopelvic stability and IT band extensibility depends on proper recruitment of the gluteus medius muscle throughout the range. Open kinetic chain gluteus medius strengthening is necessary before transferring to dynamic activity and function.

ACTIVITY: Squats (see Self-Management 20-8 in Chapter 20).

PURPOSE: Strengthen hip girdle muscles and train independent movement between hips and spine in a functional context.

RISK FACTORS: Watch for symmetric loading between extremities.

ELEMENT OF MOVEMENT SYSTEM EMPHASIZED: Base and modulator.

STAGE OF MOTOR CONTROL: Controlled mobility.

MODE: Concentric and eccentric hip girdle muscle contractions.

POSTURE: Standing with weight equally distributed between both feet, and pelvis and spine in neutral in front of a full-length mirror.

MOVEMENT: First set inner core. Slowly bend your hips and knees. Return to the start position by using quadriceps and gluteals.

SPECIAL CONSIDERATIONS: Knees should not flex beyond the length of the feet or medial to the second toes. More emphasis should be placed on gluteal muscles versus hamstring muscles. Keep the lumbopelvic region stable and bend through the hips with equal loading and avoidance of lateral pelvic tilt.

DOSAGE

Special Considerations

Anatomic: Bilateral hip girdle muscles, bilateral hip joints

Physiologic: Length-associated changes in eccentric and concentric strength and asymmetric mobility in hips

Learning Capability: Very ingrained movement pattern from a long history of high-mileage running; may require high repetitions and significant feedback in early stages of learning

Repetitions/Sets: To form fatigue, pain, or 20 to 30 repetitions

Frequency: 6 to 7 days per week

Sequence: After gluteus medius strengthening

Speed: Slowly

Environment: At home with or without a chair, depending on strength

Feedback: Initially in clinic with clinician providing tactile and verbal feedback and mirror providing visual feedback. Taper to continued use of mirror, with knowledge of results of verbal feedback after every three to four repetitions. Withdraw mirror and verbally provide knowledge of results every three to four repetitions.

FUNCTIONAL MOVEMENT PATTERN TO REINFORCE GOAL OF EXERCISE: Ascending stairs, sit to stand, walking, and running.

RATIONALE FOR EXERCISE CHOICE: This functional exercise was chosen to improve strength of hip girdle muscles and hip joint mobility. Improved hip joint mobility and force-generating capability of the gluteus maximus enables increased hip flexion and decreased knee flexion during squatting activities. Squats with shared forces at the hip and knee decrease excessive forces at the low back and knee.

ACTIVITY: Step ups (see Self-Management 20-3)

PURPOSE: Incorporate proper total-body movements in a functional context.

RISK FACTORS: Avoid hip hike patterns and hamstring dominance.

ELEMENT OF MOVEMENT SYSTEM EMPHASIZED: Base and modulator.

STAGE OF MOTOR CONTROL: Controlled mobility.

MODE: Concentric and eccentric hip girdle muscle contractions.

POSTURE: Standing in front of a 6-in step in front of a mirror.

MOVEMENT: First set inner core. Lift the right leg onto the step. Step up.

SPECIAL CONSIDERATIONS: Be sure the patient does not hike his right hip during the hip flexion phase or perform a Trendelenburg pattern during hip extension phase. The pelvis must remain level and stable throughout the entire exercise to adequately recruit iliopsoas during hip flexion and prepare to use gluteus maximus and gluteus medius muscles in their proper length-tension properties during hip extension.

DOSAGE

Special Considerations

Anatomic: Right hamstring and adductor

Physiologic: Chronic moderate strain

Learning Capability: Very ingrained movement pattern from a long history of high-mileage running; may require high repetitions and significant feedback in early stages of learning

Repetitions/Sets: To form fatigue as evidenced by hip hike, pain, or 20 to 30 repetitions, up to 3 sets

Frequency: 6 to 7 days per week

Sequence: Perform after specific exercises for psoas and gluteus medius muscle performance and squats.

Speed: Slow progressed to functional speed

Environment: At home in front of a mirror

Feedback: Initially in clinic with clinician providing tactile and verbal feedback and mirror providing visual feedback. Taper to continued use of mirror, with knowledge of results of verbal feedback after every three to four repetitions. Withdraw mirror and verbally provide knowledge of results every three to four repetitions. Progress toward skill.

FUNCTIONAL MOVEMENT PATTERN TO REINFORCE GOAL OF EXERCISE: Ascending stairs, walking, running.

RATIONALE FOR EXERCISE CHOICE: This functional exercise was chosen to replace the faulty movement with one that is correct. Faulty hip hiking does not emphasize hip flexion and efficient recruitment of the gluteus maximus and medius muscles. Trendelenburg pattern does not emphasize lumbopelvic stability. Correct step-up pattern encourages gluteus maximus and quadriceps recruitment over hamstring and gluteus medius recruitment over TFL or adductors.

COMPLETE INTERVENTION—UPPER QUADRANT
For Case Study No. 10

Following is a comprehensive exercise program for upper quadrant intervention for Peter. It is prescribed in week 3 post initial evaluation.

AT WEEK 3

ACTIVITY: Sidelying lateral rotator and posterior capsule stretch (see Self-Management 26-4)

PURPOSE: To lengthen lateral rotators of the shoulder.

RISK FACTORS: None.

ELEMENT OF MOVEMENT SYSTEM EMPHASIZED: Base.

STAGE OF MOTOR CONTROL: Mobility.

MODE: Contract-relax of the shoulder lateral rotators.

POSTURE: Sidelying with bottom arm elevated to 90 degrees and elbow flexed to 90 degrees.

MOVEMENT: Shoulder joint should rotate allowing your forearm to move toward your feet and the floor. At that point, lightly press up into the resistance of the other hand and hold for 6 to 10 seconds. Relax and gently push the bottom forearm further toward your feet and the floor. Repeat three to four times.

SPECIAL CONSIDERATIONS: Scapula should be entirely on your back rather than under your body to target the lateral rotators. If the scapula slips under your body, scapular adductors will stretch instead.

DOSAGE

> *Special Considerations*
>
> > *Anatomic:* Right shoulder lateral rotators.
> >
> > *Physiologic:* Short shoulder lateral rotators. Length-associated changes in strength; stronger in the shortened range than the lengthened range.
> >
> > *Learning Capability:* Good with specific verbal and visual instructions.
>
> *Repetitions/Sets:* Three to four repetitions; two sets
>
> *Frequency:* Three to five times per day, 7 days per week
>
> *Sequence:* Begin with this stretch followed by the rest of the exercises.
>
> *Speed:* Hold for 6 to 10 seconds
>
> *Environment:* At home on a firm surface
>
> *Feedback:* Initially in clinic with clinician providing verbal, visual, and tactile feedback. Begin with knowledge of performance for every repetition, then taper every other repetition with knowledge of results.

FUNCTIONAL MOVEMENT PATTERN TO REINFORCE GOAL OF EXERCISE: Reaching overhead without discomfort or unstable feeling.

RATIONALE FOR EXERCISE CHOICE: This stretch was chosen to improve the length of the shoulder lateral rotators. Sufficient shoulder medial rotation is needed for optimal GH congruency and to prevent anterior displacement of the humeral head.

ACTIVITY: Supine GH lateral and medial rotation.

PURPOSE: Develop motor control strategy of the rotator cuff muscles for ideal path of instant center of rotation (PICR) of the GH joint.

RISK FACTORS: Chronic subscapularis strain and tendinitis.

ELEMENT OF MOVEMENT SYSTEM EMPHASIZED: Modulator and biomechanical.

STAGE OF MOTOR CONTROL: Mobility.

MODE: Concentric and eccentric rotator cuff contractions.

POSTURE: Lying supine with arm abducted to 90 degrees and elbow flexed to 90 degrees on an even, stable surface. Right scapular spine should lie at the level of the second vertebra.

MOVEMENT: Slowly rotate arm so that your forearm moves back toward your head, then in the opposite direction so the forearm moves forward.

SPECIAL CONSIDERATIONS: The arm should move independently from the scapula spinning in its socket. The scapula should not displace forward or depress nor should the humeral head displace forward from the socket.

DOSAGE

> *Special Considerations*
>
> > *Anatomic:* Right medial and lateral rotator cuff muscles, right GH joint
> >
> > *Physiologic:* Chronic moderate strain and tendinitis, questionable instability of the right GH joint
> >
> > *Learning Capability:* Very ingrained movement pattern from a long history of high-mileage running; may require high repetitions and significant feedback in early stages of learning
>
> *Repetitions/Sets:* To form fatigue, pain, or 20 to 30 repetitions, up to 3 sets
>
> *Frequency:* 6 to 7 days per week
>
> *Sequence:* Begin with this exercise followed by the wall slide with subscapularis bias and muscle performance exercise of the serratus anterior.
>
> *Speed:* Slowly for good-quality movement.
>
> *Environment:* At home on the floor or firm bed.
>
> *Feedback:* Initially in clinic with clinician providing tactile and verbal feedback. Begin with knowledge of performance for every repetition then taper every three to four repetitions with knowledge of results.

FUNCTIONAL MOVEMENT PATTERN TO REINFORCE GOAL OF EXERCISE: Reaching behind the back without discomfort or unstable feeling.

RATIONALE FOR EXERCISE CHOICE: This exercise was chosen to improve motor control strategies of shoulder medial and lateral rotators. Independent movement of the GH joint with ideal PICR is the goal rather than faulty compensatory scapulothoracic movement.

ACTIVITY: Right arm wall slide with medial rotation bias (see Fig. 25-11B)

PURPOSE: Develop motor control strategy to encourage rotator cuff activation specifically the subscapularis as opposed to pectoralis major, latissimus dorsi, and teres major muscles for ideal PICR of the GH joint.

RISK FACTORS: Chronic subscapularis strain.

ELEMENT OF MOVEMENT SYSTEM EMPHASIZED: Modulator and biomechanical.

STAGE OF MOTOR CONTROL: Controlled mobility.

MODE: Isometric rotator cuff activation with subscapularis bias.

POSTURE: Standing with palm of the hand against the door frame. Right scapular spine should lie at the level of the second vertebra.

MOVEMENT: Slide the hand upward and downward while maintaining mild pressure into medial rotation against the door frame.

SPECIAL CONSIDERATIONS: More than mild pressure applied into medial rotation against the door frame will recruit pectoralis major, latissimus dorsi, and teres major muscles instead of subscapularis causing anterior translation of the humeral head.

DOSAGE

Special Considerations

Anatomic: Right subscapularis, right GH joint

Physiologic: Chronic moderate strain and tendinitis, questionable instability of the right GH joint

Learning Capability: Very ingrained movement pattern from a long history of high-mileage running; may require high repetitions and significant feedback in early stages of learning

Repetitions/Sets: To form fatigue, pain, or 20 to 30 repetitions, up to 3 sets

Frequency: 6 to 7 days per week

Sequence: After GH rotation but before muscle performance exercise of the serratus anterior.

Speed: Slowly for good-quality movement.

Environment: At home in a door frame.

Feedback: Initially in clinic with clinician providing tactile and verbal feedback. Begin with knowledge of performance for every repetition then taper every three to four repetitions with knowledge of results.

FUNCTIONAL MOVEMENT PATTERN TO REINFORCE GOAL OF EXERCISE: Reaching overhead and behind the back without discomfort or unstable feeling.

RATIONALE FOR EXERCISE CHOICE: This exercise was chosen to improve motor control strategies of shoulder medial rotators. Proper recruitment of the subscapularis muscle over other medial rotators provides dynamic anterior stability of the GH joint during dynamic activity. It is important that the subscapularis muscle is trained because of its anterior insertion close to the axis of rotation.

ACTIVITY: Supine serratus anterior isometric (see Self-Management 26-3, Level I)

PURPOSE: Serratus anterior neuromuscular education to promote recruitment in the shortened range with scapular upward rotation.

RISK FACTORS: Impingement of rotator cuff tendons.

ELEMENT OF MOVEMENT SYSTEM EMPHASIZED: Modulator.

STAGE OF MOTOR CONTROL: Mobility.

MODE: Isometric serratus anterior contraction.

POSTURE: Supine with arm elevated resting on pillows placed above your head.

MOVEMENT: Lightly press thumb into pillows engaging the serratus anterior muscle.

SPECIAL CONSIDERATIONS: More than mild pressure applied into the pillows will recruit muscles of the GH joint over the serratus anterior causing anterior translation of the humeral head.

DOSAGE

Special Considerations

Anatomic: Right serratus anterior, right scapulothoracic joint

Physiologic: Length associated changes in strength; stronger in the lengthened range than the shortened range

Learning Capability: May be difficult secondary to painful arc. May require a less than desirable starting point in the range

Repetitions/Sets: To form fatigue, pain, or 20 to 30 repetitions, up to 3 sets

Frequency: 6 to 7 days per week

Sequence: After wall slides and GH rotation

Speed: Hold for 10 seconds

Environment: At home on a firm surface

Feedback: Initially in clinic with clinician providing tactile and verbal feedback. Begin with knowledge of performance for every repetition then taper every three to four repetitions with knowledge of results.

FUNCTIONAL MOVEMENT PATTERN TO REINFORCE GOAL OF EXERCISE: Reaching overhead without discomfort or unstable feeling.

RATIONALE FOR EXERCISE CHOICE: This exercise was chosen to improve motor control strategies of shoulder elevator muscles. Sufficient scapular upward rotation depends on proper recruitment of the serratus anterior muscle in the shortened range with arm elevation. This method of neuromuscular re-education is necessary before translating to dynamic activity and function.

AT 3 WEEKS

ACTIVITY: Stomach lying middle and lower trapezius isometric.

PURPOSE: Middle and lower trapezius neuromuscular education to hold the scapula in a position of upward rotation.

RISK FACTORS: Impingement of rotator cuff tendons and anterior displacement of the humeral head.

ELEMENT OF MOVEMENT SYSTEM EMPHASIZED: Modulator.

STAGE OF MOTOR CONTROL: Stability.

MODE: Isometric middle and lower trapezius contraction (see Self-Management 26-2, Level I)

POSTURE: Stomach lying with both hands resting on the head. Good cervical and scapular alignment.

MOVEMENT: Barely lift your elbows keeping neck and upper trapezius muscles relaxed. Contract middle and lower trapezius muscles.

SPECIAL CONSIDERATIONS: Lifting elbows excessively will recruit posterior muscles of the GH joint and rhomboids causing anterior translation of the humeral head and scapular adduction, respectively.

DOSAGE

Special Considerations

Anatomic: Bilaterally middle and lower trapezius muscles, scapulothoracic joint

Physiologic: Weak middle and lower trapezius muscles, dominant rhomboids.

Learning Capability: May be difficult secondary to painful arc.

Repetitions/Sets: To form fatigue, pain, or 20 to 30 repetitions, up to 3 sets

Frequency: 6 to 7 days per week

Sequence: Begin with this exercise followed by stomach lying shoulder rotation and sidelying serratus anterior exercises.

Speed: Hold for 10 seconds

Environment: At home on a firm surface

Feedback: Initially in clinic with clinician providing tactile and verbal feedback. Begin with knowledge of performance for every repetition then taper every three to four repetitions with knowledge of results.

FUNCTIONAL MOVEMENT PATTERN TO REINFORCE GOAL OF EXERCISE: Reaching overhead without discomfort or unstable feeling.

RATIONALE FOR EXERCISE CHOICE: This exercise was chosen to improve motor control strategies of scapular stabilizing muscles. Scapular upward rotation about a stable PICR depends on recruitment of the middle and lower trapezius muscles with arm elevation. This method of neuromuscular re-education is necessary before translating to dynamic activity and function.

ACTIVITY: Prone GH lateral and medial rotation with 1-lb weight (see Self-Management 26-1)

PURPOSE: Develop motor control strategy of the rotator cuff muscles and scapulothoracic muscles for ideal PICR of the GH joint and scapula.

RISK FACTORS: Chronic subscapularis strain and tendinitis.

ELEMENT OF MOVEMENT SYSTEM EMPHASIZED: Modulator and biomechanical.

STAGE OF MOTOR CONTROL: Controlled mobility.

MODE: Concentric and eccentric rotator cuff contractions. Isometric contractions of the middle and lower trapezius muscles.

POSTURE: Lying prone with arm abducted to 90 degrees and elbow flexed to 90 degrees on an even, stable surface. A towel roll should be placed under the anterior shoulder joint.

MOVEMENT: Slowly rotate arm so that your forearm moves up toward your head, then in the opposite direction so the forearm moves back toward your feet.

SPECIAL CONSIDERATIONS: The arm should move independent from the scapula spinning in its socket. The scapula should not displace forward nor should the humeral head displace forward from the socket.

DOSAGE

Special Considerations

Anatomic: Right medial and lateral rotator cuff muscles, right GH joint, right middle and lower trapezius muscles, right scapula.

Physiologic: Chronic moderate strain and tendinitis, questionable instability of the right GH joint

Learning Capability: Very ingrained movement pattern from a long history of high-mileage running; may require high repetitions

Repetitions/Sets: To form fatigue, pain, or six to eight repetitions with fatigue

Frequency: 3 to 4 days per week

Sequence: Begin with this exercise followed by the wall slide with subscapularis bias and muscle performance exercise of the serratus anterior.

Speed: Slowly for good-quality movement.

Environment: At home on the floor or firm bed.

Feedback: Initially in clinic with clinician providing tactile and verbal feedback. Begin with knowledge of performance for every repetition then taper every couple of repetitions with knowledge of results.

FUNCTIONAL MOVEMENT PATTERN TO REINFORCE GOAL OF EXERCISE: Reaching behind the back without discomfort or unstable feeling.

RATIONALE FOR EXERCISE CHOICE: This exercise was chosen to improve motor control strategies of scapular stabilizers and shoulder medial and lateral rotators. Independent movement of the GH joint with ideal PICR and a stable scapula are the goals.

ACTIVITY: Sidelying serratus anterior dynamic contractions with resistive band (see Self-Management 26-3, Level II)

PURPOSE: Serratus anterior muscle strengthening throughout the range with scapular upward rotation.

RISK FACTORS: Impingement of rotator cuff tendons.

ELEMENT OF MOVEMENT SYSTEM EMPHASIZED: Modulator and biomechanical.

STAGE OF MOTOR CONTROL: Controlled mobility.

MODE: Concentric and eccentric serratus anterior contractions.

POSTURE: Sidelying with arm rested on pillows placed in front of your head and shoulders. Resistive band is attached on the upper foot and the other end grasped in the resting hand.

MOVEMENT: Slide your arm upward toward your head, keeping it in contact with the pillows. On the return, slowly lower the arm back down to the starting position against the resistance of the band.

SPECIAL CONSIDERATIONS: Keep the scapula on your back upwardly rotating about a stable PICR.

DOSAGE

Special Considerations

Anatomic: Right serratus anterior, right scapulothoracic joint.

Physiologic: Faulty eccentric motor control of serratus anterior muscle.

Learning Capability: May be difficult secondary to painful arc. May require a less than desirable starting point in the range.

Repetitions/Sets: To form fatigue, pain, or six to eight repetitions.

Frequency: 3 to 4 days per week.

Sequence: After wall slides and GH rotation.

Speed: Slowly.

Environment: At home on a firm surface.

Feedback: Initially in clinic with clinician providing tactile and verbal feedback. Begin with knowledge of performance for every repetition then taper every couple of repetitions with knowledge of results.

FUNCTIONAL MOVEMENT PATTERN TO REINFORCE GOAL OF EXERCISE: Reaching overhead and behind the back without discomfort or unstable feeling.

RATIONALE FOR EXERCISE CHOICE: This exercise was chosen to improve motor control strategies and strength of shoulder elevator muscles. Sufficient scapular upward rotation depends on proper recruitment of the serratus anterior muscle throughout the range with arm elevation. This method of neuromuscular re-education and strengthening is necessary before returning to functional activities.

 CASE STUDY NO. 11

Mr. Lawn, a 67-year-old man, had a right (R) total hip replacement (THR) 4 years ago. He also has left (L) hip degenerative joint disease (DJD). For the last 4 months he has been noticing increasing L hip pain and is beginning to have pain in the R hip as well if he attempts to play more than nine holes of golf. He states that 18 holes is usual, and he pulls his own cart. Recent muddy conditions seem to have made symptoms worse. His main concern is that R

low back pain will be triggered by R hip pain, as it has been in the past. During the last episode of low back pain, he had to sleep sitting up in his chair, because it was the only place he could get comfortable. Mr. Lawn lives with his wife, who is in the early stages of Alzheimer disease, and his golf games are his main social contact with friends. He is otherwise healthy and does all the driving, shopping, and housework.

EXAMINATION

Pain: L hip at rest 2/10, after 18 holes of golf 7/10; R hip at rest 1/10, after golf 3/10; R low back at rest 0/10, after golf 1/10

Posture: In standing: bilateral (B) supinated feet; marked B tibial bowing; B femoral internal rotation; high L iliac crest; anterior tilted pelvis; mild hip flexion; supine apparent short R leg; R iliac crest and ischial tuberosity high compared with L

Gait: Marked B trunk sidebend to side of stance leg, decreased hip and knee flexion; slight circumduction B; decreased pronation B feet; R stance time decreased compared with L

(continued)

CASE STUDY NO. 11 *(Continued)*

Active Range of Motion (open chain)

	R hip	*L hip*
Extension/flexion	5–110 degrees	5–115 degrees (pain)
Internal/external rotation	20–25 degrees	20–15 degrees (pain)
Abduction	30 degrees	20 degrees
Knee flexion/extension	2–125 B degrees	
Lumbar flexion	Hands 4 in below knees	
Lumbar extension	25% normal range (pain)	

Accessory Motion: L Hip: hypomobile in distal glide, capsular tightness in internal and external passive rotation. Lumbar spine: extension and right sidebend with overpressure restricted and painful compared with L

Palpation: B rectus femoris, iliopsoas, hip adductors, and R quadratus lumborum dense/tender

Strength Testing: Rectus femoris (B) 5/5; iliopsoas (R) 4–/5, (L) 5/5; gluteus maximus (R) 4–/5, (L) 4/5; gluteus medius (R) 4–/5, L 3+/5; quadriceps (B) 5/5; gastroc/soleus (B) 5/5; abdominals 4–/5 by leg lowering test

Balance: R single-leg stance time; 5 seconds; L single-leg stance time: 12 seconds

Neurologic Signs: Normal for L3–S1 light touch, deep tendon reflexes, and key muscle strength.

Active Movement Testing (open chain): Pain is elicited with L hip flexion. Internal rotation and abduction at end of available range in each motion. Standing lumbar sidebend and R rotation is painful. Single-leg stance (R) causes R hip pain, and closed chain testing was deferred because of initial apprehension and balance deficits.

EVALUATION: DJD-related hip muscle strength and range deficits leading to gait and pelvic asymmetry and hip joint pain and to R L5/S1 compression and irritation.

Impairment	*Functional Limitation*	*Disability*
• B hip range of motion restriction • B hip joint muscle weakness • Abdominal muscle overstretch • Frontal plane pelvic asymmetry • Sagittal plane lumbopelvic asymmetry • Decreased standing balance • Gait abnormality • Unable to maintain neutral pelvis	• Pain limits walk endurance	• Unable to play golf • Unable to socialize and restore self mentally and emotionally for wife's care

DIAGNOSIS: Condition after R hip THR; L hip DJD with muscle imbalance leading to probable R L5–S1 facet compression irritation

PROGNOSIS

Short-Term Goals (14 to 21 days)
1. Regain sagittal and frontal plane alignment in standing and walking
2. Regain at least 4/5 strength in all hip and abdominal muscle groups
3. Equalize L hip range of motion to that of R hip
4. Able to balance 30 seconds in single-leg stance (B)

Long-Term Goals (4 to 6 weeks)
1. Ambulate with normal gait pattern
2. Walk 18 holes of golf, pulling cart, without pain in hips or low back

appendix 1

Red Flags: Recognizing Signs and Symptoms

DAVID MUSNICK* AND CARRIE M. HALL

Because therapists often have consistent daily or weekly contact with patients, they may be the health professionals to recognize serious neuromusculoskeletal pathology or systemic disease requiring medical referral. A thorough history, carefully conducted interview, systems review, and screening examinations must be completed during the initial evaluation. Any red flags—signs or symptoms that signal pathologic conditions—may indicate serious somatic or visceral disease or disorders that are beyond the scope of physical therapy intervention. The information outlined in this appendix delineates signs and symptoms of somatic and visceral origin.

Physical therapists often perform interventions, such as therapeutic exercise, to alleviate pain. The physical therapist must be sure that the pain is of neuromusculoskeletal origin and is within the scope of physical therapy practice. A patient with pain that may be caused by serious pathology or referred from a visceral source should be immediately referred to a medical physician for further testing.

Visceral structures can be a source of referred pain to musculoskeletal regions, particularly to the shoulder, back, chest, hip, or groin. The mechanism by which visceral structures refer pain to musculoskeletal regions is twofold:

1. Visceral afferents that supply internal organs transmit impulses to the dorsal horn in which somatic and visceral pain fibers share second-order neurons. Impulses from visceral nerve endings arrive at similar interneuron pools as impulses from somatic origin. Visceral pain may then be felt in somatic segments and skin areas with which it shares neurons in the dorsal horn. This pattern is called referred visceral sensation. Broader pain referral from visceral structures can occur with multiple-segment overlap. Referred visceral sensation may coexist with reflex muscle spasm and vasomotor changes.
2. Visceral structures in the thoracic and abdominal cavities have free nerve endings in loose connective tissue in epithelial and serous linings and in blood vessels. Neural afferent information is transmitted along small, unmyelinated, type C nerve fibers within sympathetic and parasympathetic nerves of the autonomic nervous system. The pain is usually not well localized by the patient and is usually described as vague, deep, and aching.

Signs and symptoms associated with referred visceral pain are the most common red flags signaling the need for further evaluation. The cause of this pain is related to the pathologic function of the primary visceral structure involved. Viscera may refer pain caused by tissue ischemia, obstruction, mechanical distention, or inflammation. Tables 1 and 2 describe the sources and characteristics of somatic and visceral pain. Tables 3 and 4 review the signs and symptoms associated with referred visceral pain. Whenever a patient reports symptoms described in Tables 3 and 4, screening for systemic disease is appropriate. The decision to screen for systemic disease may be even more critical if the patient is older than 45 years of age and the symptoms have an insidious onset.

Table 5 describes systemic, visceral, or nonmechanical causes of regional musculoskeletal pain. The physical therapist should be aware of constant, severe pain with increases in intensity, nonmechanical patterns, or the symptoms or signs described in Table 4 in association with regional musculoskeletal pain. Referral of the patient to a physician is indicated when pain in a musculoskeletal region is accompanied by symptoms and signs indicating systemic or nonmechanical disease. Some types of referred visceral pain are made worse with mechanical stress. Mechanical exacerbation on examination is not 100% specific and cannot alone be used for diagnosing mechanical problems.

Female patients, persons older than 50 years of age, and children may present with symptoms about which the practitioner should be aware:

- Female patients with new-onset thoracolumbar, lumbosacral, or sacroiliac pain should be screened through a renal and reproductive history and lumbar scanning examination. Prompt medical screening is indicated if the person has fever, costovertebral angle tenderness, urinary symptoms, pelvic or suprapubic pain or tenderness, tachycardia, orthostatic changes, or an unclear diagnosis. Renal and reproductive organ disease can cause significant morbidity if not treated quickly.
- Malignant disease should be suspected in patients older than 50 years of age who have constant back pain that is increased with recumbency, history of primary tumor, pathologic fractures, night pain, or multiple painful areas in the spine. The axial skeleton is involved more commonly than the appendicular skeleton, with the lumbar and thoracic spine affected similarly (incidence of approximately 45% to 50%). Cord compression signs require immediate referral to a physician.

---

*David Musnick, MD, is an internal medicine/sports medicine physician in Seattle and Bellevue, Washington. He teaches seminars in differential diagnosis to physical therapists. He has taken numerous courses in exercise and manual therapy topics taught by physical therapists. He has written a book on functional exercise, Conditioning for Outdoor Fitness, published by Mountaineers Books in Seattle.

TABLE 1	Sources and Characteristics of Somatic and Visceral Pain

Somatic Sources

Superficial Somatic Cutaneous Pain
- Localized but may refer within 6–12 in
- Aching
- Burning
- Throbbing (e.g., abscesses)
- Neck, hip, or elbow pain with reactive lymph nodes
- Reactive lymph glands are aggravated by pressure or stretching

Deep Somatic Pain*

Muscles
- Localized or may be in referred patterns
- Increases with direct pressure on a tender area or site of lesion, locally or in a referral pattern

Joints
- Deep aching that is vague within the area (more common with peripheral joints) and a referred pattern that is felt more distally from the area (especially spinal joints)
- May decrease with rest or when stressful action has stopped
- May increase with activity
- Increases with stress testing or palpation

Ligaments
- Deep aching in the region of the ligament but may also be perceived distally
- Increases with stress testing or palpation

Neurologic Pain
- Characteristic pain referral patterns based on the site of the lesion
- May be associated with bone pain if the origin of neurologic compression is bone

Bone Pain
- Perceived close to the bone (see Table 2)
- Constant and not relieved by rest
- May be worse with walking, jumping, or other impact
- If a tumor is growing in a bone the pain will be gradually increasing and may be worse at night when the patient is trying to sleep

Visceral Sources
- Vague pain
- Deep pain
- Aching pain
- Boring pain
- Tearing pain
- If a hollow organ is involved, pain may be more colicky (i.e., crescendo and decrescendo)

---

*Pain may originate in muscles, ligaments, joints, periosteum, vessles dura, and fascia.

- Back pain is rare in patients younger than 16 years of age, especially in nongymnasts and in patients without trauma. Pediatric patients with low back pain and without history of trauma or overuse should be screened by a medical practitioner.
- Pediatric patients with hip pathology may complain of knee or hip pain or a vague pain with walking. Any pediatric patient seen for recent onset, undiagnosed limping should be evaluated with a medical history and scan of the lumbar spine, hip, knee, and lower extremity (including temperature). Patients with these complaints should be seen promptly by a medical practitioner and have an x-ray examination to evaluate the hip, if indicated.

TABLE 2	Causes of Bone Pain and Associated Signs and Symptoms

CAUSES	ASSOCIATED CONDITIONS AND SYMPTOMS
• Stress and compression fractures	• Overuse • Osteoporosis • Evaluate for menstrual and eating disorders in young females
• Avascular necrosis (wrist, femoral head, shoulders, feet)	• Corticosteroid use • Trauma
• Osteomyelitis • Hematologic disorders of the bone marrow	• Fever or other source of infection • Fatigue • Multiple areas of bone pain, especially in the spine and pelvis
• Paget disease	• Cranial neuropathies • Leg deformities • Warm bones on examination • Scoliosis if in the spine, especially in a child
• Benign tumor • Cancer (primary or metastatic)	• Symptoms of the primary cancer • Fatigue • Pain of bone origin in more than one spine site; a spine site combined with a rib or long bone site may be metastatic cancer and should be referred for evaluation

TABLE 3 Characteristics of Systemic Symptoms

DATA OBTAINED FROM THE HISTORY	CONSTITUTIONAL SYMPTOMS
• Insidious onset or no known cause (or both) • Pattern of presentation: gradual, progressive, cyclical • Constant • Intense • Bilateral • Unrelieved by rest or change of position • Night pain • History of infection • Migratory arthralgias	• Fever • Chills • Malaise • Fatigue • Night sweats • Gastrointestinal symptoms • Skin rash • Weight loss • Dyspnea (i.e., shortness of breath) • Diaphoresis at rest or with minimal exertion

TABLE 4 Visceral Symptoms and Signs Categorized by Origin

Infection
- Fever
- Chills
- Malaise
- Fatigue
- Night sweats
- Red rash
- Swelling
- Purulence
- Constant pain
- Painful, enlarged lymph nodes
- Superficial palpation or percussion tenderness
- Root or cord compression by space-occupying lesion in spine

Pulmonary
- Cough
- Sputum
- Wheezing
- Shortness of breath
- Chest pain
- Pain worsened by deep inspiration
- Hemoptysis (i.e., coughing up blood)
- Decreased aerobic exercise capacity

Cardiac
- Arrhythmia (fast >120, slow <40)
- Pauses
- Irregular pulse
- Chest, jaw, scapular, or left arm pain
- High or low blood pressure (>180 or <85)
- Dizziness
- Syncope (i.e., fainting)
- Bilateral leg and foot swelling
- Shortness of breath

Vascular
- Low-amplitude pulse
- Coldness
- Paleness
- Swelling
- Constant pain
- Tearing or boring pain
- Color change

Gastrointestinal
- Nausea
- Vomiting
- Bloating
- Weight loss
- Loss of appetite
- Change in stools
- Bloody stools
- Diarrhea
- Absence of bowel movement
- Abdominal pain
- Yellow eyes or skin
- Food may help or aggravate

Renal
- Costovertebral angle tenderness
- Hematuria (i.e., red urine)
- Painful or frequent urination

Endocrine
- Energy or temperature changes
- Urinary volume change
- Possible bone pain

Neoplastic
- Constant or night pain
- Age >45 years
- Myelopathy signs (e.g., spinal cord compression)
- Previous primary tumor
- Pathologic fracture
- Generalized weakness
- Pain in multiple bony locations

Gynecologic
- Pelvic or low back pain
- Menstrual abnormalities
- Pelvic mass

Rheumatologic
- Peripheral joint swelling
- Deformity
- Redness or pain
- Rash

TABLE 5   Systemic Disease or Visceral Pain Referred from the Musculoskeletal Region

Headache
- Intracranial tumor (U)
- Meningitis (U)
- Subarachnoid hemorrhage (U)
- Sinus infection
- Temporal arteritis; refer patients with visual problems immediately to prevent blindness (U)

Cervical Spine Region Pain

Visceral Referred Pain

Thoracic Origin
- Cardiac ischemia or infarction (U)
- Pneumomediastinum (U)
- Pericarditis (U)
- Aortic arch dissection (U)
- Pancoast tumor
- Pleuritis

Infectious Origin
- Meningitis (U)
- Epidural abscess (U)
- Osteomyelitis (U)
- Disk space infection (U)
- Transverse myelitis (U)
- Lyme disease

Neoplastic Causes
- Metastatic tumor
- Intramedullary or extramedullary tumor
- Epidural hematoma (U)

Vascular Origin
- Subarachnoid hemorrhage (U)
- Vertebral artery dissection (U)
- Carotid artery thrombosis (U)

Other Visceral Referred Pain
- Sphenoid sinusitis
- Thyroiditis
- Parotitis
- Cervical lymphadenitis (from a throat or skin source)
- Pharyngeal space infection (P) (U)
- Cysts (P)

Nonviscerogenic Referred Pain

Rheumatologic Disease
- Fibromyalgia
- Polymyalgia rheumatica
- Rheumatoid arthritis
- Ankylosing spondylitis
- Gout or other crystal-induced inflammation

Shoulder Pain

Visceral Referred Pain

Neoplastic Causes
- Metastatic lesions
- Breast
- Prostate
- Kidney
- Lung
- Thyroid
- Cervical cord or root compression
- Pancoast tumor
- Lung cancer

Cardiac Origin (left shoulder)
- Angina or myocardial infarction (U)
- Pericarditis (U)
- Aortic aneurysm (U)

Pulmonary Origin
- Empyema and lung abscess
- Pulmonary tuberculosis
- Spontaneous pneumothorax (U)
- Lung cancer

Breast Origin
- Mastodynia
- Primary or secondary cancer

Abdominal Origin
- Liver disease
- Ruptured spleen (U)
- Gallbladder disease
- Subphrenic abscess

Systemic Disease
- Collagen vascular disease
- Gout
- Syphilis, gonorrhea
- Sickle cell anemia
- Hemophilia
- Rheumatic disease

Thoracic-Scapular Region Pain

Visceral Referred Pain

Cardiac Origin
- Myocardial ischemia or infarction (U)
- Dissecting aortic aneurysm (U)

Pulmonary Origin
- Pneumonia (U)
- Pleuritis
- Pulmonary embolism (U)
- Pneumothorax (U)
- Empyema (U)

Neoplastic Causes
- Mediastinal tumors
- Pancreatic carcinoma

Neck Origin
- Esophagitis

Abdominal Origin
- Liver disease (e.g., hepatitis, cirrhosis, metastatic tumors)
- Gallbladder disease

Anterior or Lateral Chest Pain

Serious Causes (U)

Pulmonary Origin
- Pulmonary embolism
- Pneumothorax
- Pneumomediastinum
- Pneumopericardium
- Mediastinal tumor
- Asthma
- Pneumonia (if respiratory rate >20 and short of breath)

Cardiac Origin
- Pericarditis
- Dissecting coronary artery or aorta (e.g., Marfan syndrome)
- Cardiac hypertrophy

- Primary pulmonary hypertension
- Myocarditis
- Tachycardia (heart rate >140–160 at rest)
- Suspected myocardial infarction (may occur in younger patient using cocaine)

Less Serious Causes

Infectious Origin
- Herpes zoster infection
- Pneumonia (if no respiratory compromise)
- Pleurisy
- Bronchitis

Gastrointestinal Origin
- Esophageal tear
- Spasm
- Reflux

Thoracolumbar Spine and Sacroiliac Region Pain

Visceral Referred Pain

Neoplastic Causes
- Malignant tumors of the spinal cord or meninges (neurologic deficit)
- Lymphoma (night sweats, weight loss, lymphadenopathy)
- Multiple myeloma (>40 years of age, moderately severe bone pain, multiple osteopenic spine lesions, kidney disease, fatigue from excessive calcium)
- Metastatic tumors (e.g., prostate, breast, lung, kidney, thyroid, colon)
- Pediatric malignancies (e.g., Ewing sarcoma, osteosarcoma, lymphoma, leukemia, skeletal metastasis from Wilms tumor, neuroblastoma, rhabdomyosarcoma) (P)

Abdominal Origin
- Abdominal aortic aneurysm (U)
- Peptic ulcer
- Pancreatic disorders
- Pyelonephritis (U)
- Nephrolithiasis (renal stone) (U)
- Hydronephrosis
- Renal tumor
- Renal infarction (U)

Pelvic Origin
- Urinary bladder retention
- Crohn disease of the rectum
- Chronic prostatitis
- Uterine masses
- Retroverted or prolapsed uterus
- Endometriosis
- Pelvic inflammatory disease (fever, nausea, pelvic pain) (U)
- Ectopic pregnancy (missed menstrual cycle, pelvic pain) (U)
- Benign ovarian tumor
- Colon diverticulitis
- Retroperitoneal fibrosis

(continued)

TABLE 5 Systemic Disease or Visceral Pain Referred from the Musculoskeletal Region *(Continued)*

Rheumatologic Causes
- Ankylosing spondylitis
- Reiter syndrome
- Psoriatic arthritis

Infectious Origin (U)
- Osteomyelitis
- Disk space infection
- Epidural abscess
- Pyogenic sacroiliitis

Endocrine and Metabolic Causes
- Osteoporosis with compression fracture

Hip, Groin, and Thigh Pain

Visceral Referred Pain

Neoplastic Causes
- Bone tumors
- Spinal metastasis

Abdominal Origin
- Inguinal or femoral hernia
- Appendicitis (U)
- Crohn disease
- Ureteral colic

Pelvic Origin

Systemic disease
- Pelvic inflammatory disease (P)

Thrombosis Syndromes (U)
- Deep venous thrombosis with proximal extension to femoral vein and/or pelvic veins (calf pain and swelling)
- Greater saphenous vein phlebitis (superficial, may progress to DVT)

Arthritis
- Osteoarthritis
- Gout, pseudogout
- Rheumatoid arthritis
- Ankylosing spondylitis (degenerative joint disease of hip in a younger male)
- Reiter syndrome

Pediatric Hip Disease (P)
- Legg-Calvé-Perthes (proximal femoral epiphyseal blood flow interruption and necrosis; collapse of femoral head; hip pain, limp, adductor and iliopsoas spasm, possible Trendelenburg sign; child 4–8 years old)
- Slipped capital femoral epiphysis (hip, thigh, or knee pain; hip hypomobility especially in medial rotation; older child or adolescent)
- Transient synovitis (hip, thigh, or knee pain; difficulty walking and possible fever, 2–12 years of age with peak incidence at 6–7 years)

Infectious Origin
- Lymphadenitis caused by cellulitis distally or abdominal wall, perineum, or genital areas or other infections, including sexually transmitted diseases (U)
- Iliopsoas abscess (retroperitoneal infection or inflammation) (U)

P, pediatric; U, urgent.

Red Flags: Potentially Serious Symptoms and Signs in Exercising Patients

DAVID MUSNICK AND CARRIE M. HALL

Certain symptoms occurring during exercise may indicate significant medical problems and may be the reason for referral. Display 1 lists the symptoms associated with comorbidities and the tests that should be performed to exclude a medical emergency. Display 2 lists signs indicating medical problems that necessitate medical referral.

During supervised exercise, a patient may develop serious signs and symptoms. Display 3 describes the signs and symptoms related to exercise and the appropriate course of action with respect to various comorbidities:

- Asthma or other pulmonary disease
- Cough
- Cardiovascular disorders
- Syncope
- Hypoglycemia
- Allergic reactions
- Deep vein thrombosis (DVT)
- Pulmonary embolus (PE)
- Spinal cord compression from metastatic disease

◆ **DISPLAY 1**
Symptoms Associated with Medical Conditions

CONDITION	SYMPTOMS	TESTS
Bronchial or lung tissue	• Wheezing • Pleuritic pain (chest pain increased by a deep breath) • Cough • Significant shortness of breath	• Pulse • Respiratory rate • Blood pressure • Peak flow
Coronary artery, heart valve, cardiac tissue	• Tightness or pain in the left chest, jaw, scapula, or left arm • Lightheadedness • Nausea	• Pulse • Blood pressure in both arms to determine differential
Cardiac rhythm disturbance	• Lightheadedness • Fainting • Bradycardia (heart rate <50) • Pauses between beats, especially if associated with lightheadedness	• Postural pulse • Blood pressure • Neurologic screen
Cardiac or pulmonary condition	• Severe intolerance to aerobic or strength training	• Pulse • Respiratory rate • Blood pressure
Chronic fatigue or fibromyalgia	• Flare-up of fatigue after exercise • Intolerance to aerobic or strength training	• Screen for tender points
Cervical or intracerebral pathologies	• Exercise-induced headaches	• Complete neurologic and cervical screen
Neurogenic, vascular claudication, or deep venous thrombosis	• Calf pain with exercise	• Peripheral pulses • Straight-leg raise • Neurologic screen • Homans test • Calf circumference

DISPLAY 2
Signs Associated with Medical Conditions

SIGNS	CONDITION
Heart Rate Less than 50 beats per minute (unless very aerobically fit individual) Pauses >3 seconds between beats (especially if associated with lightheadedness) Moderately elevated heart rates during and after cessation of exercise Elevated heart rate before exercise Heart rate elevation >120 beats per minute, 5 minutes after exercise; if heart rate is >140 beats per minute and accompanied by chest pain, considered a medical emergency	• Bradycardia • Diseased sinus node • Serious bradycardia • Chronic pulmonary or cardiac disease • Arrhythmia • Fever • Pulmonary compromise • Hyperthyroidism • Volume depletion (from bleeding or other fluid loss) • Possible myocardial infarction • Fever • Hyperthyroidism • Arrhythmia (tachycardia) • Volume depletion
Blood Pressure Systolic blood pressure <85 mm Hg (exercise is contraindicated) Systolic blood pressure >140 (exercise not contraindicated until systolic reaches 170; isometric exercise contraindicated)	• Hypotension • Hypertension
Respiratory Rate Greater than 20 (exercise contraindicated unless there is a known chronic lung condition)	• Asthma • Pulmonary infections • Chronic lung conditions • Acute pain • Fever

---

DISPLAY 3
Common Medical Conditions that may Produce Serious Signs and Symptoms During Exercise

Asthma, Pulmonary Diseases, and Shortness of Breath
If a patient has a history of asthma, chronic pulmonary disease, or recent upper respiratory tract infection with any of the symptoms listed below during or after exercise, he or she may have an asthma flare, temporary bronchospasm, or another pulmonary problem (e.g., bronchitis, pneumonia). Any patient with active asthma should be managed by a physician and encouraged to bring his or her asthma inhaler and peak flow meter to the therapy department.

Symptoms and Signs
• Coughing
• Wheezing
• Substernal chest tightness
• Mild shortness of breath at rest or precipitated by exercise or cold weather
• Use of accessory muscles of respiration (e.g., scalenes, pectoralis minor, intercostals)
• Elevated respiratory rate (>18 breaths per minute) 5 minutes after cessation of exercise
• Low peak flow level for age, sex, and height

Clinical Actions
• Administer the patient's bronchospasm inhaler. A second inhalation should be administered after 1 to 2 minutes. Recheck signs and symptoms within 5 to 10 minutes.

• Peak flow of <80% of predicted indicates asthma or chronic obstructive pulmonary disease, indicating referral for a medical evaluation.
• Peak flow of <250 indicates severe airway obstruction and is reason for referral to the emergency room.
• Respiratory rate >24, resting heart rate >100, and a peak flow of <200 to 250 are signs of pulmonary compromise or a severe exacerbation and poor clinical response to the medication. If the patient is not improved significantly after the inhalation of medication, the patient's physician should be called immediately. If the patient appears to be in respiratory distress, he or she should be transferred to an emergency room.
• Exercise can be continued if the patient responds well to the medication. The physician should be called regarding management of the medications to prevent future exacerbations.

Cough
Associated Conditions
• Pulmonary infection (accompanied by colored sputum, fever, chills)
• Medication side effect
• Serious lung disorder
• Asthma
• Reactive airway disease
• Congestive heart failure
• Mild respiratory tract infection

(continued)

DISPLAY 3

Common Medical Conditions that may Produce Serious Signs and Symptoms During Exercise *(Continued)*

Increased intraabdominal and intrathoracic pressure induced by coughing can greatly exacerbate spine pain conditions of a mechanical nature. Patients with spinal disorders should be advised to suppress cough with over-the-counter medications and consult their physician to determine the cause and receive definitive treatment. Patients with a persistent cough should be referred to a physician.

Cardiovascular Disorders
Symptoms
- Chest, substernal, left arm, anterior neck, jaw, and periscapular pain
- Headache, blurred vision, exacerbation of neck pain (symptoms of severe hypertension)
- Uncontrolled hypertension that exacerbates headache and neck pain
- Chest pain, lightheadedness, fainting, and perceptions of strong beats or irregularity (symptoms of heart rhythm abnormalities)

Clinical Actions
- If heart rate is <45 or >150 beats per minute after cessation of exercise for more than 5 minutes, refer the patient immediately or call 911.
- If the patient has a heart rate >150 and is younger than 50 years old, an attempt to decrease the heart rate by putting slight pressure on the carotid body can be made by massaging the carotid pulse just inferior to the angle of the jaw. The radial pulse can be monitored with another hand, and if it begins to slow, pressure can be taken off the carotid body. If there is no effect within 10 to 15 seconds, this procedure should be stopped.
- If the patient has angina symptoms (i.e., severe, constricting chest pain) with known coronary disease, administer his or her own nitroglycerin while sitting or lying down. You may repeat this after 5 minutes. If no relief occurs after a total of three doses in 15 minutes, call 911.
- If systolic blood pressure is >180 or diastolic pressure is >110, the therapy appointment should be terminated and the patient referred to his physician.
- If the systolic blood pressure is >220 and the diastolic pressure is >130, the patient should go to the emergency room, and the referring physician should be called.
- High blood pressure, midline thoracic pain, and between-arm blood pressure differences of 10 mm Hg should be referred immediately.
- A patient with a history of coronary disease should be referred immediately if he or she is experiencing arrhythmia and has chest pain.
- If the patient is unconscious, call 911 and begin cardiopulmonary resuscitation.

Syncope
Syncope is defined as a sudden and reversible loss of consciousness and decrease or loss of postural muscle tone. It can be caused by transient cerebral ischemia (a total loss of cerebral flow for 10 seconds leads to a blood pressure <70) or altered chemical composition of blood flow to the brain (brain cells depend on a constant level of glucose for energy).

Symptoms
- Changes in vision
- Nausea
- Sweating
- Feeling of dizziness
- Feeling of leg or trunk postural weakness
- Palpitations or chest pain if tachycardia
- Calf or chest pain if pulmonary embolism

To determine if the syncope is caused by postural changes, the blood pressure and heart rate are taken in three positions: supine, sitting, and standing. The blood pressure is assessed in each position. If the systolic pressure lowers by more than 20 points or the heart rate elevates by more than 20 points with each positional change, the patient can be determined to have posturally related syncope.

Clinical Actions
- The patient should be positioned in supine with legs elevated for at least 3 minutes to increase venous return of blood.
- A patient with posturally related syncope and a history of vomiting or diarrhea is usually dehydrated and requires significant rehydration with more than 2 L of fluid. The patient should have arrangements made for transportation to a physician's office or a medical facility. It may be possible for the patient to take in enough fluid orally. Rehydration may be started in the therapy department, but it should not be completed in the therapy department.
- Syncope that occurs more than one time requires termination of the therapy appointment and transportation to the emergency room (unless it is clearly a vasovagal faint). A vasovagal faint is one in which there is no ongoing pathology and the blood pressure and pulse become normal after 3 to 5 minutes in all positions. Patients who faint more than one time should not be allowed to transport themselves to a medical facility.

Hypoglycemic Episodes
Hypoglycemic episodes most commonly occur in patients with diabetes. The causes vary, including improper timing of meals or snacks, excessive insulin or improper dosing or timing of insulin, and excessive or unplanned exercise coupled with inadequate food intake.

Symptoms and Signs
- Shakiness
- Weakness
- Sweaty
- Blurred vision
- Excessive anxiety
- Irritability
- Lightheadedness
- Confusion
- Decreased cognitive abilities
- Unconsciousness
- Blood sugar levels <50 to 60

All diabetes patients should be asked to bring their meters with strips to every therapy visit in case of a hypoglycemic episode. Any of the above symptoms should prompt blood sugar assessment.

(continued)

DISPLAY 3
Common Medical Conditions that may Produce Serious Signs and Symptoms During Exercise *(Continued)*

Clinical Actions

- If the glucose level is <60, and the patient is awake, give a carbohydrate snack of three glucose tablets, a tube of Insta-Glucose gel, *or* 1/2 to 1 cup of juice. Ask the patient to take a snack including carbohydrate and protein or fat.
- Do not begin any aerobic exercise.
- Recheck the serum glucose level in 30 minutes. If the patient feels significantly better, he or she can resume exercise.
- If the patient is unconscious, administer glucagon immediately. Mix the liquid in the syringe with the powder in the bottle, and then inject the whole clear solution that is in the syringe into the deltoid muscle or the quadriceps muscle. Place the patient in a sidelying position to protect the airway. When the patient awakens and is fully conscious, give a glucose snack and protein, refer the patient to the emergency room, and call the primary physician.

Instructions for Diabetic Patients Before Exercise

- If the glucose level is 100 to 180, administer 15 g of carbohydrate.
- If the glucose level is 180 to 250, it is not necessary to increase food intake.
- If the glucose level is more than 250, do not start aerobic exercise.

Allergic Reactions

Patients may develop allergic reactions to exercise that can occur for the first time in the therapy department:

- Exercise-related hives (i.e., itchy, raised skin areas filled with fluid)
- Angioedema (i.e., swelling in the subcutaneous tissues around the eyes, lips, hands, and feet, and possibly in the tongue and posterior pharynx and airway)
- Anaphylactic shock (i.e., associated with decreased blood pressure, increased pulse, sweatiness, pallor, angioedema, and asthma symptoms)

Anaphylactic shock may occur as a reaction to a medication such as antibiotics, angiotensin-converting enzyme inhibitors, aspirin, or nonsteroidal anti-inflammatory drugs. Exercise-induced anaphylaxis may occur with vigorous aerobic exercise as the only precipitating factor. Any patient with a history of exercise-induced shock should always exercise with another person and should always carry an epinephrine kit.
A patient may also develop any of these reactions in response to latex gloves or another allergen that he or she is severely allergic to that may be used in the therapy department. A patient may also react to medications.

Clinical Actions

- Hives usually do not cause emergent problems unless this condition progresses to other, more serious problems. Stop exercise, and consider having the patient take an antihistamine such as Benadryl. Call the patient's primary physician.
- Angioedema is an emergency if it involves swelling of the tongue and airway. If the patient displays difficulty controlling saliva or breathing, the treatment of choice is to administer one dose of epinephrine (0.3 mL of 1:1,000 solution) in the deltoid area. If a qualified person is not on the premises to administer this treatment, call 911.
- Anaphylactic shock is a **severe, life-threatening emergency**. Blood pressure and pulse should be taken, although blood pressure may be difficult to detect. The patient should lie down with legs elevated. A dose of epinephrine should be administered immediately and 911 called.

Deep Venous Thrombosis

Individuals at risk for DVT include those who have sustained local trauma to a vessel, have a hypercoagulable disorder, or have been immobilized by bed rest or casts. The most common locations of DVT include the calf, thigh, arms, and pelvis.

Symptoms and Signs

- Pain in the calf or thigh
- Swelling of the calf (circumferential tape measurements are indicated to verify swelling)
- Pain in the calf with walking
- Tenderness with palpation of the deep calf along the midline
- Positive Homans sign (i.e., pain on dorsiflexion of the ankle)

Any patient complaining of calf pain or swelling should be evaluated for DVT.

Clinical Actions

- Suspicion of DVT warrants referral to a physician or emergency room within the next few hours.
- The patient should walk minimally, because there is a danger of the clot breaking off from the vessel.

Pulmonary Embolus

PE is an **urgent condition** in which an area of lung is infarcted as a result of a thrombus occluding a pulmonary artery. The thrombus usually originates in a deep vein of the leg and travels through the venous return circulation into the right side of the heart and out through the pulmonary circulation to occlude a pulmonary artery. Small thrombi may progress to the periphery of the lung and infarct the peripheral lung tissue, with resultant inflammation and pleuritic pain. Large thrombi may occlude the pulmonary circulation and lead to severe cardiac compromise.

Symptoms and Signs

- Pleuritic pain with referred areas of pain
- Shortness of breath
- Fast respiratory rate
- Coughing up blood
- Rapid pulse rate

Suspicion of PE requires immediate referral to the emergency room. If not on the hospital premises, call 911.

Spinal Cord Compression and Metastatic Disease

Patients with metastatic spine lesions can develop cord compression that is manifested by sensory, motor, or bladder symptoms. For a patient with multisite bone pain and new-onset neurologic symptoms, a complete neurologic examination is indicated. If you suspect a cord compression syndrome, check for upper motor neuron (UMN) signs on examination (e.g., clonus, Babinski, hypertonicity). If UMN signs and motor, sensory, or bladder symptoms are present, refer the patient immediately.

Source: Physical Activity Readiness Questionnaire (PAR-Q). © 2002. Reprinted from the Canadian Society for Exercise Physiology. http:/www.csep.ca/forms.asp, with permission.

Physical Activity Readiness
Questionnaire - PAR-Q
(revised 2002)

PAR-Q & YOU

(A Questionnaire for People Aged 15 to 69)

Regular physical activity is fun and healthy, and increasingly more people are starting to become more active every day. Being more active is very safe for most people. However, some people should check with their doctor before they start becoming much more physically active.

If you are planning to become much more physically active than you are now, start by answering the seven questions in the box below. If you are between the ages of 15 and 69, the PAR-Q will tell you if you should check with your doctor before you start. If you are over 69 years of age, and you are not used to being very active, check with your doctor.

Common sense is your best guide when you answer these questions. Please read the questions carefully and answer each one honestly: check YES or NO.

YES	NO		
☐	☐	1.	Has your doctor ever said that you have a heart condition <u>and</u> that you should only do physical activity recommended by a doctor?
☐	☐	2.	Do you feel pain in your chest when you do physical activity?
☐	☐	3.	In the past month, have you had chest pain when you were not doing physical activity?
☐	☐	4.	Do you lose your balance because of dizziness or do you ever lose consciousness?
☐	☐	5.	Do you have a bone or joint problem (for example, back, knee or hip) that could be made worse by a change in your physical activity?
☐	☐	6.	Is your doctor currently prescribing drugs (for example, water pills) for your blood pressure or heart condition?
☐	☐	7.	Do you know of <u>any other reason</u> why you should not do physical activity?

If

you

answered

YES to one or more questions

Talk with your doctor by phone or in person BEFORE you start becoming much more physically active or BEFORE you have a fitness appraisal. Tell your doctor about the PAR-Q and which questions you answered YES.

- You may be able to do any activity you want — as long as you start slowly and build up gradually. Or, you may need to restrict your activities to those which are safe for you. Talk with your doctor about the kinds of activities you wish to participate in and follow his/her advice.
- Find out which community programs are safe and helpful for you.

NO to all questions

If you answered NO honestly to <u>all</u> PAR-Q questions, you can be reasonably sure that you can:
- start becoming much more physically active – begin slowly and build up gradually. This is the safest and easiest way to go.
- take part in a fitness appraisal – this is an excellent way to determine your basic fitness so that you can plan the best way for you to live actively. It is also highly recommended that you have your blood pressure evaluated. If your reading is over 144/94, talk with your doctor before you start becoming much more physically active.

→

DELAY BECOMING MUCH MORE ACTIVE:
- if you are not feeling well because of a temporary illness such as a cold or a fever – wait until you feel better; or
- if you are or may be pregnant – talk to your doctor before you start becoming more active.

PLEASE NOTE: If your health changes so that you then answer YES to any of the above questions, tell your fitness or health professional. Ask whether you should change your physical activity plan.

<u>Informed Use of the PAR-Q</u>: The Canadian Society for Exercise Physiology, Health Canada, and their agents assume no liability for persons who undertake physical activity, and if in doubt after completing this questionnaire, consult your doctor prior to physical activity.

No changes permitted. You are encouraged to photocopy the PAR-Q but only if you use the entire form.

NOTE: If the PAR-Q is being given to a person before he or she participates in a physical activity program or a fitness appraisal, this section may be used for legal or administrative purposes.

"I have read, understood and completed this questionnaire. Any questions I had were answered to my full satisfaction."

NAME _____

SIGNATURE _____   DATE_____

SIGNATURE OF PARENT _____   WITNESS _____
or GUARDIAN (for participants under the age of majority)

Note: This physical activity clearance is valid for a maximum of 12 months from the date it is completed and becomes invalid if your condition changes so that you would answer YES to any of the seven questions.

CS PE   © Canadian Society for Exercise Physiology   Supported by: 🍁 Health   Santé
                                                                    Canada   Canada

continued on other side...

...continued from other side

PAR-Q & YOU

Physical Activity Readiness
Questionnaire - PAR-Q
(revised 2002)

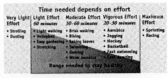

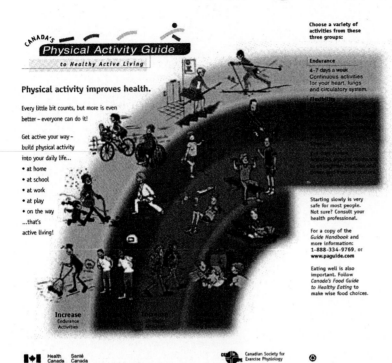

Physical activity improves health.

Every little bit counts, but more is even better – everyone can do it!

Get active your way – build physical activity into your daily life...
• at home
• at school
• at work
• at play
• on the way
...that's active living!

Increase Endurance Activities

Choose a variety of activities from these three groups:

Endurance
4-7 days a week
Continuous activities for your heart, lungs and circulatory system.

Flexibility

Starting slowly is very safe for most people. Not sure? Consult your health professional.

For a copy of the *Guide Handbook* and more information:
1-888-334-9769, or www.paguide.com

Eating well is also important. Follow *Canada's Food Guide to Healthy Eating* to make wise food choices.

Get Active Your Way, Every Day–For Life!
Scientists say accumulate 60 minutes of physical activity every day to stay healthy or improve your health. As you progress to moderate activities you can cut down to 30 minutes, 4 days a week. Add-up your activities in periods of at least 10 minutes each. Start slowly... and build up.

Time needed depends on effort

Very Light Effort	Light Effort 60 minutes	Moderate Effort 30-60 minutes	Vigorous Effort 20-30 minutes	Maximum Effort
• Strolling	• Light walking	• Brisk walking	• Aerobics	• Sprinting
• Dusting	• Volleyball	• Biking	• Jogging	• Racing
	• Easy gardening	• Raking leaves	• Hockey	
	• Stretching	• Swimming	• Basketball	
		• Dancing	• Fast swimming	
		• Water aerobics	• Fast dancing	

Range needed to stay healthy

You Can Do It – Getting started is easier than you think

Physical activity doesn't have to be very hard. Build physical activities into your daily routine.

• Walk whenever you can–get off the bus early, use the stairs instead of the elevator.
• Reduce inactivity for long periods, like watching TV.
• Get up from the couch and stretch and bend for a few minutes every hour.
• Play actively with your kids.
• Choose to walk, wheel or cycle for short trips.

• Start with a 10 minute walk–gradually increase the time.
• Find out about walking and cycling paths nearby and use them.
• Observe a physical activity class to see if you want to try it
• Try one class to start – you don't have to make a long-term commitment.
• Do the activities you are doing now, more often.

Benefits of regular activity:	Health risks of inactivity:
• better health	• premature death
• improved fitness	• heart disease
• better posture and balance	• obesity
• better self-esteem	• high blood pressure
• weight control	• adult-onset diabetes
• stronger muscles and bones	• osteoporosis
• feeling more energetic	• stroke
• relaxation and reduced stress	• depression
• continued independent living in later life	• colon cancer

Source: Canada's Physical Activity Guide to Healthy Active Living, Health Canada, 1998 http://www.hc-sc.gc.ca/hppb/paguide/pdf/guideEng.pdf
© Reproduced with permission from the Minister of Public Works and Government Services Canada, 2002.

FITNESS AND HEALTH PROFESSIONALS MAY BE INTERESTED IN THE INFORMATION BELOW:

The following companion forms are available for doctors' use by contacting the Canadian Society for Exercise Physiology (address below):

The **Physical Activity Readiness Medical Examination (PARmed-X)** – to be used by doctors with people who answer YES to one or more questions on the PAR-Q.

The **Physical Activity Readiness Medical Examination for Pregnancy (PARmed-X for Pregnancy)** – to be used by doctors with pregnant patients who wish to become more active.

References:
Arraix, G.A., Wigle, D.T., Mao, Y. (1992). Risk Assessment of Physical Activity and Physical Fitness in the Canada Health Survey Follow-Up Study. **J. Clin. Epidemiol.** 45:4 419-428.
Mottola, M., Wolfe, L.A. (1994). Active Living and Pregnancy, In: A. Quinney, L. Gauvin, T. Wall (eds.), **Toward Active Living: Proceedings of the International Conference on Physical Activity, Fitness and Health**. Champaign, IL: Human Kinetics.
PAR-Q Validation Report, British Columbia Ministry of Health, 1978.
Thomas, S., Reading, J., Shephard, R.J. (1992). Revision of the Physical Activity Readiness Questionnaire (PAR-Q). **Can. J. Spt. Sci.** 17:4 338-345.

For more information, please contact the:

Canadian Society for Exercise Physiology
202-185 Somerset Street West
Ottawa, ON K2P 0J2
Tel. 1-877-651-3755 • FAX (613) 234-3565
Online: www.csep.ca

The original PAR-Q was developed by the British Columbia Ministry of Health. It has been revised by an Expert Advisory Committee of the Canadian Society for Exercise Physiology chaired by Dr. N. Gledhill (2002).

Disponible en français sous le titre «Questionnaire sur l'aptitude à l'activité physique - Q-AAP (revisé 2002)».

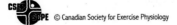 © Canadian Society for Exercise Physiology

Supported by: 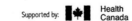 Health Canada / Santé Canada

Index